Gynecologic
Imaging

Gynecologic Imaging

JOHN C. ANDERSON, MBBS, FRACOG, DDU, COGU
Visiting Obstetrician and Gynecologist
Department of Reproductive Endocrinology and Infertility
Department of Ultrasound and Fetal Medicine
Royal Prince Alfred Hospital
King George V Memorial Hospital;
Director, Sydney Obstetric and Gynaecological Ultrasound
Sydney, New South Wales, Australia

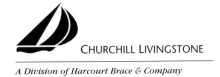

CHURCHILL LIVINGSTONE

A Division of Harcourt Brace & Company

CHURCHILL LIVINGSTONE
A division of Harcourt Publishers Limited

© Harcourt Brace & Co. Ltd. 1999
© Harcourt Publishers Limited 2000

 is a registered trademark of Harcourt Publishers Limited

First published 1999
  Reprinted 2000

ISBN 0-443-05239-5

British Library Cataloguing in Publication Data
A catalogue record for this book is available from the British Library

Library of Congress Cataloging in Publication Data
A catalog record for this book is available from the Library of Congress

Printed in Hong Kong
CTPS/02

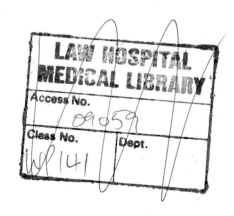

*For my mother, Margaret, my father William
and my children, Ian, Helen, Kate and Amy*

JCA

Contributors

JACQUES S. ABRAMOWICZ, MD
Associate Professor of Obstetrics and Gynecology and Radiology
Department of Obstetrics and Gynecology
University of Rochester Medical Center
Rochester, New York, U.S.A.
    *Plain Radiography and Fluoroscopy: Physical Principles and Imaging
    Techniques • Hysterosalpingography of the Endometrium • Hysterosalpingography
    of the Myometrium • Hysterosalpingography of the Fallopian Tube*

GUATAM N. ALLAHBADIA, MD, DNB, FCPS, DGO, DFP, FICMU
Honorary Assistant Consultant
Bombay Hospital and Medical Research Centre
New Marine Lines
Bombay, India
    Ultrasonography and Sonosalpingography of the Fallopian Tube

JOHN C. ANDERSON, MMBS, FRACOG, FRCOG, DDU, COGU
Visiting Obstetrician and Gynecologist
Department of Reproductive Endocrinology and Infertility
Department of Ultrasound and Fetal Medicine
Royal Prince Alfred Hospital
King George V Memorial Hospital;
Director, Sydney Obstetric and Gynaecological Ultrasound
Sydney, New South Wales, Australia
    *Ultrasound: Physical Principles and Imaging Techniques • Ultrasonography of the
    Vagina • Ultrasonography of the Endometrium • Ultrasonography of the
    Myometrium • Ultrasonography of Pathologic Pregnancy Conditions*

ANH H. AU, MD
Clinical Assistant Professor
UCLA School of Medicine; and
Chief, Section of Special Procedures
Department of Radiological Sciences
Olive View-UCLA Medical Center
Sylmar, California, U.S.A.
    *Computed Tomography and Magnetic Resonance Imaging of the Postpartum Pelvis
    and Postabortal Pelvis*

LORI L. BARR, MD
Associate Professor of Radiology and Pediatrics
University of Cincinnati College of Medicine;
Staff Radiologist
Children's Hospital Medical Center
Cincinnati, Ohio, U.S.A.
> *Ultrasonography of the Pediatric and Adolescent Pelvis*

MICHAEL W. BOURNE, BSC, MBBS, DMRD, FRCR
Consultant Radiologist
Radiology Directorate
University Hospital of Wales
Cardiff, United Kingdom
> *Ultrasonography of the Lower Urinary Tract • Magnetic Resonance Imaging of the Lower Urinary Tract*

THOMAS BOURNE
Fulham, London, United Kingdom
> *Ultrasonography of the Ovary*

JEFFREY J. BROWN, MD
Associate Professor of Radiology
Director of Clinical Research
Mallinckrodt Institute of Radiology
St. Louis, Missouri, U.S.A.
> *Computed Tomography and Magnetic Resonance Imaging of the Vagina*

MARIA HELENA S. CAMPOS, MD
Chief, Computed Tomography
Center of Diagnostic Imaging
Indaiatuba, Brazil
> *Computed Tomography, Magnetic Resonance Imaging, and Ultrasonography of Nongynecologic Pelvis Masses*

ZÉLIA M.S. CAMPOS, MD
Radiologist, Imaging Department
Emilio Ribas Institute of Infectology;
Research Associate, Department of Radiology
University of São Paulo
São Paulo, Brazil
> *Computed Tomography, Magnetic Resonance Imaging, and Ultrasonography of Nongynecologic Pelvic Masses*

DAVID CARPENTER, BE, M ENG SCI, PHD
Principal Research Scientist
Commonwealth Scientific Industrial Research Organisation
Telecommunication Industrial Physics
Sydney, New South Wales, Australia
> *Ultrasound: Physical Principles and Imaging Techniques*

JONATHAN CARTER, MBBS, DIPRACOG, FACA, FACS, FRACOG, CGO
Head, Gynecologic Oncology
Senior Lecturer, University of Sydney
King George V Memorial Hospital
Camperdown, New South Wales, Australia
Ultrasonography of Pathologic Pregnancy Conditions • Ultrasound Screening for Gynecologic Malignancy • Ultrasonography of Neoplasms Metastatic to the Female Genital Tract

GIOVANNI GUIDO CERRI, MD, PHD
Professor of Radiology and Chairman
Department of Radiology
University of São Paulo Medical School
São Paulo, Brazil
Computed Tomography, Magnetic Resonance Imaging, and Ultrasonography of Nongynecologic Pelvic Masses

HARRIS L. COHEN, MD
Cederhurst, New York, U.S.A.
Ultrasonography of the Pediatric and Adolescent Pelvis

CLÁUDIO CAMPI DE CASTRO, MD, PHD
Chief, Magnetic Resonance Imaging
Division of Diagnostic Imaging
Heart Institute (InCor)
University of São Paulo
São Paulo, Brazil
Computed Tomography, Magnetic Resonance Imaging, and Ultrasonography of Nongynecologic Pelvis Masses

SADHANA K. DESAI
Professor, Bombay Institute of Medical Sciences
Department of Obstetrics and Gynaecology
Bombay, India
Ultrasonography and Sonosalpingography of the Fallopian Tube

MICHAEL J. FULHAM, FRACP
Senior Neurologist and Director of the Department of Positron Emission Tomography
    and Nuclear Medicine
Royal Prince Alfred Hospital
Camperdown, New South Wales, Australia
Functional Imaging in Gynecologic Disease: The Role for Positron Emission Tomography, Single-Photon Emission Computed Tomography, Echo-Planar Imaging, and Magnetic Resonance Spectroscopy

SHINICHIRO FUJIWAKI
Department of Obstetrics and Gynecology
St. Marianna University School of Medicine
Kawasaki, Japan
Sonohysterography of the Endometrium

KATHARINA GRUBOECK
Lattersbarn, Tudely, Kent, United Kingdom
Three-Dimensional Ultrasound in Gynecology

HYUN KWON HA

Associate Professor, Asian Medical Center
Department of Radiology, University of Ulsan
Seoul, Korea
>   *Computed Tomography and Magnetic Resonance Imaging of Pathologic Conditions of Pregnancy*

ELISABETH HACKET

Universitaestrasse
Innsbruck, Austria
Ultrasonography of the Ovary

LYNDON M. HILL, MD

Professor of Obstetrics and Gynecology
Magee Women's Hospital
Ultrasound Division
Pittsburgh, Pennsylvania, U.S.A.
>   *Transvaginal Sonography in an Assisted Conception Program*

BUNPEI ISHIZUKA, MD

Associate Professor
Department of Obstetrics and Gynecology
St. Marianna University School of Medicine
Kawasaki, Japan
>   *Sonohysterography of the Endometrium*

MARIO P. ITURRALDE, BH, MD, DMC, DIP MIL SC, DM

Emeritus Professor
University of Pretoria
Pretoria, Republic of South Africa
>   *Radionuclide Imaging in Gynecology*

ROBERT P.S. JANSEN, MD (SYD), BSC(MED), FRACP, FRACOG, CREI

Medical Director
Sydney IVF
Clinical Professor
University of Sydney
Sydney, New South Wales, Australia
>   *Ultrasonography of the Normal Female Pelvis* • *Imaging in Gynecologic Infertility*

IAN R. JOHNSON

University of Nottingham, Queens Medical Center
Department of Obstetrics and Gynaecology
Nottingham, United Kingdom
>   *Computed Tomography and Magnetic Resonance Imaging of the Cervix*

DAVOR JURKOVIC

>   *Three-Dimensional Ultrasound in Gynecology*

SATOSHI KAWAKAMI, MD

Director, Department of Radiology
Kyoto City Hospital
Kyoto, Japan
>   *Computed Tomography and Magnetic Resonance Imaging of the Fallopian Tube*

SANJA KUPESIC

University of Zagreb;
Department of Gynaecology
Zagreb, Croatia
Color Doppler Ultrasonography in Gynecologic Malignancy

ASIM KURJAK

Medical School
University of Zagreb
Zagreb, Croatia
Color Doppler Ultrasonography in Gynecologic Malignancy

RICHARD B. KURZEL, MD, PHD

Professor of Obstetrics and Gynecology
Director of Maternal-Fetal Medicine
The Finch University of Health Sciences
The Chicago Medical School
Department of Obstetrics and Gynecology
Mount Sinai Hospital Medical Center
Chicago, Illinois, U.S.A.
Computed Tomography and Magnetic Resonance Imaging of the Postpartum Pelvis and Postabortal Pelvis

JILL E. LANGER, MD

Assistant Professor of Radiology
Department of Radiology
Hospital of the University of Pennsylvania
Philadelphia, Pennsylvania, U.S.A.
Computed Tomography: Physical Principles and Imaging Techniques • Computed Tomography of the Normal Female Pelvis

DEBORAH LEVINE, MD

Assistant Professor of Radiology
Beth Israel Deaconess Medical Center
Boston, Massachusetts, U.S.A.
Ultrasonography of the Postmenopausal Pelvis

VIVIAN LEWIS, MD

Director, Reproductive Endocrinology;
Associate Professor, Obstetrics and Gybecology
University of Rochester
Rochester, New York, U.S.A.
Plain Radiography and Fluoroscopy: Physical Principles and Imaging Techniques • Hysterosalpingography of the Endometrium • Hysterosalpingography of the Myometrium • Hysterosalpingography of the Fallopian Tube

ANDREW McLENNAN, MBBS (HONS), MRCOG, FRACOG

Department of Fetal Medicine
Royal North Shore Hospital
Sydney, New South Wales, Australia
Ultrasonography of the Postpartum Pelvis and Postabortal Pelvis

DONALD G. MITCHELL, MD

Professor of Radiology
Thomas Jefferson University Hospital
Director of Magnetic Resonance Imaging
Philadelphia, Pennsylvania, U.S.A.
Computed Tomography and Magnetic Resonance Imaging of the Myometrium

KATHRYN A. OCCHIPINTI

Fort Lauderdale, Florida, U.S.A.
Computed Tomography and Magnetic Resonance Imaging of the Ovary

RUDIGER OSMERS, MD

Obstetrician and Gynecologist
Department of Obstetrics and Gynecology
University of Goettingen
Goettingen, Germany
Ultrasonography of the Cervix

ERIK K. OUTWATER, MD

Associate Professor of Radiology
Thomas Jefferson University Hospital
Department of Radiology
Philadelphia, Pennsylvania, U.S.A.
Computed Tomography and Magnetic Resonance Imaging of the Myometrium • *Computed Tomography and Magnetic Resonance Imaging of Neoplasms Metastatic to the Female Genital Tract*

MARTIN QUINN

Department of Gynaecology
Royal Gwent Hospital
Newport, Gwent, United Kingdom
Ultrasonography of the Lower Urinary Tract • *Magnetic Resonance Imaging of the Lower Urinary Tract*

RICHARD B. RAFAL, MD

New York, New York, U.S.A.
Magnetic Resonance Imaging: Physical Principles and Imaging Techniques • *Magnetic Resonance Imaging of the Normal Female Pelvis*

PHILIPPA A. RAMSAY, MBBS, FRACOG, DDU

Fetal Medicine Unit
King George V and Royal Prince Alfred Hospitals
Camperdown, New South Wales, Australia
Ultrasonography of the Normal Female Pelvis • *Ultrasonography of the Endometrium* • *Imaging in Gynecologic Infertility*

MARY T. RICKARD, MBBS, BSC(MED), FRACR, DDU, MPH

Director/Radiologist
BreastScreen NSW, Central and Eastern Sydney
Redfern, New South Wales, Australia
Mammography and Ultrasound of the Breast

SEYED A. ROOHOLAMINI, MD

Professor of Radiological Sciences
UCLA School of Medicine;
Vice-Chairman, Director of Residency Training Program and Chief, Section of
    Computed Body Tomography
Department of Radiological Sciences
Olive View-UCLA Medical Center
Sylmar, California, U.S.A.
    Computed Tomography and Magnetic Resonance Imaging of the Postpartum Pelvis and
    Postabortal Pelvis

MICHAEL SANDBORG, PHD

Department of Radiation Physics, IMV
Linkoping University
Linkoping, Sweden
    Plain Radiography and Fluoroscopy: Physical Principles and Imaging
    Techniques • *Computed Tomography: Physical Principles and Imaging Techniques*

MARILYN J. SIEGEL, MD

Professor of Radiology and Pediatrics
Edward Mallinckrodt Institute of Radiology
Washington University School of Medicine
St. Louis, Missouri, U.S.A.
    Computed Tomography and Magnetic Resonance Imaging of the Pediatric
    and Adolescent Pelvis

CHRISTOPHER STEER

George Ward, Department of Obstetrics and Gynaecology
Orpington Hospital
Kent, United Kingdom
    Color Doppler Ultrasonography in Gynecologic Infertility

E. MALCOM SYMONDS, BSC (HONS), MBBS

Head of Department of Obstetrics and Gynaecology
Queen's Medical Centre Faculty of Medicine,
Nottingham, United Kingdom
Computed Tomography and Magnetic Resonance Imaging of the Cervix

ANIL TAILOR, BSC(HON), MBBS

Early Pregnancy Scanning Unit
Department of Obstetrics and Gynecology
King's College Hospital
London, United Kingdom
    Ultrasonography of the Ovary

MUTSUMASA TAKAHASI, MD

Department of Radiology
Kumamoto University
Kumamoto, Japan
    Computed Tomography and Magnetic Resonance Imaging of the Endometrium

MATTI VARPULA, MD
Radiologist
University Central Hospital
Imaging Center
Turku, Finland
Computed Tomography and Magnetic Resonance Imaging in the Investigation of Gynecologic Malignancy

RAMESH C. VERMA, MD
Professor and Executive Vice Chair
Department of Radiological Sciences
UCLA School of Medicine; and Chairman, Department of Radiological Sciences
Olive View-UCLA Medical Center
Sylmar, California, U.S.A.
Computed Tomography and Magnetic Resonance Imaging of the Postpartum Pelvis and Postabortal Pelvis

ELIZABETH VINING, MD, PHD
Advanced Medical Imaging
Montgomery, Alabama, U.S.A.
Computed Tomography and Magnetic Resonance Imaging of the Vagina

SHIH-CHANG WANG, BSC(MED), MBBS, FRACR
Clinical Senior Lecturer in Radiology and Senior Staff Specialist
Department of Diagnostic Radiology
Royal North Shore Hospital
Sydney, New South Wales, Australia
Magnetic Resonance Imaging of the Breast

RICHARD WAUGH, MBBS, DDR, FRACR
Department of Radiology
Royal Prince Alfred Hospital
Camperdown, New South Wales, Australia
Interventional Radiology in Gynecology

KIM M. WILSON, MD
Fellow, Thomas Jefferson University Hospital
Department of Radiology
Philadelphia, Pennsylvania, U.S.A.
Computed Tomography and Magnetic Resonance Imaging of the Myometrium

YASUYUKI YAMASHITA, MD
Associate Professor
Department of Radiology
Kumamoto University
Kumamoto, Japan
Computed Tomography and Magnetic Resonance Imaging of the Endometrium

Contents

Foreword

As awareness of women's health issues continues to increase, there is ongoing expansion of women's health centers and concomitant recognition of the importance of gynecologic imaging. In response to the demands of both health care consumers and providers, teams (in which the radiologist plays an increasingly important role) are being assembled to provide optimum gynecologic care. With the exception of ultrasonography, gynecologists have been slow to incorporate modern cross-sectional techniques. This situation is changing, however, and to be effective practitioners, clinicians need to be proficient in many different imaging modalities, including ultrasound, computed tomography, magnetic resonance imaging, and hysterosalpingography, as well as interventional procedures such as image-guided tubal ligation. Books such as GYNECOLOGIC IMAGING are essential to provide a multimodality approach to the complex imaging needs of the gynecologic patient.

Successful incorporation of new techniques and modalities into routine care depends on the skills and abilities of the physicians using them. For GYNECOLOGIC IMAGING, Dr. Anderson has recruited an international group of contributors who have provided expertise on the pathophysiology and role of imaging in the modern management of problems in gynecology. This text gives the international scope, and it is also comprehensive in its coverage of a wide variety of problems in gynecology. This text gives the international scope, and it is also comprehensive in its coverage of a wide variety of problems. This detailed and extensively illustrated text helps in providing the imaging tools which will be needed to participate successfully in the future care of women.

Introductory sections on the biophysics underlying the various imaging techniques and the imaging appearance of the normal female pelvis set the stage for detailed presentations of disorders. Special sections on the pediatric and adolescent patient, pathologic pregnancy conditions, and breast imaging supply an overview which completes the spectrum of the disease.

Each chapter provides a thorough discussion on the pathophysiology, pathology, and imaging appearance of developmental, benign, and oncologic disorders. The text is liberally illustrated, with detailed analyses of imaging findings, so that the reader has many examples of what may be found in clinical practice. Gynecologists and radiologists alike share my opinion and will find this book to be a valuable resource.

Hedvig Hricak, MD, PhD

Preface

Churchill Livingstone first asked me to edit a textbook in 1994. The topic was to be ultrasound in gynecology. The scope of the book grew to encompass all modalities that might be used to image the female pelvis. The publishers knew that there were no books on the shelves that covered this area, and that there was a need for a text that would be useful to gynecologists, radiologists, radiographers, and medical students. My brief was to cover anything that could be used to demonstrate the female pelvis other than the human eye directly, or through optic fibers. I first built a comprehensive Table of Contents and then invited experts in each area to contribute. The authors became more numerous as the content expanded until it assumed the form you see now. There are contributions from every continent on the globe except Antarctica.

One of the problems of multi-author textbooks is the variety of styles from the contributors. My aim as editor has been to produce a constant style. I have also tried to make the text clear, informative, comprehensive, and as short as possible. The final manuscript is the product of the parts and therefore I hope (as in mathematics), greater than the sum of those parts.

The book is organized systematically. It opens with a short section that covers basic physics and practical techniques. This section is not intended to be comprehensive, as other texts cover these areas in detail. It is included for the reader who is new to the field and whom wishes to learn more about a modality without the detail found in reference books. The next section of the book addresses the normal appearance of the pelvis through various imaging modalities, as one is not likely to recognize the abnormal if one cannot recognize the normal. The third section is the largest and deals with abnormal appearances. Finally, a section is included on the breast as in some parts of the world surgery of the breast is carried out by gynecologists.

My editing of both its format and expression has been fairly vigorous. Only two contributors submitted their transvaginal ultrasound images with the transducer at the bottom of the image. One contributed with some at the top and some at the bottom. In the interests of consistency I have placed the transducer at the top of the image in all chapters. This format applies almost throughout the published literature. About half of the chapters were delivered to me in time to edit them and return them to the author for review. The other half of the chapters were not delivered in time for me to do that. I consequently accept responsibility for the format and expression of the book and for any typographical errors.

I thank Mr. Geoffrey Nuttall, once publishing manager of Churchill Livingstone for his encouragement and advice, Dr. John Spurway for proofreading the final manuscript, and all of those who contributed chapters for their cooperation.

In particular I wish to acknowledge the assistance of Helen Peters in all aspects of producing this book. Without her enthusiasm and industry the book would never have been completed.

John C. Anderson

Biophysics

SECTION

I

Ultrasound: Physical Principles and Imaging Techniques

DAVID CARPENTER

JOHN C. ANDERSON

Early this century, sound waves with a frequency above the range that can be heard by the human ear were used to detect underwater objects. The first recorded use was in an unsuccessful attempt to locate icebergs after the wreck of the Titanic, although now echosounders are in common use by commercial and sport anglers. The word SONAR, which was used in early medical ultrasound units, was taken from the naval application, where it is an acronym for SOund, Navigation And Ranging. It is a method by which surface vessels can detect submarines and icebergs. The first sonars were invented during World War I by British, American, and French scientists and were called asdics (anti-submarine detection investigation committee) in Britain. The surface vessel sent a pulse of sound into the ocean below and "listened" for the echo. The time taken for the echo to return allowed the distance of the submarine from the vessel to be calculated because the velocity of sound in water was known. The direction was gauged from the position of the listening device when it received the maximum signal. Another early use was to detect flaws in metal; some of the early medical research was carried out with flaw-detecting equipment. After technical and clinical advances in the 1950s and 1960s,[1-3] ultrasound came into common medical practice in the 1970s and 1980s. In many ways, the stimulus to use ultrasound in medicine was the need in obstetrics to find a method of imaging other than using x rays; many of the applications are now in obstetrics and gynecology.

Ultrasound is operator dependent. Image quality and the accuracy of the diagnosis depend on the operator being experienced, being familiar with the equipment, and having the ability to rectify problems due to imaging artifacts. Attention to scan technique and a methodical approach are essential. The expertise of both operator and interpreter remains the basis of accurate diagnosis.

IMAGING PRINCIPLES

Sound is a form of mechanical energy. In medical imaging, high-frequency sound, or ultrasound, is generated by a transducer that rests on the tissues and that converts electrical energy into mechanical (acoustic) energy. This energy is generated for only a small fraction of a second and therefore can be described as a pulse. After generating the pulse, the transducer is still. The pulse travels rapidly through the body, and reflections occur at interfaces between tissues with different acoustic characteristics. These reflections (or echoes) return to the transducer, which is "listening" for them and converts them back to electrical energy (Fig. 1.1). This completes the pulse–echo sequence, and the transducer transmits again. It does this hundreds or thousands of times a second. Because we know the velocity of sound in tissue, the time between the transmitted signal and the received echo can then by used to calculate the distance of the interface from the transducer. The echo can then be displayed visually in a variety of ways including as a point on a video television monitor. Many factors influence the size of an echo. Points on the image do not bear simple relationships to properties of the tissue, as do images produced by some other imaging modalities.

The amplitude mode display of echoes shown in Figure 1.1 is commonly called A-mode and is rarely used nowadays, as it gives no spatial information about the echoes. Bidimensional mode, or B-mode, has almost completely superseded A-mode (Fig. 1.2). A new line of sight is displayed each time the transducer transmits. A cross-sectional image of the interfaces is constructed within the scanned area of interest. In this mode, the operator obtains a two-dimensional spatial display of the area being scanned (Fig. 1.2). The more lines of sight there are, the more complete the image becomes. This two-dimensional display has no parallax error and represents the slice of tissue that falls within the field of view of the transducer. The thickness of the slice is the width of the beam measured at right angles to the plane of the beam and is usually of the order of 1 to 5 mm (Figs 1.1 and 1.2).

ULTRASOUND: ACOUSTIC PROPERTIES AND PROPAGATION

Propagation, Velocity

Ultrasound is sound whose frequency is above the limits of human hearing. This is generally regarded as over 20 kilohertz

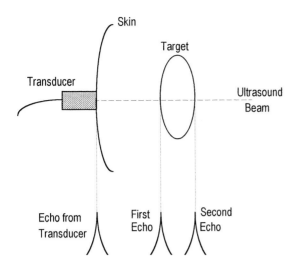

Figure 1.1 Reflections from anatomic interfaces along a single line of sight. The echoes from the target are displayed as amplitude deflections on a cathode ray tube. The information displayed refers to one dimension only.

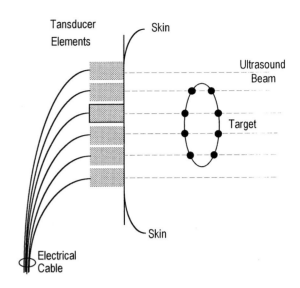

Figure 1.2 B-mode image from a number of lines of sight forms an image of the structure shown in Figure 1.1. The echoes from the front and back of the target are displayed as a point source on a television monitor. When a sufficient number of echoes are present, the outline of the target can be seen in two dimensions.

(kHz). In medical applications, the frequencies used are in the range 3 to 10 megahertz (MHz), with some special applications operating up to 30 MHz. Sound and x rays both involve the transfer of energy, but unlike x rays, sound cannot pass through a vacuum. A medium is required for its transmission. In matter, particles such as atoms or molecules tend to be held in a position of equilibrium by certain natural forces. Kinetic energy (acquired by virtue of motion) is transferred to them when they are disturbed. That kinetic energy is converted to potential energy (energy acquired by virtue of position), which is transferred to an adjacent particle as it disturbs that particle. The second particle moves a third, and so on as the energy passes through the tissue. The first particle tends to return to its position of equilibrium, developing kinetic energy from its potential energy, and it overshoots its previous position of rest. It continues to oscillate for a period of time until the potential or kinetic energy decays through friction. In liquids and soft tissues, propagation is mainly as longitudinal waves in which the energy is transferred by particle motion, which is parallel to the direction of propagation of the wave. In solids (e.g., bone), other wave modes such as shear waves can dominate.[4]

The velocity of energy transfer is determined by the density and elasticity of the tissue through which it is passing. The propagation velocity in water and soft tissues is in a small range, from 1,450 to 1,600 m/s, as shown in Table 1.1.[5] One of the assumptions that must be made for a pulse–echo imaging system to operate is that propagation velocity is constant. In medical ultrasonic imaging, the velocity commonly chosen is 1,540 m/s.

Bone has a velocity two to three times that of soft tissue, and air has a velocity one-fifth that of tissue. Air and bone cause disruption to images, and it is normal ultrasonic imaging practice to avoid them wherever possible[6] (Table 1.1).

Frequency, Wavelength

From wave theory, the relationship among velocity, frequency, and wavelength can be expressed as

$$C = f\lambda$$

where f = frequency and λ = wavelength.

An average tissue velocity of 1,540 m/s gives wavelengths between 0.44 and 0.15 mm in the frequency range of 3.5 to 10 MHz. The wavelength sets one of the resolution limits for an imaging system, and therefore it is desirable to use the highest frequency to have the shortest wavelength in order to resolve

Table 1.1 Propagation Velocities and Attenuations[4,5,7,8]

Medium	Velocity (m/s)	Attenuation (db/cm MHz)
Water (37°C)	1,523	0.002
Normal Saline (37°C)	1,560	0.002
Blood	1,560	0.18
Fat	1,460	0.4
Liver	1,550	0.55
Kidney	1,561	0.6
Brain	1,541	0.8
Muscle (Different orientations)	1,560–1,630	1.3–2.5
Bone (Different calcifications)	2,600–4,300	5–20
Air	331	1.0

small structures. As shown below, the attenuation in tissue increases with frequency. There is therefore always a dilemma between resolution and penetration. The optimal resolution is at the highest frequency, but as frequency increases, the penetration deteriorates. Ultimately, the operator will prefer the highest frequency that gives adequate penetration.

Attenuation

As ultrasound travels through tissue, there is a loss of signal due to absorption, scattering, and reflection of the wave. This loss, known as attenuation, is a complex combination of many mechanisms but causes an exponential decrease in the returned signal with increasing distance to the target. Attenuation increases in proportion to frequency (to a first approximation) and is usually expressed in dB per cm per MHz (see Table 1.1) As this attenuation affects both the transmitted pulse traveling into the body and the reflected echo returning to the transducer, the effect is doubled.

Reflection, Acoustic Impedance

In acoustics, a reflected signal is generated at the interface between two media if there is a difference in acoustic impedance between the two media. This quantity is therefore fundamental to a pulse–echo system, as the image is a plot of acoustic impedance discontinuities in the area being scanned. Acoustic impedance (Z), also called *characteristic impedance*, is analogous to electrical impedance and is defined as

$$Z = \rho c$$

where ρ = density and c = velocity.

The units of acoustic impedance are g/cm^2 sec $\times 10^{-5}$, known as *Rayls*.

The percentage of sound intensity reflected at a large (compared to the wavelength) smooth interface normal to the incident beam is given by

$$R = \left(\frac{Z_2 - Z_1{}^2}{Z_2 + Z_1}\right) \times 100\%$$

where R = percentage reflection coefficient, Z_1 = acoustic impedance of medium 1, and Z_2 = acoustic impedance of medium 2.

As shown in Table 1.1, all the biologic media, except bone and air, have a velocity close to 1,500 m/s, and as they also have a similar density (close to 1), their acoustic impedances are similar. The reflection equation takes the difference between acoustic impedances, so that in the case of reflection at soft tissue interfaces, the reflection coefficient is less than 1%.

Echo Size

There are a number of factors, other than attenuation and the reflection coefficient, that can influence the size of the echo. Surfaces that are large with respect to the wavelength (typically > 1 mm) give a "mirror-like" reflection and are called *specular reflectors*. If the target is small relative to the wavelength (typically smaller than 0.2 mm), or the large surface has small irregularities, scattering occurs and a lower signal is returned to the transducer. Any intervening air within the body or trapped between the transducer and the skin will give almost total reflection, causing a marked loss of penetration. As discussed later, the ultrasonic transducer is usually focused and a larger received echo will be obtained from targets in the focal zone compared to those in other areas of the beam.

Overlying Biologic Tissues

The overlying tissue layers of the body (skin, fat, muscle, and bone) can cause distortion of the ultrasound beam due to attenuation, beam bending, and beam broadening. These problems are overcome in some areas to a large degree by the use of an internal scanning probe such as a vaginal transducer.

TRANSDUCERS

The transducer provides the basic conversion between electrical and mechanical energy for an ultrasound system and also sets the resolution capabilities.[9,10] Certain naturally occurring substances have the property of being "piezoelectric." This means that when an electrical voltage is applied to the substance it is physically distorted and changes shape. The inverse effect also occurs. When the substance is physically distorted, an electrical voltage is produced. The substances most commonly used in medical ultrasonics are not naturally occurring but are synthetic ceramics. The ceramic materials are operated in a thickness-resonant mode. If the materials are operated directly into air, they will resonate for a considerable time after the electrical stimulus is removed because of the large impedance mismatch between the ceramic crystal and the air. To avoid this "ringing," in pulse mode operation, the transducers are built with specific backing and matching layers both to broaden their bandwidth and to improve the coupling of energy into the body.[11] The broader bandwidth gives a shorter ultrasound pulse, which improves the axial (or range) resolution of the system.[12] The other contributing factor to axial resolution is frequency, as with a higher frequency, the pulse is completed in a shorter time interval.

In virtually all medical imaging and pulsed Doppler applications, the same transducer is used to transmit and receive. The transducer geometry, its driving and receiving function, and the wavelength determine the beam characteristic. This beam pattern determines the lateral resolution, that is, the resolution at right angles to the plane of the ultrasound beam. Beam pattern characteristics are generally calculated for a circular disc transducer, and to a first order these can be applied to array transducers.

To reduce the beamwidth and hence improve the lateral resolution, focusing is generally applied. The beam may be fo-

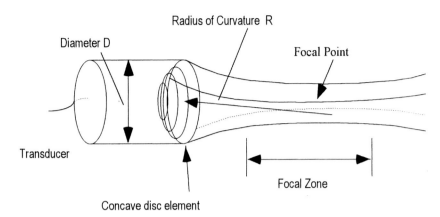

Figure 1.3 The typical beam pattern of a focused circular disc transducer. The face of the transducer is concave, allowing the beam to be focused.

cused in a number of ways, such as by using an acoustic lens on a flat transducer, by curving the disc to a concave shape, or, in the case of array transducers, by electronic delays in the transmitting and receiving circuits. Figure 1.3 shows a typical focused beam pattern.

Figure 1.4 shows a typical cross-axis beam pattern (i.e., the distribution of energy measured at right angles to the axis of the beam) at the position of focus. The beamwidth is usually defined as the distance between the two points in space where the measured output intensity has decreased by a given amount. This is typically 3 dB (reduced by a factor of 2) or 10 dB (reduced by a factor of 10) compared to the maximum output measured in the beam. The equation for the beamwidth at

focus is shown below. This equation shows that the beamwidth can be narrowed (i.e., the lateral resolution can be improved) by the use of a larger aperture and/or a higher frequency of operation (i.e., a smaller wavelength). Clearly, the beamwidth can also be narrowed by reducing the radius of curvature ("R" in Fig. 1.3), but this is usually predetermined by the depth of penetration at which the focal region is required.

$$W = \frac{2.4\lambda A}{D}$$

Where W = beamwidth at first off-axis minimum, A = radius of curvature of transducer, D = diameter of transducer aperture, and λ = wavelength.

Figure 1.4 The typical cross-axis energy distribution of a focused circular disc transducer at the focal point.

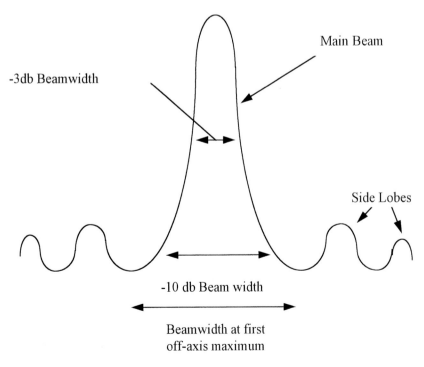

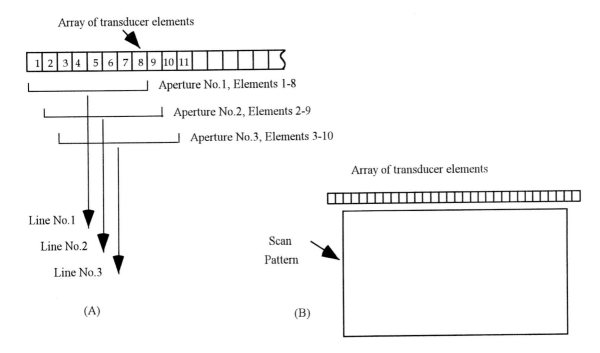

Figure 1.5 (A & B) The operation of a linear array transducer.

There is a limit on the degree of focusing that can be applied to a simple disc transducer. Increased focusing causes a reduction of the length of the focal zone, and the beamwidth away from the focal zone may be greater than with a less strongly focused transducer.[13]

Transducer Arrays

Many modern transducers use an array of small transducer elements rather than a single ceramic disc to make up the transducer aperture.[14,15] The electronic scanning and focusing of these arrays are varied and complex in modern diagnostic scanners. The array transducers are of three basic types, namely, linear array, phased array and annular array. The annular array will not be considered here, as it is a method of providing electronic focusing on a circular transducer rather than being an imaging system in its own right.

The linear array uses a long array of transducer elements, typically from 64 up to several hundred in number. A group of these elements (e.g., 8 of the 64) is selected electronically to make up the aperture for a given line of sight. This group is then switched along the array, moving by one element at a time, in sequence to make each new line of sight, as shown in Figure 1.5A. This produces a rectangular scan of an area under the transducer,[11] as shown in Figure 1.5B. Recently, curved or convex arrays have become available, as they better follow the contour of the body in many scanning applications. In these transducers, the overall array of elements follows a curve rather than being flat, but the principle of operation is the same as a linear array. This curvature may be made quite tight, such that the scan pattern produced is very similar to the sector scan of a phased array transducer (described below). These tight curved arrays are often used in vaginal probes as shown in Figure 1.6. In a vaginal probe, the center line of the array is usually offset by about 30 degrees (Fig. 1.6), so that a greater area of the pelvic contents can be scanned by rotating the probe.

Figure 1.6 The schematic design of a transvaginal probe. The scanning angle is usually offset at 15 to 30 degrees to the axis of the transducer to improve the field of view.

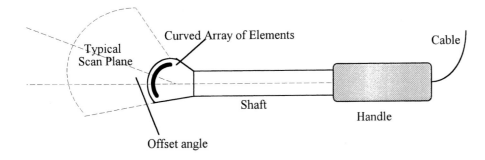

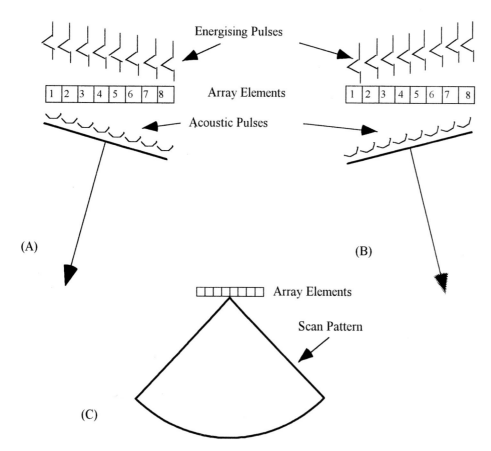

Figure 1.7 (A – C) The operation of a phased array transducer.

The phased array also uses a group of elements to make up the transducer aperture, but the transmitting signals to each element in the group have electronic delays applied such that the wavefronts from each element add to give an ultrasonic beam that is propagating at an angle to the transducer face,[15,16] as shown in Figure 1.7A. A line of sight can be produced at a different angle by the use of a different set of delays operating on the same group of elements, as shown in Figure 1.7B. Each successive line in a scan has a different set of delays to produce a different angle of propagation, and hence, a sector scan pattern is obtained (Fig. 1.7C). The advantage of this transducer is that it only needs the set of elements in the group that make up the aperture and not the long array of elements needed in the linear array. Hence, it is more compact and able to provide better access to areas of the body such as the pelvis, heart, and under the costal margin.[17] The disadvantage of the sector scan is the smaller area of anterior structures that can be imaged.

The beam can be focused in a similar manner by providing a parabolic set of delays across the aperture so that the resultant wavefront is curved, as shown in Figure 1.8. This can be applied to the group of elements making up the aperture for both a linear array and a phased array. Clearly, these electronic delays for steering and focusing must be applied to both the transmitting signals and the received echo signals to simulate the effect of mechanical scanning and focusing using a curved disc transducer.

Arrays: Advantages and Limitations

Array transducers offer a number of advantages apart from the removal of mechanics from the scan head. Electronic scanning can be carried out rapidly, with typical imaging rates of 30 frames per second, being limited only by the propagation time of the ultrasound wave in the tissue.[18] The ability to focus the beam electronically with an array transducer offers greater flexibility, as the position of focus can be varied on both transmission and reception. The receive focus can even be made to track the returning echoes so that a focused beam is obtained over almost the full depth of penetration of the scanning beam. This technique, called *dynamic focusing*, adds to the cost and complexity of the scanner but is usually employed on the more sophisticated systems because of the greater resolution. Dynamic focusing on reception does not require any operator controls, but the selection of one or more transmit focus positions is an operator control. The use of many transmit focus positions can slow down the scanning time, as each line of sight is transmitted a number of times to correspond to the number of focus positions.

The disadvantage of using an array of active elements is that there are often higher side lobe levels. Side lobes are present in any uniformly energized aperture, as shown in Figure 1.4, and are caused by diffraction effects at the edge of the aperture; however, additional lobes are generated whenever an array of elements is used to simulate an aperture. Higher side lobe levels reduce the ability to resolve low-level targets that are next to high-level ones, as signals due to the side lobe from the high-level target may be higher in amplitude than the main beam signal from the adjacent low-level target.

Apodization is a technique used in the higher-quality array scanners to reduce the level of side lobes, even though this is at the expense of a somewhat wider main beam. Apodization is achieved on transmission by applying a lower level of transmit excitation to the elements toward the edges of the aperture and on the reception by applying lower gain to these edge elements. These machines have a greater number of beam-forming channels to allow larger apertures to be used for higher resolution. In smaller portable units, the number of channels is restricted, and apodization is not often used due to the cost. Hence, these units generally cannot match the imaging quality of the more expensive machines.

Two developments are intravascular probes and surgical (or "finger") probes. Intravascular transducers are high-frequency transducers (20 to 30 MHz) that can fit inside a catheter to scan a blood vessel from within to show any plaque or deterioration of the vessel walls. Transducer probes in the 5- to 10-MHz range have been developed that are small enough to clip on the finger for use outside the body or internally during surgery.

SIGNAL PROCESSING AND DISPLAY

The signal processing in an ultrasonic scanner can be complex, but only the fundamental operations will be described. Two of the main processing functions are the time gain compensation (TGC) and the signal compression. TGC is used to compensate for the attenuation in the tissue by using an amplifier whose gain increases with increasing time after the transmit pulse, that is, for increasing depth into the body. This gain increase will compensate for the decrease in signal level due to the tissue attenuation. The controls for this amplifier are available to the operator to allow adjustment when scanning different areas of the body and when different frequencies of operation require a different rate of gain increase.

The dynamic range of echoes that reach the transducer is extremely wide (90 to 100 dB), and even though the TGC re-

Figure 1.8 Producing a focused beam by a parabolic distribution of delays to the energizing pulses applied to an array of elements.

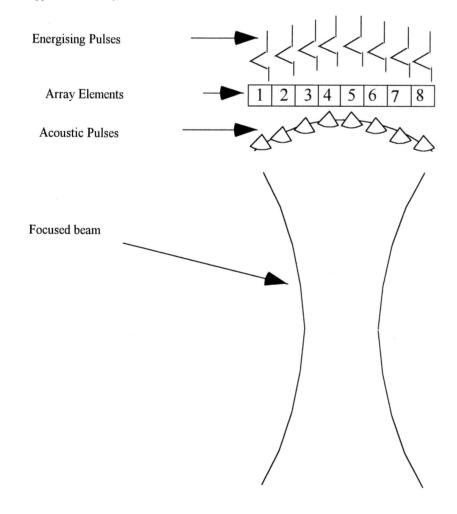

Energising Pulses

Array Elements

Acoustic Pulses

Focused beam

duces this range, it must still be compressed further to allow the full gray scale range to be displayed on a television monitor.[19] This signal compression is usually a nonlinear function, in that the higher-level echoes representing the specular reflectors around the boundary of organs are compressed most, and hence, more of the gray scale range on the display is available to the lower-level echoes from the parenchyma of organs. Different compression curves are available to the operator, and these are usually in a keyboard menu with setups for scanning different areas of the body.

A scan converter is used in the signal-processing chain to convert the transducer scan format (i.e., linear array, curved array, or sector) to a television raster format.[20] The scan converter also stores the image and allows other image processing and image measurements to be carried out. It is usual practice to digitize the signal either just after the transducer or partway through the signal chain so that a considerable amount of this processing is carried out digitally.

ARTIFACTS

Many artifacts can be generated in ultrasound images, making the information on the display not truly representative of the structures being examined.[21,22] These artifacts can be attributed to such effects as:

Multiple reflections

Attenuation and shadowing

Refraction

Beamwidth (or slice thickness)

Side lobes

Two of the more common artifacts are those due to multiple reflections and those due to refraction. Because an ultrasound pulse can be reflected from any impedance discontinuity, it can be reflected a number of times between two parallel structures such as the layers of the abdominal wall (Fig. 1.9). The echoes from the additional reflections will be displayed deeper in the body because of their later arrival time at the transducer. This phenomenon is often seen during an obstetric examination (particularly with the obese patient). It is easily recognized in the bladder, which is normally echo-free. Within the uterus, it can simulate an anterior placenta and cause a false diagnosis. Another phenomenon called "ghost or mirror images" can occur due to multiple reflections from a strong reflector.

The second artifact is that caused by refraction (or bending) of the beam by the subcutaneous tissues. It is the difference in velocity in the subcutaneous layers such as fat (1,450 m/s) and muscle (1,600 m/s) that causes refraction of the scanning beam. All scanners operate on the assumption that the acoustic pulse travels in a straight line, and this line of sight is used to display the received echo information. This echo information may have come from an adjoining structure due to refraction of the beam. The result is often seen as a double portrayal of structures. An example is display of a double bladder wall because part of the scanning beam has been refracted by a wedge of fat in the abdominal wall (Fig. 1.10).

Artifacts due to multiple reflections and side lobes can also occur in Doppler imaging and can lead to effects such as multiple vessels and reversal of colors in color Doppler imaging. There are other effects unique to Doppler such as aliasing and incorrect angulation to vessels.

The normal method of overcoming artifacts is to scan from another angle or approach. In many clinical situations, another scanning approach is not available. It is important to be able to explain the physics behind an unusual echo display before confidently calling it an artifact.

Figure 1.9 The production of a multiple-reflection artifact in the abdominal wall.

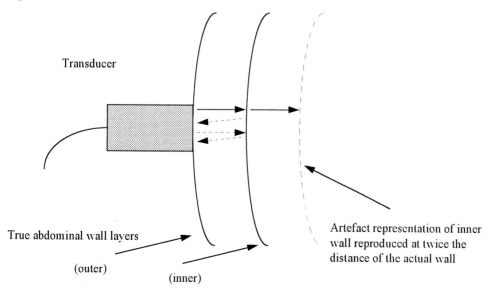

Transducer

True abdominal wall layers

(outer)

(inner)

Artefact representation of inner wall reproduced at twice the distance of the actual wall

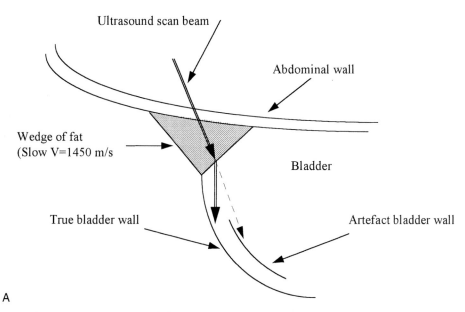

Ultrasound scan beam

Abdominal wall

Wedge of fat
(Slow V=1450 m/s

Bladder

True bladder wall

Artefact bladder wall

A

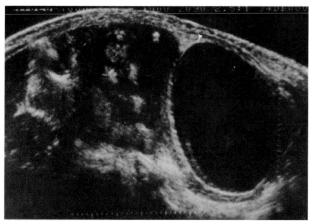

B

Figure 1.10 (A & B) Double portrayal of the bladder wall due to refraction by a wedge of fat in the abdominal wall.

DOPPLER

The Doppler effect is the shift, or change in frequency that occurs at a receiver due to the movement of the target. Ultrasonic waves are used to detect and measure movement of tissue, most commonly blood flow, using the Doppler effect.[23] The echoes returned from the red blood cells will show a shift in frequency dependent on the relative velocity between the cells and the transducer. This frequency shift is given by the classic Doppler equation.

$$F_d = \frac{Vf\cos\theta}{C}$$

where F_d = Doppler frequency shift, f = ultrasound frequency, V = velocity of targets, $\cos\theta$ = angle between the target direction and the observer (i.e., between the blood flow and the ultrasound beam), and C = velocity of sound.

Hence, by measuring this frequency shift and knowing the angle θ, the velocity of the targets (blood cells), can be determined. Signal strength is critical in a Doppler system due to

the very low level of echo signal returned from blood, compared to the echo levels from the soft tissues used in B-mode imaging.

In its simplest form, the Doppler technique uses continuous wave ultrasound with separate transmitting and receiving transducers. The frequency of the transmitted and received signals are compared, and the Doppler shift frequency is measured. The direction of flow can be determined by noting whether the received frequency is above or below the transmitted frequency. The Doppler shift is heard as an audible signal with headphones or a loudspeaker. Continuous wave Doppler equipment is relatively simple and low-cost and is used in two main applications: first, for tracing peripheral vessels in the arms or legs using a small pencil probe with transducers operating at 8 to 10 MHz and second, for fetal heart monitoring during labor using units operating at a lower frequency. The continuous wave system has the advantage of being able to measure high blood velocities, as it does not suffer from aliasing, which is a limitation of the pulsed Doppler system described below. The disadvantage is that the continuous wave system has no range resolution and will detect signals from all vessels within the crossover region of the transmit and receive beams. The pulsed Doppler technique[4,24] was developed to overcome this problem.

The pulsed Doppler technique has similarities to imaging, using B-mode ultrasound, in that a pulse of ultrasound is transmitted and the reflected echo signal received by the same transducer. The pulse used is longer than an imaging pulse, being typically 5 to 20 cycles of the ultrasound frequency in order to detect the frequency change of the echoes from consecutive transmit pulses. The pulsed Doppler system achieves range resolution by an electronic gating system that only accepts echo signals received a certain time after the transmit pulse; hence, only the Doppler shift signals from this given range are processed. This range gate system is controlled by the operator to allow the echoes from a particular vessel to be selected. Pulsed Doppler is often combined with B-mode imaging in order to image the vessel of interest and correctly place the range gate, which is highlighted on the image, within the vessel (Fig. 1.11). This is called *duplex*, as it gives a gray scale image of the vessel and a quantitative spectral display of the blood velocity.

The pulsed Doppler output is usually displayed as a spectrum of the Doppler shift frequencies. This is shown in Plate 1.1, where the spectral display on the right-hand section is taken at the point in the vessel where the range gate is highlighted in the left-hand image. The vertical axis shows the Doppler shift, and hence the blood velocity, in both positive and negative directions, while the horizontal axis displays time. The intensity, or gray scale, of the display shows how often a particular Doppler shift frequency has been measured and is therefore a type of histogram of the blood velocities. Velocities below the center line show a reversal of flow as can occur in an artery with very pulsatile flow or in a vessel in the region of a stenosis causing turbulence.

As the pulsed Doppler system only takes a sample of the blood velocity each time an ultrasound pulse is transmitted. It can give erroneous results if the blood flow changes too rapidly between pulses. This error due to the sampling effect is called *aliasing* and places an upper limit on the blood velocity that can be measured for a given rate of transmitting pulses

and a given ultrasound frequency. To avoid aliasing, the machine is set to the lowest ultrasound frequency that can be used and the highest pulsing rate frequency (PRF).

In 1985, a new development called color Doppler imaging was introduced. In this equipment, the moving targets (i.e., blood cells) are superimposed on the real-time gray scale image as color dots. An example of a spectral display and a color Doppler image of blood flow in a femoral artery is shown in Plate 1.1. Normally, red represents movement toward the transducer and blue movement away from the transducer, but this can be reversed (as is the case in the example shown). This technique is not quantitative but is proving very useful as a graphic way to determine directions and variations in blood flow for both major vessels and for perfusion in organs such as the kidney and around solid lesions to determine the nature of the lesion.

FURTHER DEVELOPMENTS: IMAGING AND DOPPLER

There have been a number of developments in medical ultrasonics both for imaging and Doppler. These include wider-bandwidth transducers, higher number of processing channels, digital processing and control, higher frequency operation, beam apodization, spectral and color Doppler imaging, dynamic focusing on reception, and multiple focal points on transmission. These have all added to the quality and diagnostic value of imaging and Doppler. Described below is a brief outline of other developments that have occurred in imaging and Doppler.

Wideband Transducers

A different construction of the transducer ceramic material has been developed in which the piezoelectric material is interspersed with a polymer filler material. This is called a *composite material* and offers a wider frequency range of operation and greater sensitivity with less reverberation artifact. This occurs because the composite is a better match to tissue than pure ceramic and hence more efficiently couples ultrasonic energy into and out of the tissue. Examples are probes that operate from 4 to 7 MHz or 5 to 10 MHz.

Signal Processing

These wideband transducers offer an advantage in the signal processing area in that the wideband echo signal that is received can be split into various frequency bands that are processed in a different manner from each other. This technique, called *parallel processing*, can assist in differentiating between tissue types and between normal and pathologic tissues.

Three-Dimensional Imaging

There has been considerable research effort into producing ultrasound images in three dimensions, and some initial systems are becoming available commercially. Systems have been de-

Figure 1.11 Duplex operation of a linear array for gray scale imaging and Doppler velocity measurement.

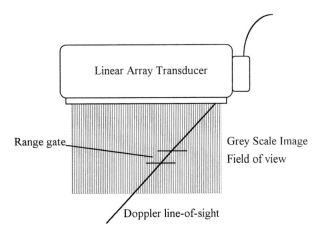

Linear Array Transducer

Range gate

Grey Scale Image
Field of view

Doppler line-of-sight

veloped using both mechanical scanners and array transducers. The major problem to overcome is production of quality images in real time because of the necessary amount of data processing. Clinical assessment is showing a benefit in images of the face and digits of the fetus and for Doppler assessment of tortuous vessels. As three-dimensional systems become more widely available, it is likely that the areas of clinical application will expand.

Power Doppler

Power Doppler is another method (akin to color Doppler) for displaying blood flow. Instead of displaying the Doppler shift, this technique displays the amplitude of the Doppler-shifted signals received from the blood. This technique is not sensitive to aliasing and offers an increased sensitivity over color Doppler, particularly in displaying flow in peripheral vessels. The display is not affected by the direction of flow but rather by the power in the signals from the moving targets. Hence, both color and power Doppler have their uses in diagnosis. This technique is given various names by different manufacturers such as Ultrasound Angio and Colour Power Angio.

Color Velocity Imaging

Color velocity imaging (CVI) is another attempt to overcome some of the limitations of color Doppler such as aliasing and at the same time to offer the ability to measure true blood flow as well as velocity. Each group of red cells in a blood vessel that returns an echo signal will have a characteristic echo pattern. CVI attempts to track this pattern from one transmit pulse to the next by correlation methods and hence determine how far the blood has moved between pulses. From this information, the velocity of the blood can be determined directly rather than by using the Doppler shift.

Contrast Agents

Contrast agents are available for use in some medical ultrasound. They are injected into the blood stream and increase the reflectivity of the blood for a few minutes. This improves the display and measurement of blood flow using the various Doppler techniques.

SAFETY AND BIOEFFECTS

There has been considerable research over the past 30 years into possible bioeffects of diagnostic ultrasound, particularly in obstetrics and gynecology.[25] This research has taken the form of epidemiology studies, animal experiments, experiments on cells, and studies of the physics of possible interactions between sound waves and tissue. The possible interactions are heating of the tissues by the sound waves and/or mechanical damage to cells by cavitation effects.[26]

The consensus is that there is no reason to withhold an ultrasound examination when its need is indicated on clinical grounds. The various ultrasound societies around the world all have statements on bioeffects that echo this consensus.[27,28] As ultrasound is a mechanical sound wave, it has never been shown to have any cumulative effects, as occurs with ionizing radiation.

In the imaging mode, heating is negligible due to the short pulses employed. In Doppler, the effects need to be considered due to the longer pulses and the higher pulsing rate. Maximum input of energy to a given area of tissue occurs when a single line of sight is being used and when the beam is not scanned. This is the case when pulsed Doppler is used to obtain a spectral display. In color or power Doppler, the beam is being scanned over an area of tissue, and hence the possibility of heating at a given point in tissue is less.

A question of safety is often raised in the use of internal probes (such as a vaginal probe) when the transducer is closer to the tissue being scanned. These probes require less power output, as the transmitted pulse and the returning echo traverse a smaller distance in tissue and hence the total attenuation is less than for a transabdominal scan. Measurements on these probes have shown that the output is much lower than that of an equivalent transabdominal probe.

Regulatory bodies, such as the Food and Drug Administration (FDA) in the United States, place limits on the output of scanners. The FDA has in the past used lower output limits for the more sensitive areas of tissue such as the eye and the developing fetus. Recently, there has been an allowance to relax these limits when a readout of a thermal index and a mechanical index is incorporated on the scanner. These indices indicate a relative risk of inducing a tissue temperature rise and/or the possibility of cavitation, if the index goes above a level of 1.[29] This allows the operator to use a higher output for special purposes but places a greater responsibility on the operator to monitor the output in use.

Although ultrasound is considered to be inherently safe, prudent operation is always recommended by using the ALARA principle (as low as is reasonably achievable) when setting the output level. Scanners should only be used by qualified personnel, and patients should only be scanned for as long as it takes to acquire the diagnostic information.

IMAGING TECHNIQUES

Transabdominal Ultrasound

Ultrasound examination of the pelvis is carried out with a distended urinary bladder to provide an "acoustic window." The distended bladder displaces bowel from the pelvis and straightens the axis of the uterus. This allows visualization of the pelvic organs and acts as a reference for evaluating cystic structures. The urinary bladder is ideally filled when it covers the fundus of the uterus. Typical preparation instructions request the patient not to empty her bladder for 3 hours and to drink three to four glasses of clear liquid 2 hours before the examination.

An overfull bladder can distort anatomy by compression, for example, by making a normal gestation sac appear irregular and flattened[30] or by producing a falsely elongated cervix with an apparent "low-lying placenta." It can also displace structures beyond the focus of the transducer, thereby limiting detail. Partial emptying of the bladder is required in these situations. This technique is limited in patients who are unable to fill their bladder, in obese patients,[31] and in patients with a retroverted uterus in which the fundus may be beyond the focal zone of the transducer.

When selecting a transducer, the highest frequency that allows adequate penetration to the area of interest at low-to-medium power is preferred. The patient is placed in the supine position. Acoustic gel is applied to the abdominal wall. The uterus and adnexa are imaged in both sagittal and transverse planes. The starting point for every scan is the midline (sagittal) plane. This will include the cervix normally, but the fundus may be deviated to one side or other even in the absence of pathology. With real-time, the pelvis should be studied by methodically sweeping the transducer vertically through the right adnexa and then through the left in parasagittal planes. The long axis of the uterus is identified in the sagittal plane. Angulation of the probe is important because the ultrasound beam must be oriented normally to the axis of the uterus for optimal demonstration of the endometrium. An off-axis plane may be necessary to display the uterus that deviates from the midline. The adnexa may be imaged by scanning obliquely from the contralateral side, thus making full use of the urinary bladder.

If hard-copy images are to be used, they should be taken every 1 cm in parasagittal planes from the midline to the pelvic sidewall. Transverse images should be recorded every 1 cm from the symphysis to the pelvic brim. Additional images should be recorded if pathology is found.

By convention, the anterior aspect of the patient is at the top of the screen, and the posterior aspect at the base of the screen. In the transverse plane, the right side of the patient appears to the left of the screen and the left side to the right side of the screen. In the sagittal plane, caudad is on the right of the screen (Fig. 1.12).

Transvaginal Ultrasound

The bladder should be empty to bring the pelvic organs into the focal zone. This also contributes to patient comfort. Transvaginal transducers range in frequency from 5 to 7.5 MHz and have a focal zone of 1 to 5 cm.

Transducers need to be disinfected between patients by washing in detergent and soaking them in liquid antimicrobial solution. A variety of liquid solutions are available, and the manufacturer's approval for decontamination must be followed.[32]

Precautions should be taken to minimize potential contamination to either patient or operator. Disposable gloves should be worn during probe insertion and during patient scanning. The transducer is prepared with ultrasound gel and covered with a latex condom or other barrier membrane after air bubbles are expelled.[33] Lubricant is then applied to the outside of the condom.

The transducer is inserted into the vagina by the patient or the operator with the patient supine with the knees partly

Figure 1.12 (**A**) Midline longitudinal (sagittal) scan of the corpus and cervix uteri and vagina using the abdominal approach through a loaded urinary bladder used to displace the bowel from the pelvis, thereby creating an "acoustic" window. Cephalad is on the left and caudad on the right. Anterior is at the top of the image. (**B**) Transverse scan through the loaded bladder. The uterine fundus is shown with the right ovary on the left of the image and the left ovary on the right.

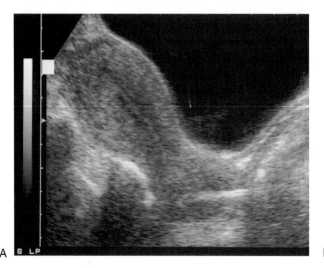

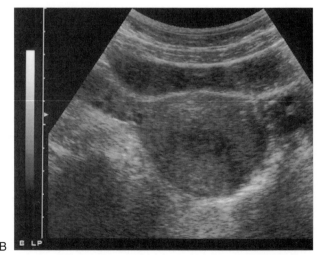

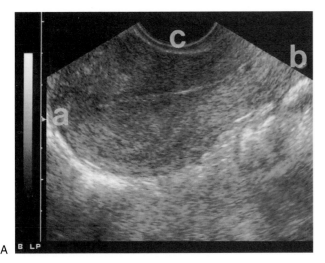 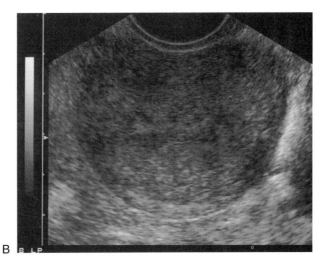

Figure 1.13 (A) Transvaginal scan of the uterus in the sagittal plane. When anteverted, the fundus is on the left and the cervix is on the right. If the bladder were seen, it would be in the upper left corner of the image. Points a, b, c in Fig. 1.13 correspond with A, B, and C on Fig. 1.14 to orient the reader. **(B)** Coronal scan through the uterine fundus. The bladder is empty, and the patient's right is on the left and vice versa. It is not possible to obtain a transverse scan transvaginally.

flexed and the hips elevated slightly resting on a pad or her own fists.

Orientation and Image Display

The display format that is now conventional is the one that was available when transvaginal transducers first became available. Ultrasound machines did not have the facility to invert the image electronically, and as a consequence, the apex of the sector wedge was the top of the screen. This format is used in current publications, is almost universally accepted, and has a superficial resemblance to the transabdominal longitudinal view.[34] It is essential that whichever method is used, each and every image needs to be labeled for correct evaluation.

All structures in the pelvis should be imaged systematically. The gain should be adjusted to give the pelvic organs uniform echo texture[35] (Fig. 1.13).

A fact to consider with transvaginal scanning is the angulation of the pelvis. The pelvis itself is tilted at an angle of 30 degrees to the long axis of the body, and the vagina runs superiorly and posteriorly with the patient supine. Almost all planes imaged are at an angle oblique to the long axis (Fig. 1.14).

The angle between the probe and the pelvic organs is continually changed to provide a detailed image of the organ on the screen. The correct marking of scanning plane, localization of a structure, and position (left or right) are crucial for later reference. "Organ-oriented" transvaginal scanning is more appropriate than anatomic pelvic planes.[36,37]

Manipulation of the transducer to obtain the appropriate images involves rotation, advancement, or retraction. These movements are often performed simultaneously to produce

optimal image. To visualize the cervix, the transducer must be pulled slightly outward away from the external os. Extreme posterior angulation may be needed to visualize the entire adnexa and the pouch of Douglas. Angulating laterally, the ovaries and adnexa will come into focus (Fig. 1.15).

Transperineal Ultrasound

The patient is examined supine. Ultrasonic gel is applied to the perineum, and the covered transducer is placed at the vaginal introitus. The beam is oriented posterosuperiorly in a sagittal plane along the direction of the vagina. The vagina lies directly away from the transducer posterosuperiorly between the bladder and the rectum, and the cervical canal typically lies at a right angle with the distal vagina.

Orientation and Image Display

The pubic bone is in the upper left-hand corner of the image. The urinary bladder is an echo-free area below the pubic bone and should be almost empty. The urethra appears as a hypoechoic tract that leaves the bladder toward the perineum at the top of the image. The vagina is located to the right of the symphysis and urethra and is seen as a vertical hypoechoic structure, corresponding to the muscular layer of the vaginal wall. The lumen is echogenic, and air can be trapped in the rugae of the vagina, causing shadowing. Behind the vagina is the rectum, which may contain various echo patterns. The cervix is below the vagina. The endocervical canal is seen as a thin, echogenic line. A rounded, hypoechoic area on each side of the canal can be seen joining the isthmus of the uterus.

To enhance tissue differentiation, the patient is asked to perform a Valsalva maneuver producing relative motion of differ-

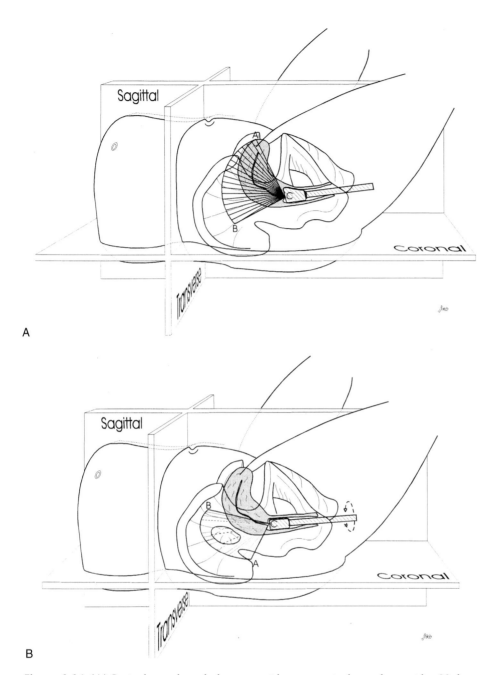

Figure 1.14 (A) Sagittal scan through the uterus with a transvaginal transducer with a 90-degree field of view offset at 15 degrees to the shaft of the transducer. Sagittal and coronal scans can be obtained. **(B)** Rotation of the transducer through 90 degrees in a counterclockwise direction permits visualization of the right adnexa and ovary. Note the reference points a, b, and c in Figure 1.13 which correspond with A, B, and C in Figure 1.14.

ent tissue layers and pelvic structures, facilitating their identification. Accurate images can be obtained from the cervix, lower uterine segment, bladder, and urethra. This technique is particularly useful in the evaluation of imperforate hymen, vaginal atresia, vaginal agenesis, masses near the cervix such as vaginal cysts, evaluation of stress incontinence,[38] cervical incompetence, suspected cord presentation, and placenta previa.[39]

Translabial scanning is limited by gas within the rectum, obscuring the external cervical os. Scanning of the patient in the left lateral decubitus position may improve visualization of the cervix in this situation.

Transrectal Ultrasound

Rectosonography is indicated for staging of cervical tumors, staging of infiltration of the bladder, assessing recurrences at the pelvic wall, and visualizing the vagina for intraoperative procedures.

Preparation requires bowel evacuation and a filled urinary

bladder. The patient is examined in the supine or lithotomy position. The covered transducer is lubricated with ultrasonic gel and inserted into the rectum. The probe is then filled with 20 to 50 ml of degassed water to provide an acoustic path for the ultrasonic waves. Images are obtained at 1-cm intervals from 2 to 15 cm from the anus. This is generally the maximal depth of the insertion that most patients can tolerate. The examination is usually of 10 to 15 minutes' duration, depending on the extent of the lesion.

DOCUMENTATION

Calibration and adjustment of monitors, printers, and recorders should be synchronized and maintained to optimize images. Individual preference for recording images will vary according to equipment, location, and cost. The principles of documentation remain the same regardless of which method is used. Three methods commonly practiced to record images are hard copy (either paper or film), video, and computer storage. Apart from the technical aspect of producing consistently accurate images reflecting the anatomy examined, the medicolegal implications should also be considered. Good documentation is imperative to avoid litigation.

SUMMARY

Accurate diagnosis by ultrasound is an interactive process involving the sonographer, the patient, and the ultrasound machine. An understanding of the physical principles such as

Figure 1.15 Scan planes showing angulation and rotation positions to view the pelvic organs. Most transducers have a field of view that is offset from the transducer centerline to improve the visibility in the adnexa.

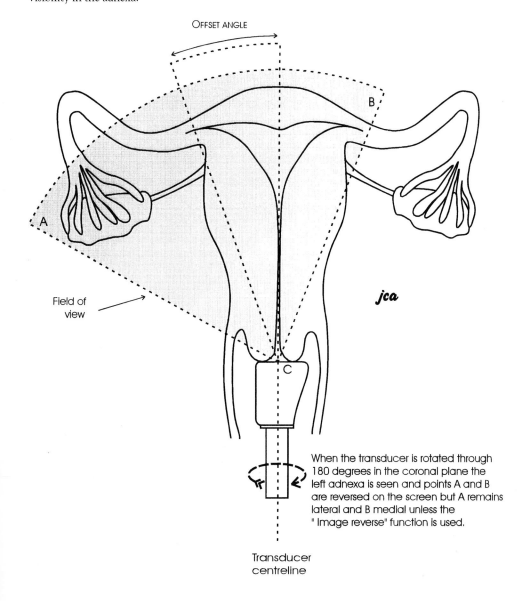

OFFSET ANGLE

B

A

jca

Field of view

When the transducer is rotated through 180 degrees in the coronal plane the left adnexa is seen and points A and B are reversed on the screen but A remains lateral and B medial unless the " Image reverse" function is used.

C

Transducer centreline

sound propagation, artifact production, safety considerations, as well as a thorough knowledge of anatomy (surface and sectional) pathology and the resulting sonographic appearances all contribute to the quality of medical care involving diagnostic ultrasonography.

REFERENCES

1. Howry JH, Bliss N. Ultrasonic visualisation of soft tissue structures of the body. J Lab Clin Med 1952;40:579

2. Donald I, Brown TG. Demonstration of tissue interfaces within the body by ultrasonic echo sounding. Br J Radiol 1961;34:539–549

3. Kossoff G, Garrett WJ, Robinson DE. An ultrasonic echoscope for visualizing the pregnant uterus. In: Kelly E, Ed. Ultrasonic Energy. University of Illinois Press, Urbana, 1965, pp 365–376

4. Wells PNT. Physical Principles of Ultrasonic Diagnosis. Academic Press, London, 1969, pp 1–2

5. deVlieger M, Ed. Handbook of Clinical Ultrasound. John Wiley & Sons, New York, 1978, pp 17–18

6. Shirley IM, Blackwell RJ, Cusick G et al. A User's Guide to Diagnostic Ultrasound. Pitman Medical, Tunbridge Wells, England, 1978, 88, pp 115–116

7. Goss SA, Johnston RL, Dunn F. Comprehensive compilation of empirical ultrasonic properties of mammalian tissues. J Acoust Soc Am 1978;64:423–457

8. Hill CR, ed. Physical Principles of Medical Ultrasonics. Ellis Horwood, Chichester, 1986, pp 175–211

9. Kossoff G. The ultrasonic transducer. Int Ophthalmol Clin Ultrasonogr Ophthalmol 1969;9:523–541

10. Hunt JW, Arditi M, Forster FS. Ultrasound transducers for pulse-echo medical imaging. IEEE Trans Biomedi Eng 1983;30:453–481

11. Carpenter DA. Ultrasonic transducers. In: Wells PNT, Ziskin MD, Eds. New Techniques and Instrumentation in Ultrasonography. Churchill Livingstone, New York, 1980, pp 31–39

12. Kossoff G. The effects of backing and matching on the performance of piezoelectric ceramic transducers. IEEE Trans Sonic Ultrasonic 1966;13:20–30

13. Robinson DE, Kossoff G. Array techniques in diagnostic ultrasound. Proceedings of the Symposium of Signal Processing for Arrays. Dept of Defence, Salisbury, South Australia, 1977, pp 2–18

14. Somer JC. Electronic sector scanning for ultrasonic diagnosis. Ultrasonics 1968;6:153–159

15. Thurstone FL, von Ramm OT. A new ultrasound imaging technique employing two-dimensional electronic beam steering. In: Green PS, Ed. Acoustical Holography and Imaging (vol. 5). Plenum Press, New York, 1974, pp 249–259

16. von Ramm OT, Smith SW. Beam steering with linear arrays. IEEE Trans Biomed Eng 1983;30:438–452

17. von Ramm OT, Thurstone FL. Cardiac imaging using a phased array ultrasound system. Circulation 1976;53:258–267

18. Wilkinson RW. Principles of real-time two-dimensional B-scan ultrasonic imaging. J Med Eng Technol 1981;5(1):21–28

19. Kossoff G, Garrett WJ, Carpenter DA et al. Principles and classification of soft tissue by grey scale echography. Ultrasound Med Biol 1976;2:89-1–5

20. Ophir J, Goldstein A. The principles of digital scan conversion and their application to diagnostic ultrasound. In: White D, Brown R, Eds. Ultrasound in Medicine. Plenum Press, New York, 1977, pp 1707–1713

21. Robinson DE, Kossoff G, Garrett WJ. Artifacts in ultrasonic echoscope visualisation. Ultrasonics 1966;4:184–194

22. Kremkau FW, Taylor KJW. Artifacts in ultrasound imaging (Review). J Ultrasound Med 1986;5:227–237

23. Burns PN. The physical principles of doppler and spectral analysis. J Clin Ultrasound 1987;15:567–590

24. Burns PN. The Physical Principles of Doppler and Spectral Analysis. Churchill Livingstone, New York, 1988

25. Ziskin MC, Petitti DB. Epidemiology of human exposure to ultrasound: a critical review. Ultrasound Med Biol 1988;14:91–96

26. Barnett SB, Kossoff G, Eds. World Federation for Ultrasound in Medicine and Biology Symposium on Safety and Standardization in Medical Ultrasound: Issues and recommendations regarding thermal mechanisms for biological effects of ultrasound. Ultrasound Med Biol 1992;18:731–810

27. Barnett SB, Kossoff G, Edwards MJ. Is diagnostic ultrasound safe? Current International Consensus on the Thermal Mechanism. Med J Aust 1994;160:33–37

28. Barnett SB, ter Harr GR, Ziskin MC et al. Current status of research on biophysical effects of ultrasound. Ultrasound Med Biol 1994;20:205–218

29. AIUM/NEMA Standard for Real-Time Display of Thermal and Mechanical Acoustic Output Indicies on Diagnostic Equipment. American Institute of Ultrasound in Medicine. Rockville, MD, 1992

30. Baker ME, Mahony BS, Bowie JD. Adverse effect of an overdistended bladder on first trimester sonography. AJR Am J Roentqenol 1985;145:597–599

31. Timor-Tritsch IE, Rottem S, Thaler I. Review of transvaginal ultrasonography: a description with clinical application. Ultrasound Q 1988;6:1–34

32. Odwin CS, Fleischer AC, Kepple DT. Probe covers and disinfectants for transvaginal transducers. J Diagn Med Sonogr 1990;6:130–135

33. Jimenez R, Duff P. Sheathing of the endovaginal ultrasound probe: is it adequate? Infect Dis Obstet Gynecol 1993;1:37–39

34. Timor-Trisch IE. Standardisation of ultrasonographic images: let's all talk the same language! Ultrasound Obstet Gynecol 1992;2:311–312

35. Baltarowich OH, Kurtz AB, Pasto ME et al. The spectrum of sonographic findings in hemorrhagic ovarian cysts. AJR Am J Roentgenol 1987;148:901–905

36. Dodson MG, Deter RL. Definition of anatomical planes for use in transvaginal ultrasonography. J Clin Ultrasound 1990; 18:239–242

37. Rottem S, Thaler I, Goldstein SR et al. Transvaginal sonographic technique: targeted organ scanning without resorting to "planes." J Clin Ultrasound 1990;18:243–247

38. Kolbl H, Bernaschek G, Wolf G. A comparative study of perineal ultrasound scanning and urethrocystography in patients with genuine stress incontinence. Arch Gynecol Obstet 1988;244:39–45

39. Mahony BS, Nyberg DA, Luthy DA et al. Translabial ultrasound of the third trimester uterine cervix. Correlation with digital examination. J Ultrasound Med 1990;9:717–723

2

Plain Radiography and Fluoroscopy: Physical Principles and Imaging Techniques

MICHAEL SANDBORG

JACQUES S. ABRAMOWICZ

VIVIAN LEWIS

The German physicist Wilhelm Conrad Röntgen (1845 to 1923) discovered x rays, for which he was awarded the first Nobel Prize for Physics in 1901. Röntgen was born in Lennep (now part of Germany) and educated at the University of Zurich. On November 8, 1895, he was studying the behavior of electrons in a Crookes', or cathode ray discharge, tube, which consisted of a glass envelope from which almost all of the air had been expelled. When a high-energy electrical discharge was passed through the tube, the remaining gas was ionized and produced a faint light.

Röntgen had enclosed the tube in a cardboard box and had darkened the room to check that no light was escaping when he noticed that a glow was coming from nearby barium platinocyanide crystals. Because of the cardboard box, he knew that the glow was not from the cathode ray tube, and he correctly hypothesized that there must be some other ray, more penetrating than ultraviolet light, responsible. He called the hitherto unknown rays "x rays" but they are now also appropriately referred to as Röntgen rays.

Imaging of the female pelvic organs and demonstration of the anatomy, physiology, and pathology are about 70 years old. Many techniques have since developed such that a multitude of imaging methods are now available: plain x ray, contrast radiography, hysterosalpingography, computed tomography (CT), ultrasonography, and magnetic resonance imaging (MRI). Each has advantages and disadvantages, and the clinician faced with a diagnostic dilemma may find it difficult to decide which to choose. A less than optimal solution, by some caregivers, is to order them all! In these times of concern regarding medical expense, the astute clinician needs to select the most appropriate test for the particular problem. The oldest and seemingly most simple technique is the plain x ray, which has survived the arrival of more sophisticated modalities and still has an important role.

IONIZING RADIATION

The Nature of X Rays

X rays are electromagnetic waves, of the same nature as light, but of a 10^4 to 10^5 times higher frequency. Alternatively, they may be thought of as individual radiation quanta, or *photons*. Each x-ray photon has a certain amount of energy, commonly expressed in the unit electron-volt, eV, (1 eV=$1.6 \cdot 10^{-19}$ J). X-ray photons used in diagnostic radiology have energy below 150 keV (1 keV=1,000 eV). When x rays enter a material, part of their energy is transferred to the material in interactions between the photons and the atoms. If the energy transfer is high enough to cause electrons to leave the atom, the radiation is called *ionizing*.

X-Ray Interactions

X-ray interaction processes in the diagnostic energy range are either absorptions or scatterings (Fig. 2.1). These processes give rise to the varying transmission of photons through the patient's body that subsequently forms the image. A photon that is absorbed is lost from the beam of primary photons emerging from the x-ray tube on its way toward the image receptor. A photon that is scattered changes its direction of motion and may lose some of its energy. The information about the patient is conveyed by the primary photons; the scattered photons, arising from interactions in the patient, reduce the image information content. Photon absorption and scattering result in energy being absorbed in the patient. The energy absorbed per unit mass is called the *absorbed dose* and is measured in J/kg or Gray, Gy (Fig. 2.1).

19

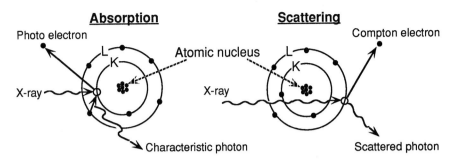

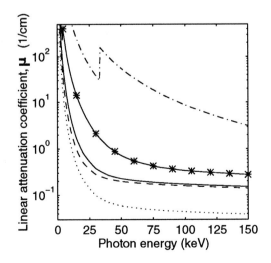

Figure 2.1 Schematic representation of x-ray photon absorption and scattering with atomic electrons. An x-ray photon interacts with an inner K-shell electron. A photoelectron escapes the atom and creates a vacancy in the K-shell, which is filled by an L-shell electron. The difference in binding energy between the K- and L-shells is transferred to a characteristic photon. When a photon is (Compton) scattered, the energy of the incoming x-ray is shared by the Compton electron and the scattered photon. Only a small fraction of the energy is transferred to the electron at the photon energies used in diagnostic radiology.

Absorption

In a photoelectric absorption event, the photon is completely absorbed by one of the inner atomic electrons that is ejected from the atom (a photoelectron). The vacancy in the electron shell is filled by an electron from an outer shell, and a new photon may be created (a characteristic photon). The energy of this photon is characteristic of the atom, and its energy equals the energy difference of the binding energy of the two atomic shells.

As the atomic number of the atom, Z, increases, the probability for absorption increases rapidly as Z^4. It decreases with increasing photon energy until the energy exceeds the binding energy of the electrons in a shell. Then more electrons can participate in the process, and the probability increases considerably. In iodine, the binding energy of the inner K-shell electrons is 33.2 keV, and this energy is called the K-edge. The probability for absorption in iodine increases by a factor of 5 at the K-edge (Fig. 2.2). Iodine absorbs many more photons than soft tissue, enhancing image contrast when used in contrast agents (Fig. 2.2).

Scattering

When an x-ray photon interacts with an atom and is scattered, the process is known as Compton scattering. The incoming photon interacts with one of the outer electrons and ejects it from the atom. Some of the energy is transferred to this (Compton) electron and the rest remains with the scattered photon. If the photon is scattered 45 degrees, the energy loss is only 5 keV for a 100-keV photon. Even if the photon is scattered backward, it cannot lose all its energy in one scattering event. This means that a photon can scatter many times before its energy is so low that it is finally absorbed or escapes the patient. The probability of Compton scattering is much less dependent on the atomic number than is absorption and the probability decreases only slowly with increasing photon energy. Scattering without energy loss is also possible.

This is known as *Rayleigh scattering* and is only important at low photon energies.

Attenuation

The number of photons of a given energy that is lost from the primary beam due to interaction with a thin material layer is proportional to the thickness of the material and the number of incident photons. The proportional constant is called the *linear attenuation coefficient*, μ, and it expresses the probability per unit length that a photon of a given energy will interact somewhere along its passage through the material. It is the sum of the two interaction processes: absorption and scattering. The value of μ depends on the energy of the x-ray photon and the material (Fig. 2.2). It is the difference in attenu-

Figure 2.2 The linear attenuation coefficient, μ for iodine –·–·–; compact bone, *———*; water (soft tissue), ———; adipose tissue (fat), - - - -; and lung tissue, ..., as a function of x-ray photon energy. The difference in attenuation coefficient, μ, between bone and soft tissue and soft tissue and adipose tissue decreases with increasing photon energy.

ation properties between tissues types in the body that gives us an image. With a large difference, the tissue type of interest will be visualized more easily in the image (larger contrast). The difference in μ-values between soft tissue and bone tissue is much larger than that between soft tissue and adipose tissue. Bone is thus easier to detect from the surrounding soft tissue in the image than is adipose tissue.

IMAGING SYSTEMS COMPONENTS

Figure 2.3 shows the components of the imaging system including x-ray tube, added filter, collimator, patient, antiscatter grid, and image receptor, each of which will be described below (Fig. 2.3).

X-ray tube

The photons generated in the x-ray tube are classed according to their origin as either continuous radiation (Bremsstrahlung) or characteristic radiation.

In the x-ray tube, electrons are emitted from the negatively charged cathode. They are focused and accelerated toward the positively charged tungsten anode target by the electric field between the cathode and anode. If the tube potential between the anode and cathode is 100 kV, the electrons receive 100 keV kinetic energy. The broad continuous spectrum of x-ray photons is generated when these high-energy electrons are slowed down in the anode. The electrons rarely lose all their energy in one interaction, so photons of all energies up to the maximum kinetic energy of the electron are generated, but low-energy photons are more common. Tungsten is chosen, since it has a high melting point and high atomic number, which increases the Bremsstrahlung production.

When the tube potential exceeds 70 kV, K-shell electrons can escape the tungsten atom. The characteristic radiation then produced is superimposed as peaks on the spectrum of continuous radiation (Fig. 2.4).

The parameters that control the exposure are the tube potential (kV) and the tube charge (mAs); the latter being the product of tube current and exposure time. The tube potential determines the energies and thus fractional transmission of the photons through the body, while the tube charge deter-

Figure 2.3 The components of the imaging system: x-ray tube, added filter, collimator, patient, antiscatter grid, and image receptor. Details of the x-ray tube housing and the image receptor are enlarged.

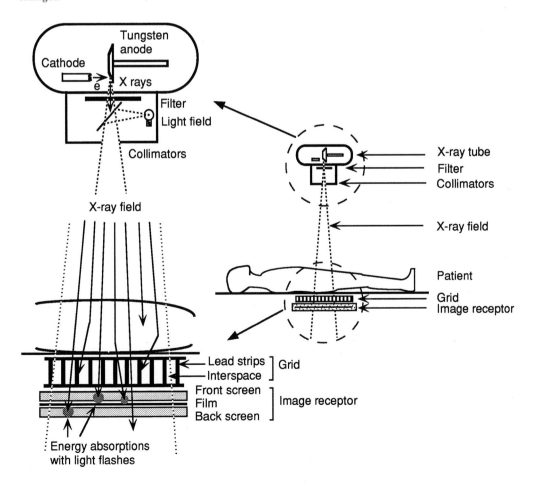

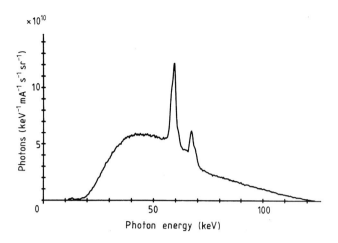

Figure 2.4 Measured absolute photon energy spectrum at 120 kV and 2.5-mm aluminium filtration. The characteristic photons from tungsten, superimposed on the Bremsstrahlung spectrum, were not completely resolved with this measuring technique. (From Matscheko and Alm Carlsson.[1] with permission.)

mines the amount of radiation that is generated in the tube. With increased tube potential, more photons will be generated per unit time as the production of x rays increases with the energy of the incoming electrons.

Filters

The applied tube potential determines the maximum energy of the x rays, whereas the lowest photon energy that can reach the patient is determined by the filtration of the beam. The photons are filtered by adding metal foils in the beam; usually, aluminium or copper. This filter should absorb low-energy photons and transmit high-energy photons, since photons of low energies are mostly absorbed at shallow depths in the patient and do not contribute to the image formation. The selection of appropriate thickness of the filter is a balance between image quality and absorbed dose in the patient. Due to the changes in the spectrum of photons passing through the filter, the average photon energy in the filtered spectrum will be higher. A higher photon energy corresponds to a lower μ-value. The radiation thus penetrates the patient more easily, thereby reducing the average dose in the patient needed to achieve a certain signal level in the image receptor (e.g., film blackness). The image contrast may be reduced, too, so a compromise has to be reached. An x-ray spectrum[1] (120-kV tube potential, 2.5-mm aluminium added filtration) is shown in Figure 2.4.

Collimators

The x rays are emitted in all directions from the focal spot in the x-ray tube. Collimators are therefore necessary to confine the x-ray field to the particular area of interest in the patient.

Two sets of separately adjustable shutters, attached to the x-ray tube, determine the field. To help align the x-ray field on the patient, a light bulb and a mirror are used to form an identical light field on the patient.

The use of an unnecessarily large x-ray field will have two disadvantages: increased patient dose and reduced image quality. The average patient dose will increase if a larger portion of the patient's body is irradiated, since the energy absorbed in the patient is proportional to the area of the field. The image quality will decrease, since excessive amounts of scattered radiation will be generated. It is therefore an essential part of good radiologic practice to use as small a field size as possible.

Contrast Agents

Image contrast agents rely on the fact that some tissues absorb more x rays than others. Since the probability for absorption increases rapidly with atomic number, contrast agents of high atomic number are used to enhance visualization of cavities, vessels, and ducts. The most frequently used water-soluble contrast agents for the extracellular space are based on the iodine atom (Z=53). Non-water-soluble contrast media containing barium (Z=56) are used to enhance the contrast of the gastrointestinal canal and used together with air in the colon.

Antiscatter Devices

If large volumes are irradiated at the same time, the number of scattered photons will outnumber the primary photons at the receptor. This will reduce the image quality (contrast). There are many ways to deal with this problem. One of the most efficient ways is to irradiate only a small part of the body at a time. This can be achieved with well-collimated beams. Another way is to use patient compression when appropriate. This technique is applied in abdominal and breast imaging (mammography) and has the further advantage of reducing the dose in the patient.

The most commonly used method is to use an antiscatter grid. A grid is made of a series of absorbing lead strips separated by a transparent interspace material usually made from aluminium or paper. It has similarities to a Venetian blind. The lead strips are aligned with the beam of primary photons so that these photons can pass the interspaces of the grid. The scattered photons are multidirectional, and most of them are absorbed by the lead strips. To work properly, the grid requires precise alignment in the x-ray beam. Misalignment will cause too many primary photons to be absorbed in the grid, which will increase patient dose and reduce image quality.

An alternative to the grid is to use an air gap between the patient and the image receptor, typically 15 to 30 cm. With increasing air-gap distance, more scattered photons will miss the image receptor. This method is most efficient in situations with a small field size and thin patients, as for instance in pediatric radiology.

Image Receptors

The outcome of an x-ray examination can be an analog or a digital image. An analog image is an image that is obtained, for example, by exposure of a film. Ordinary film contains a silver-halide that is sensitive to both light and x rays. The most frequent use of a bare film as detector is in intraoral dental x-ray examinations. By surrounding the film with two thin fluorescent screens (intensifying screens), one gets a more sensitive system that reduces patient dose. The energy absorbed in the screens by a single x-ray photon is converted into many hundreds of light photons that in turn expose the film. The film blackening is then primarily due to the light from the screens and not from direct hits of x rays. The screens are now the detector, while the film is a medium for storing and displaying the images. The active material in fluorescent screens can be made from, for example, $Gd_2O_2S{:}Tb$, $LaOBr{:}Tm$, $YTaO_4{:}Nb$ or $CaWO_4$. The screens and film are contained in a light-safe cassette. After exposure, the film is automatically removed from the cassette and fed into the film processor.

The image shows the patient anatomy with varying gray levels; dark where the x rays could easily pass through the patient (e.g., lungs and thin body parts) and light where the x rays could not (behind bones and contrast media). The characteristic curve of the film relates the blackening on the developed film to the exposure at the film (Fig. 2.5). A problem with film arises when the exposure setting is not properly chosen, that is, if the image is over- or underexposed. Then the image contrast will be much reduced, and some of the available information in the x-ray beam will be lost.

When real-time images are required, image-intensifier fluoroscopy or fluorography systems are used. In an image-intensifier system, the x rays are absorbed in a cesium iodide screen that emits light. The light then strikes a photocathode that emits low-energy photoelectrons. These electrons then gain energy from the electric field in the image intensifier vacuum tube and are focused to hit the much smaller exit screen that finally converts the high-energy electrons to many light photons that are detected by a television or film camera.

Using subtraction technique, one can subtract the data contained in an image obtained without contrast medium from an image of the same area obtained with contrast medium. The result is an image of much improved visualization of the vessels that contained the contrast medium; the contrast of other structures is much reduced and does not interfere with the interpretation of the vessels. This procedure is much facilitated by using a digital technique, in so-called digital subtraction angiography.

Digital Images

A different way of producing images is to measure values of the exposure in thousands of small areas (picture elements or pixels) in the image plane. The number of pixels in the image differs with application but can be approximately 512^2, $1,024^2$, or $2,048^2$. The pixel readings are stored in a computer and can be displayed on a monitor as different shades of gray. The number of different gray levels attainable is set by the number of bits in each pixel, for examples, 8, 10, or 12 bits, that is, 256, 1,024, and 4,096 levels of gray. All this information cannot be visualized simultaneously in one image. The storing of the images as discrete series of numbers (digits) has given this method the name *digital imaging*.

In digital radiography, processing and display of the image are separated from the process of image acquisition. There are many advantages of digital images. The images will not be under- or overexposed, and several images can be created from the same set of numbers (one single exposure of the patient) by selecting different combinations of numbers and gray levels. Image-processing techniques (e.g., edge enhancement) can easily be used to enhance certain aspects of the images that may help interpretation. With this method, all information that is detected with sufficient statistical accuracy can also be displayed in the images. Different digital image receptors have been developed such as storage phosphor image plates, selenium drums, and fluorescent screens in contact with a charge-coupled device.

Automatic Exposure Control Systems

To maintain the correct blackening at the region of interest in the image while changing the projection or orientation of the patient, the x-ray generator that controls the x-ray tube needs information about the exposure at the image receptor. By placing detectors close to the image receptor, the exposure level can be measured and the tube current and/or tube potential can be automatically adjusted. For example, the

Figure 2.5 The film characteristic curve for two x-ray films used with fluorescent screens. The curve describes the relation between film optical density (blackening) and the relative exposure of the film. At low and high optical densities, the gradient (slope or first derivative) of the film curve is low and so is the film contrast. At optical densities between 1.0 and 2.5, the film contrast is high. The maximal film contrast for film A is higher than for film B, which on the other hand has a wider latitude, that is, a range of exposure values that corresponds to a given blackening range.

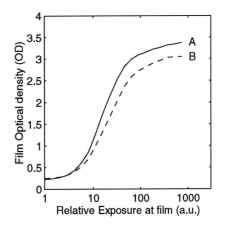

brightness of the image-intensifier output screen can be measured and used by the automatic exposure control system during fluoroscopy. The brightness is kept at a constant value by changes in tube potential and tube current.

IMAGE QUALITY

Image quality can in physical terms be expressed by the three fundamental image quality descriptors *contrast, sharpness (resolution)*, and *noise*.

The information about the patient in the x-ray image is due to different photon attenuation properties in different tissues. The contrast, and thus the information in the image, is corrupted by lack of sharpness (unsharpness) by scattered radiation, and by noise (stochastic variations) in the imaging system. The influence of contrast, sharpness, and noise on the detectability of structures of interest depends on the imaging task, that is, on the nature of the structure to be visualized. If the structure is small but has high contrast, an imaging system with high sharpness is usually preferred, but if the structure is larger but with low contrast, an imaging system with low noise would be preferred.

Contrast

Contrast is the most important image quality descriptor; without contrast there is no information. Contrast depends on object contrast, receptor contrast, and scattered radiation. The object contrast is the difference in the number of transmitted photons through the patient's body at two neighboring areas in the receptor. It depends on differences in thickness, density, and atomic composition along the rays passing the body at different positions. Obviously, a thick detail of high density will stand out more clearly in the image than a small nodule with close to unit density. If the atomic number of the detail differs significantly from the surrounding tissues and the energy of the x-ray beam is low, the difference in the attenuation (contrast) and transmission of the photons will be larger; the lower the energy (kV), the larger the contrast.

Medical x-ray film most often enhances the object contrast if the exposure is made correctly, that is, if the details of interest are located on the part of the film characteristic curve with the largest slope or gradient (Fig. 2.5). Too low or too high exposures reduce receptor contrast considerably. A film with a large slope (high gradient) enhances the contrast more than a film with a lower slope. On the other hand, a film with lower gradient will provide the opportunity simultaneously to show areas of very different attenuation or exposure levels. In digital imaging systems, contrast can be manipulated after the exposure to enhance visibility of particular details of interest. This is useful, provided the noise level is not too high.

Sharpness

Sharpness is the ability of the imaging system to depict a sharp edge. Small details are more easily detected with an imaging system with high sharpness. Different components of the imaging system contribute to reduce sharpness (increase unsharpness). These are geometric, object, and receptor unsharpness. The geometric unsharpness is caused by the finite size of the x-ray focal spot and can be minimized by keeping this spot small and the details to be imaged as close to the receptor as possible. Patient motion during exposure contributes to object unsharpness and can be minimized by using short exposure times. The receptor unsharpness is mainly caused by the lateral diffusion of the information carriers, such as the light photons in the screens before they hit the film. This can be reduced by using thin receptors, but this will reduce their ability to absorb the x rays. The search for materials that efficiently absorb the photons, but can be made thin to reduce receptor unsharpness, is important. Lenses and television cameras in image intensifiers are also a source of unsharpness.

Noise

Noise is variation in the image that does not correspond to variations in the patient's anatomy but depends on stochastic processes and imperfections in the imaging chain. The emission of x rays, their attenuation in the patient, and absorption in the receptor are stochastic processes. If an object is repeatedly irradiated in what are thought to be identical ways, the image will not be found to be exactly the same every time. The image will have an irregular, grainy appearance. These stochastic small-area variations are called *noise*. Quantum noise contributes most to the total noise in well-designed imaging systems and arises from the limited number of x-ray photons used to build up the image. The larger the number of x-ray photons that is absorbed in the receptor per unit area, the lower the quantum noise. Quantum noise can thus be reduced by increasing the irradiation (increase milliampere-second), but the dose in the patient will then increase. A schematic illustration of the influence of noise on the detection is given in Figure 2.6. It shows one line through the image of three details of increasing contrast from the background (5%, 10%, and 20%). Figure 2.6D shows three details with no noise. In Figure 2.6A to C, noise is added and the details of lower contrast are more difficult to detect (separate from the background noise). The noise decreases by a factor of 2 from Figure 2.6A to 6B and from 2.6B to 6C and the details with higher contrast are more easily separated from the noisy background (see also Ch. 3, Fig. 3.6A–C).

A measure of the accuracy in the information or the detectability of details of interest in the image is the ratio between the signal (the contrast) and the noise. This quotient, the signal-to-noise ratio (SNR), needs to be sufficiently high to separate (detect) a low-contrast detail from the noisy background. For well-designed digital imaging systems, the SNR increases with increasing irradiation of the patient. To double the SNR, the irradiation of the patient must be increased four times, all other things being equal.

RADIATION RISK
Radiologic Protection Principles

Acute radiation damage was reported soon after the discovery of x rays in 1895. From the radiologic protection point of view, the main concern today is the increased risk for stochastic effects

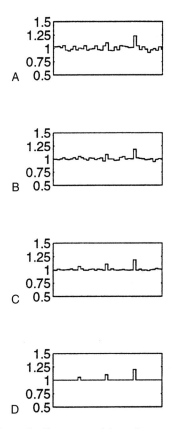

Figure 2.6 A simple illustration of the influence of noise on the detection of details. (**D**) The details without noise are shown. The contrasts (the signal) are 5%, 10%, and 20% for the leftmost, middle, and rightmost details, respectively. (**A – C**) Noise is added. The standard deviation in the noise distribution decreases from Figure A to C. The detectability of the details in the background noise, as quantified by the signal-to-noise ratio (SNR), increases from left to right in each figure, and for each contrast detail, from Figure A to C. When the SNR = 5, the details are just about detectable (right detail in Fig. A, middle detail in B, and left detail in C). When the SNR is less than 5, one is not able to say with any confidence whether or not the detail is present; when the SNR is greater than 5, the opportunity for making a correct detection increases.

such as cancer development following irradiation with absorbed doses too low to cause acute effects. The reduction of stochastic effects forms the basis of the principles of radiologic protection.[2] The first principle states that all practice with ionizing radiation should be *justified*. This means that the remitting physician must be reasonably sure that the information gained from the x-ray examination could not be found by another method, without ionizing radiation. The second principle states that all exposures should be as low as reasonably achievable. It is thus necessary to consider how best to *optimize* the examination, that is, to gain the information at the lowest patient dose. The third principle *limits doses* in individuals. Dose limits do not generally apply to patients, who should directly benefit from the examination, but are aimed at persons employed in the provision of the service.

For the individual, the radiation risks associated with the x-ray examination are small, but since the number of individuals undergoing x-ray examinations is very large, the collective absorbed dose

to the whole population will be significant. Failure to diagnose is probably the largest single risk for the patient, but for some patients, adverse effects of injected contrast media may be potentially hazardous. On the whole, correct diagnosis and proper treatment, based on the x-ray images, could lower the patient's risk.

Radiation Damage

Stochastic damage can be either hereditary or carcinogenic and have no threshold; that is, the character of the damage (e.g., cancer) does not depend on the absorbed dose. The assumption in radiologic protection is that the probability for developing cancer later in life due to the exposure increases linearly with increasing absorbed dose. This is an approximation because the radiosensitivity varies among individuals, and the link between dose and risk for radiation-induced cancer at very low doses is difficult to determine. This lack of knowledge has led to a conservative approach, not to presuppose the existence of threshold doses under which the risk is zero. Acute damage (e.g., skin erythema and cataracts of the lens), on the other hand, occurs only after a threshold dose has been exceeded.

An increased frequency of occurrence of leukemia and cancer was noted among the survivors of the nuclear bombs in Japan. These survivors were exposed to almost homogeneous total-body irradiation. By studying the frequency of cancer in this group, it has been possible to derive relative risk factors and tissue weighting factors for different organs.

Acute damage such as skin erythema has been very rare. Recently, however, in complicated interventional procedures with long-time fluoroscopy with high dose rates, skin erythema has been reported.

Dosimetric Concepts

In an x-ray examination, the patient is not homogeneously exposed to radiation. The dose decreases rapidly with depth in the patient's body and even more rapidly outside the boundaries of the radiation field. The effective dose was defined to express the stochastic risk of cancer induction and genetic injury under such circumstances.[2] It is the product of the average organ or tissue dose and the relative tissue weighting factor for that organ or tissue type, totalled over all exposed organs. The effective dose is measured in the unit Sievert, Sv. The organs that have the largest tissue weighting factor are gonads, red bone marrow, colon, lung, and stomach. The effective dose per film and the dose in the uterus and the ovaries are shown in Table 2.1 for some common x-ray examinations.[3] Reference doses for some x-ray examinations have been suggested along with image quality criteria and image technique settings.[4] If the patient dose is significantly higher than the reference dose, it is an indication that the imaging system or technique is not operating optimally.

The risk for developing fatal cancer after exposure to ionizing radiation has been estimated at 5%/Sv or 0.05%/mSv. This risk is two to four times higher for children. As a comparison, the natural background dose in Sweden, excluding exposure to radon, is about 1 mSv. It is difficult to compare risks, but smoking 60 cigarettes per day, or driving a car 5,000 km is about the same as being exposed to a dose of 1 mSv. It is not unusual to underestimate the risk for everyday activities while the risk for rare and unknown activities is overestimated.

Table 2.1 Effective Doses and Absorbed Doses in the Uterus and the Ovary for Some Common X-Ray Examinations[a]

Examination (view)	Effective Dose (mSv)	Uterus Dose (mGy)	Ovary Dose (mGy)
Chest (PA)	0.03	[b]	[b]
Thorac Spine (AP)	0.5	1.0	0.7
Pelvis (AP)	0.8	1.5	1.2
Lumbar Spine (AP)	0.9	1.9	1.5
Abdomen (AP)	1.0	2.1	1.6

Abbreviations: AP, anteroposterior; PA, posteroanterior.

[a] The data come from a survey of 20 English hospitals[3] and are averages from the patient sample measured. The effective doses have been recalculated using the new tissue weighting factors,[2] assuming 81 kV, 3.5 mm Al filtration. The doses will vary with imaging technique, such as tube potential, filtration, image receptor, field size, and field position and of course with the weight (thickness) of the patient.

[b] Absorbed dose is less than 0.01 mGy.

OPTIMIZATION OF IMAGE QUALITY AND DOSE

An optimization strategy is a procedure that searches for an imaging technique that utilizes the information most efficiently, that is, tries to maximize the ratio between image quality and radiation risk. Image quality may be difficult to quantify and is task-dependent, but the SNR has been suggested as an image quality descriptor for the detection of low-contrast details in a noisy image. Using this approach, it is then necessary to decide on the required level of image quality and then search for imaging system design and operating parameters (kilovolt, filter, field size, grid, image receptor, etc.) that fulfills these requirements at the lowest patient risk.

Digital image capture and image processing are required to take full advantage of all information in the image. This is facilitated by separating image capture and image display. CT (see Ch. 3), was introduced in the 1970s using digital image capture and is able to register small differences in attenuation (or contrast). A danger with digital techniques is that the information capture (theoretically) can be infinite. Very small details and very small tissue differences (contrasts) can be detected, provided the noise level is low and thus the irradiation of the patient is increased. With the increasing capacity of modern x-ray tubes and even smaller pixel sizes in the digital images, we can come to a point where the demands on more information (higher image quality) will lead to unacceptably high doses. More efficient utilization of the x rays could counteract this scenario.

PLAIN RADIOGRAPHY IMAGING TECHNIQUES

Plain radiography is usually begun with the patient erect after having emptied her bladder. Anteroposterior projections are obtained. Occasionally, an oblique film may be important to delineate sacrum, coccyx, feces, or gas when they are thought to be artifacts. Hysterosalpingography (HSG) is performed with the patient in the lithotomy position (Fig. 2.7). This is in contrast to the supine position of ultrasound imaging (Fig. 2.8). The presence of fluid can cause a loss of clear borders and displacement of organs and can be diagnosed by air–liquid interfaces (Fig. 2.9).

Pelvimetry

Plain radiography is still an appropriate method of assessing the bony female pelvis, even though CT has recently been described as more accurate.[5] MRI has also been used but is less practical, being much more costly and time-consuming.[6]

Figure 2.7 This patient is undergoing an HSG. While one practitioner injects dye (not shown), the radiologist operates the fluoroscopy. The monitor is positioned so that the patient, as well as the physician, can see the images.

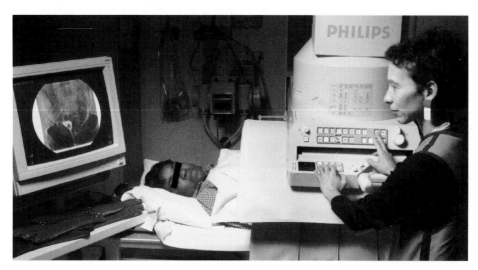

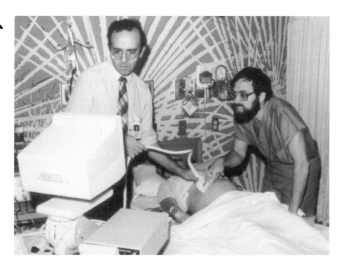

Figure 2.8 Ultrasonography in labor. The patient and her husband can watch the monitor.

Pelvic shape can be evaluated by a single anteroposterior (AP) view with the patient supine with an empty bladder. The previous "ideal" view (Thom's view) which was a superoinferior view of the inlet with the patient seated on the table, her back supported at an angle of 50 to 60 degrees, is not used now, being difficult to obtain and exposing the fetus to relatively high levels of radiation. Inserting a pad under the patient's lumbar spine may approximate the AP view to Thom's view. The widest transverse diameter of the inlet, as well as the interspinous diameter, can thus be evaluated. A lateral view with the patient erect, may, however, be the best diagnostic projection. One can measure the available conjugate, AP diameter of the midpelvis, and pubosacral distances.

Uterine Anomalies

Congenital anomalies result from abnormal in-utero development of the müllerian ducts. These anomalies can be evaluated by ultrasonography,[7] MRI, CT, and HSG,[8–10] as well as by direct visualization through the hysteroscope or laparoscope. When a congenital anomaly is suspected, HSG is probably the preferred method of making the diagnosis.[11] Other methods are either more complex, more expensive, or more invasive. However, HSG cannot differentiate between a sep-

Figure 2.9 A 74-year-old with a previous total abdominal hysterectomy, bilateral oophorectomy, and postoperative chemotherapy for stage IV poorly differentiated leiomyosarcoma. One year after surgery, the patient was admitted with cachexia and intractable abdominal pain. **(A)** The supine film shows a markedly dilated stomach and proximal duodenum. **(B)** The left lateral decubitus film shows air–fluid levels suggestive of bowel obstruction. Further treatment was refused, and the patient died the next day.

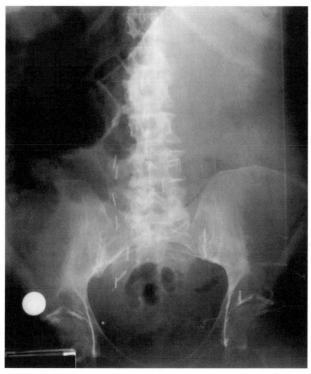

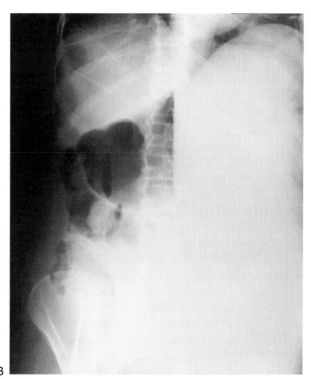

A

B

tate and a bicornuate uterus, and it will not demonstrate a noncommunicating uterine horn. Although MRI is the most expensive, it may be the most accurate.[12] Plain x ray has no place in the diagnosis of these anomalies.

Leiomyomas

Depending on the location of the leiomyomas, imaging techniques may have varied diagnostic accuracy.[13] Subserous leiomyomas will not cause changes in the contour or the size of the uterine cavity and may give some nondiagnostic blurriness on plain x ray. If pedunculated, they can be confused with other solid pelvic masses. Intramural myomas (the most common), particularly if large, will distort the uterine cavity or cause it to appear irregularly enlarged. Submucous leiomyomas distort the uterine cavity and assign it an abnormal shape. Plain x ray is usually insufficient to demonstrate distortion of the uterine cavity. Most of the time, it is also useless in demonstrating leiomyomas unless they are calcified. When considering expense and simplicity, HSG remains the method of choice to image the uterine cavity and, therefore, submucous leiomyomas, in particular.[11,13,14] When demonstrating a filling defect in the opacified uterine cavity, one needs to remember other potential diagnoses such as polyp, carcinoma, adhesions (Asherman's syndrome), pregnancy, and artifact caused by the presence of air bubbles. MRI can differentiate uterine tumor from leiomyomas as well as leiomyomas from adenomyosis. CT, particularly with intravenous contrast, will differentiate the three types of leiomyomata.

Cervical Pathology

Plain radiography of the pelvis has no role in the diagnosis of cervical pathology, but chest x-ray is valuable if metastases are suspected. CT is effective in staging invasive cervical carcinoma by assessing tumor extension to the pelvic sidewalls, lymph node involvement, and invasion of the bladder or rectum.

Intrauterine Device Localization

Intrauterine device misplacement is the major cause of failed contraception for this method. If the intrauterine contraceptive device (IUCD) string is missing on pelvic examination, it could have withdrawn into the cervical canal, or the IUCD could have perforated of the uterine wall or have been expelled unnoticed. The simplest way to demonstrate an IUCD (or any foreign body—Fig. 2.10) is by x ray with a flat AP view of the abdomen. The accuracy is 100% for presence in the pelvis but not for presence in the uterus. Other methods are either less precise or too costly. However, once the IUCD is found in the pelvis, ultrasonography is the best method of localizing it in the uterus (especially if the patient is pregnant).[15] If it is embedded in the uterine wall, ultrasonography

is less accurate and hysterosalpingogram or hysteroscopy may be necessary.[16]

OTHER RADIOGRAPHIC TECHNIQUES

Pelvic Angiography

The most common method of pelvic angiography is selective hypogastric arteriography via a transfemoral retrograde approach. Fluoroscopy is necessary to demonstrate the position of the catheter. Renographin 60% is the most commonly used medium at a rate of 15 cc per second for a total of 60 cc. A total of 16 to 20 shots at 2- to 8-second intervals are taken to show the blood vessels Angiography can demonstrate distortion of pelvic arteries by tumors, but is rarely used today. It can also be used as a therapeutic procedure for selective embolization of specific pelvic vessels in cases of intractable obstetric hemorrhage. Phlebography by retrograde pelvic, transuterine, or renal vein is resorted to in some cases of possible thrombosis.

Lymphangiography

Intra- or subdermal injection of a blue dye into the web spaces of the toes allows visualization of the lymphatics into which Ethindiol can be injected. Lymph vessels of the lower limbs, pelvis, and abdominal cavity can be demonstrated. Both AP and oblique views are obtained. Neoplastic involvement by pelvic disease or general diseases (such as Hodgkin's disease)

Figure 2.10 This 4-year-old girl had lower abdominal pain and vaginal discharge. She reported playing with a small metallic toy ring. The ring can be seen on the AP flat plate of the lower abdomen. It was removed with the patient under general anaesthesia.

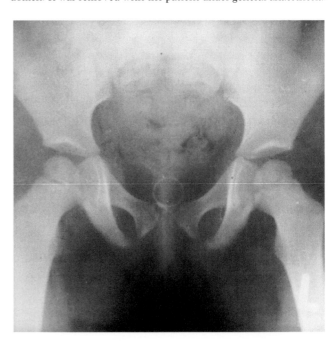

can be demonstrated in 70% to 80% of cases. Less invasive methods such as CT or MRI give similar or better results.

SUMMARY

When Röntgen discovered the x ray 100 years ago, he might have little realized the potential of his remarkable observation. Now a plain radiograph is useful for pelvimetry, to demonstrate calcification in a leiomyoma, to localize an IUCD, or to assess gastrointestinal complications of pelvic surgery. Fluoroscopy can assess the uterine cavity or tubal patency.[17] CT is a further development that Röntgen could not have foreseen when he first noticed that little glow in the dark.

REFERENCES

1. Matscheko G, Alm Carlsson G. Measurement of absolute energy spectra from a clinical CT machine under working conditions using a Compton spectrometer. Phys Med Biol 1989;34: 209–222

2. ICRP, International Commission on Radiological Protection. 1990 Recommendations of the International Commission on Radiological Protection. Annals of the ICRP, Publication 60, Pergamon, Oxford, 1991

3. Shrimpton PC, Wall BF, Jones DG et al. A national survey of doses to patients undergoing a selection of routine X-ray examinations in English hospitals. NRPB-R200. National Radiological Protection Board, Chilton, United Kingdom, 1986

4. European Guidelines on Quality Criteria for Diagnostic Radiographic Images. EUR 16260 EN, European Commission, Directorate-General XII: Science, Research and Development, Luxembourg: Office for Official Publications of the European Communities, 1996, pp 1–46

5. Christian SS, Brady K, Read JA, Kopelman JN. Vaginal breech delivery: a five-year prospective evaluation of a protocol using computed tomographic pelvimetry. Am J Obstet Gynecol 1990;163:848–855

6. van Loon AJ, Mantingh A, Thijn CJ, Mooyaart EL. Pelvimetry by magnetic resonance imaging in breech presentation. Am J Obstet Gynecol 1990;163:1256–1260

7. Daya S. Ultrasonographic evaluation of uterine abnormalities. In: Jaffe R, Pierson RA, Abramowicz JS, Eds. Imaging in Infertility and Reproductive Endocrinology. JB Lippincott, Philadelphia, 1994, pp 63–91

8. Occhipinti KA. Magnetic resonance imaging of abnormal pelvic anatomy. In: Jaffe R, Pierson RA, Abramowicz JS, Eds. Imaging in Infertility and Reproductive Endocrinology. JB Lippincott, Philadelphia, 1994, pp 249–268

9. Friedman WN, Perlman ES, Rosenfield AT. Computed tomography of normal and abnormal female pelvic anatomy. In: Jaffe R, Pierson RA, Abramowicz JS, Eds. Imaging in Infertility and Reproductive Endocrinology. JB Lippincott, Philadelphia, 1994, pp 285–305

10. Lewis V, Abramowicz JS. Hysterosalpingography of the abnormal pelvis. In: Jaffe R, Pierson RA, Abramowicz JS, Eds. Imaging in Infertility and Reproductive Endocrinology. JB Lippincott, Philadelphia, 1994, pp 321–333

11. Zhioua F, Ferchiou M, Dey F et al. Hysteroscopy and hysterosalpingography. Which examination to choose? Rev Fr Gynecol Obstet 1993;88:253–255

12. Pellerito JS, McCarthy SM, Doyle MB et al. Diagnosis of uterine anomalies: relative accuracy of MR imaging, endovaginal sonography and hysterosalpingography. Radiology 1992;183:795–800

13. Karasick S, Lev-Toaff SS, Toaff ME. Imaging of uterine leiomyomas. AJR Am J Roentgenol 1992;158:799–805

14. Simon P, Hollemaert S, Schwers J. Respective diagnostic importance of hysterography and hysteroscopy in common uterine pathology. J Gynecol Obstet Biol Reprod 1993;22:141–144

15. Piiroinen O. Ultrasonic localization of intrauterine contraceptive devices. Acta Obstet Gynecol Scand 1972;51:203–207

16. Rosenblatt R, Zakin D, Stern WZ, Kutcher R. Uterine perforation and embedding by intrauterine device: evaluation by US and hysterography. Radiology 1985;157:765–770

17. Rajah R, McHugo JM, Obhrai M. The role of hysterosalpingography in modern gynecological practice. Br J Radiol 1992;65:849–851

3

Computed Tomography: Physical Principles and Imaging Techniques

MICHAEL SANDBORG

JILL E. LANGER

In planar projected images, important anatomic details may be concealed by overlying tissues. By using a slice-imaging technique (tomography), selective morphology can be seen layer by layer.

Computed tomography (CT) is a form of ideal tomography that yields sequences of consecutive thin-slice images of the patient and allows localization in three dimensions. As distinct from conventional (classical) tomography, CT does not suffer from interference of structures that do not lie in the slice to be imaged. This is achieved by irradiating only thin sections of the patient with a fan-shaped beam. Transaxial images (tomograms) give more selective information than conventional planar projection radiographs. A CT image has superior contrast resolution; that is, it is capable of separating very small differences in tissue attenuation but has inferior spatial resolution compared to planar radiography. A contrast of less than 1% can be seen, but the spatial resolution is inferior. In conventional planar radiography, such small contrasts cannot be seen, but tiny details can.

PRINCIPLES OF OPERATION

The principle of operation of CT has two steps. The first is physical measurements of the attenuation of x rays in different directions, and the second is the mathematical calculation of the linear attenuation coefficient, μ, over the slice (see Ch. 2 for further information). The x-ray tube rotates in a circular orbit around the patient in a plane perpendicular to the length-axis of the patient (Fig. 3.1).[1] A fan-shaped beam passes through the patient. It is of variable width (1 to 10 mm). The x-ray tube is more powerful than that used for planar radiography. The image receptor is an array of several hundred small receivers. The readings from the receivers are handled in the computer and produce a tomogram, that is, a map of linear attenuation coefficients μ.

The arrangement of the x-ray tube and the receptor array

has changed over the years, and different technical solutions are labeled by generations. CT scanners used today are of the third or fourth generation (Fig. 3.1). The arrangement of the x-ray tube and the receptor array rotating together is typical of the third generation of CT scanners, whereas the fourth generation has a complete ring of receptors that remains stationary and only the x-ray tube rotates. CT scanners are now available where the x-ray tube orbits the patient, while the patient examination table moves continuously longitudinally; thus, the x-ray tube forms a spiral orbit around the patient. These are called spiral (helical) CT scanners.

CT was one of the first forms of digital radiology. The receptor array measures the x-rays coming through a slice of the patient in different positions. This forms one projection. The reading in the receptor is a measure of the attenuation in the patient along the path of that ray. Behind a homogeneous object, the receptor reading is equal to $I = I_0 e^{-\mu x}$, where I_0 is the receptor reading without object and μ is the linear attenuation coefficient for the material in the object, x is the object thickness along the path of that ray, and e is the base of the natural logarithm system ($e \approx 2.718$). The receptor reading I is an exponential function and decreases with increasing thickness of the object (patient) and with increasing attenuation of the photons in the object. The linear attenuation coefficient μ depends on the atomic composition of the material and on the photon energy. Elements with a high atomic number have a higher μ, and it decreases with increasing photon energy. For an inhomogeneous object such as a patient, the product μx is in reality a sum of all the different tissue attenuation coefficients, μ_i, such that

$$\Sigma_i \, \mu_i x_i.$$

After all the readings from the receptor array have been received by the computer, the tube moves to another angle and "looks" at the patient from a slightly different view and a new projection profile can be measured. Following a complete rotation, the table with the patient is moved a small distance and the next section imaged.

Given the data from a set of projection profiles through all

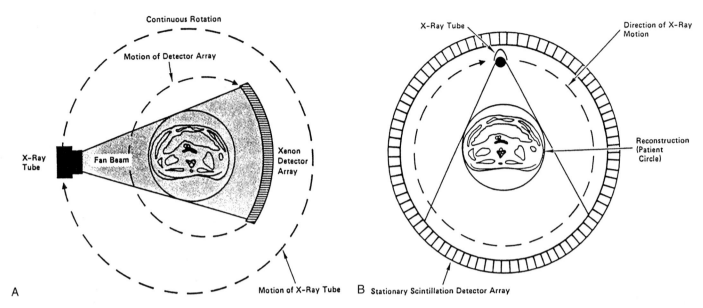

Figure 3.1 **(A)** Third-generation CT scanner. The x-ray tube and the receptor array are located on opposite sides of the patient, and both rotate around the patient during the data acquisition. The receptor array is made from about 700 pressurized Xenon detectors. **(B)** Fourth-generation CT scanner where only the x-ray tube rotates around the patient; the receptor array, which is situated in the outside perimeter of the scanning frame, remains stationary. The receptors are made from a solid-state material and are as many as 4,000. Both scanners use a fan beam and about 1,000 projections. The data acquisition time is a few seconds, and the 512×512 image matrix can be viewed just a few seconds after the data acquisition is completed. (From Huang,[1] with permission.)

volume elements (voxels) in a slice of the patient for sufficient numbers of rotation angles (projections), it is possible to calculate the average linear attenuation coefficient, μ, for each voxel. This procedure is called *reconstruction*. Each value of μ is assigned a gray scale value on the display monitor and is presented in a square picture element (pixel) of the image.

RECONSTRUCTION ALGORITHMS

The computer reconstructs an image: a matrix of μ-values for all voxels in a section (slice) perpendicular to the rotation axis. The procedure to reconstruct the image, based on the many projections at different angles, is made with a reconstruction algorithm. An algorithm is a mathematical method for solving a problem. The problem is to find the μ-values in each voxel based on all the measured data in the projection profiles.

There are several types of reconstruction algorithms available such as filtered back-projection, direct Fourier, and algebraic reconstruction techniques. The method used for medical CT scanners is filtered back-projection. Figure 3.2 shows the imaging geometry of a very simple object, such as two

discs of different diameter (d_1 and d_2) and linear attenuation coefficient (μ_1 and μ_2). The projection profiles are schematically shown at three different rotation angles (0, 24 and 48 degrees). Figures 3.3A to 3.3C show images where one profile is projected back on to the whole image matrix. The projection profile changes with the rotation angle, and Figures 3.3D to 3.3f show the tomogram images using an increasing number of projections in the back-projection procedure; 5, 25, and 125 projections in Figures 3.3D to F, respectively. In all images, the details are smeared out over the whole image area. Even with many projections, this effect will occur. If each projection is filtered (using a specific mathematical filter) before the back-projection procedure, the details and all μ's will be correctly reconstructed. Figures 3.3G to 3.3I shows an example of filtered back-projection for the same object. The filtering procedure removes the smearing out of the detail. One needs approximately 1.5 times more projections than there are pixels along one side of the reconstructed image. An insufficient number of projections can cause the streak-shaped artifact seen in Figures 3.3D, E, G, and H.

Typical medical CT scanners today use a fan beam, have about 700 receptors (third generation) or 4,000 receptors (fourth generation), take 1,000 projections, and complete data acquisition in approximately 1 to 2 seconds. They take only a few seconds to reconstruct the 512×512 image matrix with 12 or 16 bits' depth.

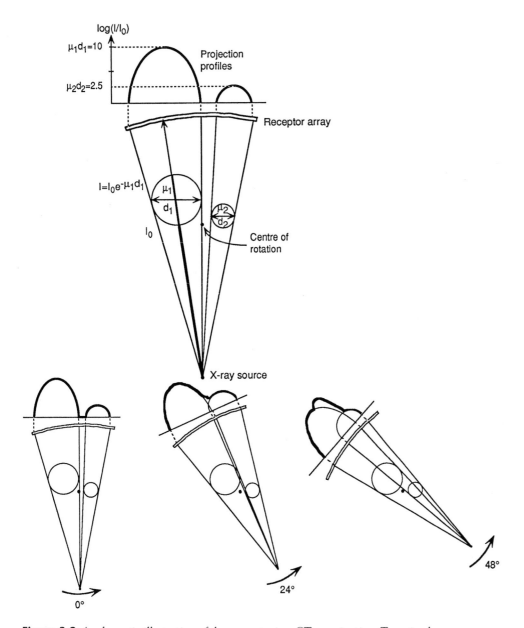

Figure 3.2 A schematic illustration of the geometry in a CT examination. Two circular objects—discs—are imaged, and their projection profiles, measured with the receptor array, are shown for three different rotation angles: 0,24, and 48 degrees. The disks have different diameters (d_1=10 cm, d_2=5 cm) and linear attenuation coefficients (μ_1=1 cm^{-1}, μ_2=0.5 cm^{-1}). I_0 is the reading in the receptor without the object, and $I_0\,e^{-\mu_1 d_1}$ the reading with the object.

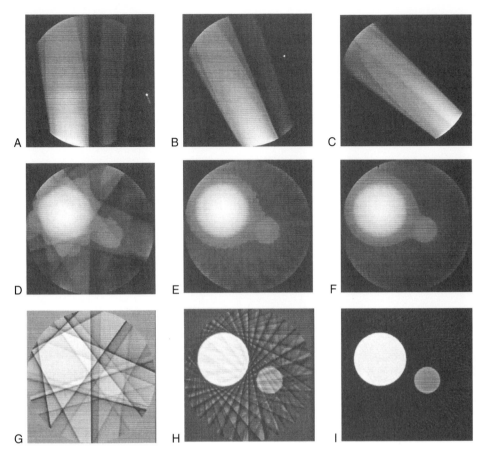

Figure 3.3 An example of an image reconstruction of the two circular discs in air in Figure 3.2 using unfiltered (**D – F**) and filtered (**G – I**) back-projection. (**A – C**) Images of the projections at 0, 24 and 48 degrees. (**D – F**). The reconstructed CT scans using an increasing number of projections in the unfiltered back-projection procedure: 5, 25, and 125 projections, respectively. A large number of projections are required for a scan of high quality. With unfiltered back-projection, the image of the discs is concentrated in the right position but also smeared out over the whole image, regardless of the number of projections used. (**G – I**) The same discs are reconstructed using filtered back-projection. The filtering procedure corrects for the smeared-out information, provided sufficient number of projections were used in the reconstruction.

DISPLAY OF CT NUMBERS

In the display, the measured μ-values can be distributed over a gray scale with the lowest μ black and the highest μ white. In plain radiography, the four so-called x-ray elements—gas, fat, soft tissue and bone—are distinguishable (see Ch. 2, Fig. 2.2). Most soft tissues have linear attenuation coefficients very similar to that of water over a large photon energy interval. This is the reason for a CT number, N_{CT}, defined by

$$N_{CT} = 1,000 \left(\frac{\mu - \mu_w}{\mu_w} \right)$$

where μ is the average linear attenuation coefficient for the material in a given voxel and μ_w is that for water. N_{CT} is given in the dimensionless unit Hounsfield, H (after Godfrey N.

Hounsfield, who won the 1979 Nobel Prize laureate in Physiology in Medicine for the development of computer-assisted tomography). The CT number scale has two fixed values independent of photon energy. For a vacuum (approximately air or body gas)

$$N_{CT,vac} \equiv - 1,000 \text{ and for water}$$
$$N_{CT,water} \equiv 0.$$

Alternatively, the μ-values may be graphically displayed. Figure 3.4 shows the variation of N_{CT} with photon energy. The normalization with μ_w in the equation above diminishes the variation of N_{CT} with energy, especially for material with an atomic number similar to that of water. Different kinds of soft tissues, such as muscle, liver, brain, blood, and cartilage, attenuate photons in the energy interval 40 to 150 keV simi-

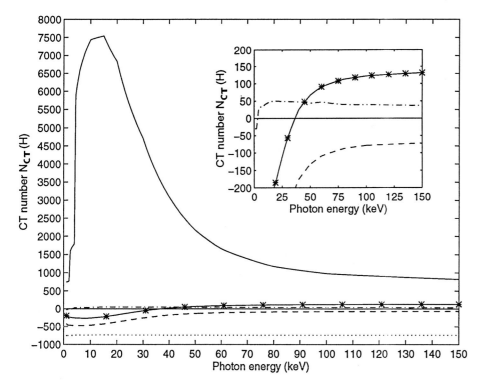

Figure 3.4 The variation of CT numbers, N_{CT}, with photon energy. The N_{CT} are normalized to water, which substantially reduces the variation of N_{CT} with energy, especially for materials with atomic number similar to that of water. The N_{CT} are therefore the same for all CT scanners. The N_{CT} for fat and especially for bone vary with the application. Compact bone (ρ=1.85 g/cm³), ___; adipose tissue (ρ=0.93 g/cm³), ---; muscle (ρ=1.05 g/cm³), ·—·; lung tissue (ρ=0.26 g/cm³), ...; water (ρ=1.00 g/cm³), the solid line at N_{CT}=0. Plexiglas, *___*, is a common phantom material used for testing the performance of the scanner. Its higher density (ρ=1.17 g/cm³) yields an N_{CT} larger than zero for photon energies above 40 keV. The insert shows the N_{CT} in an expanded scale.

larly to water, and thus their N_{CT} will be close to zero. This means that the N_{CT} of these tissues may be the same for all users including the spectra used in clinical CT scanners. The N_{CT} of fat and especially bone vary more with photon energy (Fig. 3.4).

IMAGE DISPLAY

Images can be digitally processed to meet a variety of clinical requirements in order to distinguish medically important features. The assignment of gray values on a display monitor to the CT numbers in the computer memory can be adjusted to suit special application requirements. A lookup table lists the relationship between stored (input) CT numbers and their corresponding (output) gray scale values (Fig. 3.5).

Contrast can be increased by covering just a narrow part of the CT numbers on the whole gray scale on the display mon-

itor. This is called *window technique*. The range of CT numbers displayed on the whole gray scale is called the *window width*. The average value is called the *window level*. Change in window width alters the contrast, and change in window level selects the structures in the image that are displayed on the gray scale (Fig. 3.5). As the window width is made narrower, a part of the image is displayed over the whole gray scale but only over the window width centered around the window level. These structures benefit from the higher contrast, whereas structures on the lower and higher sides of the window width (low and high CT numbers) are either completely black or white. As the window width is made even narrower, the contrast of the structures displayed increases but over an even more narrow range of CT numbers.

Combinations of these techniques enable small differences in tissue attenuations and composition to be visualized, provided the precision in the measured CT numbers is high enough, that is, if the image quality is sufficient.

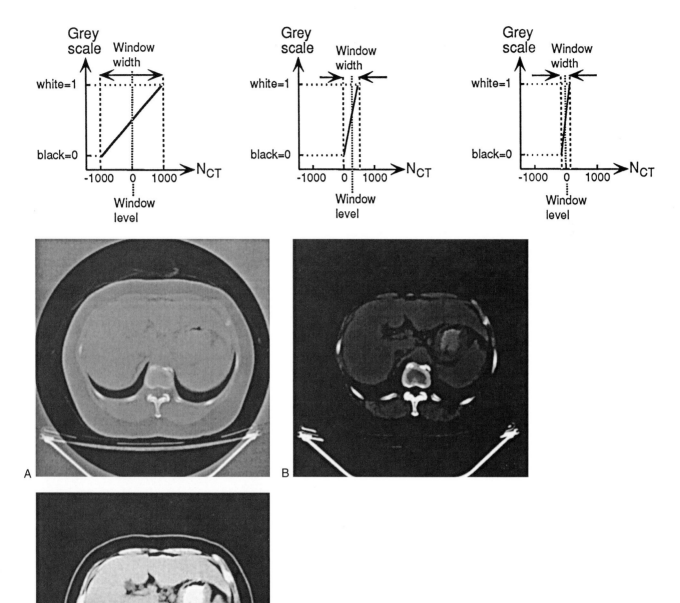

Figure 3.5 CT scans of the thorax showing the effect from changes in window width and window level. **(A)** A wide range of CT numbers between $-1,000 \leq N_{CT} \leq 1,000$ is shown, and the contrast is low. **(B)** CT numbers between $0 \leq N_{CT} \leq 500$, which displays some soft tissue and bone, are shown. **(C)** A narrow range of CT numbers between $-100 \leq N_{CT} \leq 100$, which displays soft and adipose tissue and the skin with higher contrast, is shown. As the window width is narrowed, the contrast of tissues centered around the window level increases. Structures outside the window width are displayed either completely black or white (see schematic diagrams of lookup tables above the CT images.

IMAGE QUALITY

In a digital imaging system, image quality and patient absorbed dose are interrelated. Image quality can be expressed in terms of quantum noise, contrast, and resolution. The contrast (primarily determined by differences in CT numbers) can be manipulated as discussed in the previous section. Scat-

tered photons are not the large problem that they are in planar radiography, since only a thin slice of the body is irradiated at a time.

The precision in the measurement of CT numbers is limited by quantum noise. The stochastic nature of quantum noise can be shown by inspecting a tomogram of a homogeneous object. All pixels do not have the same CT number, but a random spread in CT numbers is found. This is because attenuation and absorption of x-ray photons are stochastic processes, and only a limited number of x-ray photons are absorbed in the receptor and used to build the image. The larger the number of x-ray photons that is absorbed in the receptors, the larger the precision and the lower the quantum noise. Figure 3.6A to 3.6C shows tomograms of a cylinder-shaped Plexiglas container containing water and disc-shaped details of varying contrast and diameter. The number of photons used in the reconstruction of the image decreases 10 times from Figure 3.6A to 3.6B and 3.6B to 6C. The detectability of the small low-contrast details is significantly reduced when fewer x-ray photons are used, since the quantum noise increases.

The number of x-ray photons absorbed in the receptors depends on the x-ray tube charge (the product of x-ray tube current and exposure time) and on the energy spectra of the photons. The number will increase if the patient is thinner and the tube potential is higher and if the receptor absorbs a larger fraction of the photons (e.g., is made thicker or with a larger area).

The receptor area is proportional to the section thickness and voxel size and is therefore related to the resolution in the image. If the resolution in the images is doubled, the number of x-ray quanta required to retain the same noise level as with the larger voxels would need to be increased $2^4 = 16$ times. This means that in order to make full use of the increased spatial resolution, one needs to increase the dose to the patient 16 times.

For a patient who is 25 cm from skin to skin, the pixel size in the patient for a 256×256 matrix would be just below 1.0 mm and for $512 \times 512 \times$ matrix 0.5 mm. A less noisy image would be achieved by changing from a $512 \times 512 \times$ to 256×256 matrix, at the expense of a loss in spatial resolution.

ARTIFACTS

Practical CT is based on physical measurements followed by mathematical computations. The computations are based on idealized assumptions that do not entirely correspond to physical reality. This creates artifacts or errors in the measurement and reconstruction of the μ-values.

Artifacts in the image are patterns that do not correspond to the patient's anatomy. An example is shown in Figure 3.6d. The streak patterns originate from the high-absorbing steel detail in the water. Such artifacts are caused by metal or other

Figure 3.6 CT scans of a cylinder-shaped Plexiglas container (1-cm-thick wall) containing 20 cm water and low-contrast details of increasing contrast (1%, 2%, 4%, 8%, 16% higher) and diameter (0.5, 1.0, 1.5, 2.0, 2.5 cm). **(A – C)** The number of x-ray photons used in the reconstruction of the image is decreased a factor of 10 between each scan, which reduces the detectability of the small, low-contrast details (at the lower left in the images). The quantum noise in the projection data in Figures a, b, and c are 0.1%, 0.316%, and 1%, respectively. **(D – G)**. Examples of artifacts are shown. **(D)** Partial volume effect (due to a 3-mm-diameter steel pin in the upper left corner). **(E)** Ring artifacts (due to poorly calibrated receptors). **(F)** Beam-hardening effect in an 8-cm disc of bone (darkening toward the disc center). **(G)** With a lower window level, the beam-hardening effect in the surrounding water is also visualized. Note also the partial volume effect in water in the vicinity of the water–bone boundary.

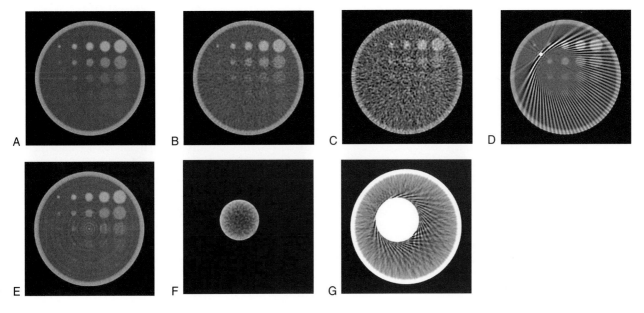

A B C D

E F G

high-density objects (bone) in the slice. If the detail in one projection is covered by one receptor (one ray) and not in another projection, the voxel will be assigned the wrong μ-value. This is called *partial volume effect* and is a particular problem in CT of the head. It can be reduced by using smaller receptor areas.

Concentric rings in the image may be caused by poorly calibrated or malfunctioning receivers (Fig. 3.6e).

Beam-hardening artifacts are found when a spectrum of photon energies are used. As the beam traverses the patient, the low-energy photons are more likely to be absorbed in the patient, and this increases the mean energy of the beam. An increased mean energy corresponds to a lower μ-value, and if a homogenous object is imaged, the central parts of the object are assigned too low an N_{CT} and thus seem less dense (blacker). Figure 3.6f and g show this effect when a bone cylinder in the water phantom is imaged. The effect is accentuated if the length of the path is long or if a material has a high atomic number. To reduce this effect, the x-ray spectrum (see Ch. 2, Fig. 2.4) is additionally filtered before reaching the patient with thick aluminium or copper filters.

Scattered radiation creates artifacts similar to that of beam hardening. To minimize this problem, the fraction of scattered photons should only be about 1% of the total radiation but will in reality be more.

Patient movement during exposure will cause artifacts, and it is therefore important to reduce the exposure time. With ultrafast CT scanners, subsecond data acquisition time can be achieved to image cardiac motion. This type of scanner is sometimes referred to as fifth-generation CT scanner.

ABSORBED DOSES

The patient-absorbed dose in CT examinations constitutes a large portion (about 20%) of the total dose from medical diagnostic x-ray examinations. This is due to the increased number of CT scanners in operation. The number of sections per patient has increased, since the time to perform and reconstruct the image has become much shorter. The dose per section, however, has not been reduced. Improved image quality has been achieved in part by reducing the quantum noise. Much of this reduced quantum noise has come about by increasing the irradiation of the patient.

To assess doses in CT, the dose in the center of the gantry is measured. Tables are available[2] to convert this dose to the effective dose[3] in the patient (see Ch. 2 for Table 2-1).[4] The quotient of the effective dose in these examinations using conventional (planar) radiography procedures to the effective dose in CT are also given in Table 3.1. When the effective doses are compared, one should remember that the information retrieved from conventional radiography and CT examinations is different. In view of the relatively high doses in CT, the United Kingdom Royal College of Radiology and the National Radiological Protection Board[5] suggest that all CT

Table 3.1 The Effective Dose in Common Routine CT Examination and the Relative Frequency for These Examinations*

Examination	Frequency (%)	Effective Dose, E (mSv)	E_{CR}/E_{CT}
Head	34.9	1.8	0.06
Abdomen	11.6	7.2	0.16
Chest	7.9	8.3	0.01
Pelvis	5.6	7.3	0.13

* The data originates from a survey of 20 English hospitals.[5] The quotient, E_{CR}/E_{CT}, is the ratio between the effective dose in the patient from a conventional radiography (CR) examination and the effective dose in CT.

examinations should be individually referred to a radiologist who will advise on whether CT is appropriate.

CT TECHNIQUE

CT continues to be well suited and valuable for the evaluation of the female pelvis because the solid organs are often outlined by extraperitoneal fat, opacification of the gastrointestinal and genitourinary tract can be easily achieved, and image quality is relatively unaffected by body habitus or bowel peristalsis. Furthermore, advances in CT technology have allowed the rapid acquisition of high-resolution images, improving CT imaging of the female genital tract attention to technique and adequate patient preparation are essential to ensure the highest quality images for optimal visualization.

CT relies on differences in x-ray beam attenuation, since the inherent attenuation difference of the pelvic soft tissue structures is small, and technique that will accentuate this difference will therefore improve visualization and discrimination of those structures.[6,7] In abdominopelvic CT, this is accomplished with the use of intravenous contrast, a class of clinical compounds that contain iodine, which produces marked attenuation of the x-ray beam. All current iodinated intravenous contrast agents are water soluble and hyperosmolar relative to plasma. Contrast agents are generally divided into two classes: the conventional high osmolar agents, which may be up to eight times as osmolar as plasma, and the newer, but more costly, lower osmolar agents, which are two to three times as osmolar as plasma[8,9] (Fig. 3.7). Adverse side effects from the administration of intravenous contrast media vary from minor physiologic disturbances to severe, life-threatening reactions. Adverse reactions have been reported to occur in 5% to 12% of all intravenous injections with ionic high-osmolar contrast media and in 1% to 3% with nonionic low-osmolar contrast media.[9–13] While most reactions are mild or

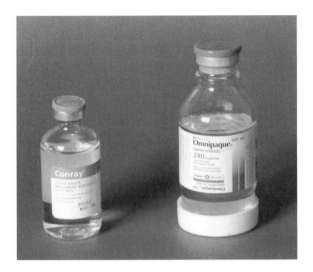

Figure 3.7 Intravenous contrast. The intravenous contrast agents administered to patients undergoing CT examination are typically packaged in small glass bottles containing 50 or 100 ml. This allows individual dosing per patient and the possibility of warming the solution prior to administration to reduce its viscosity. The contrast agent shown on the left is an ionic contrast agent (Conray; Mallinckrodt, St. Louis, MO), and the one on the right is a nonionic agent (Omnipaque; Nycomed, Princeton, NJ)

agents,[15] they are used selectively in patients at high risk because of their cost. Although serious adverse side effects are infrequent, the information to be gained from the administration of intravenous contrast must be weighed against its potential side effects for each patient requiring imaging evaluation. A knowledge of the side effects and their treatment is essential[9] (Fig. 3.8).

Following injection, intravascular contrast agents are distributed in both the vascular and extravascular spaces.[16–18] Various tissues will demonstrate different features of contrast media enhancement related to their different vascular supply and physiology, which will help to accentuate the existing small attenuation differences of normal and abnormal tissue.[8,16,19,20] Factors affecting the resultant attenuation of any tissue will depend on the rate, method, and amount of contrast administered, its rate of redistribution from the vascular to the extravascular space, and the timing of the imaging sequence.[8,17–23] The goal is to scan rapidly through the body part to be imaged when the arteriovenous contrast difference is greatest.[16] In general, the delivery of contrast by a rapid bolus infusion is the method of administration that has shown the highest levels of parenchymal contrast enhancement.[16–18] The initiation and duration of the scan acquisition should be carefully timed to image the pelvis during this parenchymal phase of contrast enhancement, when the soft tissue contrast is highest, to facilitate the detection of the differential enhancement patterns of both normal and abnormal tissue.[6,20,24–26] (Fig. 3.9).

A scanning protocol designed to image the pelvis during the optimal phase of enhancement is therefore recommended for patients presenting with known or suspected gynecologic pathology or those in whom the abdominal pelvic CT suggests an abnormality.[24,26] This dedicated protocol may be per-

moderate, severe contrast reactions can lead to patient morbidity, with an estimated risk of fatality of 0.9 per 100,000 noncardiac uses.[14] Research has shown the nonionic contrast agents to be less cardiotoxic and neurotoxic and has shown that the risk of mild, moderate, and severe nonfatal reactions is less than with ionic contrast.[9–14] Since no studies have demonstrated a decreased mortality with nonionic contrast

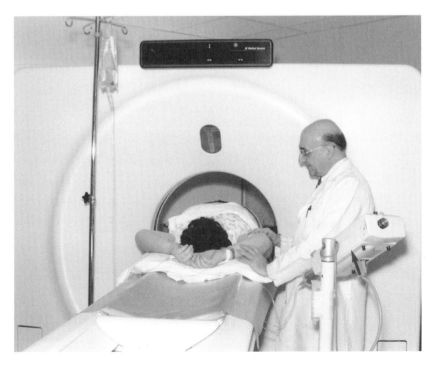

Figure 3.8 Patient monitoring. A 55-year-old woman with pelvic pain is undergoing an abdominopelvic CT examination. The patient is initially placed supine on the CT table, which will move through the CT gantry during the imaging sequence. The intravenous contrast will be administered via a mechanical injector (arrow), which is programmed to deliver contrast with a prescribed timing and rate dosage schedule. A CT technologist (or other appropriately trained person) should be present, palpating the injection site for any potential extravasation of contrast and monitoring the patient for a potential contrast reaction during the early phase of contrast administration, before the CT imaging sequence has begun.

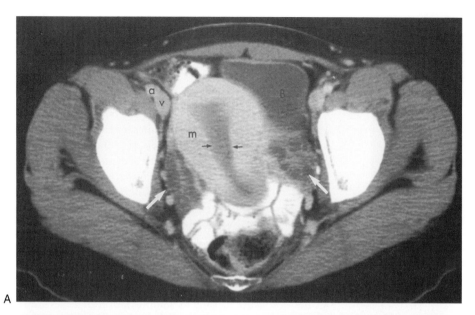

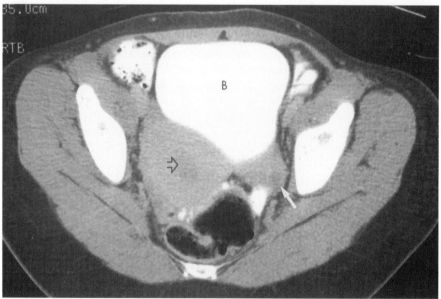

Figure 3.9 The parenchymal phase of contrast enhancement. **(A)** CT examination of the pelvis performed during rapid intravenous bolus contrast administration in a 21-year-old woman demonstrates the normal endometrial canal (black arrows) as a central area of low attenuation relative to the myometrium (m), which enhances as densely as the pelvic vessels due to its rich vascular supply. Multiple small, rounded, low-attenuation areas within the ovaries (white arrows) are identified, representing follicular cysts. (a, external iliac artery; v, external iliac vein. B, bladder. **(B)** An image obtained approximately 5 minutes later in the same patient at a slightly more cephalad level demonstrates the urinary bladder (B) to be filled with excreted contrast. The full urinary bladder has pushed the uterus posteriorly. Soft tissue contrast is poor, since these images were not acquired during the parenchymal enhancement phase of intravenous contrast enhancement. The endometrial cavity (open arrow) is just barely visible within the uterus, and the follicular pattern of the left ovary (white arrow) is no longer appreciated.

formed as the initial imaging sequence, or following the survey of the abdomen, since it is often clinically relevant to examine the upper abdomen as well as the pelvis. Our protocol is a biphasic, split-dose injection technique that is performed on a helical CT scanner. The upper abdomen from the level of the diaphragms to the iliac crests is examined helically with the patient supine (one breathhold; 7 mm collimation; pitch 1.0 to 1.3:1 and mAs ≥ 280). An initial intravenous contrast injection of 100 ml is delivered by a power injector at the rate of 2 ml/s, and scanning is initiated 60 seconds following the onset of contrast injection. This phase allows the upper abdominal organs especially the liver to be examined during its parenchymal phase of enhancement. A second bolus is administered via a mechanical injector at a rate of 1 ml/s, and scanning of the pelvis begins 30 seconds following the initiation of this phase of contrast administration to obtain images of the pelvis during the parenchymal phase of enhancement. The pelvis is then imaged from the iliac crests through the symphysis pubis (or lower if clinically indicated) by an axial cluster aquisition using 5 mm collimation at 8 mm intervals (15 second breathhold; 8-second intergroup delay; ≥ 320 mAs). Thin collimation, 5 mm or smaller, is recommended for this phase of the examination to minimize volume averaging of the small pelvic structures[24,27,28] (Fig. 3.10). Rectal air insufflation is routinely used as part of our dedicated pelvis protocol or in conjunction with an additional imaging series of the pelvis, if there is suspicion of an abnormality seen on a routine abdominopelvic CT. Before the pelvis is imaged the patient is placed in the prone position on the CT table, and approximately 15 to 20 puffs of air are then instilled into the patient's rectum via a soft red rubber catheter connected to a bulb. Large bowel distension is often useful when assessing the rectosigmoid colon, which is often affected by neoplastic and inflammatory gynecologic disease processes[22,24] (Fig. 3.11). Air insufflation is contraindicated in patients with radiation enteritis, profound neutropenia, and clinically severe colitis.[29] The patient also receives 0.5 cc of glucagon intravenously to reduce any rectosigmoid spasm.

Optimization of the pelvic CT examination also requires patient preparation. The gastrointestinal tract occupies a portion of the pelvic cavity and is best evaluated maximally opacified and distended. For routine CT, the gastrointestinal tract is opacified by an orally ingested suspension of dilute barium (Fig. 3.12). This oral contrast may be administered via a nasogastric tube or other indwelling enteric tube if the patient is unable to swallow. The aim is to have the entire gastrointestinal tract from stomach to rectum opacified at the time of the CT. This avoids misinterpreting unopacified bowel loops as masses, abscesses, or enlarged lymph nodes[30,31] (Fig. 3.13). We give about 1,000 ml of a 2% barium sulfate solution (Readi-CAT 2; E-Z-EM, Inc., Westbury, NY) in equal aliquots over a 45-minute to 1-hour interval before the CT examination. In preoperative and trauma patients as well as in those patients with suspected bowel perforation, diatrizoate meglumine, an iodine-containing solution suitable for oral administration, is given to avoid the potential noxious effects

Figure 3.10 Thin-section collimation. **(A)** An image from a CT scan performed with 10-mm collimation on a 67-year-old woman with acute diverticulitis demonstrates circumferential bowel wall thickening of the descending colon (black arrow) and linear stranding within the adjacent pericolic fat (open white arrow), representing perienteric inflammation. **(B)** An image obtained at almost exactly the same level as Figure A with 5-mm collimation demonstrates the additional finding of a microabscess (arrow) at the site of perforation. The thinner collimation reduced the volume average effect and allowed visualization of this small structure.

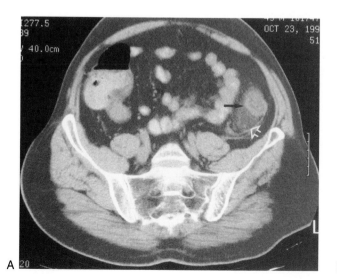
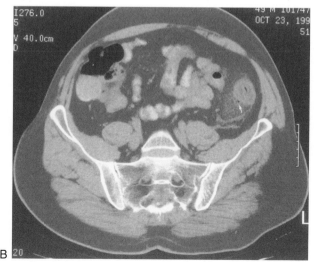

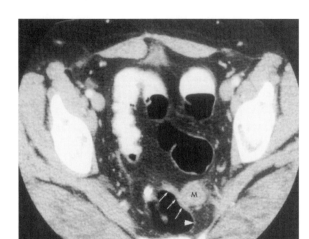

Figure 3.11 Rectal air insufflation. An image through the pelvis in a patient being evaluated for potential ovarian carcinoma was performed in the prone position with rectal air insufflation. An approximately 1-cm soft tissue mass (M) is identified adjacent to the rectosigmoid colon, which at second-look laparotomy proved to be recurrent ovarian carcinoma along the pelvic floor. There is also eccentric thickening of the wall of the rectosigmoid colon (small arrows), indicating serosal metastatic disease. The distension of the bowel achieved by air insufflation demonstrates the normal bowel wall to be pencil thin (arrowhead), thereby facilitating the detection of the focal wall thickening.

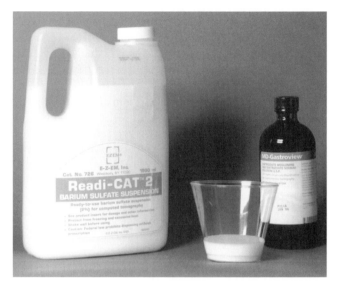

Figure 3.12 Oral contrast. Approximately 1,000 ml of the dilute barium solution (shown here in plastic cup) is placed in three or four styrofoam cups, and patients are asked to sip the contrast via a drinking straw. Approximately 30 ml of distrizoate meglumine solution (MD-Gastroview; Mallinckrodt, St. Louis. MO) is diluted in 1,000 ml of a noncarbonated beverage or water for patients unable to receive barium contrast.

Figure 3.13 Unopacified bowel loops. **(A)** CT examination in a 46-year-old woman with lymphoma shows a soft tissue mass adjacent to the right common iliac vein (v), which is suggestive of an enlarged lymph node (white arrow). (*Figure continues*)

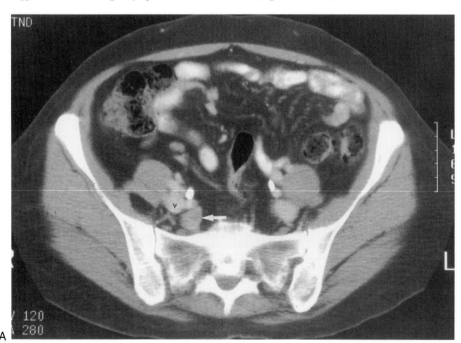

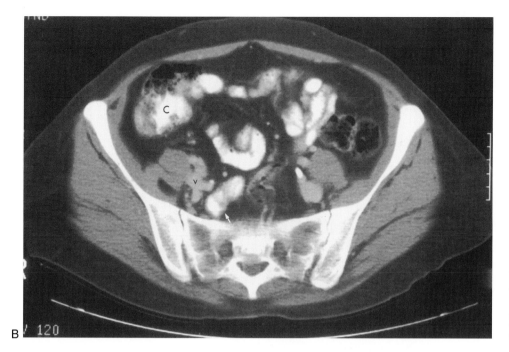

Figure 3.13 (*Continued*) **(B)** CT at the same location 1 year earlier shows the "mass" to represent small bowel loops (white arrow) opacified with orally ingested contrast. On this examination, the oral contrast has opacified the entire bowel and can be seen within the cecum (C).

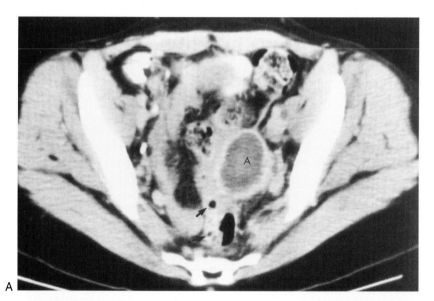

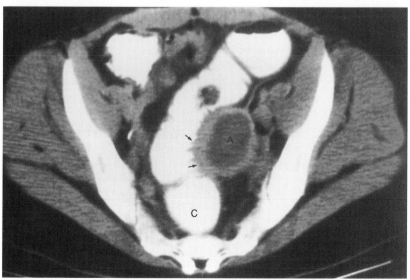

Figure 3.14 Rectal contrast. **(A)** An image from a CT performed on a 38-year-old woman who had fever and pelvic pain following hysterectomy reveals an encapsulated fluid collection with an enhancing rim (A) consistent with a pelvic abscess. On this examination, it was uncertain whether the few foci of air (arrows) behind the abscess represented an additional air-containing abscess or if they were merely within the collapsed unopacified rectosigmoid colon. **(B)** Following the instillation of rectally administered contrast, the pelvis was rescanned. The rectosigmoid colon (C) is distended and contrast filled. The few foci of air are no longer seen, proving they were within the colon rather than within an extraluminal collection. The distension of the rectosigmoid colon demonstrates spiculation (arrows) along the serosa of the bowel adjacent to the abscess secondary to the inflammatory process.

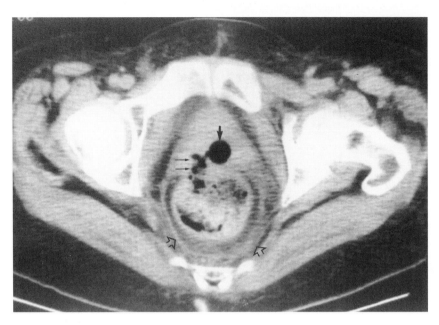

Figure 3.15 Use of a vaginal tampon. Irregular dots of air (arrows) are seen tracking from the rectum to the vagina in this patient who developed a rectovaginal fistula following pelvic irradiation for cervical carcinoma. An air-filled tampon (arrow) is present, delineating the vaginal cavity. Note the thickening of the uterosacral ligaments (open arrows), a common postradiation finding.

of barium contacting the peritoneal surfaces should there be a disruption of the integrity of the bowel wall. A 10-mg dose of metoclopromide, a peristaltic-stimulating drug, may be administered orally with the first cup of barium solution to expedite small bowel transit. Metoclopromide is contraindicated in patients with known or suspected pheochromocytoma, bowel obstruction, bowel perforation, or gastrointestinal bleeding. In patients in whom the distal large bowel is poorly opacified, contrast may be instilled rectally via a red rubber catheter. Dilute gastrographin (approximately 30 cc in 1,000 ml of water) is placed in a large plastic bag and given slowly until the patient experiences discomfort, and the pelvis is then immediately rescanned in the supine position (Fig. 3.14).

Imaging of the pelvis is generally best performed with distension of the urinary bladder with urine or saline.[7,24] The distended urinary bladder displaces the small bowel loops out of the pelvis, helps to orient the ante- or retroflexed uterus into a more cranial caudal orientation, displaces the adnexal structures laterally, and makes the paravesical peritoneal reflections more easily defined. Intrinsic bladder abnormalities may be obscured by high attenuation excreted intravenous contrast and are often better seen when a bladder is distended by unopacified urine or saline[32] (Fig. 3.9). In patients with a suspected enterovesical fistula, imaging should be carried out after oral and rectal contrast but before the administration of intravenous contrast.[30] This sequence helps to ensure that renal contrast excretion into the urinary bladder does not obscure small amounts of oral contrast entering the bladder via a fistulous tract.

A tampon may be inserted before scanning to see the vagina.[33] This may be especially helpful in the postoperative pelvis where visualization of the normal tissue planes may be difficult (Fig. 3.15). In patients with a suspected rectovaginal fistula, rectal contrast may be helpful. Presumably, the increased pressure and distension facilitate the migration of contrast from the rectum along the fistulous tract to the vagina.

SUMMARY

CT is valuable for imaging of the female pelvis, and further improvements will see an increase in its use in gynecology.

REFERENCES

1. Huang HK. Elements of Digital radiology: A Professional Handbook and Guide. Prentice Hall, Upper Saddle River, NJ: 1987
2. Jones DG, Shrimpton PC. Survey of CT Practice in the UK Part 3: Normalised Organ Doses Calculated Using Monte Carlo Techniques. NRPB-R250. National Radiological Protection Board, Chilton, United Kingdom, 1991
3. ICRP, International Commission on Radiological Protection. 1990 Recommendations of the International Commission on Radiological Protection. Ann ICRP, Publication 60. Pergamon, Oxford, 1991
4. Shrimpton PC, Jones DG, Hillier MC et al. Survey of CT Prac-

tice in the UK Part 2: Dosimetric Aspects. NRPB-R250. National Radiological Protection Board, Chilton, United Kingdom, 1991

5. NRPB, National Radiological Protection Board. Patient Dose Reduction in Diagnostic Radiology. Report by the Royal College of Radiologists and the National Radiological Protection Board (vol. 1, No. 3). National Radiological Protection Board, Chilton, United Kingdom, 1990

6. Kormano MJ, Goske MJ, Hamlin DJ. Attenuation and contrast enhancement of gynecologic organs and tumours on CT. Eur J Radiol 1981;1:307–311

7. Gross BH, Moss AA, Mihara K et al. Computed tomography of gynecologic disease. AJR Am J Roentgenol 1983;141:765–773

8. Stolberg HO, McClennan BL. Ionic versus nonionic contrast use In: Keats TE, Bragg DG, Evens RG et al. Eds. Current Problems in Diagnostic Radiology. Mosby Year Book, St. Louis, 1991, pp 51–58

9. Manual on Iodinated Contrast Media. Am Coll Radiol Bull 1991;3–16

10. Palmer FJ. The RACR survey of intravenous contrast media reactions: Final report. Australas Radiol 1988;32:426–428

11. Wolf GL, Arenson RL, Cross AP. A prospective trial of ionic vs nonionic contrast agents in routine clinical practice: comparison of adverse effect. AJR Am J Roentgenol 1989;152:939–944

12. Katamaya H, Yamaguchi K, Kozuka T et al. Adverse reactions to ionic and nonionic contrast media. Radiology 1990;175:621–628

13. Bettman MA. Ionic versus nonionic contrast agents for intravenous use: are all the answers in? Radiology 1991;175:616–618

14. Carro JJ, Trindale E, McGregor M. Risks of death and severe nonfatal reactions with high-vs low-osmolity contrast media: a meta-analysis. AJR Am J Roentgenol 1991;156:825

15. Levin DC, Gardiner GA, Karasick, et al. Cost containment in the use of low-osmolar contrast agents: effect of guidelines, monitoring, and feedback mechanisms. Radiology 1993;189:753–757

16. Burgener FA, Hamlin DJ. Contrast enhancement in abdominal CT: bolus versus infusion. AJR Am J Roentgenol 1991;137:351–358

17. Foley WD, Berland LL, Lawson TL et al. Contrast enhancement technique for dynamic hepatic computed tomographic scanning. Radiology 1983;147:797–803

18. Foley WD. Dynamic hepatic CT scanning. AJR Am J Roentgenol 1989;152:272–274

19. Kormano M, Dean PB. Extravascular contrast material: the major component of contrast enhancement. Radiology 1976;121:379–382

20. Hamlin DJ, Burgener FA, Beecham JB. CT of intramural endometrial carcinoma: contrast enhancement is essential. AJR Am J Roentgenol 1981;137:551–554

21. Berland LL, Lee JY. Comparison of contrast media injection rates and volumes for hepatic dynamic incremental computed tomography. Invest Radiol 1988;23:918–922

22. Miller Dl, Simmons JT, Chang R et al. Hepatic metastasis detection. Comparison of three CT contrast enhancement methods. Radiology 1987;165:785–790

23. Dean PB, Kivisaari L, Kormano M. The diagnostic potential of contrast enhancement pharmacokinetics. Invest Radiol 1978;13:533–540

24. Foshager MC, Walsh JW. CT anatomy of the femal pelvis: a second look. Radiographics 1994;14:51–66

25. Silverman PM. Pharmacokinetics on contrast enhancement in body CT. In: Fishman EK, Jeffrey RB, Jr, Eds.: Spiral CT: Principle, Techniques and Clinical Applications. Raven Press, New York, 1995, pp 11–24

26. Zeman RK, Silverman PM. Abdomen and pelvis. In: Zeman RK, Brink JA, Costello P et al, Eds. Helical/Spiral CT: A Practical Approach. McGraw-Hill, New York, 1994, pp 153–220

27. Megibow AJ, Bosniak MA, Ho AG et al. Accuracy of CT detection of persistent or recurrent ovarian carcinoma: correlation with second-look laparotomy. Radiology 1988;166:341–345

28. Scoutt LM, McCarthy SM, Moss AA. Computed tomography and MRI of the pelvis. In: Moss AA, Gamsu G, Genant HK Eds. Computed Tomography of the Body with MRI (2nd ed.). WB Saunders, Philadelphia, 1992, pp 1183–1265

29. Jacobs JE, Birnbaum BA. CT of inflammatory disease of the colon. Semin Ultrasound CT MR 1991;16:91–101

30. Megibow AJ, Zerhouni EA. Techniques of gastrointestinal computed tomography, In: Megibow AJ, Balthazar EJ (eds). Computed Tomography of the Gastrointestinal Tract. CV Mosby, St. Louis, 1986, pp 1–32

31. Marks WM, Goldberg HI, Moss A et al. Intestinal pseudotumors: a problem in computed tomography solved by directed techniques. Gastrointests Radiol 1980;5:155–160

32. Arger PH, Coleman BG, Mintz MC. Lower urinary tract computed tomography. Semin Ultrasound CT MR 1986;7:287–297

33. Cohen WN, Seidelman FE, Bryan PJ. Use of a tampon to enhance vaginal localization in computed tomography. AJR Am J Roentgenol 1977;128:1064–1154

Magnetic Resonance Imaging: Physical Principles and Imaging Techniques

RICHARD B. RAFAL

There are several reasons for the small number of magnetic resonance imaging (MRI) examinations performed in gynecology. Referring physicians may be unfamiliar with the principles of MRI and with its clinical indications. There is a wide variation in the quality and thoroughness of pelvic MRI, and it is expensive.[1] Few studies have been performed to analyze outcomes using MRI compared with other imaging modalities. This chapter addresses these issues.

MRI ADVANTAGES

MRI is noninvasive[2,3] and suited to examination of the pelvis. It is particularly advantageous due to the natural contrast of the pelvic fat, bowel gas, and urine in the bladder.[4,5]

Its resolving power, global views, and lack of operator dependence[6] are favorable characteristics for any imaging modality. Compared with computed tomography (CT) or ultrasound, MRI possesses superior soft tissue contrast resolution.[1,2,7–10] MRI can detect morphologic and physiologic changes. Morphologic changes, similar to those seen on other imaging modalities, can be evaluated, and signal intensity alterations, unique to MRI, also yield valuable information.[5,9,11] Physiologic changes can also be assessed, that is, changes in hormonal status during the menstrual cycle, pregnancy, and the menopause.[9]

A major advantage of MRI is its direct multiplanar capability, which means that it has the ability to display anatomy in any plane. This yields a more precise demonstration of anatomy and pathology.[2,4–6,8,10] Different planes can be imaged without moving the patient (Fig. 4.1). Multiplanar imaging of the pelvis is especially useful in evaluation of the base and dome of the bladder, which are difficult to see on axial views.[4] This facilitates the evaluation of the bladder, uterus, and rectum, despite their close proximity. Multiple planes are also useful in assessment of the levator ani muscle[4] and urogenital diaphragm,[6] and help assess both anteroposterior (AP) and craniocaudad components.[11]

CT can directly image in only the transverse (or axial) plane. Although CT can reconstruct images in other planes, these reformatted images are of poor quality when compared with the axial views from which they are derived.[4,8] Direct sagittal and coronal imaging on CT requires awkward patient positioning, which is often impossible in the weak or the elderly.[4]

There is little respiratory movement of pelvic structures, so motion artifact is less of a problem in MRI of the pelvis than in the chest or abdomen.[2,4,8] Bowel gas can cause artifacts on CT or ultrasound, but is not a problem on MRI.[7]

MRI does not utilize ionizing radiation.[2,6,7] This allows family members to stay in the room during imaging to allow monitoring and obviates the risks associated with ionizing radiation. MRI causes no known harmful effects[6,8] on the fetus, embryo, or reproductive organs,[1] and is apparently safe in pregnancy.[10]

No special patient preparation is required,[7,8,10] and in general, there is no requirement for intravenous contrast during routine pelvic MRI,[8] as is the case with CT. MRI is therefore useful in cases for which iodinated contrast is contraindicated, such as allergic patients or those at risk of the nephrotoxic effects associated with the contrast used with pelvic CT.[5] MRI differentiates vessels from solid structures without the use of intravenous contrast,[2,7,10] since moving blood, in general, produces no signal (the "signal void").

MRI DISADVANTAGES

The perception that MRI is expensive limits its use in pelvic disease.[5,10,12,13] The test alone is expensive, but there are indirect benefits and cost savings from MRI. Other disadvantages of MRI include its limited availability compared to ultrasound or CT,[12] possible unknown risks, and the lack of a bowel contrast. Absence of bowel contrast can lead to difficulty in separating soft tissue lesions, collections, and normal

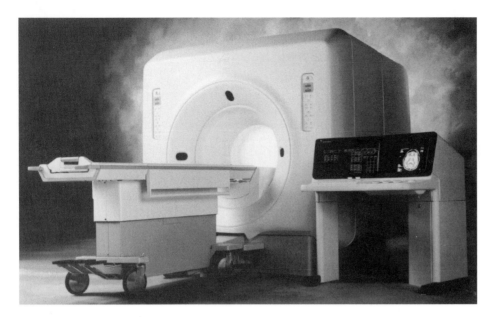

Figure 4.1 Signa Horizon MRI scanner. (Courtesy of GE Medical Systems, Milwaukee, WI.)

adnexa from bowel loops.[5,7,14] Additionally, cortical bone and calcification may not be detected due to their lack of mobile protons and long T1 relaxation times.[7] MRI does not reliably visualize adhesions,[15] and it cannot always distinguish between malignant and inflammatory changes, which decreases specificity.[11] This can be a problem with most imaging techniques.

There are numerous disadvantages related to the long scanning times required for MRI (especially when compared with CT).[2,4,7] The increased scanning times allow greater degradation of the images from movement and more cooperation from patients is required. It is uncomfortable to remain still for long periods, and sometimes claustrophobia[5,13] can be a problem.

Uniquely problematic to MRI are magnetic materials, which can cause artifacts that distort the image. Offenders are surgical clips and metal prostheses, which can also cause artifacts with CT or ultrasound, and it may be necessary to use several techniques to evaluate a given region. MRI is contraindicated in patients with cardiac pacemakers, intracranial aneurysm clips, cochlear implants,[2] and metal fragments in the eye.

MRI VS. CT VS. ULTRASOUND

Sonography excels for screening the pelvis and for diagnosis of pelvic masses.[1] Tissue differentiation and localization of abnormalities are superior with MRI,[2,14] which has a larger field of view and is better for surveying the retroperitoneum and for evaluating higher stage cervical disease.[12] Although ultrasound allows direct multiplanar imaging, this capability is more flexible with MRI, since ultrasound is limited by available sonographic windows.[1] Ultrasound is inexpensive,[12] and

scanning times are short,[8] allowing analysis of arterial and venous waveforms while scanning.[1]

Disadvantages of ultrasound include operator dependence, limited field of view,[12] diminished utility in obese patients, poor tissue characterization,[2] and shadowing by bowel gas.[14] It is not known whether MRI is better than transvaginal ultrasound with Doppler for adnexal mass characterization.[1] MRI is useful for evaluation of pelvic masses that are indeterminate at sonography.[1] Uterine and adnexal masses can usually be differentiated when ultrasound is inconclusive.[3,15] MRI is especially useful in those patients for whom ultrasound is suboptimal, such as in obese patients, or in those with excessive bowel gas.[14] Like CT, abnormalities are detected on ultrasound mainly as morphologic changes.[12] Depth of tumor invasion confined to the cervix or uterus is difficult to assess on ultrasound.[12] CT is not without problems during pelvic imaging. It uses ionizing radiation and is prone to distortion secondary to metallic clips, which can be a problem in postoperative patients. Optimal pelvic examination requires intravenous contrast[13] and an associated risk to both patient and attendant.[2] CT is limited to the transverse plane and has less soft tissue contrast,[1,5] and with CT, it is difficult to distinguish among the urethra, vagina, and rectum.[11] As with ultrasound, abnormalities on CT are detected principally by morphologic criteria, and the extent of tumor invasion is hard to evaluate.[12]

CT is quicker than MRI. Conventional CT can have a 2-second scan time, and spiral techniques can scan the entire pelvis in less than a minute. This minimizes the image-degrading effects of movement and maximizes patient tolerance. Ovaries can be inseparable from neighboring bowel (and uterus) on MRI,[2,5,7,14] but bowel contrast during CT scanning can help overcome this. As opposed to MRI, CT produces excellent images of calcium and cortical bone. CT also has good spatial resolution,[8] is more readily available[5,12] and cheaper than MRI. CT, similar to MRI but unlike ultrasound, allows evaluation of the entire pelvis in a single scan, including the peritoneum and lymph nodes.[1] MRI is similar to CT in detection of lymph node involvement.[12]

MRI gives pelvic anatomic detail of greater quality compared to CT or sonography.[5] In the urethra, for example, the soft tissue contrast of MRI permits differentiation between the muscular sheath and the submucosa.[16] MRI detects abnormalities by both morphology and signal intensity changes.[12] In general, more T2 weighting gives improved contrast between normal tissue and most neoplasms,[5] but these longer sequences necessitate longer imaging times and produce a low signal.[5]

There are few diagnoses made on MRI that cannot be made on CT or ultrasound, but MRI can combine the benefits of CT and ultrasound in one examination.[1] With large fields of view, CT and MRI can show the entire pelvis. Contrast can be used in both CT and MRI to detect solid masses, necrosis, or cysts. Special MRI pulse sequences permit tissue characterization beyond cystic, fatty, or solid.[1] MRI can help determine the origin of a pelvic mass, since it usually clearly shows the cavity of the uterus.[14]

MRI compares favorably with other modalities used to evaluate the vagina. Vaginography only shows the luminal contents, without evaluating the vaginal wall.

INTRODUCTORY PHYSICS

Nuclear magnetic resonance is the name given to the occurrence of electromagnetic energy absorption or emission that some nuclei experience in a static magnetic field.[7] MRI uses this phenomenon to produce images. The physics of MRI is a complicated topic beyond the scope of this book; however, a brief overview follows for those desiring an introduction to the subject.

MRI signal intensity depends on proton density, T1 and T2 relaxation times, and blood flow.[8] Strong signals are produced by high proton concentration, short T1 values, and long T2 values. The changes in signal intensity produced by each of these can vary depending on the radiofrequency (RF) pulse sequence used.[4] By convention, structures with strong signals are displayed as white on MRI. Tissues with absent or weak signals appear as black on MRI. Intermediate-strength signals are shades of gray,[4,7] therefore, tissues with a high concentration of mobile protons yield a high signal and are bright on MRI. For example, fat has a rapid relaxation time, giving a strong signal and therefore appears as white on MRI.[7] Low proton density structures emit a weak signal and appear black on MRI.[8] Calcification, in general, produces no signal and appears as a signal void or black when surrounded by signal producing tissues, but calcification may not be visible on MRI if surrounded by tissues that do not produce much signal.[7]

The conventional MRI gray scale gives the lowest signal intensity (i.e., darkest or black) to air and cortical bone. Along the gray scale, increasing signal intensity is then in the following order: ligaments and tendons, striated muscle, smooth muscle, viscera, brain, spinal cord, bone marrow, and fat.[6] Fat has the highest signal intensity (i.e., brightest or white) on a spin echo (SE) MRI[6] and is the reason that pelvic fat provides MRI with good natural contrast that separates organs and tissue planes.[7]

Nuclear particles possess intrinsic angular momentum, or spin, and nuclei with uneven numbers of neutrons or protons have a magnetic moment. Hydrogen nuclei (protons) are one example. When placed in a static magnetic field, the spinning protons tend to align parallel to the field and produce a net magnetic moment. This can be shown diagrammatically by a vector in the direction of the magnetic field.

The protons exhibit a complex wobbling motion along the axis of the magnetic field termed *precession*. The precessional frequency depends on intrinsic properties of the nuclei and the gyromagnetic ratio and is directly proportional to the magnetic field strength. After alignment with the magnetic field, the protons can be excited via an RF pulse applied at the precessional frequency. This perturbation can tip the net magnetic moment from its axis along the static field. During MRI, RF pulses are supplied that tip the spins 90 degrees (or perpendicular to the field) or 180 degrees (or antiparallel to the field). After a 90-degree RF pulse, the proton spins precess together in the transverse plane and emit an RF signal at the precessional frequency; this can be detected by a receiver coil. Over time, this signal decreases, as the spins return to realign with the static magnetic field. The T2 relaxation time is a rate constant that describes the time over which this signal disappears and is dependent on the loss of synchrony of the spins secondary to interactions of the spinning nuclei with neighboring nuclei. The T1 relaxation time is another rate constant that reflects the time required to realign with the static magnetic field. This constant reflects the spin's ability to give energy up to its neighbors and return to its original alignment with the magnetic field.[7]

Since T1 and T2 values of soft tissue vary to a greater extent than the x-ray coefficient of the same tissue, MRI has inherently superior soft tissue contrast resolution when compared with CT. Using conventional SE techniques, variations of the repetition time (TR) and excitation time (TE) will differentiate between different tissues as a consequence of their relative T1 and T2 relaxation times.[6]

Spatial localization of the emitted RF signal is crucial to using the phenomenon of nuclear magnetic resonance to yield MRI. This signal is detected by a receiver coil. Spatial localization can be obtained by the application of low field strength magnetic field gradients at the time of acquiring the signal. The gradients locally alter the resonance frequency at different points in the sample. Sequences of RF excitation pulses in different magnetic field gradients produce RF signals related to the position within this sample. Computer interpretation of the signal, after digitization of the data, yields spatial localization of the sources of the signals, which can then be displayed as an image.[7]

TR is the time between RF pulses applied to the image volume to excite the nuclei.[6] TE is the time elapsed from excitation of the nuclei by the RF pulse and the receipt of the signal from the nuclei.[6] T1-weighted sequences utilize short TR and short TE; with this technique, the T1 effect predominates, so that tissues with a short T1 value have a high signal, while structures with a long T1 give a weak signal.[8] T1-weighted images show poor soft tissue contrast other than in tissues that contain fat, yet are useful, since they are motion-free images that detail bone marrow and fat planes[10] and can demonstrate lymph nodes, since nodes are usually surrounded by fat.[10] T1-weighted sequences help show areas of hemorrhage and/or fat within organs and tissues by the characteristic high signal of blood and lipid.[10] Comparison of both T1- and T2-weighted images is usually necessary to distinguish between various tissues and to separate normal from abnormal structures.

On T2-weighted sequence (generally, an SE technique with long TR and long TE), the T2 effect is emphasized. Structures with a long T2 value emit high signal, and tissues with a short T2 yield weak signal intensity.[8] These images demonstrate MRI's excellent intrinsic soft tissue contrast in the pelvis, such as that seen in the zonal anatomy of the uterus and cervix, and by the demonstration of follicles in the ovaries.[10]

The TRs of neoplastic tissues are usually longer than those of normal tissue. Contrast between normal and abnormal areas can be emphasized by use of different pulse sequences as in both T1- and T2-weighted images.[7] Differences in signal intensity can then be detected. Absolute measurements of T1 and T2 TRs can be obtained with the MRI scanner. Care should be taken during image interpretation, since an overlap of signal intensities and relaxation times can be found in both benign and malignant conditions.[7,8,14]

Generally, MRI has been limited to hydrogen nuclei, since they are in great abundance in biologic tissues and yield a strong nuclear magnetic resonance signal.[7] Conventional MRI reflects the distribution of hydrogen, and hydrogen is mainly in water and fat in the body. Since water content is fairly constant between tissues, the density and distribution of protons is not the main factor determining contrast in MRI. Most important are the effects of T1 and T2 TRs and blood motion. By varying the RF pulse sequences, the clinician can produce images that emphasize T1 and T2 information.[7]

MRI tissue contrast depends on magnetic field strength and imaging techniques and the intrinsic characteristics of a given tissue.[6] Technical variables include the type of pulse sequence (e.g., SE inversion recovery, fast spin echo, etc.), and the particular parameters used within the pulse sequence (such as the TR and TE).[6]

Hardware

Surface Coils

A *surface coil* is an RF coil used to obtain high-resolution images of a limited area. The coils are of different shapes and sizes, depending on the area of the body to be examined. Surface coils are usually placed directly over the area of interest and applied close to the skin surface. They function as receiver coils only. The body coil, which surrounds the patient and usually is permanently inside the MRI scanner, transmits the RF excitation pulses.[17]

With surface coils, most of the signal that is received originates from superficial structures, since they are close to the coil. Tissues distant from the surface coil usually cannot be adequately imaged. Optimum image quality is obtained when the area of interest is as close as possible to the receiving coil. This is a major advantage of a surface coil, since the standard body coil is distant from the patient and, hence, the internal pelvic structures.[12] Note that images obtained using only the body coil are of less than optimal resolution, since they must be obtained with large fields-of-view in order to maintain an adequate signal-to-noise ratio (SNR).[10]

With surface coils, areas close to the coil have a marked improvement in the SNR when compared with standard body coils.[17] This permits the use of thinner slices and smaller fields of view and they have higher resolution compared with whole-volume body coils.[10,18,19] Smaller diameter surface coils permit increased SNRs, and this is used to advantage in both endoluminal coils and multiple arrays of external surface coils.[10] These improved SNRs allow both decreased acquisition times and enhanced resolution.[12] Surface coils have only a small sensitive region and can yield only small field of view images when used singly. "Multicoils" consist of multiple separate surface coils used at the same time, allowing large field of view (FOV) images with a markedly increased SNR to be obtained. Each coil in the multicoil acts independently in the receive-only mode.[10,17]

The pelvic phased array coil is a type of multicoil. Signal from each receiver produces separate sets of data that are reconstructed into a single image composite.[10] Each coil has a smaller effective diameter than would be normally used to image a given area, allowing the composite image to cover a wider area with the benefit of the equal or increased SNR made possible by the small diameter surface coils.[10] This substantially increased SNR, when compared with the body coil, helps produce high-resolution images.[17,20]

The multicoil shows anatomic details not previously seen on MRI.[17] Improved image quality demonstrates far greater detail and visualization of the zones of the cervix and uterus, ovarian stroma and follicles in the ovaries, and nabothian cysts, and identification of the individual veins of the perivaginal and periurethral venous plexus.[17] The high-resolution imaging parameters possible with a multicoil cannot be duplicated when using a body coil, since the image quality of the body coil would suffer due to a lower SNR.[17,21]

Artifacts are more pronounced with the phased array coil,[17] which can offset the advantage of increases in SNR. The smaller FOV possible with the phased array coil improves the image quality compared to those obtained with the body coil.[21] Such high-resolution and small FOV images are not obtainable in the body coil.[21]

The General Electric pelvic phased array coil consists of

two adjacent anterior coils and two adjacent posterior coils. Data from each coil are combined into one composite image.[10] The phased array coil has the advantage of the high sensitivity of smaller coils without compromising the larger volume coverage possible with the larger coils.[22] These coils share all the disadvantages of all local receiver coils mentioned previously, such as the steep signal loss away from the coil.[10] There are also problems with the reconstructions obtained with the coil; for example, tissues close to the surface (and therefore close to the coil) yield bright signal intensity and can be minimized by use of in field saturation pulses[17] or image intensity correction algorithms.[10] Another problem is the poor suppression of phase ghost artifacts, which allows them to be propagated along the whole image. This artifact, caused by the bright signal from subcutaneous fat adjacent to the surface coil, can be minimized by using in-field saturation pulses,[17] changing the phase encoding direction, using fat suppression, or using physical restriction of the anterior pelvic wall.[10] Theoretically, the decreased voxel size and imaging times used with high-resolution sequences can lead to image degradation; however, no perceptible worsening of motion artifact was detected when using a multicoil and fast spin echo (FSE) technique, also known as turbo spin echo (TSE), in one study.[17] Other limitations of the multicoil include their expense,[17] increased memory requirements, and lengthened reconstruction times.[10] In obese, large, or pregnant patients, the improved SNR (compared with the conventional body coil) may be lost secondary to a drop off in sensitivity of the coils toward the middle of the imaging volume.[10] To achieve an adequate SNR in these patients, one might have to increase the FOV or decrease the matrix size,[17] which will decrease image quality. Alternatively, body coil images can be substituted.[1]

Other Surface Coils

Intravaginal surface coils have been used to image the cervix. A solenoid receiver coil that envelops the cervix can yield images of greater detail and resolution than those obtained with the body coil[18,19] and more precisely demonstrates cervical zonal anatomy.[19] Enhancement patterns can also be more clearly delineated. In one study, this coil required only simple digital insertion, without the use of a speculum or sedation, and caused only minor discomfort when the coil was passed through the introitus.[18] Use of the coil may prove problematic in patients whose cervix is enlarged by disease, since proper positioning may not be possible.[18] The coil may prove most useful in stage I disease. It is recommended that patients with large masses or more advanced disease be imaged with the standard body coil, pelvic phased array coil, or endorectal coil.[18] The body receiver coil is more useful for detecting lymph node involvement and the extent of large masses.[19]

Endorectal coils can assess the cervix, parametrium, and rectum with higher resolution than the standard body coil, but suffer from a drop-off of signal anteriorly.[10,18] This can lead to suboptimal visualization of the anterior cervix, vagina,

and base of the bladder. Due to these limitations, images with endoluminal coils should be obtained in conjunction with larger field of view standard body coil images. Endorectal coils consist of a coil loop of small diameter that is surrounded by a balloon or latex cover.[10] The enveloping cervical ring gives uniform signal from the cervix and surrounding tissues and may be especially useful for visualizing early cervical tumors and local invasion.[18,19] The multicoil can be used along with the endorectal coil to give the benefits of both: high local SNR of the endorectal coil and the larger volume coverage and higher SNR of the multicoil.[10] Certain intracavitary (rectal/vaginal) surface coils have also been used to obtain high-resolution images of the urethra.[23]

Helmholtz-type surface coils consist of two electrically connected flat rings (standard surface coils), located anteriorly and posteriorly, which provide a limited FOV.[12,20] One study reviewed the use of such coils utilizing fast gradient echo pulse sequences during dynamic MRI, producing high-resolution images of the whole uterus during a single breath-hold.[20] Advantages of such a coil include increased SNR, optimization of image acquisition in the region between the coils, and improved resolution and contrast.[12,20] Disadvantages of Helmholtz coils include a nonuniform gray scale across the image secondary to signal loss caused by the distance from the region of interest to the ring coil surface. This effect can be minimized by using a larger diameter Helmholtz-type coil or a phased array coil.[20] Images with this coil can demonstrate individual uterine arteries and the venous plexus in the parametrial or perivaginal areas, and dynamic images obtained with this coil have been shown to help differentiate tumor from necrosis, secretion, or debris.[20]

Field Strength

Field strength refers to the intensity of the static magnetic field. In general, a "low field strength" scanner is 0.3 Tesla (T) or less. A "mid field strength" machine is 0.3 to 1.0 T. "High field strength" scanners range are those ≥ 1.0 T or more. Each type has its strengths and weaknesses, although each can generally perform diagnostic examinations of the pelvis. Quality surface coils can compensate for lower field strength. Field strength is apparently not crucial in tumor detection, lymph node involvement, or parametrial invasion and is not a vital factor in the determination of tumor staging, size, or extent.[12]

Higher field strength machines can be advantageous in pelvic imaging, especially for specialized imaging such as chemical shift imaging which offers the potential benefit of adnexal mass characterization.[10] Higher field strength magnets have inherently increased SNRs, which theoretically allow higher resolution.[12] Increasing the SNR is beneficial to a point, but further increasing this ratio results in only a small image improvement.[17] High field strength magnets yield better spatial resolution and also decrease image acquisition times. Quicker scanning allows for more patients to be scanned in a given amount of time, decreases motion artifact, and improves patient tolerance.[12]

Disadvantages of high field strength scanners include their high cost, expensive maintenance, and stricter siting requirements. Images obtained with these magnets also exhibit proportionately increased susceptibility to chemical shift artifact,[12] and higher incidences of flow and motion artifacts.

Lower field strength magnets have their advantages including improved contrast. These machines are cheaper and have lower operating costs, but they take longer to scan.

Pulse Sequences

Pulse sequences are the set of RF pulses and the time intervals between the pulses. The usual shorthand designations of various common pulse sequences are as follows:

SE, spin echo

IR, inversion recovery

FSE, fast spin echo

GRE, gradient recalled echo

The timing parameters of the sequence are generally listed after the above shorthand designations, in the following order: TR, TI (inversion time), then TE. An example is "SE 750/30," which means a spin echo sequence utilizing a TR of 750 ms, and a TE of 30 ms.

Conventional (SE) pulse sequences obtain echoes at given times after each 90-degree excitation pulse. Each excitation pulse is section-selective. Images acquired with long TRs are usually obtained with multiple echoes at the same location, typically yielding the proton density and T2-weighted images at a given slice location. The phase encoding for each echo at a given location is identical.[24] The major disadvantage of conventional SE imaging is its long imaging time.[25] Because of this, images are often degraded by artifacts due to movement.[20]

FSE techniques allow more rapid acquisition times and can improve image quality.[24,25] This can be as much as 16 times faster than conventional SE imaging. During FSE imaging, the initial 90-degree pulse is followed by the acquisition of 2 to 16 echoes (representing the echo train length, ETL). Each of these echoes is obtained at a different phase encoding value, as opposed to SE techniques.[24,25] Multiple 180-degree pulses in rapid succession generate the multiple echoes.[24] FSE sequences reduce imaging time by a factor equal to ETL.[24] For example, FSE sequences obtained with an ETL of 16 are 16 times faster than SE T2-weighted sequences. Imaging time for FSE sequences can be calculated by the following equation:

$$(TR) \text{ (No. signals averaged) (No. phase encodings)}/ETL$$

Advantages of accelerating image acquisition times include the use of longer TR and TE values (which allows increased T2 weighting and increases contrast), larger matrices[1,10,25] (increased spatial resolution), more signal averages (increased overall image quality), and faster scanning times (increased patient throughput, better patient tolerance, decreased physiologic motion artifact[24]). Fat saturation techniques are better employed with FSE techniques, as discussed below.

Quicker T2-weighted acquisitions make practical the performance of T2-weighted sequences in multiple planes,[1] and the acquisition of thinner sections;[10] doing either with conventional SE imaging can make the examination prohibitively long. Even after the use of fat suppression, or longer TRs or TEs, or larger matrices, FSE techniques are generally three to four times faster than conventional T2-weighted images.[25] T2-weighted FSE images, in general, have contrast similar to SE images. One exception is the increased signal from fat.[10,25] However, FSE imaging with longer effective TEs compared with those used during conventional SE imaging) yields images with less fat signal intensity and can improve the detection of tumors and edema.[10] Combining FSE with fat saturation makes more conspicuous edema as well as pathologic lesions with long T2 values.[25] An "edge enhancement effect" has been described with FSE, contributing to increased sharpness of the images[25] and is seen as increased conspicuity and sharpness of fluid collections and cysts on FSE images obtained with long effective TEs (> 120 ms).[10]

Disadvantages to FSE imaging include lack of respiratory compensation, which allows respiratory ghosting artifacts to be prominent, and increased motion sensitivity to FSE sequences. The ghosting artifacts can be diminished via fat suppression of the abdominal wall fat with or without the use of a pelvic binder.[25] Another disadvantage is that fewer slices can be acquired during slice acquisitions, since a greater portion of the TR is devoted to the echo train. The result is that FSE sequences necessitate a longer TR to image the same number of slices and can be overcome by decreasing the ETL and echo spacing. FSE images also have increased susceptibility to "cross talk," and edge blurring is noted with short effective TEs and a long ETL.[10]

Fat saturation sequences allow selective decrease in signal from fatty tissues and can be obtained to detect and evaluate fat-containing masses. This technique is also useful for suppressing signal from fat on contrast-enhanced images, since both fat and contrast-enhanced structures will be bright without fat saturation. Both normal anatomy and pathology are often better delineated with fat suppression.[10] Fat-sensitive techniques include short time inversion recovery (STIR), frequency-selective fat saturation, and phase-sensitive chemical shift. The use of fat saturation can increase imaging time and is best used in conjunction with FSE sequences, since the time savings associated with FSE techniques help compensate for this problem. In addition, since lipid has high signal on FSE images (compared with SE images), fat suppression has greater importance in FSE imaging.[25]

Gradient echo (GE) images have utility in determining blood vessel patency and in distinguishing lymph nodes from vascular structures. GE imaging allows the use of excitation pulses of less than 90 degrees, and short TRs, permitting rapid image acquisition. GE images have increased SNRs per unit time over conventional SE techniques. These sequences are more sensitive to magnetic field inhomogeneities and are not particularly diagnostic in the evaluation of the female pelvis.[26]

STIR completely suppresses signal from normal bone marrow. It is best in the pelvis for evaluation of bone marrow abnormalities and muscular edema. STIR techniques suppress all tissues with a T1 value approximating that of fat and is therefore not chemical shift specific and therefore should not be used to distinguish between fat and blood within pelvic masses; signal from both types will be suppressed to a similar degree on such images, since the T1 values of each can overlap. STIR images have low SNRs and limited T2 contrast, limiting their application to pelvic MRI of soft tissue structures.[10]

Chemical shift imaging takes advantage of the fact that fat and water protons have different resonant frequencies and are therefore susceptible to RF pulses applied at these given frequencies.[10] Chemical shift imaging allows differentiation between blood and lipid-containing lesions. This distinction can otherwise be difficult, since both types of tissues can appear bright with conventional SE techniques. Chemical shift imaging allows a definitive diagnosis of dermoid cysts.[1] Fat saturation techniques help identify small hemorrhagic lesions (such as endometriomas) that, on conventional scans, can be difficult to distinguish from bright pelvic fat. Fat saturation imaging also helps during gadolinium-enhanced scanning of the pelvis by making enhancing lesions more conspicuous.[1,10]

Two main chemical shift techniques are frequency-selective fat saturation and phase-sensitive chemical shift. Frequency-selective fat saturation can be applied to T1- or T2-weighted images to suppress fat signal in the imaging volume, but this technique is sensitive to inhomogeneities in the magnetic field.[10]

An example of phase-sensitive chemical shift is the opposed phase technique. The physics are complicated, but suffice it to say that they depend on differences in the waveforms of the signals from fat and water protons, and the respective waveforms are out of phase at the time of signal recording. Proper interpretation of opposed phase imaging sequences requires an in-phase reference image to determine which areas have signal loss secondary to a mixture of fat and water protons. This technique, which can be performed with standard SE or GE sequences, is sensitive to fat- and water-containing voxels. In those volumes that contain 50% of the signal due to lipid, and 50% due to water, complete loss of signal is seen. It is useful for detecting fat in a dermoid, since the sebaceous lipid is usually mixed with water protons. Both the above chemical shift imaging techniques can be used together in what are known as "hybrid" techniques. This results in maximal suppression of fat signal.[10] There are many uses for chemical shift imaging in pelvic MRI:

1. Differentiating fat-containing masses from other masses with high signal intensity on T1-weighted images, such as dermoids and endometriomas.[10]

2. In conjunction with gadolinium-enhanced scans (see above).

3. In conjunction with T1- or T2-weighted imaging to increase the sensitivity to small contrast differences based on T1 and T2 values.[10]

4. To minimize chemical shift artifacts.[10]

Artifacts

Entire textbooks have been written about artifacts during MRI. Outlined in this section is a general overview of the most common artifacts that affect MRIs.

Patient motion is common, but pelvic MRIs are not as affected by motion as are MRIs of the chest wall and abdomen.[10] Motion artifacts can be minimized by using short TR/short TE sequences (which lessen imaging time) and multiple data collections.[5] Reassurance is important with all patients, and sedation is beneficial in some. Judicious use of anterior and posterior saturation pulses can minimize abdominal wall motion artifacts on sagittal and axial images. Breath-hold imaging sequences can be used to eliminate this artifact.[20]

Respiratory motion can also degrade MRIs but is less of a problem with pelvic MRI, since the pelvis is distant from the chest wall. Respiratory compensation and breath-hold techniques can help overcome this problem to some extent.

Peristalsis can be lessened by use of glucagon or with faster imaging techniques including breath-hold acquisitions.[20,26] Cardiovascular motion[4] can cause artifacts, although it is less problematic with pelvic MRI.

Chemical shift artifact is caused by a chemical shift difference between the resonant frequency between water and fat. The effect on the images is to produce a bright rim on one side of an organ (where there is overlap of fat and water) and a corresponding dark rim on the other side of the organ (where fat and water separate).[27]

Flow-related enhancement is an effect that is most pronounced in the image section that is first entered by the blood. This slice receives protons that have not undergone RF excitation and hence will display maximal signal intensity and appear bright on the MRI. Subsequent sections show decreased or absent signal, as the protons were perturbed in the previous section.[6] In the typical axial multislice sequence obtained from superior to inferior, flow-related enhancement of arterial blood will appear in the most cranial section (also called "entry phenomenon"), while blood in the veins will demonstrate this enhancement on the most caudad section.[6] This effect is important when evaluating the first and last slices from an MRI examination, to avoid confusing this phenomenon with arterial or venous thrombosis. Other flow-related artifacts can occur adjacent to vessels in the direction of the phase-encoding gradient. Saturation pulses and gradient moment nulling can suppress artifact from flowing blood.[26]

Magnetic susceptibility artifacts are caused by variations in susceptibility in an object, which can lead to spatial mismapping, and are observable at interfaces between air and soft tissue.

Aliasing, or wrap around artifact, occurs when the diameter of the object being scanned is greater than the field of view. This can be solved by using a surface coil and/or increasing the field of view.

Metallic artifacts can occur in the region of metallic surgical clips, implants, dental work, or metal clothing snaps or hairpins that have not been removed from the patient before scanning. Such artifacts can be seen as a central area of low signal intensity surrounded by an area of high signal intensity, and the degree of image distortion can vary considerably. Ferromagnetic materials cause this by distorting the magnetic field.

Truncation artifact (Gibbs artifact) appears as multiple concentric rings in regions of marked transitions in signal intensity and is due to computer errors in Fourier transformation. This effect can be lessened by use of various filters.

CONTRAST AGENTS

Gadolinium is an example of a paramagnetic substance. Paramagnetic substances usually possess an unpaired electron; these include atoms or ions of rare earth elements, transition elements, and some metals and molecules like free radicals. They also possess small local magnetic fields, which decrease the relaxation times of surrounding protons. This effect leads to a signal intensity change via shortening of T1 and T2 TRs of the surrounding tissues. For use in contrast material, gadolinium can be chelated to diethylenetriaminepenta acetic acid (DTPA) (as in Magnevist), since free gadolinium is toxic.

Each available MRI contrast agent has been approved for central nervous system indications in adults. Magnevist (gadopentate dimeglumine) is the MRI contrast agent with the longest history; other approved MRI contrast agents, all of which are administered intravenously, include Omniscan (gadodiamide) and Prohance (gadoteridol). Magnevist is an ionic compound and is also approved for pediatric (above the age of 2) and body imaging indications. Omniscan is a non ionic agent and has been approved for pediatric (above the age of 2) and body imaging studies. Prohance is also non ionic and has been approved for imaging of the central nervous system and head and neck in adults and children over the age of 2. Hence, presently, Prohance is not approved for pelvic imaging.

The recommended dosage for each of the agents, according to the package inserts, is 0.1 mmol/kg. No known contraindications exist, making these agents good choices in patients with allergies to iodinated contrast agents (used during CT scanning) or those in renal failure.

Adverse reactions are uncommon and include nausea, headache, dizziness, and taste perversion, and the majority of these effects are of mild-to-moderate severity. Magnevist is excreted in low concentrations in human breast milk. It is therefore recommended that nursing females refrain from breast-feeding and express for 36 to 48 hours after contrast injection.[28]

The usual indications for giving intravenous contrast during pelvic CT include the identification of vessels and ureters and the characterization of collections and tissue. Vascular and ureteral localization in MRI of the pelvis can usually be readily accomplished without contrast administration. Contrast-enhanced pelvic MRI may be indicated for the staging of gynecologic and bladder neoplasms.[10,12] Often, non-contrast-enhanced T2-weighted images suffice, since these sequences usually provide enough contrast between tumors and normal structures.[10] Differentiation between cystic and solid masses is usually readily apparent on non-contrast MRI studies. Uncomplicated fluid is generally uniformly dark on T1-weighted images and hyperintense on T2-weighted images. Sometimes, the contents of a cyst, or cystic components of a neoplasm, present a confusing MRI due to high mucin content, blood products, or cellular debris. These lesions may be bright on conventional T1-weighted images, and intermediate in signal intensity on T2-weighted images. Gadolinium administration can help in separating areas of solid components, fluid, and necrosis, since simple fluid collections should not enhance. In pelvic imaging, this can be beneficial in imaging the adnexa and characterizing adnexal masses.[10]

If contrast is used, both pre-and post-contrast-enhanced T1-weighted images should be obtained to assess for contrast enhancement. The use of fat saturation during this imaging aids in searching for regions of contrast enhancement, since fat, if not suppressed, is bright on T1-weighted images (as is contrast) and is therefore difficult to separate from contrast enhancement. This is especially useful in trying to detect peritoneal spread of tumor.[10]

Contrast enhancement can help demonstrate margins of tumor, since both tumor and surrounding edematous tissue can be bright on T2-weighted images, and noncontrast images may not be able to make this distinction. Theoretically, contrast should enhance only the tumor.[12] Contrast enhancement helps detect vascularized, solid tissue in ambiguous areas on noncontrast images. Such ambiguity may be present if judged solely on morphologic criteria or signal intensity characteristics on noncontrast T1- or T2-weighted images.[1] Noncontrast MRI often has difficulty distinguishing between omental masses and normal bowel, since both are hyperintense on T2-weighted images; contrast administration can make the distinction, since only the omental mass should enhance.[10]

In the uterus, contrast can help distinguish between necrosis, endometrial secretions, and viable tumor, as all can be bright on noncontrast T2-weighted images, only tumor should enhance. It should be noted that MRI contrast enhancement patterns seen in the uterus vary with the menstrual cycle.[29,30]

Characterization of adnexal masses is facilitated by use of gadolinium-DTPA (Gd-DTPA), since contrast helps demonstrate areas of necrosis, solid components, papillary projections, internal septa, and omental and peritoneal involvement.[1,22] Contrast helps distinguish vascularized tissue from clot and debris.[1]

Dynamic pelvic MRI scanning includes the bolus injection of contrast and repeated imaging through the suspected lesion or structure. Fast GE sequences, coupled with contrast administration via an intravenous tube entering the magnet bore during imaging, enables one to obtain repeated images through a given slice, or through an entire organ, during the injection. The pattern and speed of contrast enhancement can then be assessed to help evaluate lesions, define the border of tumors, and formulate a differential diagnosis.[10,12] Ideally, during dynamic MRI, spatial resolution is highest when the SNR is kept near a given threshold and when images are obtained within a short measurement time.[20]

An example protocol for dynamic scanning of the cervix is as follows: After a contrast bolus (0.1 mmol of Gd-DTPA), acquire images immediately and every 30 seconds thereafter up to 4 minutes. One study showed a marked difference in the rate of contrast enhancement of tumor and normal uterine and cervical tissue in the early phase (30 to 60 seconds after injection) with little or no difference later.[12,30]

The normal cervical stroma enhances slightly and in a gradual fashion compared with normal myometrium.[30] Carcinoma of the cervix has been shown to enhance dramatically in the dynamic phase, and early in this phase (at 30 to 60 seconds) it is easily distinguished from cervical stroma and myometrium. Contrast between the normal cervix and tumor using the dynamic technique is greater than with noncontrast T2-weighted images or with conventional static contrast-enhanced T1-weighted images. Parametrial invasion may also be better assessed using dynamic techniques than with T2-weighted images. Other features of cervical carcinoma that are better evaluated with dynamic scanning include tumor size and amount of stromal invasion.[30] Each of these features may be better assessed on dynamic scans than on noncontrast T2-weighted images, which are in turn better than postcontrast T1-weighted images.

Uterine carcinoma shows more gradual and less intense enhancement than cancer of the cervix.[30] One study using dynamic technique for the uterus showed that contrast between tumor and myometrium was maximal at 120 seconds after injection.[29] This distinction was better than on static postcontrast T1-weighted images and on noncontrast T2-weighted images.[29]

Disadvantages of dynamic scanning are that it usually can only be done in few imaging planes, since the number of slices is necessarily limited in such short time frames, spatial resolution is decreased compared with routine SE images,[30] and that the MRI examination becomes complicated and prolonged.[1]

Gastrointestinal MRI contrast agents have not seen widespread use, since an ideal agent has yet to be developed. Investigators are evaluating both "positive" (which brighten bowel contents on MRI) and "negative" (causes the bowel contents to be dark) bowel contrast agents for MRI. Lack of bowel opacification during MRI can be a problem when compared with CT, since bowel contrast agents definitively identify bowel loops. This avoids confusion with other soft tissue lesions and helps in the evaluation of peritoneal, intraluminal, or bowel wall abnormalities. Such agents are less important for MRI than for CT, since intraluminal content tends to have different signal intensity from most pathologic lesions. This distinction can often be made by location, morphology, and connection to known bowel loops elsewhere in the pelvis.[10]

PATIENT PREPARATION

It is important to screen patients properly before MRI. Careful questioning of the patient to exclude contraindicated devices (e.g., cardiac pacemakers, metal intraocular foreign bodies, or magnetic cerebral aneurysm clips) should be undertaken. In the pelvis, some hip prostheses may cause image artifact near the area of interest, but this does not prevent the acquisition of diagnostic images.

It is beneficial for the referring physician to be familiar with the MRI examination because a description is reassuring to the patient. Patients are generally imaged while supine and breathing quietly.[3,8] Occasionally, some images are obtained while the patient is prone[10] or after rectal air insufflation.[3] Prone imaging decreases motion artifact of the anterior pelvic wall during respirations but is not tolerated as well as the supine position.[10] It is preferred that the bladder be half distended during pelvic MRI, as this helps displace bowel loops outside the pelvis and improves evaluation of the adnexa and uterus.[3,8] Glucagon (1 mg intramuscularly or intravenously) can be used to decrease bowel peristalsis.[10,22] Tampons may obscure vaginal anatomy and are not recommended.[3,9] Routine pelvic MRI does not require suspended inspiration. A respiratory bellows can limit the degrading effects of motion of the anterior pelvic wall.[10]

Claustrophobic patients may need sedation, as the patient's body (and head) are usually inside the gantry, and a special MRI-compatible pulse oximeter may be required. Imaging in "open" MRI scanners may be better tolerated. Reassurance and piped music are helpful in anxious patients. Loud thumping noises may be heard at different times; ear plugs are usually supplied to the patient before scanning to minimize this problem and to prevent damage to the ear.

No special patient preparation is required before MRI.[7,8,10] The patient is questioned about possible contraindications and is generally asked to complete a questionnaire to help determine if MRI is indicated. A consent form may be signed before the procedure. Patients are dressed in a gown (without snaps), since both snaps and clothing can create image artifact. Hairpins, jewelry, watches, and so on should be removed from the patient, since some can act as projectiles, cause artifact, and/or be damaged in the magnetic field. Some sites have the patient pass through a metal detector before entry into the scanner room. Once in the scanner, the patients are informed that they are constantly being observed and that they can be heard via a microphone in case there is a problem. The technologists can talk with them through a speaker in the "tunnel." Pelvic MRI usually takes about 1 hour, and the patient must remain completely still during imaging. This may not be possible for patients in severe pain or those with involuntary motion.

MAGNETIC RESONANCE ANGIOGRAPHY/VENOGRAPHY

Magnetic resonance angiography or venography (MRA/MRV) provides a gross demonstration of the major vessels of the pelvis showing patency, stenoses, or encasement, and the state of grafts.[10] MRA images obtained with the body coil are markedly inferior to those obtained during contrast angiography. Although the multicoil allows smaller FOVs and improved resolution, the high signal of the stationary tissue next to the coil causes problems with the reconstruction algorithms of the maximum intensity pixel reconstruction unless it is removed during interactive postprocessing of the data.[10] MRA also tends to overestimate stenotic lesions.

The two major techniques used for MRA are time-of-flight (TOF) and phase contrast (PC). Generally, two-dimensional TOF techniques are preferable in the pelvis compared with PC sequences. This is not only due to the fact that two-dimensional TOF allows rapid acquisition times. Since the main direction of blood flow direction in the pelvis is from head to toe, this is the ideal environment to obtain the axial two-dimensional TOF acquisitions that compose two-dimensional TOF MRA images.[10]

Cost Considerations

MRI is costlier than other imaging methods, but it is cheaper than diagnostic laparoscopy or exploratory laparotomy.[15] Several studies indicate that while the charge for MRI itself is more expensive than most other modalities, use of MRI may decrease total medical expenditures and be cost-effective in certain patients.[1] Optimization of preoperative therapeutic regimens and surgical planning can lead to shorter recovery time, reduced hospitalisation, and earlier resumption of normal activity.[12] In some patients, the need for surgery may be obviated entirely.[15]

Schwartz et al.[15] compared treatment plans for patients before and after MRI results were made known. The results showed that pelvic MRI can alter treatment, allowing nonsurgical therapy or less invasive surgery, reducing overall health care costs.[15]

Lessler et al.[13] demonstrated that in patients who are at high risk for nephrotoxic effects of iodinated contrast material, unenhanced MRI of the abdomen and pelvis performed for a specific indication actually decreases overall hospital costs when compared with enhanced CT. Overall, unenhanced MRI was the least costly imaging technique in this patient group, irrespective of whether high- or low-osmolality CT contrast agents were used.[13] Because of these results, MRI might be the procedure of choice in patients with mild-to-moderate renal failure, congestive heart failure, or diabetic nephropathy.[1]

REFERENCES

1. Outwater EK, Dunton CJ. Imaging of the ovary and adnexa: clinical issues and applications of MR imaging. Radiology 1995;194:1–18
2. Hricak H. MRI of the female pelvis: a review. AJR Am J Roentgenol 1986;146:1115–1122
3. Olson MC, Posniak HV, Tempany CM, Dudiak CM. MR imaging of the female pelvic region. Radiographics 1992;12:445–465
4. Bryan PJ, Butler HE, LiPuma JP et al. NMR scanning of the pelvis: initial experience with a 0.3 T system. AJR Am J Roentgenol 1983;141:1111–1118
5. Council on Scientific Affairs. Magnetic resonance imaging of the abdomen and pelvis. JAMA 1989;261:420–433
6. Hricak H, Alpers C, Crooks LE, Sheldon PE. Magnetic resonance imaging of the female pelvis: initial experience. AJR Am J Roentgenol 1983;141:1119–1128
7. Thickman D, Kressel H, Gussman D et al. Nuclear magnetic resonance imaging in gynecology. Obstet Gynecol 1984;149:835–840
8. Picus D, Lee JK. Magnetic resonance imaging of the female pelvis. Urol Radiol 1986;8:166–174
9. Hricak H, Chang YC, Thurnher S. Vagina: evaluation with MR imaging. Part I. Normal anatomy and congenital anomalies. Radiology 1988;169:169–174
10. Outwater EK, Mitchell DG. Magnetic resonance imaging techniques in the pelvis. Magn Reson Imaging Clin N Am 1994;2:161–188
11. Hricak H, Secaf E, Buckley DW et al. Female urethra: MR imaging. Radiology 1991;178:527–535
12. Mezrich R. Magnetic resonance imaging applications in uterine cervical cancer. Magn Reson Imaging Clin N Am 1994;2:211–243
13. Lessler DS, Sullivan SD, Stergachis A. Cost-effectiveness of unenhanced MR imaging vs contrast-enhanced CT of the abdomen or pelvis. AJR Am J Roentgenol 1994;163:5–9
14. Dooms GC, Hricak H, Tscholakoff D. Adnexal structures: MR imaging. Radiology 1986;158:639–646
15. Schwartz LB, Panageas E, Lange R et al. Female pelvis: impact of MR imaging on treatment decisions and net cost analysis. Radiology 1994;192:55–60
16. Klutke C, Golomb J, Barbaric Z, Raz S. The anatomy of stress incontinence: magnetic resonance imaging of the female bladder neck and urethra. J Urol 1990;143:563–566
17. Smith RC, Reinhold C, McCauley TR et al. Multicoil high-resolution fast spin-echo MR imaging of the female pelvis. Radiology 1992;184:671–675
18. deSouza NM, Hawley IC, Schwieso JE et al. The uterine cervix on in vitro and in vivo MR images: a study of zonal anatomy and vascularity using an enveloping cervical coil. AJR Am J Roentgenol 1994;163:607–612
19. Baudouin CJ, Soutter WP, Gilderdale DJ, Coutts GA. Magnetic

resonance imaging of the uterine cervix using an intravaginal coil. Magn Reson Med 1992;24:196–203

20. Ito K, Fujita T, Uchisako H et al. MR imaging of the uterus: findings from high-resolution multisection dynamic imaging with a surface coil. AJR Am J Roentgenol 1994;163:873–879

21. McCauley TR, McCarthy S, Lange RC. Volume phased array coils: do they have diagnostic utility in pelvic MR imaging? J Magn Reson Imaging 1991;1:198

22. Outwater EK, Schiebler ML. Magnetic resonance imaging of the ovary. Magn Reson Imaging Clin N Am 1994;2:245–274

23. Yang A, Mostwin JL, Yang SS, Zerhouni EA. High-resolution MR imaging of female and male urethras with intracavitary surface coils and body coils. J Magn Reson Imaging 1991;1:197–198

24. Smith RC, Reinhold C, Lange RC et al. Fast spin-echo MR imaging of the female pelvis. Part I. Use of a whole-volume coil. Radiology 1992;184:665–669

25. Nghiem HV, Herfkens RJ, Francis IR et al. The pelvis: T2-weighted fast spin-echo MR imaging. Radiology 1992;185:213–217

26. McCarthy S. Magnetic resonance imaging of the normal female pelvis. Radiol Clin North Am 1992;30:769–775

27. Fisher M, Hricak H, Crooks LE. Urinary bladder MR imaging. Part I. Normal and benign conditions. Radiology 1985;157:467–470

28. Kanal E. Pregnancy and the safety of magnetic resonance imaging. Magn Reson Imaging Clin N Am 1994;2:309–317

29. Yamashita Y, Harada M, Sawada T et al. Normal uterus and FIGO stage I endometrial carcinoma: dynamic gadolinium-enhanced MR imaging. Radiology 1993;186:495–501

30. Yamashita Y, Takahashi M, Sawada T et al. Carcinoma of the cervix: dynamic MR imaging. Radiology 1992;182:643–648

Imaging of the Normal Female Pelvis

SECTION

II

5

Ultrasonography of the Normal Female Pelvis

PHILIPPA A. RAMSAY

ROBERT P. S. JANSEN

The position and relationship of the female pelvic organs vary with posture and with the distension of bladder and bowel. The size and structure of the pelvic organs also change with reproductive age and with the stage of the ovarian cycle.

An awareness of the clinical setting, an understanding of the cyclic changes in the ovaries and endometrium, and sometimes serial ultrasound examinations can be needed to make sense of ultrasonographic findings during ultrasound examination of the female pelvis.

UTERUS

Position

The uterus is a reliable landmark in the female pelvis because it is centrally located, comparatively large, and recognizably pear-shaped. The cervix is anchored in the midline by the uterosacral ligaments and is thus less mobile than the body. The position and flexion of the uterus are important for access for various procedures, such as curettage or insertion of an intrauterine contraceptive device. The uterus is described as anteverted if it projects from the anterior vaginal fornix and extends anterosuperiorly to the uterine fundus (Fig. 5.1A). It is retroverted if it projects from the posterior vaginal fornix and extends posterosuperiorly (Fig. 5.1B). It can be difficult to demonstrate the fundus of a retroverted, retroflexed uterus on transabdominal ultrasound. Although a full bladder will displace bowel loops upward, the retroflexed uterus can still be obscured behind the interposed cervix. Anteflexion is present if the uterine body is angled forward in relation to the axis of the cervix; retroflexion if the body is angled backward. Rarely, the uterus might be anteverted but retroflexed (Fig. 5.1C) or retroverted but anteflexed (Figs. 5.1D and 5.2D).

On transvaginal scanning (Fig. 5.2), with the transducer pressed on the flexed cervical–corporeal junction (and the image oriented with the transducer at the superior apex of the screen), an anteverted uterus is most commonly imaged with the fundus to the left of the screen, with anteversion concave upward (Fig. 5.2A); in the retroverted uterus, the fundus will be directed to the right, with retroflexion now concave upward (Fig. 5.2B). (This orientation came about because transvaginal ultrasound was introduced in the days before most ultrasound machines had the ability to invert the image electronically.) If the uterus is lying in the same axis as the vagina and cervix, then transvaginal scanning of the endometrium, no longer perpendicular to the ultrasound beam, is less informative (Fig. 5.2C).

There is often slight deviation of the uterus to the right or left; this can be normal, but more substantial deviations might be caused by a pelvic mass or by peritoneal adhesions. Position and deviation of the uterus can be altered transiently by bladder fullness, rectal fullness, or the patient's posture, and by manual pressure from the transvaginal transducer in the anterior or posterior vaginal fornices.

Shape, Size, and Echo Texture

The dimensions of the uterus in the longitudinal and anteroposterior direction can be accurately measured with transabdominal ultrasound;[1] extrapolation to uterine volume using the conventional prolate ellipse formula, however, is not accurate because the shape of the uterus does not approximate an ellipsoid.[2] The normal size of the uterus, its shape, the ratio of cervical length to body length, and, especially, the appearance of the endometrial lining or mucosa depend on the age of the patient and her parity.

The endometrial cavity is flat from front to back, so appears slit-like in sagittal section, with the anterior and posterior surfaces touching (Figs. 5.1 and 5.2). In coronal section, it is roughly triangular, as it opens up from the cervical canal to the two lateral uterine angles, which receive the fallopian tubes via the internal tubal ostia at the uterotubal junctions. This view corresponds to the typical anteroposte-

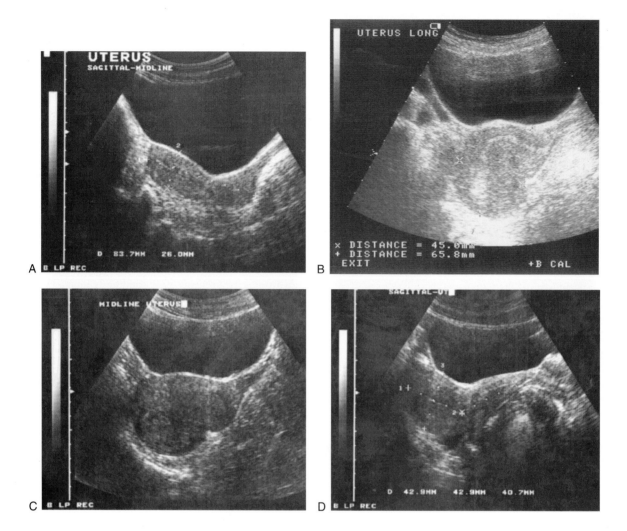

Figure 5.1 Transabdominal, transvesical scanning of the adult cervix and uterus. **(A)** Anteverted uterus indenting the bladder from behind. The uterine corpus and cervix have a 2:1 length ratio, and the uterus is in anteflexion. **(B)** Retroverted uterus. **(C)** Anteverted but retroflexed uterus (the axis is angulated backward). **(D)** Retroverted but anteflexed uterus (the axis is angulated forward).

rior view of the uterine cavity on hysterosalpingography. Figure 5.3 shows the equivalent views on hysteroscopy.

The bulk of the imaged uterus consists of the myometrium that constitutes the uterine wall. The muscle of the uterine body is ultrasonically continuous with the fibrous substance of the cervix. Normal myometrium is homogeneously echodense, with a moderately fine echo texture (Figs. 5.1 and 5.2). The uterine walls are approximately 1.5 to 2 cm in thickness. The inner, junctional layer of myometrium can be slightly less echogenic (Fig. 5.2A);[3] the border with the endometrial lining is normally smooth and well demarcated. This junctional zone of the myometrium, not always so clearly visible on ultrasound (Fig. 5.2A), is dramatically visible on magnetic resonance imaging.

Small circular hypoechoic spaces may be seen in the outer layers of myometrium, representing arcuate vessels in cross-

section. They show slow nonturbulent blood flow with color Doppler imaging. The walls of these vessels can become calcified and echogenic with age (Fig. 5.4).[4]

The development of the endometrial mucosa, between the myometrium and the uterine cavity, is exquisitely sensitive to circulating estrogens and progestogens.[5] The thickness and echotexture of the mucosa depend on the quantitative, qualitative, and temporal exposure to these ovarian steroids.

Newborn and Prepuberty

The newborn uterus and prepubescent uterus are tubular in shape, with little differentiation of body and cervix, which have a 1:1 length ratio (Fig. 5.5). Just before puberty, the uterus measures approximately 3 cm long, 2 cm wide, and 2 cm deep; the size of the uterine corpus is similar to that of the cervix, with a length ratio of 1:1, as in the newborn. Differentiation into the adult configuration occurs during puberty, with enlargement of the corpus to a bulbous shape that tapers to the cervix.

Adult

The adult nulliparous uterus measures approximately 7.5 × 5 × 2.5 cm. Normal uterine size varies greatly in parous women, but in general all dimensions stabilize at an increase of about 1.5 cm following involution after the first pregnancy.[6]

During the reproductive years, the pelvic organs are under the control of the ovarian cycle, resulting in cyclic changes in their dimensions and echogenicity, particularly the uterus. The normal menstrual cycle averages 28 days in length, with about equal time for the (preovulatory) follicular and (postovulatory) luteal phases, but it is important to appreciate that the duration of these phases, especially the follicular phase,

can normally vary, with further variation possible in abnormal states. Menstrual cycle length in women of normal fertility can range between about 25 and 36 days,[7] with most of the variation arising from the follicular phase (corresponding with the proliferative phase in the endometrium), while the luteal phase (the endometrial secretory phase) takes about 14 days, with a normal range of 11 to 16 days, whatever the follicular phase length.[7] Approaching the menopause, the follicular phase typically becomes shorter, thereby shortening the whole cycle as the time of ovulation is brought forward.

Proliferative Phase

As menstruation ceases, the functional layer of the endometrium soon responds to small amounts of estrogen secreted by the ovary. As estrogen production rises with follic-

Figure 5.2 Transvaginal scans of the uterus. (**A**) Anteverted, anteflexed uterus. The fundus is to the left of the image. (**B**) Retroverted, retroflexed uterus. The fundus is to the right of the image. (**C**) Slightly retroverted (or "vertical") uterus, in line with the transducer, and showing a resultant technical deterioration of the endometrial image. (**D**) Retroverted but remarkably anteflexed uterus.

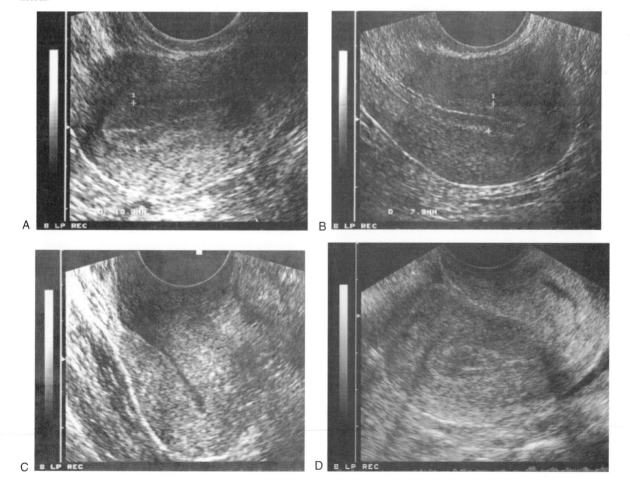

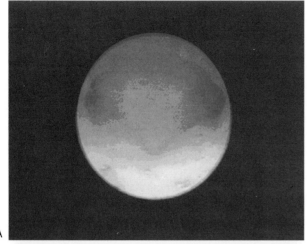

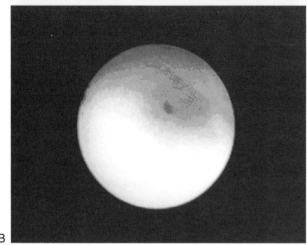

Figure 5.3 Hysteroscopy of the normal uterus. **(A)** The endometrial cavity imaged by hysteroscopy from the cervix; the internal tubal ostia are out of sight at the lateral angles of the cavity. **(B)** With the hysteroscope in the left uterine angle, the internal tubal ostium (uterotubal junction) is visible.

ular development (Fig. 5.6), the endometrial glands proliferate, lengthen, and become tortuous (Fig. 5.7A). On ultrasound, the endometrium thickens quantitatively with the accumulating action of estradiol, the double layer, midsagittal endometrial thickness measurement increasing from 1 or 2 mm to up to 12 mm. Qualitatively, one thin echogenic line is seen from menstruation for the first few days of endometrial growth (Fig. 5.8A); then as the proliferative phase progresses, the endometrium becomes less echogenic than the surrounding myometrium (Fig. 5.8B), and a change to three echogenic lines is soon observed (Figs. 5.8B & C). The outer lines represent the myometrial–endometrial interface, and the central line represents the apposition of the anterior and posterior endometrial layers. The endometrial tissue between thickens and remains hypoechoic for most of the proliferative phase,[8] but, as estrogen exposure continues, the basal echogenic line widens inward (Fig. 5.8C), eventually to join the central echogenic zone (Fig. 5.8D).

Categorization of and terminology for the sequential qualitative echogenic appearances of the endometrium have been notably inconsistent among authors (Table 5.1).[9–12] Quantitatively, care should be taken in reporting endometrial thickness from myometrium to myometrium (averaging around 1 cm at ovulation) and in distinguishing it from the less conventionally reported thickness from myometrium to midline, which is half that measurement.

Successful implantation and pregnancy are said to be uncommon among endometria with a full-thickness measurement at ovulation of less than 7.5 mm and rare with a thickness less than 5 mm.[13] Qualitatively, many authors have reported that implantation is most common if a triple-line pattern has been seen,[14] although it is unwise to give a prognosis for pregnancy on echographic appearances and measurements of the endometrium alone.

Secretory Phase

After ovulation, the progesterone secreted during the ovarian luteal phase (Fig. 5.6) stops epithelial and stromal proliferation in the endometrium; the endometrial glands differentiate and secrete glycoproteins (Fig. 5.7B).[15] On ultrasound, blurring of the three lines typical of late proliferative endometrium by a generalized change to echogenicity (Fig. 5.8D) precedes typical secretory changes on histology. This uniformly echogenic appearance can reflect the prolonged action of estrogen alone, presumably as glycogen accumulates,[5,16] and, if it is accompanied by further or abnormal endometrial thickening (in the absence of a luteal structure imaged in either ovary), it should suggest endometrial hyperplasia. An echogenic appearance of the endometrium is therefore consistent with, but not diagnostic of, ovulation. In some cases, echolucency is seen within a generally echodense, highly developed endometrium (Fig. 5.8E).[17]

Figure 5.4 Calcified uterine artery branches (arrows) within the myometrium.

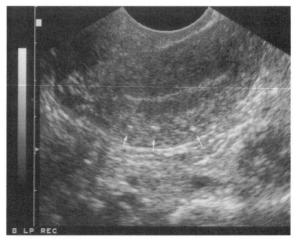

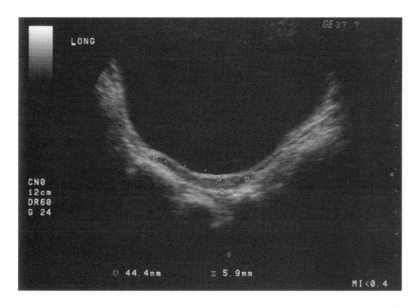

Figure 5.5 Transabdominal scan of the newborn uterus; the fundus is to the left; the cervix with a fundus: cervix ratio of approximately 1:1; the vagina is clearly seen to the right.

The changes in endometrial appearances in the proliferative phase are ultrasonically conspicuous despite comparatively minor qualitative changes histologically, whereas the echogenic appearances of secretory endometrium mask a wealth of histopathologic development (Fig. 5.7B). Seven days after ovulation, when the endometrium has long been thick and echogenic, secretion is fully developed. The appearance on ultrasound does not change further as the stroma on histology exhibits first edema and then the predecidual reaction. With pregnancy, echogenicity and thickness are maintained as the decidual reaction to implantation takes place (Fig. 5.8F). If pregnancy does not ensue, the growth of the endometrium be-

Table 5.1 Categories and Terminology for Echogenic Appearances of the Endometrium

Image	Description (Relative to Myometrium)	Mono-follicular Development	Bald, 1983[53]	Sydney, IVF, 1986[54]	Smith et al.,[9] 1989	Gonen et al.,[10] 1989	Germar-Martinez et al.,[11] 1990	Sher et al.,[12] 1991	Endometrial Histology
Fig. 5.8A	Thin hyperechoic center	<1 cm	Type 1	Type I	Grade D	Type A			Menstrual, early proliferative
	Isoechoic	1.0–1.7 cm	Type 2, 3	Type II	Grade C	Type B	Type I		Midproliferative
Fig. 5.8B	Isoechoic, hyperechoic rim early "triple line"	1.6–1.9 cm	Type 4	Type II	Grade B	Type B to C	Type I	Grade II	Midproliferative
Fig. 5.8C	Late "triple line"	1.9–2.6 cm	Type 5	Type III	Grade A	Type C	Type II	Grade II	Late proliferative
Fig. 5.8D	Thick, diffuse hyperechoic	Corpus luteum	Type 6	Type IV			Type III	Grade I	Late proliferative, secretory, or hyperplastic
Fig. 5.8E	v. thick, hyperechoic, center hypoechoic		Not described	Type V					Late proliferative, secretory; or hyperplastic

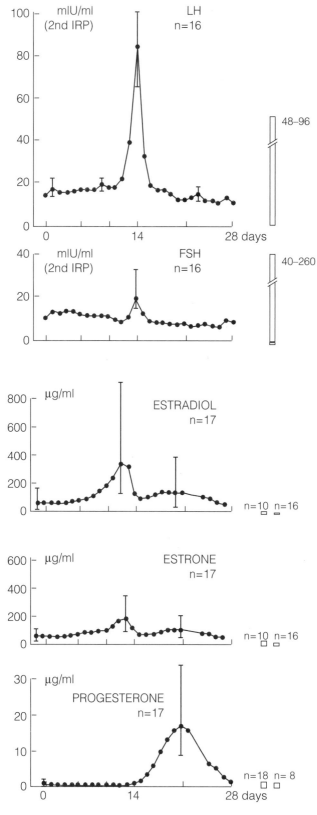

Figure 5.6 Changes in circulating gonadotropic and ovarian steroid hormone concentrations through the menstrual cycle; the LH peak (top) occurs at midcycle. FSH shows a small but important rise at the end of the cycle, with a progressive fall through the following follicular phase. Estradiol rises with follicular development before falling sharply with ovulation, as progesterone comes to be secreted by the ovary; progesterone dominates the second half of the cycle. (From Jansen,[51] with permission.)

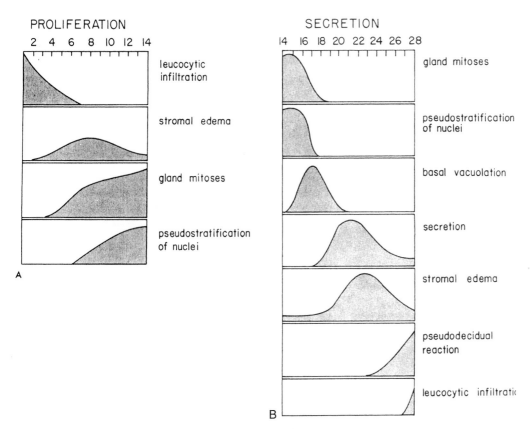

PROLIFERATION

2 4 6 8 10 12 14

leucocytic infiltration

stromal edema

gland mitoses

pseudostratification of nuclei

A

SECRETION

14 16 18 20 22 24 26 28

gland mitoses

pseudostratification of nuclei

basal vacuolation

secretion

stromal edema

pseudodecidual reaction

leucocytic infiltration

B

Figure 5.7 Diagramatic description of endometrial changes. **(A)** The proliferative phase. **(B)** The secretory phase. Echogenicity in "type IV" endometrium masks numerous functionally important endometrial events. (Courtesy of Dr. E. Friedrich, Milwaukee, Wisconsin and from Friedrich,[52] with permission.)

gins to regress,[8,18] decreasing in thickness but maintaining echogenicity. As circulating levels of progesterone (and estradiol) drop at the end of the ovarian cycle (Fig. 5.6), the functional layers of the endometrium break down and separate off with menstruation—generally a brightly echogenic event ultrasonically.

Menstrual Phase

During menstruation, blood clot and endometrial fragments can be seen in the endometrial cavity as echogenic debris. The remaining endometrial lining is irregular until regeneration begins in the proliferative phase of the new cycle.

Postmenopausal State

After menopause the size of both the cervix and body of the uterus reduces gradually and steadily, with the total length decreasing from 6.5 to 3.5 cm with time.[19]

In postmenopausal women, the ovaries are usually quiescent, and the endometrium is normally thin and atrophic, exhibiting no temporal or cyclic changes. The mean endometrial thickness is 2.3 ± 1.8 mm.[20] Normal ovaries after the menopause might not secrete estrogen but still produce androgens, which along with androgens derived from the adrenal glands are converted to estrogens by peripheral adipose tissue. The resulting estrogen levels depend on both the absolute amount of adipose tissue and the age of the woman. Estrogen from these sources can be enough to cause endometrial thickening and, histologically, proliferative changes that range through to hyperplasia or neoplasia. Fatter women thus tend to have thicker endometrium,[20] even within the normal range. Once the endometrial thickness is greater than 5 mm, endometrial hyperplasia or malignancy must be considered.

Subendometrial Myometrial Waves

With real-time transvaginal scanning, and especially with the help of fast-forward video playback, myometrial waves that affect the endometrium have been documented. These contractions are seen in the slightly hypoechoic junctional zone of the myometrium immediately adjacent to the endometrial lining—a region considered to have special physiologic importance[21] and thought to help propel sperm to the fallopian tubes before ovulation and later perhaps to position the pre-embryo properly for implantation. The waves require exposure to estrogen and, as a result, the frequency, amplitude, and direction of these waves appear to depend on the balance of the hormonal milieu. Progesterone secretion in the luteal phase eventually causes this activity to abate.

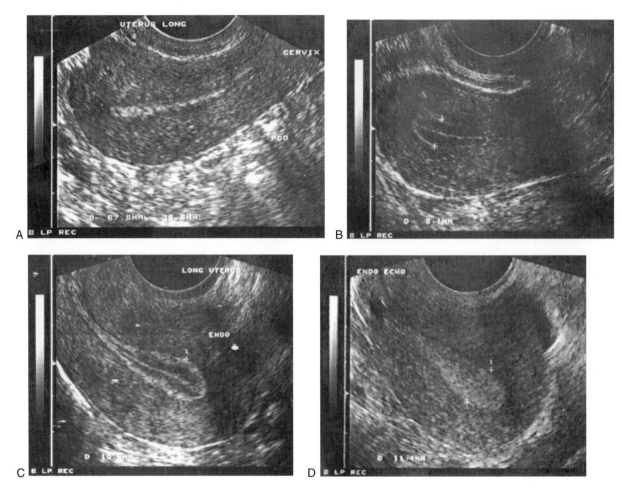

Figure 5.8 Qualitative and quantitative alterations in endometrial echoes during the ovarian or menstrual cycle. Sydney IVF classification of endometrial development (see Table 5.1). (Note: The uterus is retroverted in Figures C, D, and F.) **(A)** Menstrual or early follicular phase. The endometrium is thin and echogenic (type 1). **(B)** Midfollicular phase. The endometrium is lucent compared with myometrium; an echo demarcates the endometrium from the junctional layer, and a third line is visible at the point of contact between front and back mucosal surfaces (type II). The lucency might correlate with midfollicular stromal edema. **(C)** Late follicular phase. Echogenicity is spreading from the front and back basal layer toward the mucosal surface (type III). **(D)** Periovulatory and luteal phase. Echogenicity is uniform (type IV). The same picture can be obtained from non secretory, hyperplastic endometrium. (*Figure continues.*)

CERVIX

The uterine cervix is a canal that measures approximately 2.5 cm or more in length. The site of the internal os is inferred to be where the uterine body turns away from the cervix on ultrasound examination; if the uterus is anteflexed, this point is visualized as an indentation in the anterior wall (see Figs. 5.1A and 5.2D). The epithelium of the cervical canal does not respond histologically or sonographically to ovarian hormonal changes. The mucus in the endocervical canal is highly viscous and echogenic in its interface with the cervical mu-

cosa, except at the time of ovulation, when it has a higher water content and may be seen as an echolucent space on ultrasound (Fig. 5.9A).

Nabothian cysts are retention cysts of the cervical glands that form within the ectocervix as it undergoes metaplasia from simple columnar to stratified squamous epithelium with age. The cysts can protrude into the vagina or into the lower endocervix, where they can distort the endocervical canal. They are thin-walled and spheric, measuring up to about 10 mm in diameter, and contain echolucent fluid. Even when large and multiple (Fig. 5.9B), they are of no clinical importance.

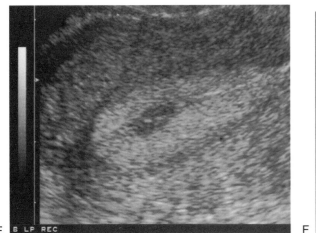 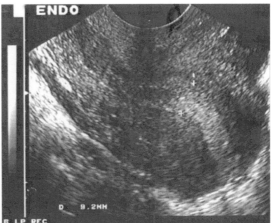

Figure 5.8 *(Continued)*.
(E) A variant of echogenic endometrium in which a central lucent area has formed (sometimes called type V). **(F)** Echogenic early pregnancy endometrium with artifactual enhancement distal to reflective tissues.

The ectocervix is best seen when surrounded by fluid in the vaginal fornices (Fig. 5.9C).

THE VAGINA

The vagina is thin-walled and potentially tubular. It runs anteroinferiorly from the uterine cervix to the perineum, posterior to the bladder and urethra, and anterior to the rectum. It can be imaged with a transabdominal ultrasound transducer directed caudally, utilizing a full bladder to displace confounding echoes from the bowel (Fig. 5.10). The vaginal walls are usually 3 mm in thickness and, because of their fibromuscular nature, are hypoechoic. Apposition of the epithelial mucosal layers results in a bright reflection in the midsagittal plane. During menstruation, blood can occasionally pool in the vagina. Urine can collect in the vagina in a woman with incontinence who lies supine with a distended bladder for the ultrasound examination. Ultrasound determinations of length are not reliable because of the variable degree of bladder distention.

Paradoxically, transvaginal ultrasound is often less able to demonstrate the vaginal wall than is transabdominal scanning, because the wall is then closer than the focal zone of the transducer. Transperineal ultrasound can circumvent this problem, but frequently the vaginal walls lie at an angle along the ultrasound beam, which reduces the resolution and can cause posterior acoustic shadow artifacts.

FALLOPIAN TUBES

The origin of the fallopian tubes at the lateral uterine angles can reliably be demonstrated by transvaginal echography. The endometrial cavity is first demonstrated by tangential coronal scanning; the origin of the tube is then resolved with an oblique sagittal view. If the tube is to be cannulated for an assisted conception procedure[22] or for sonosalpingography, the cannula can be imaged within the intramural part of the tube with views in the correct, oblique plane.

The fallopian tubes are approximately 10 to 12 cm long, just a few millimeters wide, and are only occasionally seen on ultrasound (Fig. 5.11A). They lie outward and backward from the lateral uterine angles toward the corresponding ovary, abutting (and generally offering no echographic contrast to) loops of bowel. Visualization of one or other tube becomes possible if it is distended with fluid (as a hydrosalpinx) (Fig. 5.11B), transfused with an echogenic substance such as air or a cannula, or thrown into ultrasonic relief by chance suspension in abundant peritoneal fluid (Fig. 5.11C).[23]

OVARIES

Both transabdominal and transvaginal scanning might be needed to identify the ovaries properly; however, the superior resolution and closer focusing possible with transvaginal scanning is much preferable for accurate ultrasonic assessment (Fig. 5.12A & B).

Position

The normal position of the ovaries is on each side of the cervix, close to the lateral wall of the pelvis, and imaged adjacent to the iliac vessels (Fig. 5.13A). Normal ovaries are mobile and transducer pressure often influences their position. An ovary might be found in the cul-de-sac (pouch of Douglas) (Fig. 5.13B), in front of the uterus, high in the pelvis above the uterus, or in the abdomen. Ovaries fixed by adhe-

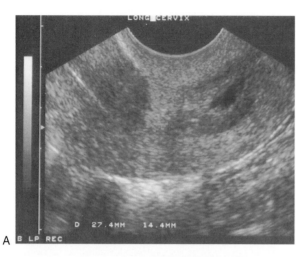

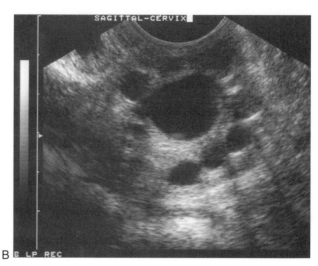

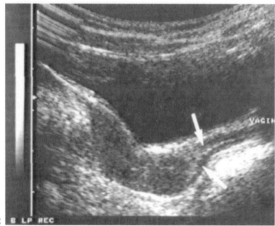

Figure 5.9 (A) Transvaginal scan of the cervix revealing abundant, echolucent mucus in the cervical canal. (B) Transvaginal scan of the cervix displaying mucus gland retention cysts (nabothian follicles). (C) Transabdominal scan of the ectocervix (arrows show anterior and posterior vaginal fornices).

sions from previous pelvic inflammatory disease can be in normal or unusual situations. They are commonly fixed close to the lateral fornices of the vagina and are thus easily found with transvaginal scanning.

Size, Shape, and Echo Texture

Normal ovaries are ellipsoid in shape, despite asymmetric development of ovarian follicles (Fig. 5.12), and ovarian volume is estimated using the prolate ellipse formula: volume = length × width × depth × 0.523. Variability using this method with transvaginal ultrasound is low,[24] and the correlation with ovarian volumes measured at or after laparotomy is excellent.[1]

The ovarian stroma has a coarse echotexture and is slightly less echo-dense than myometrium. Ovarian follicles contain echolucent fluid and are easily demonstrated. They usually appear more or less spheric and vary in size from 2 mm (in fact, the resolving power of the equipment) to 25 mm in diameter. The great majority of ovarian follicles are microscopic in size and cannot be demonstrated with ultrasound.

Ovarian Cycle

Oocyte-containing follicles are present by the millions in the ovaries of female fetuses—about 7 million being present at about 20 weeks of gestation (Fig. 5.14).[25] All ovarian follicles that the ovaries will ever contain are formed by this stage of fetal life. These follicles are overwhelmingly primordial, microscopic in size, and metabolically quiescent. At any subsequent time, whether during relative ovarian quiet in childhood, cyclic activity in later years, or during ovarian suppression by oral contraception or pregnancy, follicles grow out of the primordial pool by becoming primary; then secondary; and then (still microsocopic) tertiary follicles, with formation of a fluid-filled antrum that pushes the oocyte off to one side. If endocrine conditions permit, ambient follicle stimulating hormone (FSH) levels drive further growth of these tertiary follicles into the realm of ultrasonic visibility. If endocrine conditions are not so supportive, the follicles undergo atresia, with apoptosis of their cells, including the oocyte, and permanent loss from the follicular oocyte pool. By menopause, few follicles (in the range 100 to 1,000) are left.

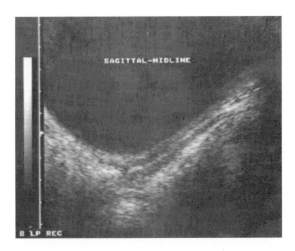

Figure 5.10 Transabdominal scan showing the lucent walls of the vagina on each side of a conspicuous mucosal surface echo; the patient has had a hysterectomy.

In the meantime, only a tiny fraction of ovarian follicles will ever have ovulated; the vast majority having been lost through atresia.[26]

Newborn

In the newborn infant, the many follicles that are developing remain mostly small and invisible to ultrasound resolution. The ovaries can be difficult to demonstrate with ultrasound because of their small size, the need for an abdominal approach for scanning, and difficulty in securing a full bladder to displace the intestines. For all these reasons, failure to demonstrate the ovaries in the newborn infant is common and does not imply ovarian dysgenesis. The ovaries decline further in size for the first two years of childhood, making their identification ultrasonographically even more difficult.[27,28] In one study, the mean ovarian volume was 1.2 cm³ (range 0.7 to 3.6 cm³) among girls up to 3 months old; 1.1 cm³ (range 0.2 to 2.7 cm³) among girls 4 to 12 months old; and 0.7 cm³ (range 0.1 to 1.7 cm³) among girls 13 to 24 months old.[27] Sometimes, the presence of a cyst or an unusually large follicle can enable what

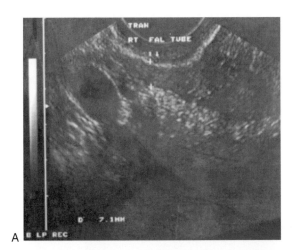

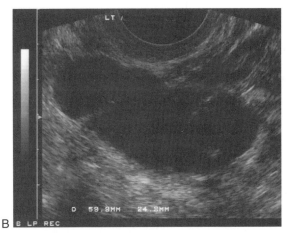

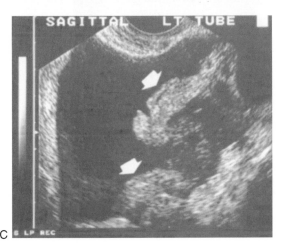

Figure 5.11 Ultrasound images of the fallopian tube. (**A**) Uncommon image of the right fallopian tube's medial part, in continuity with the lateral angle of the uterus. (**B**) Hydrosalpinx accumulating fluid at midcycle. (**C**) The fallopian tube thrown into ultrasound relief by suspension in abundant peritoneal fluid. The tube (arrows) appears thickened and might be abnormal.

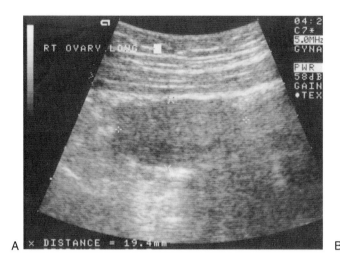
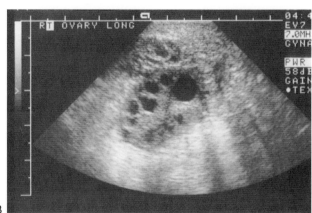

Figure 5.12 Ultrasound of the ovary showing the superior resolution on transvaginal screening. **(A)** Transabdominal scan at 5.0 MHz. **(B)** Transvaginal scan at 7.0 MHz, revealing follicular activity.

would otherwise be an unidentifiable ovary to be distinguished. Ovarian cysts were seen in 84% of all identified ovaries in one childhood series,[7] and 18% were larger than 9 mm in diameter.

Childhood

The ovaries grow slowly but steadily through later childhood,[29] increasing from a mean ovarian volume of 0.5 cm³ at the age of 3 to a mean ovarian volume of 2.8 cm³ at the age of 18 years. There are two periods of rapid growth: The first, at around 8 years of age, occurs at the time of adrenarche and during a time of gradually rising levels of FSH, and the second occurs before and during puberty, when FSH levels rise further. Constitutionally tall girls with no known hormonal imbalance have been found to have ovaries larger than average.[29]

Adolescence and Adulthood

The appearance of the ovary changes considerably during the ovarian cycle. The normal sequence comprises development of a follicular cohort in the first week; dominance of one follicle as others regress during the second week; collapse of the greater than 2-cm diameter dominant follicle with ovulation; formation of the corpus luteum; and then the regression of the corpus luteum if pregnancy does not happen. The details of these normal follicular and luteal developments follow. Interruption of this ovulatory sequence is common in both the early and the late reproductive years, resulting in functional (or dysfunctional) follicular or luteal cysts—cysts that can be cause or effect of menstrual irregularity.

Accurate measurement of ovarian stromal volumes is difficult during the ovarian cycle, because the follicles distort the otherwise elliptic shape of the ovary. There are conflicting re-

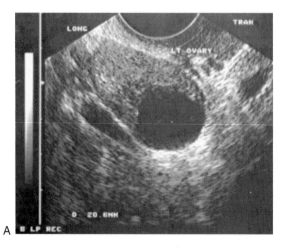
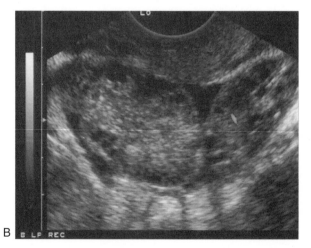

Figure 5.13 **(A)** The ovary alongside the pelvic side wall, marked by the (here obliquely imaged) internal iliac artery. **(B)** The two ovaries occupying the pouch of Douglas (cul-de-sac).

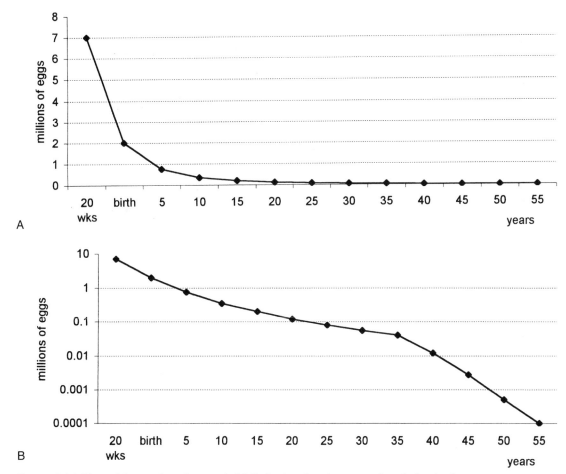

Figure 5.14 Plots of the number of primordial follicles found in the ovaries from before birth until menopause. The number of follicular "recruits" visible in normal early follicular phase ovaries will be roughly proportional to the number of primordial follicles remaining in the ovaries.
(A) There is an exponential decline from before birth independent of cyclic ovarian activity.
(B) A logarithmic plot reveals that oocyte loss follows a biexponential pattern, with an increased rate of loss from about the age of 38, corresponding with a sudden and permanent decline in fertility clinically (Data adapted from Faddy et al.[25] With permission of Oxford University Press.)

ports on whether ovarian stromal volume remains the same through the cycle[30] or whether the active, ovulating ovary shows an increase in stromal volume through the follicular phase.[31]

The number of small, hormone-responsive antral follicles reaching the size of ultrasound definability is directly related to the number of follicles still present in the ovaries and therefore is inversely proportional to the woman's age (Fig. 5.14). It is the variable state of development of some ovarian follicles in women of reproductive age from primordial, microscopic dimensions to fluid-filled antral (tertiary) follicles 1 or 2 cm in size that accounts for the variable appearance and dimensions of the ovaries in adolescence and adulthood. By the menopause, such responsive follicles are almost depleted. In the years immediately preceding menopause, the supply of follicles reaching endocrine sensitivity and discernible dimensions becomes so patchy that cycle irregularity becomes apparent clinically.

Follicular Phase

The transient rise in serum levels of FSH that occurs at the end of each ovarian cycle (see Fig. 5.6) "recruits" whatever small antral follicles happen to have reached a size of 1 or 2 mm—the threshold of transvaginal 7.5-MHz ultrasound resolution—at the time of menstruation. This "cohort" of antral follicles has the opportunity of growing further instead of undergoing atresia. As they respond to FSH with growth, during the early follicular phase of the new ovarian cycle, they secrete the estrogen estradiol and the peptide hormone inhibin, which have a negative feedback effect on pituitary gonadotropic function, reducing FSH production as the follicular phase progresses. The drop in FSH levels causes the smaller of the recruits to regress, the larger and more self-sufficient follicles growing regardless. By the end of the first week of the follicular phase, one follicle (sometimes two) (Fig. 5.15A) has become dominant. The others, by this point, have

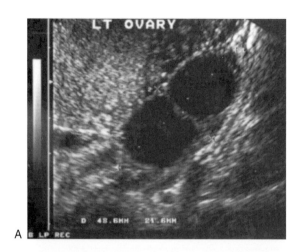
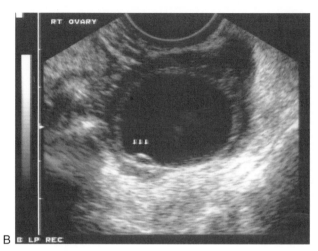
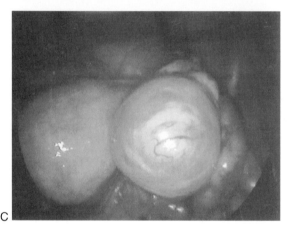

Figure 5.15 Preovulatory follicle. **(A)** Preovulatory ovary containing two dominant follicles. **(B)** A "hillock" in the dominant follicle interpreted by some observers to be the mucus-like cumulus oophorus surrounding the preovulatory oocyte (arrows). **(C)** Laparoscopic image of a preovulatory follicle showing new blood vessel growth on the follicular surface. (See also Plate 45.1)

functionally been lost through atresia, though they will still be visible and might still grow somewhat, particularly in the dominant ovary.[32] The dominant follicle produces substantial and increasing amounts of estradiol as it grows (see Fig. 5.6).

Follicles grow through increase in the number of follicle cells and by the production of the fluid that swells the antrum. The dominant (or Graafian) follicle's diameter increases at a rate of 2.5 mm/day until it reaches about 2 cm in size, after which, the two-dimensional growth slows to 1.3 mm/day.[33] According to some authors, the oocyte and surrounding cumulus oophorus protrude into the follicular antrum to be seen as a small papillary projection from the wall of the follicular antrum on transabdominal ultrasound (Fig. 5.15B). Others, using especially high-resolution transvaginal transducers, have not confirmed this assertion.[34] The side of ovulation in successive cycles is apparently not affected by the side of ovulation in the preceding cycle.[35]

Follicular development is not always sustained: ovulation does not always follow dominant follicular development. Particularly in the early reproductive years, one follicle can take another's place without ovulation, giving follicular phases (and hence menstrual cycles) that are long and irregular, extending to qualify for the designation oligomenorrhea, or even amenorrhea. The variable persistence of differently sized

developing follicles, some functioning and some atretic, enlarges the ovaries and gives the ultrasound picture of "multifollicular" ovaries,[36–39] distinguishable from polycystic ovaries by the central as well as peripheral location of the follicles and by the relative lack of echogenic ovarian stroma. Although the multifollicular appearance can be normal during adolescence, and is seen during recovery from weight loss, we believe that a similar picture involving fewer follicles in older women might be associated with significantly disordered ovulation of primarily ovarian origin and even with impending ovarian failure.

Ovulation

By the time it reaches approximately 2.1 cm in diameter (range 1.6 to 3.3 cm),[40] the dominant follicle is ready to ovulate. High estrogen effect increases fallopian tube fluid secretion, and there is transudation of water across the follicle, both of which contribute to an increase in free peritoneal fluid that can be visible on ultrasound. At midcycle, the pituitary responds to high circulating estrogen levels with a surge of luteinizing hormone (LH) (see Fig. 5.6). Ovulation will take place about 38 hours after the LH surge starts or about 20 hours from the time LH levels peak. During this time, as the preovulatory follicle begins to luteinize and to secrete progesterone, there is a rapid development of new blood vessels around the follicle (Fig. 5.15C)—a phenomenon that can easily be observed with color Doppler (Plate 5.1). Ovulation occurs with dissolution of part of the follicle wall and escape of follicular fluid into the peritoneal cavity. The ultrasonically recognizable events consist of a more-or-less sudden disappearance of the lucent dominant follicle, perhaps with an appearance of increased peritoneal free fluid, and then, several days later, the development of a usually complex corpus luteum (Fig. 5.16A and Plate 5.2). Ovulation pain (Mittelschmerz) may have been experienced about 24 hours before ovulation. Endocrinologically, after ovulation, serum levels of progesterone rise (Fig. 5.6) to reflect the corpus luteum's maturation into a solid-to-cystic, steroid-producing tissue (Figs. 5.16 and see Fig. 5.17).

If ovulation does not occur, the follicle can continue to grow to become a follicular cyst (see Fig. 5.18). Such follicular cysts are typically simple, with sharply marginated thin walls and echolucent fluid. They can grow to be 6 cm or more, but are typically 3 to 4 cm in diameter and eventually regress if left alone. They might or might not continue to produce estrogen, resulting in further, generally echogenic, endometrial proliferation.

Luteal Phase

After extrusion of the follicular contents, the wall of the follicle collapses, the tissue is invaded by exuberant new blood vessels (Fig. 5.16B), and the follicular/granulosa cells luteinize, accumulating fat and secreting progesterone. The old cavity may fill with transudated serum or blood (Fig. 5.17A) as fragile proliferating capillaries invade the theca interna and zona granulosa. On transvaginal ultrasound, the corpus luteum might at first be barely visible among the variegated echoes of the ovarian stroma. As it matures, however, it can often first be seen as a solid dimple on the surface of the ovary, about 2 cm in diameter, then with rather thick,

echogenic walls that have a crenated appearance and enclose a hypoechoic center (Fig. 5.17A). Neovascularization—having commenced during the 24 hours leading up to ovulation and being detectable with color Doppler imaging (Plate 5.2)—persists for the functional life of the corpus luteum, especially if there is pregnancy.

Occasionally, after ovulation, the follicle seals up and fills with blood, to form a cystic or hemorrhagic corpus luteum (Fig. 5.17B). A cystic corpus luteum can expand to be 5 or 6 cm in diameter, with ultrasound appearances that can mimic an endometrioma. Alternatively, a corpus luteum can fill with serous fluid and in some circumstances persist beyond the normal 2 weeks' life of a normal corpus luteum, when it is then called a *corpus luteum cyst*. Luteal cysts typically have thicker walls than follicular cysts, owing to the relative health of the luteinized granulosa cell (follicular cell) layer, but the distinction can often be impossible without prior ultrasound or hormonal documentation of ovulation. Luteal cysts are more likely to cause pain than follicular cysts, especially if there is pregnancy, due to further stimulation of the cyst by chorionic gonadotropin. If cysts persist for more than a month or two, in the absence of pregnancy, endocrine function will have long ceased, and characterization is not possible hormonally or histopathologically: the label "functional" (or dysfunctional) then suffices for the cyst (Fig. 5.18).

The natural history of luteal cysts, as for follicular cysts, is to resolve with time. Reassessment of a suspicious ovarian lesion 6 to 8 weeks later, preferably just after menstruation to avoid the diagnostically confounding effect of a new corpus luteum, usually confirms their disappearance.[41] The diagnostic confusion that the range of appearances a normal corpus luteum might have on ultrasound, including the findings on color Doppler examination, means that evaluation of ovarian masses and cysts is best done during the follicular phase—or during ovarian suppression with progestogens.

If an ovulatory stimulus occurs that is sufficient to luteinize the follicle but not to release follicular fluid and the oocyte,

Figure 5.16 Early corpus luteum. **(A)** Fresh hemorrhagic corpus luteum. **(B)** Laparoscopic image of a newly vascularized corpus luteum.

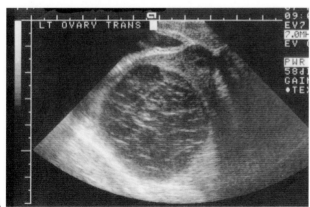

A

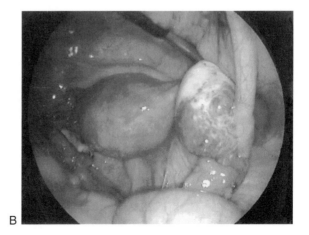

B

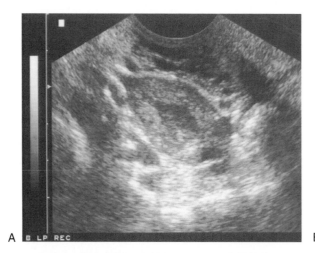

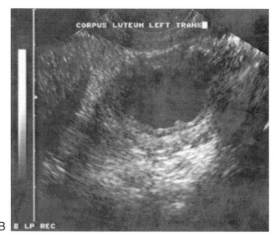

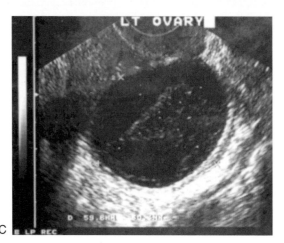

Figure 5.17 Range of appearances of the established normal corpus luteum. Differential diagnosis from potentially important ovarian cysts is difficult and thus is best carried out in the follicular phase or during ovarian suppression with progestogens. **(A)** Predominantly solid, established corpus luteum. **(B)** Cystic corpus luteum with fleshy wall composed of luteal tissue. **(C)** Blood clot within a corpus luteum.

the follicle will continue to grow toward a diameter of about 3 cm with echogenic or clear contents—a phenomenon known as the luteinized unruptured follicle (Fig. 5.18).[42,43] Progesterone production is less than in a normal luteal phase, and the luteal phase can be shorter than normal.[44] Luteinized unruptured follicles occur in about 5% of apparently normal menstrual cycles[45] and in a higher percentage of abnormal ones.[46] It can also occur if there is a strong ovulatory stimulus but the follicle is too small or immature to respond fully with ovulation. In this circumstance, hemorrhage into the follicle is usual, resulting in a corpus hemorrhagicum, with relatively echo-dense contents; progesterone production rises only marginally, and the "luteal" phase might last just a few days.[47,48]

Perimenopausal and Postmenopausal State

As ovarian follicular depletion progresses, the availability of antral follicles a few millimeters in diameter for recruitment diminishes, production of follicular inhibin is low, and levels of FSH begin to rise sooner during the usual phase of antral follicle recruitment, the late luteal phase. The result is that

Figure 5.18 Follicular cyst of the ovary. Such a cyst might or might not be producing estradiol and effecting endometrial proliferation. A recent luteinized unruptured follicle can present the same appearance.

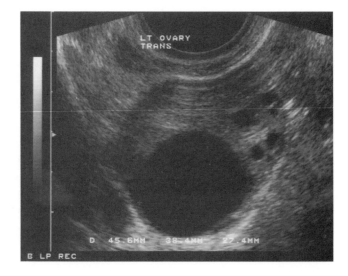

follicular development of such recruits is prone to start earlier and earlier in the previous ovarian or menstrual cycle, before menstruation has actually begun and thus before a new ovarian cycle is seen to start. The result is that the apparent length of the follicular phase (and hence the menstrual cycle more generally) gets shorter as menopause gets closer. The ovaries must make do with less than perfect follicles, and follicular growth is often disordered or delayed, with sporadic long cycles interspersed among the generally shortened ones, and predisposing to the phenomenon of luteinized unruptured follicles. During the perimenopausal years, it is common to have functional cysts on the ovaries, sometimes with a multifollicular overall appearance.

Menopause itself is a clinical event not closely related to a particular appearance of the ovaries beyond a relative absence of developing follicles. Estrogen and inhibin production fails, and levels of FSH are high. By 3 years after menopause, follicles are truly depleted ultrasonically and histologically. The ovaries become small and homogeneous in echo texture, and with a lack of contrasting features; they can, as in young girls, be difficult or impossible to find among the complex abdominal and pelvic ultrasonic noise reflected by peristaltic bowel.

BLADDER

The bladder is a thin-walled reservoir, which when full can be well delineated by ultrasound. Normally, it assumes a characteristic shape that is roughly triangular in the longitudinal sagittal view (Fig. 5.19A) and a rounded rectangle in the transverse plane (Fig. 5.19B). However, the shape also depends on pressure from surrounding structures; the fundus of the uterus often indents it posteriorly (Fig. 5.19A). The bladder, because of its typical shape and central, anterior position, ought not be confused with other pelvic cysts, which are usually spheric and located asymmetrically.[49] Images should be compared before and after micturition or, bladder catheterization if there is any doubt. The bladder has urine filling it regularly from the ureters, so another way to prove that a cystic structure is the bladder is to demonstrate these fluid ureteric jets with color Doppler. (The ureters themselves are not evident on ultrasound unless they are abnormally distended.)

A partially empty bladder is seen as a collapsed triangular structure close to the symphysis pubis (Fig. 5.19C). On

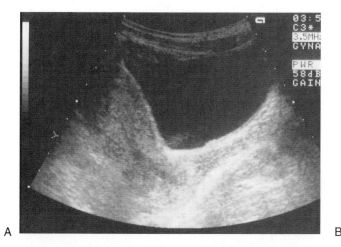

A

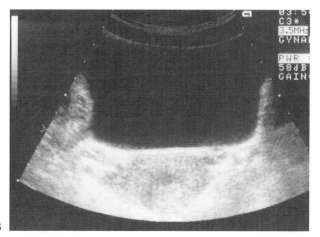

B

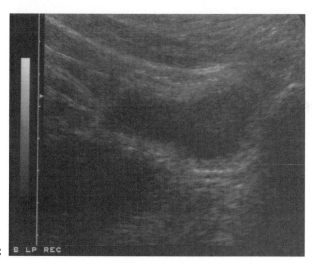

C

Figure 5.19 Imaging the normal bladder. The uterus normally indents the posterior aspect of the distended bladder. (**A**) Sagittal section of the normal distended bladder on transabdominal scanning reveals a triangle. (**B**) Transverse section of the normal distended bladder on transabdominal scanning reveals a rounded rectangle. (**C**) Partially empty bladder.

transvaginal ultrasound, the wall of a partially empty bladder becomes irregular and thick, and it can resemble the papillary projections of a tumor. Re-examination with a distended bladder should show the walls stretched and thin and resolve any diagnostic difficulty.

Some clinicians examine the patient rectally at the same time as the abdominal ultrasound to demonstrate that an apparent mass consists of feces in the rectum; others carry out a water enema to demonstrate the change in rectal appearances. Alternatively, re-examination a few days after administration of an aperient might show that an innocent bowel mass has gone.

RECTOSIGMOID COLON

The rectum and sigmoid colon lie posterior and to the left of the uterus. Like the loops of small intestine that surround the pelvic organs, the rectosigmoid can contain any combination of solid and fluid fecal material and gas (Fig. 5.20), with the consequence that image artifacts from reflection, refraction, and reverberation are traps for the unwary. The appearances of bowel contents are so variable that they can mimic adnexal masses, particularly a dermoid cyst of the ovary. If on transvaginal ultrasound two normal ovaries are identified separate to the mass, then the mass in question is probably bowel. Bowel masses can be identified positively if they show peristalsis or if their dimensions change during observation.

PERITONEAL SPACES

Free fluid in the pelvis and abdomen collects in dependent peritoneal spaces. Most commonly, it collects in the pouch of Douglas, which is posterior to the uterus and anterior to the rectum (Fig. 5.21); less commonly, it collects in the uterovesical pouch between uterus and bladder. Transvaginal ultrasound is a sensitive test for free peritoneal fluid: just 25 ml of fluid is enough to be reliably discerned by ultrasound.[50] Such a quantity of fluid is common after ovulation—or after rupture of a cyst—but can be present before follicular rupture (see above), especially when the ovaries have been stimulated.

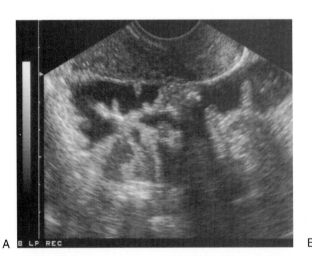

A   B LP REC

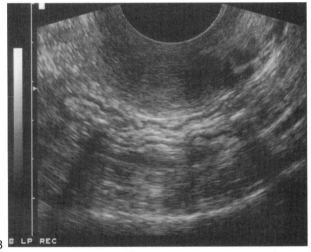

B   B LP REC

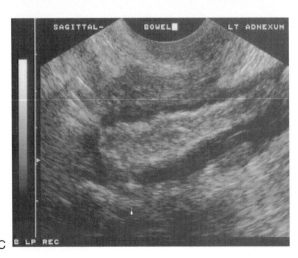

SAGITTAL-   BOWEL   LT ADNEXUM

C   B LP REC

Figure 5.20 Ultrasound of the bowel. (**A**) Complex echoes from the rectosigmoid colon in the pelvis (**B**) Outlining of the appendix. (**C**) View of the colon in a patient with chronic severe constipation

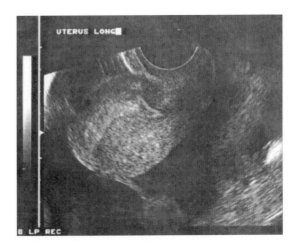

Figure 5.21 Free peritoneal fluid in front of and behind the uterus, respectively, in the uterovesical pouch (to the left) and in the cul-de-sac, or pouch of Douglas (to the right).

Serous fluid is usually echolucent, whereas blood is commonly faintly echogenic.

A small amount of free fluid in the pelvis is often an indication that an ovary is functioning. It is not seen in postmenopausal women with inactive ovaries. In asymptomatic postmenopausal women with no indication of ovarian abnormality in one study,[20] free fluid was found in only 1 of 300 postmenopausal subjects, and she had a hepatic cause for ascites.

PELVIC BLOOD VESSELS

Internal Iliac Vessels

The common iliac artery bifurcates into the external and internal iliac arteries at the pelvic brim, with the internal iliac artery coursing along the pelvic sidewall. The arteries are accompanied by the relevant veins. The external iliac vessels are larger and are easily imaged at the pelvic brim with transvaginal ultrasound. The internal iliac artery is 5 to 7 mm in diameter (Fig. 5.13A). It is straight, tubular, and pulsates with expansion of the walls. The blood within it is faintly echogenic on gray scale imaging and, unlike a dilated ureter or a hydrosalpinx, lights up brightly with color Doppler. The internal iliac vein is approximately 10 mm in diameter and does not pulsate. It also contains blood, but the slow flow within is not as impressive on color Doppler imaging. Unless special care is taken, the iliac veins in transverse ultrasonic section can be confused with ovarian follicles during transvaginal follicle aspiration for assisted conception.

REFERENCES

1. Saxton DW, Farquhar CM, Rae T et al. Accuracy of ultrasound measurements of female pelvic organs. Br J Obstet Gynaecol 1990;97:695–699

2. Wiener JJ, Newcombe RG. Measurements of uterine volume: a comparison between measurements by ultrasonography and by water displacement. J Clin Ultrasound 1992;20:457–460

3. Wakeling AE, Wyngarden LJ. Prostaglandin receptors in the human, monkey and hamster uterus. Endocrinology 1974;95:55–64

4. Occhipinti K, Kutcher R, Rosenblatt R. Sonographic appearance and significance of arcuate artery calcification. J Ultrasound Med 1991;10:97–100

5. Jansen RPS. Endocrine response in the female genital tract. In: Shearman RP, Ed. Clinical Reproductive Endocrinology. Churchill Livingstone, Edinburgh, 1985, pp 109–164

6. Gross BH. Ultrasound of the uterus. In: Callen PW, Ed. Ultrasonography in Obstetrics and Gynaecology. WB Saunders, Philadelphia, 1983; p 249

7. Vollman RF. The Menstrual Cycle. WB Saunders, Philadelphia, 1977, pp 19–190

8. Bakos O, Lundkvist O, Bergh T. Transvaginal sonographic evaluation of endometrial growth and texture in spontaneous ovulatory cycles—a descriptive study. Hum Reprod 1993;8:799–806

9. Smith B, Porter R, Ahuja K, Craft I. Ultrasonic assessment of endometrial changes in stimulated cycles in an in-vitro fertilization and embryo transfer program. (Abstract.) J In Vitro Fert Embryo Transf 1989;1:233–238

10. Gonen Y, Casper RF, Jacobson W, Blankier J. Endometrial thickness and growth during ovarian stimulation: a possible predictor of implantation in in vitro fertilization. Fertil Steril 1989;52:446–450

11. Germar-Martinez [sic], Okai T, Masuda H et al. Transvaginal sonographic assessment of the endometrium in spontaneous and induced cycles. Asia-Oceania J Obstet Gynaecol 1990; 16:239–246

12. Sher G, Herbert C, Maassarani G, Jacobs MH. Assessment of the late proliferative phase endometrium by ultrasonography in patients undergoing in-vitro fertilization and embryo transfer (IVF/ET). Hum Reprod 1991;6:232–237

13. Abdalla HI, Brooks AA, Johnson MR et al. Endometrial thickness: a predictor of implantation in ovum recipients. Hum Reprod 1994;9:363–365

14. Serafini P, Batzofin J, Nelson J, Olive D. Sonographic uterine predictors of pregnancy in women undergoing ovulation induction for assisted reproductive treatments. Fertil Steril 1994;62:815–822

15. Jansen RPS, Turner M, Johannisson E et al. Cyclic changes in human endometrial surface glycoproteins: a quantitative histochemical study. Fertil Steril 1985;44:85–91

16. Gompel C. The ultrastructure of the human endometrial cell studied by electron microscopy. Am J Obstet Gynecol 1962;84:1000–1009

17. Welker BG, Gembruch U, Diedrich K et al. Transvaginal sonography of the endometrium during ovum pickup in stimulated cycles for in vitro fertilization. J Ultrasound Med 1989;8:549–553

18. Lenz S, Lindenberg S. Ultrasonic evaluation of endometrial growth in women with normal cycles during spontaneous and stimulated cycles. Hum Reprod 1990;5:377–381

19. Miller EI, Thomas RH, Lines P. The atrophic postmenopausal uterus. J Clin Ultrasound 1977;5:261–263

20. Andolf E, Dahlander K, Aspenberg P. Ultrasonic thickness of the endometrium correlated to body weight in asymptomatic postmenopausal women. Obstet Gynecol 1993;82:936–940

21. Brosens JJ, de Souza NM, Braker FG. Uterine junctional zone: function and disease. Lancet 1995;346:558–560

22. Jansen RPS, Anderson JC. Catheterisation of the fallopian tubes from the vagina. Lancet 1987;2:309–310

23. Rottem S, Thaler I, Goldstein SR et al. Transvaginal sonographic technique: targeted organ scanning without resorting to "planes." J Clin Ultrasound 1990;18:243

24. Higgins RV, Van Nagell JR, Jr, Woods CH et al. Interobserver variation in ovarian measurements using transvaginal sonography. Gynecol Oncol 1990;39:69–71

25. Faddy MJ, Gosden RG, Gougeon A et al. Accelerated disappearance of ovarian follicles in mid-life: Implications for forecasting menopause. Hum Reprod 1992;7:1342–1346

26. Khan I, Devroey P, Van den Bergh M et al. The effect of pneumoperitoneum gases on fertilization, cleavage and pregnancy in human in-vitro fertilization and gamete intrafallopian transfer. Hum Reprod 1989;4:323–326

27. Cohen HL, Shapiro MA, Mandel FS, Shapiro ML. Normal ovaries in neonates and infants: a sonographic study of 77 patients 1 day to 24 months old. Am J Roentgenol 1993; 160:583–586

28. Haber HP, Mayer EI. Ultrasound evaluation of uterine and ovarian size from birth to puberty. Pediatr Radiol 1994;24:11–13

29. Bridges NA, Cooke A, Healy MJR et al. Standards for ovarian volume in childhood and puberty. Fertil Steril 1993;60:456–460

30. Cohen HK, Tice HM, Handel FS. Ovarian volumes measured by US: bigger than we think. Radiology 1990;177:189–192

31. Merce LT, Andrino R, Barco MJ, de la Fuente F. Cyclic changes of the functional ovarian compartment: echographic assessment. Acta Obstet Gynecol Scand 1990;69:327–332

32. Mendelson EB, Fiedman H, Neiman HL et al. The role of imaging in infertility management. Am J Radiol 1985;144:415–420

33. Rossavik IK, Gibbons WE. Variability of ovarian follicular growth in natural menstrual cycles. Fertil Steril 1985; 44:195–199

34. Zandt-Stastry D, Thorsen MK, Middleston WB et al. Inability of sonography to detect imminent ovulation. Am J Radiol 1985;152:91–95

35. Check JH, Dietterich C, Houck MA. Ipsilateral versus contralateral ovary selection of dominant follicle in succeeding cycles. Obstet Gynecol 1991;77:968–970

36. Adams J, Franks S, Polson DW et al. Multifollicular ovaries: clinical and endocrine features and response to pulsatile gonadotropin releasing hormone. Lancet 1985;2:1375–1379

37. Treasure JL, Gordon PAL, King EA et al. Cystic ovaries: a phase of anorexia nervosa. Lancet 1985;2:1379–1382

38. Anonymous. Follicular multiplicity. Lancet 1985;2:1404

39. Futterweit W, Yeh H-C, Mechanick JI. Multifollicular ovaries in weight-loss-related amenorrhoea. Lancet 1986;1:796

40. Hamilton CJCM, Evers JLH, Tan FES, Hoogland HJ. The reliability of ovulation prediction by a single ultrasonographic follicle measurement. Hum Reprod 1987;2:103–107

41. Okai T, Kobayashi K, Ryo E et al. Transvaginal sonographic appearance of hemorrhagic functional ovarian cysts and their spontaneous regression. Int J Gynecol Obstet 1994;44:47–52

42. Marik J, Hulka J. Luteinized unruptured follicle syndrome: a subtle cause of infertility. Fertil Steril 1978;29:270–274

43. Katz E. The luteinized unruptured follicle and other ovulatory dysfunctions. Fertil Steril 1988;50:839–850

44. Coutts JRT, Adam AH, Fleming R. The deficient luteal phase may represent an anovulatory cycle. Clin Endocrinol 1982;17:389–394

45. Kerin JF, Kirby C, Morris D et al. Incidence of the luteinized unruptured follicle phenomenon in cycling women. Fertil Steril 1983;40:620–625

46. Liukkonen S, Koskimies AI, Tenhunen A, YI"stalo P. Diagnosis of luteinized unruptured follicle (LUF) syndrome by ultrasound. Fertil Steril 1984;41:26–30

47. Strott CA, Cargille CM, Ross GT, Lipsett MB. The short luteal phase. J Clin Endocrinol Metab 1970;30:246–251

48. Beard RW, Reginald PW, Wadsworth J. Clinical features of women with chronic lower abdominal pain and pelvic congestion. Br J Obstet Gynaecol 1988;95:153–161

49. Witschi E. Overripeness of the egg as a cause of twinning and teratogenesis. Cancer Res 1952;12:763–786

50. Steinkampf MP, Blackwell RE, Younger JB. Visualisation of free peritoneal fluid with transvaginal sonography. J Reprod Med 1991;36:729–730

51. Jansen RPS. Oncological endocrinology. In: Coppleson M, Ed. Gynecologic Oncology (2nd ed.). Churchill Livingstone, Edinburgh, 1992, pp 135–171

52. Novak ER, Woodruff JD. Histology of the endometrium. In: Novak ER, Woodruff, Eds. Gynecologic and Obstetric Pathology (8th ed.) WB Saunders, Philadelphia, 1979, p 179

53. Bald, R. Studien über die sonografischen Endometriumdarstellung. Inaugural-Dissertation, Marburg. In: Deichert, U., Hackelöer, B.J., and Daume, E. The sonographic and endocrinologic evaluation of the endometrium in the luteal phase. Human Reproduction 1986;1:219–222

54. Sydney IVF, 1986 (unpublished data)

6

Computed Tomography of the Normal Female Pelvis

JILL E. LANGER

Computed tomography (CT) continues to be valuable for the evaluation of the female pelvis. Recent technologic improvements in CT allow the expeditious acquisition of high-resolution images, improving imaging of the genital tract. Assessment of pathologic conditions affecting the female pelvis as well as the ability to establish a confident diagnosis of a normal study depend on a thorough understanding of normal and variant anatomy as visualized by CT.

TECHNIQUE

Careful attention to CT technique is essential to ensure the highest quality images for optimal visualization of pelvic anatomy and abnormalities. Scan acquisition should be performed during the administration of intravenous contrast by rapid bolus to obtain intense parenchymal enhancement of the pelvic organs and to opacify the pelvic blood vessels[1-5] (Fig. 6.1). Collimation of 10-mm or smaller slices may be used selectively to reduce volume averaging of the small pelvic structures or to examine an area of suspected abnormality.[3,4]

Patient preparation involves the administration of oral contrast to opacify the pelvic small bowel loops and the colon. Patients should be scanned with a distended urinary bladder, which displaces small bowel loops out of the pelvis.[2,6-8] Insertion of a tampon before scanning often helps to delineate the vaginal canal, a technique that is especially helpful in the assessment of the postoperative female pelvis.[9]

ANATOMY

The pelvis is defined anatomically as a complex structure composed of an osseous ring with numerous attached muscles that supports the vertebral column and facilitates ambulation. Anatomically, the pelvis can be divided into two parts by an imaginary plane that extends obliquely from the sacral promontory along the anterior border of S1 to the symphysis pubis.[10] The false or greater pelvis is defined as that portion of the pelvis above this plane and contains the ascending, descending, and sigmoid colon; small bowel; and major vascular bifurcations (Figs. 6.2 and 6.3). The true or lesser pelvis is situated below the imaginary plane and contains the reproductive organs, rectum, bladder, pelvic ureters, and small bowel loops (Figs. 6.4 to 6.6). The pelvic diaphragm, a muscular sling composed of the levator ani and coccygeal muscles, forms the floor of the true pelvis and separates the pelvic viscera from the perineum (Fig. 6.7). The inferior portion of the peritoneal cavity, the anterior and posterior pararenal spaces, and occasionally the lesser sac may extend into the pelvis.[11]

MUSCULOSKELETAL PELVIS

The osseous pelvis consists of four bones. The two paired innominate bones lie anteriorly and laterally, forming most of the osseous boundary of the pelvis. The sacrum and coccyx lie posteriorly and insert like a triangular wedge between the two innominate bones. The innominate bone is composed of three bones that fuse between the fifteenth and twentieth year of life; the ileum superiorly, the ischium posteroinferiorly, and the pubis anteroinferiorly.[10-14] At the level of the sacral promontory, the pelvis has a somewhat elliptic shape with the long axis oriented mediolaterally. This is because the relative forward projection of the junction of the lumbar spine with the sacrum narrows the antero posterior (AP) dimension of the pelvis. Just a few centimeters lower, the geometry changes to that of an ellipse, with the long axis oriented in the AP dimension because of the relative horizontal orientation of the upper sacral segments[10] (Fig. 6.4). This elliptical shape persists throughout the lower pelvis (Fig. 6.5 to 6.7).

On CT, the cortical bone of the pelvis has high attenuation and appears as a uniform white rim. Small lucent linear structures representing nutrient grooves may sometimes be seen. The central medullary portion of bone is less dense, since it contains the bone marrow elements, which have a large amount of fat and less compact trabecular bone.[12] When assessing osseous abnormalities, the image should be viewed with a high CT level and a wide window setting. This so-

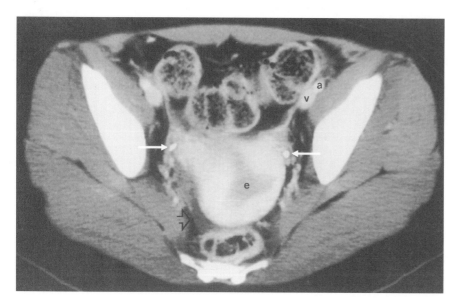

Figure 6.1 Use of rapid bolus intravenous contrast. This CT scan obtained during bolus intravenous contrast enhancement shows a retroverted uterus projecting into the posterior cul-de-sac in a 36-year-old woman. There is enhancement of the normal myometrium, approaching that of the pelvic vasculature, distinguishing it from the normal lower attenuating endometrial cavity (e). A small amount of fluid (open arrow) is present within the rectouterine pouch, probably due to ovulation. a, external iliac artery; v, external iliac vein; arrows; ureters.

Figure 6.2 CT of the pelvis, iliac crest level. An image obtained at the most superior aspect of the pelvis shows the left iliac bone but not the right, secondary to asymmetric positioning of the patient. This image is just below the aortic bifurcation into the common iliac arteries (A). The left ovarian artery (medium black arrow) and vein (curved black arrow) are seen adjacent to the unopacified ureter (small black arrow). V, inferior vena cava; P, psoas; AC, ascending colon; DC, descending colon; TC, transverse colon; I, Iliac bone; L4/5; intervertebral disc at the L4–5 level; sb, small bowel.

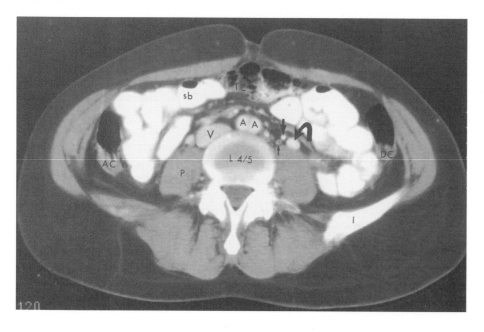

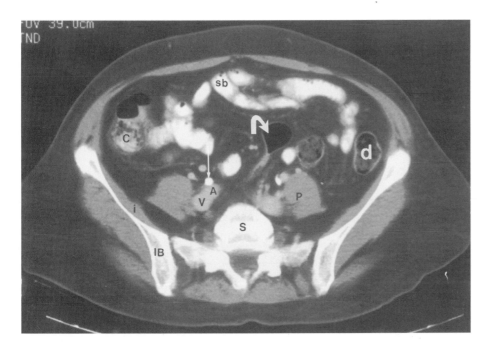

Figure 6.3 CT of the pelvis, sacral promontory level. The plane dividing the false pelvis from the true pelvis begins at this level and extends obliquely anterioinferiorly to the symphysis pubis. The curved white arrow indicates sigmoid colon, straight white arrow indicates the ureter. C, cecum; d, descending colon; sb, small bowel; V, common iliac vein; A, common iliac artery; P, psoas; i, iliacus; S, body of S 1; IB, iliac bone.

Figure 6.4 CT of the pelvis, sacroiliac joint level. The pelvic ureter (open white arrow) is seen crossing just anterior to the common iliac artery on the left. The right iliac vessels have bifurcated into the internal and external iliac arteries and veins. C, cecum; d, descending colon; sb, small bowel; p, psoas muscle; i, iliacus; gma, gluteus maximus; gme, gluteus medius; gmi, gluteus minimus; S, sacrum; IB, iliac bone; V, common iliac vein; VI, internal iliac vein; VE, external iliac vein; AE; external iliac artery; AI, internal iliac artery, white arrow rectosigmoid colon black arrows; sacroiliac joint: black arrow, sacral plexus; black arrowheads, gonadal veins.

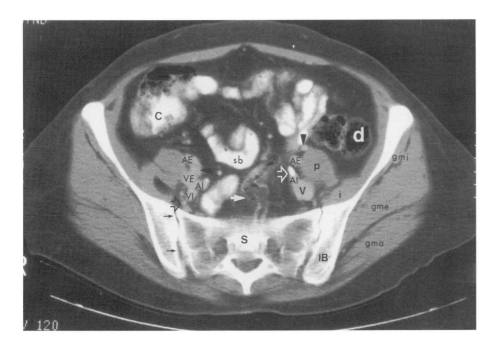

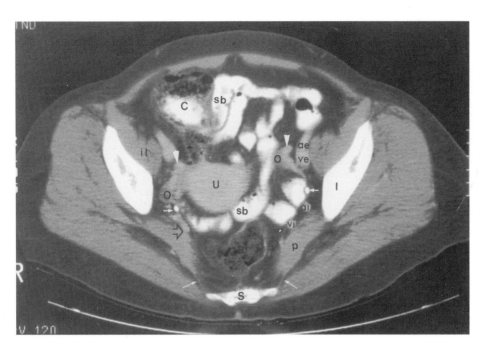

Figure 6.5 CT of the pelvis, sciatic foramen level. The fundus of the uterus (U) and the adjacent adnexal structures are well seen. Ureters are indicated by the short white arrows, sacral plexus is indicated by the open black arrows, ovarian vessels are indicated by the white arrowheads, sacrospinous ligament is indicated by the long white arrows. C, cecum; R, rectosigmoid colon; sb, small bowel; O, ovaries; I iliac bone; S, sacrum; il, iliopsoas; p, piriformis; ae, external iliac artery; ve, external iliac vein; ai, internal iliac artery; vi, internal iliac vein.

Figure 6.6 CT of the pelvis; acetabular roof level. The distal ureters (black arrows) are angling medially at the base of the broad ligament just before entering the bladder. An enlarged right inguinal lymph node (n) is probably present within the deep chain. The white arrows indicate the obturator internus muscles along the pelvic sidewall. A surgical clip is noted in the left adnexa (arrowhead). C, cervix; a, common femoral artery; v, common femoral vein; F, femoral head; gma, gluteus maximus; gme, gluteus medius; ip, iliopsoas; t, tensor fascia lata; s, sartorius; Co, coccyx; A, anterior column of the acetabulum; P, posterior column of the acetabulum; sb, small bowel.

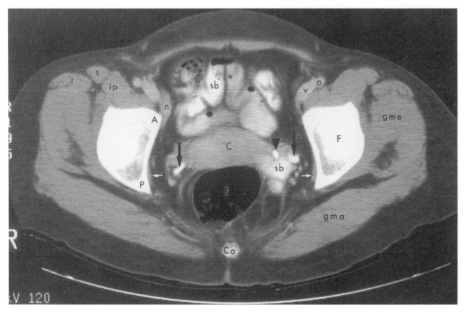

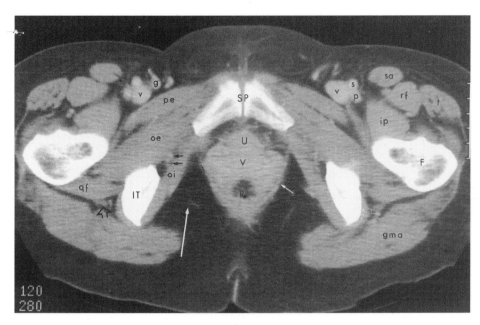

Figure 6.7 CT of the pelvis, symphysis pubis level. The urethra (U), vagina (V), and rectum (R) are leaving the pelvis through the pelvic diaphragm as it separates the pelvic floor from the perineum at this level. The obturator artery, vein, and nerve are seen (short black arrows) between the obturator internus (oi) and obturator externus (oe). The levator ani is indicated by the short white arrow, the sciatic nerve is indicated by the open arrow, and the ishiorectal fossa is indicated by the long white arrow. IT, ischial tuberosity; SP, symphysis pubis; ip, iliopsoas muscle; pe, pectineus; qf, quadriceps femoris; t, tensor fascia lata; sa, sartorius; rf, rectus femoris; gma, gluteus maximus; v, common femoral vein; p, profunda femoral artery; s, superficial femoral artery; g, greater saphenous vein.

called "bone window" provides the contrast needed to assess the cortical bone.

The pelvic muscles are well delineated on CT. They are symmetric and are of uniform soft tissue attenuation. The principle muscles of the false pelvis are the psoas and iliacus. The psoas is a fusiform muscle that originates from the lumbar vertebral bodies and their transverse processes. The iliacus is fan shaped and originates from the upper, inner aspect of the ileum and sacral ala. These muscles join to form the iliopsoas muscle, which leaves the pelvis to insert on the lesser trochanter of the femur.

The muscles of the true pelvis can be divided into those of the lower limbs, which arise in the pelvis, and those of the pelvic diaphragm. The pelvic sidewall is lined by the obturator internus and piriformis muscles and their covering fasciae (Figs. 6.5 and 6.6). The obturator internus muscle extends from the anterolateral walls of the true pelvis along the inner aspect of the acetabulum and extends outside the pelvis to insert on the greater trochanter. The piriformis is a flat triangular-shaped muscle, which extends from the lateral aspect of the sacrum through the greater sciatic foramen to insert on the greater trochanter of the femur[10,12] (Fig. 6.5). The pelvic musculature along with its investing fasciae provide a potential pathway for the spread of infectious, neoplastic, and hemorrhagic processes from the retroperitoneum and pelvis to the hip and thigh, and vice versa.[11]

The true pelvis is bounded inferiorly by the pelvic diaphragm, the main support of the pelvic floor, which is a hammock-like structure composed of the levator ani and coccygeus muscles and their covering fasciae (Figs. 6.7 to 6.9). The urethra, vagina, and rectum pass through the pelvic diaphragm from the pelvic cavity to the perineum. The levator ani is seen on CT as a V-shaped structure surrounding the rectum, extending anteriorly from the superior surface of the pubic rami, and medially from the inner aspect of the ischium to insert posteriorly on the inferior coccygeal segments and the anococcygeal raphe. The coccygeus is a triangular muscle that extends from the ischial spine to the coccyx.

The perineum is a diamond-shaped space that lies below the pelvic floor. It is bounded by the symphysis pubis anteriorly and by the inferior pubic ramus and the inferior aspect of the ischium laterally. A line drawn between the ischial tuberosities divides this space into an anterior (or urogenital) triangle containing the external urinary and genital organs, and the posterior (or anal) compartment. The fatty ischiorectal fossa is present on either side of the midline[4,10,12,14–16] (Fig. 6.10).

The greater sciatic foramen begins just beneath the sacroiliac joint. Superiorly, it contains the piriformis muscle and the sacral plexus, which can be seen as an oval soft tissue attenuation structure lying in the fascial plane just anterior to the piriformis muscle (see Fig. 6.5). The sciatic nerve runs through the inferior aspect of the greater sciatic foramen, leaving the pelvis behind the sacrospinous ligament near its attachment to the ischial spine. The sciatic nerve is a circular structure just lateral and posterior to the ischial spine, or it may be seen more distally along its course, dorsal to the ten-

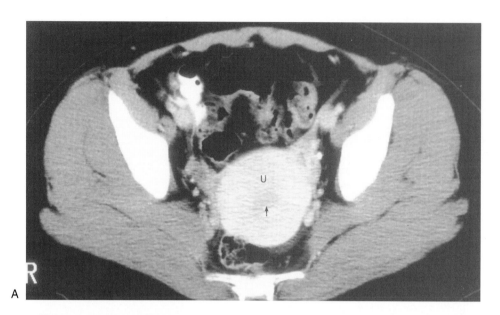

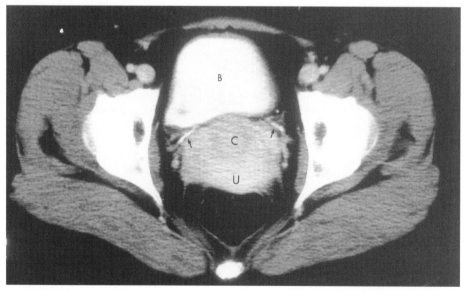

Figure 6.8 Apparent uterine enlargement. **(A)** An image obtained in a 48-year-old during dynamic scanning shows marked myometrial enhancement of the uterine body (U) and slightly lower attenuation of the endometrial cavity (arrow) centrally. **(B)** An image obtained slightly inferior to Figure A, at the level of the junction of the lower uterus (U) and the cervix (C), shows the uterus to be retroflexed, since the cervix is anterior relative to the uterine body. This image may give a false impression of uterine or cervical enlargement, since the angulation of the uterine body relative to the cervix in the AP plane causes both the cervix and lower uterus to appear at the same level on the axially oriented CT image. Arrows, the ureters; B, bladder.

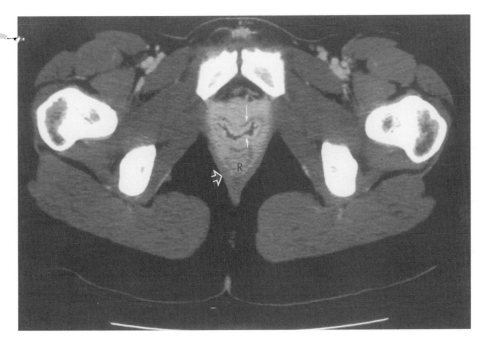

Figure 6.9 Normal vagina. An axial image through the lower vagina during dynamic intravenous contrast administration shows the densely enhanced vaginal epithelium (short arrow) and the less enhanced muscular wall (long arrow). The levator ani (open arrow) is seen surrounding the rectum (R).

Figure 6.10 Urethra. An axial image obtained during dynamic CT shows dense enhancement of the periurethral tissues (open arrowhead). The vagina is just posterior (curved arrow) and shows enhancement of its epithelium. Two calcified phleboliths (arrowhead) are noted adjacent to the vagina. R, rectum.

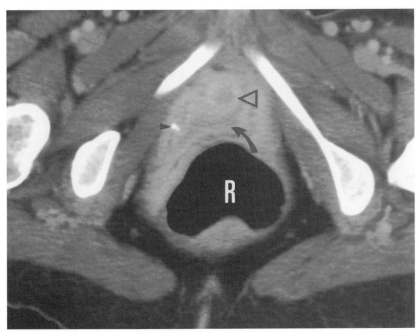

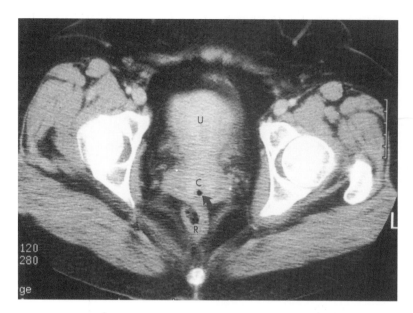

Figure 6.11 Anteverted uterus. Marked anteversion in this 53-year-old has caused the entire uterus to be tipped into a coronal orientation on this axial image. A small dot of air (arrow) is present within the cervical canal from a pelvic examination performed before the CT. The uterine body (U) to-cervix (C) ratio is approaching 1:1 in this patient nearing menopause. R, rectum.

don of the obturator internus muscle, covered by the gluteus maximus[17–19] (Fig. 6.11).

THE REPRODUCTIVE ORGANS

Uterus

The uterus is in the midline behind the bladder and the rectum (Fig. 6.12). There is great variation in the size and morphology of the normal uterus on CT.[6,7,12,20] The nulliparous uterus measures 7.7 to 9 cm in length, 4 to 6 cm in width, and 3 to 4 cm in AP diameter.[14,21] Multiparous dimensions are about 1 to 2 cm greater.[10] The uterine body is twice the length of the cervix during the reproductive years. A body-to-cervix ratio approaching 1:1 occurs in the premenarcheal and postmenopausal years. The postmenopausal uterus atrophies, decreasing to 4 to 6 cm in length. The most rapid decline in volume occurs over the first 10 years following menopause, with a more gradual decline occurring in the next 10 years.[22,23]

When the uterus is anteverted, it is seen along the superior and posterior aspect of the bladder (Fig. 6.11). When retroverted or retroflexed, it projects into the cul-de-sac. Also, the cervix may be midline, with the uterine body deviating to one side of the pelvis. The degree of bladder distension may also affect the position of the uterus.[6,14,20] A markedly anteverted or retroverted uterus often appears abnormally enlarged, since the entire length of the uterus will be imaged on a single axially oriented CT image (Fig. 6.11).

The walls of the normal uterus should appear smooth in contour and uniform in attenuation.[24–28] The normal myometrium enhances more than other pelvic soft tissues fol-

lowing the administration of intravenous contrast secondary to its rich vascular supply.[6,14,15,29] Examining the uterus during dynamic contrast enhancement allows identification of lesions arising within the wall and the less-enhancing endometrial cavity[29–32] (Figs. 6.13 and 6.14). When imaged in cross-section, the cavity appears as a circular area of low attenuation. If the uterine orientation is such that it is imaged coronally, the "T" shape of the endometrial cavity may be apparent (Fig. 6.15). In women of reproductive age, the endometrium appears as a central region of lower attenuation, typically 5 to 15 mm in thickness.[13,24,32,33]

The spectrum of normal cervical enhancement during CT has yet to be defined. The central "inner zone" of the cervix may show intense enhancement corresponding to the richly vascular cervical epithelium, while the more peripheral fibrous stroma may only show intermediate enhancement[2] (Fig. 6.16).

Vascular calcifications within the intrauterine arterial vessels may be present in the outer myometrium, possibly as a consequence of cystic medial necrosis within the arcuate arteries. This may be related to senescent change in the elderly patient or to hypertension, diabetes, or calcium metabolism abnormalities in women of any age.[34] These calcifications appear as small linear or branching structures, most commonly noted peripherally within the myometrium in the distribution of the arcuate artery (Fig. 6.17). Focal or globular calcifications suggest the presence of a myoma or foreign body.[6,24–26]

The anterior surface of the uterus is apposed to the urinary bladder. It is covered with peritoneum that is reflected forward to cover the posterior wall of the bladder at the level of the cervix. The vesicouterine pouch or anterior cul-de-sac,

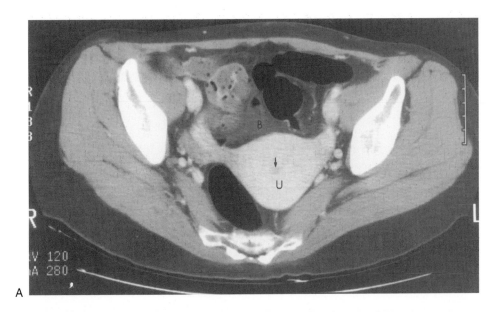

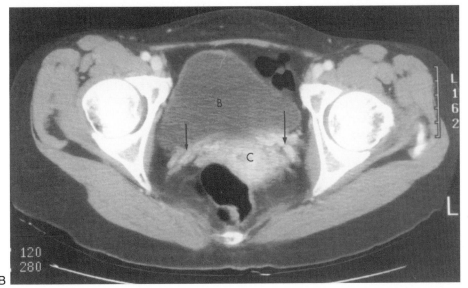

Figure 6.12 Normal uterus. **(A)** The pelvis of a 38-year-old shows the uterus (U) in a neutral position. The endometrial cavity is seen as a small region of low attenuation (arrow) within the densely enhancing myometrium. The most superior aspect of the urine-filled bladder (B) is seen just anterior to the uterus. **(B)** An image approximately 5 cm caudal to Figure A shows a normal cervix (C). Note the rounded shape of the cervix and the approximate 2:1 ratio of the uterine body to cervix in this patient of reproductive age. Arrows indicate the paracervical venous plexus. B, bladder.

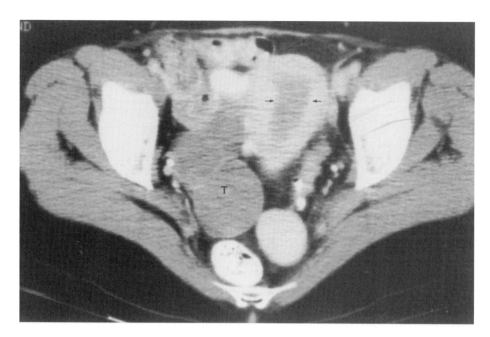

Figure 6.13 Prominent endometrial cavity. The low-attenuation endometrial cavity (arrows) measured over 1 cm in this postmenopausal patient who presented with dysfunctional uterine bleeding. The abnormal endometrial proliferation was related to a hormonally active right ovarian tumor (T).

Figure 6.14 Differential temporal enhancement of arteries and veins. This CT scan obtained in the arterial phase of contrast enhancement demonstrates enhancement of the common femoral arteries (a), while the adjacent femoral veins (v) are not yet opacified. The enhanced vessels (small white arrows) along the lateral aspect of the uterus therefore correspond to the uterine arterial network, while the adjacent unopacified vessels (large white arrows) represent the uterine veins. Similarly, the left ovarian arterial supply can be seen as enhanced vessels (small black arrow) adjacent to the left ovary (O). A myoma (m) is present within the uterus.

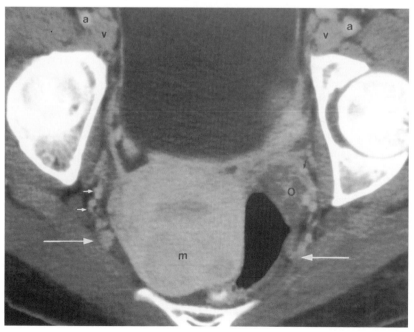

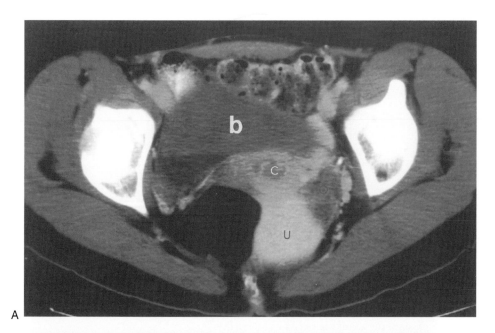

A

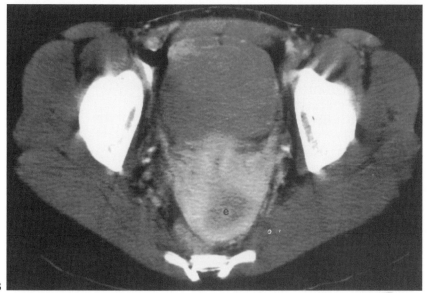

B

Figure 6.15 Retroflexed uterus. (**A**) This image of a retroflexed uterus shows the more triangular appearance of the uterine body (**u**) compared with the more circular shape of the cervix (**c**). The degree of flexion is such that the cervix is imaged in cross-section, while the uterine body is imaged coronally. A physiologic cyst is present within the left ovary (**o**). b, bladder. (**B**) A retroflexed uterus in a patient in the secretory phase of her menstrual cycle shows the lower attenuating endometrial cavity (**e**) in coronal orientation.

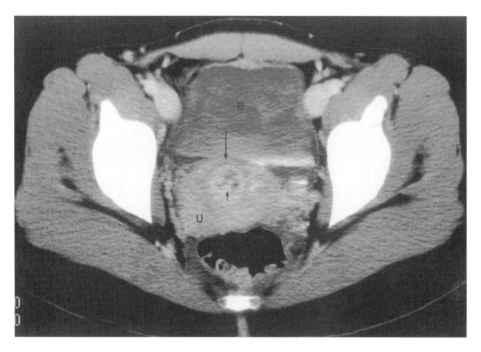

Figure 6.16 Cervical enhancement. Dynamic CT scan through a normal cervix shows normal central enhancement of the cervical epithelium (short arrow). The peripheral fibrous cervical stroma enhances to a lesser degree (long arrow). The cervix and lower uterine body are imaged at the same level, similar to the appearance in Fig. 6.15, since the uterus was tipped slightly to the right and retroverted. B, bladder; U, uterine body.

Figure 6.17 Arcuate artery calcification. Calcification is present in a circumferential distribution (arrows) throughout the myometrium in this 89-year-old patient with a small postmenopausal uterus. This is probably calcification within the intrauterine arcuate arteries, and based on its rather symmetric and peripheral distribution, it can be distinguished from other causes of calcifications within the uterus.

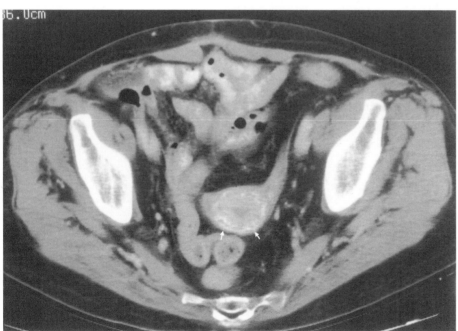

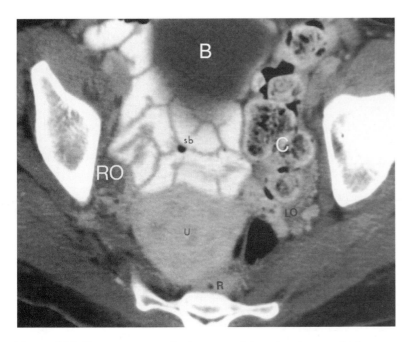

Figure 6.18 Vesicouterine pouch. An image of the pelvis shows multiple contrast-filled small bowel loops (sb) posterior to the bladder (B) and anterior to the uterus (U) within the vesicouterine pouch. The right (RO) and left ovary (LO) can be identified by their low attenuation secondary to multiple follicles. R, rectum.

the recess that is formed by this peritoneum between the bladder and uterus, is usually empty but may occasionally contain small bowel loops[12,15] (Fig. 6.18). The posterior aspect of the uterus is covered with peritoneum that continues onto the cervix and upper portion of the vagina before reflecting backward onto the rectum. This forms the rectouterine pouch (posterior cul-de-sac or pouch of Douglas), which is the most dependent and caudal portion of the peritoneal cavity. It often contains bowel loops as well as a small amount of fluid. A small amount of fluid is frequently seen in patients during ovulation and may occasionally be seen in asymptomatic postmenopausal women[6,12,21] (Fig. 6.19).

Figure 6.19 Rectouterine pouch. A moderate amount of ascitic fluid (arrows) is present dependently within the rectouterine pouch, posterior to the atrophic uterus (U) and anterior to the rectum (R), in this postmenopausal patient with severe liver disease. The broad ligaments (arrowheads) are well seen, as they are outlined by the adjacent fluid.

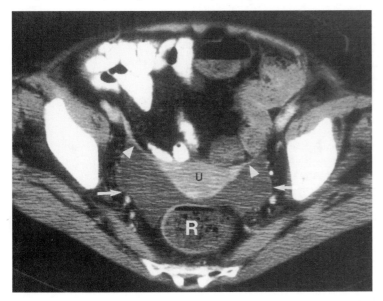

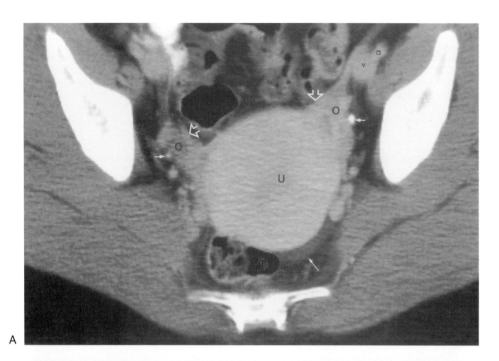

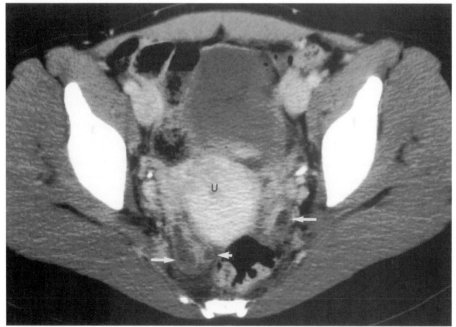

Figure 6.20 Normal ovaries. **(A)** CT scan through the pelvis of a 33-year-old woman demonstrates the ovaries (O) as slightly heterogeneously enhanced oval-shaped soft tissue structures immediately adjacent to the uterus (U). Note the origin of the round ligaments (white open arrows) just anterior to the ovary and the pelvic ureters just laterally (short white arrows). A small amount of fluid is present in the posterior cul-de-sac (long white arrow). v, external iliac vein; a, external iliac artery. **(B)** The ovaries are posterolateral to the uterus in this patient of menstruating age and lying within the posterior cul-de-sac. Several rounded and oval areas of low attenuation. probably follicles (arrows), are seen within each ovary.

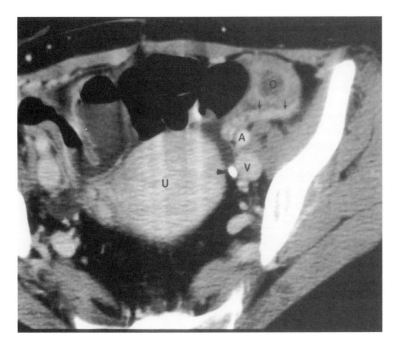

Figure 6.21 Ovarian vessels. CT scan shows an enhancing curvilinear vessel (arrows) surrounding the left ovary (O), which represents ovarian branches of the uterine vessels passing through the left ovarian ligament. Note the position of the ovary anterior to the external iliac vessels, an anatomic variant that occurs due to ligamentous laxity. U, uterus; A, internal iliac artery; V, external iliac vein; arrowhead, the ureter.

Ovary

Normal ovaries are often visualized on CT, particularly when thin collimation is used. Often, the ovaries are seen within the ovarian fossa between the external iliac arteries anterolaterally and the pelvic ureter posteriorly. However, their position within the pelvis is variable due to ligamentous laxity, so that the normal ovary may be seen in the cul-de-sac, pelvic inlet, iliac fossa, or lower abdomen[7,15,22] (Figs. 6.20 and 6.21). They are usually of soft tissue attenuation; often, small cystic areas representing normal follicles may be seen (Figs. 6.19 and 6.20). Larger benign ovarian cysts are often seen in women of repro-

Figure 6.22 Normal vagina. At the level of the vaginal fornices, the vagina (v) surrounding the cylindric portion of cervix (c) is seen. The ureters (large arrows) enter the bladder just anterior to the anterior fornices. Uneven mixing of contrast excreted by the ureters into the bladder (small arrows) with the unopacified urine gives the impression of a lesion along the anterior bladder wall (open arrow). r, rectum.

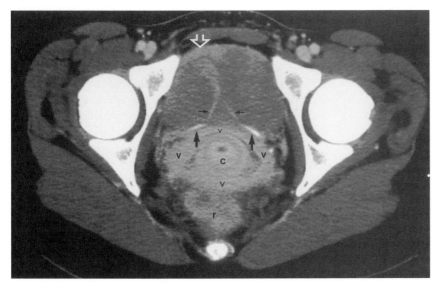

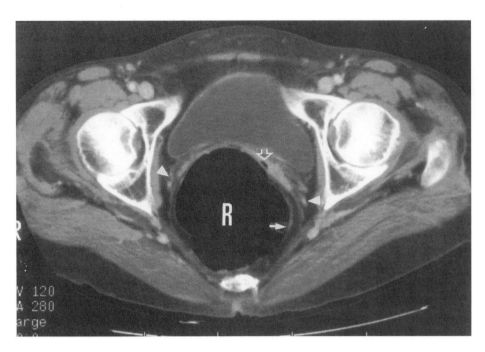

Figure 6.23 Air in the vagina. A small dot of air (open arrow) is noted in the left vaginal fornix of an elderly women undergoing CT examination of the pelvis. The absence of distension of the vagina and the small amount of air indicate that this is not clinically significant. The rectum (R) is distended with air, revealing its normal thin wall (arrow). Enhanced vessels in the paravaginal plexus are indicated by the arrowheads.

ductive age.[6,24,35] These characteristically are of fluid attenuation and have smooth walls on CT; however, single internal septa and slight wall irregularity are often present.[24,35] Further characterization of more complex adnexal cysts detected by CT may require ultrasound evaluation to exclude a neoplasm.[35–37] Their small size makes premenarchal and postmenopausal ovaries difficult to see on CT, and they are often not identified.

Vagina

The vagina is a fibromuscular tube that extends inferiorly from the uterus to the vestibule (the cleft between the labia minora). The vagina lies between the bladder and urethra anteriorly and the rectum and anus posteriorly. Superiorly, the vagina surrounds the cervix, creating anterior, lateral, and posterior fornices[10,38] (Fig. 6.22). A tampon in the vagina may be displaced to one side by the cervix, an appearance that should not be mistaken for a mass.[38]

The central aspect of the vagina may enhance intensely, likely reflecting the vascular epithelium, while the more muscular walls of the vagina enhance poorly[2] (see Fig. 6.9). A prominent venous plexus surrounding the vagina can be seen with dynamic intravenous contrast enhancement. A small amount of air within the vagina is normal[39] (Fig. 6.23). Marked distension of the vagina by air or gas, however, should arouse suspicion of an enterovaginal fistula.

After hysterectomy, CT shows the vaginal cuff (localized by a tampon) as a symmetric oval soft tissue structure behind the bladder, usually surrounded by fat[40,41] (Fig. 6.24).

Fallopian Tubes

The fallopian tubes arise from the back of the uterus at the junction of the fundus and the body. They pass along the superior aspect of the broad ligament, suspended by the mesosalpinx, toward the ovaries. The normal fallopian tube is infrequently imaged by CT.[10] If the tubes fill with fluid, they may be seen as serpiginous structures in the adnexa.[42]

PELVIC LIGAMENTS

Several ligaments supporting the genitalia can be identified on CT. The broad ligament is a winglike fold of peritoneum that surrounds the uterus and extends laterally to the pelvic sidewall (Fig. 6.25). Between the two leaves are the fallopian tube, round ligament, ovarian ligament, uterine and ovarian vessels, nerves, lymphatics, mesonephric remnants, and the loose extraperitoneal connective tissue and fat known as the parametrium[10,38] (Fig. 6.26). At its upper end, the broad ligament encircles the tube and extends to the pelvic sidewall as the infundibulopelvic ligament (see Figs. 6.19 and 6.20). The ureter is intimately associated with the inferior aspect of the broad ligament.[2,6] The broad ligament itself is rarely seen on CT, but its position can be determined by the structures that it contains or abuts. The cardinal or transcervical ligament

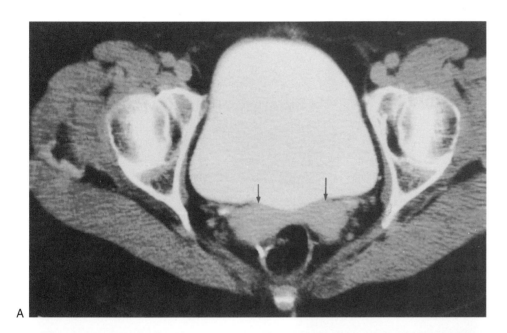

A

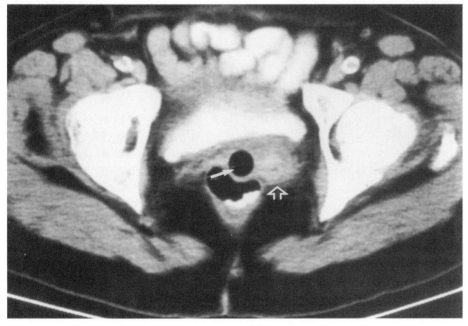

B

Figure 6.24 Normal and abnormal vaginal cuff. **(A)** Note the symmetric bowtie configuration of a normal vaginal cuff (arrows) immediately behind the bladder in this patient after total hysterectomy for benign disease. **(B)** A tampon (arrow) helps delineate the borders of the vagina. While slight asymmetry may be present following hysterectomy, the marked discrepancy in the appearance of the left vaginal cuff (open arrow) was secondary to recurrence of cervical carcinoma in this patient.

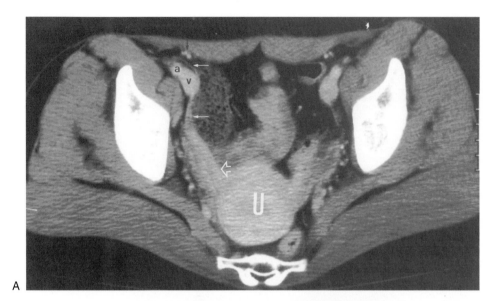

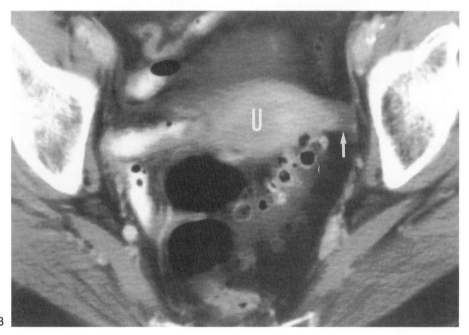

Figure 6.25 Broad ligament. **(A)** CT scan through a retroverted uterus (U) in a women of reproductive age demonstrates the broad ligament (open arrow) as a broad-based soft tissue band arising from the lateral aspect of the uterine fundus. The round ligament on the right (white arrows) is seen as it emerges from the broad ligament to cross just in front of the external iliac artery (a) and vein (v) to enter the internal inguinal ring. The black arrow indicates the inferior epigastric vessels. **(B)** A scan at the level of the uterine fundus (U) in a postmenopausal woman shows the left broad ligament (arrow) extending to the pelvic sidewall.

forms the base of the broad ligament and provides the primary ligamentous support for the uterus and upper vagina. This ligament extends from the cervix and upper vagina to merge with the fascia of the obturator internus. There is a wide variation in the shape, contour, and thickness of the normal cardinal ligament, which often appears triangular with tapered or occasionally squared off ends.[2,38] Sometimes, the cardinal ligament is not seen as a discrete band of connective tissue but instead

as an irregular network of nerves, blood vessels, and loose connective tissue (Fig. 6.27). The uterine artery runs along the superior aspect of the ligament (Fig. 6.28).

The uterosacral ligaments are folds of peritoneum with scant amounts of connective tissue containing some nerve fibers. They arise posteriorly from the lateral aspect of the cervix and arc posteriorly to extend to the anterior body of the sacrum at the S2 or S3 level. Medially, they fuse with those of the

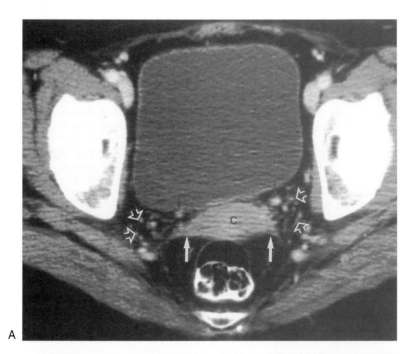

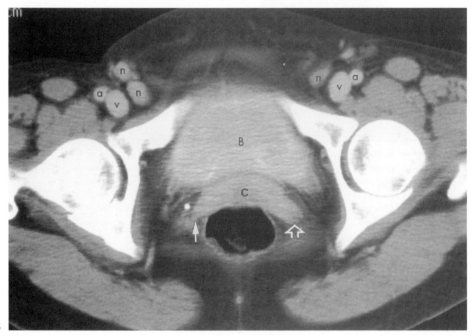

Figure 6.26 Normal cardinal ligaments. **(A)** CT scan at the level of the cervix (C) in a post-menopausal patient shows the triangular cardinal ligaments (white arrows), which gradually taper into thin bands of soft tissue extending toward the pelvic sidewall. Several small tubular and dot-like structures (open white arrows) representing vessels, nerves, lymphatics, and fibrous tissue are present in the adjacent parametrial fat within the broad ligament. The distal ureters are seen (black arrows) passing through the cardinal ligament. **(B)** CT image through the cervix (C) of a 40-year-old shows an asymmetry of the cardinal ligaments, a common finding. The right cardinal ligament has a more typical triangular appearance (arrow), while the left cardinal ligament (open arrow) has a square appearance and ends more abruptly without obvious tapering within the parac-ervical fat. A phlebolith is present in the right paracervical fat (arrow). Enlarged superficial inguinal lymph nodes (n) are present in this patient with lymphoma. v, common femoral vein; a, common femoral artery; B, bladder.

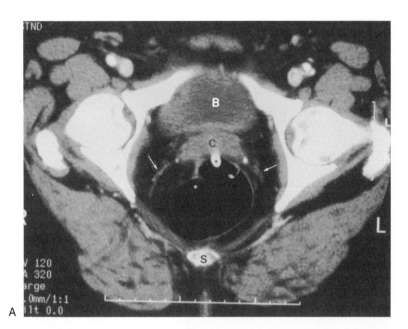

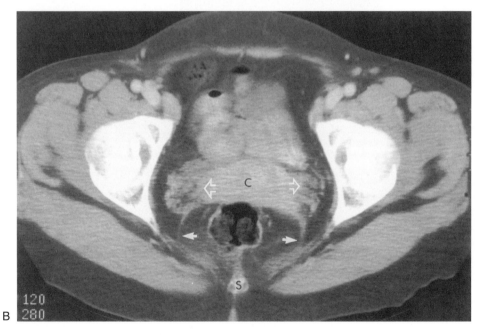

Figure 6.27 Normal uterosacral ligaments. **(A)** CT scan with 5-mm collimation through the pelvis and rectal air insufflation in a patient with possible recurrent ovarian carcinoma showing the typical appearance of the uterosacral ligaments (arrows) extending from the posterolateral aspect of the cervix (C) toward the sacrum (S). These very fine ligaments may be difficult to see on CT examinations, particularly when larger collimation is used. The bladder (B) is not distended and is collapsed anteriorly. **(B)** The uterosacral ligaments (arrows) are seen as bands of soft tissue extending from the cervix (C) toward the sacrum (S) in a different patient. The cardinal ligaments (open arrows) are not detectable as a discrete structure but rather as a network of connective tissue within the parametrium.

cardinal ligaments. Although only a few millimeters in thickness, the uterosacral ligaments are often seen with high-resolution CT, as they are outlined by the perirectal fat[2,38] (Fig. 6.27).

The round ligaments are bands of fibromuscular tissue extending from the anterolateral aspect of the uterus to the internal inguinal ring, terminating in the labia majora. At the uterine attachment, these ligaments may have a broad-based triangular configuration, which gradually tapers as it extends across the pelvis[2] (Fig. 6.29).

The ovary has two supporting ligaments, which are often not appreciated on CT. The ovarian ligament arises from the uterus just below and behind the origin of the fallopian tubes

and extends to the ovary. The suspensory ligament of the ovary extends from the ovary anterolaterally to the pelvic sidewall, fusing with the connective tissue overlying the psoas muscles. Rather than being a true ligament, this is a peritoneal fold containing the ovarian artery and vein[2] (Fig. 6.30).

LYMPH NODES

On CT, lymph nodes appear as rounded or oval structures of soft tissue attenuation. Occasionally, the fatty hilum of a normal lymph node may be appreciated. They are best seen after

Figure 6.28 Normal uterine and cervical vessels. **(A)** An enhanced image in a patient of childbearing age with a retroflexed uterus (U) shows the right uterine artery (white arrow) arching over the distal right ureter (black arrow) to the cervix (open arrow). The left uterine artery (open white arrow) is seen as well. **(B)** Slightly inferior to Figure A, the cervical vascular plexus, an enhancing network of thin vessels (white arrows) is just lateral to the cervix and within the paracervical fat. The ureters (curved arrows) are entering the bladder. A phlebolith is seen (short black arrow) within the paracervical venous plexus.

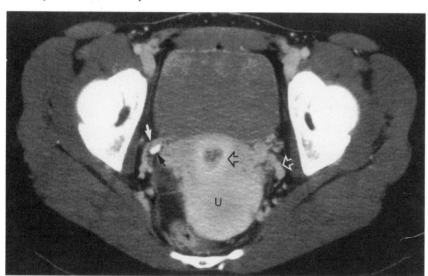

A

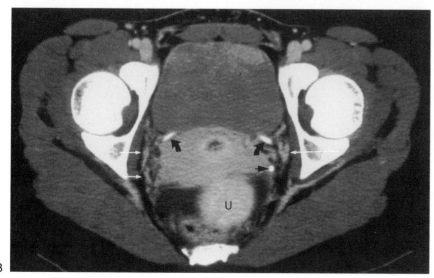

B

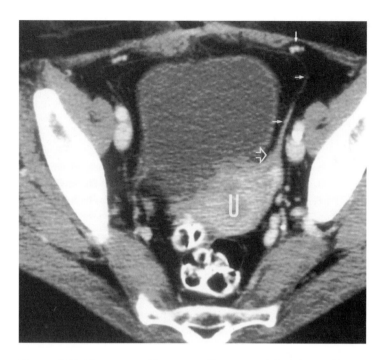

Figure 6.29 Normal round ligaments. The course of the left round ligament is seen in this axial image at the level of the uterus (U) of a postmenopausal patient. The ligament (white arrows) has a triangular origin (open arrow), then tapers into a thin soft tissue band extending anteriorly toward the inferior epigastric vessels (white arrowhead).

Figure 6.30 Normal ovarian ligaments. CT scan through the uterus (U) shows the left ovarian ligament (open arrow), also called the round ligament of the ovary, extending between the body of the uterus and the ovary (O). The densely enhancing structures (white arrows) just lateral the left ovary, are probably the ovarian vessels within the suspensory ligament of the ovary, a ligament that is rarely seen on CT. Two metallic clips are present below the ovarian ligament.

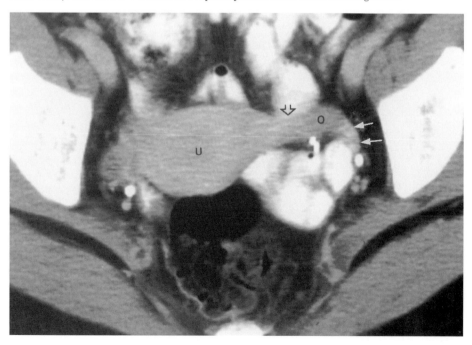

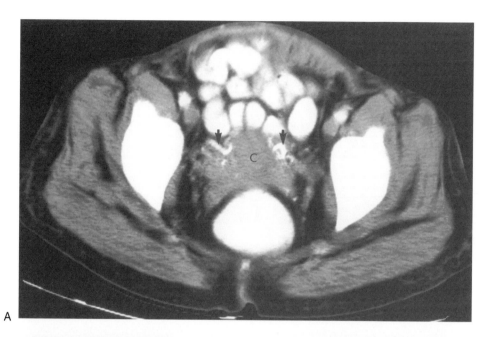

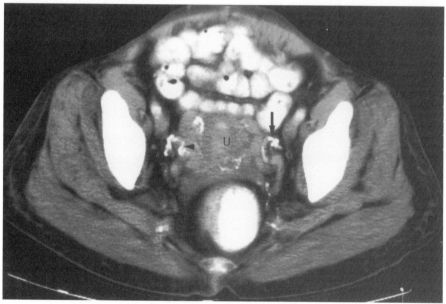

Figure 6.31 Calcified uterine artery. **(A)** CT scan at the level of the cervix (C) in an elderly diabetic shows marked calcification of the tortuous uterine arteries (arrows). **(B)** A slightly more cephalad image than that in Figure A near the uterine fundus shows the calcified uterine arteries giving rise to branches that penetrate the uterus (arrowhead) as well as branches to the adnexa (arrow). U, uterus. *(Figure continues.)*

intravenous contrast that distinguishes blood vessels and lymph nodes.[12,43] Pelvic nodes are identified by their relationship to normal vascular structures. The common iliac nodes lie dorsal and lateral to the common iliac arteries. The external iliac nodes are on the lateral, anterior, and medial borders of the external iliac artery and vein. The obturator nodes, along the lateral pelvic sidewalls adjacent to the obturator internus muscles, are considered part of the medial chain of the external iliac nodes[4,43–46] (Fig. 6.31). The internal iliac lymph nodes or hypogastric nodes parallel the branches of the internal iliac artery. Nodes at the junction between the internal and external vessels are sometimes referred to as the *junctional nodes*.[45] The obturator and internal iliac lymph nodes are often the first nodes to be involved by pelvic malignancies such as cervical and bladder carcinoma.[43,45] The inguinal nodes can be divided into superficial and deep chains. The superficial inguinal nodes are located in the subcutaneous tissue anterior to the inguinal ligament accompanying the superficial femoral and saphenous veins[45] (see Fig. 6.26b). This group receives lymphatic drainage from the perineum. The

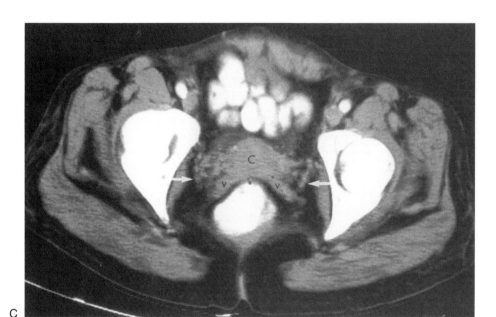

C

Figure 6.31 *(Continued).* **(C)** The cervical and vaginal venous plexus (arrows) appear as a network of vessels within the parametrial tissue. (C, cervix; v, vaginal fornices.)

deep inguinal nodes are medial to the femoral artery and vein within the femoral sheath (see Fig. 6.6). A group of nodes along the posterior iliac crest have also been described[43,47] (Fig. 6.32). Normal lymph node size varies with location. Pelvic lymph nodes are less than 1.5 cm in diameter.[10,43,44,46] Since intranodal architecture cannot be assessed by CT, enlargement is the only criterion of pathology.

BLOOD VESSELS

At the pelvic level, the major arteries and veins follow a similar course with the artery located just anterior to the vein. The aorta bifurcates at the level of the fourth lumbar vertebra, giving rise to the common iliac arteries (see Fig. 6.2). The common iliac arteries are approximately 5 cm in length and bifurcate at about the level of the lower sacro iliac joint, near the point of fusion of the iliopsoas muscles, into the internal and external iliac arteries (see Fig. 6.4). The external iliac continues along the medial border of the iliopsoas, leaving the pelvis beneath the inguinal ligament to form the common femoral artery. The external iliac artery carries the blood supply to the lower extremity. The internal iliac artery continues along the posterior aspect of the pelvis and gives rise to vessels that supply the pelvic viscera.[10,12,43]

The paired uterine arteries arise from the anterior (visceral) trunk of the internal iliac artery to provide the primary blood supply to the uterus. The uterine artery travels within the base of the broad ligament crossing anterior to the pelvic ureter to reach the cervix, where it divides into a large uterine branch and a smaller cervicovaginal branch

(see Figs. 6.14, 6.28 and 6.31). Each of these branches is tortuous and forms extensive vascular networks within the soft tissues lateral to the uterus. At the level of the upper uterus, the uterine branch trifurcates, sending branches to the fallopian tube, the uterine fundus, and the ovary via the ovarian ligament. The ovaries also receive direct arterial supply from the ovarian arteries that arise from the aorta just below the origin of the renal arteries (see Fig. 6.2). At the level of the pelvis, the ovarian artery enters the broad ligament via the suspensory ligament of the ovary. These small vessels are infrequently visualized on CT. Occasionally, tortuous uterine arteries and veins adjacent to the uterus cannot be clearly seen. Imaging performed early in the arterial phase, however, will demonstrate enhancement of the arterial supply only[2,12] (Fig. 6.31). In patients of advanced age or with arteriosclerosis, calcification of the uterine arteries can be seen.

Venous drainage of the uterus, cervix, upper vagina, and ovaries is via an extensive plexus of thin-walled veins within the parametrium (see Figs. 6.12, 6.15, 6.23, and 6.28). This plexus eventually forms veins that parallel the arterial supply, with the exception of the left ovarian vein that drains into the left renal vein instead of the inferior vena cava (see Fig. 6.7). The appearance of the veins will depend on the rapidity with which the contrast was administered and the timing of imaging. If images are taken during the arterial phase of contrast administration, the venous plexus and veins may be unopacified. When opacified, the venous plexus appears as a delicate network of small vessels along the lateral aspect of the cervix and vagina. The larger draining veins will appear as more prominent well-defined vessels paralleling the arteries. The periuterine veins may be promi-

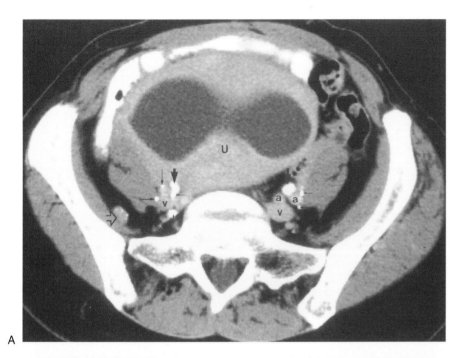

A

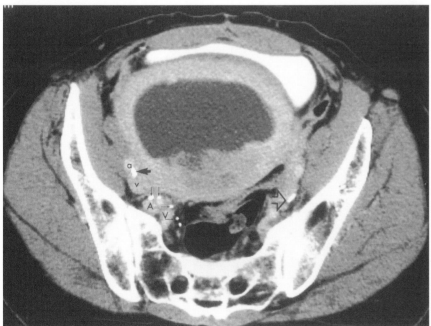

B

Figure 6.32 Lymph nodes. CT of the pelvis of a 46-year-old with cervical carcinoma and an obstructed fluid-filled uterus (U). Contrast from a previous lymphangiogram identifies the normal-sized pelvic nodes. **(A)** The common iliac lymph nodes (small arrows) are seen dorsally and laterally relative to the common iliac vessels. There is dilatation of the ureters (larger arrows) secondary to compression from the enlarged uterus. The left common iliac artery is just bifurcating at this level. Also, an enlarged retroperitoneal node (open arrow) is present just anterior to the iliacus muscle. a, left external and internal iliac arteries; v, common iliac vein. **(B)** An image 3-cm caudal relative to Figure A has multiple internal iliac nodes (small arrows) and an external iliac node (large arrow) adjacent to their respective vessels. The left ureter is indicated by the open arrow. V, internal iliac vein; A, internal iliac artery; a, external iliac artery; v, external iliac vein. *(Figure continues.)*

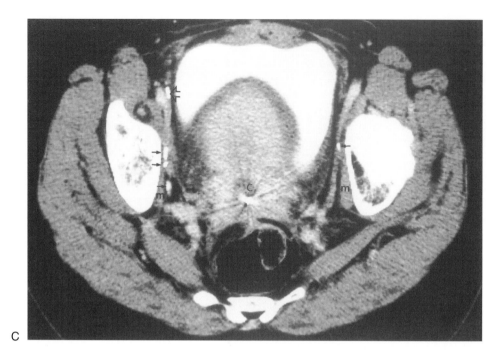

C

Figure 6.32 *(Continued).* **(C)** At the level of the cervix (C), which has a surgical clip in place, obturator nodes (small arrows) are seen adjacent to the obturator internus muscles (m) bilaterally. An external iliac node (open arrow) is seen as well.

Figure 6.33 Normal bladder and distal ureter. An image of the bladder during a spiral CT in a 41-year-old following trauma. A ureteral jet (open arrow) is formed when opacified urine propelled by ureteral peristalsis enters the nonopacified bladder. Since the excreted contrast is denser than urine, it will gravitate within the bladder. Note the normal angulation of the distal ureter (black arrow) as it enters the bladder. The bladder wall (small white arrow) is seen best where it is outlined by the unopacified urine.

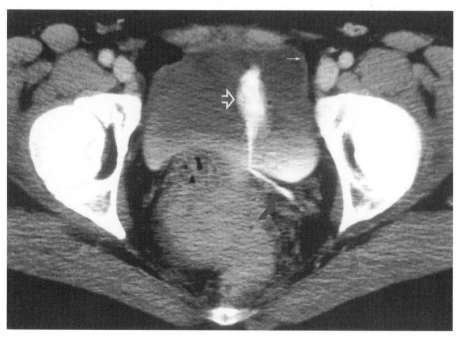

nent, especially in women of reproductive age. Occasionally, large pelvic varicies may be present. Uneven mixing of unopacified and opacified venous return at the junction of the larger veins may cause apparent intraluminal filling defects, which should not be mistaken for thrombosis. This is common at the common femoral vein–greater saphenous vein junction within the pelvis. Phleboliths are common within the pelvis and are of no clinical consequence (see Figs. 6.10 and 6.28).

GASTROINTESTINAL TRACT

Part of the alimentary tract lies within the pelvis (see Figs. 6.2 to 6.6). The cecum lies in the right iliac fossa, anterior to the right psoas muscle, but in some patients may descend lower into the pelvis. The descending colon lies in the left iliac fossa and curves medially to join the sigmoid colon, which lies in the midpelvis at the level of the true pelvic inlet. The sigmoid colon may ascend into the abdominal cavity before descending to the level of S2 or S3 to become the rectum. The rectum is approximately 12 cm long and leaves the pelvis through the anal hiatus at the level of the pelvic diaphragm (see Fig. 6.7). Normal bowel wall should have homogeneous attenuation. When the small bowel and colon are distended and imaged axially, the normal wall thickness is 2 to 3 mm. The rectal wall may have a thickness of up to 6 mm because of its thicker musculature[12,48] (see Fig. 6.23).

GENITOURINARY STRUCTURES

The ureters enter the pelvis by crossing the pelvic inlet anterior to the bifurcation of the common iliac arteries (see Fig. 6.3 and 6.4). They then pass posteroinferiorly over the obturator internus, forming the posterior boundary of the ovarian fossa (see Figs. 6.5 and 6.20). As the ureter runs forward toward the bladder, it passes through the cardinal ligament in the base of the broad ligament below the uterine arteries (see Fig. 6.6, 6.26, and 6.28). It then passes lateral to the anterior fornix before entering the bladder (Fig. 6.33). When empty, the bladder tends to be thick walled, flattened against the pubis, and confined to the true pelvis (see Fig. 6.27). As it distends, it expands to fill more of the true pelvis and across the plane of the pelvic inlet into the lower abdomen.[8] The outer margin of the bladder wall is smooth and well outlined by fat. The bladder wall is normally 2 to 5 mm thick and is best evaluated on unenhanced images where it appears as a rim of soft tissue whose inner margin is outlined by the adjacent low attenuation urine (Fig. 6.33). After contrast, the ureter is usually visualized as an enhanced dot on axial CT images (see Fig. 6.3 to 6.5). The distal ureter appears more tubular as it travels in the plane of section near the bladder (Fig. 6.33). Ureteral jets are a common finding on spiral CT when contrast from the opacified ureters is entering the urine-filled bladder (Fig. 6.33). When the jet extends to the anterior bladder wall, it can create a false impression of a mass[5] (see Fig. 6.22). The urethra is approximately 4 cm in length.

On CT, it is not well delineated from its surroundings, because of similar attenuation. The periurethral tissues may show enhancement with dynamic scanning[4] (see Fig. 6.10).

REFERENCES

1. Zeman RK, Silverman PM. Abdomen and pelvis. In: Zeman RK, Brink JA, Costello P et al, Eds. Helical/spiral CT: a practical approach. McGraw-Hill, New York, 1994, pp 153–220
2. Foshager MC, Walsh JW. CT anatomy of the female pelvis: A second look. Radiographics 1994;14:51–66
3. Megibow AJ, Bosniak MA, Ho Ag et al. Accuracy of CT in detection of persistent or recurrent ovarian carcinoma: correlation with second look laparatomy. Radiology 1988;166:341–345
4. Scoutt LM, McCarthy SM, Moss AA. Computed tomography and MRI of the pelvis. In: Moss AA. Gamsu G, Genant HK, Eds. Computed Tomography of the Body with MRI 2nd eds. WB Saunders, Philadelphia, 1992, pp. 1183–1265.
5. Silverman PM. Pharmacokinetics of contrast enhancement in body CT. In: Fishman EK, Jeffrey RB, Jr, Eds. Spiral CT: Principle, Techniques and Clinical Applications. Raven Press, New York, 1995, pp 11–24
6. Gross BH, Moss AA, Mihara K et al. Computed tomography of gynecologic disease. AJR Am J Roentgenol 1983;141:765–773
7. Redman HC. Computed tomography of the pelvis. Radiol Clin North Am 1977;25:441–448
8. Arger PH, Coleman BG, Mintz MC. Lower urinary tract computed tomography. Semin Ultrasound CT MR 1986;7:287–297
9. Cohen WN, Seidelman FE, Bryan PJ. Use of a tampon to enhance vaginal localization in computed tomography. AJR Am J Roentqenol 1977;128:1064–1154
10. Schneck CD, Friedman AC, Petersen RO. Embryology, anatomy, and histology. In: Friedman AC, Radecki PD, Lev-Toaff AS, Hilpert PL, Eds. Clinical Pelvic Imaging: CT, Ultrasound and MRI. CV Mosby, St. Louis, 1990, pp 1–60
11. Meyers MA. Pathways of extrapelvic spread of disease. In: Meyers MA, Eds. Dynamic Radiology of the Abdomen: Normal and Pathologic Anatomy (2nd ed,). Springer-Verlag, New York, 1982, pp 342–352
12. Gore RM. Computed tomography In: Fisher MR, Kricun ME, Eds. Imaging of the Pelvis. Aspen Publications, Rockville MD, 1989, pp 247–281
13. Bryan PJ, Cohen WN, Seidelman FE. The pelvis. In: Haaga JR, Alfidid RJ, Eds. Computed Tomography of the Whole Body. CV Mosby, St. Louis, 1983, pp 786–834
14. Lee JKT, Marx MV. Pelvis. In: Lee JKT, Sagel SS, Stanley RJ, Eds. Computed Body Tomography. Raven, New York, 1989, pp 851–897
15. Ammann AM, Walsh JW. Normal anatomy and technique of examination. In: Walsh JW, ed. Computed Tomography of the Pelvis. Churchill Livingstone, New York, 1985, pp 1–25
16. Tisnado J, Amendola MA, Walsh J et al. Computed tomography of the perineum. AJR Am J Roentgenol 1981;136:475–481
17. Gebarski KS, Gebarski SS, Glazer GN et al. The lumbosacral plexus: anatomic-radiologic-pathologic correlation using CT. Radiographics 1986;6:401–425
18. Lanzieri CF, Hilal SK. Computed tomography of the sacral

plexus and the sciatic nerve in the greater sciatic foramen. AJR Am J Roentgenol 1984;143:165–168

19. Pech P, Haughton V. A correlative CT and anatomic study of the sciatic nerve. AJR Am J Roentgenol 1985;144:1037–1041

20. Korobkin M, Callen PW, Fisch AE. Computed tomography of the pelvis and retroperitoneum. Radiol Clin North Am 1979;17:301–319

21. Kurtz AB, Rifkin MD. Normal anatomy of the female pelvis: ultrasound with computed tomography correlation. In Sanders RC, James AV, Eds. The Principles and Practice of Ultrasonography in Obstetrics and Gynecology. Appleton-Century-Crofts, New York, 1985

22. Miller EI, Thomas RH, Lines P. The atrophic postmenopausal uterus. J Clin Ultrasound 1977;4:261–263

23. Platt JF, Bree FL, Davidson D. Ultrasound of the normal nongravid uterus: correlation with gross and histopathology. J Clin Ultrasound 1990;18:15–19

24. Sawyer RW, Walsh JW. CT of gynecologic pelvic diseases. Semin Ultrasound CT MRI 1988;9:122–142

25. Casillas J, Joseph RC, Guerra JJ Jr. CT appearance of uterine leiomyomas. Radiographics 1990;10:999–1007

26. Tada S, Tsukioka M, Ishii C et al. Computed tomographic features of uterine myoma. J Comput Assist Tomogr 1981;5:866–869

27. Togashi K, Nishimura K, Nakano Y et al. Cystic pedunculated leiomyomas of the uterus with unusual CT manifestations. J Comput Assist Tomogr 1984;10:642–644

28. Langer JE, Dinsmore BJ. Computed tomography of benign and inflammatory disorders of the female pelvis. Radiol Clin North Am 1992;30:831–842

29. Kormano MJ, Goske MJ, Hamlin DJ. Attenuation and contrast enhancement of gynecologic organs and tumors on CT. Eur J Radiol 1981;1:307–311

30. Walsh JW, Goplerud DR. Computed tomography of primary, persistent, and recurrent endometrial malignancy. AJR Am J Roentgenol 1982;139:1149–1154

31. Hamlin DJ, Burgener FA, Beecham JB. CT of intramural endometrial carcinoma: contrast enhancement is essential. AJR Am J Roentgenol 1981;137:551–554

32. Balfe DM, VanDyke J, Lee JKT et al. Computed tomography in malignant endometrial neoplasms. J Comput Assist Tomogr 1983;7:677–681

33. Scott W, Rosenshein N, Siegelman S, Sanders R. The obstructed uterus. Radiology 1981;141:767–770

34. Occhipinti K, Kutcher R, Rosenblatt R. Sonographic appearance and significance of arcuate artery calcification. J Ultrasound Med 1991;10:97–100

35. Sawyer RW, Vick CW, Walsh JW, McClure PH. CT of benign ovarian masses. J Comput Assist Tomogr 1985;9:784–789

36. Fukada T, Ikeuchi M, Hashimoto H et al. Computed tomography of ovarian masses. J Comput Assist Tomogr 1986;10:990–996

37. Williams AG, Mettler FA, Wicks JD. Cystic and solid ovarian neoplasms. Semin Ultrasound 1983;4:166–183

38. Vick CW, Walsh JW, Wheelock JB, Brewer WH. CT of the normal and abnormal parametria in cervical cancer. AJR Am J Roentgenol 1984;143:597–603

39. Nokes SR, Martinez CR, Arrington JA, Davito R. Significance of vaginal air on computed tomography. J Comput Assist Tomogr 1986;10:997–999

40. Kasales CJ, Langer JE, Arger PH. Pelvic pathology after hysterectomy: a pictorial essay. Clin Imaging 1995;19:210–217

41. Heiken JP, Lee JK. Recurrent pelvic malignancy. In Walsh JW, Ed. Computed Tomography of the Pelvis. Churchill Livingstone, New York, 1985, pp 185–209

42. Togashi K, Mishimura K, Itoh K et al. Computed tomography of hydrosalpinx following tubal ligation. J Comput Assist Tomogr 1986;10:78.

43. Patten RM, Shuman WP, Jeffrey RB. Retroperitoneum and lymphovascular structures. In: Moss AA, Gamsu G, Genant HK, Eds. Computed Tomography of the Body with MRI (2nd ed.), WB Saunders, Philadelphia, 1992, pp 1091–1138

44. Walsh JW, Amendola MA, Kronerding KF et al. Computed tomographic detection of pelvic and inguinal lymph node metastasis from primary and recurrent pelvic malignant disease. Radiology 1980;137:157–166

45. Park JM, Charnsangavej C, Herron DH et al. Pathways of nodal metastasis from pelvic tumors: CT demonstration. Radiographics 1994;14:1309–1321

46. Lee JKT, Stanley RJ, Sagel SS, McClennan BL. Accuracy of CT in detecting intra-abdominal and pelvic lymph node metastases from pelvic cancers. AJR Am J Roentgenol 1978;131:675–679

47. Castellino RA. Lymph nodes of the posterior iliac crest: CT and lymphographic observations. Radiology 1990;175:687–689

48. Balthazar EJ. The colon. In: Megibow AJ, Balthazar EJ, Eds. Computed Tomography of the Gastrointestinal Tract. Churchill Livingstone, New York, 1988, pp 279–331

7

Magnetic Resonance Imaging of the Normal Female Pelvis

RICHARD B. RAFAL

Magnetic resonance imaging (MRI) allows an excellent demonstration of anatomy and pathology of the female pelvis. To understand MRI abnormalities of this region, it is essential to be familiar with the appearance of the normal female pelvis. Findings considered normal one day can be abnormal on another. MRI of the female pelvis is dependent on numerous factors. In order to detect and diagnose pathology, the radiologist needs to be armed with each patient's clinical, gynecologic, and surgical history. Since the appearance of the female pelvic organs is dynamic and changes with the age and hormonal status, clinical history is vital to proper MRI interpretation (Table 7.1). A labeled atlas of typical images, seen in coronal, axial, and sagittal planes, is included for reference (Fig. 7.1 to 7.3). Also outlined are the changes seen with MRI at different stages of life in the female, as well as the variations noted during the phases of the normal menstrual cycle.

PELVIC SUPPORT STRUCTURES

Bones

The bones of the pelvis, like bones elsewhere in the body, have a characteristic MRI appearance. Cortical bone has low signal intensity and therefore appears dark on all pulse sequences (Fig. 7.1f). This is secondary to its small number of mobile protons.[1,2] Bone marrow, on the other hand, is bright due to its fat content.[1] Since fat has a very short T1 relaxation time and a relatively long T2 relaxation time, it is bright in intensity on both T1- and T2-weighted images.[2]

Muscle

Skeletal muscle in the pelvis displays a low-to-intermediate signal intensity, which is seen on T1-weighted MRI as a shade of gray (Fig. 7.1 to 7.3).[2,3] Since striated muscle has moderately long T1 and short T2 relaxation times, it has low signal intensity on T1-weighted images, and on T2-weighted images, becomes decreased in signal compared to adjacent soft tissues.[1]

Blood Vessels

The signal intensity of flowing blood is dependent on many factors, including the relaxation time of blood, its velocity and direction, the pulse sequence, slice location, and the imaging plane used. Analysis of images obtained in each plane may be necessary to detect flow.[1,2]

However, in general, flowing blood has no signal and is therefore black on conventional MRI (the so-called "flow void phenomenon").[1-3] This helps differentiate vascular structures from solid or soft tissue structures without the use of intravenous contrast.[4]

Lymph Nodes

Lymph nodes and blood vessels have similar soft tissue attenuation, and contrast-enhanced CT is often required to make the distinction. Since lymph nodes on MRI appear as intermediate signal-producing masses, and blood vessels appear as "signal voids,"[1-3] MRI differentiation between lymph nodes and vessels is possible without the use of intravenous contrast material. This is useful in allergic patients and avoids the risks of contrast administration.

UTERUS

Demonstration of the parts of the uterus is dependent on the pulse sequences used[1] and is best seen with T2-weighted images[5] in the sagittal plane (Fig. 7.4). On conventional spin echo (SE) T1-weighted images, the corpus has a homogeneous, moderate signal intensity, similar to or slightly stronger than that of skeletal muscle.[3,6] On these images, the difference in signal intensity between endometrium and myometrium is negligible,[1] since both have similar T1 relaxation times[7] (Fig. 7.5). T2-weighted images show three layers of uterine signal intensity. Centrally, there is the high-signal endometrium; peripherally, a zone of medium intensity characteristic of the majority of the smooth muscle of the myometrium; and separating these layers, a thin, low-intensity

Table 7.1 Clinical Information Required
Before MRI of the Female Pelvis

1. Clinical problem being evaluated
2. Age
3. Menstrual status
4. Surgical history
5. Medication/hormone therapy

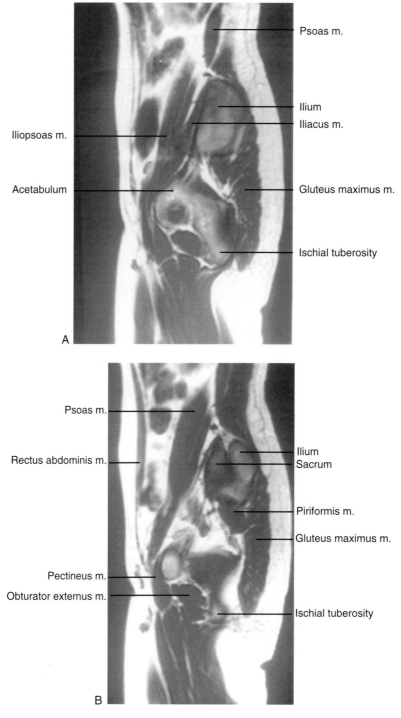

Figure 7.1 (**A – H**) T1-weighted spin echo (TR600/TE16; body coil) sagittal images. (*Figure continues.*)

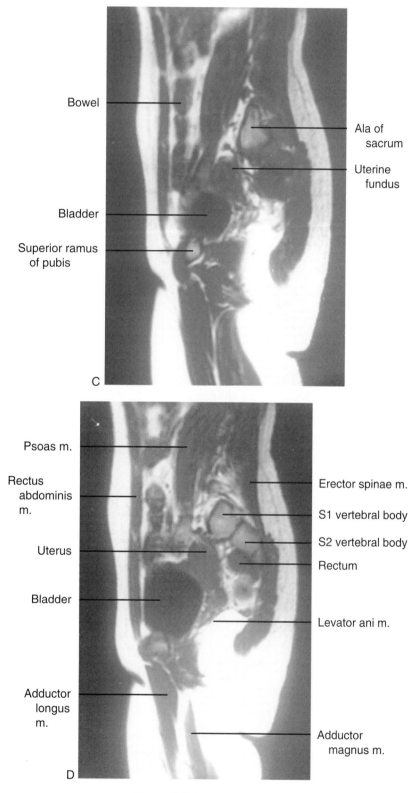

Figure 7.1 (*Continued*).

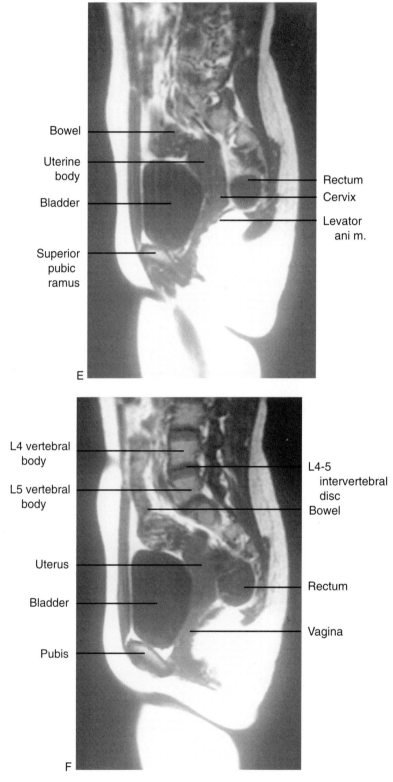

Bowel

Uterine body

Bladder

Superior pubic ramus

Rectum

Cervix

Levator ani m.

E

L4 vertebral body

L5 vertebral body

Uterus

Bladder

Pubis

L4-5 intervertebral disc

Bowel

Rectum

Vagina

F

Figure 7.1 *(Continued)*.

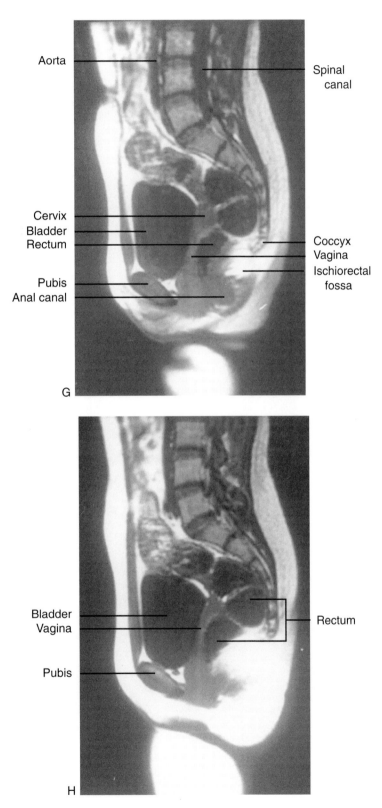

Figure 7.1 *(Continued)*.

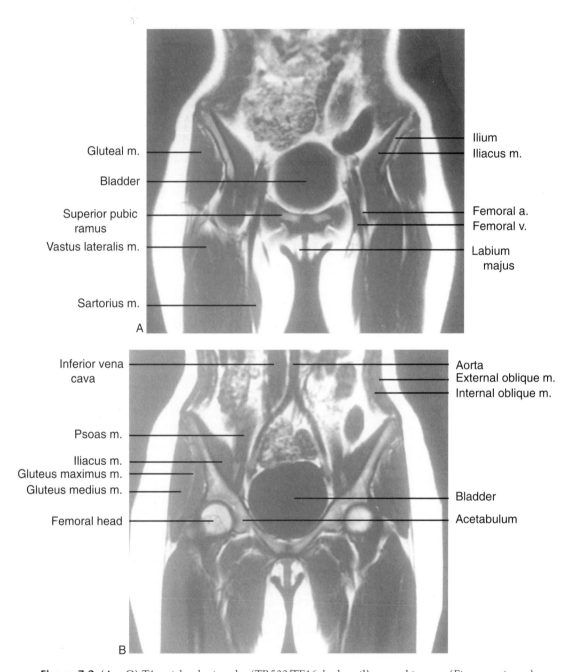

Gluteal m.
Bladder
Superior pubic ramus
Vastus lateralis m.
Sartorius m.

Ilium
Iliacus m.
Femoral a.
Femoral v.
Labium majus

A

Inferior vena cava
Psoas m.
Iliacus m.
Gluteus maximus m.
Gluteus medius m.
Femoral head

Aorta
External oblique m.
Internal oblique m.
Bladder
Acetabulum

B

Figure 7.2 (A – G) T1-weighted spin echo (TR500/TE16; body coil) coronal images. (*Figure continues.*)

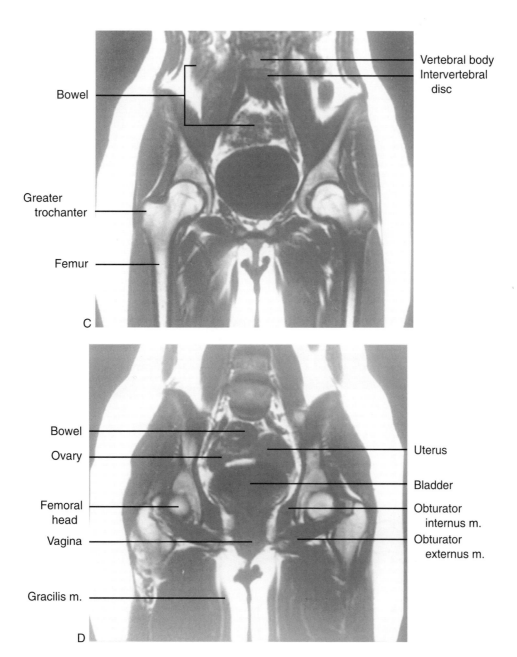

Figure 7.2 *(Continued)*.

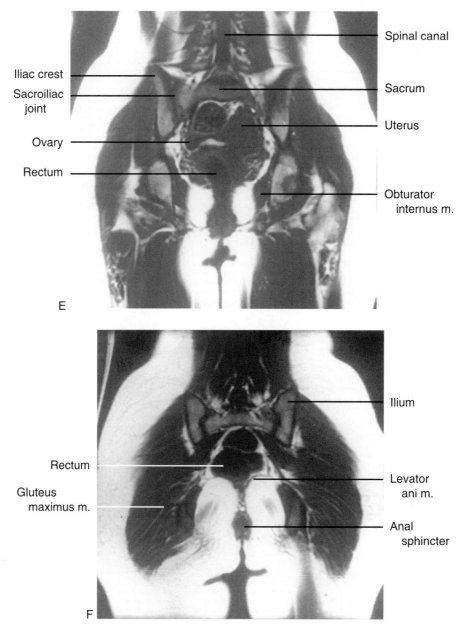

Spinal canal

Iliac crest

Sacroiliac joint

Sacrum

Ovary

Uterus

Rectum

Obturator internus m.

E

Rectum

Ilium

Gluteus maximus m.

Levator ani m.

Anal sphincter

F

Figure 7.2 *(Continued)*.

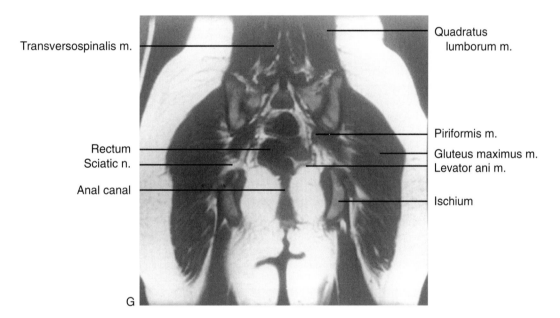

Figure 7.2 (*Continued*).

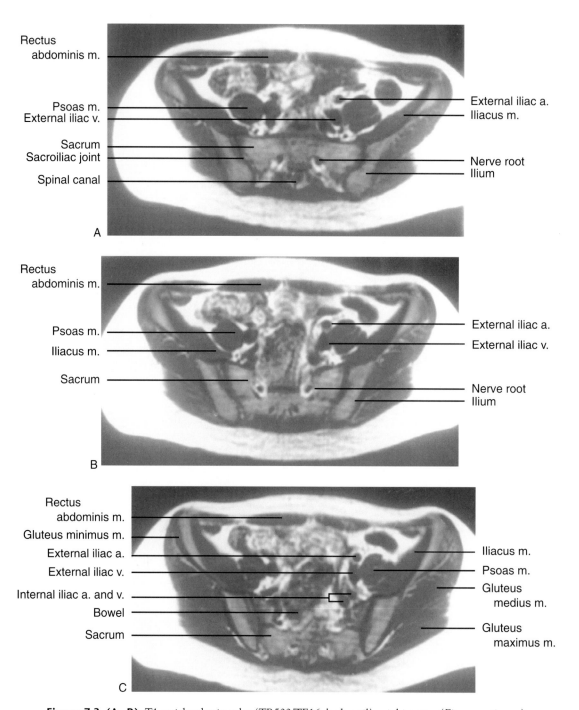

Figure 7.3 (A–P) T1-weighted spin echo (TR500/TE16; body coil) axial images. (*Figure continues.*)

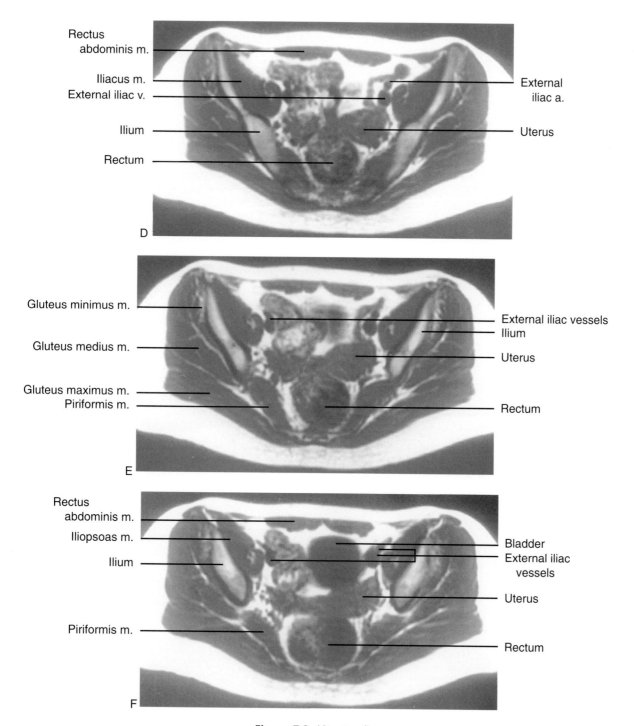

Rectus abdominis m.
Iliacus m.
External iliac v.
Ilium
Rectum
External iliac a.
Uterus
D

Gluteus minimus m.
Gluteus medius m.
Gluteus maximus m.
Piriformis m.
External iliac vessels
Ilium
Uterus
Rectum
E

Rectus abdominis m.
Iliopsoas m.
Ilium
Piriformis m.
Bladder
External iliac vessels
Uterus
Rectum
F

Figure 7.3 *(Continued)*.

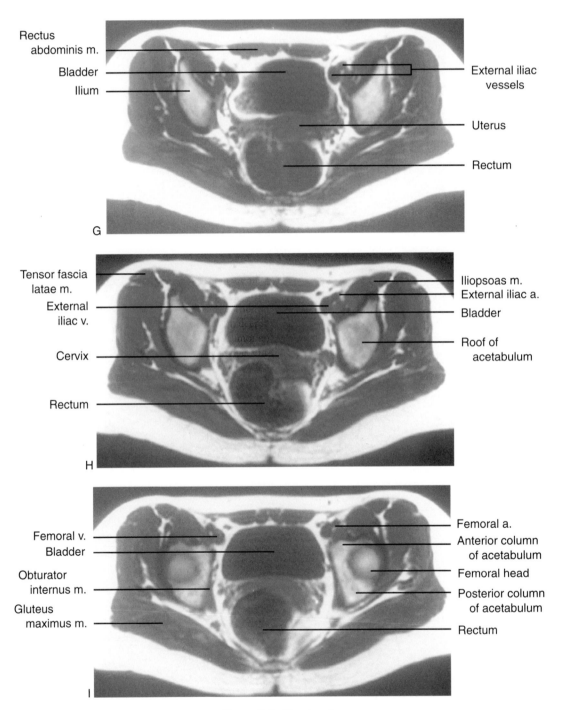

Figure 7.3 *(Continued)*.

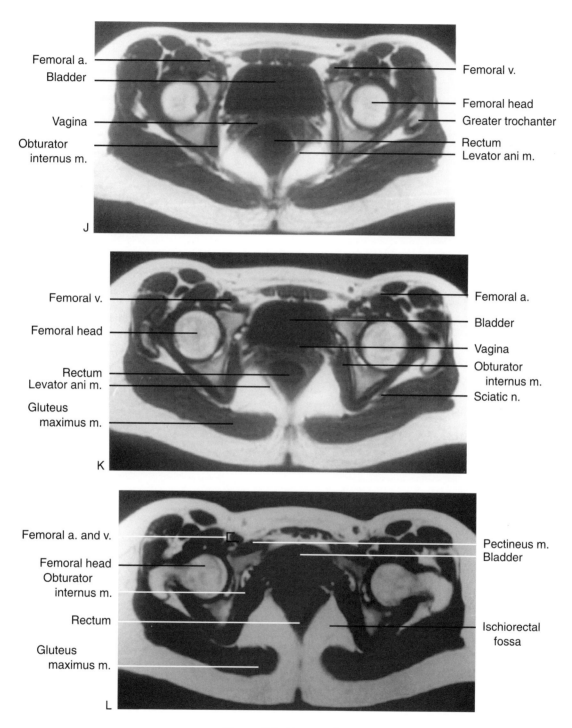

Femoral a.
Bladder
Vagina
Obturator internus m.
Femoral v.
Femoral head
Greater trochanter
Rectum
Levator ani m.

J

Femoral v.
Femoral head
Rectum
Levator ani m.
Gluteus maximus m.
Femoral a.
Bladder
Vagina
Obturator internus m.
Sciatic n.

K

Femoral a. and v.
Femoral head
Obturator internus m.
Rectum
Gluteus maximus m.
Pectineus m.
Bladder
Ischiorectal fossa

L

Figure 7.3 *(Continued).*

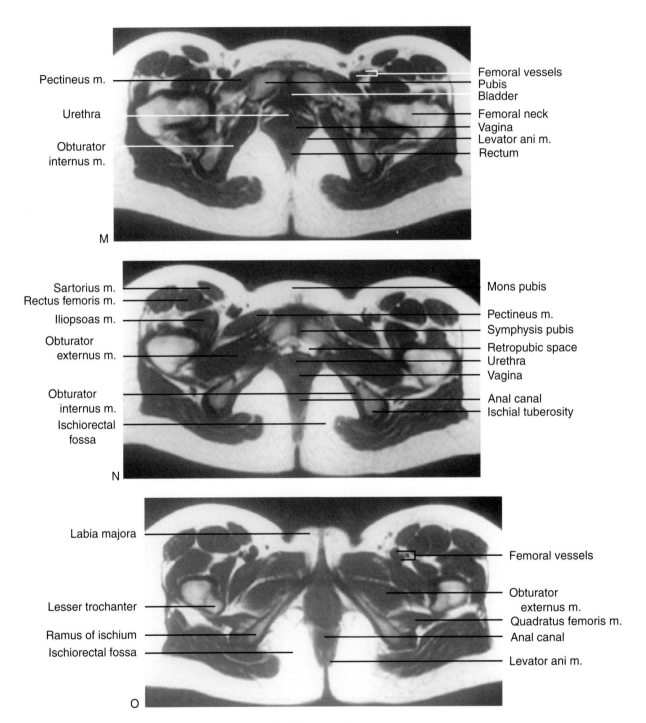

Figure 7.3 (*Continued*).

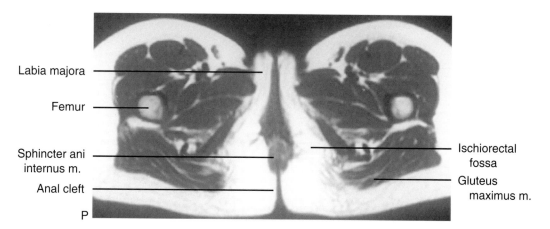

Labia majora

Femur

Sphincter ani
internus m.

Anal cleft

P

Ischiorectal
fossa

Gluteus
maximus m.

Figure 7.3 *(Continued)*.

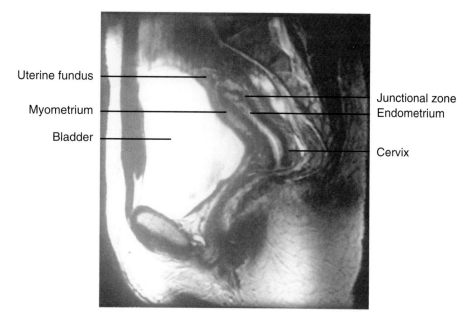

Uterine fundus

Myometrium

Bladder

Junctional zone
Endometrium

Cervix

Figure 7.4 T2-weighted fast spin echo (FSE) (TR6000/TE108; pelvic coil) sagittal image with a distended bladder. Compare the position and configuration of the uterus to that seen in Figure 7.6A.

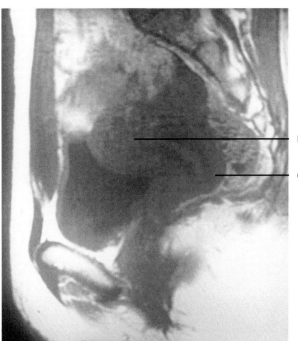

Uterine
fundus

Cervix

Figure 7.5 T1-weighted (TR600/TE16) sagittal view demonstrates little difference in signal intensity between the uterine zones and cervix.

band known as the *junctional zone*[2,8–12] (Fig. 7.6). Myometrium on SE T1-weighted images is generally of homogeneous medium signal intensity, slightly higher than the striated muscles of the pelvic side walls.[1,2,5] The myometrium increases in intensity with increased T2 weighting, giving a marked contrast between striated muscle and the smooth muscle of the uterus.[1]

Each part of the uterus changes in MRI appearance during the menstrual cycle,[2] and other more gradual changes occur in the endometrium and myometrium during the patient's lifetime. In women of reproductive age, MRI shows thick, bright endometrium on T2-weighted images[1,9] (Fig. 7.6). The bright signal from endometrium may be indistinguishable from that of intraluminal blood, so endometrial measurement on MRI can be inaccurate.[7] The myometrium is also affected by hormones, although its thickness does not change.[12] On T2-weighted images, its signal intensity is highest in the secretory phase. Total uterine volume is also highest during the secretory phase. Visualization of the arcuate vessels of the myometrium is maximal at the midsecretory phase.[5,13]

Women on oral contraceptives show poor separation between the myometrium and endometrium, endometrial atrophy, and inconsistent visualization of the junctional zone. The thin endometrium does not significantly change in thickness during the menstrual cycle in these patients. The uterus appears globular or swollen, although long-term use of oral contraceptives can lead to a decrease in the size of the corpus. The myometrium is of slightly higher signal intensity

compared with those not on oral contraceptives and probably reflects the higher water content found with myometrial edema. The uterus of patients on gonadotropin releasing hormone (GnRH) resembles that of postmenopausal women with a decrease in size, myometrial and endometrial atrophy, and a decrease in myometrial signal intensity.[5,7,8,12–14]

Premenarchal and postmenopausal females show a relatively featureless and small uterine corpus and absent or atrophic cycling endometrium. Zonal anatomy is less distinct, and the signal intensity of the myometrium on T2-weighted images can be lower than that seen in reproductive aged females.[2,5,12,13]

In the postmenopausal group, the central endometrial layer of high intensity should be thin, never exceeding 2 to 5 mm in width.[1,2,5] In addition, this bright area should only be seen on the T2-weighted sequence; if noted on T1-weighted images, lesions such as endometrial carcinoma should be excluded.[5] Postmenopausal females on exogenous estrogen therapy are an exception, since they have uteri similar in MRI appearance to those seen in reproductive aged women[5,8,12] with a thicker endometrium than is normally found in untreated postmenopausal women.

The junctional zone is a low signal intensity band separating the intermediate signal intensity of the outer two-thirds of the myometrium from the bright endometrial signal, which becomes darker in intensity on T2-weighted images. It is always seen in reproductive aged women but may be absent after the menopause[5,6,8,15] and in premenarchal patients. On average, the width of this zone is 5 mm, with little variation

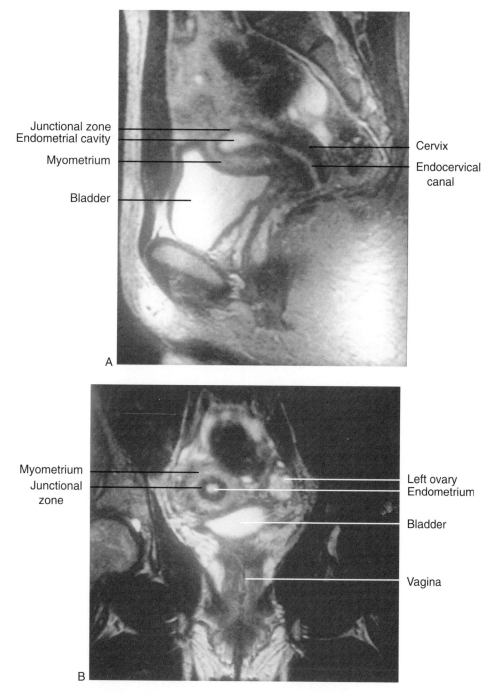

Junctional zone
Endometrial cavity
Myometrium
Bladder
Cervix
Endocervical canal

A

Myometrium
Junctional zone
Left ovary
Endometrium
Bladder
Vagina

B

Figure 7.6 (**A**) T2-weighted SE (TR2500/TE80; pelvic coil) sagittal image. (**B**) T2-weighted FSE (TR6000/TE108; pelvic coil) coronal views nicely show the three zones of the uterus. Note the slightly lower intensity of the fibromuscular stroma of the cervix seen in Figure A and the configuration of the uterus with a relatively nondistended bladder in Figure B.

during the menstrual cycle.[9] Histologically, the junctional zone represents the innermost (one-third) of the myometrium.[11,12,16]

Dynamic MRI using gadolinium contrast has been described.[15,17] Early (arterial) and delayed (venous) phases can help distinguish arteries and veins. Myometrial enhancement is maximal at 120 seconds after contrast injection and decreases over time. The pattern of enhancement is dependent on the menstrual cycle and the hormonal status of the patient. Only slight enhancement of the endometrium is seen in the early phase, while marked enhancement is noted on more delayed images.

CERVIX

The internal os of the cervix forms a constriction in the contour of the uterus, at the point of transition from medium-to-low signal intensity, which occurs between the smooth muscle of the corpus and the predominantly fibrous tissue of the cervix.[7,18] This fibrous tissue accounts for the characteristic hypointense or dark appearance of the normal cervical stroma on MRI, since only 10% to 15% of the cervix consists of smooth muscle.[19] The isthmus is the junction of the corpus and cervix uteri. The cervix consists of vaginal and supravaginal parts.[6] The external os is located at the lower limit of the vaginal part. The parametrium consists of cellular connective tissue and blood vessels. It extends along the sides of the cervix, separating the supravaginal cervix from the bladder.

As is seen with MRI of the uterus, the cervix has a homogeneous hypointense-to-isointense signal, seen as a shade of gray on noncontrast T1-weighted images[2,6,8,20] (Fig. 7.1e). Its internal architecture is best seen on T2-weighted images[6] (Fig. 7.7). Three cervical zones have been described on MRI. The outer zone is of medium signal intensity on T1-weighted images, becoming high in intensity on T2-weighted sequences.[1] This layer is continuous with the myometrium and of slightly lower intensity. The middle zone is a homogeneous, wide, low-intensity band, due to the fibrous cervical stroma.[5] This is continuous with the junctional zone but is of slightly lower intensity. Centrally, there is high signal intensity, consisting of epithelium[19] and glandular and intraluminal mucus in the canal. This layer is of similar intensity and continuous with the endometrium.

Techniques using phased array coils allow high-resolution scans that reveal another zone in the cervix immediately outside the central bright signal.[21,22] This zone is of slightly lower intensity and may represent mucosa. Alternatively, it may correspond to partial volume averaging of the hyperintense mucus within the plica palmatae (cervical glands filled with mucus) with the low signal intensity of the fibromuscular stroma.[19] Fast spin echo (FSE) (also known as turbo spin echo, TSE) images show a serrated central zone of high intensity surrounded by a band of slightly lower intensity cervical stroma. The serrations correspond to the folds of the plicae palmatae. These observations are best appreciated on multicoil FSE images.[21] Nabothian cysts are seen so often that they are regarded as normal.[5] They are seen in far greater detail on multicoil images (Fig. 7.8).

High-resolution studies with intravaginal surface coils show that the cervical mucosa is smooth and regular in the nulliparous patient, while in the parous patient, it tends to have a more irregular and indented margin and sometimes contains dilated, secretion-filled glands.[23,24] The two layers of the fibromuscular stroma of the cervix differ in signal intensity due to differences in nuclear area. This probably reflects increased numbers of cells rather than larger nuclei in the inner zone.[19]

The parametrium has medium-to-high signal intensity, making it easy to distinguish from the low-intensity cervical stroma.[5] T2-weighted images generally show moderate signal intensity[8] but can show high signal intensity from slow-flowing blood in the parametrium.[5] The ligaments supporting the uterine corpus and cervix are difficult to identify with any cross-sectional imaging modality.[6]

Figure 7.7 T2-weighted FSE (TR6000/TE108; pelvic coil) coronal image shows the hypointense cervical stroma surrounding the bright endocervical canal. Note the presence of bright adnexal cysts bilaterally.

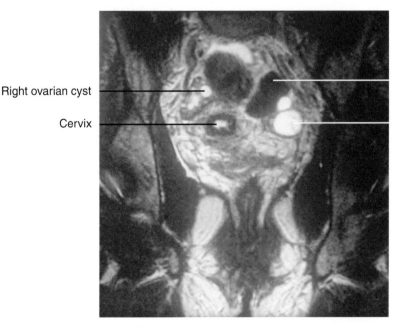

Right ovarian cyst

Cervix

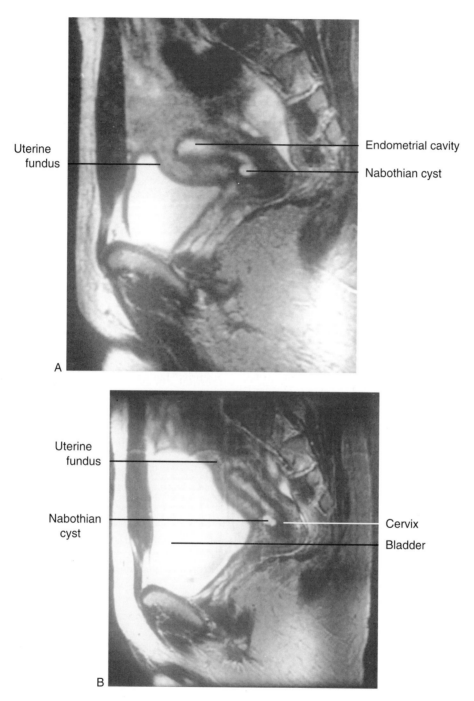

Figure 7.8 **(A)** T2-weighted SE (TR2500/TE80; pelvic coil MRI. **(B)** T2-weighted FSE (TR6000/TE108) sagittal MRI. **(C)** T2-weighted SE (TR2500/TE80) axial views show the bright nabothian cyst adjacent to the endocervical canal. (*Figure continues.*)

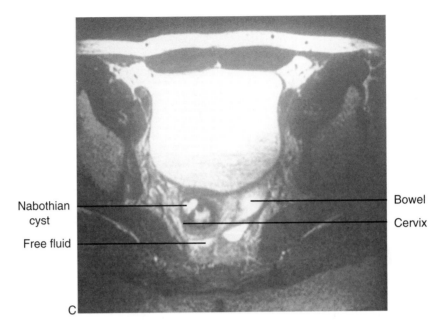

Nabothian cyst

Free fluid

Bowel

Cervix

C

Figure 7.8 *(Continued)*.

The MRI appearance of the cervix changes with the menstrual cycle.[2] Cyclic variations in the cervix are seen as changes in the width of the central zone. Overall cervical dimensions do not vary with the cycle or with use of oral contraceptives[7] but do change with age and parity.[1] Dynamic studies show rapid enhancement of the endocervical mucosa with contrast, peaking at 120 seconds. The outer fibromuscular stroma of the cervix enhances more gradually. This discrepancy is due to differences in vascularity.[23]

ADNEXA

The MRI appearance of the ovary is variable. The signal intensity depends on the pulse sequence used[1] as well as the menstrual status of the patient.[25] Typically, in premenopausal females, on conventional T1-weighted images, the ovaries are homogeneously low to medium in signal intensity (similar in signal to myometrium or skeletal muscle).[6,8,20] The ovary increases in brightness with increased T2 weighting.[26] The stroma becomes isointense with fat on conventional T2-weighted SE images, and the follicles become hyperintense[6,8] (Figs. 7.6b and 7.9).

Since the ovary can get quite bright on conventional SE T2-weighted images, differentiation from surrounding fat can be difficult, as the ovarian stroma can be approximately the same signal intensity as fat. This can create problems in locating the ovaries and in delineating them from surrounding fat. In these cases, more T1-weighted images,[1,2,26] or FSE images,[25] can be useful, since these sequences better differentiate ovary from fat. FSE images show higher fat signal intensity than conventional SE images. With T2-weighted FSE images, contrast is increased between the ovaries and surrounding fat

compared to conventional SE T2-weighted images, because on T2-weighted FSE, images the ovarian stroma is significantly lower in signal intensity than surrounding fat.

On T1-weighted images, ovarian cysts appear as smooth, well-circumscribed, and hypointense following water in signal intensity. On more T2-weighted images, they become hyperintense. When located in the periphery of the ovary, their walls are smooth and almost undetectable.[26] These thin walls are especially apparent after gadolinium contrast injection.[25] MRI can show the development of the dominant follicle.[6] After ovulation on MRI, borders of the follicle become irregular, and its contents show a slightly heterogeneous decrease in intensity. The corpus luteum is seen as a partly collapsed structure, which is usually fluid filled (but can be hemorrhagic and indistinguishable from endometriomas on MRI).[27] There is intense enhancement of the wall due to vascularization after gadolinium.[25]

Axial or coronal MRI, or a combination of the two, is the most useful to demonstrate the ovaries.[2,5,20,26] In one study, normal ovaries were seen in only one-half of patients imaged in the sagittal plane.[26] Axial or coronal contiguous slices (i.e., without interval gaps) can be beneficial,[5,26] and high-resolution images with a phased array coil can identify ovaries not seen on routine body coil images.[21]

VAGINA

The vagina is seen on MRI as a narrow band between the rectum and bladder (Fig. 7.10).[2] Anatomic divisions of the vagina are best separated on axial scans. The upper third of the vagina is at the level of the lateral fornices[5,6] (Fig. 7.11a). The middle third is at the level of the bladder base (Fig.

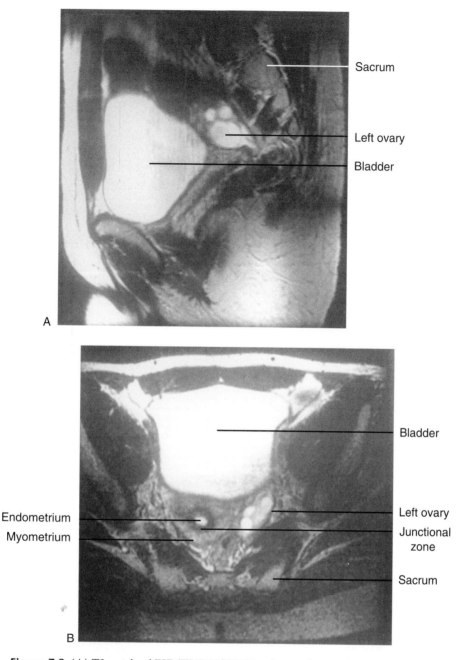

Sacrum

Left ovary

Bladder

A

Bladder

Endometrium

Myometrium

Left ovary

Junctional
zone

Sacrum

B

Figure 7.9 (A) T2-weighted FSE (TR6000/TE108; pelvic coil) sagittal MRI. **(B)** T2-weighted (TR2500/TE80; pelvic coil) axial images show round, bright ovarian follicles.

7.11b). The lower third is that part seen in the axial plane below the bladder, the urethra is noted anteriorly at this level (Fig. 7.11c). Although the axial plane is optimal for the evaluation of the vagina, its relationship with the cervix is best seen on coronal and sagittal images.[2] Slice thickness of 5.0 mm is preferred for studying the vagina on MRI. A tampon obscures details of the vaginal wall and should not be used in MRI.[28]

On T1-weighted images, the vagina has a hypointense signal similar to the uterus and cervix (see Fig. 7.1f).[1,2] On T2-weighted images, the signal intensity of the vaginal wall is medium to low (compared with the higher intensity uterus),[1] and the vagina is best separated from neighboring structures on T2-weighted images (see Fig. 7.6b). The canal has high signal intensity on T2-weighted images, due to mucus and vaginal epithelium.[5,8] A venous plexus of high signal intensity on T2-weighted images surrounds the vagina.[6]

The MRI appearance of the vagina varies with the hormonal status of the patient. The contrast seen on T2-weighted images between the vaginal wall and central canal is most marked in the early follicular and late secretory phases of the menstrual cycle.[6,28] The central epithelial layer is

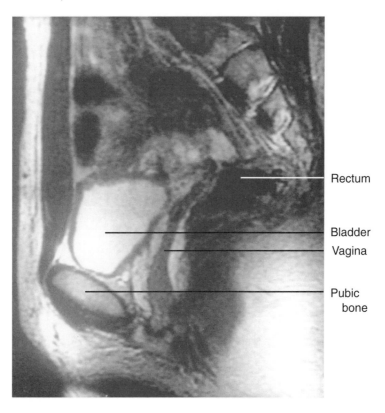

Figure 7.10 T2-weighted (TR2500/TE80; pelvic coil) sagittal view shows the vagina as a dark, tubular structure between the bladder and rectum.

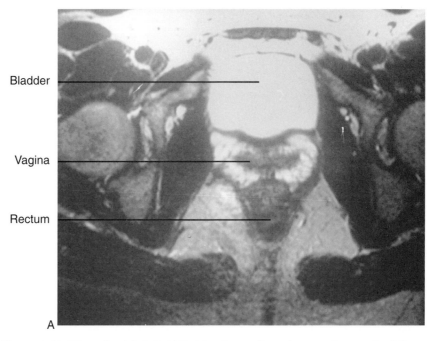

Figure 7.11 T2-weighted (TR6700/TE108; pelvic coil) axial images showing the different parts of the vagina. **(A)** Upper third. **(B)** Middle third. **(C)** Lower third. (*Figure continues.*)

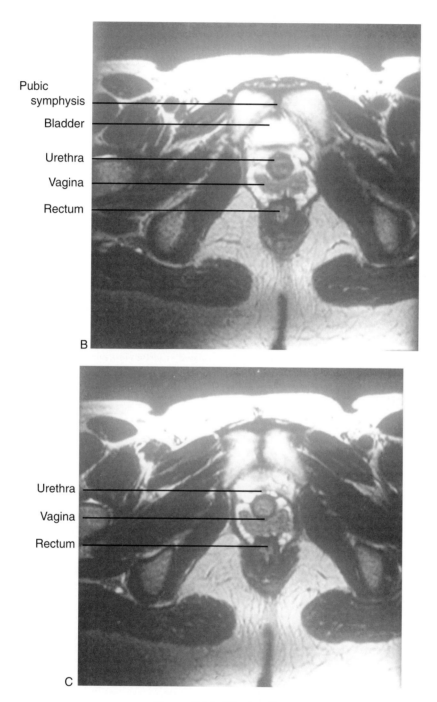

Pubic symphysis

Bladder

Urethra

Vagina

Rectum

B

Urethra

Vagina

Rectum

C

Figure 7.11 (*Continued*).

thickest in pregnancy, the midsecretory phase, and in newborns, reflecting estrogen levels. The signal intensity of the vaginal wall depends on water content, which also varies with the hormonal status of the patient. Increased brightness on T2-weighted images reflects edema that is seen in pregnancy and in the midsecretory phase of the menstrual cycle. Relatively low signal intensity of the wall is seen during the early proliferative and late secretory phases of the cycle.[8,28] Since the MRI appearance of the vagina changes with the hormonal status of the patient, one should endeavor to schedule patients in the early proliferative or late secretory phases of the menstrual cycle, if possible.

The MRI appearance of the vagina in premenarchal patients (apart from newborn infants) and of postmenopausal women (not on estrogen therapy) is that of a very thin layer of high signal intensity on T2-weighted images, indicative of low estrogen levels.[28]

BLADDER

Urine consists mostly of water, which has long T1 and T2 relaxation times.[1,2] Therefore, urine has a low signal on noncontrast T1-weighted or inversion recovery MRI (see Fig. 7.5). The long T2 of urine makes it bright on T2-weighted images[2,3] (see Figs. 7.6 and 7.9b). Normally, the bladder wall is thin and smooth and is best imaged when moderately distended,[1] since this enables more accurate demonstration of its thickness.[1,3] The bladder wall is generally seen equally well in the sagittal, axial, and coronal planes,[29] although the base and dome are best seen in sagittal images.

Normal bladder muscle, similar to muscle elsewhere, has relatively low signal intensity on both T1- and T2-weighted images. This helps differentiate normal bladder wall from tumor, since tumor is generally brighter on T2-weighted images.[20] However, since both urine and the bladder wall have low signal on T1-weighted images, very little if any contrast is seen between bladder tumors and bladder wall on this sequence.[30] The muscularis of the wall is best seen on the T2-weighted images. Scans obtained this way show the urine to be bright, in contrast to the darker bladder wall,[29,30] since the muscular bladder wall darkens with increasing T2-weighting.

Gadolinium causes thin enhancement of the bladder mucosa/submucosa, which can be detected as a bright lining to the inner bladder wall on contrast-enhanced T1-weighted images.[30]

URETHRA

MRI can consistently demonstrate urethral anatomy. Noncontrast T1-weighted images show homogeneous intermediate signal in the area of the urethra; this signal is similar to that of striated muscle. On the T1-weighted sequence, one cannot differentiate urethra from vagina or rectum (see Fig. 7.3M&N).[31] Axial T2-weighted images of the normal female urethra show a characteristic zonal anatomy that appears as a "target" consisting of three layers (see Fig. 7.11C):

1. outer ring, low signal intensity muscular layer
2. middle zone, higher signal intensity submucosal layer
3. center area, low signal intensity dot representing the mucosa

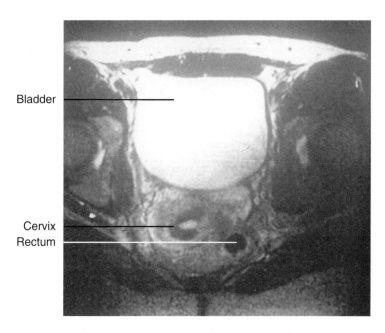

Bladder

Cervix
Rectum

Figure 7.12 T2-weighted SE (TR2500/TE80; pelvic coil) image demonstrates the posterior location of the air-filled rectum.

This superior soft tissue differentiation gives MRI an advantage over computed tomography or ultrasound evaluation of the urethra. MRI's ability to differentiate between the muscular ring of the urethra, its submucosal layer, and mucosa is important in evaluating urinary incontinence.[14]

The MRI appearance of each of these zones depends on the level of the urethra being imaged, as well as the age of the patient. For example, in the distal third of the urethra, the target-like appearance is seen in only 30% of women. The outer muscular layer is most prominent in the middle of the urethra and can be incomplete posteriorly or less prominent in postmenopausal females. Also, the low signal intensity central dot was not seen in 20% of normal females in one study. After contrast administration, a "target" is evident on T1-weighted images, with marked enhancement of the middle zone.[31]

Modified intracavitary rectal/vaginal coils have been used for high-resolution imaging of the urethra.[32]

BOWEL

Bowel gas has very low or absent signal on MRI.[2,3] The rectum is localized by its position and appears donut shaped, with central low intensity secondary to intraluminal air (Fig. 7.12).[4]

REFERENCES

1. Hricak H, Alpers C, Crooks LE, Sheldon PE. Magnetic resonance imaging of the female pelvis: initial experience. AJR Am J Roentgenol 1983;141:1119–1128
2. Picus D, Lee JK. Magnetic resonance imaging of the female pelvis. Urol Radiol 1986;8:166–174
3. Bryan PJ, Butler HE, LiPuma JP et al. NMR scanning of the pelvis: initial experience with a 0.3 T system. AJR Am J Roentgenol 1983;141:1111–1118
4. Thickman D, Kressel H, Gussman D et al. Nuclear magnetic resonance imaging in gynecology. Am J Obstet Gynecol 1984;149:835–840
5. Hricak H. MRI of the female pelvis: a review. AJR Am J Roentgenol 1986;146:1115–1122
6. McCarthy S. Magnetic resonance imaging of the normal female pelvis. Radiol Clin North Am 1992;30:769–775
7. McCarthy S, Tauber C, Gore J. Female pelvic anatomy: MR assessment of variations during the menstrual cycle and with use of oral contraceptives. Radiology 1986;160:119–123
8. Olson MC, Posniak HV, Tempany CM, Dudiak CM. MR imaging of the female pelvic region. Radiographics 1992;12:445–465
9. Haynor DR, Mack LA, Soules MR et al. Changing appearance of the normal uterus during the menstrual cycle: MR studies. Radiology 1986;161:459–462
10. Mitchell DG, Schonholz L, Hilpert PL et al. Zones of the uterus: discrepancy between US and MR images. Radiology 1990;174:827–831
11. Brown HK, Stoll BS, Nicosia SV et al. Uterine junctional zone: correlation between histologic findings and MR imaging. Radiology 1991;179:409–413
12. Kier R. Magnetic resonance imaging of the uterus. Magn Reson Imaging Clin N Am 1994;2:189–210
13. Demas BE, Hricak H, Jaffe RB. Uterine MR imaging: effects of hormonal stimulation. Radiology 1986;159:123–126
14. Klutke C, Golomb J, Barbaric Z, Raz S. The anatomy of stress incontinence: magnetic resonance imaging of the female bladder neck and urethra. J Urol 1990;143:563–566
15. Yamashita Y, Harada M, Sawada T et al. Normal uterus and FIGO Stage I endometrial carcinoma: dynamic gadolinium-enhanced MR imaging. Radiology 1993;186:495–501
16. Scoutt LM, Flynn SD, Luthringer DJ et al. Junctional zone of the uterus: correlation of MR imaging and histologic examination of hysterectomy specimens. Radiology 1991;179:403–407
17. Ito K, Fujita T, Uchisako H et al. MR imaging of the uterus: findings from high-resolution multisection dynamic imaging with a surface coil. AJR Am J Roentgenol 1994;163:873–879
18. Mezrich R. Magnetic resonance imaging applications in uterine cervical cancer. Magn Reson Imaging Clin N Am 1994; 2:211–243
19. Scoutt LM, McCauley TR, Flynn SD et al. Zonal anatomy of the cervix: correlation of MR imaging and histologic examination of hysterectomy specimens. Radiology 1993;186:159–162
20. Magnetic resonance imaging of the abdomen and pelvis. Council on Scientific Affairs. JAMA 1989;261:420–433
21. Smith RC, Reinhold C, McCauley TR et al. Multicoil high-resolution fast spin-echo MR imaging of the female pelvis. Radiology 1992;184:671–675
22. Smith RC, Reinhold C, Lange RC et al. Fast spin-echo MR imaging of the female pelvis. Part I. Use of a whole-volume coil. Radiology 1992;184:665–669
23. deSouza NM, Hawley IC, Schwieso JE et al. The uterine cervix on in vitro and in vivo MR images: a study of zonal anatomy and vascularity using an enveloping cervical coil. AJR Am J Roentgenol 1994;163:607–612
24. Baudouin CJ, Soutter WP, Gilderdale DJ, Coutts GA. Magnetic resonance imaging of the uterine cervix using an intravaginal coil. Mag Reson Med 1992;24:196–203
25. Outwater EK, Schiebler ML. Magnetic resonance imaging of the ovary. Magn Reson Clin N Am 1994;2:245–274
26. Dooms GC, Hricak H, Tscholakoff D. Adnexal structures: MR imaging. Radiology 1986;158:639–646
27. Janus CL, Wiczyk HP, Laufer NL. Magnetic resonance imaging of the menstrual cycle. Magn Reson Imaging 1988;6:669–674
28. Hricak H, Chang YC, Thurnher S. Vagina: evaluation with MR imaging. Part I. Normal anatomy and congenital anomalies. Radiology 1988;169:169–174
29. Fisher MR, Hricak H, Crooks LE. Urinary bladder MR imaging. Part I. Normal and benign conditions. Radiology 1985; 157:467–470
30. Outwater EK, Mitchell DG. Magnetic resonance imaging techniques in the pelvis. Magn Reson Imaging Clin N Am 1994;2:161–188
31. Hricak H, Secaf E, Buckley DW et al. Female uethra: MR iaging. Radiology 1991;178:527–535
32. Yang A, Mostwin JL, Yang SS, Zerhouni EA. High-resolution MR imaging of female and male urethras with intracavitary surface coils and body coils. J Magn Reson Imaging 1991; 1:197–198

Imaging of the Abnormal Female Pelvis

SECTION

III

8

Ultrasonography of the Vagina

JOHN C. ANDERSON

The vagina is normally examined by visual inspection, but in some cases, for instance in children, this may not be appropriate, and in cases of imperforate hymen, it may not be possible. Even when visual examination of the vagina is possible, there will be times when a transabdominal pelvic ultrasound includes incidental features that should be recognized. The vagina is easily demonstrated on abdominal views of the pelvis, but occasionally, lesions of the vagina or related structures are seen on transvaginal scans when they may cause some diagnostic concern.

DEVELOPMENTAL ABNORMALITIES

The female genital tract originates embryologically from the paired müllerian ducts. The proximal portions of these ducts form the fallopian tubes. The distal portions fuse to form the uterus, cervix, and vagina. Developmental arrest or failure in fusion of the ducts gives rise to a spectrum of anomalies of the genital tract often accompanied by anomalies of the urinary tract.[1] They may be associated with infertility, recurrent abortion, and prematurity.[2] All morphologic abnormalities occur between the 55th and 68th day of fetal life.

Vertical Fusion Defects

Defects of vertical fusion can occur at any level of the vagina, resulting in a transverse septum (Fig. 8.1). Forty-six percent of ventrical fusion defects are reported to be high in the vagina, whilst 35% cases in the mid portion, and 19% are low.[3] A transverse vaginal septum prevents loss of menstrual blood, with consequent cryptomenorrhea. Patients present as teenagers with cyclic abdominal pain and a hematocolpos. Associated pressure symptoms of urinary frequency and/or retention may also be a feature.

Ultrasound shows a simple fluid filled swelling due to a hematocolpos, which can be large and displace the uterus so much that it may not be seen. A hematometra may form. The most important factor in making the diagnosis is a high index of suspicion. If one is not conscious of this possibility, an erroneous diagnosis of ovarian cyst may be made.

Imperforate Hymen

The hymen vaginae is a thin fold of mucous membrane situated at the orifice of the vagina. The internal surfaces of the fold are normally in contact with each other, and the vaginal orifice appears as a cleft between them. The hymen varies much in shape and extent and has no known function. It may be absent or may form a complete septum across the lower end of the vagina, the latter is known as an imperforate hymen. Classically, an imperforate hymen forms a thin bulging membrane between the labia.[4] Imperforate hymen and other congenital disorders may occur in isolation or be associated with other congenital abnormalities, especially of the urinary tract. Hymenal bands, posterior and anterior openings, and folded hymens may all interfere with free vaginal discharge and require investigation for other genital malformations.[5]

Hematocolpos results from a collection of menstrual blood in the vagina. Hydrocolpos is a collection of secretions. The location of the retained secretions or menstrual blood depends on the level and duration of the obstruction and the amount of accumulated fluid. Magnetic resonance imaging may differentiate hematocolpos from hydrocolpos because blood has a different signal intensity.

Imperforate hymen results in hematometrocolpos at puberty.[6] Pubertal age patients present with amenorrhea, pelvic discomfort or pain, back pain, abdominal distension, palpable pelvic mass, and urinary tract obstruction. Sonographic features include:

1. An ovoid or pear-shaped sonolucent midline mass with acoustic enhancement behind the urinary bladder.
2. Low-level internal echoes may be scattered throughout the mass, or the mass may be anechoic.
3. The uterus may be displaced superiorly.
4. The lesions can be lobulated or tubular if there is extension of the hemorrhage into the cervix and uterus.

Hematometrocolpos is a uterus and vagina filled with blood. Echogenic clotted blood may be present in the dependent portion of the uterine cavity. Sonographic measurements can estimate of the volume of retained blood.[7]

Lateral Fusion Defects

These patients are usually asymptomatic, and the incidental finding of a vaginal septum is diagnosed during pregnancy when an excision is required to allow vaginal delivery. Dys-

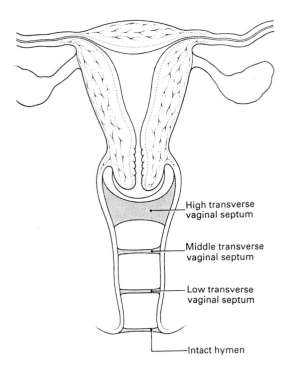

Figure 8.1 Diagrammatic representation of vertical fusion defects. (From Edmunds,[52] with permission.)

pareunia caused by the septum can occur, as in most cases one vaginal canal is larger than the other and intercourse may have occurred partially successfully in the larger side. In unilateral vaginal obstruction, patients usually present with abdominal pain and hematometra and hematocolpos. The confusing sign is the associated menstruation from the other side, and the diagnosis may be missed if careful examination is not performed (Fig. 8.2).

Vaginal Atresia

Absence of the endocervical canal occurs when there is abnormal development of the müllerian duct and may cause vaginal obstruction.[8] Vaginal atresia presents at puberty with complicated or uncomplicated primary amenorrhea. The Mayer-Rokitansky-Kuster-Hauser syndrome comprises vaginal atresia, rudimentary bicornuate uterus, normal fallopian tubes and ovaries, and broad and round ligaments. Patients may have vague pelvic discomfort or pain.

Ultrasound is useful in determining the cause and extent of obstructed uterovaginal anomalies.[9] Transperineal scanning can be useful in evaluating patients with hydro/hematocolpos whose obstruction is low lying. Identification of the level of the obstruction and the thickness of the obstructing septum can be made. The study of vaginal atresia is performed with a standoff to improve the imaging of superficial structures. The distance from the perineum to the caudal aspect of the distended vagina is then measured to decide the best method of surgical reconstruction.[10]

BENIGN CONDITIONS

Wolffian Duct Remnant Cysts

Gartner's duct cysts arise from the mesonephric remnants of the distal wolffian duct within the mesovarium. Single or multiple cysts form along the lateral anterolateral vaginal wall. They are simple tubular cysts within the vagina on ultrasound and are usually an incidental finding (Fig. 8.3).

Gartner's duct cysts are best seen by inserting the tip of the transducer only a short distance into the vagina. Unlike physiologic ovarian cysts, remnant duct cysts show no cyclic changes. They range in size from 1.5 to 19 cm[11] and mostly are anechoic, although some contain internal echoes due to hemorrhage[12] Other cystic vaginal masses include paraurethral cysts, inclusion cysts, and paramesonephric (müllerian) duct cysts. They are usually indistinguishable from wolffian duct remnant cysts on ultrasound.

Solid Lesions

True vaginal polyps are rare and not readily identifiable by ultrasound. The diagnosis is made by visual inspection. Leiomyoma is the most common mesenchymal neoplasm of the vagina.[13,14] They can occur at any adult age but are most commonly detected around 40 years. They are usually submucous and can occur anywhere in the vagina (Fig. 8.4). Grossly and microscopically, they are similar to their uterine counterpart.[15] Rhabdomyomas have rarely been reported arising in the vagina.[16–19] They are benign and can be safely excised. An extremely rare case of benign vaginal rhabdomyoma was

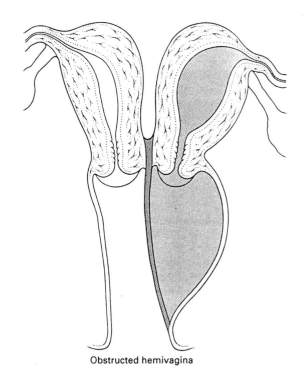

Obstructed hemivagina

Figure 8.2 When the failure of vertical fusion affects only one side, the symptoms are confusing because menstruation is normal from the nonobstructed side. (From Edmunds,[52] with permission.)

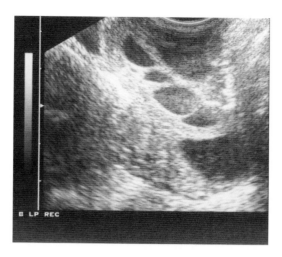

Figure 8.3 Gartner's duct cysts are shown along the lateral anterolateral vaginal wall. This is a transvaginal scan low in the vagina, and the interface between anterior and posterior walls of the vagina cannot be seen.

reported in a 35-year-old healthy woman in whom it presented as a pedunculated polyp measuring 1.2 cm in diameter in the anterior wall of the vagina.[20] A case of extraovarian Brenner tumor of the vagina in a postmenopausal woman who presented with a vaginal polyp has been described.[21] Neurofibromas of the vagina are solid, uncommon, and benign.[22]

MALIGNANT CONDITIONS

Vaginal Cancer

Ultrasonography is not used for diagnosis of carcinoma of the vagina, but it may play a role in staging, and it is possible that these conditions could be seen incidentally during examinations for other reasons. Vaginal carcinoma is primarily a disease of women over 50. Vaginal and vulval cancers frequently occur in association with epithelial neoplasms of other anogenital sites, including the cervix, anus, urethra, and bladder.[23–26] These tumors are seen as low-level, echo-producing masses, continuous with the clear zone of the vagina. They may appear as thickening of the vaginal wall or as an obvious mass invading surrounding tissue. Carcinoma of the cervix invading the upper vagina has the same appearance as a primary vaginal carcinoma. Aggressive angiomyxoma of the vagina has presented as a mass arising within the vaginal wall and extending to the perineum. The mass appeared cystic on ultrasound. This condition mainly affects the soft tissues and perineum; it is neither encapsulated nor circumscribed and has a tendency for local recurrence.[27]

Diethylstilbestrol Exposure

Carcinoma of the vagina (usually clear-cell carcinoma) usually occurs in women with a history of in utero exposure to diethylstilbestrol (DES). About 9% of primary vaginal carci-

nomas are adenocarcinomas, and they affect a younger population of women, regardless of whether exposure to DES in utero has occurred or not.[28] Adenocarcinomas may arise in areas of vaginal adenosis, particularly in patients exposed to DES in utero, but they probably also arise in wolffian rest elements, periurethral glands,[29] and foci of endometriosis. Secondary tumors from sites such as the colon, endometrium, or ovary should be considered when vaginal adenocarcinoma is diagnosed. DES (a synthetic estrogen) was used from 1940 until 1971 to maintain high-risk pregnancies in women suffering from recurrent miscarriage, hypertension, diabetes mellitis, threatened abortion, previous stillbirth, and a history of premature labor. It is estimated that at least 2 million women were exposed to DES.[30]

In 1971 an association was observed between DES administration during pregnancy and the development years later of a clear cell adenocarcinoma of the vagina in the female offspring exposed in utero.[31–33] Various structural and cytologic abnormalities of the reproductive system have since been described and characterized.[34–36] DES exposure in utero can cause structural changes to the cervix and vagina that include a transverse vaginal septum, a cervical collar, a cockscomb (a raised ridge, usually on the anterior cervix), or cervical hypoplasia. The malformations associated with DES exposure include the classic T-shaped uterus with widening of the interstitial and isthmic portions of the fallopian tubes and narrowing of the lower two-thirds of the uterus.[37] Hysterosalpingography, shows a variety of abnormalities including irregular endometrium, synechiae, constrictions, and a T-shaped uterus.[38] Ultrasound may show a small T-shaped uterus lacking the normal bulbous nature of the uterine fundus.[39,40]

Rhabdomyosarcoma

The most common primary malignant neoplasm is the rhabdomyosarcoma. It can arise from the uterus or vagina, al-

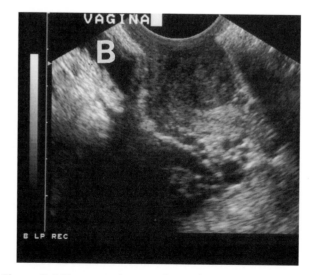

Figure 8.4 Transvaginal scan with transducer low in the vagina shows a 2-cm solid nodule in the wall of the vagina. This proved to be a leiomyoma. The bladder (B) is seen to the left.

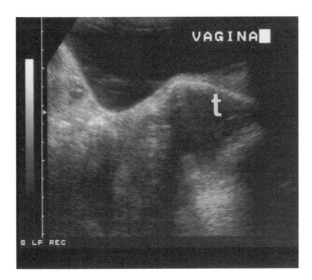

Figure 8.5 A tampon (t) in the vagina viewed through the urinary bladder appears as a bright leading edge with posterior shadow due to enclosed air.

though uterine involvement is more frequent by direct extension from a vaginal tumor. It is commonly found in children 6 to 18 months of age with vaginal bleeding or protrusion of a polypoid cluster of masses (sarcoma botryoides) through the introitus. It often arises from the anterior wall of the vagina near the cervix but can also be found in the distal vagina or labia. Direct extension of the tumor into the bladder neck is common, but rarely does it extend into the rectum posteriorly. Ultrasonically, these tumors appear as solid, homogenous masses that fill the vaginal cavity or cause enlargement of the uterus with an irregular contour.[41,42]

Endodermal Sinus (Yolk Sac) Tumor

Endodermal sinus tumors are rare germ cell tumors that are occasionally found in extragonadal sites such as the vagina. Leverger et al.[43] reported 11 cases (average age 10 months) presenting with vaginal bleeding. The ultrasound appearance is predominantly that of echogenic masses that may contain anechoic to hypoechoic areas from hemorrhage or necrosis.

INFLAMMATORY CONDITIONS

Foreign Bodies

The role of ultrasonography in locating foreign bodies (especially in children) is well established. The sonographic signs include varying echogenicity, acoustic shadowing, and indentation of the posterior bladder wall.[44] Foreign bodies present in the vagina for long periods of time are infrequent but potentially serious. Serious injury can occur to the bowel, bladder, or other pelvic structures due to ulceration.

Tampon

A vaginal tampon appears on ultrasound as a linear bright leading edge echo with posterior shadowing. This is because the tampon contains much air and therefore does not transmit the sound beam. The posterior bladder wall may be indented slightly (Fig. 8.5).

Intrauterine Contraceptive Device

An IUCD expelled into the vagina has the ultrasound appearance of a bright linear specular reflection with complete posterior shadowing along the vaginal canal (Fig. 8.6).

Ring Pessary

A case is reported of a neglected pessary. After erosion through the anterior vaginal and bladder walls, the device came to rest entirely within the bladder.[45]

Vaginal Calculi

Vaginal stones may form around foreign material such as surgical suture material[46] and inadvertently unremoved medical gauze.[47]

POSTOPERATIVE APPEARANCE

Vaginal Vault Posthysterectomy

The vaginal cuff is normally less than 2.1 cm in diameter.[48] An unusually large cuff or a cuff that contains a definite mass should be suspected for malignancy. Nodular areas in the vaginal cuff may reflect postradiation fibrosis.

Ultrasound is useful in the assessment of complications of

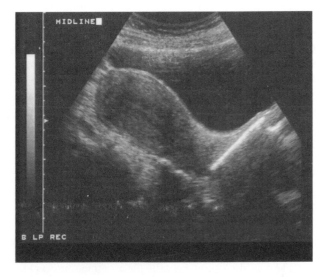

Figure 8.6 An intrauterine contraceptive device that has been expelled into the vagina.

vaginal hysterectomy such as vaginal cuff hematomas[49] and vaginal vault hematomas.[50,51]

Summary

Ultrasound examination of the vagina is usually best carried out abdominally through the loaded bladder. Occasionally, examination by endovaginal transducer will give the clue to diagnosis, for instance, in the case of remnant duct cysts.

REFERENCES

1. Malini S, Valdes C, Malinak LR et al. Sonographic diagnosis and classification of anomalies of the female genital tract. J Ultrasound Med 1984;3:397

2. Cooperberg PL, Kidney MR. Ultrasound evaluation of the uterus. In: Callen PU, Ed. Ultrasonography in Obstetrics and Gynecology. WB Saunders, Philadelphia, 1988, pp 393–412

3. Rock JA, Zacur HA, Dlugi AM et al. Pregnancy success following surgical correction of imperforate hymen and complete transverse septum. Obstet Gynecol 1982;59:448–454

4. Sawhney S, Gupta R, Berry M, Bhatnager V. Hydrometrocolpos: diagnosis and follow-up by ultrasound—a case report. Australas Radiol 1990;34:93–94

5. Mor N, Merlob P, Reisner SH. Types of hymen in the newborn infant. Eur J Obstet Gynecol Reprod Biol 1986;22:225–228

6. Radman HM, Askin JA, Kolodner LJ. Hydrometrocolpos and hematometrocolpos. Obstet Gynecol 1966;27:2–6

7. Ali GM, Kordoff R, Franke D. Ultrasound volumetry in hematometrocolpos. JCU J Clin Ultrasound 1989;17:257–259

8. Nguyen L, Youssef S, Guttman FM et al. Hydrometrocolpos in neonate due to distal vaginal atresia. J Paediatr Surg 1984;19:510–514

9. Blask AR, Sanders RC, Rock JA. Obstructed uterovaginal anomalies: demonstration with sonography. Part II. Teenagers. Radiology 1991;179:84–88

10. Scanlan K, Pozniak M, Fagerholm M, Shapiro S. Value of transperineal sonography in the assessment of vaginal atresia. AJR Am J Roentgenol 1990;154:545–548

11. Hagspiel KD. Giant Gartner duct cyst: magnetic resonance imaging findings. Abdom Imaging 1995;20:566–568

12. Alpern MB, Sandler MA, Madrazo BL. Sonographic features of paraovarian cysts and their complications. AJR Am J Roentgenol 1984;143:157

13. Bennett HG, Ehrlich HM. Myoma of the vagina. Am J Obstet Gynecol 1941;42:314

14. Fu YS, Reagan JW. Pathology of the Uterine Cervix, Vagina and Vulva. WB Saunders, Philadelphia, 1989, pp 336–379

15. Tavassoli FA, Norris HJ. Smooth muscle tumors of the vagina. Obstet Gynecol 1979;53:689–693

16. Carinelli SG, Carinelli I, Merlo D-N. Mucinous cysts of the vulva. Cervix & l.f.g.t. 1984;2:143–148

17. Gad A, Eusebi V. Rhabdomyoma of the vagina. J Pathol 1975;115:179–181

18. Gold JH, Bossen EH. Benign vaginal rhabdomyoma. A light and electron microscopic study. Cancer 1976;37:2283–2294

19. Leone PG, Taylor HB. Ultrastructure of a benign polypoid rhabdomyoma of the vagina. Cancer 1973;31:1414–1417

20. Lopez JI, Brouard I, Eizaguirre B. Rhabdomyoma of the vagina. Eur J Obstet Gynecol Reprod Biol 1992;45:147–148

21. Rashid AM, Fox H. Brenner tumour of the vagina. J Clin Pathol 1995;48:678–679

22. McCarthy S, Taylor KJW. Sonography of vaginal masses. AJR Am J Roentgenol 1983;140:1005–1008

23. Newman W, Cromer JK. The multicentric origin of carcinomas of the female anogenital tract. Surg Gynecol Obstet 1959;108:272

24. Marcus SL. Multiple squamous carcinomas involving the cervix, vagina, and vulva: the theory of multicentric origin. Am J Obstet Gynecol 1960;80:802

25. Stern BD, Kaplan L. Multicentric foci of carcinomas arising in structures of cloacal origin. Am J Obstet Gynecol 1969;104:255

26. Jones RW, McLean MR. Carcinoma in situ of the vulva: a review of 31 treated and five untreated cases. Obstet Gynecol 1986;68:499–503

27. Amr SS, el-Mallah KO. Aggressive angiomyxoma of the vagina. Int J Gynecol Obstet 1995;48:207–210

28. Ballon SC, Lagasses LD, Chang NH et al. Primary adenocarcinoma of the vagina. Surg Gynecol Obstet 1979;53:218

29. Frick HC, Jacox HW, Taylor HC. Primary carcinoma of the vagina. Am J Obst Gynecol 1968;101:695

30. Senekjian E. Reproductive function in DE-exposed women. Female Patient 1988;13:12

31. Herbst AL, Ulfelder H, Poskanzer DC. Adenocarcinoma of the vagina: association of maternal stilbestrol therapy with tumor appearance in young women. N Engl J Med 1971;284:878

32. Herbst Al, Poskanzer DC, Robboy SJ et al. Prenatal exposure to stilbestrol: a prospective comparison of exposed female offspring with unexposed controls. N Engl J Med 1975;292:334

33. Burke L, Antonioli D, Rosen S. Vaginal and cervical squamous cell dysplasia in women exposed to diethylstilbestrol in utero. Am J Obstet Gynecol 1978;132:537

34. Kaufman RH, Binder GL, Gray PM, Jr, Adam E. Upper genital tract changes associated with exposure in utero to diethylstilbestrol. Am J Obstet Gynecol 1977;128:51

35. Haney AF, Hammond CB, Soules MR, Creasman WT. Diethylstilbestrol-induced upper genital tract abnormalities. Fertil Steril 1979;31:142

36. Kaufman RH, Adam E, Grey MP, Gerthoffer E. Urinary tract changes associated with exposure in utero to diethylstilbestrol. Obstet Gynecol 1980;56:330

37. Kaufman RH, Adam E, Binder GL, Gerthoffer E. Upper genital tract changes and pregnancy outcome in offspring exposed in utero to DES. Am J Obstet Gynecol 1980;137:299–306

38. Nunley WC, Pope TL, Bateman BG. Upper reproductive tract radiographic findings in DES exposed female offspring. AJR Am J Roentgenol 1984;142:337

39. Viscomi GN, Gonazalez R, Taylor KJW. Ultrasound detection of uterine abnormalities after diethylstilbestrol (DES) exposure. Radiology 1980;136:733

40. Lev-Toaff AS, Toaff ME, Friedman AS. Endovaginal sonographic appearance of a DES uterus. J Ultrasound Med 1990;9:661–664

41. Kangarloo H, Sarti DA, Sample WF. Ultrasound of the pediatric pelivs. Semin Ultrasound 1980;1:51–60

42. Schneider M, Grossman H. Sonography of the female chid's reproductive system. Pediatr Ann 1980;9:180–186

43. Leverger G, Flamant F, Gerbaulet A et al. Tumors of the vitelline sac located in the vagina in children. Arch Fr Pediatr 1983;40:85

44. Caspi B, Zalel Y, Katz Z et al. The role of sonography in the detection of vaginal foreign bodies in young girls: the bladder indentation sign. Pediatr Radiol 1995;25 (suppl):S60–61

45. Goldstein I, Wise GJ, Tancer ML. A vesicovaginal fistula and intravesical foreign body. A rare case of the neglected pessary. Am J Obstet Gynecol 1990;163:589–591

46. Lukacs T, Mohammed S. Giant secondary vaginal calculus. Orv Hetil 1989;130:2537–2538

47. van Oorschot FH, Mallens WM, van Helsdingen PJ. A secondary vaginal stone. A case report. Diagn Imaging Clin Med 1986;55:157–160

48. Schoenfeld A, Levavi H, Hirsch M et al. Transvaginal sonography in postmenopausal women. J Clin Ultrasound 1990; 18:350–358

49. Lev-Gur M, Patel S, Greston WM, McGill F. Pararenal hematoma as a complication of vaginal hysterectomy. A case report. J Reprod Med 1987;32:68–71

50. Kuhn RJ, de Crespigny LC. Vault haematoma after vaginal hysterectomy: an invariable sequel? Aust N Z J Obstet Gynaecol 1985;25:59–62

51. Demos TC, Churchill R, Flisak ME et al. The radiologic diagnosis of complications following gynecologic surgery: radiography, computed tomography, sonography and scintigraphy. Crit Rev Diagn Imaging 1984;22:43–94

52. Edmunds DK. Sexual differenciation–normal and abnormal. In: Shaw RW, Souter WP, Stanton SL, Eds. Gynaecology. Churchill Livingstone, New York, 1992, p 166–167

Computed Tomography and Magnetic Resonance Imaging of the Vagina

ELIZABETH VINING

JEFFREY J. BROWN

Computed tomography (CT) and magnetic resonance imaging (MRI) can help to resolve many diagnostic problems of vaginal disorders. CT has high spatial resolution and relatively rapid scanning time. MRI has better soft tissue contrast, can image in many planes, and has no ionizing radiation. This chapter describes CT and MRI techniques for imaging the vagina.

TECHNIQUE

CT of the vagina is usually performed as part of a CT examination of the pelvis. About 450 ml of dilute oral contrast material should be taken by the patient 3 to 4 hours before scanning. Additional rectal contrast material can be administered to mark the rectum and sigmoid colon. A tampon can be inserted to mark the vagina. Intravenous contrast material (60% iodinated) is useful for differentiating blood vessels from lymph nodes, opacifying the ureters and bladder, defining the extent of an inflammatory process, and determining whether a mass has cystic components. Typically, a pelvic CT to evaluate the vagina consists of sequential axial 5 to 10 mm thick sections obtained from the iliac crests to the inferior pubic symphysis with the addition of thinner slices (2 mm) through any detected masses. Scanning can be continued caudally, if necessary, to obtain complete anatomic coverage of the vagina. CT examinations using oral and intravenous contrast have superseded barium enemas and intravenous urograms for staging of gynecologic malignancies.

An MRI examination of the vagina should include transaxial T1- and T2-weighted images and sagittal T2-weighted images. Coronal T1-and T2-weighted images provide additional diagnostic information in some patients. Gradient echo transaxial images can be acquired to evaluate the pelvic veins or help differentiate blood vessels from lymph nodes. Image slice thickness can vary from 5 to 10 mm. Thinner slices can be used in conjunction with surface coils for high spatial resolution. Fast (or turbo) spin echo (FSE) pulse sequences have largely replaced conventional spin echo (SE) sequences for T2-weighted imaging with reductions in image acquisition time. Initially, MRI of the vagina was performed with circumferential transmit–receive body coils. Recently, phased-array coil systems (Fig. 9.1A) have been used increasingly for imaging the female pelvis. These coils result in substantial increases in signal-to-noise ratio. By using FSE imaging in conjunction with phased-array surface coils, high spatial resolution images can be acquired within a reasonable imaging time. Endorectal and endovaginal surface coils (Fig. 9.1b) have also been used for vaginal imaging but are still being evaluated.

Intravenous contrast material is not administered routinely for MRI of the female pelvis but is useful in certain clinical situations. For example, gadolinium enhancement should be considered in patients with suspected pelvic masses or inflammatory conditions. Like the iodinated contrast agents used for CT scanning, the gadolinium chelates equilibrate rapidly with the extracellular fluid and are eliminated primarily by glomerular filtration. Several oral MRI contrast agents designed to mark the gastrointestinal tract are currently being evaluated and should be available in the future. Frequency-selective fat saturation can be used with either T1-or T2-weighted sequences to help distinguish fat from hemorrhage. Glucagon (1 to 2 mg) intramuscularly or intravenously minimizes bowel peristalsis, and respiratory compensation reduces motion artifacts. Finally, MRI angiography is useful for visualizing the vascular system and distinguishing flow from thrombosis.

NORMAL ANATOMY

On CT scans, the normal vagina (Fig. 9.2) appears as a circular or oval area of soft tissue attenuation between the urethra and the rectum. It can be followed as a continuous structure on sequential transaxial images from the proximal vaginal fornices to the introitus. The level of transition from vagina to

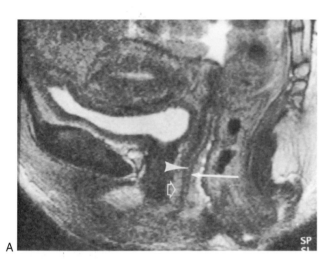

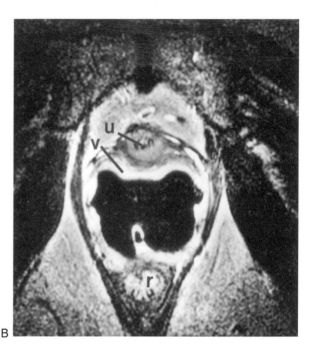

Figure 9.1 MRI of the normal vagina. (**A**) The vaginal layers are also readily identified on the sagittal image (FSE TR 4416/TE 99) arrowhead, vaginal canal; open arrow, anterior vaginal wall; long arrow, posterior vaginal wall. (**B**) A transaxial T1-weighted (TR 683/TE 11) image acquired with an endovaginal surface coil. u, urethra; v, vaginal wall; r, rectum.

cervix is inferred from changes in contour of the soft tissue, that is, widening at the level of the cervix. Lateral to the vagina, fat provides tissue contrast between the vagina and the normal structures of the pelvic walls.

On T1-weighted MRIs, the vagina has low-to-intermediate signal intensity and is difficult to distinguish from the urethra anteriorly, the rectum posteriorly, and the levator ani muscles laterally due to the similar signal intensities of these

Figure 9.2 CT of the normal vagina. transaxial CT scan of the pelvis in an adult at the level of the pubic symphysis shows a normal vagina (arrow). A Foley catheter is present in the urethra (arrowhead)

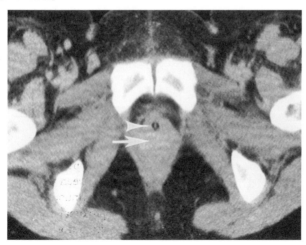

structures (Fig. 9.3A). However, on T2-weighted images, the vagina is clearly visualized as a distinct structure (Fig. 9.3B). Three discrete vaginal anatomic layers can be distinguished on T2-weighted images. The vaginal smooth muscle (tunica muscularis), which has low-to-intermediate signal intensity, forms the middle layer.[1] The inner layer represents vaginal mucosa and appears bright on T2-weighted images. The outer layer, which is also bright, consists of connective tissue and a prominent venous plexus.[1] These layers are usually most clearly visualized on transaxial images.

In women of reproductive age, the appearances of the layers of the vagina change with the menstrual cycle. During the early proliferative phase of the menstrual cycle, T2-weighted images of the vagina show a distinct mucosal layer of high signal intensity and a surrounding wall of low signal intensity.[1] During the mid-secretory phase, the tissue contrast on T2-weighted images is less distinct between the central mucosal layer and the surrounding vaginal wall.[1] By the late secretory phase, the layers of the vagina again become more distinct and have an appearance similar to that seen during the proliferative phase.[1] Generally, the inner mucosal layer is most prominent in women of reproductive age and in neonates (under the influence of maternal estrogen). The mucosal layer can be inconspicuous or imperceptible in postmenopausal women.[1]

A potential pitfall in vaginal imaging of children with CT or MRI is that urine can reflux into the vagina during voiding and may simulate hydrocolpos (Fig. 9.4). Delayed images can be obtained to confirm the presence of a normal vagina.

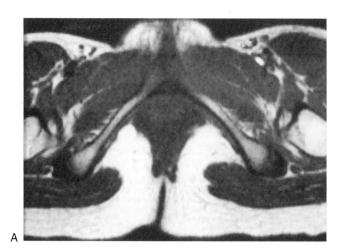 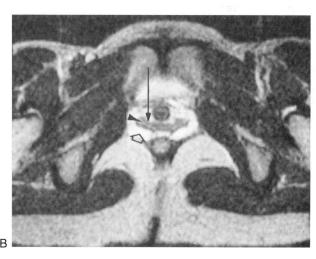

A   B

Figure 9.3 (**A**) Transaxial T1-weighted image (TR 450/TE 15) of the normal vagina in an 18-year-old woman. The vagina cannot be distinguished from the urethra (anteriorly) or the rectum (posteriorly). (**B**) Transaxial T2-weighted image (TR 1,800/TE 80) in the same patient shows clear demarcation of the vagina from the urethra and the rectum. Three distinct vaginal layers are identified including the mucosa (arrowhead), the smooth muscle layer (long arrow), and the outer connective tissue layer, which appears bright due to slow-flowing blood within the vaginal venous plexus (short open arrow).

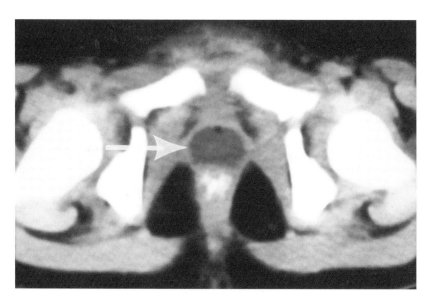

Figure 9.4 Transaxial CT scan of the pelvis in a child shows a dilated fluid-filled vagina (arrow) secondary to reflux of urine during voiding. Oral contrast material is present in the rectum. Delayed scans demonstrated a normal vagina.

CONGENITAL ANOMALIES

Accurate diagnosis of congenital vaginal and uterine anomalies is important because they are associated with an increased incidence of menstrual disorders, infertility, and obstetric complications including spontaneous abortion and preterm delivery. Uterine anomalies are also associated with renal agenesis and renal ectopia. Patients with suspected congenital anomalies can be evaluated with sonography, MRI, hysterosalpingography(HSG), and laparoscopy. Sonography is usually the appropriate initial test; however, it is limited in some patients due to body habitus. MRI, unlike HSG and laparoscopy, is noninvasive and provides a global demonstration of the uterine anatomy. CT has little or no role in the evaluation of congenital anomalies. In a recent study, MRI had slightly greater accuracy than endovaginal sonography for diagnosing müllerian duct anomalies.[2] Sonography evaluation of genitourinary tract congenital anomalies is discussed in Chapter 8.

Cloacal Malformation

The upper two thirds of the vagina forms from fusion of the müllerian ducts, while the lower one-third forms from the urogenital sinus.[3] Cloacal malformation results from the failure of separation of the urogenital sinus into the urethra, vagina, and the rectum, resulting in a single perineal opening. This is readily demonstrated on MRI (Fig. 9.5). Internally, the vagina may be divided by a septum or be fused distally. When fused distally, hydrometrocolpos will result. The uterus can be normal or abnormal in children with cloacal malformation. These patients often have sacral defects and associated upper urinary tract anomalies.[4] MRI can be used to define the anatomy for surgical planning and to detect associated abnormalities.

Vaginal Duplication

Vaginal duplication results from failure of fusion of the lower paramesonephric ducts.[3] Nonfusion of the müllerian ducts can also result in duplication of the upper vagina. *Uterus didelphys* refers to complete uterine duplication in association with a vertical septum in the upper vagina. MRI is predominantly used for evaluating the uterus in patients with müllerian duct anomalies. Duplication of the vagina is well demonstrated (Fig. 9.6). In one patient (illustrated), there is also duplication of the cervix and uterus, that is, uterine didelphys (Fig. 9.6 C&D).

Vaginal Agenesis

Vaginal agenesis (partial or complete) is a congenital anomaly of the müllerian ducts affecting 1 in 4,000 to 5,000 girls.[4] Management of these patients depends on the length of vagina, the presence of a functioning cervix, and the presence of endometrium. The goal of treatment, in addition to vagin-

oplasty, is to preserve the capacity for a full-term pregnancy.[5] MRI is helpful for surgical planning to assess the length of the vagina, its relationship to the uterus, and the presence of endometrial tissue.[1,6,7] MRI is used to detect associated anomalies such as uterine agenesis (Mayer-Rokitansky-Kuster-Hauser syndrome) and unilateral renal agenesis. Figure 9.7 shows a patient with agenesis of the lower vagina.

Imperforate Hymen

Failure of recanalization of the vaginal plate results in imperforate hymen or more rarely a transverse vaginal septum. Excessive secretions(blood, mucus) produce dilatation of the proximal vagina and cervix (hematocolpos, hydrocolpos)(Fig. 9.8). These patients often do not come to medical attention until menarche, when they present with amenorrhea and abdominal distension. The dilatation is relieved by incision of the hymen. MRI shows dilatation of the vagina proximal to the imperforate hymen.

Androgen Insensitivity

Patients with androgen insensitivity (46, XY chromosomes, androgen receptor defect) have external female phenotypic characteristics and an absent or short blind-ending vagina. The uterus and ovaries are absent, and undescended testes may be present. The vagina is abnormally small, in the absence of estrogen stimulation. Compare the MRI of the vagina in a patient with androgen insensitivity in Figure 9.9 to the normal MRI appearance of the vagina in Figure 9.1. In particular, note the much less prominent mucosal layer in the abnormal vagina. The testes are often surgically removed in these patients due to an increased incidence of testicular cancer. Localization of the testes before surgical removal can be performed with CT[8] or MRI[9] (Fig. 9.9C).

Cysts

Bartholin's glands are located in the vulvovaginal area. Cysts of the Bartholin's glands form secondary to blockage of their ducts and accumulation of secretions. They are found at physical examination in approximately 2% of women.[10] Kier[11] reported a prevalence of Bartholin's cysts of 1.3% on MRI examinations. Most Bartholin's cysts are unilocular and are caused by blockage of the main duct, but multilocular cysts can also form secondary to occlusion of deeply placed minor ducts or the ductal acini.[10] They typically range from 1 to 4 cm in diameter. They are usually asymptomatic but can become painful if secondarily infected. On CT scans, Bartholin's cysts appear as well-defined low-attenuation masses (Fig. 9.10A). Infected or hemorrhagic cysts can have high-attenuation values. On MRI, Bartholin's cysts appear as well-defined round or oval masses in the vulvovaginal area with variable signal intensity on T1-weighted images (depending on the protein content) and high signal intensity on T2-weighted images (Fig. 9.10B).[11]

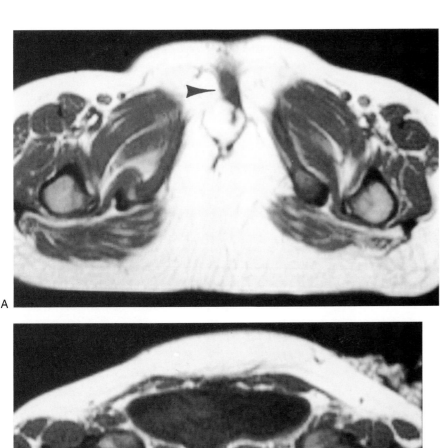

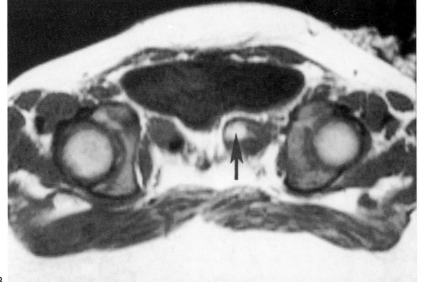

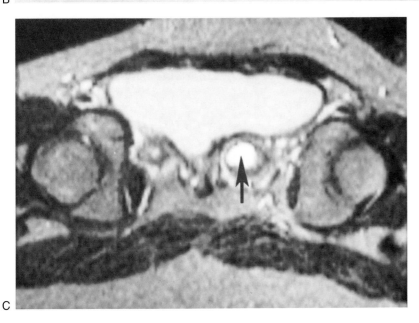

Figure 9.5 Cloacal malformation. (**A**) Transaxial T1-weighted (TR 575/TE 10) image shows a single perineal opening (arrowhead). (**B**) Transaxial T1-weighted (TR 575/TE 10) image at a more superior level shows a slightly dilated vagina (arrow). No distinct rectum is seen. The patient has a colostomy (not shown). (**C**) Transaxial T2-weighted (TR 2,600/TE 90) in the same patient at a slightly more cranial level shows a mild dilatation of the endocervical canal (arrow).

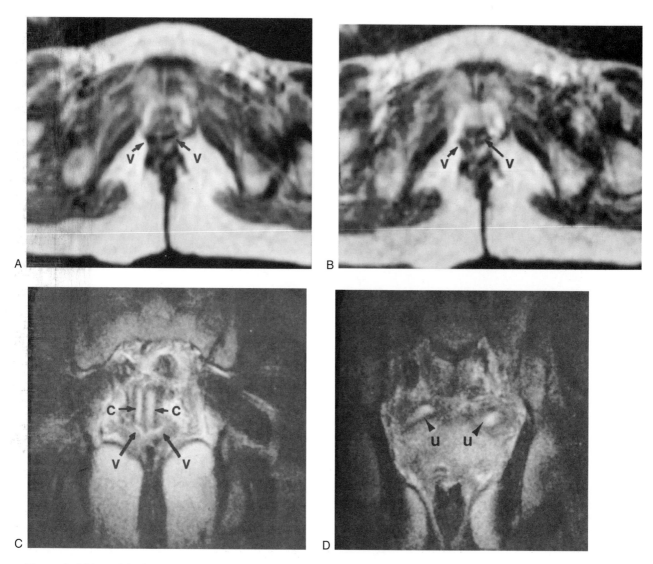

Figure 9.6 Vaginal duplication in two patients. (**A & B**) Transaxial proton density (TR 2,500/TE 30) and T2-weighted (TR 2,500/TE 90) images in a 9-year-old girl demonstrate a duplicated vagina (v). This was confirmed on physical examination. This patient had a single cervix and uterus. (**C & D**) Coronal T2-weighted (TR 2,100/TE 90) images in a different patient with uterus didelphyis. There is duplication of the vagina (v), cervical canal (c), and uterus (u).

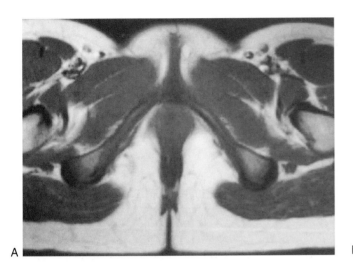
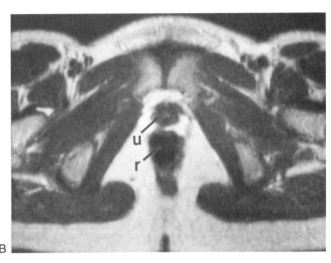

Figure 9.7 Partial vaginal agenesis in a 12-year-old girl with abdominal distension. (**A**) Transaxial T1-weighted (TR 600/TE 15) and (**B**) T2-weighted (TR 3,900/TE 90) images demonstrates urethral and rectal perineal openings. No vaginal opening or lower vagina is identified. u, urethra; r, rectum.

Figure 9.8 (**A**) Coronal T2-weighted (TR 4,000/TE 90) and (**B**) sagittal T1-weighted (TR 600/TE 15) images show a markedly dilated upper vagina (v) and left fallopian tube (ft). The high signal intensity of the fluid on the T1-weighted image is consistent with subacute hemorrhage.

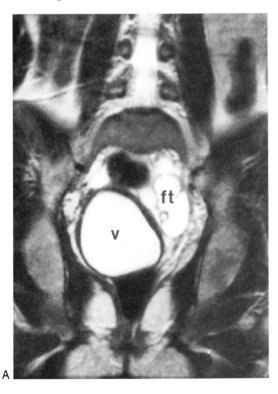
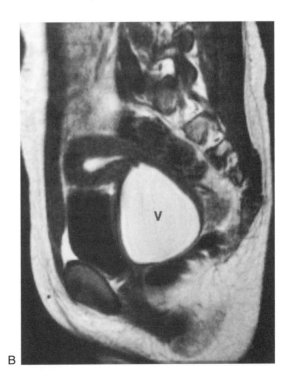

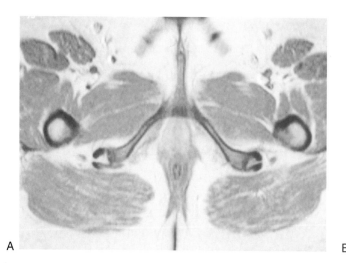

A

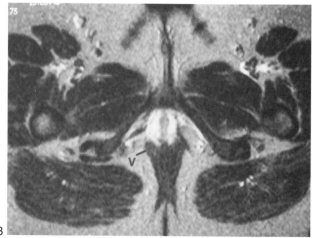

B

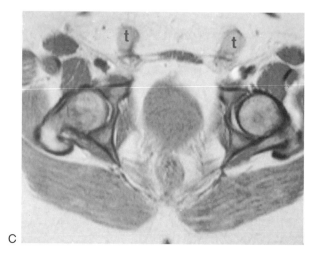

C

Figure 9.9 Androgen insensitivity in a 20-year-old patient. (**A**) Transaxial proton density-weighted (TR 2,600/TE 20) and (**B**) T2-weighted (TR 2,600/TE 90) images show a diminutive vagina (v). The normal vaginal layers are indistinguishable. (**C**) Transaxial proton density-weighted image (TR 2,600/TE 20) shows the testes (t) within the inguinal canal.

Figure 9.10 Bartholin's cyst. (**A**) A CT scan shows a well-defined oval mass of low attenuation at the left vulvovaginal junction (arrow). This appearance is characteristic of a Bartholin's gland cyst. (**B**) Sagittal FSE image (TR 3,550/TE 90) shows a 2-cm Bartholin's cyst at the anterior aspect of the lower vagina (arrow). The patient has had a hysterectomy, and a small amount of free intraperitoneal fluid is present above the vaginal cuff (arrowhead).

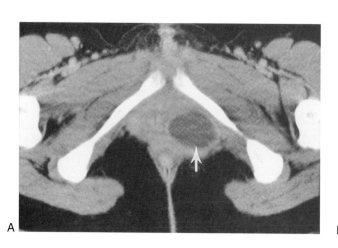

A

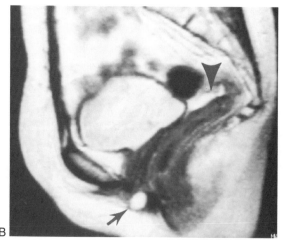

B

Gartner's duct cysts (remnants of the wolffian ducts) are small, benign fluid-filled cysts in the anterolateral wall of the vagina.[10] On CT scans, they can appear as low-attenuation masses in the wall of the vagina, typically smaller than 2 cm in diameter. Like Bartholin's cysts, they have variable signal intensity on T1-weighted images and high signal intensity on T2-weighted images.[11]

INFLAMMATION

The vagina is relatively resistant to primary inflammation or infection. Inflammatory changes of the vagina are usually secondary to adjacent inflammatory bowel disease, diverticulitis, or radiation therapy (most often for cervical cancer). In the early stages, inflammation causes ill-defined thickening of the vaginal wall and loss of distinct perivaginal tissue planes. Over time, vaginal wall thickening diminishes as fibrosis occurs. The clinical course can be complicated by fistula formation. No contrast material should be seen within the vagina unless there has been a recent vaginogram or reflux from voiding after intravenous contrast administration. Otherwise, intravaginal contrast indicates the presence of a fistula. Other findings on CT or MRI suggestive of fistulas include air and/or fluid within the vagina.[12] Figure 9.11 demonstrates CT scans of two patients, both with fistulas secondary to inflammation. The accuracy of CT scanning for detecting vaginal fistulas has been shown to be 60% compared

to a 28% accuracy for contrast enemas, vaginography, cystoscopy, and colonoscopy.[12]

Fistulas can also be demonstrated on MRI.[13] They appear as high signal intensity linear tracts on T2-weighted images with low-to-intermediate signal intensity on T1-weighted images. A fistulous tract extending posteriorly from the vagina is shown in Figure 9.12. Injection of 2 to 30 ml of saline into a fistula before MRI can help show its course and extent.[14]

NEOPLASM

Benign masses of the vagina include leiomyoma (the most common benign neoplasm of the vagina in adults), rhabdomyoma, fibroepithelial polyps, papillomas (squamous and müllerian), benign mixed tumors (histologically similar to benign mixed tumors of salivary glands), endometriomas, and adenosis.[15] Other tumors and tumor-like processes have been sporadically reported. On CT and MRI examinations, these masses can fill the vagina, cause focal thickening of the vagina walls, or extend outward from the vagina. The surrounding tissue planes are usually preserved. An example of angiomatosis of the vagina and cervix is shown on CT in (Fig. 9.13). There is nodular enlargement of the vagina and the other involved structures. Phleboliths are also present within the tumor mass. A large fibroma is shown invading the left wall of the vagina in a young woman who complained of pain with intercourse (Fig. 9.14).

Figure 9.11 Vaginal fistulas on CT. (**A**) Rectovaginal fistula secondary to radiation therapy for cervical cancer. There is intravaginal contrast material (arrow) consistent with a vaginal fistula. The presence of a rectovaginal fistula was confirmed with a contrast enema. High attenuation in the bladder is secondary to intravenous contrast material. (**B**) A CT scan in a patient with vesicovaginal and rectovaginal fistulas secondary to extensive rectal cancer. Stool extends from the area of the rectum to the vagina (arrow) and into the bladder (arrowhead).

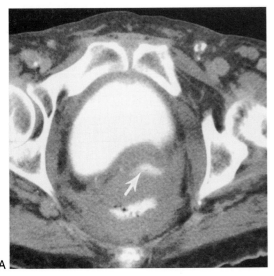
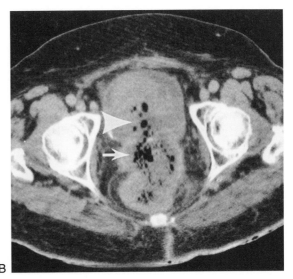

A   B

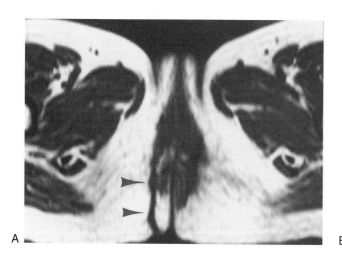

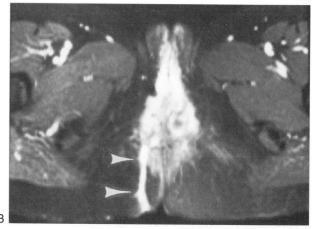

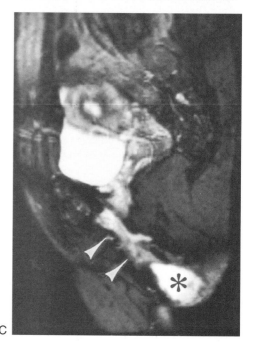

Figure 9.12 Vaginal fistula on MRI. (**A**) Transaxial T1-weighted (TR 600/TE 10) and (**B**) fat-suppressed T1-weighted with gadolinium (TR 748/TE 8) images shows a fistula (arrowheads) extending posteriorly from the right side of the vagina into the posterior soft tissues. (**C**) Sagittal fat-suppressed T2-weighted image (FSE TR 8,099/TE 90) shows the fistulous tract (arrowheads) extending from the vagina posteriorly and inferiorly to an abscess collection (asterisk). The cause of the fistula in this patient was unknown.

Figure 9.13 Vaginal angiomatosis. (**A & B**) CT scans show a nodular soft tissue mass (arrows) involving the left side of the vagina. Several phleboliths appear as punctate calcifications within the mass. The circular area of air density represents a vaginal tampon (t).

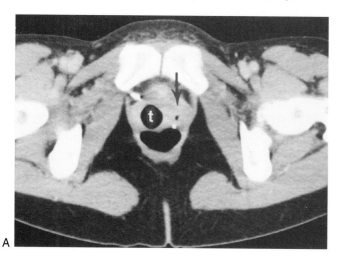

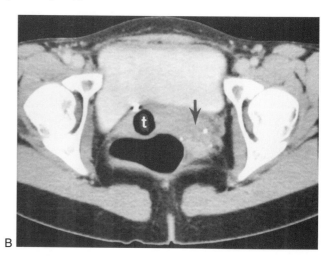

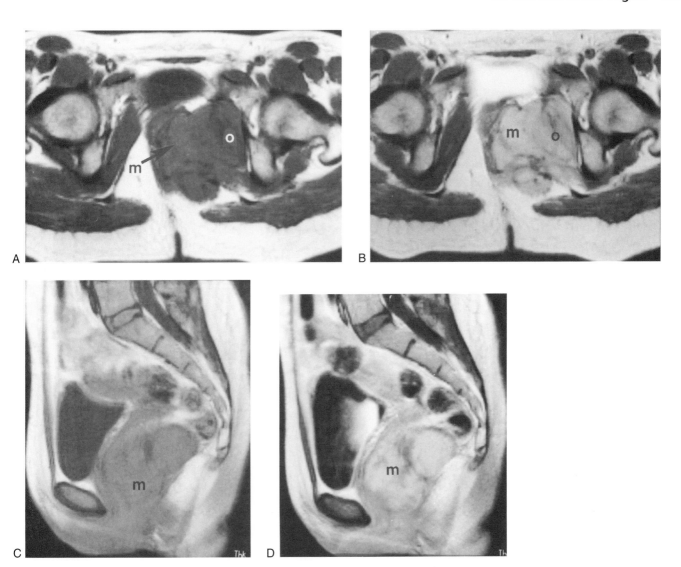

Figure 9.14 Vaginal fibromatosis. (**A & B**) Transaxial T1-weighted images (TR 630/TE 15) acquired before and after gadolinium injection show a large mass (m) involving the left side of the vagina, rectum, and obturator internus muscle (o). The mass shows marked enhancement on the postcontrast image (B). (**C & D**) Parasagittal T1-weighted images (TR 630/TE 15) obtained before and after contrast administration help delineate the size and extent of the tumor.

Primary vaginal malignant neoplasms are rare in adults, accounting for only 1% to 2% of all gynecologic malignancies.[16] Most of these (90%) are squamous cell carcinomas or primary adenocarcinoma (including clear cell carcinoma). Rarer forms of primary vaginal cancer include verrucous squamous cell carcinoma, primary melanoma, lymphoma, and hemangiopericytoma. The most common presenting complaints include a palpable or visible vaginal mass and/or bloody vaginal discharge. Clinically, these masses can block drainage of normal fluid from the cervical canal causing uterine dilatation. On CT (Fig. 9.15A&B) and MRI (Fig. 9.15C), primary vaginal neoplams can focally enlarge the vagina and cause distortion of the surrounding tissues. These masses typically enhance with intravenous contrast and appear bright on

T2-weighted images. Internal nonenhancing areas indicate regions of necrosis or cystic change. With MRI, vaginal masses can be evaluated in multiple planes (usually transaxial and sagittal), thereby improving detection and extent. Direct sagittal and coronal reconstructions can also be obtained with helical CT. Preliminary reports suggest that MRI is an accurate means of staging primary vaginal cancers.[17] The FIGO clinical stages of vaginal cancer are shown in Table 9.1.

Of the other primary vaginal cancers, clear cell adenocarcinoma deserves special mention. It is a rare tumor associated with in utero exposure to diethylstilbestrol (DES). The risk of developing this tumor for a woman exposed to DES is 1 per 1,000 up to the age of 34.[18] The most common clinical presentation is a bloody vaginal discharge followed by dyspar-

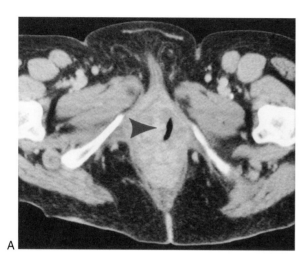

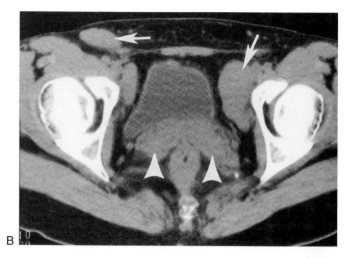

Figure 9.15 Malignant vaginal neoplasms. (**A**) Contrast-enhanced CT scan shows a heterogeneously enhancing vaginal mass that was found to be a primary vaginal carcinoma. Note that the vaginal introitus is shifted to the left by the mass. (**B**) Lymphomatous involvement of the vagina. A CT scan shows an abnormal bulky appearance of the vagina (arrowheads). Enlarged lymph nodes are also identified (white arrows) (**C**) Recurrent cervical carcinoma after hysterectomy. Sagittal proton density-weighted image (TR 2,500/TE 25) shows a mass involving the upper vagina (arrowhead) consistent with recurrent tumor.

eunia and leukorrhea.[18] Gilles et al.[19] described the MRI appearance of six cases of clear cell adenocarcinoma of the vagina. In this study, the tumor was best delineated after the insertion of a vaginal tampon and following the injection of intravenous Gd-DOTA. Clear cell adenocarcinoma showed evidence of gadolinium enhancement on T1-weighted images and increased signal intensity on T2-weighted images. The authors concluded that the signal characteristics of clear cell adenocarcinoma were similar enough to cervical carcinoma with infiltration of the vagina to make them indistinguishable.[19]

Direct invasion of the vagina by adjacent neoplasm (cervical, endometrial, ovarian, or rectal carcinoma) or by metastatic disease (melanoma, lymphoma, etc.) (Fig. 9.15B) is more common than primary vaginal carcinoma.[16] MRI has been shown to be highly accurate for demonstrating metastatic disease involving the vagina.[17]

The vagina is the most common site of recurrent gynecologic malignancy after hysterectomy.[20] Brown et al.[21] describe the MRI appearance of the vaginal cuff after hysterectomy. A normal vaginal cuff (no tumor recurrence) demonstrates a well-defined low signal intensity muscularis on T2-weighted

Table 9.1 1978 FIGO Staging of Primary Vaginal Cancer

Stage	Description
I	Limited to the vaginal wall
II	Involvement of the subadjacent tissues but not extending to the pelvic walls
III	Extends to one or both pelvic walls
IV	Tumor extending into the bladder or rectum or beyond the true pelvis

images (see Fig. 9.10B). Tumor recurrence at the vaginal cuff results in obliteration of the muscularis layer and increased signal intensity on T2-weighted images (Fig. 9.15C). A high signal intensity mass is often seen on T2-weighted images at the site of recurrence.

NEOPLASMS IN CHILDREN

Primary neoplasms of the vagina in children include embryonal rhabdomyosarcoma (Fig. 9.16) endodermal sinus tumor, and clear cell adenocarcinoma (associated with in utero exposure to DES).[4] Sarcoma botryoides, a variant of embryonal rhabdomyosarcoma, produces grape-like clusters that protrude from the vagina. It is generally seen before the age of 3 years.[4] Endodermal sinus tumor more frequently involves infants and is usually located in the posterior wall of the upper vagina.[4]

POSTSURGICAL AND TRAUMATIC CHANGES

CT and MRI are both excellent techniques for evaluating postoperative and traumatic changes including hematoma, lymphocele, and urinoma. Acute hemorrhage has a characteristic appearance on CT scans (high attenuation values), while subacute and chronic hemorrhage have characteristic features on MRI (bright signal intensity on T1-weighted images and dark signal on T2-weighted images, respectively). MRI angiographic techniques can be used to evaluate the vascular system.

Vaginal Hysterectomy

The number of vaginal hysterectomies has increased with the rise in laparoscopically assisted surgery. Hemorrhage occurs in up to 2.6 per 1,000 gynecologic laparoscopic procedures, with an overall serious complication rate of approximately 15.4 per

Figure 9.16 Rhabdomyosarcoma of the vagina. (**A & B**) CT scans in a child demonstrate a soft tissue mass (arrows) in the expected location of the vagina. Oral contrast is seen within the rectum. (**C & D**) Rhabdomyosarcoma in a different patient. Transaxial proton density-weighted (TR 2,000/TE 20) and T2-weighted (TR 2,000/TE 80) images show a high signal intensity mass (arrows) replacing the normal vagina.

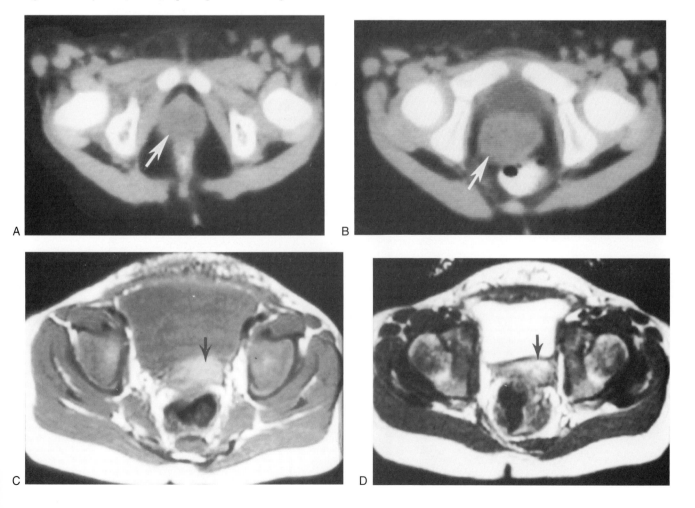

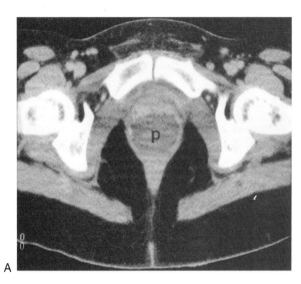

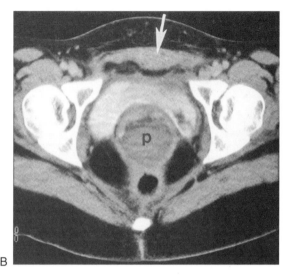

A   B

Figure 9.17 Posthysterectomy CT. (**A & B**) CT scans show a dilated vagina filled with fluid-soaked packing material (p) in a patient with persistent vaginal bleeding 48 hours after laparoscopic-assisted surgery. There is a left rectus abdominus muscle hemotoma (arrow) at the site of the laparoscopically puncture wound.

Figure 9.18 Vaginal colpopexy. (**A**) This CT scan shows the proximal end of a Gortex tube (black arrow) sewn onto the sacral periosteum. (**B**) At a more caudal level, the Gortex tube (white arrow) is suspended within the pelvis. (**C**) Sutures are noted (small arrows) at the vaginal fornices.

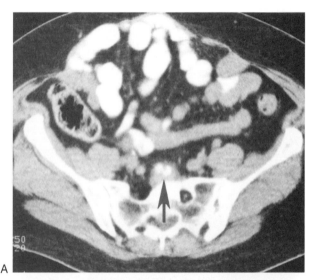

A

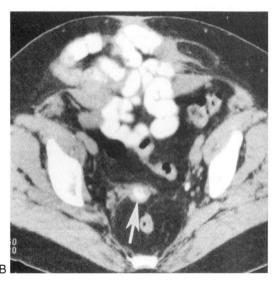

B

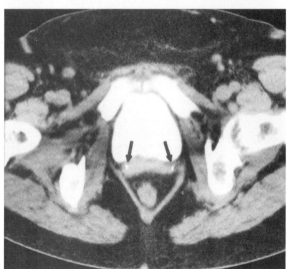

C

1,000 procedures.[22] After hysterectomy, the vagina is often filled with packing material (Fig. 9.17A&B).

Vaginal Vault Prolapse

Vaginal vault prolapse is a rare sequela to hysterectomy affecting approximately 900 to 1200 women per year in the United States.[23] Patients present with protrusion of the vagina, a feeling of increased pressure, difficulty walking, and impaired intercourse.[23] This condition can be treated with sacral colpopexy, whereby mesh is sutured to the superior vaginal remnant and brought through the periosteum to the anterior sacrum (Fig. 9.18).[24]

Neovagina

Vaginal reconstruction is performed after vaginectomy for cancer, trauma, or infection.[25] Several techniques are used including split-thickness skin grafts and myocutaneous pedicle flaps (from the gracilis or rectus abdominis muscles). Vaginal reconstructions can be imaged with either CT or MRI (Fig. 9.19).[26,27]

Trauma

Most traumatic vaginal injury occurs during vaginal delivery. On CT and MRI examinations, a vaginal laceration can appear as an air or fluid-filled tract extending from the vagina into the surrounding perineal fat (Fig. 9.20).

Foreign Bodies

The most common vaginal foreign body is the vaginal tampon, which appears as a column of air within the lower vagina on CT and MRI examinations (Fig. 9.21). Postsurgical packing material within the vagina can have a similar appearance, although the packing material may be fluid soaked and therefore have intermediate attenuation on CT scans (see Fig.

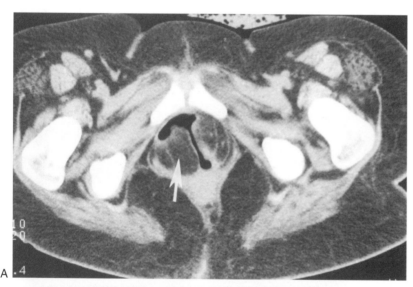

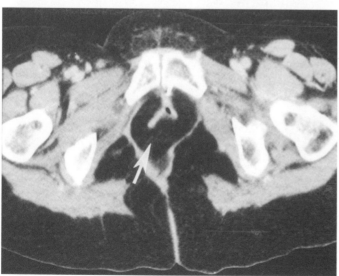

Figure 9.19 CT appearance of neovagina. (**A** & **B**) Vaginal reconstructions in two patients. Note the fat attenuation (arrow) within the neovagina. Air is present within the vaginal lumen.

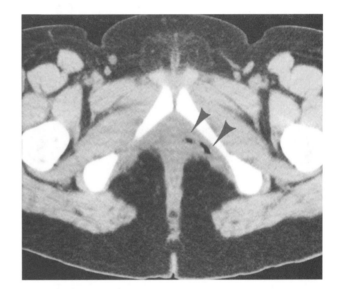

Figure 9.20 Vaginal trauma. This CT scan in a 25-year-old woman 2 days after vaginal delivery shows an air-filled tear (arrowheads) extending from the left vaginal sulcus into the adjacent soft tissues.

Figure 9.21 Vaginal tampon. (**A**) This CT scan shows a tampon (arrow) as a round area of air attenuation (black) within the vagina. (**B & C**) Transaxial T2-weighted (TR 2,640/TE 90) and sagittal T2-weighted (TR 2,500/TE 90) images show a tampon as a column of intravaginal air (signal void) (arrows).

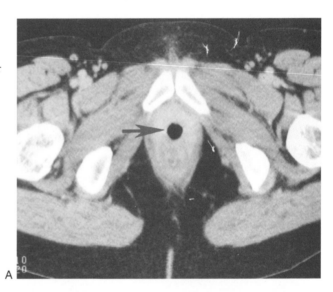

A

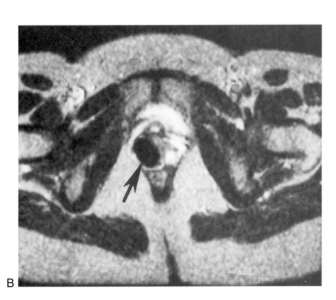

B

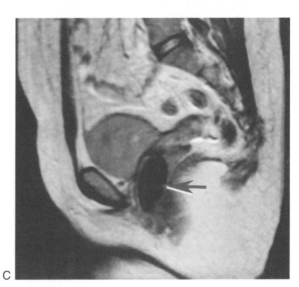

C

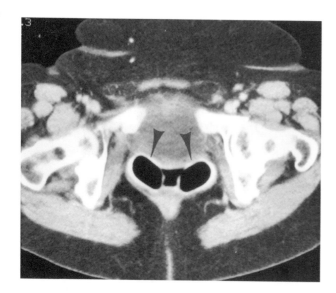

Figure 9.22 Pessary. This CT scan shows a thin high attenuation ring in the upper vagina representing a pessary (arrowheads).

9.17) and intermediate-to-bright signal intensity on T2-weighted MRIs.

Pessaries are also seen occasionally on CT scans and MRI. They typically have the appearance of a high attenuation ring in the upper vagina on CT scans (Fig. 9.22). They are less obvious on MRIs but may be visualized as a black ring at the level of the cervix.

Intravaginal catheters, used to drain pelvic fluid collections, can also be seen on CT and MRI. Figure 9.23 shows a drainage catheter extending from a pelvic abscess into the vagina. The catheter is seen as a small linear area of high at-

tenuation. Detection of catheters is usually difficult on MRIs. Fluid-filled catheters appear as tubular areas of bright signal intensity on T2-weighted images, while air-filled catheters produce a signal void on T1- and T2-weighted images.

REFERENCES

1. Hricak H, Chang YC, Thurnher S. Vagina: evaluation with MR imaging. Part I. Normal anatomy and congenital anomalies. Radiology 1988;169:169–174
2. Pellerito JS, McCarthy SM, Doyle MB et al. Diagnosis of uterine anomalies: relative accuracy of MR imaging, endovaginal sonography, and hysterosalpingography. Radiology 1992;183:795–800
3. Ramsey EM. Embryology and developmental defects of the female reproductive tract. In: Danforth DN, Scott JR, Eds. Obstetrics and Gynecology. JB Lippincott, Philadelphia, 1986 pp 78–105
4. Currarino G, Wood B, Majd M. Abnormalities of the genital tract. Section 2. Abnormalities of the female genital tract. In: Silverman FN, Kuhn JP, Eds. Caffey's Pediatric X-ray Diagnosis: An Integrated Imaging Approach (9th ed.). CV Mosby, St. Louis, 1993, pp 1384–1389
5. Mattingly RF, Thompson JD. Surgery for anomalies of the müllerian ducts. In: Mattingly RF, Thompson JD, Eds. Te Linde's Operative Gynecology (6th ed.). JB Lippincott, Philadelphia, 1985, pp 345–380
6. Togashi K, Nishimura K, Itoh K et al. Vaginal agenesis: classification by MR imaging. Radiology 1987;162:675–677
7. Vainwright JR, Jr, Fulp CJ, Jr, Schiebler ML. MR imaging of vaginal agenesis with hematocolpos. J Comput Assist Tomogr 1988;12:891–893

Figure 9.23 Vaginal drainage catheter. (**A**) This CT scan demonstrates the catheter tip (white arrow) looped within a pelvic fluid collection. (**B**) The distal end of the catheter passes through the vagina (arrow). A Foley catheter is present in the urethra.

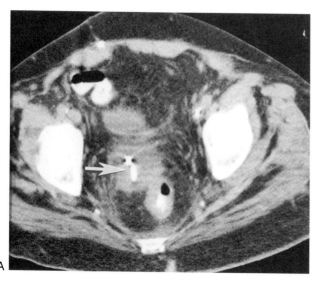
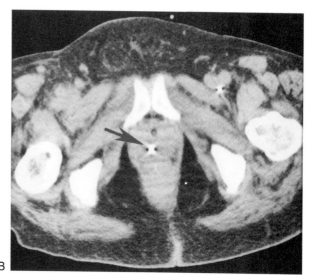

8. Lee JKT, McClennan BL, Stanley RJ, Sagel SS. Utility of computed tomography in the localization of the undescended testis. Radiology 1980;135:121–125

9. Kier R, McCarthy S, Rosenfield AT et al. Nonpalpable testes in young boys: evaluation with MR imaging. Radiology 1988; 169:429–433

10. Kaufman RH, Friedrich EG, Gardner HL. Benign Diseases of the Vulva and Vagina (3rd ed.). Yearbook Medical, Chicago, 1989, p 269

11. Kier R. Nonovarian gynecologic cysts: MR imaging findings. AJR Am J Roentgenol 1992;158:1265–1269

12. Kuhlman JE, Fishman EK. CT evaluation of enterovaginal and vesicovaginal fistulas. J Comput Assist Tomogr 1990;14: 390–394

13. Outwater E, Schiebler ML. Pelvic fistulas: findings on MR images. AJR Am J Roentgenol 1993;160:327–330

14. Myhr GE, Myrvold HE, Nilsen G, et al. Perianal fistulas: use of MR imaging for diagnosis. Radiology 1994;191:545–549

15. Zaino RJ, Robboy SJ, Bentley R, Kurman RJ. Diseases of the vagina. In: Kurman RJ, Ed. Blaustein's Pathology of the Female Genital Tract (4th ed.). Springer-Verlag, New York, 1994, pp 152–156

16. Cramer DW, Cutler SJ. Incidence and histopathology of malignancies of the female genital organs in the United States. Am J Obstet Gynecol 1974;118:443–460

17. Chang YC, Hricak H, Thurnher S, Lacey CG. Vagina: evaluation with MR imaging. Part II. Neoplasms. Radiology 1988; 169:175–179

18. Herbst AL, Anderson D. Clear cell adenocarcinoma of the vagina and cervix secondary to intrauterine exposure to diethylstilbestrol. Semin Surg Oncol 1990;6:343–346

19. Gilles R, Michel G, Chancelier MD et al. Case report: a clear cell adenocarcinoma of the vagina: MR features. Br J Radiol 1993;66:168–170

20. Morrow PC, Townsend DE. Tumors of the endometrium. In: Morrow PC, Townsend DE, Eds. Synopsis of Gynecologic Oncology (3rd ed.). Churchill Livingstone, New York, 1987, pp 159–205

21. Brown JJ, Gutierrez ED, Lee JKT. MR appearance of the normal and abnormal vagina after hysterectomy. AJR Am J Roentgenol 1992;158:95–99

22. Peterson HB, Hulka JF, Philips JM. American Association of Gynecologic Laparoscopists' 1988 membership survey in operative laparoscopy. J Repro Med 1990;35:587–589

23. Dunton CJ, Mikuta JS. Posthysterectomy vaginal vault prolapse. Postgrad Obstet Gynecol 1988;8:1

24. Timmons MC, Addison WA. Abdominal sacral colpopexy for management of vaginal vault prolapse. In: Baden WF, Walker T, Eds. Surgical Repair of Vaginal Defects. JB Lippincott, Philadelphia, 1992, pp 138–139

25. Burghardt E, Webb MJ, Monaghan JM et al. In: Burghardt E, Ed. Surgical Gynecologic Oncology. Thieme Medical, New York, 1993, p 663

26. Nichols DH, Randall CL. Vaginal Surgery (3rd ed.). Williams & Wilkins, Baltimore, Md, 1989, pp 415–416

27. Sadove RC, Horton CE. Utilizing full-thickness skin grafts for vaginal reconstruction. Clin Plast Surg 1988;15:443–438

Ultrasonography of the Cervix

RUDIGER OSMERS

Although the cervix can be easily seen by visual inspection, its various appearances are worth demonstrating on ultrasound, as it is incidentally imaged on all abdominal and transvaginal scans.

NORMAL ANATOMY OF THE NONPREGNANT CERVIX

Imaging the cervix is often more difficult than imaging of the corpus, due to artifacts caused by proximity of the transducer to the cervix. Drawing the probe back a little from the cervix often moves it into the focal zone. When the cervix is demonstrated sonographically, the internal and external os should be included in the image (Fig. 10.1). The fibrous part of the cervix uteri is of intermediate echo texture. The cervix changes in appearance during the menstrual cycle. During menstruation, a hypoechoic area due to blood may be seen (Fig. 10.2). The appearance of the cervix does not change until the midfollicular phase. Initially, the anterior and posterior walls are adjacent, appearing as an echogenic line. Around the time of ovulation, the cervical canal is of reduced echogenicity, due to mucus accumulation in the canal (Fig. 10.3). This reaches a maximum thickness of 5 mm by ovulation and disappears by the second postovulatory day. These changes are seen in spontaneous cycles and in women on hormone replacement therapy (HRT).[1] In some women, there is no preovulatory transformation of the ectocervix (no cervical plug is seen), although serum estradiol levels are normal.

In many patients on long-term oral contraceptives, there is a typical ultrasound appearance of the cervix. In response to progestagenic stimulation, a narrow anechoic strip of mucus is seen in the canal. This is associated with a symmetrically thickened echogenic mucosal layer adjacent to a broad hypoechoic submucosal layer (Fig. 10.4). Similar changes are described in microglandular endocervical hyperplasia (MEH). This benign condition occurs in women on oral contraceptives or in pregnant and older postpartum patients.[2–4] Persistence of MEH for a long time after contraceptive usage or pregnancy suggests that increased hormones are needed for its induction but not for its maintenance.[3] However, several cases are recorded in which there was no hormonal association.[4,5]

After menopause, the mucosa of the cervix in women not on HRT appears as a 1 to 2 mm echoic layer with a small hypoechoic submucosal layer. In postmenopausal women on HRT, there is thickening of both the cervical mucosa and the hypoechoic submucous layer.

BENIGN DISEASES OF THE CERVIX

Most polyps are of increased echogenicity (Fig. 10.5), but some can be of reduced echogenicity (Fig. 10.6 and Plate 10.1) Occasionally, they occupy a cavity in the stroma of the cervical wall. In that case, they may not prolapse into the canal and can be difficult to see (Fig. 10.7).

Cervical fibroids are rare and account for only 8% of uterine myomas. They vary considerably in appearance. Some are echogenic (Figs. 10.8 and 10.9) while necrotizing fibroids have hypoechoic or anechoic areas. Those with rapid growth and good vascularization appear homogenously hypoechoic (Fig. 10.10 and Plate 10.2)

Nabothian cysts are common in the cervix. They form when the mouth of an endocervical gland becomes occluded by the proliferating surface squamous epithelium (Fig. 10.11). They range up to about 3 cm in size. Epithelial inclusion cysts are similar in appearance. They are solitary and unilocular and measure 1 to 2 cm in diameter. Both nabothian and epithelial inclusion cysts are anechoic round cysts adjacent to the epithelium of the ectocervix or the cervical canal.

Mesonephric remnant cysts are found in about 1% of cervices[6] (Fig. 10.12). Very rarely, an endometriotic cyst is seen (Fig. 10.13), which, as in the myometrium, has homogenous contents. Occasionally, endometriotic cysts in the cervical stroma or myometrium are surrounded by an echogenic capsule due to fibrosis.

Other benign cervical tumors that are rarely reported by ultrasound include an extensive multicystic mass described as adenoma malignum of the cervix,[7] hemangioma,[8] and cervical pheochromocytoma.[9] A hematocervix can occur rarely after the external os becomes occluded, usually secondary to surgery. It is unknown why these patients do not develop a hematometra (Fig. 10.14). It can be difficult to differentiate clinically between a hematocervix and a partial hematocolpos in the case of an occluded vagina.

SONOGRAPHY IN THE PATIENT WITH A POSITIVE SMEAR

Suren and co-workers[10] carried out a clinical examination and transvaginal scan on 215 women with a positive cervical smear, suggestive clinical findings, or a known cervical cancer. Ultrasound appearances and clinical pelvic examination were correlated with staging after further investigation—cystoscopy, sigmoidoscopy, computed tomography, and cone biopsy—when necessary. Any echogenic, asymmetrically thickened cervical mucosa distinct from the normal cervical storma was regarded as a possible proliferative process and considered suggestive. In a group of 54 patients with clinically and sonographically normal cervices in whom cone biopsy was performed due to positive cytology, histology revealed cervical intraepithelial neoplasia (CIN) 0–2 in 26 cases and CIN 3 in 19 cases (where CIN 0 includes normal histology, inflammatory atypia, squamous atypia, and human papillomavirus atypia on cytology). Overall, in 22 of 41 cases with CIN 3, ultrasound appearances were suggestive (Table 10.1). Of invasive cancers, 33% of stage I, 14% of stage II, and 6% of stage III were not detected clinically. All of these patients had changes in cervical appearance on transvaginal sonography (TVS).[10] On the other hand, four cases of stage Ia, three cases of stage Ib, and two cases of stage IIa were not detected on TVS (Table 10.1). Only three cervical cancers (stage Ia) were not detected by either palpation or sonography (Table 10.2). Examples of CIN 3 and early stage I cervical carcinomas are shown in Figures 10.15 to 10.18.

Degenhardt and co-workers[11] reported 35 women with a suspicious ultrasound appearance of the cervix and 21 with ultrasonically normal cervices. Of those with ultrasonically suspicious cervices, histology revealed 8 with CIN 1–2 lesions, 16 with CIN 3 lesions, 6 invasive cancers, and 5 false-positives (Fig. 10.19). Of those with ultrasonically normal cervices, there were 10 CIN 1–3 lesions and 1 early invasive cancer. The sensitivity was 30.8% and specificity 59% in detecting cervical lesions after a suggestive smear. The authors concluded that the application of vaginal ultrasound was limited in the detection of preinvasive cancer of the cervix.

Because of its low sensitivity and specificity, (TVS) is not the most appropriate method to detect early cervical cancer, but combined with cytology, it may contribute to staging and management of the patient.

SONOGRAPHY IN THE PATIENT WITH CERVICAL CANCER

Development of transvaginal and transrectal high-resolution probes allows classification and localization of a tumor, its size, and extension onto the pelvic side wall or adjacent organs.[12–28] Transvaginal and transrectal sonography may be helpful in staging cervical cancer.[19,20,29,30] The transrectal transducer is further from the cervix and less affected by near-field artifacts.

When cancer produces morphologic change it alters the sonographic appearance of the cervix. Heterogeneous areas are often seen (Fig. 10.20 and Plate 10.3). If the epithelium is involved, the bright reflection line of the cervical canal is interrupted or not seen. Most cervical tumors are predominantly hypoechoic, although hyperechoic masses have also been reported, especially in the early stages.[10,26] Tumor infiltration into the cervical wall, vagina, and the parametrium can be evaluated by transvaginal and transrectal ultrasound.[19,20,29,30] If the tumor extends to the parametrium, the mainly hypoechoic tumor can be seen as irregularly protruding, solid masses (Fig. 10.21). Larger abscess cavities, due to necrosis, frequently are of increased echogenicity, provided there are no bacteria forming gas. Infiltration into the urinary bladder can be seen by both TVS and transabdominal sonography (Fig. 10.22).

Preoperative detection of parametrial involvement is difficult, as differentiation between malignancy and inflammation is not possible.[31–36] In some cases, ultrasound-guided biopsies from the parametrium are helpful.[37,38] For the detection of pelvic and para-aortic lymph node spread, CT or magnetic resonance imaging are more suitable modalities than ultrasound.[39–43]

Sonography is preferred for detecting urinary obstruction and for excluding recurrence. Transrectal sonography can be useful for the patient with a stenosed vagina secondary to surgical or radiation changes.[44–47] Recurrent disease appears as a hypoechoic mass in the pelvis. In some cases, color Doppler can be helpful to differentiate recurrence from fibrous scars in the pelvis.

The advantage of adding color Doppler to B-mode is being investigated. Some authors have described differences in blood flow between patients with cervical malignancy and healthy women.[48–50] Breyer and co-workers[50] were not able to visualize cervical blood flow in 17% of either healthy women or those with cervical cancer. They found a lower resistance index and pulsatility index in cervical malignancies than in normal cervices but no difference in the peak-systolic velocity.[50] In our experience, color Doppler is only helpful in selected cases. Increased vascularity with a loss of cervical architecture can be another clue to the diagnosis of cervical malignancy or recurrence (Fig. 10.23 and Plate 10.4) Further investigations are required to clarify whether color Doppler is useful for the diagnosis of cervical disease.

SUMMARY

TVS permits detailed evaluation of the cervix and demonstration of the surrounding tissues. It may be helpful in the assessment of clinically apparent masses.

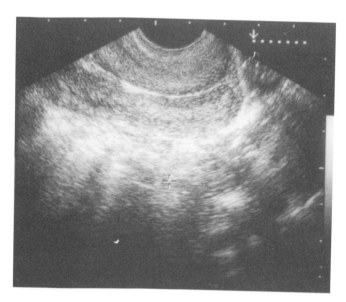

Figure 10.1 Longitudinal scan of the cervix. The external and internal os are included in this image.

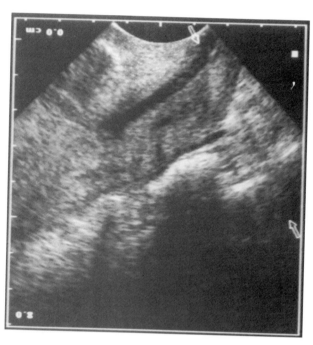

Figure 10.2 A hypoechoic area in the cervical canal due to menstruation.

Figure 10.3 Midcycle mucus produces a hypoechoic area in the canal. This vanishes by the second postovulatory day when the cervix appears closed again.

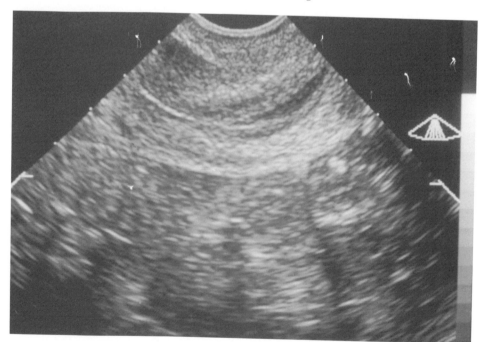

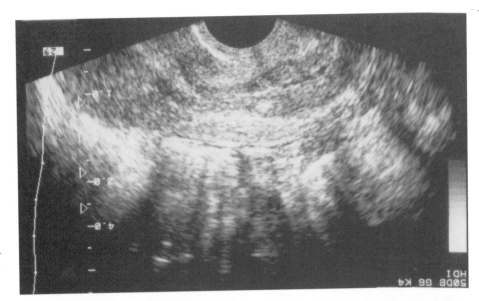

Figure 10.4 The mucosal layers in the cervical canal are hypoechoic and thickened in a patient on long-term oral contraceptives.

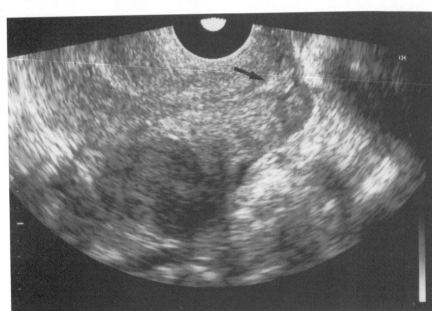

Figure 10.5 This polyp at the external os is hyperechoic (arrow) (see also Plate 10.1).

Figure 10.6 A large hypoechoic cervical polyp (arrow) (see also Plate 10.1).

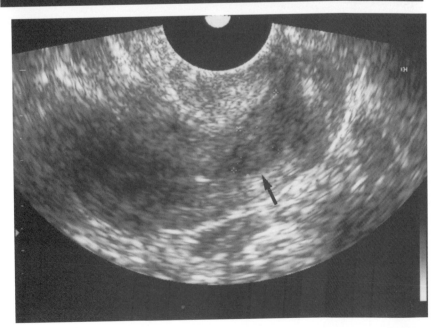

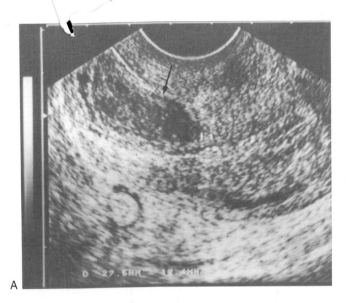

A

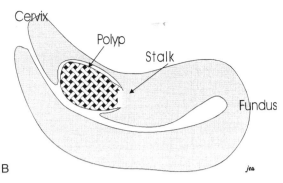

B

Figure 10.7 (**A**) A large hypoechonic intracervical polyp (arrow) in the posterior wall of a retroverted uterus. The polyp did not prolapse into the canal and is difficult to see. (**B**) Diagram of the polyp as found in the gross specimen. (Courtesy of Dr. J. Schmidt, Sydney, Australia).

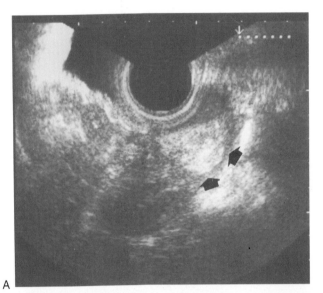

A

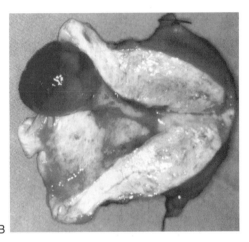

B

Figure 10.8 (**A**) A hyperechoic fibroid in the cervix (arrows). (**B**) The gross specimen shows a pedunculated fibroid from the uterine cavity.

Figure 10.9 This hyperechoic cervical myoma (arrows) has caused a small amount of fluid to collect in the uterus.

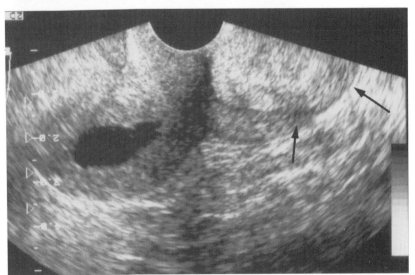

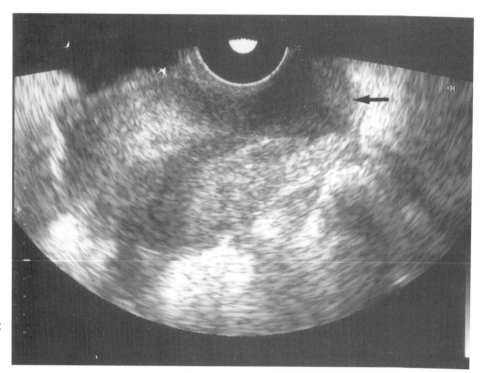

Figure 10.10 Hypoechoic fast growing pedunculated fibroid in the cervix (arrow) (see also Plate 10.2).

Figure 10.11 An anteverted uterus with a nabothian cyst ("follicle").

Figure 10.12 This mesonephric remnant cyst is in the cervical stroma and appears similar to a nabothian cyst.

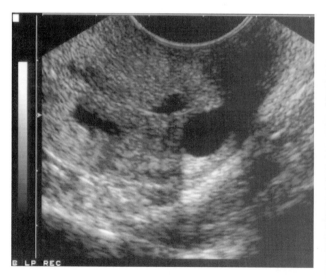

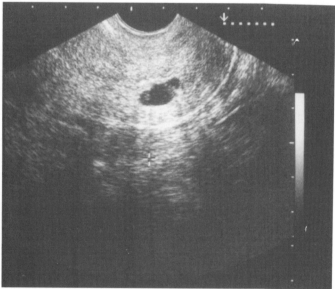

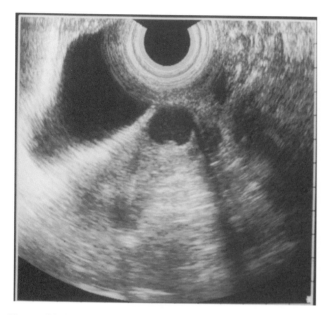

Figure 10.13 This cyst with a tiny solid component deep in the cervical stroma proved to be an endometrioma.

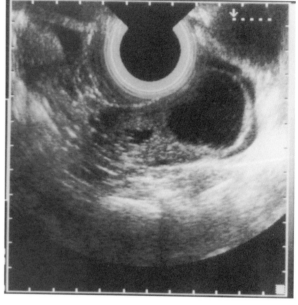

Figure 10.14 A rare case of hematocervix. The uterine cavity shows only a small hematometra. Two years previously, the patient had a cone biopsy.

Table 10.1 Comparison of Pathologic Staging and TVS Evaluation of the Cervix Uteri

Histology	TVS Appearance	
	Normal	Suspicious
CIN 0	13	0
CIN 1	3	1
CIN 2	10	4
CIN 3	19	22
Stage Ia	4	7
Ib	3	40
II	—	3
IIa	2	21
IIb	—	27
III	—	10
IIIa	—	21
IIIb	—	1
IV	—	4
Total (N = 215)	54	161

Table 10.2 Comparison of Palpation and Sonographic Evaluation of the Cervix Uteri

Clinical Examination	TVS of the Cervix	
	Not Suggestive (Cancers)	Suggestive (Cancers)
Not suggestive (cancers)	47 (3)	55 (27)
Suggestive (cancers)	7 (6)	106 (106)
Total (N = 215)	54 (9)	161 (133)

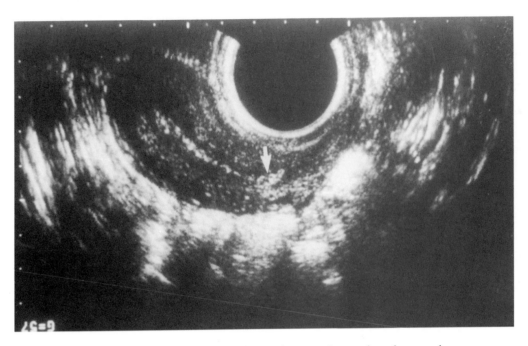

Figure 10.15 Sagittal scan of the uterus with a hyperechoic area distinct from the normal cervical stroma (white arrow). The patient had carcinoma in situ.

Figure 10.16 Sagittal scan of the uterus with a small hyperechoic zone adjacent to the external os of the cervical canal. The patient had carcinoma in situ (arrow).

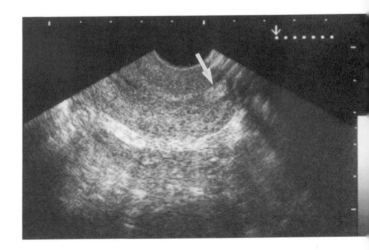

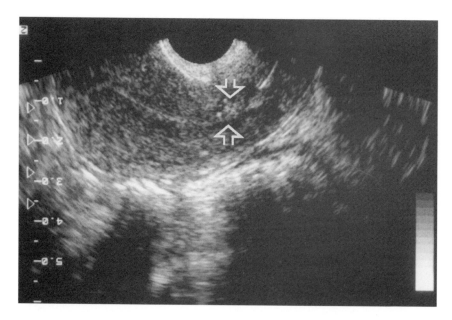

Figure 10.17 Sagittal scan of the uterus with a stage Ia carcinoma (open arrows).

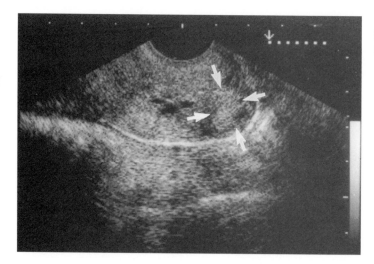

Figure 10.18 Sagittal scan of a small stage Ib cervical cancer (white arrows).

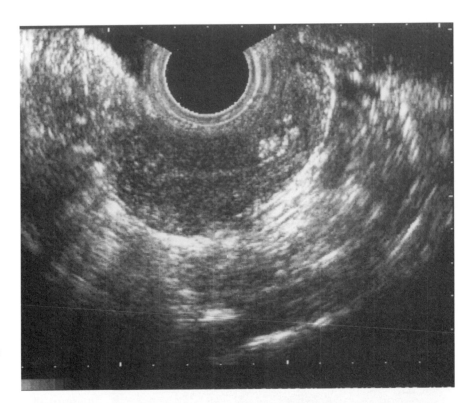

Figure 10.19 A hyperechoic area adjacent to the cervical mucosa gives a false positive appearance for cervical neoplasia. Notice the short distance to the mucosa. It is a small scar after several insertions of an intrauterine contraceptive device.

Figure 10.20 A sagittal scan shows a large hypoechoic cervical cancer (see also Plate 10.3).

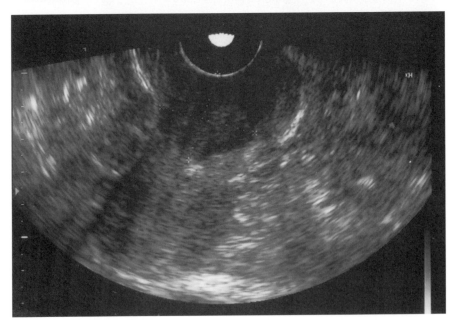

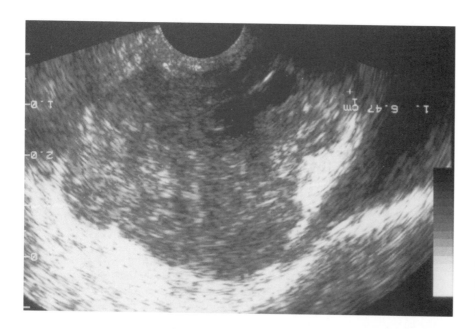

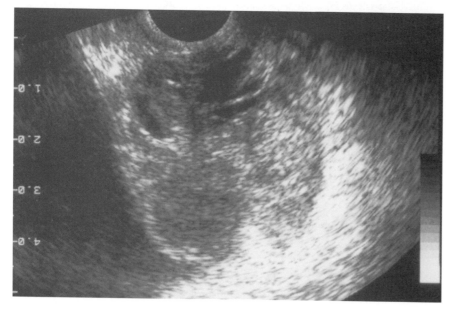

Figure 10.21 This scan shows irregularly protruding hypogenic tumor masses infiltrating the parametrium in a case of cervical cancer.

Figure 10.22 Cervical cancer infiltrating the wall of the urinary bladder.

Figure 10.23 A large cervical carcinoma in a longitudinal scan of the uterus. The irregular tumor is difficult to define from the surrounding tissue (see also Plate 10.4).

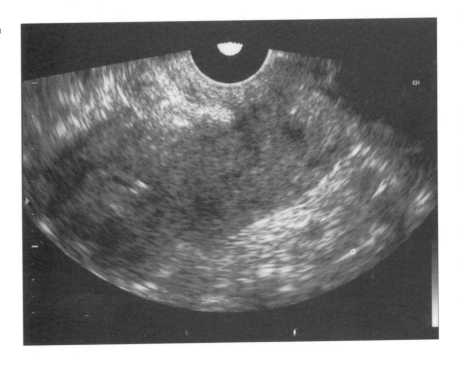

REFERENCES

1. Eppel W, Schurz B, Knogler W. Sonographische Darstellung funktioneller Zervixveranderungen im Rahmen der Sterilitatsabklarung. In: Hansmann M, Koischwitz D, Lutz H, Trier HG, Eds. Ultraschalldiagnostik 86. Springer-Verlag, Berlin, 1987, pp 306–308

2. Candy J, Abell MR. Progestogen-induced adenomatous hyperplasia of the uterine cervix. JAMA 1968;203:323–326

3. Nicols TM, Fidler HK. Microglandular hyperplasia in cervical cone biopsies taken for suspicious and positive cytology. Am J Clin Pathol 1971;56:424–429

4. Wilkinson E, Dufour DR. Pathogenesis of microglandular hyperplasia of the cervix uteri. Obstet Gynecol 1976;47:189–195

5. Tsukada Y, Piver MS, Barlow JT. Microglandular hyperplasia of the endocervix following long-term estrogen treatment. Am J Obstet Gynecol 1977;127:888–889

6. Scherrick JC, Vega JG. Congenital intramural cysts of the uterus. Obstet Gynecol 1962;19:486–495

7. Tsuruchi N, Tsukamoto N, Kaku T et al. Adenoma malignum of the uterine cervix detected by imaging methods in a patient with Peutz-Jeghers syndrome. Gynecol Oncol 1994;54:232–236

8. Hawes DR, Hemann LS, Cornell AE, Yuh WT. Hemangioma of the uterine cervix: sonographic and MR diagnosis. J Comput Assist Tomogr 1991;15:152–154

9. Becker G, Jockenhovel F, Bauer R et al. Cervical pheochromocytoma: a rare localization and a difficult diagnosis. J Endocrinol Invest 1991;15:767–770

10. Suren A, Dietrich M, Osmers M, Osmers R. Transvaginal sonography in patients with pathological cervical exfoliative cytology or histologically verified cervical carcinoma. Int J Gynecol Obstet 1994;47:141–145

11. Degenhardt F, Bohmer S, Schneider J. Vaginal ultrasound follow-up of suspicious smears of the cervix uteri. Ultraschall Med 1991;12:139–142

12. Suren A, Puchta J, Osmers R. Sonographic evaluation of the cervix uteri. In: Osmers R, Kurjak A, Eds. Ultrasound and the Uteri. Parthenon, London, 1995, pp 13–18

13. Innocenti P, Pulli F, Savino L et al. Staging of cervical cancer: reliability of transrectal US. Radiology 1992;185:201–205

14. Artner A, Bosze P, Gonda G. The value of ultrasound in preoperative assessment of the myometrial and cervical invasion in endometrial carcinoma. Gynecol Oncol 1994;54:147–151

15. Barrilot I, Horiot JC, Maingon P et al. Maximum and mean bladder dose defined from ultrasonography. Comparison with ICRU reference in gynecological brachytherapy. Radiother Oncol 1994;30:231–238

16. Belloso RM, Miquilarena RE, Ayala LA et al. Carcinoma of the colon metastatic to the cervix uteri. Review of unusual metastases and report of one case. GEN (Venezuela) Jan–Mar 1990;44:63–66

17. Besson P, Constant M, Besson-Proye F. Transvaginal echography in gynecologic oncology. Ann Radiol Paris 1993;32: 435–440

18. Bidzinski M, Lemieszczuk B. The value of transvaginal ultrasonography (TVS) in the assessment of myometrial and cervical invasion in corpus uterine neoplasma. Eur J Gynaecol 1993; 14:86–91

19. Carter J, Carson LF, Elg S et al. Transvaginal sonography as an aid in the clinical staging of carcinoma of the cervix. J Clin Ultrasound 1992;20:283–287

20. Cobby M, Browning J, Jones A et al. Magnetic resonance imaging, computed tomography and endosonography in the local staging of the carcinoma of the cervix. Br J Radiol 1990; 63:673–679

21. Genolet PM, Hanggi W, Dreher E. Evaluation of tumor extension in invasive cancer of the uterine cervix. Diagnostic evaluation of cervix cancer. Gynakol Geburtshilfliche Rundsch 1993; 33:180–184

22. Gitsch G, Deutinger J, Bernaschek G. The diagnostic value of rectal ultrasound in the assessment of parametrial infiltration of cervix cancer. Geburtshilfe Frauenheilkd 1992;52:412–414

23. Kochi T, Akamatsu N, Sekiba K. Ultrasonic assessment of efficacy of radiotherapy in cases of carcinoma of the cervix uteri by using rectosonography. Eur J Gynaecol Oncol 1989;10:367–378

24. Levenback C, Dershaw DD, Rubin SC. Endoluminal ultrasound staging of cervical cancer. Gynecol Oncol 1992;46:186–190

25. Magee BJ, Logue JP, Swindell R, McHugh D. Tumour size as a prognostic factor in carcinoma of the cervix: assessment by transrectal ultrasound. Br J Radiol 1991;64:812–815

26. Osmers R, Bergholz M, Kuhn W. Vaginal sonographic visualization of a cervical carcinoma. Int J Gynecol Obstet 1989; 28:283–285

27. Prefontaine M, Demianczuk N. Vaginal probe ultrasound in malignancy involving the uterine cervix. Eur J Gynaecol Oncol 1993;14:455–460

28. Soyer P, Michel G, Masselot J. Imaging of cancer of the uterine cervix. J Radiol 1990;71:681–689

29. Bernaschek G, Deutinger J, Bartl W, Janisch H. Endosonographic staging of carcinoma of the uterine cervix. Arch Gynecol 1986;239:21–26

30. Yuhara A, Akamatsu N, Sekiba K. Use of transrectal radial scan ultrasonography in evaluating the extent of uterine cervical cancer. J Clin Ultrasound 1987;15:507–517

31. Bernadino ME, Dodd GD. Imaging of the pelvic contents in the female oncologic patient. Cancer 1981;48:504–510

32. Fleischer AC, Walsh JW, Jones HW, 3d et al. Sonographic evaluation of pelvic masses: method of examination and role of sonography relative to other imaging modalities. Radiol Clin North Am 1982;20:397–412

33. Hansmann M. Pathologie des Genitales. In: Hansmann MB, Hackeloer BJ, Staudach A, Eds. Ultraschalldiagnostik in Geburtshilfe und Gynakologie. Lehrbuch und Atlas, Springer, Berlin, 1985, pp 367–384

34. Kurtz AB, Rubin CS, Kramer FL Goldberg BB. Ultrasound evaluation of the posterior pelvic compartment. Radiology 1979; 132:677–682

35. Sanders RC. Ultrasound in pelvic malignancy. In: Steel WB, Cochrane WJ, Eds. Gynecologic Ultrasound. Churchill Livingstone, New York, 1991, pp 215–231

36. Gitsch G, Deutinger J, Reinthaller A et al. Effect of inflammatory stromal reaction on the value of rectal sonography in assessment of parametrial infiltration of cervix cancer. Gynakol Gerburtshilfliche Rundsch 1992;32:133

37. Bernaschek G, Janisch H. Method for recording the parametrial situation in cases of carcinoma of the cervix uteri. Geburtshilfe Frauenheilkd 1983;43:498–500

38. Lemieszczuk B, Bidzinski M, Zielinski J, Sikorowa L. Clinical value of transvaginal, sonographically guided fine needle aspiration biopsy of parametria in recurrent cervical carcinoma. Eur J Gynaecol Oncol 1993;14:68–76

39. Bruneton JN, Merran D, Balu-Maestro C et al. Echography and computed tomography in the evaluation and follow-up of uterine cancers. Bull Cancer 1990;77:689–694

40. Chen JT, Yamashiro T, Shimizu Y et al. Comparison of ultrasound and computed tomography (CT) for the diagnosis of paraaortic lymph node metastases in patients with gynecologic malignancies. Nippon Sanka Fujinka Gakkai Zasshi 1989;41:55–60

41. Heller PB, Maletano JH, Bundy BN et al. Clinical-pathologic study of stage IIB, III and IVA carcinoma of the cervix: extended diagnostic evaluation for paraaortic node metastasis—a Gynecologic Oncology Group study. Gynecol Oncol 1990;38: 425–430

42. Scheidler J, Heuck A, Reiser M. MR tomography in staging of carcinoma of the uterus. Radiologe 1994;34:377–383

43. Wu N. Computed tomography and ultrasonography of lymphoma involving urogenital systems. Chung Hua Chung Liu Tsa Chih 1990;12:383–388

44. Bernaschek G, Tatra G, Janisch H. Rectal sonography—an expansion of the diagnosis of recurrent cervical neoplasms. Geburtshilfe Frauenheilkd 1984;44:495–497

45. Giovannini M, Rosello R, Seitz JF et al. Intrarectal echography in the evaluation of locoregional extension of female genital cancers. Presse Med 1989;18:128–129

46. Meanwell CA, Rolfe EB, Blackledge G et al. Recurrent female pelvic cancer: assessment with transrectal ultrasonography. Radiology 1987;162:278–281.

47. Squillaci E, Salzani MC, Grandinetti ML et al. Recurrence of ovarian and uterine neoplasms: diagnosis with transrectal US. Radiology 1988;169:355–358

48. Kurjak A, Zalud I, Jurkovic D et al. Transvaginal color Doppler for the assessment of pelvic circulation. Acta Obstet Gynecol Scand 1989;68:131–135

49. Zalud I, Kurjak A. The assessment of luteal blood flow in pregnant and non-pregnant women by transvaginal color Doppler. J Perinat Med 1990;18:215–221

50. Breyer B, Despot A, Kurjak A. Blood flow in malignancy of the uterine cervix. In: Kurjak A. An Atlas of Transvaginal Color Doppler. The Current State of the Art. Parthenon, London, 1994, pp 329–333

Computed Tomography and Magnetic Resonance Imaging of the Cervix

E. MALCOLM SYMONDS

IAN R. JOHNSON

ANATOMY

The cervix is divided into an upper, supravaginal portion and a lower vaginal portion. The vaginal skin consists of stratified squamous epithelium and covers the cervix up to the squamocolumnar junction.

The cervix does not undergo cyclic changes. It is cylindric in shape and varies with parity and pregnancy. In pregnancy, it increases in size and vascularity and becomes more edematous. The canal is fusiform in shape and is generally flattened from front to back. The cervix lies between the bladder and the rectum and is supported by the cardinal and uterosacral ligaments and the pubocervical fascia. The ligaments supporting the cervix consist of fibrous tissue with some smooth muscle, nerves, blood vessels, and lymphatics. The histologic differences are reflected in the response to magnetic resonance imaging (MRI) and are therefore important in any description of appearances.

The ectocervix is covered with stratified squamous epithelium, but this changes at the squamocolumnar junction, where it becomes columnar. The glandular appearance of the endocervix is due to longitudinal folds in the canal (Fig. 11.1).

The blood supply to the cervix arises from the cervicovaginal branch of the uterine artery, the uterine artery, and the vaginal artery. The cervicovaginal branch leaves the uterine artery at the level of the internal os and descends to the lateral margin of the cervix. There is a rich anastomosis between all three arteries. The terminal vessels consist of freely anastomosing vessels in the stroma, a zone of vessels running perpendicularly toward the epithelium, a palisade zone terminating near the epithelium, and a basal plexus of terminal capillaries in the subepithelial tissues. Lymphatic drainage occurs to lymph nodes along the external and internal iliac vessel and finally to the common iliac nodes.

MRI OF THE NORMAL CERVIX

The uterus is easy to distinguish from surrounding structures, although the signal intensity from both uterus and cervix is intermediate and uniform regardless of whether T1 or T2 elements are dominant. The bowel and bladder are distinctive. Gas in the rectum and urine in the bladder have low signal intensity, whereas pelvic fat has a high intensity both on T1- and T2-weighted sequences (Fig. 11.2).

The uterine body has an outer serosal layer, a muscular middle layer, and an internal endometrial lining. The cervix is lined with mucous epithelium. With long T2-weighted sequences, the cervix and the corpus uteri have a very distinctive phenomenon specific to MRI. There is an inner band of low signal intensity—a "black" nonresonant band that runs into the cervix as far as the external os. This low-intensity band is still apparent on T1-weighted sequences, although less pronounced because of the relative low-intensity of the outer zone of the cervix or myometrium. Short-term inversion recovery sequences (STIR) enhance the appearance of the low resonant band because it enhances the appearance of the endometrium and the outer part of the myometrium. Thus, the cervix can be clearly seen. The endocervical epithelium is distinct from the substance of the cervix and is separated from it by the nonresonant band. The cervical canal can be measured in its length and shape, and the internal and external os clearly defined. The best views of the cervix are obtained from sagittal sections. The cervix shows little change throughout the menstrual cycle, but approaching menstruation, there is some dilatation of the canal and some increase in signal intensity. The cervix in the postmenopausal woman decreases in size. Whereas the low-intensity band tends to disappear from the body of the uterus, it can still be seen in the cervix.

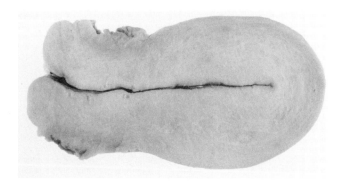

Figure 11.1 Sagittal section through the cervix and corpus uteri removed at hysterectomy shows the structure of the cervical canal and the ectocervix. The cervix is on the left, and the fundus of the uterus is on the right. (Courtesy of Dr. Jane Johnson, Nottingham, England.)

Figure 11.2 Sagittal MRI of a normal pelvis. The uterus is visible between bladder and bowel. The myometrium has intermediate density, but the endometrium and endocervical endothelium in this sequence have a harsh white appearance. The nonresonant band external to the endometrium can be seen to extend into the cervix.

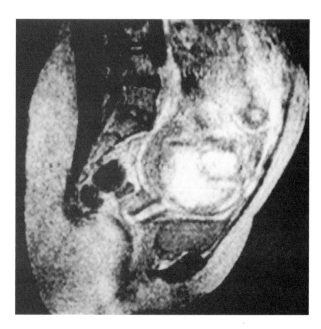

Figure 11.3 The trilaminar structure of the cervix is seen in pregnancy in this MRI. The fetal brain is apposed to the internal os.

Figure 11.4 An MRI demonstrating central placenta previa. The placenta can be seen on both anterior and posterior uterine walls. The internal cervical os is covered by the placenta.

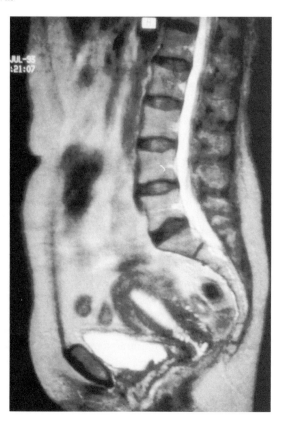

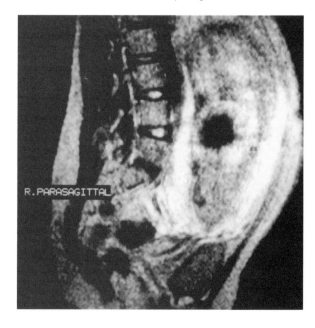

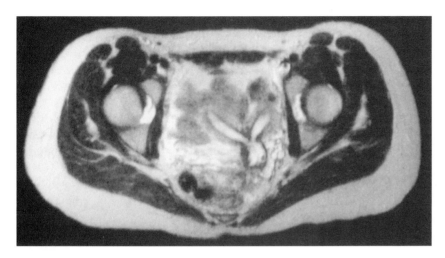

Figure 11.5 Transverse MRI image midpelvis in uterus bicornis unicollis. The uterine cavities can be seen merging into the single cervical canal.

The Cervix in Pregnancy

The features of the cervix become even more prominent in the first trimester as the cervix enlarges (Fig. 11.3). There is a distinctive trilaminar structure, which can be seen until cervical effacement occurs. High intensity in the center of the cervix reflects the mucus and mucus-secreting epithelium. The trilaminar configuration of the cervix allows identification of the internal and external os and therefore accurate localization of the placenta with MRI (Fig. 11.4). Apparent migration of the placenta in relation to the internal cervical os has been demonstrated.[1] This occurs only where the placenta previa is marginal.

BENIGN CONDITIONS OF THE CERVIX

Fibroids of the cervix have similar imaging characteristics to normal myometrium. Congenital abnormalities of the cervix can also be identified (Fig. 11.5). MRI is not used to identify cervical polyps, but they are occasionally seen during examinations for other purposes (Fig. 11.6).

On computed tomography (CT), the cervix is homogenous and separate from the parametrium. Identification of the cervix and surrounding structures is easier if a vaginal tampon is inserted. CT has potential in evaluating carcinoma of the cervix but is not appropriate for investigating benign conditions.

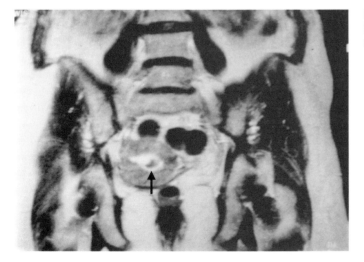

Figure 11.6 Coronal MRI section of pelvis. A small polyp can be seen protruding into the lower part of the uterine cavity near the internal cervical os.

THE EVALUATION OF CERVICAL INCOMPETENCE

MRI produces high-quality images of the cervix. It is therefore surprising that so little published work has appeared on the assessment of cervical incompetence by MRI. In one large and definitive study, 41 volunteers were investigated prospectively in random order.[2] Twenty had normal cervices, 11 were known to have cervical incompetence, and 10 had small cervices related to the maternal ingestion of diethylstilbestrol (DES) during pregnancy. The length of the canal was the same in both the normal and the incompetent cervices. However, the internal os was wider in the incompetent cervix group (4.5 mm) than in the normal group (3.3 mm). In the group exposed to DES, the canal was shorter (22.9 mm) than in normal women (33.0 mm).

CARCINOMA OF THE CERVIX

Two features are required of any imaging in relation to carcinoma of the cervix. First, the technique should identify the extent and volume of local tumor invasion. Second, it should be able to identify secondary tumor, particularly lymph node deposits.

CT of Carcinoma of the Cervix

CT has been used to assess carcinoma of the cervix. Five features have been investigated; the identification of the primary tumor of the cervix, volumetric analysis of tumors, evaluation of parametrial or vaginal involvement, estimation of lymph node involvement, and evaluation of tumor recurrence.

Identification of tumor confined to the cervix is difficult, if not impossible. Tumor and normal cervix are isodense on CT, and unless surrounding tissues are distorted, cancers cannot be identified and the thickness of stromal involvement cannot be seen on CT.[3,4]

In a retrospective study of 56 patients treated for cancer of the cervix with radical radiotherapy, tumor bulk was measured on CT.[5] Tumor depth and width were related to survival and node involvement, and it was found, not surprisingly, that both were related. If the depth of the tumor on CT was greater than 4 cm, there was an increase in node involvement and reduced survival. Collins et al.[6] also showed a relationship between involved lymph nodes and tumor depth of greater than 3.8 cm. However, Arimoto,[7] in a prospective study of 87 patients, all but one with stage IIB or IIIB cancer of the cervix, found that initial tumor volume as measured on CT was not significantly related to survival after radiother-

apy. The tumor volume measured immediately after radiotherapy was related to 3- and 5-year survival rates. The CT measurement of tumor volume after response to radiotherapy may be of prognostic value.

It is in the identification of parametrial involvement and nodal secondaries that CT has been most used to study cancer of the cervix. There is no doubt that parametrial extension of tumor and involvement of surrounding structures can be identified using CT. Figure 11.7 shows a mass involving the cervix with some asymmetry suggesting spread into the right parametrium and possibly also the left. There is involvement of the vault of the vagina and some infiltration of paracervical fat. Figure 11.8 shows a large cervical/uterine mass extending into the parametrium on the right and to the pelvic sidewall on the left. There is infiltration of the paravaginal and pararectal fat. These figures show parametrial involvement in stage II and stage III tumours. However, even here success is limited. Kim et al.[4] studied 99 patients with cancer of the cervix who had CT and MRI in the 2 weeks before operation. Of the 17 patients found to have parametrial involvement at histology, 80% were identified by CT and 87% on MRI. Genolet et al.[8] found that CT was no better than rectal and vaginal clinical examination in the prediction of tumor stage. A review of the American experience of CT and cancer of the cervix, found that CT was no more accurate than clinical examination in staging early disease.[9] CT is of value in estimating the extent of parametrial disease and has been used successfully to plan radiotherapy.[10] Clinical evaluation of lymph node involvement is not possible. When CT was introduced, it was hoped that it would provide a more effective and less invasive technique than lymphangiography. In practice, CT can lead to false-positives and particularly false-negatives. Brennah et al.[11] found a false-negative rate of 33% with a false positive rate of 8%, and Genolet et al.[8] calculated a positive predictive value of only 36%. Moore et al.[12] assessed how CT might change management and affect survival. They found that in the 171 cases who had CT before treatment only 8 had their management changed to their benefit, but a further 8 patients had unnecessary surgery. They concluded that CT made little difference to the outcome. Others have claimed greater success, finding CT to be comparable to MRI, having an 80% to 90% accuracy in identifying node involvement.[13] Where lateral invasion involves the ureter, the resultant hydronephrosis and hydroureter can be clearly demonstrated (Fig. 11.9).

Tumor recurrence is identifiable using CT, although distinguishing fibrosis from recurrence can be difficult. In general, accuracy in identification of recurrence is a factor of the size of the recurrence rather than any other feature. CT evaluation of cancer of the cervix is probably no more useful than clinical examination in terms of staging but may have a place in planning radiotherapy. MRI is superseding CT as the modality of choice.

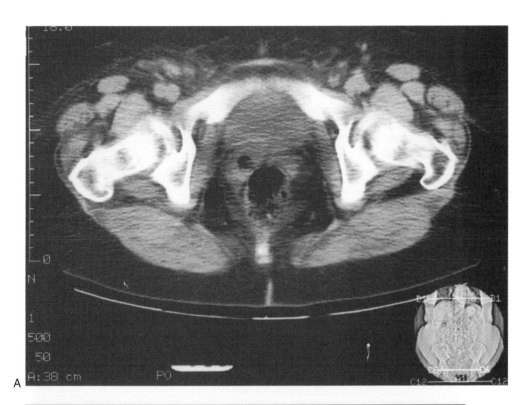

A

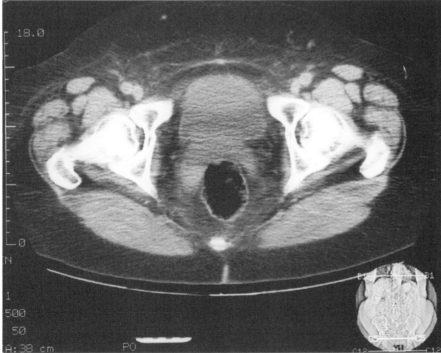

B

Figure 11.7 (**A**) Transaxial CT image through the vault of the vagina. The large dark area centrally placed is air in the rectum. Anterior, and to the right, is a smaller dark circle representing air in the vagina. Tumor is seen involving the vault of the vagina. (**B**) Transaxial CT image through the lower part of the cervix. Tumor extends partly into the left parametrium but more extensively to the right. In neither case is tumor extending to the pelvic sidewall. (*Figure continues*.)

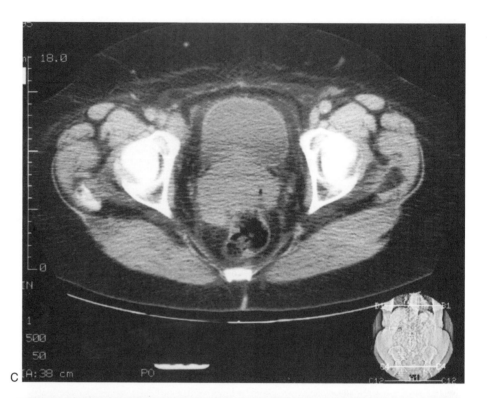

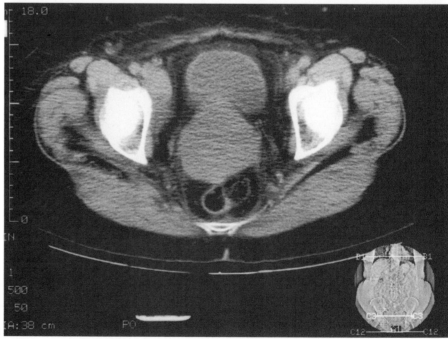

Figure 11.7 (*Continued*). (**C**) Transaxial CT image through the upper part of the cervix. The cervix is replaced by a bulky asymmetric tumor, more pronounced on the right than the left, extending into the parametria and posteriorly into pararectal fat on the right. (**D**) Transaxial CT image through the lower pole of the body of the uterus. No further involvement of parametria or bowel is seen at this level.

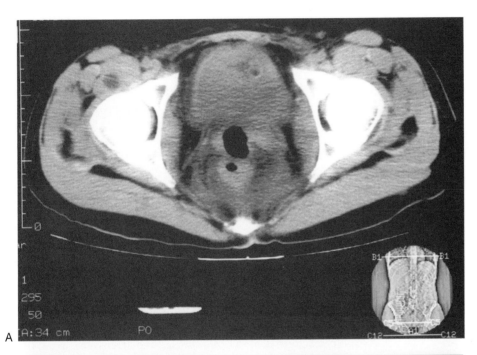

A

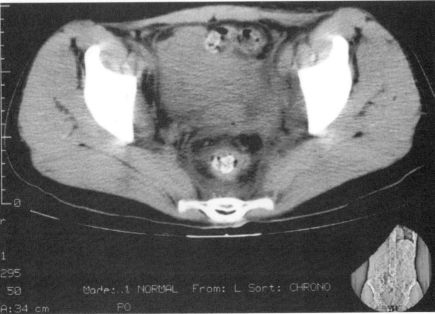

B

Figure 11.8 (**A**) Transaxial CT image through vault of vagina. The large dark area is air and a tampon in the vagina. To either side, tumor is seen infiltrating the vaginal vault and the perirectal fat (surrounding the smaller air shadow in the rectum). (**B**) Transaxial CT image through the cervix. Tumor extends into the parametrium on the right and out to the pelvic side wall on the left.

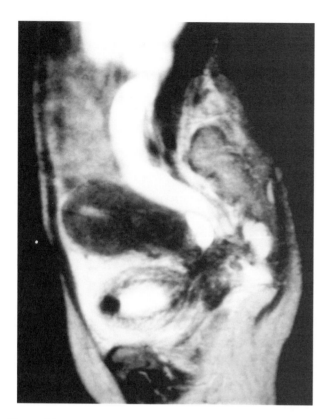

Figure 11.9 Sagittal MRI view of tumor invasion causing ureteric obstruction with resultant hydronephrosis and hydroureters.

MRI of Carcinoma of the Cervix

Unlike endometrial carcinoma, squamous cell carcinoma on a T1/T2-weighted sequence is similar to the surrounding myometrium. The lengthening of T2 weighting increases the differentiation between tumor and surrounding normal tissue. A pseudocapsule can be seen defining the tumor (Fig. 11.10). The imaging characteristics do not change with the differentiation of the tumor. Tumor necrosis is reflected by areas of

Figure 11.10 MRI in cervical carcinoma. Sagittal view demonstrates disruption of the posterior cervical wall through to the pouch of Douglas. The tumor does not appear to have invaded into the rectum.

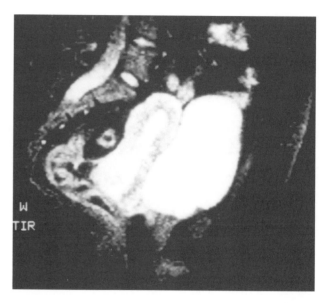

Figure 11.11 STIR sequence that highlights the tumor mass in cervical carcinoma. There is loss of tissue definition in the surrounding structure.

low intensity. The STIR sequence enhances the appearance of the tumor mass but at the price of reduced imaging quality of normal tissue (Fig. 11.11). It has been shown that T1-weighted images generally have an intermediate signal compared to that of smooth muscle.[1,14,15] Transverse axial T1-weighted images are essential in establishing tumor invasion into the broad ligament (Fig. 11.12). The use of the STIR sequence highlights the tumor signal, but there is a loss of definition of the surrounding normal tissues.

Adenocarcinoma of the Cervix

The signal intensities are different in cervical adenocarcinoma compared with squamous cell carcinoma. The signal intensity on T2-weighted sequences resembles that of endome-

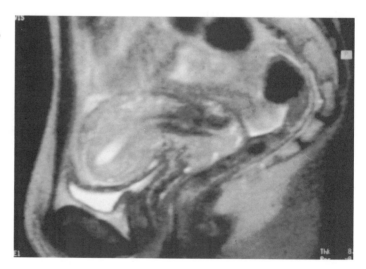

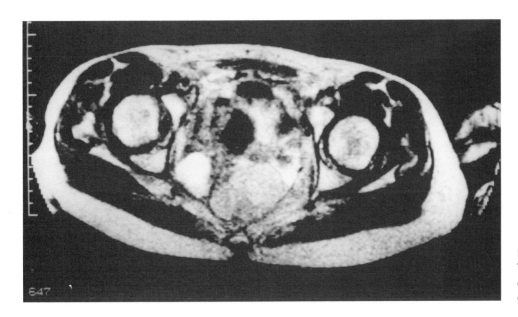

Figure 11.12 Transverse axial T1-weighted image in cervical carcinoma demonstrating invasion out to the lateral pelvic wall.

trial adenocarcinoma, and therefore the assessment of tumor staging is easier. Hawnaur et al.[16] examined 45 patients before radical hysterectomy and showed that the accuracy of staging was 84%, which is better than CT. They demonstrated a specificity of 88% in predicting node involvement. In an assessment of parametrial invasion, 21 patients were examined with CT and MRI.[17] All were thought to have invasive cervical cancer, and after surgery the specimens were examined histologically. CT was shown to have an accuracy of 62% in detecting parametrial invasion with 63% sensitivity and 60% specificity. MRI had 81% accuracy with 69% sensitivity and 80% specificity. Williams et al.[18] in a comparative study assessing recurrence in 20 patients, found that CT and MRI were equally effective. Cobby et al.[19] compared ultrasound, CT, and MRI in 37 patients with carcinoma of the cervix and showed that MRI and ultrasound were more accurate than CT in the assessment of local tumor invasion.

Lymph Node Invasion

Despite the nonspecific nature of secondary tumor deposits, it is possible to identify lymph node deposits using MRI. Greco et al.[20] examined 46 patients with carcinoma of the cervix using a 0.5-T magnet. All patients underwent lymphadenectomy and radical hysterectomy. In the detection of nodal involvement, the accuracy of MRI was 76%, and the accuracy of determining tumor size approached 100%. Assessment of parametrial and vaginal involvement had an accuracy of 85% and 100%, respectively. Waggenspack et al.[21] examined 20 consecutive patients with primary untreated carcinoma of the

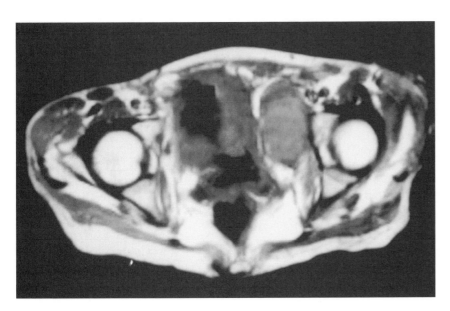

Figure 11.13 Transverse axial MRI of recurrent tumor mass in cervical carcinoma. The volume and extent of recurrent disease can be assessed.

cervix. These were patients with predominantly clinical stage IB. MRI was useful in detecting metastatic lymphadenopathy. Lymph nodes, greater than 1.5 cm in diameter, were present on MRI in the three patients for whom this was proven after lymphadenectomy. In summary, MRI is useful in detecting lymph node involvement, and the sensitivity is likely to improve in the future.

Recurrent Disease

Recurrent cervical carcinoma has similar MRI characteristics to the primary tumor. Signal intensity increases with T2 weighting, and tumor tissue can be highlighted using the STIR sequence. Powell et al.[22] reported 26 women with suspected recurrent cervical cancer. Fifteen had large central or sidewall masses, and in 6 the tumor involved large bowel. MRI provided information about the tumor recurrence (Fig. 11.13).

SUMMARY

MRI has proven to be useful for staging tumor and for assessing recurrence. The cervical canal was found to be wider but not shorter in cervical incompetence and shorter in women exposed to DES than in those not exposed.

REFERENCES

1. Powell MC, Buckley JH, Price H et al. Magnetic resonance imaging and placenta praevia. Am J Obstet Gynecol 1986; 154:565–569
2. Hricak H, Chang YC, Cann CE, Parer JT. Cervical incompetence: preliminary evaluation with MR imaging. Radiology 1990;174:821–826
3. Russell AH, Anderson M, Walter J et al. The integration of computed tomography and magnetic resonance imaging in treatment planning for gynecologic cancer. Clin Obstet Gynaecol 1992;35:55–72
4. Kim SH, Choi BI, Han JK et al. Pre-operative staging of uterine cervical carcinoma: comparison of CT and MRI in 99 patients. J Comput Assist Tomogr 1993;17:633–640
5. Shepherd SF, Collins CD, Fryatt IJ et al. Computerized axial tomographic scan measurements as prognostic indicators in patients with cervical carcinoma. Br J Radiol 1995;68:600–603
6. Collins CD, Constant O, Fryatt I et al. Relationship of computed tomography tumour volume to patient survival in carci-

noma of the cervix treated by radical radiotherapy. Br J Radiol 1994;67:252–256
7. Arimoto T. Significance of computed tomography-measured volume in the prognosis of cervical carcinoma. Cancer 1993; 72:2383–2388
8. Genolet PM, Hanggi W, Dreher E. Evaluation of tumour extension in invasive cancer of the uterine cervix. Diagnostic evaluation of cervix cancer. Gynakol Geburtshilfliche Rundsch 1993; 33:180–184
9. McGonigle KF, Berek JS. Early stage squamous cell and adenocarcinoma of the cervix. Curr Opin Obstet Gynaecol 1992;4: 109–119
10. Kim RY, McGuinnis LS, Spencer SA et al. Conventional four-field pelvic radiotherapy technique without computed tomography-treatment planning in cancer of the cervix: potential geographic miss and its impact on pelvic control. Int J Radiat Oncol Biol Phys 1995;31:109–112
11. Brennah DE, Whitley NO, Prempree T, Villasanta U. An evaluation of the computed tomographic scanner for the staging of carcinoma of the cervix. Cancer 1982;50:2323
12. Moore DH, Dotters DJ, Fowler WC, Jr. Computed tomography: does it really improve the treatment of cervical carcinoma? Am J Obstet Gynecol 1992;167:768–821
13. Subak LL, Hricak H, Powell CB et al. Cervical carcinoma: computed tomography and magnetic resonance imaging for pre-operative staging. Obstet Gynecol 1995;86:43–50
14. Togashi K, Nishimura K, Itoh K et al. Uterine cervical cancer: assessment with high-field MR imaging. Radiology 1986; 160:431–435
15. Kim SH, Choi BI, Lee HP et al. Uterine cervical carcinoma: comparison of CT and MR findings. Radiology 1990;175:45–51
16. Hawnaur JM, Johnson RJ, Buckley CH et al. Staging volume estimation and assessment of nodal status in carcinoma of the cervix: comparison of magnetic resonance imaging with surgical findings. Clin Radiol 1994;49:443–452
17. Sironi S, Zanello A, Radighiero MG et al. Invasive carcinoma of the cervix uteri (stage IB–IIB). Comparison of CT and MR for the assessment of the parametrium. Radiol Med 1991;81: 671–677
18. Williams MP, Husband JE, Heron CW, et al. Magnetic resonance imaging in recurrent carcinoma of the cervix. Br J Radiol 1989;62:544–550
19. Cobby M, Browning J, Jones A et al. Magnetic resonance imaging, computed tomography and endosonography in the local staging of carcinoma of the cervix. Br J Radiol 1990;63:673–679
20. Greco A, Mason P, Leung AW et al. Staging of carcinoma of the uterine cervix: MRI–surgical correlation. Clin Radiol 1989;40: 401–405
21. Waggenspack GA, Ampara EG, Hannigan EV. MR imaging of uterine cervical carcinoma. J Comput Assist Tomogr 1988;12: 409–414
22. Powell MC, Worthington BS, Symonds EM, Eds. Carcinoma of the cervix. In: Magnetic Resonance Imaging in Obstetrics and Gynaecology. Butterworth Heinemann, Oxford, UK, 1993, p 60

12

Ultrasonography of the Endometrium

JOHN C. ANDERSON

PHILIPPA A. RAMSAY

The endometrium undergoes remarkable histologic change during the menstrual cycle. It is sensitive to endogenous estrogen and progesterone, which are produced principally by the ovary. In the preovulatory (or follicular) phase of the cycle, the stromal and glandular elements undergo proliferation influenced by estradiol. In the postovulatory (or luteal) phase, progesterone inhibits this proliferation and stimulates a secretory change in which the glands become tortuous and there is a prominent development of the spiral arterioles. Although these changes are histologic, they influence the thickness and texture of the endometrium enough to be seen on ultrasound (see Ch. 5).

At any time of life, the endometrium can be influenced by medications, the most common of which are the oral contraceptive in the reproductive years and hormone replacement therapy after the menopause. Hormone therapy can now be administered via a skin patch, and even estrogen vaginal creams can be absorbed easily, so a systemic effect is common. Other medications that have an endometrial effect are danazol, which is used to treat endometriosis, and tamoxifen, which is prescribed to reduce the recurrence risk of breast cancer.

Rarely, the source of the estrogen is endogenous, as in a granulosa cell tumor of the ovary.

An appearance that is normal in reproductive life may be abnormal after the menopause. For example, normal premenstrual endometrium in a young woman can look similar to hyperplastic endometrium in an older woman. It is therefore impossible to determine whether an image is normal or abnormal without knowing the patient's age, menstrual history, and recent medications.

When measuring the thickness of the endometrium on ultrasound studies, it is standard practice to include both anterior and posterior layers. This is because the junction between the endometrium and myometrium is often easier to define than the interface between the anterior and posterior surfaces of the endometrium. Unless there is a major interruption like an endometrial polyp, the whole surface of the endometrium is usually similar in thickness, so if the endometrial thickness is reported as 10 mm, the anterior layer and the posterior layers are each probably 5 mm thick.

THE EFFECT OF DRUGS

Oral Contraceptives

The most common drugs to affect the endometrium are oral contraceptives. Now they usually consist of ethinylestradiol plus a progestogen in a single pill taken daily for 21 days followed by a placebo for 7 days. They work in most cases by preventing ovulation with a negative feedback mechanism on the hypothalamus by progesterone, which suppresses the luteinizing hormone surge. The estrogen is included to stimulate some growth and stability of the endometrium to prevent breakthrough bleeding during the cycle. The dose of ethinylestradiol has progressively been reduced over the years to reduce the side effects but maintain efficacy. The endometrial effect seen on ultrasound examination is predictable. The changes depend on the length of time that the woman has been receiving therapy. In the first cycle, there is a marked stromal edema, but in later cycles this becomes decidual, and finally, after long-term use, the endometrium becomes atrophic and consequently thin[1] (Fig. 12.1).

Hormone Replacement Therapy in Menopausal Women

Many postmenopausal women are now being prescribed hormone replacement therapy to alleviate the symptoms of the menopause and to reduce the risk of osteoporotic fractures and coronary vascular disease.[2,3] Estrogen is the effective agent but when given alone endometrial hyperplasia occurs within 2 years in 40% of women,[4] and there is an increased incidence of endometrial carcinoma.[5] Therefore, continuous combined estrogen and progesterone regimens are used in a dose sufficiently high to induce the beneficial effects but low enough to leave the endometrium in an atrophic state in almost all women.[6] Consequently, the endometrium in menopausal women on optimized hormonal therapy should have a normal atrophic appearance on ultrasound.

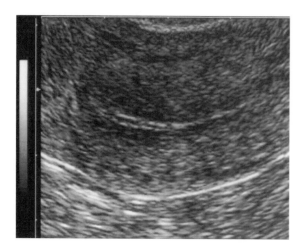

Figure 12.1 Transvaginal view of sagittal section of the endometrium of a 32-year-old woman after 4 years receiving combined oral contraceptives scanned on day 14 of the cycle. Note the thin endometrium.

Danazol

Another exogenous substance in use is danazol, a synthetic derivative of ethisterone, used for the treatment of endometriosis. Danazol itself has no significant estrogenic or progestogenic effects but is mildly androgenic. Danazol causes the endometrium to atrophy by inhibiting proliferation.

Tamoxifen

Tamoxifen is a nonsteroidal estrogen antagonist that has some agonistic properties. It is used in the treatment of breast cancer and has been suggested for protection against breast cancer in women at risk on the basis of heredity. It inhibits breast cancer but, paradoxically, stimulates endometrial growth, suggesting a tissue-specific action. It has been implicated in a variety of endometrial problems including uterine polyps, endometrial hyperplasia, and adenocarcinoma.[7–11] Annual vaginal sonography and endometrial biopsy have been suggested for surveillance in women on tamoxifen.[12–14] The endometrium has been shown to be thickened to more than 7 mm in some cases and to be homogeneously hyperechoic in others. Small cystic spaces are often seen, but on sonohysterography they are seen to lie in the subendometrial myometrium.[15] It has been shown that the endometrium of asymptomatic menopausal women is not usually atrophic if they are on tamoxifen.[16] In the same study, the endometrial thickness was increased to about 10 mm in these women, and about one third of them had polyps. The image of the endometrium among women on tamoxifen can be quite variable, and therefore curettage is often required to rule out hyperplasia or malignancy (Fig. 12.2 and Plate 12.1).

Clomiphene Citrate

Clomiphene citrate is a nonsteroidal compound similar in structure to stilbestrol. Since the early 1970s, it has been used to induce ovulation in anovulatory women. The principal site of action is the pituitary, where it increases the output of gonadotrophins, which in turn stimulate the maturation of ovarian follicles. On clomiphene, normal cyclic endometrial changes usually take place, but clomiphene may exert an antiestrogenic effect on the endometrium, which slows its growth in the periovulatory period[17] and delays maturation in the luteal phase.[18] These changes may be observed with ultrasound, and they could interfere with implantation.

Human Menopausal Gonadotropin

Human menopausal gonadotropin is most commonly used for in vitro fertilization (IVF) and other forms of assisted conception, to increase the number of developing follicles. The endometrium often develops normally during these IVF cycles, though the length of the cycles can vary enormously according to the drug doses and the ovarian response.

RU486 Mifepristone

RU486 is a synthetic steroid that blocks the action of progesterone on the endometrium. Its uses include termination of pregnancy, medical curettage in blighted pregnancy, and postcoital contraception. It causes bleeding, and on ultrasound examination the appearances are usually of a disorganized menstrual endometrium. There is potential for daily administration of RU486 to be effective as a contraceptive. It has been shown to retard endometrial maturation, and it may

Figure 12.2 Transvaginal scan of a coronal section of the uterus of an asymptomatic 71-year-old receiving tamoxifen for 8 years because of previous breast cancer. The endometrium appears irregularly cystic.

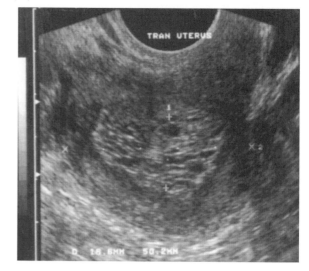

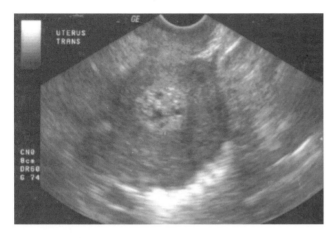

Figure 12.3 A 60-year-old receiving cyproterone acetate for 2 years presented with vaginal bleeding after forgetting her medication for 1 month. Note the thickened endometrium with occasional small cystic spaces.

prevent implantation and be effective for fertility control.[19] The endometrial appearances in this situation have not yet been ascertained. It may be that ultrasound assessment of endometrial thickness will be a measure of contraceptive effectiveness in each woman, allowing the best selection of the appropriate dose.

Cyproterone Acetate

Cyproterone acetate is a potent antiandrogen that has some progestational effect. It is used in the treatment of hirsutism in women and prostatic cancer in men. It can cause some thickening and echogenicity of the endometrium (Fig. 12.3).

BENIGN CONDITIONS

Endometrial Hyperplasia

Women with endometrial hyperplasia usually present with abnormal bleeding, but occasionally endometrial hyperplasia is detected during infertility investigation either by curettage or ultrasonography. The infertile women are usually anovulatory, obese, and hirsute and have polycystic ovaries (Stein-Leventhal syndrome). Ample evidence suggests that hyperplasia of the endometrium occurs secondarily to the trophic influence of excessive endogenous estrogen or to unopposed exogenous estrogen. Furthermore, there is an association between hyperplasia and adenocarcinoma of the endometrium which is also associated with estrogen. It is not absolutely certain, however, that hyperplasia is an essential transitional stage between normal endometrium and carcinoma, although it seems likely. Histologically, there are three types of hyperplasia that are regarded as being associated with, or precursors of, carcinoma of the endometrium. These are cystic, adenomatous, and atypical hyperplasia.[20] These all show histologic structural changes in the glands and stroma (Figs 12.4 to 12.6) that cannot be differentiated from each other on ultrasound. They are all seen as thickened, echogenic endometrium. (Fig. 12.7) Carcinoma in situ also shows histologic changes in the glands (Fig. 12.8), but the ultrasound appearance is indistinguishable from hyperplasia. Therefore, the diagnosis of carcinoma in situ from hyperplasia requires histologic assessment. Similarly, the ultrasound appearances of decidual change in the endometrium in the presence of an ectopic gestation are indistinguishable from hyperplasia. For this reason, it is essential to obtain an accurate history from the patient.

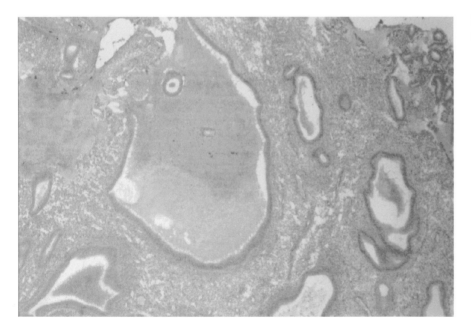

Figure 12.4 Histopathologic section of cystic hyperplasia at low power.

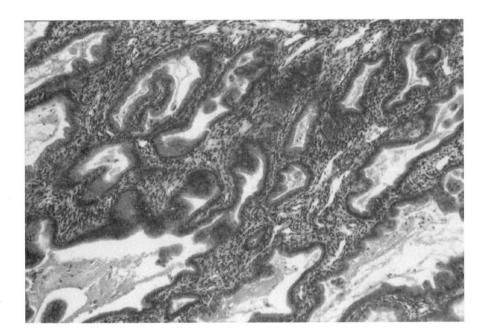

Figure 12.5 Histopathologic section of adenomatous hyperplasia.

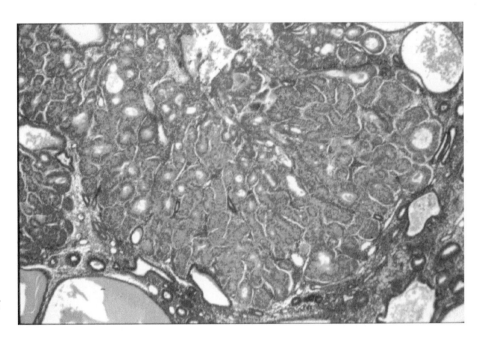

Figure 12.6 Histopathologic section of atypical hyperplasia.

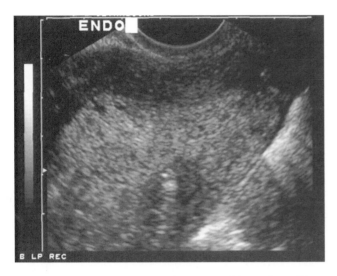

Figure 12.7 Transvaginal scan of endometrial hyperplasia. (Courtesy of Dr. J. Spurway, Sydney, Australia.)

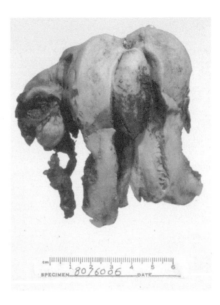

Figure 12.9 Gross appearance of an endometrial polyp in a hysterectomy specimen.

Endometrial Polyps

Endometrial polyps occur most commonly in women of 35 to 50 years, and they usually present with intermenstrual bleeding or menorrhagia. They may cause infertility by interfering with implantation of the blastocyst,[21–23] so they are often found by ultrasound during investigation of infertility or during the follicle tracking of an IVF cycle.

Macroscopically, polyps of the endometrium are often multiple, can be broad based or pedunculated, and range in size from a few millimeters to several centimeters in diameter. The surface may be ulcerated, often at the tip,[21] (Fig. 12.9). They are thought to develop as localized overgrowths of the basal zone of the endometrium and continue to be supported

through the stalk by their straight artery, which enlarges as they grow.[20]

On ultrasound examination, they appear as a well-circumscribed echogenic mass in the endometrial cavity (Figs. 12.10 to 12.16). To be confident of the diagnosis, the physician should see the endometrium on either side of the polyp, and the pedicle between polyp and endometrium should be demonstrated.

Polyps are not responsive to cyclic hormonal changes, and their echo texture therefore remains constant during the menstrual cycle. The best time to demonstrate a polyp is in the proliferative phase of the cycle when the surrounding en-

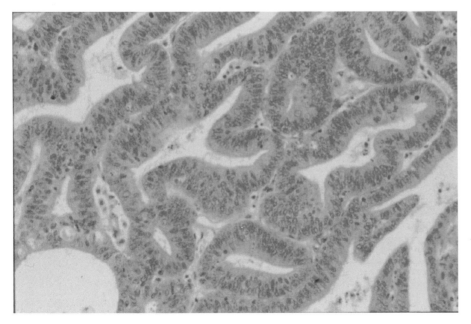

Figure 12.8 Histopathologic section of adenocarcinoma in situ.

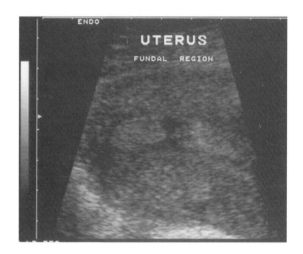

Figure 12.10 Transabdominal scan of an endometrial polyp.

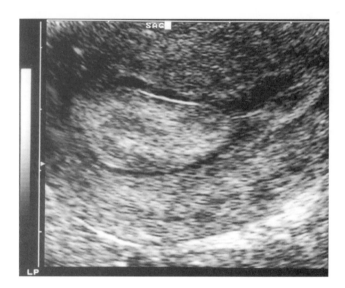

Figure 12.12 Transvaginal scan of a large endometrial polyp filling the uterine cavity.

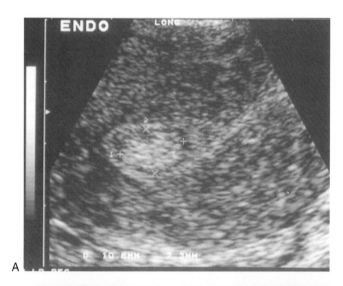

A

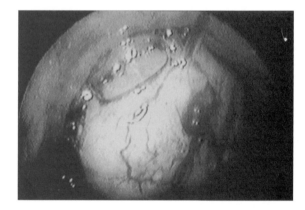

Figure 12.13 View of the endometrial polyp as seen through the hysteroscope.

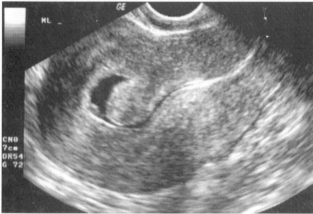

B

Figure 12.11 **A** Transvaginal scan of an endometrial polyp showing the superior resolution obtained from this approach. This 44-year-old complained of menorrhagia. (**B**) Sonohysterogram of the same patient showing the polyp even more clearly. (Courtesy of Dr. A. Boogert, Sydney, Australia.)

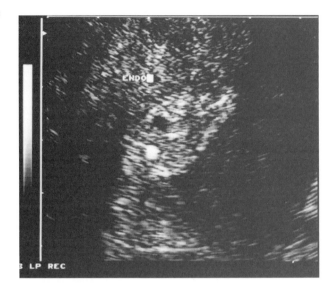

Figure 12.14 Occasionally, polyps can assume an atypical appearance. This scan in a 41-year-old with irregular menses was considered to be that of endometrial hyperplasia, but hysteroscopy showed a large endometrial polyp. The echogenic focus may have been a clue to the diagnosis.

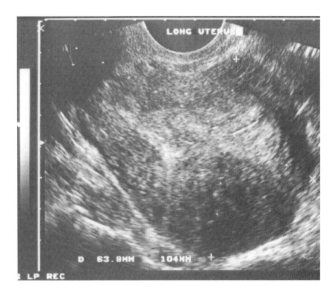

Figure 12.16 Endometrium may occasionally assume a polypoid appearance. This sonogram from a 39-year-old woman complaining of dyspareunia seemed to be irregular in outline, and, in some places, echo texture. Hysteroscopy showed a polypoid appearance, but histology described it as an exuberant secretory change, with no true polyps, hyperplasia, or neoplasia. (Courtesy of Dr. Cecilia Senior, Sydney, Australia.)

dometrium is thin and hypoechoic and contrasts most with the polyp. They are also easier to see if surrounded by fluid during bleeding (Fig. 12.17).

The most common cause of diagnostic difficulty is the appearance of the endometrium in the periovulatory phase of the cycle when there can be a small area of focal change to se-

cretory endometrium (Fig. 12.18). This appearance only lasts for a very short time, perhaps hours, as the rest of the endometrium then changes from late proliferative to secretory. It is sometimes possible to distinguish the secretory change by showing that the echogenic focus is in the endometrial layer

Figure 12.15 Another example of an atypical appearance assumed by a polypoid endometrium. This 49-year-old presented with menorrhagia. Although the sonogram looked as though it could have been hyperplastic, as it was thickened to 2.5 cm and was slightly echogenic, pathology showed a polypoid endometrium with stromal hyalinization and pseudodecidualization and no hyperplasia was seen.

Figure 12.17 A 39-year-old woman presented with a history of severe metrostaxis for years. Several D&Cs had failed to alleviate her problem. Transvaginal scan shows an endometrial polyp highlighted in surrounding blood in sagittal section. It is hyperechoic in comparison with the surrounding myometrium.

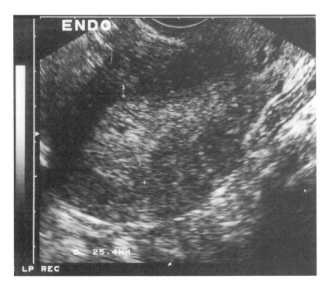

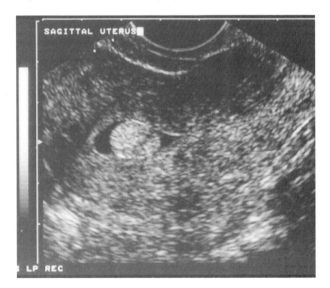

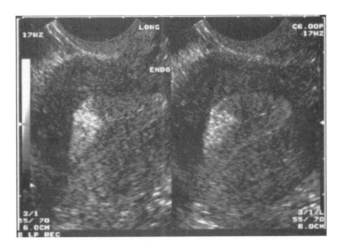

Figure 12.18 Focal secretory change is occasionally seen at the periovulatory stage of the cycle. This could be confused with an endometrial polyp if imaged in one plane only, as seen here in the sagittal plane.

itself rather than in the cavity. This may be demonstrable in one plane but not another. The differential diagnosis also includes submucous myomata, which may protrude into the cavity. Polyps tend to be hyperechoic, while myomata are hypoechoic and tend to have a broader base and a component that is clearly intramural.

Polyps are known to be rather frequent in uteri containing endometrial carcinoma,[24,25] but this is probably due to a common etiology, i.e. estrogens.[26] They are probably not premalignant, as carcinoma in situ is no more frequent in the glands of the polyp than in the surrounding nonpolypoid endometrium.[27] The incidence of carcinoma arising in a polyp is thought to be less than 1%,[26,28] but removal seems prudent. This is best done with direct visualization by hysteroscopy, as polyps on a pliable stalk can be missed with blind curettage alone.

Endometrial Atrophy

The endometrium of postmenopausal women is normally atrophic due to the low levels of circulating estrogen. Atrophic endometrium can also occur in women on oral contraceptive therapy when the endometrium is inadequately supported by estrogen. Other situations that can result in reduced estrogen levels and consequent atrophic endometria are premature ovarian failure, surgical removal of the ovaries, or radiation therapy for cervical cancer. The most common histologic appearance in postmenopausal women complaining of vaginal bleeding is endometrial atrophy. Most women complaining of postmenopausal bleeding have either atrophic or hyperplastic endometria. Only 10% to 20% of women with postmenopausal bleeding have cancer.[29] Microscopically, atrophic endometrium is thin and composed of variably sized glands with compact but reduced stroma. On ultrasound, the endometrium is less than 5 mm thick. Many studies have shown that endometria less than 5 mm are associated with at-

rophic endometritis and curettage usually yields only scant, if any, tissue.[29–32] Thus, if the endometrium is less than 5 mm on transvaginal scanning, diagnostic curettage is probably not necessary.

MALIGNANT CONDITIONS

Endometrial Carcinoma

Endometrial carcinoma is the most common invasive neoplasm of the female genital tract. Patients with endometrial carcinoma usually present with abnormal vaginal bleeding. Most are postmenopausal. Only 3% of patients with endometrial carcinoma present under the age of 40 years, and there have been only 21 cases reported below the age of 30 years.[33] In younger women, nulliparity and obesity are predisposing factors.

The most recent histologic classification of endometrial carcinoma by the World Health Organization in 1994 is shown in Table 12.1.[34] This classification is based on the microscopic appearance of the endometrium, but a histologic diagnosis cannot be achieved on ultrasound examination. The malignancy arises in the glandular elements of the endometrium and is therefore usually an adenocarcinoma. Because there is marked glandular activity in the endometrium, there are echogenic secretions and an increased number of reflective interfaces that are sonographically visible. The sonographic appearance can be indistinguishable from that of secretory endometrium or decidua unless it is advanced and invades the myometrium. In postmenopausal women, the appearance can be indistinguishable from endometrial hyperplasia.

Asymptomatic Patients

Unlike cervical cancer, screening asymptomatic patients for endometrial cancer is not readily practiced. Tissue for a histopathologic diagnosis is normally obtained in symptomatic patients by dilatation of the cervix and curettage of the

Table 12.1 Classification of Endometrial Cancer*

Endometrioid adenocarcinoma
Villoglandular
Secretory
Ciliated cell
Endometrioid adenocarcinoma with squamous differentiation
Serous carcinoma
Clear cell carcinoma
Mucinous carcinoma
Squamous carcinoma
Mixed types of carcinoma
Undifferentiated carcinoma

* Modified from World Health Organization and International Society of Gynecological Pathologists Histologic Classification of Endometrial Carcinoma.

endometrium (D&C), which requires general anesthesia, and thus its use is unsuitable as a screening procedure. Attempts at predicting the presence of endometrial cancer from cytologic study of cells found in cervical smears have been disappointing.[35] A wide variety of mechanical devices has been developed for cytologic sampling of the endometrium without general anesthesia, but none has been found to be sensitive enough. Shipley and co-workers,[35] in a study of 50 asymptomatic postmenopausal women, compared transvaginal scanning with nondirected endometrial biopsy as a screening method. Women with abnormal endometrial patterns on ultrasound were further investigated by hysteroscopy and biopsy or D&C. They found that the sensitivity of transvaginal sonography in identifying endometrial pathology was 80%, whereas that of nondirected endometrial biopsy was only 30%.[35] Another study by Rullo and others[36] found that the sensitivity of transvaginal ultrasound in the early detection of endometrial pathology was 95.8%, compared to a diagnostic accuracy of hysteroscopy of 100%. However, because sonography was so well accepted by the patients, the authors suggested that high-risk patients undergo transvaginal sonographic screening annually to select patients who may benefit from hysteroscopy and, if necessary, directed biopsy.[36] D&C has also been used as the diagnostic test after ultrasound screening. Osmers and co-workers[37] carried out transvaginal sonography in a prospective study of 155 asymptomatic postmenopausal women not on hormone replacement therapy and found seven endometrial cancers and one cervical cancer.

Symptomatic Patients

Patients with carcinoma of the endometrium usually present with unusual vaginal bleeding. A lesion of the cervix is ex-

Figure 12.19 Transvaginal sagittal view of endometrial carcinoma in a 35-year-old obese (160-kg) woman who presented with irregular vaginal bleeding. The echogenic endometrium is 3.7 cm thick and appears to be encroaching on the myometrium. It was histologically an endometrioid adenocarcinoma FIGO (International Federation of Gynecologists and Obstetricians) stage I with grade 2 nuclear features. (Courtesy of Dr. Kenneth Atkinson, Sydney, Australia.)

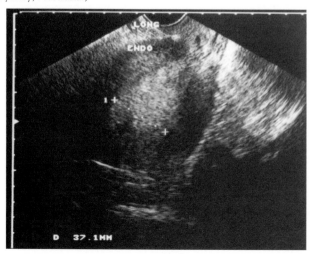

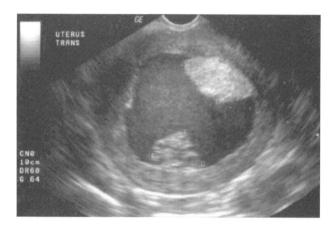

Figure 12.20 This 47-year-old was asymptomatic. An enlarged uterus was found on a routine check. The irregular echo texture of the endometrium has extended 3.5 cm through the myometrium. Histology showed a well-differentiated endometrioid carcinoma. (Courtesy of Dr. Trevor Hyde, Sydney, Australia.)

Figure 12.21 (A & B) This 69-year-old presented with vaginal spotting. Hysterosonography showed irregularity of the endometrium posteriorly with a polypoidal mass in the left cornual region (arrows). Histopathology of an endometrial biopsy confirmed a well-differentiated endometrioid carcinoma.

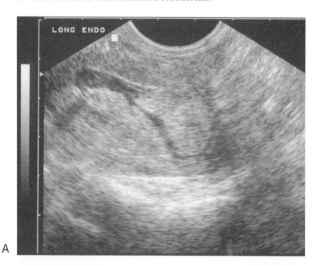

A

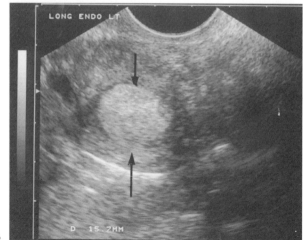

B

cluded by speculum examination, and tissue for histologic examination of the endometrium can be obtained by uterine curettage. It has been suggested that transvaginal ultrasound replace uterine curettage in the investigation of postmenopausal bleeding.[38] Ultrasound examination of carcinoma of the endometrium shows echogenic endometrium that is thickened depending on the stage of the disease (Figs. 12.19 to 12.21 and Plate 12.2). About 90% of women with postmenopausal bleeding do not have endometrial carcinoma, and many reports have shown that when the endometrium is thin, the histopathology is invariably benign and atrophic. The cutoff levels suggested have ranged from 3 to 8 mm.[38–43] Granberg and co-workers[29] found no endometrial carcinomas in 205 women with postmenopausal bleeding if the endometrium was less than 9 mm thick. However, Dorum and colleagues,[44] in a study of 100 women with postmenopausal bleeding found that 3 of 54 patients with an endometrial thickness of less than 5 mm had endometrial carcinoma. The sensitivity and negative predictive value in their view is not high enough for ultrasound to replace histologic examination of the endometrium. It seems likely that with high-resolution transvaginal ultrasound a histologic diagnosis is not mandatory in women who have an endometrial thickness of less than 5 mm.

Color Doppler Imaging

Transvaginal color Doppler may identify the few patients who have endometrial carcinoma even though the endometrium is thin.[45] Malignant tumors show signs of altered vascularization and a low pulsatility index (mean 0.49, range 0.29 to 0.92).[45] In general, hyperplastic endometria do not have the increased spiral arteriole vascularity which is seen in most endometrial cancers, so there is no change in pulsatility, and the pulsatility index remains over 1.0.

INFLAMMATORY CONDITIONS

Acute Endometritis

In health, the cervix acts as a barrier to ascending infection from the vagina. This barrier is compromised during menstruation, abortion, parturition, and curettage or insertion of an intrauterine contraceptive device. The usual organisms responsible are hemolytic *Streptococcus* and *Staphylococcus species*, *Neisseria gonorrhea*, and *Clostridium perfringens* (Fig. 12.22). Patients with acute endometritis usually complain of pelvic pain and a purulent vaginal discharge. The uterus is tender to palpation. If the condition becomes chronic, the patient may become asymptomatic.

The ultrasonic appearances are variable, ranging from normal to thickened, echogenic endometrium with echogenic fluid resembling pus within the cavity.

Chronic Endometritis

Chlamydia trachomatis is a recognized cause of infertility. It causes an acute or chronic salpingitis but also can infect the endometrium. *Mycoplasma* species are also thought to be responsible for infertility and fetal loss.[46–48] Tuberculous endometritis caused by *Mycobacterium tuberculosis* is part of systemic disease. It can manifest as a pelvic mass with lower abdominal pain or during the investigation of infertility. It reaches the endometrium from the fallopian tubes, which in turn are infected by hematogenous or, rarely, lymphatic spread from the lungs or gastrointestinal tract.[49]

Parasitic infections and viral infections are rare causes of endometritis in developed countries, but schistosomiasis is endemic in Central America, Africa, and the East.[50–54] Toxoplasmosis (*Toxoplasma gondii*) produces a nonspecific inflammation of the endometrium (Fig. 12.23).

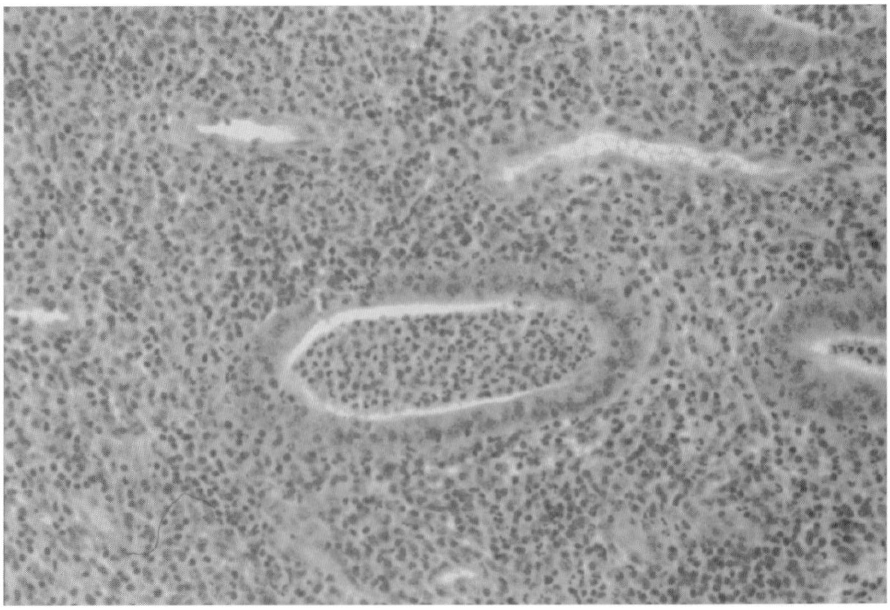

Figure 12.22 Histologic section of acute gonococcal endometritis.

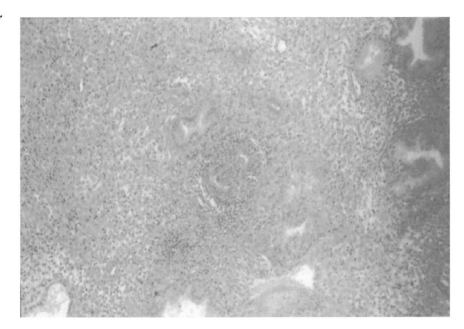

Figure 12.23 Histopathologic section of chronic nonspecific endometritis.

POSTOPERATIVE CONDITIONS

Endometrial Resection (Ablation)

Ablation of the endometrium has become popular in the treatment of menorrhagia, as it avoids hysterectomy. The cervix is dilated sufficiently to allow the introduction of a hysteroscope, and then under direct vision, the endometrium is either resected with loop diathermy or ablated with a diathermy rollerball. In the first days postprocedure, it is common to see fluid in the cavity, presumably blood or distending medium, and fluid in the pelvis, as it can drain there during the procedure via the fallopian tubes (Fig. 12.24A).

The aim is tissue destruction to a depth of 4 to 5 mm so that the endometrium does not regenerate; if this is achieved, then months or years later, the endometrium may still be indiscernible or immeasurably thin. If some endometrium remains, it may regenerate and cause menstruation once again. The endometrium can look irregular. If menstrual blood cannot drain because of adhesions inferior to the sloughing endometrium, then small areas of hematometra can occur. They are usually small irregularly shaped collections of blood, and

Figure 12.24 **(A)** Transvaginal scan through the uterus 2 days postendometrial ablation showing a small amount of fluid trapped in the cavity. **(B)** Transvaginal scan through the uterus 6 months after endometrial ablation for menorrhagia. The effect was incomplete, and endometrial adhesions can be seen separating areas of blood. Menorrhagia persisted, and the patient underwent hysterectomy 4 months later. (Courtesy of Dr. Trevor Hyde, Sydney, Australia.)

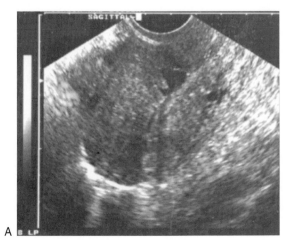

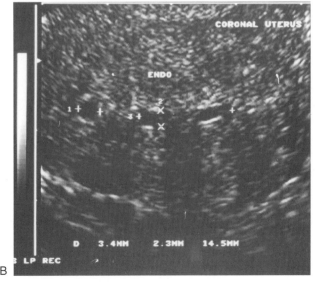

they are often multiple (Fig. 12.24A). The patient may report cyclic pain and bleeding, and the treatment is either repeat ablation or more commonly, hysterectomy.

Dilatation of Cervix and Curettage of Uterus

Various degrees of disorganization of the endometrial cavity are seen immediately after curettage, depending on how complete the procedure has been. Burks and colleagues[55] recognized echogenic foci along the inner myometrium in 35 of 80 patients who had undergone much earlier dilatation and curettage or biopsy and only 2 of 174 patients who had no prior instrumentation (Fig. 12.25). These foci are linear, nonshadowing, and lie adjacent to the endometrium and myometrium. They are thought to be due to calcification of retained products of conception and can occur in any parous woman;[56] however, calcification can be seen after any form of intrauterine instrumentation presumably in areas of trauma and fibrosis. These foci have no known clinical consequence.

Asherman Syndrome

Asherman syndrome presents as amenorrhea or marked hypomenorrhea, due to intrauterine adhesions. It usually follows vigorous curettage of the soft parous uterus resulting in resection of almost the entire endometrium and adhesion formation between the anterior and posterior walls of the uterus. The cavity can be entirely obliterated. On ultrasound, the endometrium may be partially or entirely invisible. If some endometrium remains, joined by intrauterine synechiae, they appear as bands that extend from the anterior to the posterior endometrial surface, sometimes with small collections of fluid

trapped in between. Sonohysterography can be used to identify the location and extent of intrauterine synechiae.

The best treatment of Asherman syndrome is hysteroscopic division of adhesions followed by estrogen therapy to allow endometrium to regenerate from the glandular elements that remain and once again resurface the entire endometrial cavity. In some cases, even a hysteroscope cannot detect the location of the original cavity, and in these cases, transabdominal ultrasound guidance is invaluable to prevent uterine perforation during the procedure. Some operators also place an intrauterine contraceptive device (IUCD) in the cavity after the procedure to try to prevent further adhesion formation.

INTRAUTERINE CONTRACEPTIVE DEVICE

IUCDs are easily identified with ultrasound. They cause a bright specular reflection with complete posterior shadowing (Fig. 12.26). Their shape and location can be determined by correlation of images from different planes, the Lippes loop is particularly characteristic (Fig. 12.27), as is the Graafenberg ring (Fig. 12.28). To prevent implantation of the blastocyst, they must be located in the cavity of the uterus, toward the fundus. Symptoms such as pain and bleeding can occur if they are placed too low in the cavity, in the myometrial wall, or through the wall into the adnexa (Figs 12.29 and 12.30). If the IUCD is within the field of view, it can be seen outside the uterus in the adnexa (Fig. 12.31) or pouch of Douglas; however, care must be taken not to confuse it with a linear pattern of gas in the surrounding bowel (Fig. 12.32). If the IUCD cannot be seen, it may of course have fallen out vagi-

Figure 12.25 Osseous dysplasia (calcification) in old fragments of placenta. This can often be seen in healthy parous women, as was the case with this 54-year-old. The calcified fragments may lie in the deeper layers of the endometrium than is seen here, and they are not usually as prominent.

Figure 12.26 A normally situated IUCD in a well 49-year-old woman. The uterus is a little bulky, and the myometrium anteriorly is mildly heterogenous in echo texture, possibly indicating diffuse adenomyosis.

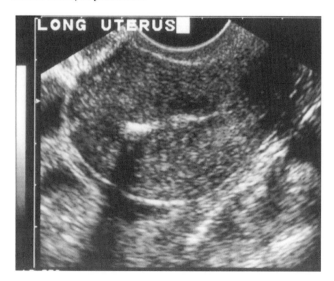

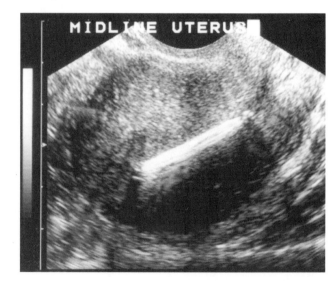

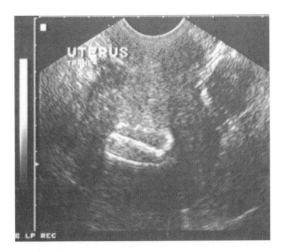

Figure 12.27 The Lippes loop produces a characteristic appearance.

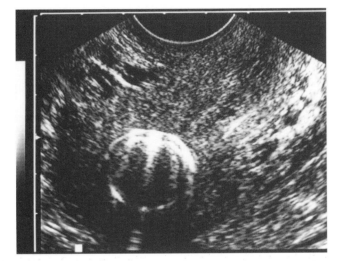

Figure 12.28 An unusual intrauterine device nowadays: a Graffenburg ring in situ for 25 years.

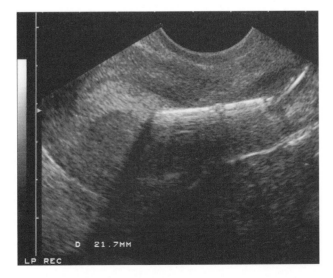

Figure 12.29 An IUCD situated low in the uterine cavity.

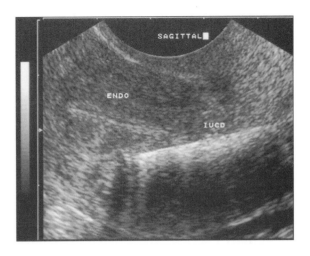

Figure 12.30 The IUCD is embedded in the myometrium.

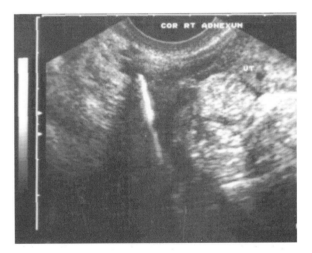

Figure 12.31 The IUCD can be seen in the left adnexa.

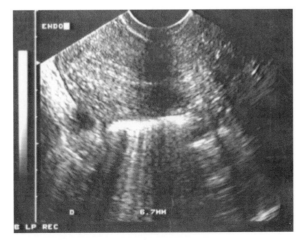

Figure 12.32 Bowel gas behind the uterus can produce an image suggestive of an IUCD. On real-time imaging, however, it will be seen to move with peristalsis.

nally, without the patient noticing. If the misplaced IUCD is clearly seen on ultrasound examination, it can be predicted whether retrieval should be attempted hysteroscopically or laparoscopically by its location and proximity to the uterine cavity.

IUCDs produce profound histologic changes in the endometrium,[57] but they are not noticeable on ultrasound examination, as the normal endometrial cyclic changes continue. Only those IUCDs that release progesterone produce changes which are seen on ultrasound examination, as the endometrium becomes atrophic.

OTHER CONDITIONS

Submucosal Leiomyoma

Leiomyomata (fibroids) have a characteristic appearance on ultrasound as rounded encapsulated myometrial masses that are homogeneously echo-dense and usually slightly hypoechoic compared to surrounding myometrium. Submucosal fibroids lie just beneath the mucosal (endometrial) layer of the uterus and often indent the overlying endometrium. As they enlarge, they may bulge into the endometrial cavity. Occasionally, they can become pedunculated and prolapse through the cervix. (Figs 12.33 to 12.37). They can cause menorrhagia, but many are asymptomatic and some are only discovered during investigation for infertility, as, like polyps, they are thought to impair implantation. Excellent views of submucosal fibroids are given by transvaginal ultrasound, which can be used to plan myomectomy; fibroids that are less than 5 cm in diameter and predominantly intracavitary are often resectable hysteroscopically.

Fluid in the Endometrial Cavity

Fluid may be seen in the endometrial cavity without vaginal bleeding or discharge. This is due to stenosis of the cervical canal, which can be caused by surgical or obstetric trauma. It can also be due to cervical carcinoma or radiation-induced fibrosis, and if it distends the uterus, it may warrant the label

Figure 12.33 Macroscopic appearance of a submucous myoma, in a uterus with diffuse adenomyosis.

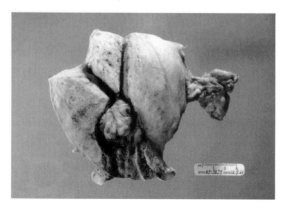

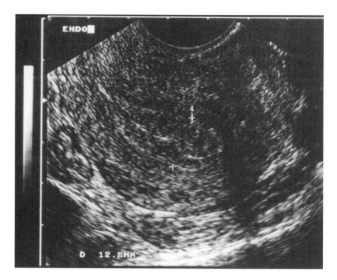

Figure 12.34 Transvaginal sonogram on day 14 of the cycle of a submucous myoma about 1 cm in diameter. The woman was aged 34 and presented because of infertility. The myoma could not be seen on hysteroscopy. (Courtesy of Dr. Robert Lyneham, Sydney, Australia.)

hydrometra, pyometra, or hematometra. But a small amount of fluid in asymptomatic postmenopausal women can be a normal variant or can accompany pathology such as ovarian, tubal, endometrial, or cervical cancer.[58] However, Goldstein[40] studied 51 asymptomatic postmenopausal women with fluid in the uterine cavity and reported that all had some degree of cervical stenosis and that if the surrounding endometrium was thin then it was invariably atrophic and no further investigation was required. In three patients, the surrounding endometrium was more than 3 mm in thickness, and of these, one had an endometrial polyp, while the other two had simple hyperplasia. Histologic diagnosis was considered mandatory if the uterine cavity contains fluid and the sur-

Figure 12.35 A larger (3 cm) submucous myoma distorts the endometrial cavity, causing menorrhagia. Quite small myomas can cause menorrhagia when they distort the endometrial cavity.

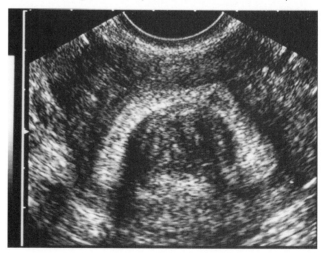

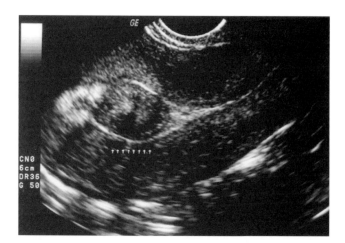

Figure 12.36 A 40-year-old woman presented with persistent menorrhagia after D&C. A 2-cm intracavitary myoma distorts the uterine cavity. Its echogenicity is similar to that of the myometrium. (Courtesy of Dr. Russell Millard, Sydney, Australia.)

rounding endometrium is more than 3 mm thick.[40] A careful search for other gynecologic malignancies is also wise.

SUMMARY

Unlike any other tissue, the endometrium undergoes extraordinary change in health and disease, in youth and old age. It is influenced by cyclic and noncyclic, endogenous and exogenous hormones. It is subject to infection and malignancy. With the advent of transvaginal ultrasound, these dynamic

Figure 12.37 A 69-year-old woman presented with left iliac fossa pain. The uterine cavity is distended to over 2 cm, and the endometrium appears to be heterogeneous. This could have been a possible malignant change. Hysteroscopy revealed small submucosal lieomyomata, and histopathology showed atrophic endometrium without evidence of hyperplastic or neoplastic change.

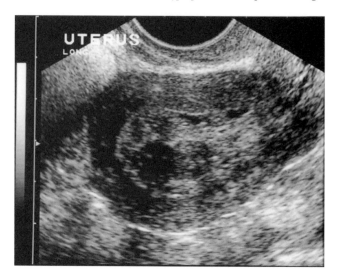

changes can now be scrutinized noninvasively. And unlike curettage and histopathology, transvaginal ultrasound does not disrupt the tissue we strive to understand.

ACKNOWLEDGEMENT

The histopathologic sections and photomicrographs of gross specimens were provided courtesy of Professor Peter Russell, (Sydney, Australia).

REFERENCES

1. Kurman RJ. Benign diseases of the endometrium. In: Blaustein's Pathology of the Female Genital Tract (4th ed.). Springer-Verlag, New York, 1994
2. Dawson-Hughes B. Calcium supplementation and bone loss: a review of controlled clinical trials. Am J Clin Nutr 1991;54:274S–280S
3. Evans RA, Somers NM, Dunstan CR et al. The effect of low-dose cyclical etidronate and calcium on bone mass in early postmenopausal women. Osteoporos Int 1993;3:71–75
4. Clisham PR, Cedars MI, Greendale G et al. Long-term transdermal estradiol therapy: effects on endometrial histology and bleeding patterns. Obstet Gynecol 1992;79:196–201
5. Voigt LF, Weiss NS, Chu J, et al. Progestagen supplementation of exogenous oestrogens and risk of endometrial cancer. Lancet 1991;338:274–277
6. Moyer DL, de Lignieres B, Driguez P, Pez JP. Prevention of endometrial hyperplasia by progesterone during long-term estradiol replacement: influence of bleeding pattern and secretory changes. Fert Steril 1993;59:992–997
7. Hulka CA, Hall DA. Endometrial abnormalities associated with tamoxifen therapy for breast cancer: sonographic and pathologic correlation. AJR Am J Roentgenol 1993;160:809–812
8. Deligdisch L. Effects of hormone therapy on the endometrium. Mod Pathol 1993;6:94–106
9. Kedar RP, Bourne TH, Powles TJ et al. Effects of tamoxifen on uterus and ovaries of postmenopausal women in a randomised breast cancer prevention trial. Lancet 1994;343:1318–1321
10. van Leeuwen FE, Benradt J, Coebergh JW et al. Risk of endometrial cancer after tamoxifen treatment of breast cancer. Lancet 1994;343:448–452
11. Segna RA, Dottino PR, Deligdisch L, Cohen CJ. Tamoxifen and endometrial cancer. Mt Sinai J Med 1992;59:416–418
12. Uziely B, Lewin A, Brufman G et al. The effect of tamoxifen on the endometrium. Breast Cancer Rest Treat 1993;26:101–105
13. Cohen I, Rosen DJ, Shapira J et al. Endometrial changes in postmenopausal women treated with Tamoxifen for breast cancer. Br J Obstet Gynaecol 1993;100:567–570
14. Seoud MA, Johnson J, Weed JC, Jr. Gynecologic tumours in tamoxifen-treated women with breast cancer. Obstet Gynecol 1993;82:165–169
15. Goldstein SR. Unusual ultrasonographic appearance of the uterus in patients receiving tamoxifen. Am J Obstet Gynecol 1994;170:447–451

16. Lahti E, Blanco G, Kauppila A et al. Endometrial changes in postmenopausal breast cancer patients receiving tamoxifen. Obstet Gynecol 1993;81:660–664

17. Wolman I, Sagi J, Pauzner D et al. Transabdominal ultrasonographic evaluation of endometrial thickness in clomiphene citrate-stimulated cycles in relation to conception. J Clin Ultrasound 1994;22:109–112

18. Massai MR, de Ziegler D, Lesobre V et al. Clomiphene citrate affects cervical mucus and endometrial morphology independently of the changes in plasma hormone levels induced by multiple follicular recruitment. Fertil Steril 1993;59:1179–1186

19. Batista MC, Cartledge TP, Zellmer AW et al. Delayed endometrial maturation induced by daily administration of the antiprogestin RU 486: a potential new contraceptive strategy. Am J Obstet Gynecol 1992;167:60–65

20. Vellios F. Endometrial hyperplasia, precursors of endometrial carcinoma. In: Pathology Annual 1972. Appleton-Century-Croft, New York, p 201

21. Kurman RJ. Benign disease of the endometrium. In: Blaustein A, Ed. Pathology of the Female Tract. Springer-Verlag, New York, 1982, p 279

22. Foss BA, Horne HW, Hertig AT. The endometrium and fertility. Fertil Steril 1958;9:193

23. Wallach EE. The uterine factor in infertility. Fertil Steril 1972;23:138–158

24. Gray LA, Robertson RW, Jr, Christopherson WM. Atypical endometrial changes associated with carcinoma. Gynecol Oncol 1974;2:93–100

25. Hertig AT, Sommers SC. Genesis of endometrial carcinoma. Study of prior biopsies. Cancer 1949;2:964

26. Peterson WF, Novak ER. Endometrial polyps. Obstet Gynecol 1956;8:40

27. Gore H, Hertig AT. Carcinoma in situ of endometrium. Am J Obstet Gynecol 1966;94:134–155

28. Wolfe SA, Mackles A. Malignant lesions arising from benign endometrial polyps. Obstet Gynecol 1962;20:542

29. Granberg S, Wikland M, Karlsson B et al. Endometrial thickness as measured by endovaginal ultrasonography for identifying endometrial abnormality. Am J Obstet Gynecol 1991;164:47–52

30. Goldstein SR, Nachtigall M, Snyder JR, Natchigall L. Endometrial assessment by vaginal ultrasonography before endometrial sampling in patient with postmenopausal bleeding. Am J Obstet Gynecol 1990;163:119–123

31. Sheth S, Hamper UM, Kurman RJ. Thickened endometrium in the postmenopausal woman: sonographic–pathologic correlation. Radiology 1993;187:135–139

32. Nasri MN, Coast GJ. Correlation of ultrasound findings and endometrial histopathology in postmenopausal women. Br J Obstet Gynaecol 1989;96:1333–1338

33. Fluhmann CF: Squamous epithelium in the endometrium in benign and malignant conditions. Surg Gynecol Obstet 1928;47:309

34. Scully RE, Poulson H, Sobin LH. International Histological Classification and Histologic Typing of Female Genital Tract Tumours. Springer-Verlag, Berlin, 1994

35. Shipley CF, 3rd, Simmons CL, Nelson GH. Comparison of transvaginal sonography with endometrial biopsy in asymptomatic postmenopausal women. J Ultrasound Med 1994;13:99–104

36. Rullo S, Piccioni MG, Framarino dei Malatesta ML et al. Sonographic, hysteroscopic, histological correlation in the early diagnosis of endometrial carcinoma. Eur J Gynaecol Oncol 1991;12:463–469

37. Osmers R, Volksen M, Rath W, Kuhn W. Vaginosonographic detection of endometrial cancer in postmenopausal women. Int J Gynaecol Obstet 1990;32:35–37

38. Wikland M, Granberg S, Karlsson B. Replacing diagnostic curettage by vaginal ultrasound. Eur J Obstet Gynecol Repord Biol 1993;49:35–38

39. Botsis D, Kassanos D, Pyrgiotis E, Zourlas PA. Vaginal sonography of the endometrium in postmenopausal women. Clin Exp Obstet Gynecol 1992;19:189–192

40. Goldstein SR. Postmenopausal endometrial fluid collections revisited: look at the doughnut rather than the hole. Obstet Gynecol 1994;83:738–740

41. Karlsson B, Granberg S, Wikland M et al. Endovaginal scanning of the endometrium compared to cytology and histology in women with postmenopausal bleeding. Gynecol Oncol 1993;50:173–178

42. Nasri MN, Shepherd JH, Setchell ME et al. The role of vaginal scan in measurement of endometrial thickness in postmenopausal women. Br J Obstet Gynecol 1991;98:470–475

43. Smith P, Bakos O, Heimer G, Ulmsten U. Transvaginal ultrasound for identifying endometrial abnormality. Acta Obstet Gynecol Scand 1991;70:591–594

44. Dorum A, Kristensen GB, Langebrekke A et al. Evaluation of endometrial thickness measured by endovaginal ultrasound in women with postmenopausal bleeding. Acta Obstet Gynecol Scand 1993;72:116–119

45. Bourne TH, Campbell S, Steer CV et al. Detection of endometrial cancer by transvaginal sonography with color flow imaging and blood flow analysis: a preliminary report. Gynecol Oncol 1991;40:253–259

46. Brudenell JM. Chronic endometritis and plasma cell infiltration of the endometrium. J Obstet Gynecol Br Emp 1955;62:269

47. Taylor-Robinson D, McCormack WM. The genital mycoplasmas. N Engl J Med 1980; 302:1003–1010

48. Taylor-Robinson D, McCormack WM. The genital mycoplasmas. N Engl J Med 1980;302:1063–1067

49. Hendrickson MR, Kempson RL. The approach to endometrial diagnosis: a system of nomencalature. In: Bennington JL, (Ed.) Surgical Pathology of the Uterine Corpus. WB Saunders, Philadelphia, 1980, pp 99–157

50. Berry A. A cytopathological and histopathological study of bilharziasis of the female genital tract. J Pathol Bacteriol 1966;91:325–328

51. Mouktar M. Functional disorders due to biharzial infection of the female genital tract. J Obstet Gynaecol Br Commonw 1966;73:307

52. Williams AO. Pathology of schistosomiasis of the uterine cervix due to S. haematobium. Am J Obstet Gynecol 1967;98:784–791

53. Schenken JR, Tamisica J. Enterobious vermicularis (pinworm) infection of the endometrium. Am J Obstet Gynecol 1956; 72:913

54. Weicker ML, Kaneb GD, Goodale RH. Primary echinococal cyst of the uterus. N Engl J Med 1940;223:574

55. Burks DD, Stainken BR, Burkhard TK, Balsara ZN. Uterine inner myometrial foci. Relationship to prior dilatation and curettage and endocervical biopsy. J Ultrasound Med 1991;10:487–492

56. Fleischer A. Transvaginal sonography of the endometrium. In: Fleischer AC, Romero R, Manning FA, Jeanty P, Eds. The Principles and Practice of Ultrasonography in Obstet and Gynecology (4th ed). Appleton & Lange Norwalk, CT 1991

57. Moyer DL, Mishell DR, Jr. Reactions of human endometrium to the intrauterine foreign body. II. Long-term effects on the endometrial histology and cytology. Am J Obstet Gynecol 1971;111:66

58. Carlson JA, Jr, Arger P, Thompson S, Carlson EJ. Clinical and pathologic correlation of endometrial cavity fluid detected by ultrasound in the postmenopausal patient. Obstet Gynecol 1991;77:119–123

13

Sonohysterography of the Endometrium

BUNPEI ISHIZUKA

SHINICHIRO FUJIWAKI

Transvaginal sonography allows us to visualize the endometrium as never before. The interface between the anterior and posterior surface of the endometrium, and changes during the menstrual cycle are well seen.[1,2] Sonohysterography gives even greater detail because there is liquid contrast between the surfaces. This is similar to the detail seen when imaging the fetus at 18 weeks when it is surrounded by amniotic fluid, compared with the difficulty encountered when the membranes are ruptured and there is no fluid. It is a simple matter to instill liquid into the uterine cavity to separate the sonographic interfaces and clarify the echo texture of any enclosed lesion. Sonohysterography demonstrates intrauterine lesions more clearly than does transvaginal ultrasound, especially in cases of leiomyomata, endometrial polyps, and endometrial carcinoma with myometrial invasion.[3]

METHOD

Sonohysterography can be performed using any ultrasound imaging system with a transvaginal transducer of good quality and resolution. A 5.5 or 8-French flexible catheter with balloon is suitable for filling the uterine cavity. We initially inflated the uterine cavity with a catheter whose balloon was at the internal os. However, the balloon catheter interferes with the image of the endometrium in the inferior part of the endometrial cavity. Therefore, we changed to a method of inflating the cavity with the balloon fixed in the cervical canal. Satisfactory inflation of the uterine cavity can also be achieved using a simple catheter with a bulb tip such as the 3-French Jansen Anderson embryo transfer cannula supplied by Cook IVF (K-JET 3200). The catheter in this case is passed through the cervical canal. Using either method, the endometrial cavity is slightly distended with 5 to 10 ml of 10% glucose (or any clear sterile isotonic aqueous solution or gel)[4] while being recorded on transvaginal ultrasound (Fig. 13.1).

SEPTATE UTERUS

Usually, the separate parts of the uterine cavity can be seen on transvaginal sonography. On a coronal scan, the cavities can be identified (Fig. 13.2). With contrast, however, the thickness of the wall of the septum can be measured. This condition can also be seen on magnetic resonance imaging (MRI).

SURGICAL SCAR

With sonohysterography, a surgical scar, which otherwise would be impossible to visualize, can be seen (Fig. 13.3). This patient had undergone an operation to excise a left rudimentary horn of the uterus with an incision on the left side of the remaining right horn.

INTRAMURAL LEIOMYOMA

When the leiomyoma is intramural, it may distend the endometrial cavity. This can be difficult to demonstrate on transvaginal scanning, but on sonohysterography, the boundaries can be distinguished in relationship to the endometrial cavity (Fig. 13.4).

SUBMUCOSAL LEIOMYOMA

It is frequently difficult to decide whether a small myoma is pedunculated, submucosal, or intramural[5] (Fig. 13.5). The distinction can be important in the case of infertility or in women complaining of menorrhagia. Instillation of the uter-

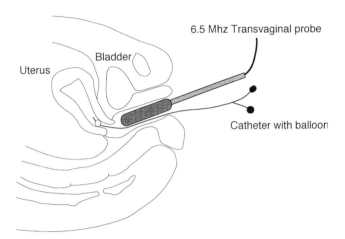

Figure 13.1 Schematic drawing of sonohysterography: The balloon at the tip of the catheter is placed at the internal os or in the cervical canal.

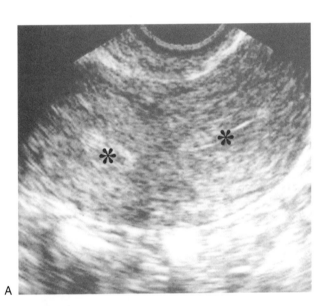

A

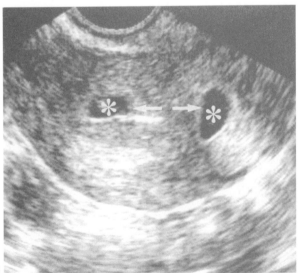

B

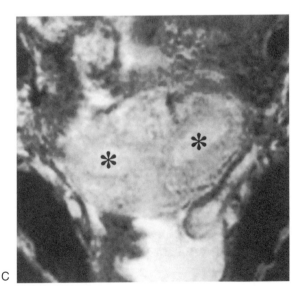

C

Figure 13.2 Septate uterus. (**A**) Transvaginal ultrasound: Two hyperechoic endometrial echoes (asterisks) are seen. (**B**) Sonohysterography: Two endometrial cavities (asterisks) are shown. Therefore, it is possible to measure the thickness of the septum (arrows). (**C**) MRI, T2-weighted image: The two endometria are of high signal intensity (asterisks).

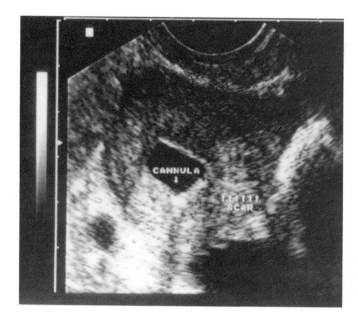

Figure 13.3 Surgical scar. Transvaginal sonohysterogram showing a coronal view of the remaining horn of the uterus. This patient had a left rudimentary horn removed, leaving the right horn with a transverse scar. This scar could not be seen using conventional transvaginal ultrasound, but with contrast, the scar is well demonstrated (arrows). The scar is quite sound.

ine cavity outlines the fibroid, indicating that it is submucosal. Hysteroscopy will confirm that the mass is submucosal if not pedunculated.

secretory endometrium or submucus fibroids (Fig. 13.6). With contrast, the endometrial polyps become quite obvious. These polyps were confirmed on hysterosalpingography.

ENDOMETRIAL POLYP

Perhaps the greatest use of sonohysterography is in the demonstration of endometrial polyps.[3] Without contrast, endometrial polyps can be very difficult to distinguish from

SUBMUCOSAL LEIOMYOMA AND ENDOMETRIAL POLYP

In other cases where the pathology of endometrial masses is unclear (Fig. 13.7), it is possible to resolve the condition with

Figure 13.4 Intramural leiomyoma. (**A**) Transvaginal ultrasound: The leiomyoma (asterisk) is seen in the uterus, but its position in relationship to the cavity cannot be determined. (**B**) Sonohysterography: With an expanded fluid-filled endometrial cavity (arrowheads), the leiomyoma (asterisk) is localized. It can be seen in the myometrium.

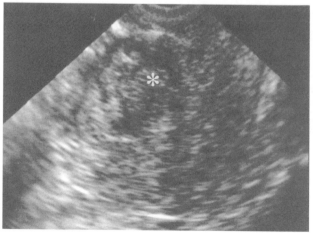

A

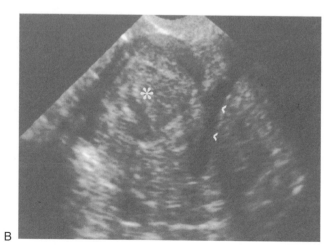

B

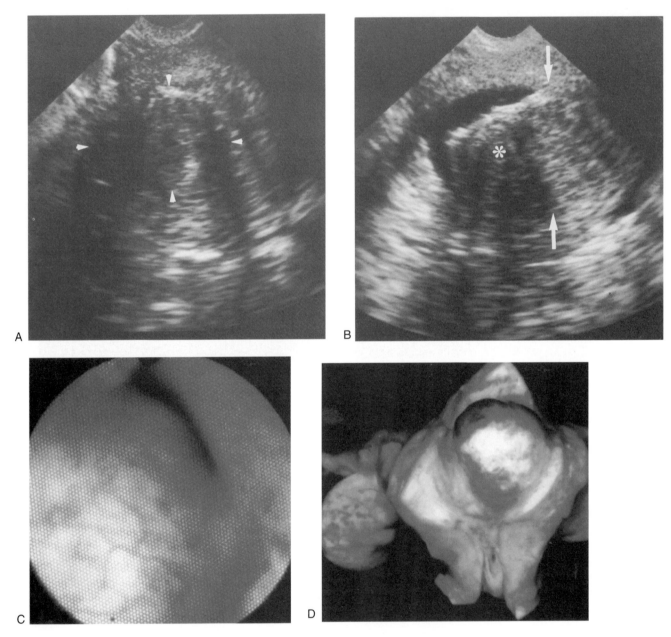

Figure 13.5 Submucosal leiomyoma. (**A**) Transvaginal ultrasound: Sagittal section of the mass in the uterus (arrowheads) shows it as a homogenous area of low echogenecity. (**B**) Sonohysterography: The same section shows that the mass (asterisk) in the endometrial cavity originates from the myometrium (arrows). (**C**) Hysteroscopy: The mass is seen in the uterine cavity. The mass is submucosal and almost pedunculated. (**D**) Macroscopic specimen: The leiomyoma originates from the posterior wall of the uterus, as seen on sonohysterography.

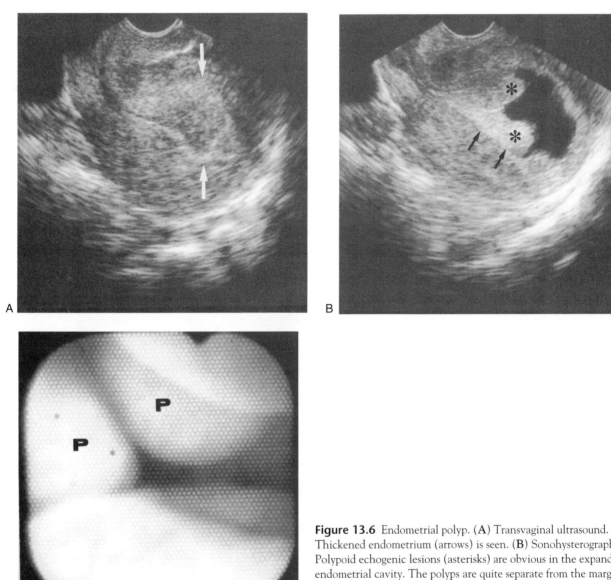

Figure 13.6 Endometrial polyp. (**A**) Transvaginal ultrasound. Thickened endometrium (arrows) is seen. (**B**) Sonohysterography: Polypoid echogenic lesions (asterisks) are obvious in the expanded endometrial cavity. The polyps are quite separate from the margin of the myometrium (arrows). (**C**) Hysteroscopy: The polyps are seen top left and top right (P).

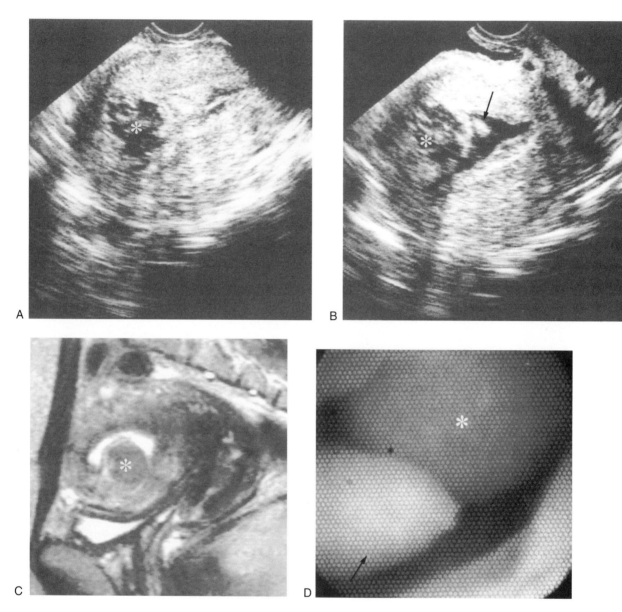

Figure 13.7 Coexisting submucosal leiomyoma and endometrial polyp. (**A**) Transvaginal ultrasound: A heterogenous echo complex (asterisk) and hyperechoic endometrium are seen in the uterus, but resolving the pathology is difficult. (**B**) Sonohysterography: The heterogenous mass originating from myometrium (asterisk) and a small echogenic lesion arising from the endometrium, (arrow) are seen in the endometrial cavity. (**C**) MRI, T2-weighted image: An isointense mass (asterisk) originating from myometrium is present in the endometrial cavity, consistent with the submucosal leiomyoma. (**D**) Hysteroscopy. The endometrial polyp (arrow) is at the lower left. The submucosal myoma (asterisk) is at the posterior aspect of the polyp.

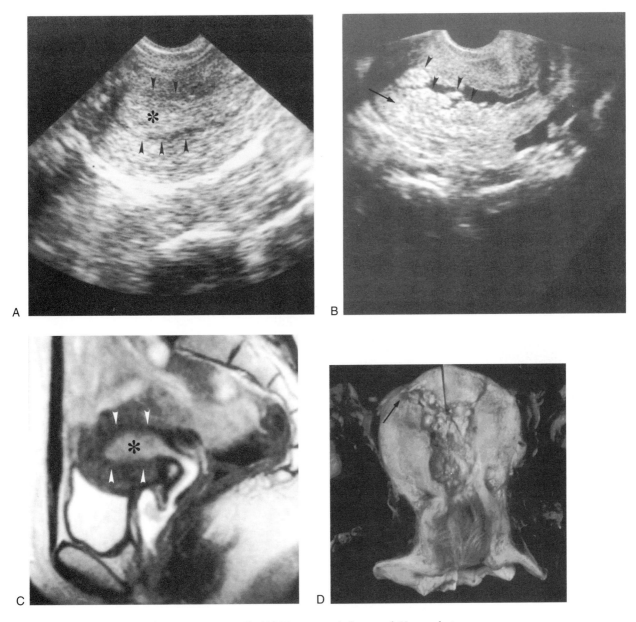

Figure 13.8 Endometrial carcinoma, stage 1b. (**A**) Transvaginal ultrasound: Hyperechoic endometrium (asterisk) is present. There is a halo (arrowheads) around it, suggesting that any lesion is confined. (**B**) Sonohysterography: The endometrium has irregular edges and thick hyperechoic areas (arrowheads). The endometrium in the posterior wall of the uterus is invading into the outer half of the myometrium (arrow). (**C**) MRI, T2-weighted image: The endometrium (asterisk) has high signal intensity. The halo (arrowheads) is again clearly visualized. Myometrial invasion is not seen. (**D**) Macroscopic specimen: The polypoid mass (arrow) invaded the outer half of myometrium.

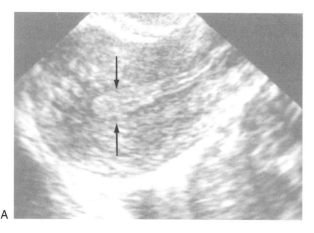

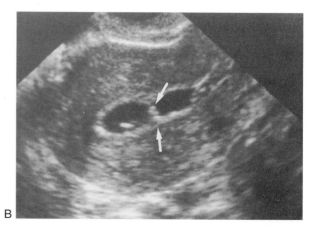

Figure 13.9 Intrauterine adhesion. (**A**) Transvaginal ultrasound: The endometrium (arrows) is normally visualized. (**B**) Sonohysterography: A linear echo extends from anterior to posterior endometrium (arrows).

contrast. In this case, a submucosal leiomyoma and a polyp coexist. The image without contrast fails to resolve the lesions. With contrast, a small polyp is seen in addition to a submucus leiomyoma. On a T2-weighted MRI, the leiomyoma was the only mass to be seen. Both lesions are confirmed on hysteroscopy.

ENDOMETRIAL CARCINOMA

Distinguishing early endometrial carcinoma from endometrial hyperplasia or even from an exaggerated secretory change is usually impossible on transvaginal ultrasound (Fig. 13.8). With contrast, the irregular endometrial surface becomes evident, and even the extent of invasion can be estimated.[6–9] On MRI, the invasion of the endometrium is not seen. The lesion was confirmed at hysterectomy (Fig. 13.8D).

INTRAUTERINE ADHESIONS

Transvaginal sonography of the uterine cavity is normal in most cases with adhesions.[6,7] It is usually not possible to identify the small areas where the anterior and posterior walls adhere (Fig. 13.9A). With contrast, the adhesions become quite obvious (Fig. 13.9B).

SUMMARY

Sonohysterography is a form of contrast-enhanced transvaginal ultrasound. It has proved to be simple and repeatable. It can differentiate intrauterine lesions with higher specificity compared to transvaginal ultrasound, hysterosalpingography, and MRI.

REFERENCES

1. Fleischer AC, Kalemeris GC, Entman SS. Sonographic depiction of the endometrium during normal cycles. Ultrasound Med Biol 1986;12:271–277
2. Forrest TS, Elyaderani MK, Muilenburg MI et al. Cyclic endometrial changes: US assessment with histologic correlation. Radiology 1988;167:233–237
3. Deichert U, van de Sandt M, Lauth G, Daume E. Transvaginal contrast hysterosonography. A new diagnostic procedure for the differentiation of intrauterine and myometrial findings. Geburtshilfe Frauenheikd 1988;48:835–844
4. Klug PW. Vaginal sonographic contrast imaging of the endometrium with gel. Geburtshilfe Frauenheilkd. 1991;51:469–473
5. Fukuda M, Shimizu T, Fukuda K et al. Transvaginal hysterosonography for differential diagnosis between submucous and intramural myoma. Gynecol Obstet Invest 1993;35: 236–239
6. Parsons AK, Lense JJ. Sonohysterography for endometrial abnormalities: preliminary results. J Clin Ultrasound 1993;21: 87–95
7. Goldstein SR. Use of ultrasonohysterography for triage of perimenopausal patients with unexplained uterine bleeding. Am J Obstet Gynecol 1994;170:565–570
8. Becker H, Hotzinger H. Hysterosonography and its significance in the diagnosis of endometrial cancer. Gerburtshilfe Frauenheilkd 1986;46:693–696
9. Sahakian V, Syrop C, Turner D. Endometrial carcinoma transvaginal ultrasonography prediction of depth of myometrial invasion. Gynecol Oncol 1991;43:217–219

Computed Tomography and Magnetic Resonance Imaging of the Endometrium

YASUYUKI YAMASHITA

MUTSUMASA TAKAHASHI

Ultrasound is the preferred method of imaging the endometrium, but computed tomography (CT) and magnetic resonance imaging (MRI) are useful for investigating abnormalities that are equivocal on ultrasonography and for assessing malignancy, especially in patients unsuitable for surgery.

Although CT has been widely used for pretreatment assessment of endometrial cancer, it is not an accurate method for determining the depth of myometrial invasion.[1] MRI is preferred for demonstrating deep myometrial or cervical invasion.[2–4] In the management of uterine malignancies, CT is used primarily for evaluating metastatic or recurrent disease. Pretreatment staging with CT or MRI is used to determine the extent of myometrial invasion and influences whether or not the patient has preoperative intracavitary radiation.[2–8] CT can be used to study patients with suspected advanced disease if they are unsuitable for surgery.[1–9] In clinical practice, various benign conditions may mimic endometrial cancer and should be differentiated from it. This is often difficult on MRI or CT alone.

BENIGN CONDITIONS

Polyps, hyperplasia, and carcinoma usually appear as a thickening of the endometrium.[10,11] Normal secretory change and decidual change in early or ectopic pregnancy can also cause the endometrium to be thickened. In one study of 18 patients with endometrial carcinoma detected by sonography, the average endometrial thickness was 17.7 mm ± 5.8 mm.[11] The thickening of the endometrium when hyperplastic is seen in Figure 14.1. In endometrial carcinoma confined to the endometrium, a similar and indistinguishable thickening may be the only finding on MRI or on CT.[12] Carcinoma in situ can produce a completely normal MRI, or it can have a thickened appearance, as is seen in Figure 14.2. Patients with endometrial atrophy have an endometrium less than 8 mm in thickness. The thicker the endometrium, the more likely it is to be abnormal.

Endometrial Polyps

Endometrial polyps are not true neoplasms but are circumscribed foci of hyperplasia.[13] They are common incidental findings and typically appear as diffuse or focal thickening of the endometrium. They are indistinguishable from endometrial carcinomata or hyperplasia on CT or MRI unless histologic examination is performed. On T2-weighted MRI the signal intensity is variable and indistinguishable from that of the adjacent myometrium (Fig. 14.3), while submucosal leiomyomata typically have a signal intensity lower than or the same as that of the adjacent myometrium (Fig. 14.4). When an endometrial polyp is of medium signal intensity on a T2-weighted image, it may be indistinguishable from a submucosal leiomyoma. With contrast, endometrial polyps usually appear less enhanced (Fig. 14.3). Although contrast improves the detection of endometrial polyps, the pattern of enhancement is nonspecific, and differentiation from other endometrial abnormalities (atypical polypoid adenomyoma, endometrial hyperplasia, polypoid endometrial carcinoma, or submucosal leiomyoma) may be difficult.[14,15]

Adhesions

Endometrial adhesions can follow vigorous curettage, and when oligomenorrhea or amenorrhea result, the condition is known as Asherman syndrome.[16] Although best diagnosed with hysteroscopy or hysterosalpingography, endometrial adhesions have occasionally been observed with T2-weighted MRI as irregularities or bridges within the endometrial cavity.[17] They are better seen during menstruation, or following distension of the uterine cavity with contrast.[18]

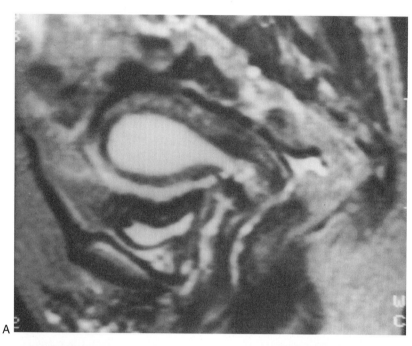

A

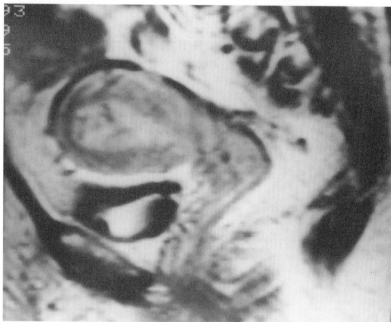

B

Figure 14.1 Endometrial hyperplasia in a 76-year-old. **(A)** This sagittal T2-weighted image shows a relatively large uterus for age with distension of the endometrial cavity. The junctional zone is clearly seen. **(B)** Postcontrast T1-weighted image: An irregular enhanced area is seen in the distended endometrial cavity, indistinguishable from superficial endometrial carcinoma.

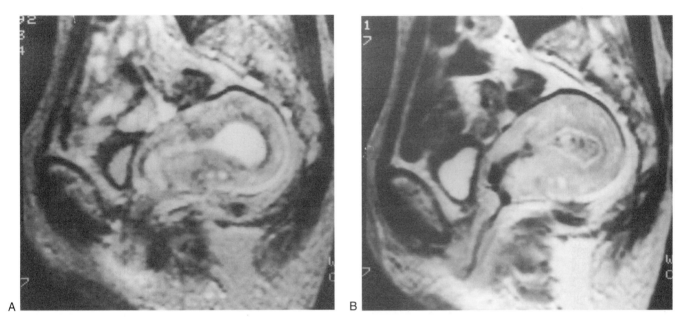

Figure 14.2 Carcinoma in situ in a 80-year-old. **(A)** This sagittal T2-weighted image shows a retroverted uterus with thickening of the endometrium due to carcinoma in situ. Although 80 years of age, the uterus is large and the junctional zone is visible, suggesting an estrogenic state. **(B)** Postcontrast T1-weighted image: An irregular enhanced area is seen due to the thickened endometrium.

Figure 14.3 Endometrial polyp in a 41-year-old. **(A)** The T2-weighted image shows the cervical canal distended by a lesion of intermediate signal intensity. The polyp appears to be sessile (arrow). **(B)** The postcontrast T1-weighted image also shows a slightly enhancing sessile tumor (arrow).

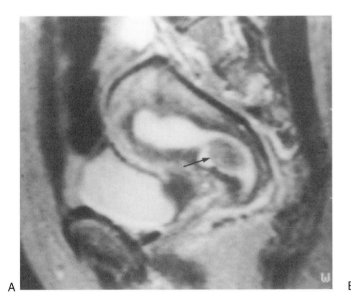

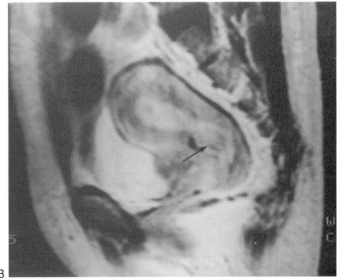

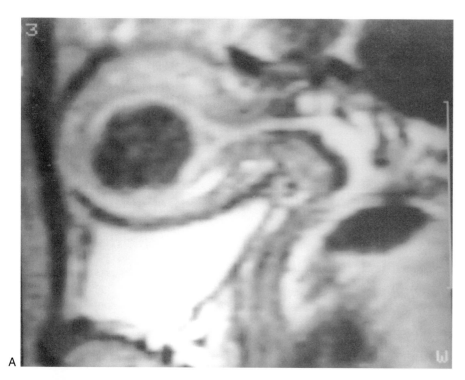

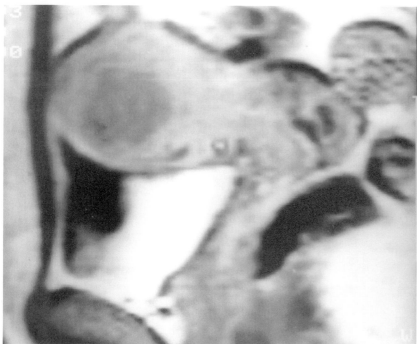

Figure 14.4 Submucosal leiomyoma in a 43-year-old. (**A**) This sagittal T2-weighted image shows a submucosal leiomyoma of very low intensity compared to the myometrium. (**B**) The postcontrast T1-weighted image demonstrates the slight degree of enhancement after contrast. Contrast enhancement pattern does not allow differentiation between endometrial polyp and submucosal leiomyoma.

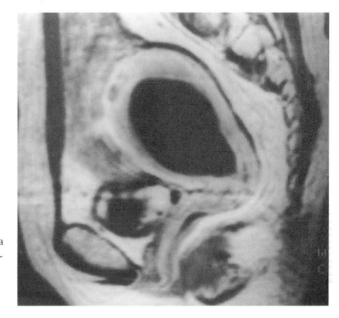

Figure 14.5 Endometrial pyometra due to endometrial carcinoma in a 55-year-old. On postcontrast T1-weighted image, the endometrial cavity is distended due to pyometra. Tumor is not visualized. On pathologic examination, superficial tumor obstructed internal os, causing pyometra. (From Yamashita et al,[8] with permission.)

Figure 14.6 Atypical polypoid adenomyoma in a 30-year-old. **(A)** Sagittal T2-weighted MRI (2,000/80) shows a heterogeneous lesion of similar signal intensity with thickened myometrium. Hyperintense areas are seen within the tumor (arrowheads). **(B)** Postcontrast T1-weighted image: Gadolinium-diethylenetriaminepentaacetic acid-enhanced MRI reveals irregular enhancement of the tumor. Hyperintense areas on T2-weighted images showed contrast enhancement as did endometrium (arrowheads).

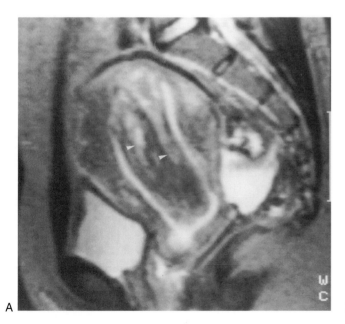

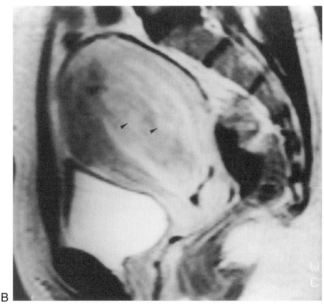

Endometrial Fluid

Small amounts of normal fluid can be retained in the endometrial cavity temporarily in women with acute anterversions or retroversions, especially after periods of inactivity. Larger amounts of fluid such as blood or pus can be retained more permanently in women with congenital vaginal or cervical atresia, cervical stricture, obstructive uterine masses, including malignancy, or pelvic inflammatory disease.[19–21]

On T2-weighted MRI, fluid is similar to hyperintense endometrial thickening and may be difficult to distinguish from endometrial carcinoma. With contrast enhancement, simple fluid or a pyometra becomes obvious in the endometrial cavity (Fig. 14.5). In patients with hematometra, the blood is hyperintense on T1-weighted imaging.

Intrauterine Contraceptive Device

Both metallic and non metallic intrauterine contraceptive devices (IUCDs) are better visualized with transvaginal ultrasound or CT than with MRI. On ultrasound, an IUCD forms a highly echogenic and reflective interface within the endometrial cavity.[22] MRI and CT have little role in the detection of IUCDs.

Endometrial Hyperplasia

When hyperplastic, the endometrium is thickened on T2-weighted MRIs.[12] MRIs are similar to those of superficial endometrial carcinoma, making the distinction difficult (see Figs. 14.1 and 14.2). In both endometrial hyperplasia and stage Ia endometrial carcinoma, the junctional zone appears normal. With contrast, hyperplasias appear as slightly enhancing masses. The degree of enhancement is more intense in hyperplasia than in invasive carcinomas.

Atypical Polypoid Adenomyoma

When endometrial polyps have smooth muscle fibers in addition to glands and stroma, they are described as polypoid adenomyomata, or its variant, the atypical polypoid adenomyoma.[23–25]

Atypical polypoid adenomyoma is a benign form of mixed epithelial and mesenchymal tumor of the uterus, most frequently seen in the endometrial cavity. Some atypical polypoid adenomyomata occur in women with Turner syndrome who have been on estrogen therapy.[26] They usually present in women with abnormal uterine bleeding and can occasionally contain an adenocarcinoma. Central necrosis may be present. The glands occurring between the endometrial stroma and smooth muscle exhibit varying degrees of hyperplasia and atypia. T2-weighted MRIs show a polypoid mass in the uterine cavity (Fig. 14.6). The signal intensity is similar to that of adenomyosis. Multiple hyperintense areas are seen, corresponding to islands of metaplastic endometrial foci. With contrast, the pattern of enhancement of these areas is similar to that of the endometrium (Fig. 14.6).

MALIGNANT CONDITIONS

Endometrial Carcinoma

The 1971 staging system for endometrial cancer devised by the International Federation of Gynecology and Obstetrics (FIGO) was a *clinical* system. This staging system is shown in Table 14.1. It depended on examination under anesthesia, sounding of the uterus, endocervical (fractional) curettage, hysteroscopy, cystoscopy, proctoscopy, and x ray of the lungs and skeleton. It is only used now for patients unsuitable for surgery. This system was shown to understage a number of patients when compared to surgical staging,[27–32] and consequently, in 1988 FIGO changed to a system based on staging after surgery. This system is shown in Table 14.2. MRI was evaluated as a tool for preoperative staging in a National Cancer Institute study. The accuracy for diagnosing the depth of myometrial invasion was 66%, and imaging was considered adequate for the evaluation of para-aortic nodes in 8% of cases.[33] Preoperative evaluation of endometrial cancer with MRI therefore has a limited role in the preoperative evaluation of endometrial cancer.

CT has been used to detect endometrial carcinoma and follow the effects of therapy, and there have been reports suggesting that MRI, including conventional T2-weighted spin echo and contrast-enhanced techniques[2,4,6,8,34–41] and transvaginal sonography,[42–48] may be preferred in this role.

Computed Tomography

Endometrial carcinomas usually produce focal or global enlargement of the uterine body. They are seen on contrast CT

Table 14.1 1971 FIGO Clinical Staging for Endometrial Carcinoma

Stage 0	Carcinoma in situ
Stage I	The carcinoma is confined to the corpus
Stage Ia	The length of the uterine cavity is 8 cm or less
Stage Ib	The length of the uterine cavity is more than 8 cm
Stage I cases should be subgrouped with regard to the histologic grade of the adenocarcinoma as follows:	
Grade 1	Highly differentiated adenomatous carcinoma
Grade 2	Moderately differentiated adenomatous carcinoma with partly solid areas.
Stage II	The carcinoma has involved the corpus and the cervix but not extended outside the uterus.
Stage III	The carcinoma has extended outside the uterus but not outside the true pelvis.
Stage IV	The carcinoma has extended outside the true pelvis or has obviously involved the mucosa of the bladder or rectum. A bullous edema as such does not permit a case to be allocated to Stage IV.
Stage IVa	Spread of the growth to adjacent organs
Stage IVb	Spread to distant organs

Table 14.2 1988 FIGO Surgical Staging
for Endometrial Cancer

Stage Ia	G123	Tumor limited to the endometrium
Stage Ib	G123	Invasion to less than one-half the myometrium
Stage Ic	G123	Invasion to more than one-half the myometrium
Stage IIa	G123	Endocervical gland involvement only
Stage IIb	G123	Cervical stromal invasion
Stage IIIa	G123	Tumor invades serosa and/or adnesa and/or positive peritoneal cytology
Stage IIIb	G123	Vaginal metastases
Stage IIIc	G123	Metastases to pelvic or para-aortic lymph nodes
Stage IVa	G123	Tumour invasion of bladder and/or bowel mucosa
Stage IVb		Distant metastases including intraabdominal and/or inguinal lymph nodes

Rules related in staging:
1. Because corpus cancer is now staged surgically, procedures previously used for determination of stages are no longer applicable such as the findings from fractional D&C to differentiate between stage I and stage II.
2. It is appreciated that there may be a small number of patients with corpus cancer who will be treated primarily with radiation therapy. If that is the case, the clinical staging adopted by FIGO in 1971 would still apply but designation of that staging system would be noted.
3. Ideally, width of the myometrium should be measured along with the width of tumor invasion.

as hypodense areas surrounded by well-enhanced normal myometrium[49,50] (Fig. 14.7). Carcinomas extending to the cervix may occlude the internal os, resulting in a hydrometra, hematometra, or pyometra.[20] In these conditions, CT shows a symmetrically enlarged uterus containing a central water-density mass but does not distinguish hydrometra from pyometra unless gas is present.[51] The hypodense area represents a tumor with variable necrosis. Attenuation of an endometrial carcinoma on precontrast CT scans is often indistinguishable from those found in submucosal leiomyomas of the uterus. Calcification and/or fatty degeneration in a uterine mass suggests a benign leiomyoma, although calcification is sometimes seen in an endometrial carcinoma[51] (Fig. 14.8).

Diagnosis of cervical involvement of endometrial carcinoma is very difficult with axial CT. Although CT has been the preferred method of assessing advanced endometrial cancers, MRI has been shown to be more accurate in evaluating local disease.[2–4] CT is useful in assessing recurrent disease (Fig. 14.9) and for the assessment of omental, peritoneal, skeletal, and hepatic metastases.

Magnetic Resonance Imaging

The most common finding on MRI in patients with a small tumor of the endometrium is widening of the cavity due to the tumor or an associated fluid collection[2,4,8,52,53] (see Fig. 14.2). On T2-weighted images, myometrial invasion by an endometrial carcinoma appears as a mass of high or heterogenous signal intensity that invades the junctional zone and disrupts the intermediate signal intensity of the outer myometrium (Fig. 14.10). The carcinoma and adjacent endometrium or myometrium are frequently indistinguishable, because the MRI signal intensity of these tissues is sometimes similar[2,6,8,38,52,54,55] (Fig. 14.11). The distinction between viable tumor and uterine secretion or necrotic tissue is often difficult on T2-weighted images (Fig. 14.12).

Enhanced MRI is superior to conventional T2-weighted MRI in the assessment of endometrial carcinoma because of the greater contrast between tumor and myometrium or between tumor and endometrium.[15,34,36,39] Tumors usually enhance somewhat less than myometrium after gadolinium-diethylenetriamine pentaacetic acid (Gd-DTPA) (Figs. 14.11 and 14.13). Early-phase Gd-DTPA-enhanced imaging also differentiates vascularized tumor from nonenhanced necrosis or residual secretion (Fig. 14.12). Gd-DTPA identifies tumor volume and small lesions and better enhances the subendometrial and myometrial layers than postcontrast T1-weighted images[34] (Fig. 14.12). Unenhanced T1-weighted images usually offer no additional information about the endometrial cavity. Although MRI is suitable for assessing endometrial carcinoma, it is too time-consuming and expensive to be used as a screening test for endometrial cancer.[54] Transvaginal sonography is much more operator dependent than MRI but is less expensive and more widely available.

The most reliable sign of myometrial invasion on MRI is focal or segmental disruption of the junctional zone[2,6,7,38,52] (Figs. 14.10 and 14.14). Myometrial invasion is best imaged in two planes[2] (Figs. 14.14 and 14.15). A distinct junctional zone is not always seen in postmenopausal women. Focal thinning of the myometrium or irregularity of the tumor–myometrial interface is another sign of myometrial invasion[2,52] (Figs. 14.12 and 14.15). Assessment of depth of invasion is often difficult on T2-weighted images, because signal contrast between tumor and residual myometrium is not obvious.[8,34,56] Enhanced MRI may be useful because contrast between tumor and residual myometrium is more marked[8,34] (Figs. 14.11 and 14.13).

With T2-weighted MRIs, accuracy of 74% to 87% in assessing myometrial invasion has been reported.[4,8,34–39] Transvaginal sonography and conventional T2-weighted MRI have been found to be comparable. Contrast-enhanced MRI is more accurate in detecting myometrial invasion than transvaginal sonography and conventional T2-weighted images.[8]

Stage IIA disease can be seen in Figures 14.15 and 14.16. On T2-weighted images, there is dilatation of the internal os, which may occur with or without visualization of a mass of

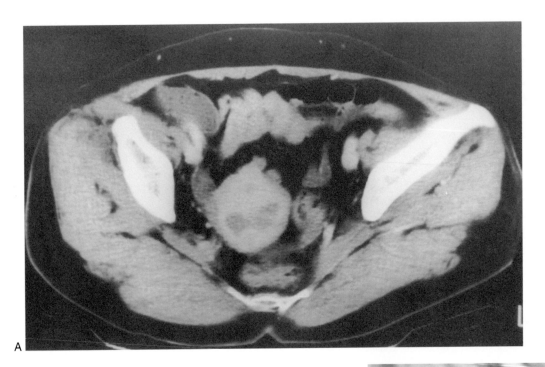

Figure 14.7 Endometrial carcinoma in a 62-year-old. **(A)** Contrast-enhanced CT shows a hypodense lesion within well-enhanced myometrium. Anterior wall of the uterus is thick. **(B)** This T2-weighted MRI shows widening of the endometrium. Adenomyosis is seen in the anterior wall.

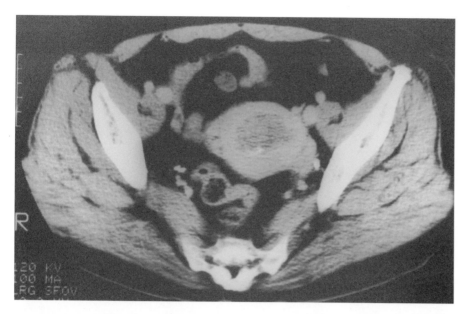

Figure 14.8 Endometrial carcinoma in a 62-year-old. Contrast-enhanced CT shows a hypodense lesion within well-enhanced myometrium. A small focus of calcification is seen.

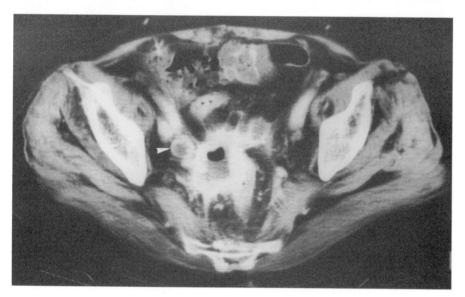

Figure 14.9 Recurrent endometrial cancer in a 66-year-old. On CT, a solid pelvic mass with cavitation is seen. The margin of the tumor is irregular, indicating invasion to the surrounding tissues. Right internal iliac lymph node swelling is seen (arrowhead).

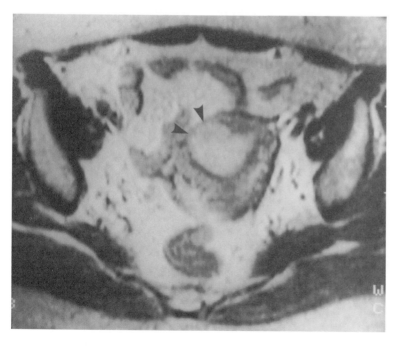

Figure 14.10 Endometrial carcinoma (stage Ic) in a 76-year-old. An axial T2-weighted image shows a high-intensity mass distending the endometrial cavity. There is disruption of the junctional zone and high-intensity tumor deep in the myometrium (arrowheads).

219

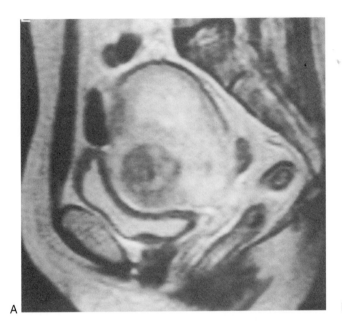
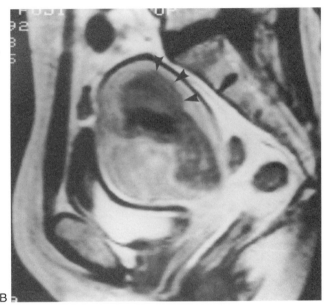

Figure 14.11 Endometrial carcinoma (stage Ic) in a 60-year-old. **(A)** A T2-weighted image shows diffuse hyperintensity in the myometrium, representing deep invasion. However, the carcinoma and adjacent endometrium or myometrium are frequently indistinguishable, because the MRI signal intensity of these tissues is similar. A myoma nodule is seen in the anterior wall. **(B)** On the postcontrast T1-weighted image, the tumor was seen as a hypointense area compared with well-enhanced myometrium, deeply invading the posterior myometrial wall (arrowheads). The contrast between the tumor and myometrium or endometrial cavity is apparently superior in the enhanced image. Gd-DTPA is seen in the bladder. (From Yamashita et al,[8] with permission.)

Figure 14.12 Endometrial carcinoma (stage IB) in a 53-year-old. **(A)** A T2-weighted image of the sagittal plane shows a heterogeneous high signal intensity in the endometrial cavity. The intensity at the center of the tumor is irregular, the junctional zone is irregularly observed, and the anterior portion has disappeared. The central unenhanced area in the endometrial cavity is consistent with necrotic debris of the tumor (asterisk). (*Figure continues.*)

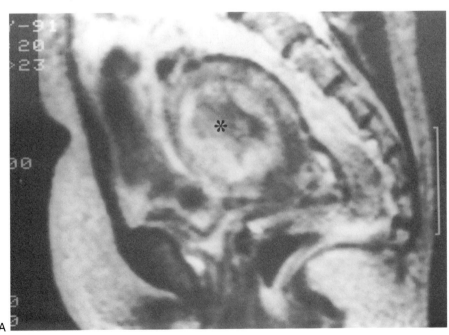

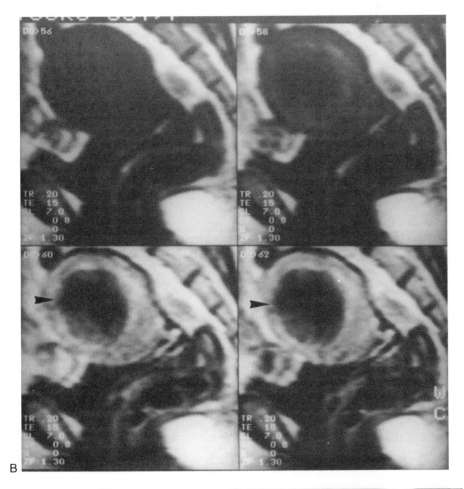

B

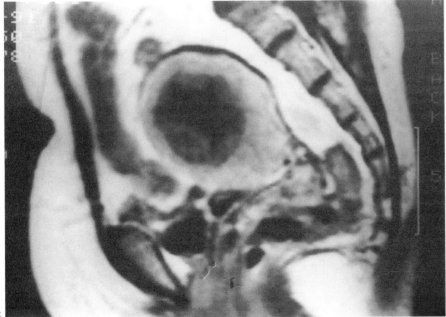

C

Figure 14.12 (*Continued*). **(B)** Dynamic MRIs. Upper left, before, upper right, 30 seconds; lower left, 60 seconds; lower right, 90 seconds. **(C)** Postcontrast T1-weighted image. At 60 and 90 seconds of dynamic images, the tumor is seen as intermediate signal intensity comparing with well-enhanced myometrium. Because subendometrial enhancement is irregularly interrupted and myometrium is thin in the anterior wall (arrowheads), myometrial invasion is suspected. Histologically, papillary tumor extended superficially to the entire endometrium, and there was 50% invasion of the myometrium. (From Yamashita et al,[34] with permission.)

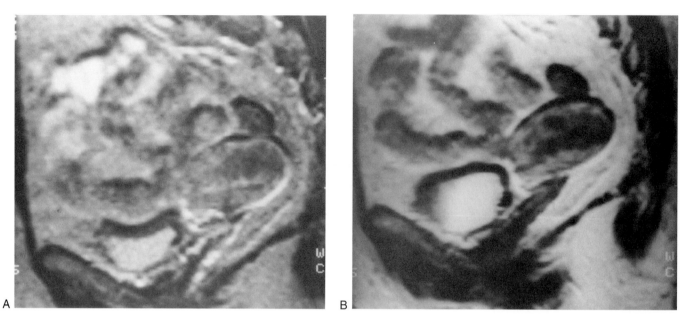

Figure 14.13 Endometrial carcinoma (stage IC) in a 60-year-old. **(A)** A T2-weighted image shows irregular hypointensity in the anterior myometrium, although hyperintensity of the endometrium appears to be preserved. The tumor was thought to represent deep invasion. **(B)** Postcontrast T1-weighted image. The tumor was seen as a hypointense area compared with well-enhanced myometrium, invading the full thickness of the myometrial wall. (From Yamashita et al,[8] with permission.)

Figure 14.14 Endometrial carcinoma (adenoacanthoma Ib) in a 36-year-old. **(A)** Sagittal T2-weighted image. The endometrium has a homogeneous hyperintense signal, protruding into the anterior myometrium. (*Figure continues.*)

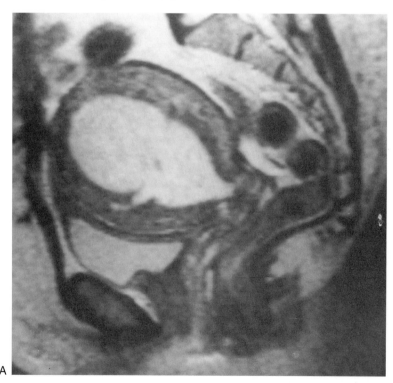

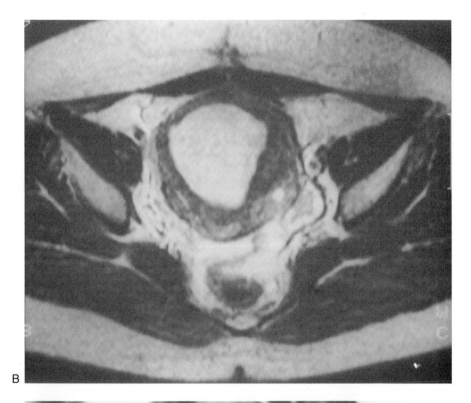

B

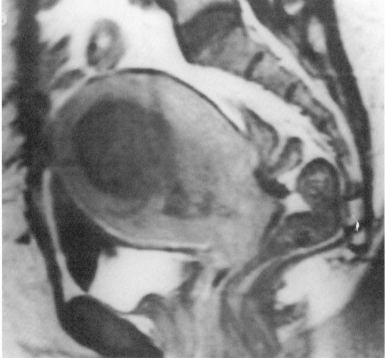

C

Figure 14.14 (*Continued*). **(B)** Axial T2-weighted image. On the right side, the myometrium is thin. The junctional zone is not clearly seen. **(C)** A sagittal postcontrast T1-weighted image shows a slightly enhanced mass distending the endometrial cavity.

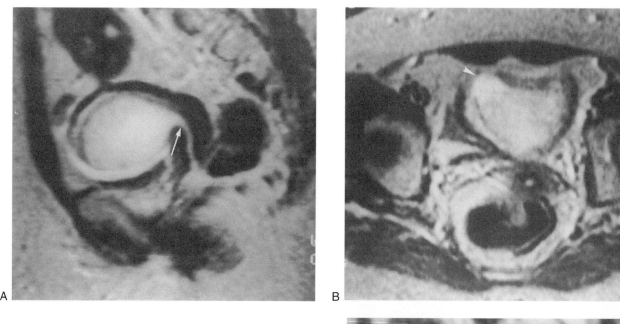

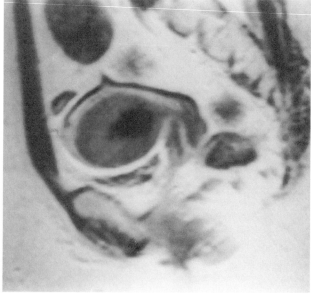

Figure 14.15 Endometrial carcinoma (stage IIa) in a 60-year-old. **(A)** T2-weighted image (sagittal). Marked distension of the endometrial cavity is seen. The residual myometrium is thin. The internal os is widened because of tumor extension (arrow). **(B)** T2-weighted image (axial). Although the junctional zone is not seen, deep myometrial invasion is apparent in right fundus (arrowhead). **(C)** This postcontrast T1-weighted image clearly shows carcinoma, with a necrotic area within the tumor and the residual myometrium.

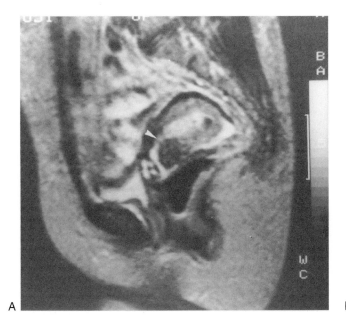 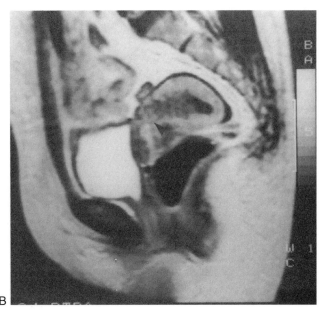

Figure 14.16 Endometrial carcinoma (stage IIa) in a 55-year-old. **(A)** T2-weighted image (sagittal): A heterogeneous intense lesion is seen extending into the endocervical canal (arrowhead). **(B)** The postcontrast T1-weighted image also shows the mass extending to the internal os (arrowhead).

similar intensity to the primary tumor.[4] Stage IIB disease can be seen on T2-weighted images when a mass invades and disrupts the low signal intensity of the fibrous cervical stroma.[2,38,52] The accuracy of stage II disease on MRI is reported to be 85% to 90%.[53,57]

Assessment of stage III or IV disease requires examination of the adnexa, uterine and cervical ligaments, pelvic lymph nodes, bladder, and rectal walls.[2,5–7,52] The accuracy of MRI for assessing stage III and IV tumors is less clear because the number of patients reported is small, although MRI has been reported to compare favorably with CT.[2] Microscopic spread of disease to lymph nodes, ovaries, parametria, or cervices, as well as small (<2 cm) peritoneal or omental implants, are not usually identified on MRI examination.[2,3,52] The sensitivity for the detection of stage III or IV disease by MRI was only 17%, and the positive predictive value for findings suggestive of advanced disease was only 50% in one study.[6]

Direct extension of the tumor through the serosal surface of the uterus disrupting the signal intensity of the parametrial fat indicates parametrial spread.[2,3] Ovarian metastases usually appear as lobulated, triangular, occasionally large masses of intermediate signal intensity rather than the normal signal intensity of the ovarian stroma[2,3,52] (Fig. 14.17). Peritoneal or omental tumor implants are usually of intermediate signal intensity on T1-weighted images and higher signal intensity on T2-weighted images. The presence of normal pelvic fat planes does not exclude extrauterine spread of microscopic foci of tumor. The criterion for diagnosing lymph node metastases by tumor is a length greater than 1.5 cm in the pelvic or para-aortic regions. The determination of lymphadenopathy is by size and number with criteria similar to CT and suffers from similar lack of accuracy.[6]

Recurrent Endometrial Carcinoma

Recurrent endometrial carcinomas are most frequently seen in the vagina, uterus, pelvic, and para-aortic lymph nodes and lung. Recurrent lesions develop outside the pelvis in 75% of patients[58] and when present in the pelvis may cause low back pain, sciatic pain, leg edema, or obstructive uropathy. CT has been preferred to MRI in detection of persistent and recurrent endometrial carcinomas.[1,9,59] CT features include a central pelvic mass with or without an intact uterus (Fig. 14.18), pelvic and para-aortic lymph node metastases, and mesenteric, peritoneal, omental, and liver metastases.[9] CT is sensitive in detecting both pelvic and abdominal metastases. MRI may be useful in distinguishing recurrent tumor from posttreatment fibrosis. Recurrent tumor may be seen as a mass of higher signal intensity than pelvic side wall or fat.[60,61] The signal intensity of radiation changes may vary with time. Recent radiation change produces high signal intensity on T2-weighted images. With time, late fibrosis can be expected to have a lower signal intensity.[60] This information is essential before suggesting further surgery, radiotherapy, or chemotherapy. Most false-positive results are related to postradiation changes that simulate recurrent tumor. Although the role of MRI in recurrent disease has not been established, MRI may be useful in differentiating these two conditions.

Malignant Mixed Müllerian Tumor

Malignant mixed müllerian tumors, derived from the totipotential endometrial stromal cell, are the most common uterine sarcomas (75% of all sarcomas). Malignant tumors derived from only endometrial stromal elements are endome-

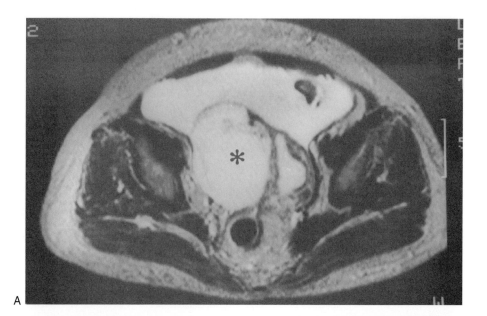

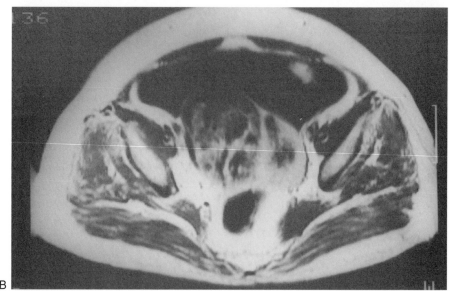

Figure 14.17 Endometrial carcinoma with right ovarian metastasis in a 76-year-old. **(A)** This T2-weighted image shows slight thickening of the endometrium. A large right ovarian mass (asterisk) is observed adjacent to the uterus. A large amount of ascites is seen anterior to the uterus. **(B)** The postcontrast T1-weighted image shows both endometrial mass and ovarian mass to have irregular internal architecture.

Figure 14.18 Recurrent endometrial cancer in a 65-year-old. A CT image demonstrating a calcified solid mass in the pelvis. The uterus had been removed.

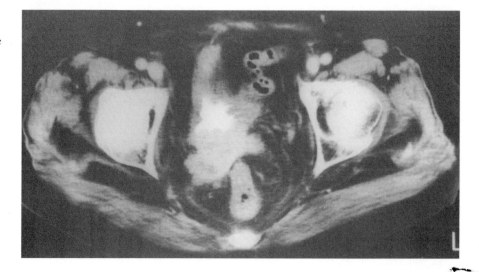

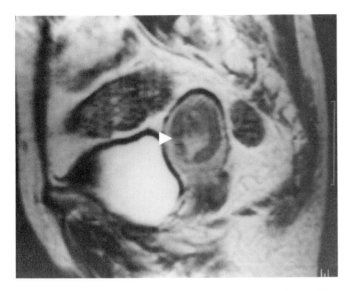

Figure 14.19 Malignant mixed müllerian tumor in a 66-year-old. This postcontrast T1-weighted spin echo image shows marked enhancement of the central portion of the tumor as well as the residual outer myometrium. At pathologic examination, a polypoid tumor invading the myometrium is demonstrated. (From Yamashita,[63] with permission).

trial stromal sarcomas. Both sarcomas usually manifest as a large mass at the initial presentation. Although the majority of mixed müllerian tumors and stromal sarcomas are aggressive, some mixed müllerian tumors are less aggressive, usually presenting as a polypoid mass (Fig. 14.19).

It has been reported that the MRI signal-intensity characteristics of these tumors are not unique and that they cannot be differentiated from endometrial carcinoma.[4,7,62] In Figure 14.20, an aggressive stromal sarcoma has a heterogeneous medium and high-intensity signal on a T2-weighted image, the highest signal being necrosis and hemorrhage[62] (Fig. 14.20). The distinction of the tumor and myometrium is more obvious with contrast; the degree of enhancement appears to be slight compared with myometrium, although the enhancement pattern is heterogeneous (Fig. 14.19).[63] Unenhanced and contrast-enhanced MRI appearances are nonspecific and can simulate those of invasive endometrial cancer or leiomyosarcoma.

SUMMARY

MRI has emerged as the most accurate imaging modality for the evaluation of endometrial abnormality. High-field MRI provides unique diagnostic information to guide therapy of various endometrial diseases. T2-weighted imaging is the most diagnostic sequence in the evaluation of endometrial abnormalities. Contrast-enhanced high-field MRI may be indicated to interpret correctly the myometrial invasion for preoperative assessment of endometrial carcinoma and mixed müllerian tumors. Although lymphadenopathy and metastatic tumors may be detected with CT, its current role is limited compared with MRI.

Figure 14.20 Stromal sarcoma in a 76-year-old. **(A)** A sagittal T2-weighted image shows enlargement of the uterus without zonal structure. The signal of the uterus is irregularly hyperintense. **(B)** A postcontrast T1-weighted image shows an irregularly contrast-enhanced mass in the endometrial cavity. The myometrium is distended.

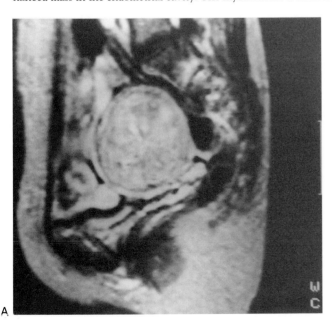

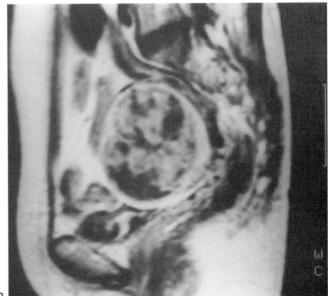

A   B

REFERENCES

1. Balfe DM, Van Dyke J, Lee JK et al. Computed tomography in malignant endometrial neoplasms. J Comput Assist Tomogr 1983;7:677–681

2. Hricak H, Stern JL, Fisher MR et al. Endometrial carcinoma staging by MR imaging. Radiology 1987;162:297–305

3. Javitt MC, Stein HL, Lovecchio JL. MRI in staging of endometrial and cervical carcinoma. Magn Reson Imaging1987;5:83–92

4. Worthington JL, Balfe DM, Lee JK et al. Uterine neoplasms: MR imaging. Radiology 1986;159:725–730

5. Hahn PF, Saini S, Stark DD et al. Intraabdominal hematoma: the concentric-ring sign in MR imaging. AJR Am J Roentgenol 1987;148:115–119

6. Hricak H, Rubinstein LV, Gherman GM, Karstaedt N. MR imaging evaluation of endometrial carcinoma: results of an NCI cooperative study. Radiology 1991;179:829–832

7. Togashi K, Konishi J. Magnetic resonance imaging in the evaluation of gynecologic malignancy. Magn Reson Q 1990;6:250–275

8. Yamashita Y, Mizutani H, Torashima M et al. Assessment of myometrial invasion by endometrial carcinoma: transvaginal sonography vs contrast-enhanced MR imaging. AJR Am J Roentgenol 1993;161:595–599

9. Walsh JW, Goplerud DR. Computed tomography of primary, persistent, and recurrent endometrial malignancy. AJR Am J Roentgenol 1982;139:1149–1154

10. Goldstein SR, Nachtigall M, Snyder JR, Nachtigall L. Endometrial assessment by vaginal ultrasonography before endometrial sampling in patients with postmenopausal bleeding. Am J Obstet Gynecol 1990;163:119–123

11. Granberg S, Wikland M, Karlsson B et al. Endometrial thickness as measured by endovaginal ultrasonography for identifying endometrial abnormality. Am J Obstet Gynecol1991;164:47–52

12. Malpani A, Singer J, Wolverson MK, Merenda G. Endometrial hyperplasia: value of endometrial thickness in ultrasonographic diagnosis and clinical significance. J Clin Ultrasound 1990;18:173–177

13. Rosai J, Ed. Female reproductive system/uterus-corpus. In: Ackerman's Surgical Pathology, (vol. 2) CV Mosby, St. Louis, 1989, pp 1050–1097

14. Hricak H, Finck S, Honda G, Goranson H. MR imaging in the evaluation of benign uterine masses: value of gadopentetate dimeglumine-enhanced T1-weighted images. AJR Am J Roentgenol 1992;158:1043–1050

15. Hricak H, Hamm B, Semelka RC et al. Carcinoma of the uterus: use of gadopentetate dimeglumine in MR imaging. Radiology 1991;181:95–106

16. Mendelson EB, Bohm-Velez M, Joseph N, Neiman HL. Endometrial abnormalities: evaluation with transvaginal sonography. AJR Am J Roentgenol 1988;150:139–142

17. Dykes TA, Isler RJ, McLean AC. MR imaging of Asherman syndrome: total endometrial obliteration. J Comput Assist Tomogr 1991;15:858–1860

18. van Roessel J, Wamsteker K, Exalto N. Sonographic investigation of the uterus during artificial uterine cavity distention. J Clin Ultrasound 1987;15:439–450

19. Laing FC, Filly RA, Marks WM, Brown TW. Ultrasonic demonstration of endometrial fluid collections unassociated with pregnancy. Radiology 1980;137:471–474

20. Scott WW, Jr, Rosenshein NB, Seigelman SS, Sanders RC. The obstructed uterus. Radiology 1981;141:767–770

21. Breckenridge JW, Kurtz AB, Ritchie WGM, Macht EL, Jr. Post menopausal uterine fluid collection: indicator of carcinoma. AJR Am J Roentgenol 1982;139:529–534

22. Fleischer AC, Kepple DM. Benign conditions of the uterus, cervix, and endometrium. In: Nyberg DA, Hill LM, Bohm-Velez M, Mendelson EB, Eds. Transvaginal Ultrasound. Mosby Year Book, St. Louis, 1992, pp 21–41

23. Young RH, Treger T, Scully RE. Atypical polypoid adenomyoma of the uterus. A report of 27 cases. Am J Clin Pathol 1986;86:139–145

24. Silverberg SG, Kurman RJ, Eds. Mixed Epithelial–Nonepithelial Tumors. Armed Forces Institute of Pathology, Washington, DC, 1992 pp 153–157

25. Mazur MT. Atypical polypoid adenomyoma of the endometrium. Am J Surg Pathol 1981;5:473–482

26. Clement PB, Young RH. Atypical polypoid adenomyoma of the uterus associated with Turner's syndrome. A report of three cases, including review of "estrogen-associated" endometrial neoplasms and neoplasms associated with Turner's syndrome. Int J Gynecol Pathol 1987;6:104–113

27. Musumeci R, De Palo G, Conti U et al. Are retroperitoneal lymph node metastases a major problem in endometrial adenocarcinoma? Cancer 1980;46:1887–1892

28. Tiitinen A, Forss M, Aho I et al. Endometrial carcinoma: a clinical outcome in 881 patients and analysis of 146 patients whose deaths were due to endometrial cancer. Gynecol Oncol 1986;25:11–19

29. Cowles TA, Magrina JF, Masterson BJ, Capen CV. Comparison of clinical and surgical-staging in patients with endometrial carcinoma. Obstet Gynecol 1985;66:413–416

30. Lotocki RJ, Copeland LJ, DePetrillo AD, Muirhead W. Stage I endometrial adenocarcinoma: treatment results in 835 patients. Am J Obstet Gynecol 1983;146:141–145

31. Boronow RC, Morrow CP, Creasman WT et al. Surgical staging in endometrial cancer; clinical-pathologic findings of a prospective study. Obstet Gynecol 1984;63:825–832

32. Creasman WT, Morrow CP, Bundy BN et al. Surgical pathologic spread patterns of endometrial cancer. A Gynecologic Oncology Group Study. Cancer 1987;60:2035–2041

33. Hricak H, Rubinstein LV, Gherman GM, Karstaedt N. MR imaging evaluation of endometrial carcinoma: results of an NCI cooperative study. Radiology 1991;179:829–832

34. Yamashita Y, Harada M, Sawada T et al. Normal uterus and FIGO stage I endometrial carcinoma: dynamic gadolinium-enhanced MR imaging. Radiology 1993;186:495–501

35. Saigo PE, Cain JM, Kim WS et al. Prognostic factors in adenocarcinoma of the uterine cervix. Cancer 1986;57:1584–1593

36. Sironi S, Taccagni G, Garancini P et al. Myometrial invasion by endometrial carcinoma: assessment by MR imaging. AJR Am J Roentgenol 1992;158:565–569

37. Sironi S, Mellone R, Vanzulli A et al. Assessment of the myometrial infiltration of endometrial carcinoma (FIGO stage I–II). The accuracy of magnetic resonance (1.5 T). Radiol Med 989;77:386–390

38. Yazigi R, Cohen G, Munoz AK, Sandstad J. Magnetic resonance imaging determination of myometrial invasion in endometrial carcinoma. Gynecol Oncol 1989;34:94–97

39. Lien HH, Blomlie V, Trope C et al. Cancer of the endometrium:

value of MR imaging in determining depth of invasion into the myometrium. AJR Am J Roentgenol 1991;157:1221–1223

40. Sironi S, Colombo E, Villa G et al. Myometrial invasion by endometrial carcinoma: assessment with plain and gadolinium-enhanced MR imaging. Radiology 1992;185:207–212

41. Yamashita Y, Torashima M, Takahashi M et al. Hyperintense uterine leiomyoma at T2-weighted MR imaging: differentiation with dynamic enhanced MR imaging and clinical implications. Radiology 1993;189:721–725

42. Cacciatore B, Lehtovirta P, Wahlstrom T, Ylostalo P. Preoperative sonographic evaluation of endometrial cancer. J Obstet Gynecol 1989;160:133–137

43. Fleischer AC, Gordon AN, Entman SS, Kepple DM. Transvaginal sonography (TVS) of the endometrium: current and potential clinical applications. Crit Rev Diagn Imaging 1990; 30:85–110

44. Conte M, Guariglia L, Benedetti Panici P et al. Transvaginal ultrasound evaluation of myometrial invasion in endometrial carcinoma. Gynecol Obstet Invest 1990;29:224–226

45. Gordon AN, Fleischer AC, Reed GW. Depth of myometrial invasion in endometrial cancer: preoperative assessment by transvaginal sonography. Gynecol Oncol 1990;39:321–327

46. Mendelson EB, Bohm-Velez M. Transvaginal ultrasonography of pelvic neoplasms. Radiol Clin North Am 1992;30:703–734

47. Schoenfeld A, Levavi H, Hirsch M et al. Transvaginal sonography in postmenopausal women. JCU 1990;18:350–358

48. Varner RE, Sparks JM, Cameron CD et al. Transvaginal sonography of the endometrium in postmenopausal women. Obstet Gynecol 1991;78:195–199

49. Hamlin DJ, Burgener FA, Beecham JB. CT of intramural endometrial carinoma: contrast enhancement is essential. AJR Am J Roentgenol 1981;137:551–554

50. Dore R, Moro G, D'Andrea F et al. CT evaluation of myometrium invasion in endometrial carcinoma. J Comput Assist Tomogr 1987;11:282–289

51. Scoutt LM, McCarthy SM, Moss AA. Computed tomography and magnetic resonance imaging of the pelvis. In: Moss AA, Gamsu G, Genant HK, Eds. Computed Tomography of the Body with Magnetic Resonance Imaging (2nd ed., vol. 3). WB Saunders, Philadelphia 1992; pp 1183–1265

52. Posniak HV, Olson MC, Dudiak CM et al. MR imaging of uterine carcinoma: correlation with clinical and pathologic findings. Radiographics 1990;10:15–27

53. Thorvinger B, Gudmundsson T, Horvath G et al. Staging in local endometrial carcinoma. Assessment of magnetic resonance and ultrasound examinations. Acta Radiol 1989;30:525–529

54. Gordon AN, Fleischer AC, Dudley BS et al. Preoperative assessment of myometrial invasion of endometrial adenocarcinoma by sonography (US) and magnetic resonance imaging (MRI). Gynecol Oncol 1989;34:175–179

55. Powell MC, Womack C, Buckley J, et al. Pre-operative magnetic resonance imaging of stage 1 endometrial adenocarcinoma. Br J Obstet Gynaecol 1986;93:353–360

56. Togashi K, Nishimura K, Kimura I et al. Endometrial cysts: diagnosis with MR imaging. Radiology 1991;180:73–78

57. Belloni C, Vigano R, del Maschio A et al. Magnetic resonance imaging in endometrial carcinoma staging. Gynecol Oncol 1990;37:172–177

58. Currie JL. Malignant tumors of the uterine corpus. In: Thompson JD, Rock JA, Eds. Te Linde's Operative Gynecology. JB Lippincott, Philadelphia, 1992, pp 1253–1302

59. Franchi M, La Fianza A, Babilonti L et al. Clinical value of computerized tomography (CT) in assessment of recurrent uterine cancers. Gynecol Oncol 1989;35:31–37

60. Ebner F, Kressel HY, Mintz MC et al. Tumor recurrence versus fibrosis in the female pelvis: differentiation with MR imaging at 1.5T. Radiology 1988;166:333–340

61. Weber TM, Sostman DH, Spritzer CE et al. Cervical carcinoma: determination of recurrent tumor extent versus radiation changes with MR imaging. Radiology 1995;194:135–139

62. Shapeero LG, Hricak H. Mixed müllerian sarcoma of the uterus: MR imaging findings. AJR Am J Roentgenol 1989;153:317–319

63. Yamashita Y, Takahashi M, Miyazaki K, Okamura H. Contrast-enhanced MR imaging of malignant mixed müllerian tumor of the uterus. AJR Am J Roentgenol 1993;160:1150–1151

15

Hysterosalpingography of the Endometrium

VIVIAN LEWIS

JACQUES S. ABRAMOWICZ

Hysterosalpingography (HSG) is the established examination for determining fallopian tube patency, and it also provides information about the uterine cavity. Bubbles, catheter configuration, blood clots, cervical mucus in the cavity, and uterine contractions can cause artifacts (Fig. 15.1). Linear or small filling defects are probably artifacts in patients with no history suggestive of pathology.[1,2] Patients with abnormal bleeding, an intrauterine contraceptive device (IUCD), pelvic infection, or previous uterine instrumentation are more likely to have an abnormal HSG and hysteroscopy.

ENDOMETRIAL NEOPLASIA

Hyperplasia, metaplasia, polyps, and carcinomas are seen in women of reproductive years. These are histologic diagnoses, but the HSG and the clinical picture may warrant further investigation by hysteroscopy or endometrial biopsy.

Polyps may cause intermenstrual bleeding, metrostaxis, or infertility. Small polyps are usually asymptomatic. The HSG typically shows a rounded or sessile projection into the cavity (Fig. 15.2).[3,4] A tissue diagnosis from hysteroscopy or curettage is necessary, although polyps are usually benign.

Endometrial metaplasia is generally asymptomatic and of no clinical significance. Various heterologous elements have been described in the endometrium, including cartilage, bone, glial tissue, skin, retina, and kidney.[3] There is a common association with previous abortion and endometritis, suggesting that some of these elements are probably fetal tissue rather than true metaplasia. However, there are series in which the patients give no such history and the heterotopic tissue appears mature, suggesting true metaplasia.[3,5] Osseous metaplasia sometimes shows endometrial calcification on HSG (Fig. 15.3).

HSG can suggest carcinoma of the endometrium, though this is hardly the best way to make the diagnosis. Endometrial cancer is relatively rare in patients of reproductive age, since 95% are postmenopausal at diagnosis. Because of the association between ovulatory dysfunction and endometrial cancer, occasional carcinomas will be found on HSG.[6] Retrospective data suggest that patients with polycystic ovary syndrome have a threefold increase in the incidence of endometrial carcinoma.[7] The radiographic appearance is rather nonspecific and easily confused with endometrial hyperplasia or polyps. In localized tumors, a well-defined mass can protrude into the cavity. More commonly, irregular, diffuse defects are seen in the cavity.[6,8] Efforts to use HSG or sonographic appearance to predict myometrial invasion have not proven to be accurate.[9]

INFLAMMATORY CONDITIONS

Infection of the endometrial cavity usually results from the transport of pathogens from the lower genital tract. Hematogenous spread of tuberculosis and echinoccocal diseases are two notable exceptions. Local factors in the cervix usually act to prevent this but can be compromised during menstruation, surgery, childbirth and IUCD insertion. Acute endometritis usually occurs in puerperal or postabortion patients, in whom HSG would not be performed. From studies of patients who undergo diagnostic laparoscopy and endometrial biopsy, chronic endometritis is often a component of pelvic inflammatory disease. However, endometritis can also occur in asymptomatic patients, in whom it is probably an intermediate stage of infection between cervicitis and salpingitis. Chronic inflammation is found on endometrial biopsy for abnormal uterine bleeding in 3% to 10% of specimens.[10–12]

The most common causative organism is *Chlamydia trachomatis*, which is likely to be responsible for 50% to 60% of the cases of salpingitis in Western countries. *Neisseria gonorrhea*, *Escherichia coli*, and various gram-negative anaerobic organisms are also common pathogens. Certain Mycoplasma strains (*Ureaplasma urealyticum* in particular) have been associated with infertility and repetitive spontaneous abortions;

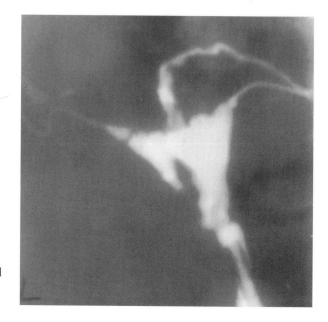

Figure 15.1 This 36-year-old gravida 1, para 0 had unexplained infertility and a filling defect in the endometrial cavity on HSG. Hysteroscopy was within normal limits.

Figure 15.2 This 34-year-old infertile woman had an oval filling defect in the left cornual region of the uterus, which corresponded to the area where a polyp was found at hysteroscopy.

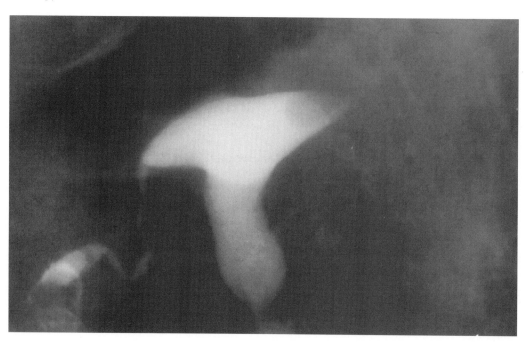

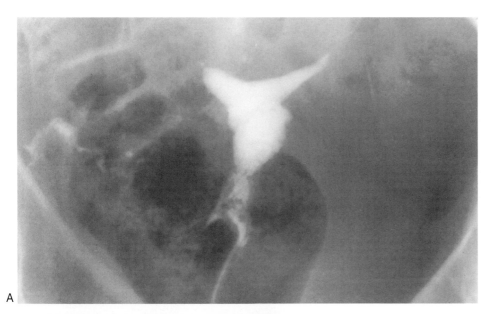

A

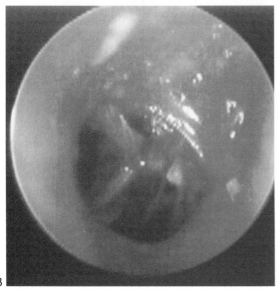

B

Figure 15.3 A 38-year-old, infertile woman with a history of a single spontaneous abortion, at 6 weeks' pregnancy. (**A**) The lower uterine segment appeared quite irregular on HSG. (**B**) Hysteroscopy showed calcified bands in the lower uterine segment. Biopsy showed osseous metaplasia and endometritis.

however, the data have been conflicting.[10,13] Actinomycetes can cause endometritis and salpingitis, usually in association with an IUCD. It is sometimes identified on a Papanicoloau smear and generally causes chronic, rather than acute, infection.[14] Identification of the causative organism must be made by culture and, at times, serologic techniques along with the clinical picture. HSG cannot distinguish between etiologic agents.

Lost IUCDs can be located by HSG. Clinically, an IUCD cannot be located if the string is not seen at the external os. Ultrasound usually shows that the IUCD remains within the uterus. HSG requires intrauterine injection of dye to demonstrate the cavity. If the IUCD is seen outside, removal will be either by laparoscopy or laparotomy (Fig. 15.4).

Inflammation can cause intrauterine adhesions, or Asherman syndrome. The classic picture occurs in patients who undergo dilatation and curettage for pregnancy termination or retained products of conception. However, adhesions can also result from infection, myomectomy, or intrauterine foreign body.[15] Data from prospective studies suggest that about 15% of patients with spontaneous abortion and curettage will form intrauterine adhesions.[16] Symptoms include hypomenorrhea, amenorrhea, dysmenorrhea, and infertility. The diagnosis can be made by HSG, hysteroscopy, or sonohysterography. HSG will show a small irregular cavity in severe cases or intrauterine filling defects in milder cases (Fig. 15.5). However, findings at HSG may not correspond with clinical findings. In one series, 30% of patients with severe scarring on HSG had minimal or no adhesions at hysteroscopy.[17] Treatment of choice is the hysteroscopic resection of the adhesions. Laparotomy for transfundal lysis of adhesions has been performed but is more likely to result in obstetric complications such as placenta accreta and uterine rupture.[18,19] D&C is an alternative but is less successful than hysteroscopy in terms of resumption

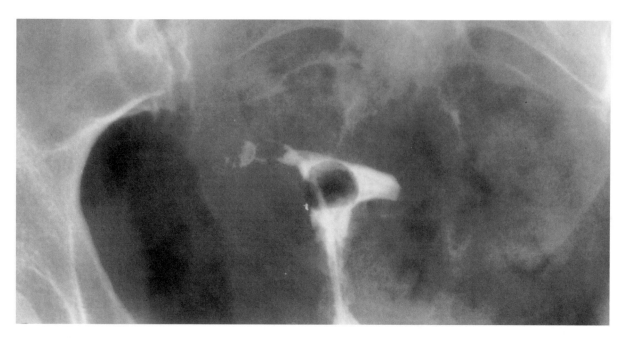

Figure 15.4 A 35-year-old gravida 3, para 0 presented with recurrent spontaneous abortion and infertility. The uterine cavity showed some irregularities thought to be either endometrial hyperplasia or endometritis. Hysteroscopy showed a Copper-7 IUCD (denuded of the copper). She thought she had expelled the device shortly after insertion, 10 years previously.

of menstruation and return of normal fertility. Some authors recommend insertion of an IUCD or Foley catheter temporarily to prevent reapposition of the uterine walls. This is followed by a course of estrogens to promote proliferation of

Figure 15.5 This 37-year-old nulligravida had menorrhagia and a 16-week-sized uterus, with multiple myomata. The largest tumor was considered partly intramural and partly submucosal in location. The pathology report showed partial resection of the endometrium. The patient presented 18 months after surgery with hypomenorrhea and infertility. HSG shows a small and irregular cavity.

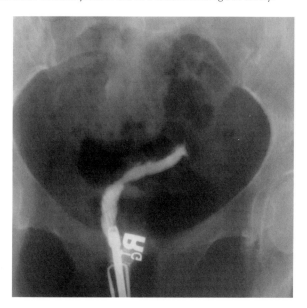

the endometrium. Most patients resume spontaneous menstruation.

CONGENITAL DEFECTS

HSG is very helpful in detection of congenital uterine anomalies. The overall incidence is probably about 1 in 200.[20] Although many of these patients are diagnosed during investigation of fertility problems, many remain asymptomatic.[21,22] Normal in utero development of the müllerian ducts begins with paired solid structures, closely associated with the urinary system. In the midtrimester, these ducts fuse, and the caudal portion canalizes to become the uterus and upper third of the vagina. If fusion, canalization, or development fails or is incomplete, the syndromes of müllerian dysgenesis can result. Duplication of uterus, vagina, or cervix is fairly common and results from complete failure of fusion of the müllerian ducts. Examples of canalization failure include noncommunicating uterine horn and cervical or vaginal agenesis. Absence of the uterus and unicornuate uterus are examples of nondevelopment of part of the müllerian system. The concurrent in utero development of the urinary system explains the high incidence of renal anomalies. Most anomalies are classified according to the system proposed by Buttram and Gibbons[23] and later adopted by the American Society for Reproductive Medicine (Fig. 15.6). Nonetheless, there are patients who elude the usual classification system. Clinical judgment and experience are necessary for their management (Fig. 15.7).[23–26]

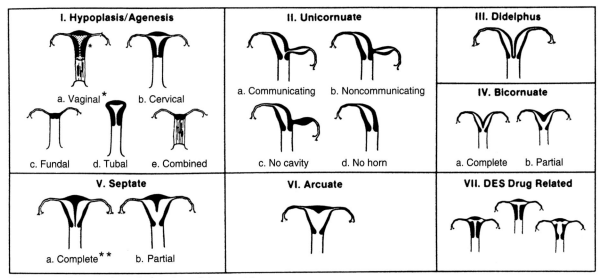

* Uterus may be normal or take a variety of abnormal forms.
** May have two distinct cervices

Figure 15.6 The American Society for Reproductive Medicine (formerly the American Fertility Society) classification of müllerian anomalies. *Uterus may be normal or take a variety of a normal forms. **May have two distinct cervices. (From American Fertility Society.[25] With permission of the American Society for Reproductive Medicine.)

Septate uterus is one of the most common anomalies (class V, Fig. 15.6). Although most patients are asymptomatic, this anomaly can be associated with an increased rate of spontaneous abortions and premature deliveries. The septum comprises abnormal myometrium and fibrous tissue with decreased vascularity and a poorly developed overlying endometrium.[22] Pregnancies that implant on the septum tend to miscarry.[27] Breech presentation may also be more common.[20] HSG is excellent for the diagnosis of septate uterus; however, other studies are needed to distinguish this from bicornuate uterus. MRI or transvaginal ultrasound can sometimes determine the difference; otherwise, laparoscopy is required.[28-30] Hysteroscopic resection of the septum has a good prognosis and low morbidity.[31] Studies of asymptomatic patients show that most patients have normal pregnancies.[32] Patients who are already infertile, particularly if they are older, should not necessarily have to wait until they have three miscarriages before hysteroscopic resection (Fig. 15.8).

The septate uterus and the bicornuate uterus (class IV, Fig. 15.6) were frequently grouped together in the older literature, but symptoms and treatment differ (Fig. 15.9). Premature birth, dystocia, and postpartum hemorrhage are more frequently seen in these patients.[20] Recommended treatment is the Strassman metroplasty, which results in improved pregnancy outcome.[31] Many authors also recommend concurrent cervical cerclage.[21,24,33]

Uterus didelphys (class III, Fig. 15.6) is a rare condition in which there is duplication of the uterus, part or all of the cervix, and at times vaginal structures (Fig. 15.10). The clinical significance is controversial, but most series find an in-creased rate of miscarriage (33% to 43%) and prematurity (25% to 45%). These figures are based on small numbers, making treatment recommendations difficult.[21,24,33]

Unicornuate uterus (class II, Fig. 15.6), in which one fallopian tube and uterine cornual area is absent, is even less common than didelphys (Fig. 15.11). It is thought that the vascularity is poorly developed, resulting in an increased risk of spontaneous abortion, premature birth, and breech presentation.[23,34] Intrauterine growth retardation may also be more common. The literature is divided on the question of cerclage.[24,33-35] Certainly, these patients tend to be high risk and should be monitored appropriately. In some patients, there is an associated rudimentary horn (class IIa–c, Fig. 15.6), which may increase the chance of ectopic pregnancy and endometriosis.[20,36] Diethylstilbestrol (DES) was once used to prevent recurrent abortion. Exposure to it in utero is responsible for class VII anomalies. Although the incidence is declining, women of reproductive age continue to present with this complication. The impact on fertility is controversial. Many of the studies are done on small numbers of patients in which statistical significance may not be reached. However, infertility, ectopic pregnancy, spontaneous abortion, and premature labor have all been cited as complications of DES exposure.[37-39]. Some women will be quite aware of DES exposure, whereas others will have the typical cervical or vaginal changes. In either case, HSG may show a hypoplastic uterine cavity, T-shaped uterus, and periosteal constriction bands (Fig. 15.12) and see Figs. 21.3 and 21.12. Some authors also describe widening or lengthening of the lower uterine segment and irregular borders of the cavity similar to adhesions.

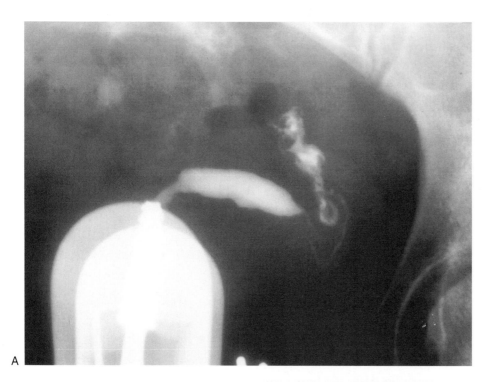

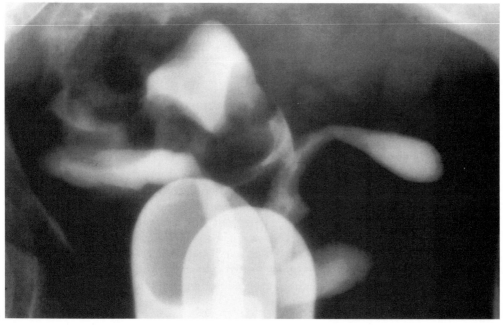

Figure 15.7 A 34-year-old nulligravida with infertility and severe dysmenorrhea. (**A**) The initial film appeared to show a unicornuate uterus with patent tube. (**B**) A later view showed a similar structure on the left. At laparoscopy, there were two apparent uterine cavities, with a communication near the junction of the uterus and cervix. There were also two cervices. However, the left cervix was quite small and connected to a small blind pouch which was opened surgically, relieving the dysmenorrhea.

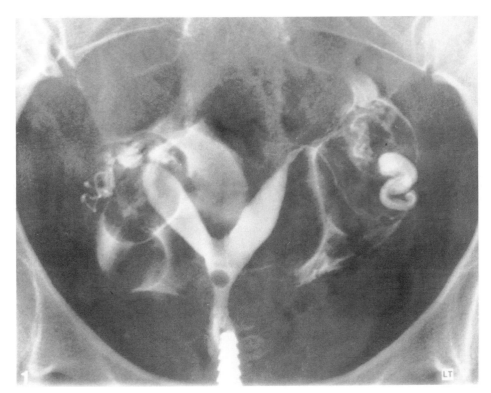

Figure 15.8 A 40-year-old nulligravida had infertility due to severe male factor. The uterine septum shown in this HSG was resected hysteroscopically before the patient's planned in vitro fertilization cycle to optimize her chances for embryo implantation.

Figure 15.9 This 30-year-old nulligravida woman underwent HSG as part of an infertility evaluation. The widely divergent angle of the uterine cornual area is highly suggestive of bicornuate uterus.

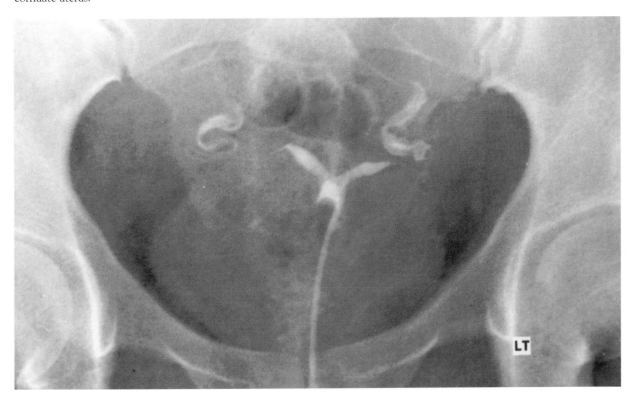

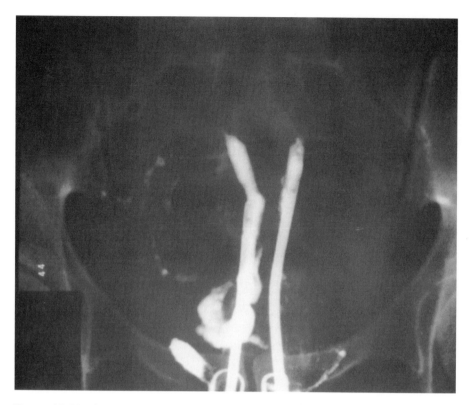

Figure 15.10 This HSG shows the separate cannulation of each cervix and the two separate, noncommunicating cavities. (From Lewis and Abramowicz,[15] with permission.)

Figure 15.11 Unicornuate uterus with patent tube. (Courtesy of Dr. Mark Adams, Rochester, New York.)

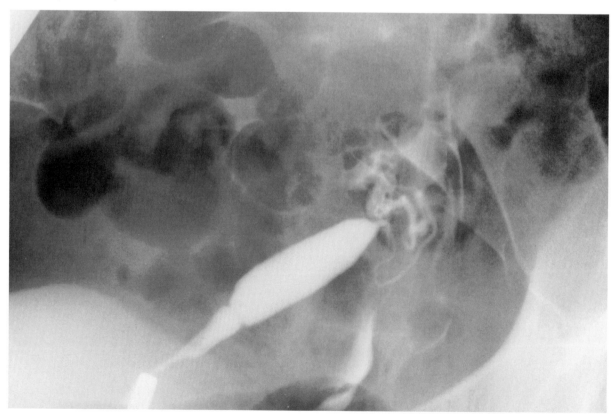

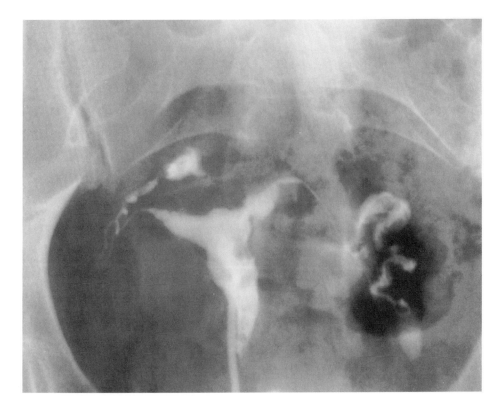

Figure 15.12 This 30-year-old woman had been exposed to DES and had a history of metrorrhagia and infertility. The uterine cavity shows irregular borders and a widened lower uterine segment. Hysteroscopy was normal.

Figure 15.13 A 27-year-old woman whose husband has suffered a spinal cord injury. HSG was performed after several cycles of failed insemination with sperm obtained from electro-ejaculation. The arcuate configuration of the uterus, shown here, was considered insignificant. The couple's first cycle of in vitro fertilization was successful.

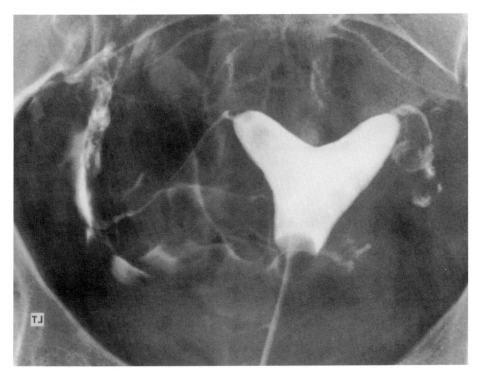

Women who have physical stigmata of exposure evident on pelvic examination are more likely to have the upper tract changes seen on HSG. According to Kaufman et al.,[38] patients with an abnormal HSG are more likely to have reproductive failure. Furthermore, data from in vitro fertilization suggest that there may be underlying endometrial abnormalities that cause reduced embryo implantation rates.[40]

Patients with müllerian hypoplasia and agenesis (class I, Fig. 15.6) usually present as adolescents with primary amenorrhea or pelvic pain.[26] HSG does not help in making the diagnosis, but ultrasound and MRI may demonstrate functional endometrial tissue. Infertility due to many of these anomalies cannot be treated without surrogacy. Class VI müllerian anomalies consist of patients with arcuate uterus (Fig. 15.13). These patients are fairly common and have a good prognosis.[24]

REFERENCES

1. Snowden EU, Jarrett JC, 2nd, Dawood MY. Comparison of diagnostic accuracy of laparoscopy, hysteroscopy and hysterosalpingography in evaluation of female infertility. Fertil Steril 1984;41:709–713.

2. Stovall DW, Christman GM, Hammond MG, Talbert LM. Abnormal findings on hysterosalpingography: effects on fecundity in a donor insemination program using frozen semen. Obstet Gynecol 1992;80:249–252.

3. Kurman RJ, Mazur MT. Benign diseases of the endometrium. In: Kurman RJ, Ed. Blaustein's Pathology of the Female Genital Tract (4th ed.). Springer-Verlag, New York, 1994, pp 367–499

4. Winfield AC, Wentz AC. The uterine cavity. In: Diagnostic Imaging in Infertility 2nd ed. Williams & Wilkins, Baltimore, 1992, pp 96–116

5. Roth E, Taylor HB. Heterotopic cartilage in uterus. Obstet Gynecol 1966;27:838–844

6. Yoder IC, Hall DA. Hysterosalpingography in the 1990's. AJR Am J Roentgenol 1991;157:675–683

7. Coulam CB, Annegers JF, Kranz JS. Chronic anovulation syndrome and associated neoplasia. Obstet Gynecol 1983;61:403–407

8. Menczer J, Frenkel Y, Serr DM. Hysterosalpingography in young infertile patients with unsuspected endometrial adenocarcinoma. Am J Obstet Gynecol 1980;138:352–353

9. Hoetzinger H. Hysterosonography and hysterography in benign and malignant diseases of the uterus: a comparative in vitro study. J Ultrasound Med 1991;10:259–263

10. Westrom L, Joesoef R, Reynolds G et al. Pelvic inflammatory disease and fertility. A cohort study of 1,844 women with laparoscopically verified disease and 657 control women with normal laparoscopic results. Sex Transm Dis 1992;19:185–192

11. Paavonen J, Aine R, Teisala K et al. Comparisons of endometrial biopsy and peritoneal fluid cytologic testing with laparoscopy in the diagnosis of acute pelvic inflammatory disease. Am J Obstet Gynecol 1985;151:645–650

12. Greenwood SM, Moran JJ. Chronic endometritis: morphological and clinical observations. Obstet Gynecol 1981;58:176–184

13. Toth A, Lesser ML, Brooks C, Labriola D. Subsequent pregnancies among 161 couples treated for T-mycoplasma genital tract infection. N Engl J Med 1983;308:505–507

14. Burkman R, Schlesselman S, McCaffrey L et al. The relationship of genital tract actinomycetes and the development of pelvic inflammatory disease. Am J Obstet Gynecol 1982;143:585–589

15. Lewis V, Abramowicz JS. Hysterosalpingography of the abnormal pelvis. In: Jaffe R, Pierson RA, Abramowicz JS, Eds. Imaging in Infertility and Reproductive Endocrinology. JB Lippincott, Philadelphia, 1994, pp 321–333

16. Adoni A, Palti Z, Milwidsky A, Dolberg M. The incidence of intrauterine adhesions following spontaneous abortion. Int J Fertil 1982;27:117–118

17. March CM, Israel R, March AD. Hysteroscopic management of intrauterine adhesions. Am J Obstet Gynecol1978;130:653–657

18. Friedman A, De Fazio J, De Cherney A. Severe obstetric complications after aggressive treatment of Asherman syndrome. Obstet Gynecol 1986;67:864–867

19. Jewelewicz R, Khalaf S, Neuwirth RS et al. Obstetric complications after treatment of intrauterine synechiae (Asherman's sydrome). Obstet Gynecol 1976;47:701–705

20. Rock JA, Schlaff WD. The obstetric consequences of uterovaginal anomalies. Fertil Steril 1985;43:681–692

21. Golan A, Langer R, Bukovsky I, Caspi E. Congenital anomalies of the müllerian system. Fertil Steril 1989;51:747–755

22. Abramovici H, Faktor JH, Pascal B. Congenital uterine malformations as indication for cervical suture (cerclage) in habitual abortion and premature delivery. Int J Fertil 1983;28:161–164

23. Buttram VC, Jr, Gibbons WE. Mullerian anomalies: a proposed classification. (An analysis of 144 cases). Fertil Steril 1979;32:40–46

24. Buttram VC, Jr. Müllerian anomalies and their management. Fertil Steril 1983;40:159–163

25. The American Fertility Society classifications of adnexal adhesions, distal tubal occlusion, tubal occlusion secondary to tubal ligation, tubal pregnancies, müllerian anomalies and intrauterine adhesions. Fertil Steril 1988;49:944–955

26. Stassart JP, Nagel TC, Prem KA, Phipps WR. Uterus didelphys, obstructed hemivagina and ipsilateral renal agenesis. Fertil Steril 1992;57:756–761

27. Candiani GB, Fedele L, Zamberletti D et al. Endometrial patterns in malformed uteri. Acta Eur Fertil 1983;14:311–318

28. Fedele L, Dorta M, Brioschi D et al. Pregnancies in septate uteri: outcome in relation to site of uterine implantation as determined by sonography. AJR Am J Roentgenol 1989;152:781–784

29. Pellerito JS, McCarthy SM, Doyle MB et al. Diagnosis of uterine anomalies: relative accuracy of MR imaging, endovaginal sonography, and hysterosalpingography. Radiology 1992;183:795–800

30. Reuter KL, Daly DC, Cohen SM. Septate versus bicornuate uteri: errors in imaging diagnosis. Radiology 1989;172:749–752

31. De Cherney AH, Russell JB, Graebe RA, Polan ML. Resectoscopic management of müllerian fusion defects. Fertil Steril 1986;45:726–728

32. Simon C, Martinez L, Pardo F et al. Müllerian defects in women with normal reproductive outcome. Fertil Steril 1991;56:1192–1193

33. Makino T, Umeuchi M, Nakada K et al. Incidence of congenital uterine anomalies in repeated reproductive wastage and prognosis for pregnancy after metroplasty. Int J Fertil 1992;37:167–170

34. Heinonen PK, Saarikoski S, Pystynen P. Reproductive performance of women with uterine anomalies. An evaluation of 182 cases. Acta Obstet Gynecol Scand 1982;61:157–162

35. Bider D, Kokia E, Seidman DS et al. Cervical cerclage for anomalous uteri. J Reprod Med 1992;37:138–140

36. Fedele L, Zamberletti D, Vercellini P et al. Reproductive performance of women with unicornuate uterus. Fertil Steril 1987;47:416–419

37. Barnes AB, Colton T, Gundersen J et al. Fertility and outcome of pregnancy in women exposed in utero to diethylstilbestrol. N Engl J Med 1980;302:609–613

38. Kaufman RH, Adam E, Binder G, Gerthoffer E. Upper genital tract changes and pregnancy outcome in offspring exposed in utero to diethylstilbestrol. Am J Obstet Gynecol 1980;137:299–308

39. Senekjian EK, Potkul RK, Frey K, Herbst AL. Infertility among daughters either exposed or not to diethylstilbestrol. Am J Obstet Gynecol 1988;158:493–498

40. Karande VC, Lester RG, Muasher SJ et al. Are implantation and pregnancy outcome impaired in diethylstilbestrol-exposed women after in vitro fertilization and embryo transfer? Fertil Steril 1990;54:287–291

16

Ultrasonography of the Myometrium

JOHN C. ANDERSON

This chapter discusses various conditions that affect the development and appearance of the myometrium. Ultrasound is particularly suitable for evaluation and diagnosis of myometrial disorders.

DEVELOPMENTAL ABNORMALITIES

Complete failure of development of the lower part of the müllerian (paramesonephric) ducts causes absence of the uterus and upper part of the vagina with consequent primary amenorrhea and infertility. True duplication of the müllerian ducts with doubling of the reproductive organs on one or both sides is extremely rare. Most developmental anomalies of the reproductive tract are due to fusion defects, or atresia of part or all of the paramesonephric ducts. Many congenital abnormalities of the uterus are due to in utero exposure to diethylstilbestrol,[1] or to endogenous hormones associated with abnormal gonads or chromosome abnormalities.

Fusion Defects of Müllerian Ducts

The uterus and vagina normally develop by fusion of the paired müllerian ducts followed by degeneration of the resulting common wall. If a failure of fusion is the predominant pathologic process, then a uterus didelphys, uterus bicornis, uterus arcuatus, or subseptate uterus will form, depending on the degree of failure (Fig. 16.1). Scanning patients with suspected defects in the müllerian ducts is best performed in the secretory phase of the cycle, as the endometrium is at its most echogenic (Fig. 16.2).

Atresia of the Müllerian Ducts

All degrees of atresia may be encountered. Bilateral complete atresia (Rokitansky-Küster-Hauser syndrome) is often associated with renal abnormalities. The cause of atresia is poorly understood, although a genetic influence is occasionally apparent, as siblings[2] can be affected, and an autosomal recessive and dominant patterns of inheritance have been described.[3,4] Diagrammatic examples of developmental anomalies due to atresia of the müllerian ducts are shown in Figure 16.3. An example of a noncommunicating horn is shown in Figure 16.4.

BENIGN CONDITIONS

Adenomyosis and Adenomyoma

Adenomyosis is a common condition, especially in pre- and perimenopausal women. The usual symptom is dysmenorrhea, but abnormal bleeding is also reported. The uterus becomes mildly enlarged, particularly on the posterior wall where adenomyosis is generally most extensive. Under the microscope, islands of endometrial glands and stroma can be seen within the myometrium where they often form hemorrhagic foci. An adenomyoma is a circumscribed, nodular aggregate of smooth muscle, endometrial glands, and stroma that usually originates in the myometrium.

The diagnosis on ultrasound is difficult[5–8] because there are no pathognomonic signs and fibroids frequently coexist.[9] The diagnosis is favored if the uterus is bulky in size with the posterior wall being slightly thicker than the anterior.[10]

The myometrium in patients with adenomyosis is heterogeneous, with patchy areas of increased or decreased echodensity and occasionally, small myometrial cysts. Using these criteria, Reinhold et al.[11] were able to diagnose adenomyosis in 25 of 29 patients with adenomyosis and exclude it in 61 of 71 patients who did not have it. Some cases are described as having a "rain-in-the-forest" pattern[12] (Fig. 16.5).

Magnetic resonance imaging (MRI) is probably superior to ultrasound in the diagnosis of adenomyosis. Ascher and colleagues[13] correctly diagnosed adenomyosis in 15 of 17 patients with MRI, but only 9 of the 17 were diagnosed using ultrasound.

Nonetheless, because of its widespread availability and patient tolerance, transvaginal sonography (TVS) remains the primary method for imaging the female pelvis. MRI is appropriate for cases in which sonography cannot detect adenomyosis.[14]

Leiomyoma

Leiomyomas are a common benign tumor that arise from the myometrium of the uterus. They are composed principally of smooth muscle, but they also contain small amounts of connective tissue. They are usually called "fibroids," although strictly speaking, this term is incorrect on histologic grounds. The term *myoma* is also used sometimes. Fibroids are spheric or ovoid and are of firm consistency to the touch. They have a light gray, whorled appearance when cut with a scalpel.

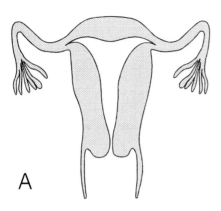
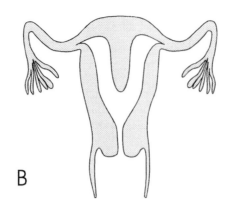
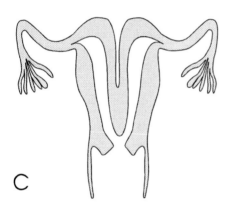
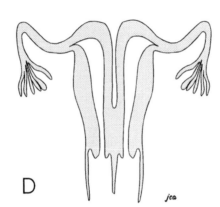

Figure 16.1 Fusion defects of the paramesonephric (müllerian) duct. (A) Uterus arcuatus.
(B) Septate uterus. (C) Uterus bicornis unicollis. (D) Uterus didelphis with double vagina.
In Figures A and B, the uterus appears externally normal. In Figure D, the cavities do not
communicate.

Usually multiple and of different sizes ranging upward from
less than a grain of rice, they are classified as intramural, subserosal, submucous, and cervical according to their position.

Intramural (or *interstitial*) fibroids lie within the uterine
wall, enclosed in a thin layer of connective tissue that separates them from adjacent myometrium. *Subserosal* fibroids
project outward from the peritoneal surface of the uterus.
These fibroids can attain huge proportions and sometimes become pedunculated (Fig. 16.6). Occasionally, they have been
known to develop an independent blood supply from the
omentum and then become separated from the uterus when
they become known as "parasitic" fibroids. *Submucous* fibroids
project into the uterine cavity and are partially covered with
endometrium. These fibroids can develop a stalk and occasionally prolapse through the cervix. *Cervical* fibroids are the
least common. They can be difficult to excise due to their
proximity to the bladder and ureters.

Microscopic Appearance

Microscopically fibroids consist of whorled, anastomosing fas-
cicles of uniform, fusiform smooth muscle cells. There is also
a variable amount of connective tissue. Due to the poor blood
supply, degenerative changes can occur in fibroids. *Hyaline*
degeneration is the most common, but *cystic* degeneration can
occur if they liquefy. *Red* degeneration occurs almost exclusively during pregnancy if there are vascular changes. It can
cause localized pain and tenderness. *Calcification* occurs in
some women after the menopause due to circulatory impair-
ment, and *sarcomatous* degeneration is a serious but, fortu-
nately, rare complication.

Etiology

The etiology of fibroids is unknown. They are thought to be
dependent on estrogen, as they do not occur before the

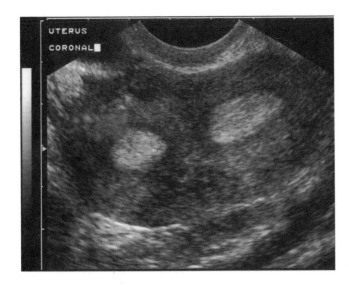

Figure 16.2 A coronal section through the uterine fundus shows two endometrial cavities surrounded by myometrium.

menarche and they regress after the menopause. It has also been found that they regress during the hypo estrogenic state induced by the agonists of luteinizing hormone releasing hormone (LHRH),[15] a fact not lost on those concerned with their treatment. Six months' treatment with LHRH can be expected to reduce the fibroids by about 50% in size. Unfortunately, they rapidly return to their previous size after cessa-

tion of therapy, so this treatment is usually used as a forerunner to surgery to make the operation technically easier.[16,17]

Appropriate doses of currently available LHRH agonists include goserelin 3.6 mg by monthly subcutaneous depot injection or intranasal buserelin 900 to 1,200 μg daily in divided doses. Receptors of both estrogen and progesterone have been shown to be present in higher concentrations in fibroids than

Figure 16.3 Atresia of the paramesonephric (müllerian) duct. (A) Communicating rudimentary horn. (B) Noncommunicating rudimentary horn. (C) Atresia of the cervix. (D) Atresia of the vagina. These conditions may be associated with renal anomalies including absence of the kidney on the atretic side. Complete atresia of the ducts results in the Rokitansky-Küster-Hauser syndrome.

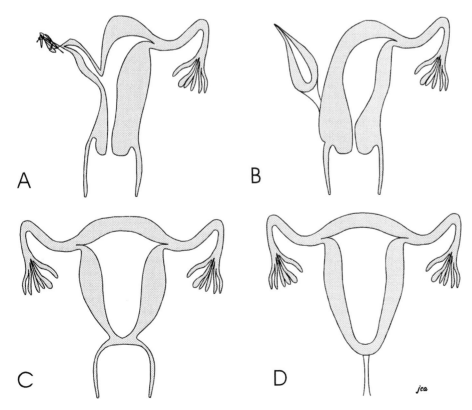

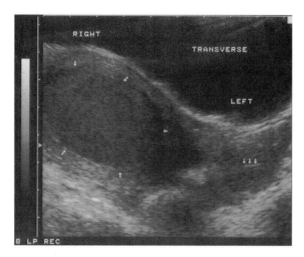

Figure 16.4 Transverse abdominal scan through the fundus of a double uterus in which the right horn is noncommunicating and is filled with blood. The left horn is empty (three small arrows).

in the surrounding myometrium,[18] but the role of progesterone remains unknown.

Symptoms

Many fibroids are asymptomatic and discovered incidentally at interval pelvic examination. When they do cause symptoms, they relate to their size and position in the uterus. If they affect the endometrial cavity, they may cause menorrhagia.[19] How they do this remains unclear. It may be due to an increase in the surface area of the endometrium or to vascular or hormonal factors. Whatever the mechanism, it is now known that fibroids can cause menorrhagia (albeit less severe) regardless of their position. Other symptoms such as pelvic discomfort and urinary symptoms are due to pressure. Pain is not usually a symptom unless the fibroid undergoes red de-

Figure 16.5 Diffuse adenomyosis. Sagittal view through the uterine fundus on a transvaginal scan in a 42-year-old woman who had a bulky, tender, retroverted uterus on bimanual palpation. Note the heterogeneous myometrium with tiny focal cystic spaces and the series of acoustic shadows described as "rain-in-the-forest."

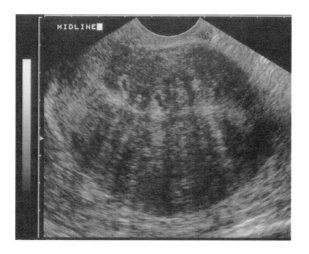

generation or torsion. Some fibroids present during the course of investigation for infertility.[20] The association between fibroids and infertility is not as strong as that between infertility and pelvic inflammatory disease, but this may be at least partly due to the fact that women being investigated for infertility and those with fibroids are of an older age group.

Variants

Several rare variants of leiomyoma may occasionally be of importance when imaging the uterus. *Benign metastasizing leiomyoma* is an enigmatic condition in which "metastatic" smooth muscle tumor deposits in the lung, lymph nodes, or abdomen appear to be derived from a benign leiomyoma of the uterus, often removed years before.[21] Some of these may represent misdiagnosed leiomyosarcomas, and others may be a multifocal smooth muscle proliferation involving the uterus and extragenital sites.[22] Yet others may simply be a primary smooth muscle tumor in a woman with a history of leiomyoma.[23] *Disseminated peritoneal leiomyomatosis* is a rare condition in which multiple small nodules up to 1 cm in diameter are scattered on the peritoneal surfaces of the abdomen and uterus and its adnexa. The nodules are composed of smooth muscle and myofibroblastic tissue, and the condition usually occurs during pregnancy and regresses afterward.[24–27] *Intravenous leiomyomatosis* is characterized by nodules of benign smooth muscle cells growing within venous channels.[28,29] The growth commences within the vessels of the uterus but can extend to the pelvic veins and even to the inferior vena cava and the heart.[28,30,31] Treatment is surgical and includes total hysterectomy with bilateral salpingo-oophorectomy and excision of more distant extensions including those in the lungs.[32,33] A *lipoleiomyoma* is a leiomyoma that contains much fat. It can be assumed that the imaging characteristics are consistent with those of fat elsewhere. A *vascular leiomyoma* contains numerous large-caliber vessels with muscular walls. The distinction between a hemangioma (Plate 16.1) or an arteriovenous malformation may be impossible on imaging the uterus, although the vascular leiomyoma tends to be sharply circumscribed by comparison.

Lymphangioma

Congenital intramural cysts of the uterus are rare. The differential diagnosis includes intramyometrial mesenchymal cysts (a developmental müllerian anomaly), marked degenerative change in a fibroid, benign cystic teratoma, and lymphangioma and hydatid disease.[34–36] A lymphangioma that presented incidentally with a coexistent early blighted pregnancy is demonstrated in Figure 16.7 and Plate 16.2. Hydatid cysts of the uterus are shown in Figure 16.8.

Hemangioma and Arteriovenous Malformation

Ultrasound examination has proved useful in providing diagnostic information in a number of cases of arteriovenous malformation.[37–39] Classical features include tortuous vessels of greater than normal calibre with real time sonography show-

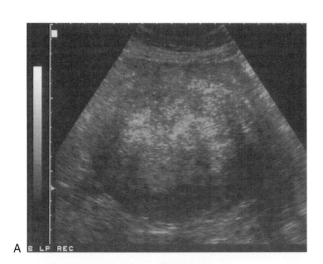

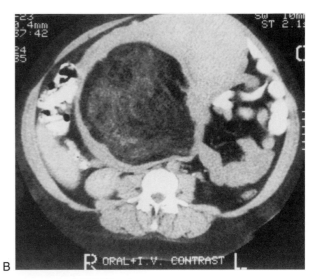

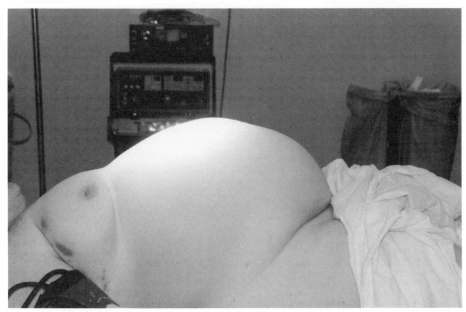

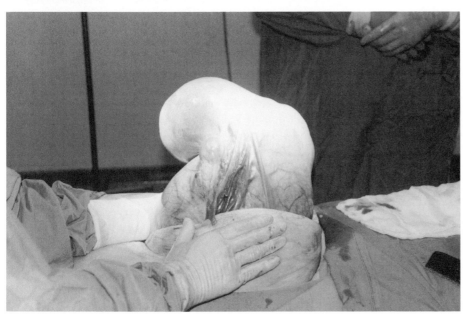

Figure 16.6 (**A**) A 42-year-old presented with abdominal distenstion gradually increasing over many years. A coronal view of a transvaginal scan shows a huge dense mass over 25 cm in diameter. It is typical of uterine fibroids in appearance. (**B**) A CT scan confirms the presence of a huge mass but led to the erroneous diagnosis of an ovarian dermoid. This may have been due to the fact that a large component of the mass was ultimately found to be a lipoleioma on histologic examination. (**C**) The patient's abdomen before surgery. (**D**) The massive fibroids delivered from the abdomen before hysterectomy. Interestingly, the patient's identical twin presented 3 months later with the same problem. (Courtesy of Dr. Victor O'Toole, Sydney, Australia.)

Figure 16.7 (**A**) A 34-year-old woman presented in early pregnancy with occasional bleeding. TVS showed an intrauterine blighted pregnancy (arrow), and to the left of this, a 5-cm-diameter intramural cyst with numerous complex trabeculated walls. (**B**) CT scan through the uterus showing the blighted pregnancy (2) and the complex cyst (1). The blighted pregnancy was dealt with by suction curettage. (Courtesy of Dr John Korber, Sydney, Australia.) (see also Plate 16.2). (Fig. A Courtesy of Dr Mark Beale, Sydney, Australia.)

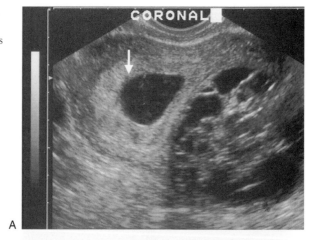

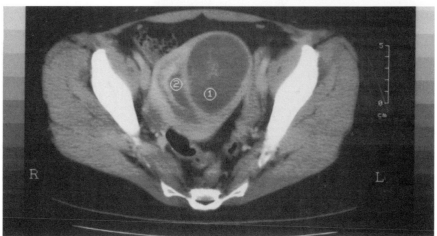

ing a bounding pulse and colour Doppler confirming the presence of numerous blood vessels.

Lipoma

Lipomatous uterine masses are uncommon hyperechoic pelvic neoplasms composed partly of adipose tissue. As a result of the high level of echogenicity, these uterine masses can produce a sonographic appearance strikingly similar to the "dermoid plug" that is considered characteristic of benign cystic teratomas. The key to distinguishing the two tumors is to ascertain the parent organ: the lipomatous uterine mass should clearly originate from the myometrium (Fig. 16.9).[40]

MALIGNANT CONDITIONS

Leiomyosarcoma

Leiomyosarcoma is responsible for about 1.3% of uterine malignancies. Less than 1% of women thought to have fibroids prove to have a leiomyosarcoma.[41] Most leiomyosarcomas are intramural, solitary, and occur in a uterus that does not contain benign fibroids.[42,43] They are generally soft and fleshy with poorly described margins, and they may contain areas of

hemorrhage.[44] No other features are likely to be helpful in distinguishing them from fibroids by ultrasound. *Endometrial stromal sarcomas* are rare and not likely to be diagnosed other than on histology.

POST UTERINE PERFORATION

Perforation of the uterus at operation by a uterine probe or sharp curette is not usually a diagnostic problem, because the operator generally recognizes the injury. In most cases, no action is required other than observation to confirm that there is no bleeding or infection. Nevertheless, occasionally ultrasound is requested on these patients. The track of the instrument is difficult to see on the scan and in any case is usually of no clinical significance. It is important, however, to ensure that there is no internal bleeding that would be indicated by blood collecting in the pouch of Douglas.

SUMMARY

Ultrasound is well suited to evaluation of the myometrium and associated disorders using the complementary techniques of transabdominal and transvaginal ultrasound.

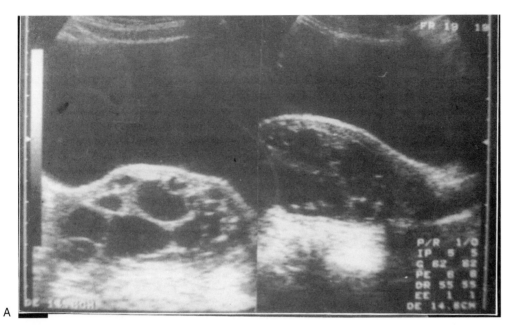

A

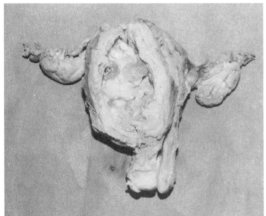

B

Figure 16.8 (**A**) A 55-year-old gravida 5, para 5 presented with irregular bleeding for 2 months. On abdominal ultrasonography, a large septated and cystic mass (8 × 5 cm) was seen on the left side of the uterus. (**B**) After hysterectomy, a yellow-colored irregular cystic mass measuring 6 × 4 × 3 cm was found under the serosa and within the myometrium. This was confirmed histologically to be hydatid disease (*Taenia echinococcus*). (Courtesy of Dr. Y. Okumus, Kayseri, Turkey.)[36]

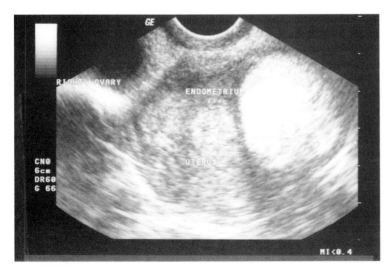

Figure 16.9 Lipoma of the uterus. Myometrium can be seen to surround the lesion to the right. (From Hertzberg BS, Kliewer MA, George P et al: Lipomatous uterine masses potential to mimic ovarian dermoids on endovaginal sonography. J Ultrasound Med 1985,14:689–692, with permission.)

REFERENCES

1. Kaufman RH, Binder GL, Gray PN et al. Upper genital tract changes associated with exposure in utero to diethylstilbestrol. Am J Obstet Gynecol 1977;128:51

2. Jones HW Jr, Mermut S. Familial occurrence of congenital absence of the vagina. Am J Obstet Gynecol 1972;114:1100–1101

3. Winter JD, Kohn G, Mellinin WJ et al. A familial syndrome or renal, genital, and middle ear anomalies. J Pediatr 1968;72:88

4. Shokeir MHK. Aplasia of the müllerian system. Evidence of

probable sex limited autosomal dominant inheritance. Birth Defects 1978;14:147–151

5. Bohlman ME, Ensor RE, Sanders RC. Sonographic findings in adenomyosis of the uterus. AJR Am J Roentgenol 1987;148: 765–766

6. Seidler D, Laing FC, Jeffrey RB, Jr, Wing VW: Uterine adenomyosis—a difficult sonographic diagnosis. J Ultrasound Med 1987;6:345–349

7. Togashi K, Ozasa H, Konishi I et al. Enlarged uterus: differentiation between adenomyosis and leiomyoma with MRI. Radiology 1989;171:531–534

8. Popp LW, Schwiedesses JP, Gaetje R. Myometrial biopsy in the diagnosis of adenomyosis uteri. Am J Obset Gynecol 1993; 169:546–549

9. Damirov MM, Bakuleva LP, Shabanov AM, Sliusar NN. A clinico-morphological comparison of the ultrasonic criteria of adenomyosis. Akush Gynekol 1994;2:40–42

10. Brozens JJ, de Souza NM, Barker FG et al. Endovaginal ultrasonography in the diagnosis of adenomyosis uteri: identifying the predictive characteristics. Br J Obstet Gynaecol 1995; 102:471–474

11. Reinhold C, Atri M, Mehio A et al. Diffuse uterine adenomyosis: morphologic criteria and diagnostic accuracy of endovaginal sonography. Radiology 1995;197:609–614

12. Timor-Tritsch IE. Relevant pelvic anatomy In: Goldstein SR, Timor-Tritsch IE, (Eds). Ultrasound in Gynecology. Churchill Livingstone, New York, 1995, p 67

13. Ascher SM, Arnold LL, Patt RH et al. Adenomyosis: prospective comparison of MRI and transvaginal ultrasonography. Radiology 1994; 190:803–806

14. Arnold LL, Ascher SM, Schruefer JJ, Simon JA. The nonsurgical diagnosis of adenomyosis. Obstet Gynecol 1995;86:461–465

15. West CP. LHRH analogues in the management of uterine fibroids, premenstrual syndrome and breast malignancies. Clin Obstet Gynecol 1988;2:689–709

16. Perry CM, Brogden RN. Goserelin. A review of its pharmacodynamic and pharmacokinetic properties, and therapeutic use in benign gynaecological disorders. Drugs 1996,51:319–346

17. Benagio G, Kivinen ST, Fadini R et al. Zoladex (goserelin acetate) and the anaemic patient: results of a multicentre fibroid study. Fertil Steril 1996:66;223–229

18. Wilson EA, Yang F, Rees ED. Estradiol and progesterone binding in uterine leiomyomata and in normal uterine tissues. Obstet Gynecol 1980;55:20–24

19. Rybo G, Leman J, Tibblin R. Epidemiology of menstrual blood loss. In: Baird DT, Michie EA, Eds. Mechanisms of Menstrual Bleeding. Raven Press, New York, 1985, pp 181–193

20. Buttram RC, Reiter RC. Uterine leiomyomata: etiology, symptomatology and management. Fertil Steril 1981;36:433–445

21. Zaloudek C, Norris HJ. Mesenchymal tumours of the uterus. In: Kurman RJ, Ed. Blaustein's Pathology of the Female Genital Tract (4th ed.). Springer-Verlag, New York, 1994, p 497

22. Cho KR, Woodruff JD, Epstein JI. Leiomyoma of the uterus with multiple extrauterine smooth muscle tumours: a case report suggesting multifocal origin. Hum Pathol 1989;20:80–83

23. Gal AA, Brooks JJ, Pietra GG. Leiomyomatous neoplasms of the lung: a clinical, histologic, and immunohistological study. Mod Pathol 1989;2:209–216

24. Aterman K, Fraser GM, Lea RH. Disseminated peritoneal leiomyomatosis. Virchows Arch (A) 1977;374:13–26

25. Dryer L, Simson IW, Sevenster CB, Dittrich OC. Leiomyomatosis peritonealis disseminata. A report of two cases and a review of the literature. Br J Obstet Gynecol 1985;92: 856–861

26. Goldberg MF, Hurt WG, Frable WJ. Leiomyomatosis peritonealis disseminata: report of a case and review of the literature. Obstet Gynecol 1977;49:46s–52s

27. Tavassoli FA, Norris HJ. Peritoneal leiomyomatosis (leiomyomatosis peritonealis disseminata): a clinicopathologic study of 20 cases with ultrastructural observations. Int J Gynecol Pathol 1982;1:59–74

28. Clement PB. Intravenous leiomyomatosis of the uterus. Pathol Annu 1988;23:153–183

29. Nogales FF, Navarro N, Martinez de Victoria JM et al. Uterine intravascular leiomyomatosis: an update and report of seven cases. Int J Gynecol Pathol 1987;6:331–339

30. Cooper MM, Guillem J, Dalton J et al. Recurrent intravenous leiomyomatosis with cardiac extension. Ann Thorac Surg 1992;53:139–141

31. Timmis AD, Smallpiece C, Davies AC et al. Intracardiac spread of intravenous leiomyomatosis with successful surgical excision. N Engl J Med 1980;303:1043–1044

32. Evans AT, III, Symonds RE, Gaffey TA. Recurrent pelvic intravenous leiomyomatosis. Obstet Gynecol 1981;57:260–264

33. Norris HJ, Parmley T. Mesenchymal tumors of the uterus. V. Intravenous leiomyomatosis. A clinical and pathological study of 14 cases. Cancer 1975;36:2164–2178

34. Gardner GH, Greene RR, Peckham BM. Myometrial cysts. Am J Obstet Gynecol 1948;55:917–939

35. Sherick V. Congenital intramural cysts of the uterus. Obstet Gynecol. 1962:19;486–493

36. Okumus Y, Tayyar M, Patiroglu T, Aygen E. Uterine hydatid cyst. Int J Gynecol Obstet 1994;45:51–53

37. Diwan RV, Brennan JN, Selim MA et al. Sonographic diagnosis of arteriovenous malformation of the uterus and pelvis. J Clin Ultrasound 1983;11:295–298

38. Manolitsas T, Hurley V, Gilford E. Uterine arteriovenous malformation—a rare cause of uterine haemorrhage. Aust NZ J Obstet Gynaecol 1994;34:197–199

39. Shanberge JN. Hemangioma of the uterus associated with hereditary hemorrhagic telangiectasia. Obstet Gynecol 1994; 84:708–710

40. Hertzberg BS, Kliewer MA, George P et al. Lipomatous uterine masses potential to mimic ovarian dermoids on endovaginal sonography. J Ultrasound Med 1985;14:689–692

41. Leibsohn S, d'Ablaing G, Mischell DR, Jr, Schlaerth JB. Leiomyosarcoma in a series of hysterectomies performed for presumed uterine leiomyomas. Am J Obstet Gynecol 1990;162: 968–974

42. Burns B, Curry RH, Bell ME. Morphologic features of prognostic significance in uterine smooth muscle tumors. A review of eighty-four cases. Am J Obstet Gynecol 1979;135:109–114

43. Evans HL, Chawla SP, Simpson C, Finn KP. Smooth muscle neoplasms of the uterus other than ordinary leiomyoma. A study of 46 cases, with emphasis in diagnostic criteria and prognostic factors. Cancer 1988;62:2239–2247

44. Barter JF, Smith EB, Szpak CA et al. Leiomyosarcoma of the uterus: clinicopathologic study of 21 cases. Gynecol Oncol 1985;21:220–227

Computed Tomography and Magnetic Resonance Imaging of the Myometrium

ERIC K. OUTWATER

KIM M. WILSON

DONALD G. MITCHELL

Magnetic resonance imaging (MRI) is playing an increasing role in the evaluation of pelvic and myometrial abnormalities, because it provides greater intrinsic soft tissue contrast than either computed tomography (CT) or ultrasound. The multiplanar capability of MRI becomes particularly important for imaging the myometrium because of the variable orientation of the uterus. The use of MRI is limited by claustrophobia in some people, and it is contraindicated in patients with pacemakers, metal in the retina, some aneurysm clips, and certain other biomedical devices.[1]

BENIGN CONDITIONS

MRI is better than CT at showing soft tissue contrast between smooth muscle proliferation and the surrounding myometrium. T2-weighted images are essential for displaying the contrast between leiomyomas or adenomyosis and the myometrium. Multiple planes are often necessary to show the extent of leiomyomas relative to the serosa and endometrium. Contrast-enhanced T1-weighted sequences usually do not help to evaluate leiomyomas, except for characterizing myomas.

Leiomyomas

Patients with submucosal leiomyomas may have menorrhagia because the leiomyomas lie immediately beneath the endometrium (Fig. 17.1). Subserosal leiomyomas can grow away from the uterus while attached by a thin stalk, becoming pedunculated (Fig. 17.2). These may present as adnexal masses and can undergo torsion, causing acute abdominal pain (Fig. 17.3). A subserosal leiomyoma that loses its uterine blood supply and adheres to another pelvic structure is called a parasitic leiomyoma.[2] MRI is useful for demonstrating the loca-

tion of a leiomyoma, for instance, when it prolapses into the vagina (Fig. 17.4).[3,4]

Leiomyomas have a variety of appearances on CT.[5–7] Leiomyomas are easily recognized on CT if they contain coarse focal calcifications, but very few do.[8] In general, the poor soft tissue contrast between leiomyomas and adjacent myometrium weakens the diagnostic capability of CT (Fig. 17.5).[6,7] When leiomyomas are large, CT may not show their origin, and they may be mistaken for adnexal masses (Fig. 17.6). Subserosal leiomyomas may be difficult to recognize, or they may appear as a pelvic mass separate from the uterus.[9] Submucosal and intramural leiomyomas also may be difficult to distinguish. Foci of degeneration or necrosis may appear as areas of low attenuation and decreased enhancement (Fig. 17.5). Rarely, myomas become infected, and enclosed gas suggests the diagnosis (Fig. 17.7).[10]

The signal intensity of leiomyomas on T1- and T2-weighted images parallels that of densely packed cellular smooth muscle, such as the junctional zone of the uterus, bladder wall, and the rectal muscle. The signal intensity of myomas on T2-weighted images is low and similar to that of skeletal muscle (Fig. 17.3). The internal structure appears as globules of low intensity with thin interspersed strands of higher signal intensity due to vascular channels or loose connective or myxoid tissue. Unlike adenomyosis, myomas are sharply demarcated from the remainder of the myometrium. This interface is often poorly defined by CT or ultrasound. The sharpness of the myometrial interface is an important diagnostic feature between leiomyomas and adenomyosis.[11] A high signal intensity rim is often present around leiomyomas on T2-weighted sequences. This corresponds to dilated lymphatic vessels, dilated veins, or edema.[12]

Myomas undergo internal changes that affect MRI. Hyalinization is characterized by replacement of muscle fibers with dense concentrations of proteinaceous material. Hyaline degeneration has a low signal on T2-weighted sequences,[13] similar to undegenerated tumors, and hyaline degeneration

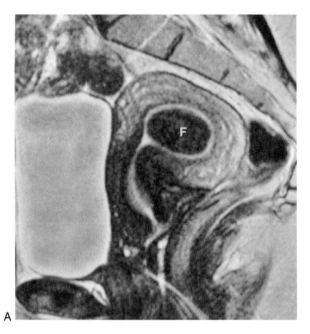
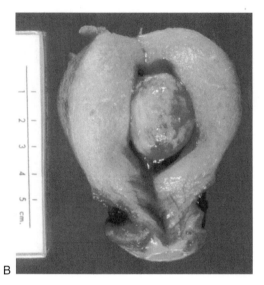

A

B

Figure 17.1 Submucosal fibroid in a patient with menorrhagia. (**A**) A T2-weighted fast spin echo (FSE) image through the midline of the uterus shows the submucosal fibroid (F) surrounded by high signal intensity endometrium. Note the typical three-layered structure of the cervix with a palmitate plicae. (**B**) Gross specimen.

does not enhance, unlike undegenerated leiomyomas. Cystic change, myxoid degeneration, and necrosis are less frequent than hyaline degeneration.[13] Because of the higher water content in these types of degeneration, they show very high signal intensity on T2-weighted images (Fig. 17.8).[13,14] Hemorrhage is infrequent with leiomyomas. One form of hemorrhagic degeneration called carneous or red degeneration occurs in leiomyomas in pregnant or postpartum women.

In addition to the common types of degeneration, several variants of leiomyomas occur. Cellular leiomyomas are distinguished from usual leiomyomas because they have increased cellular density compared to surrounding myometrium.[15] Symplastic leiomyomas contain particular large cells, which may resemble those of a leiomyosarcoma, and epithelioid smooth muscle tumors are composed of polygonal cells of various types resembling epithelial cells.[15] These histologic types have no particular radiologic significance, except that their increased cellularity results in higher than usual signal intensity on T2-weighted images (Fig. 17.4) and increased enhancement with contrast agents.[13,16]

Dynamic contrast-enhanced MRI is useful for distinguishing cellular leiomyomas, which respond to hormonal therapy, from degenerated tumors.[13,16] Some forms of degeneration as well as highly cellular tumors have a higher signal on T2-weighted sequences. Cellular tumors show marked early enhancement, compared with spotty enhancement of degenerate leiomyomas. However, unless the patient is a candidate for treatment with gonadotropin releasing hormone analogs, gadolinium enhancement is not necessary. Contrast enhancement does not increase the sensitivity or specificity of

MRI for detecting these tumors.[17] MRI can also be used to evaluate treatment with gonadotropin releasing hormone analogs.[18]

MRI is more sensitive and more specific than hysterosalpingography or ultrasound in detecting leiomyomas.[19,20] MRI is also more sensitive than ultrasound for identifying submucosal fibroids (see Fig. 17.1).[21] A problem with the ultrasound evaluation of women with large myomatous uteri is the identification of the ovaries and the endometrial pattern, but MRI is useful for delineating these structures. In 23 patients with myomas, the endometrium was visualized by ultrasound in only 2 women but was visualized in all patients by MRI.[19] MRI provides a more comprehensive evaluation of the pelvis in the patient with symptomatic or complicated leiomyomas. In addition, identification of the exact submucosal extent is necessary to plan a myomectomy and to judge the degree of myometrial defect that may result from excision of these tumors. MRI is particularly useful for localization of fibroids in pregnancy.[22–26] (Fig. 17.9).

Metastasizing and Venoinvasive Benign Smooth Muscle Tumors

A variety of extra uterine smooth muscle tumors can be associated with leiomyomas of the myometrium. These include intravenous leiomyomatosis, benign metastasizing leiomyoma, and leiomyomatosis peritonealis disseminata. Histologic evidence of venous invasion is an uncommon finding in leiomyomas, and extension of apparently benign leiomyoma into the pelvic veins, inferior vena cava, or heart is also rare.

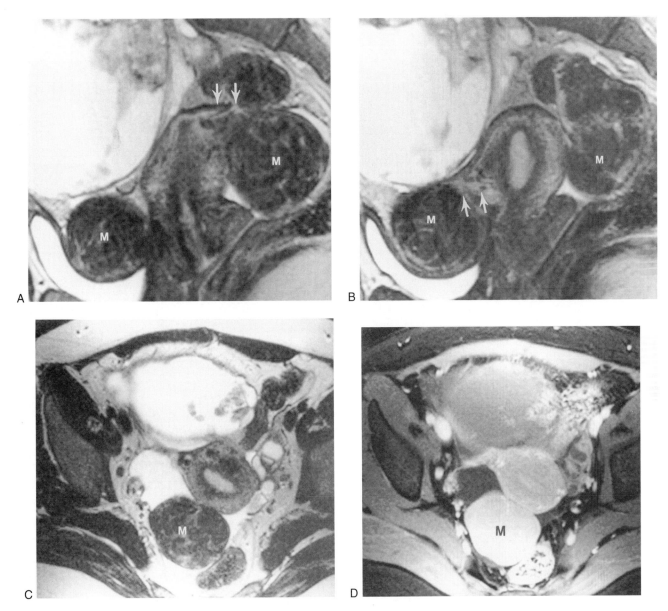

Figure 17.2 Complex leiomyomas. T2-weighted FSE (**A** & **B**) sagittal and (**C**) axial MRI show two low signal intensity masses (M) over the dome of the bladder and in the cul-de-sac. Although these masses lie outside the uterus, the stalks (arrows) to the pedunculated leiomyomas can be identified. (**D**) A gadolinium-enhanced fat-suppressed image shows marked enhancement of the cul-de-sac fibroid (M), thus establishing its solid nature and preventing any confusion with bowel. A large adnexal mass (immature teratoma) is incidentally noted above and anterior to the uterus in all images. (From Mayer and Shipilov,[69] with permission.)

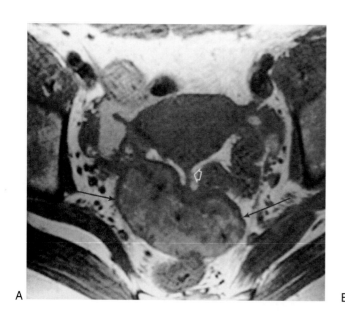

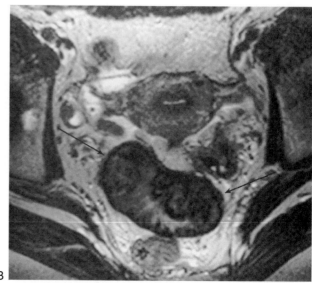

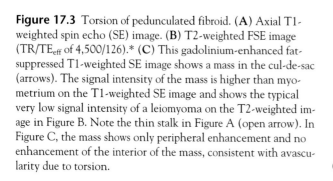

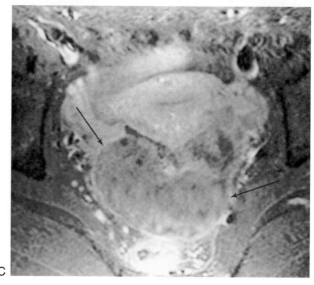

Figure 17.3 Torsion of pedunculated fibroid. (**A**) Axial T1-weighted spin echo (SE) image. (**B**) T2-weighted FSE image (TR/TE_eff of 4,500/126).* (**C**) This gadolinium-enhanced fat-suppressed T1-weighted SE image shows a mass in the cul-de-sac (arrows). The signal intensity of the mass is higher than myometrium on the T1-weighted SE image and shows the typical very low signal intensity of a leiomyoma on the T2-weighted image in Figure B. Note the thin stalk in Figure A (open arrow). In Figure C, the mass shows only peripheral enhancement and no enhancement of the interior of the mass, consistent with avascularity due to torsion.

---

* The TE for FSE sequences is expressed as effective TE (TE_eff) to mark that signals from different phase-encoded steps do not have the same TE. Effective TE is determined by the position of the low-order phase-encoded signals in k-space.

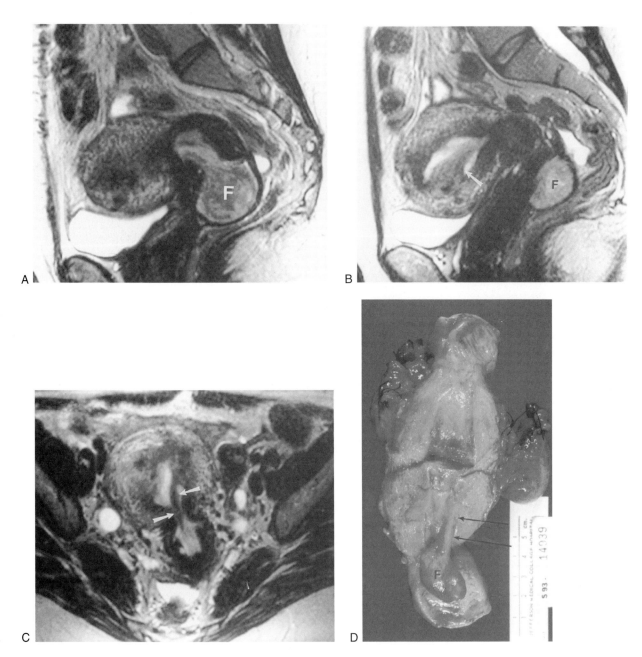

Figure 17.4 Prolapsed pedunculated submucosal leiomyoma. (**A & B**) These sagittal T2-weighted FSE images (TR/TE_eff = 4,500/108) show a submucus fibroid (F) protruding through the endocervical canal into the vagina. The stalk of the mass (white arrows) attaches to the upper myometrium junctional zone in Figure B. (**C**) A T2-weighted FSE image shows the stalk (white arrows) attached to the left side of the myometrium and passing through the endocervical canal. A low signal intensity stalk (arrows) attaches to the left side of the myometrium. (**D**) This gross photograph from a similar patient shows a pedunculated fibroid (F) in the endocervical canal. (From Mayer and Shipilov,[69] with permission.)

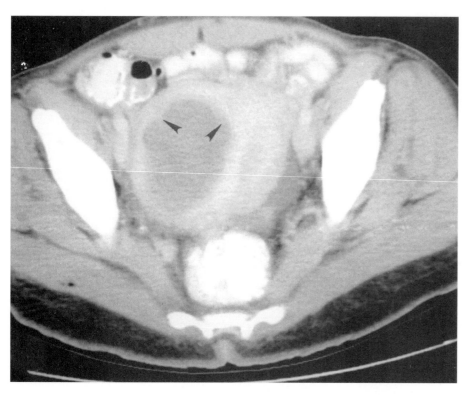

Figure 17.5 Leiomyoma. This contrast-enhanced CT image shows a focal bulge in the right side of the uterus with an irregular nonehancing area. Leiomyomas are generally demonstrable on CT only if they produce a contour defect, are calcified, or produce differential enhancement when compared to the remainder of the myometrium. The inner border of the area of lesser enhancement (arrowheads) is somewhat irregular. This does not allow distinction between leiomyomas and sarcomas.

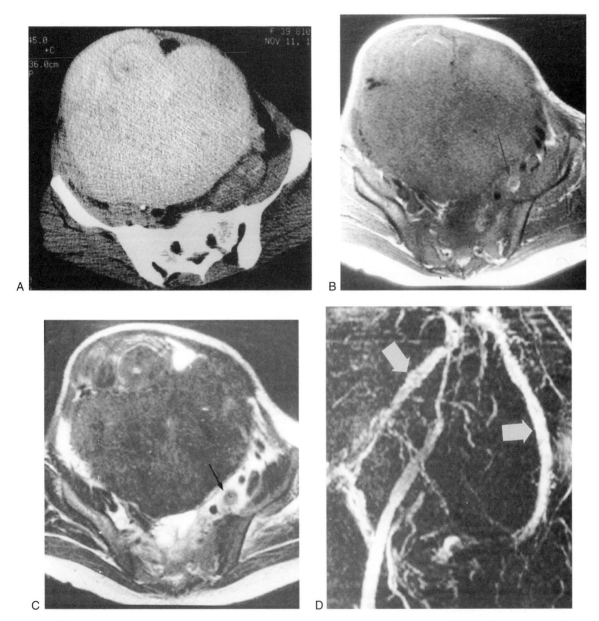

Figure 17.6 Massive leiomyomas. (**A**) CT shows a solid mass filling the pelvis. It was difficult to ascertain whether the mass was arising from the uterus or adnexa. (**B**) T1-weighted SE image. (**C**) This T2-weighted FSE image shows that it has very low signal intensity on the T2-weighted image, and, therefore, it is probably due to massive leiomyomas. Note the high signal intensity left common iliac thrombosis, which was not apparent on CT (long arrow). (**D**) A maximum intensity projection reconstruction from two-dimensional axial time-of-flight images shows occlusion of the left common iliac, external iliac, and common femoral veins due to the thrombosis visualized in Figures B and C. The large gonadal veins (arrows) drain the massively enlarged uterus. MRI was more useful for characterizing the pelvic mass. (From Outwater,[61] with permission.)

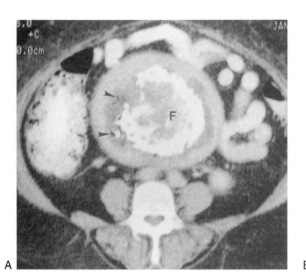
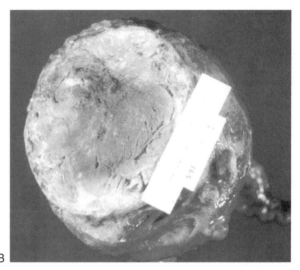

Figure 17.7 Infected fibroid. (**A**) CT through a densely calcified large fibroid (F) shows multiple small foci of air (arrowheads) within a low attenuation area near the fibroid. Infection is a rare complication of uterine fibroids and is difficult to detect unless gas is present. (**B**) This gross specimen shows that the inner portion of the mass is hemorrhagic and necrotic, leading to the poor enhancement evident on CT.

Figure 17.8 Myxoid changes in a broad ligament leiomyoma. (**A**) An axial T2-weighted FSE image shows a large low signal intensity mass (F) adjacent to the uterus. This leiomyoma arose within the broad ligament, as can be inferred from the intact serosal surface of the uterus adjacent to the mass (small arrows). The mass contains numerous lobules of high intensity (long arrows) representing myxoid change. (**B**) A T1-weighted axial image fails to distinguish between fibroid and uterus. However, signal voids from large feeding vessels of the leiomyoma can be seen arising from the broad ligament (arrows). (*Figure continues.*)

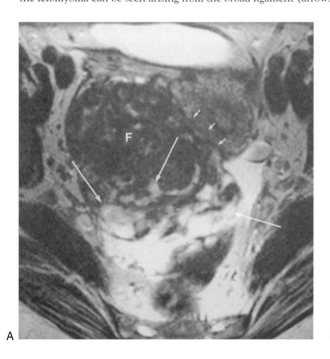
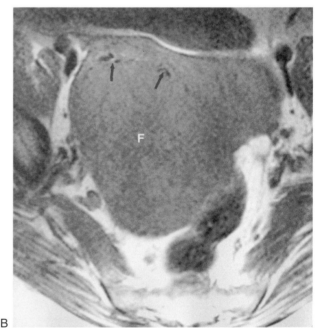

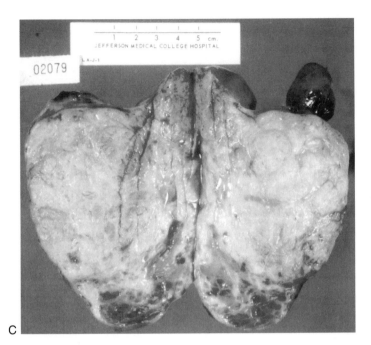

C

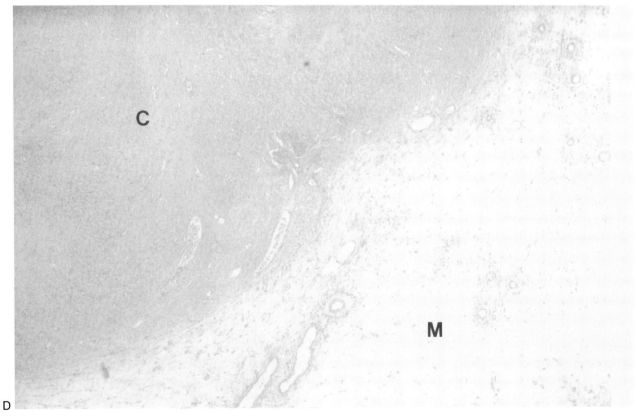

D

Figure 17.8 (*Continued*). (**C**) Gross specimen. The ovary is separate from the mass. (**D**) A photomicrograph of the tumor shows the cellular areas of leiomyoma (C) and the loose myxoid tissue (M) representing the high signal intensity areas seen in Figure A.

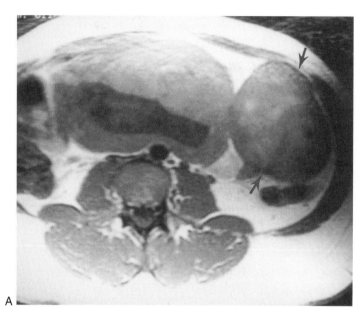

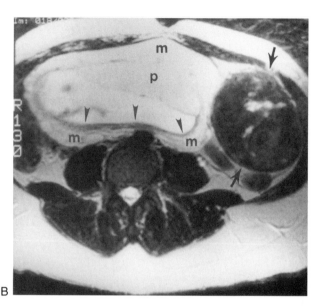

Figure 17.9 A left adnexal mass, shown on ultrasound to be partially solid, in pregnancy. (**A**) An axial SE image (TR/TE$_{eff}$ of 700/12) shows a large mass (arrows) lying to the left of the gravid uterus. (**B**) An axial T2-weighted FSE image (TR/TE$_{eff}$ of 3,800/126) shows that the mass produces very low signal intensity, indicating a pedunculated leiomyoma. Patchy areas of slightly high signal intensity within this mass indicate hemorrhage or carneous degeneration, which is a common finding in leiomyomas during pregnancy or in the post-partum period. In contrast, malignant masses have higher signal intensity on T2-weighted images. Note the appearance of the gravid uterus in Figure B, with high signal intensity outer myometrium (m), placenta (p), and a preserved junctional zone (arrowheads). (From Outwater,[61] with permission.)

A number of reports have described how valuable MRI or CT can be for identifying venous invasion.[27] On CT, distended tangled tubular structures represent intravenous tumor in myometrial veins.[27] Tumor may extend into pelvic veins, the inferior vena cava, and even the right atrium.[28–30]

MRI is particularly well suited for identifying the intravascular component of leiomyomas.[27,28,30] On T1-weighted spin echo images, the intravascular tumor can be seen as a soft tissue extension from the uterus into the pelvic veins and inferior vena cava, surrounded by signal void of the flowing blood. Gradient echo images can be used to visualize the flow as high signal intensity around the low signal intensity intraluminal filling defect. Recognition of this intravascular extension is important, so that intravascular tumor is not inadvertently transected during hysterectomy or myomectomy.

Benign metastasizing leiomyoma is associated with the unusual occurrence of apparent metastases, usually to the lungs, sometimes years after removal of a benign uterine leiomyoma.[31] Histologically, these tumors are benign, although some consider them to be a low-grade sarcoma.[15] Slow-growing lung nodules are found more frequently than metastases to the mediastinum, pelvic lymph nodes, and other soft tissue sites.[2] Leiomyomatosis peritonealis disseminata is a related entity consisting of multiple implants of histologically benign leiomyomas throughout the peritoneum.[32–35] No specific signs separate this entity from metastatic sarcoma.

Fat-containing uterine tumors are uncommon but can be identified before surgery. Pure lipomas as well as mixed tumors (with smooth muscle and/or fibrous cells) have been reported.[36] Fatty elements within a myometrial mass can be identified by low-attenuating areas on CT that have negative Hounsfield unit measurements.[36–38] With MRI, chemical shift imaging definitively identifies lipid-containing structures.[39,40]

Adenomyosis

In adenomyosis, small islands of endometrial glandular tissue become embedded within the myometrium. In superficial adenomyosis, the islands will be found within the inner myometrium (i.e., junctional zone). In diffuse adenomyosis, the islands will be found throughout the myometrium. Large masses, called adenomyomas, may form (Fig. 17.10). The endometrial glands are surrounded by whorled, densely packed smooth muscle cells that form the stromal response around the islands of endometrium. It is this stromal reaction that forms the basis of the MRI appearance of adenomyosis.[41] Because the smooth muscle surrounding the endometrial islands is densely packed like the junctional zone, it has similar signal intensity.

CT of adenomyosis usually shows a diffusely or focally enlarged uterus, but features are nonspecific.[8] The focal abnor-

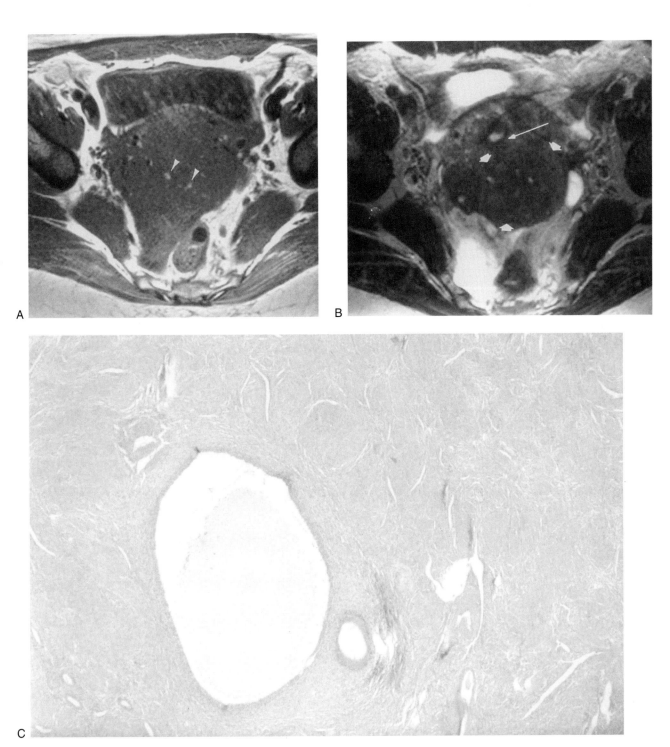

Figure 17.10 Masslike adenomyosis. (**A**) An axial SE T1-weighted image shows uterine enlargement with small punctate high signal intensity foci (arrowheads). (**B**) An axial T2-weighted FSE image shows the adenomyosis as an ill-defined mass (short arrows) of low signal intensity within the myometrium. Several punctate high signal intensity foci represent the embedded glands. The adenomyosis focally obscures the junctional zone posteriorly (long white arrow). (**C**) A photomicrograph of the adenomyotic glands shows the endometrial lined glands surrounded by a small amount of endometrial stroma and the dense whorled myometrial reaction that gives rise to the low signal intensity of the adenomyosis. (From Outwater,[61] with permission.)

mality within the myometrium has similar attenuation to the myometrium.

On MRI, adenomyosis appears as a poorly defined mass with decreased signal intensity similar to, and often blending with, the junctional zone (Fig. 17.10). Unlike leiomyomas, the interface between the myometrium is ill-defined and infiltrative.[11,41,42] Microscopically, the foci of endometrium are often surrounded by myometrial hypertrophy, which is low in signal on MRI. Tiny islands of endometrium within the hypertrophied myometrium account for the foci of increased signal intensity sometimes seen on T2-weighted sequences.[41,42] Foci of high intensity that are likely to be secondary to hemorrhage may be seen on T1-weighted images. Diffuse adenomyosis may appear as thickening of the junctional zone to over 12 mm, which has been suggested as the upper limit of normal (Fig. 17.11).[43]

Figure 17.11 Diffuse adenomyosis. (**A**) Sagittal T2-weighted FSE images through the uterus show diffuse thickening of the junctional zone. The junctional zone posteriorly measures more than 12 mm, which is strongly suggestive of diffuse adenomyosis. Note the punctate high signal intensity foci lying beneath the endometrium representing the islands of endometrium within the myometrium. (**B**) A photomicrograph shows foci of endometrial glands and stroma surrounded by dense smooth muscle whorls. (From Outwater and Schiebler,[70] with permission.)

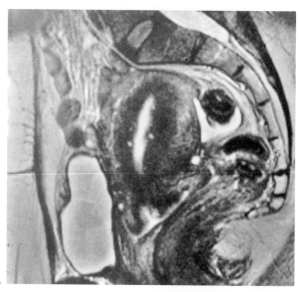

A

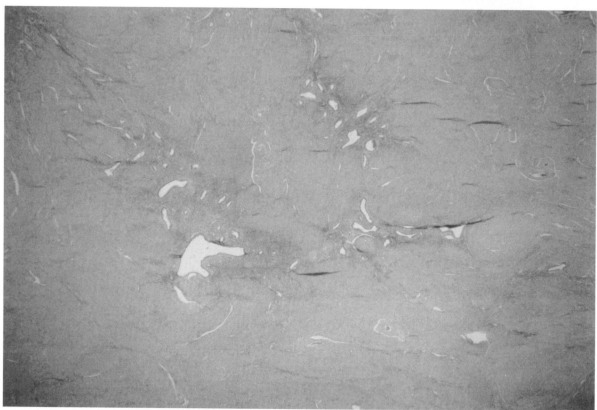

B

Other Conditions

Endometrial stromal nodules are the benign form of endometrial stromal sarcoma. These are usually solitary, often incidental findings on hysterectomy. In one series of 60 endometrial stromal nodules, the mean size was 4 cm. They are sharply circumscribed from the surrounding myometrium. The majority are totally within the myometrium, but they may involve the endometrium as well. Unlike low-grade endometrial stromal sarcomas, they do not invade the lymphatic or vascular systems.[44] The MRI and CT appearances of these tumors have not yet been reported. Because they are cellular, they can be expected to have higher signal intensity on T2-weighted sequences than leiomyomas.

Cavernous hemangiomas and arteriovenous malformations (AVMs) of the uterus are rare,[45,46] but they can be dangerous, particularly during pregnancy. Hysterectomy to control bleeding[47] is often required. Unlike the normal vessels seen on T2-weighted images within the myometrial wall, vessels associated with AVMs show signal voids because of their fast blood flow. The flow can be visualized with gradient echo sequences to take advantage of time of flight effects and flow-related enhancement to demonstrate the flow in AVMs as a high signal intensity. The venous component of AVMs and hemangiomas shows a slower flow and is of high signal intensity on the T2-weighted sequences.[48] Vessels showing flow void can be seen in AVMs, gestational trophoblastic disease, or sometimes as vessels feeding large leiomyomas.

MALIGNANT MYOMETRIAL NEOPLASMS

Primary Malignancies

Sarcomas account for less than 3% of all invasive uterine malignancies[45,49,50] and are difficult to distinguish clinically and radiologically from the benign smooth muscle proliferations. Leiomyosarcoma, malignant mixed müllerian tumor, and endometrial stromal sarcoma are the types most often encountered.[50] Malignant mixed müllerian tumor, while containing sarcomatous elements, behaves as a variant of endometrial carcinoma[51] and has indistinguishable imaging features.[52]

Leiomyosarcoma is the most common purely mesenchymal sarcoma that affects the uterus. It is usually large when diagnosed because of the difficulty of distinguishing it from the far more common leiomyoma. The diagnosis of leiomyosarcoma is usually made by histologic examination of a mass believed to be a leiomyoma or pelvic malignancy. Leiomyosarcomas do not arise from leiomyomas, so patients with leiomyomas are not at an increased risk for the development of sarcomas.[15,45]

There are no radiographic features of leiomyosarcomas that allow them to be differentiated from large or degenerate leiomyomas.[5,7,9] On CT, leiomyosarcoma is a heterogeneously enhancing mass with areas of low attenuation due to hemorrhage or necrosis (Fig. 17.12).[36,53] Calcification is uncommon.[53] This appearance mimics that of leiomyomas that have undergone myxoid or cystic degeneration.[5,7,9] A strongly suggestive diagnosis of leiomyosarcoma cannot usu-

Figure 17.12 Uterine leiomyosarcoma. (**A**) A CT image through the uterine corpus shows an irregular mass protruding into the endometrial cavity. Irregular enhancement of the tumor is seen (arrowheads). It is difficult to distinguish nonenhancing areas of the tumor from fluid, although at pathologic examination, no fluid was present. Note the deep invasion through the myometrium (arrow). (**B**) The pedunculated tumor attached to the uterine fundus. Pathologic examination showed poorly differentiated leiomyosarcoma.

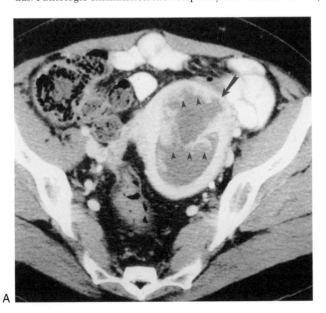
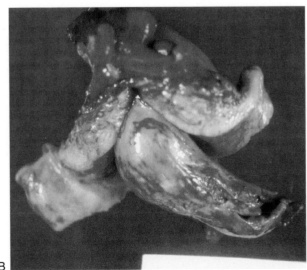

A

B

ally be made by radiologic imaging.[54] Support for the diagnosis is provided by lymphatic, hematogenous, or peritoneal spread in the presence of a dominant myometrial mass.[55] CT in suspected leiomyosarcoma is useful for evaluation of metastatic disease. Because sarcomas metastasize via the bloodstream, CT of the chest is important to exclude pulmonary metastases. Similarly, the periaortic area should be evaluated for lymphatic metastases. Unlike the peritoneal spread of carcinomas, peritoneal spread of leiomyosarcoma is not associated with ascites.[56]

Leiomyosarcomas are nearly always hypercellular compared with the surrounding myometrium,[15] suggesting that sarcomas can be differentiated from most leiomyomas on MRI. Most leiomyomas are typically hypocellular compared with myometrium, are predominantly low signal intensity on T2-weighted images, and do not enhance well with gadolinium chelates.[13,17] Cellular leiomyomas, however, show a homogeneously increased signal intensity on T2-weighted images and enhance rapidly and to a greater degree, features that overlap with sarcomas.[13] In general, leiomyosarcomas have higher signal intensity than myometrium on T2-weighted images and are necrosed or hemorrhagic (Fig. 17.13).[54,57,58]

Endometrial stroma neoplasms are tumors of the myometrium or endometrium that have the characteristics of endometrial stromal cells beneath the endometrial mucosa.

Most endometrial stroma sarcomas are low-grade neoplasms.[15,44,59] They can present a striking gross appearance in some patients, with wormlike extensions permeating the surrounding myometrium,[45] previously called endolymphatic stromal myosis. Presenting symptoms are nonspecific, but menorrhagia and other abnormal uterine bleeding are common.[44] The growth of endometrial stromal sarcomas is generally indolent, with a 5-year survival for stage I patients of 98%.[59] The few endometrial stromal sarcomas that have been described have shown diffuse high signal intensity on T2-weighted sequences with some showing necrosis and hemorrhage (Fig. 17.14).[60,61] This appearance is quite different from that of the vast majority of leiomyomas.[60,61]

Malignancies Arising From the Endometrial Cavity

Endometrial adenocarcinoma and cervical carcinoma and choriocarcinoma are the most frequent malignant neoplasms to affect the myometrium.[62] Invasion of the myometrium can be evaluated with MRI. When choriocarcinoma involves the myometrium without extending to the endometrium, endometrial curettage may show only secretory changes in a patient with elevated human chorionic gonadotropin. CT may

Figure 17.13 Uterine leiomyosarcoma. This T2-weighted SE image through the pelvis demonstrates a very large heterogeneous mass filling the pelvis. The mass has intermediate-to-high signal intensity, with several foci of very high signal intensity (n) representing necrosis. Note the intact cervix posteriorly (long white arrow). The intermediate high signal intensity of the mass indicates a cellular neoplasm such as a uterine sarcoma. Cellular leiomyomas can have similar intermediate signal intensity but generally do not show the irregular foci of necrosis. Compare the intensity of this mass with that of the mass of fibroids in Figure 17.2

Figure 17.14 Endometrial stromal sarcoma. An axial T2-weighted FSE image shows the normal junctional morphology of the uterus anteriorly with a high signal intensity myometrium and a large posterior cul-de-sac mass. Central very high signal intensity within the mass (n) indicates necrosis. The uterine serosa (white arrows) is stretched over the mass, indicating its myometrial origin. The intermediate signal intensity of much of the mass is not typical for leiomyoma and indicates a more cellular neoplasm such as a cellular leiomyoma or a sarcoma. (From Outwater,[61] with permission.)

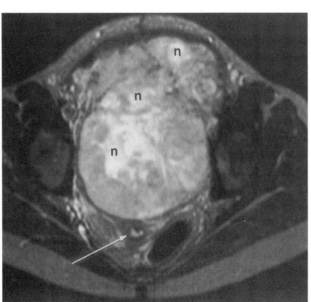

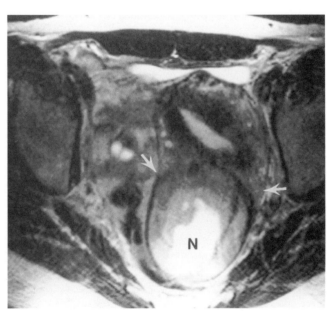

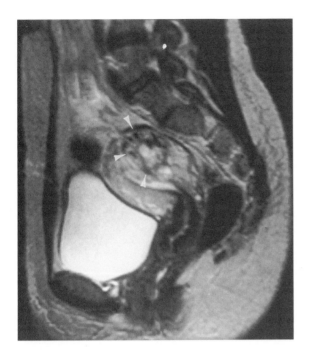

Figure 17.15 Invasive gestational trophoblastic disease in the myometrium. A heterogeneous mass within the myometrium on this T2-weighted FSE image (TR 4,000/TE108) shows punctate signal voids (arrowheads) representing enlarged vessels. Surrounding flow voids and hyperintensity on T1-weighted images are typical features of gestational trophoblastic disease.

show nonspecific uterine enlargement, with or without areas of hypoattenuating tumor within the endometrial cavity or myometrium.[5,63] Good arterial opacification may show the enlarged peritumoral vessels. On MRI, choriocarcinoma and invasive trophoblastic disease have high signal intensity on T2-weighted images.[64] High signal masses disrupt the low-intensity junctional zone when invading the myometrium (Fig. 17.15). On T1-weighted images, foci of hemorrhage are often seen in these tumors.[64] The punctate or rounded signal voids surrounding the tumor, representing flow voids in feeding or draining vessels, are distinctive (Fig. 17.15).[62,64,65]

IMAGING FEATURES OF FISTULAS

Fistulas appear on T2-weighted MRI as high signal intensity tracts surrounded by a low signal intensity from the fibrous wall.[66] Fluid within fistulas are seen as low signal tracts on gadolinium-enhanced images. Fistulas to the uterus commonly produce a fluid collection within the endometrial cavity, which may become infected or may contain air if it connects to the gastrointestinal tract (Fig. 17.16).[66,67] CT has an advantage over MRI in that contrast can sometimes show the site of the tract, but these fistulas do not always fill with contrast material.[68]

Figure 17.16 A rectouterine fistula. (**A**) A T2-weighted SE image through the midline of the uterus shows irregular high signal intensity filling the uterine cavity, representing an abscess (F). The myometrium (short white arrows) is irregular, and the junctional anatomy is obscured. There is a focal break in the myometrium posteriorly (long white arrows), communicating with the rectum, representing a fistulous tract. Note the fluid-filled balloon, in the center of the endometrial cavity, of a drainage catheter. (**B**) This gadolinium-enhanced T1-weighted sagittal image shows the outer myometrium enhancing and the necrotic abscess cavity (F) without enhancement. The enhancing thickened rectal wall posteriorly (curved arrow) communicates with the endometrial cavity. (*Figure continues.*)

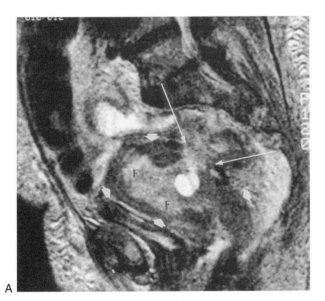

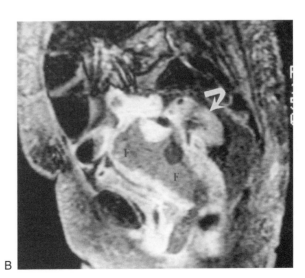

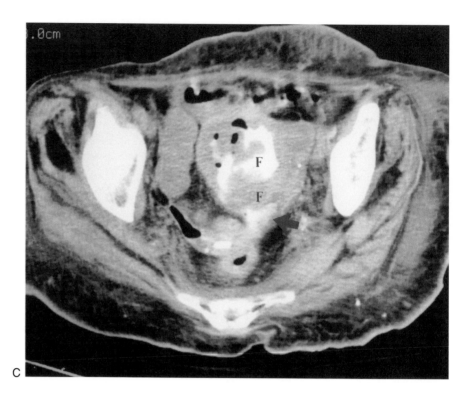

Figure 17.16 (*Continued*). (**C**) CT shows air and contrast within the endometrial cavity (F) as a result of the fistula (arrow). **C**

SUMMARY

CT and MRI can provide additional information about abnormalities that affect the myometrium that may not be readily apparent on transvaginal ultrasonography. Because of its multiplanar capabilities and the zonal anatomy displayed, MRI is the imaging modality of choice for identifying most benign disorders of the myometrium. CT can be useful for complete evaluation of the abdomen and pelvis if malignant disease is suspected.

REFERENCES

1. Shellock FG, Morisoli S, Kanal E. MR procedures and biomedical implants, materials and devices: 1993 update. Radiology 1991;189:587–599
2. Silverberg SG, Kurman RJ. Tumors of the uterine corpus and gestational trophoblastic disease. In: Rosai J, Aovin L, Eds. Atlas of Tumor Pathology (vol. 3). Armed Forces Institute of Pathology, Washington, DC, 1992, pp 113–151
3. Hricak H, Tscholakoff D, Heinrichs L et al. Uterine leiomyomas: correlation of MR, histopathologic findings, and symptoms. Radiology 1986;158:385–391
4. Panageas E, Kier R, McCauley TR, McCarthy S. Submucosal uterine leiomyomas: diagnosis of prolapse into the cervix and vagina based on MR imaging. AJR Am J Roentgenol 1992; 159:555–558
5. Walsh JW. Computed tomography of gynecologic neoplasms. Radiol Clin North Am 1992;30:817–830
6. Casillas J, Joseph RC, Guerra JJ, Jr. CT appearance of leiomyomas. Radiographics 1990;10:999–1007
7. Sawyer RW, Walsh JW. CT in gynecologic pelvic disease. Semin Ultrasound CT MR 1988;9:122–142
8. Tada S, Tsukioka M, Ishii C et al. Computed tomographic features of uterine myoma. J Comput Assist Tomogr 1981;5: 866–869
9. Togashi K, Nishimura K, Nakano Y et al. Cystic pedunculated leiomyomas of the uterus with unusual CT manifestations. J Comput Assist Tomogr 1986;10:642–644
10. Fuller AF, Scully RE. Case records of the Massachusetts General Hospital: Case 23–2985. N Engl J Med 1985;312:1505–1511
11. Mark AS, Hricak H, Heinrichs LW et al. Adenomyosis and leiomyoma: differential diagnosis with MR imaging. Radiology 1987;163:527–529
12. Mittl RL, Jr, Yeh TT, Kressel HY. High-signal-intensity rim surrounding uterine leiomyomas on MR images: pathologic correlation. Radiology 1991;180:81–83
13. Yamashita Y, Torashima M, Takahashi M et al. Hyperintense uterine leiomyoma at T2-weighted MR imaging: differentiation with dynamic enhanced MR imaging and clinical implications. Radiology 1993;189:721–725
14. Okizuka H, Sugimura K, Takemore M et al. MR detection of degenerating uterine leiomyomas. J Comput Assist Tomogr 1993; 17:760–766
15. Kempson RL, Hendrickson MR. Pure mesenchymal neoplasms of the uterine corpus. In: Fox H, Ed. Haines and Taylor Obstetrical and Gynecological Pathology (vol. 1) Churchill Livingstone, London, 1987, pp 411–456
16. Swe TT, Onitsuka H, Kawamoto K et al. Uterine leiomyoma: correlation between signal intensity on magnetic resonance imaging and pathologic characteristics. Radiat Med 1992;10: 235–242
17. Hricak H, Finck S, Honda G, Goranson H. MR imaging in the

evaluation of benign uterine masses: value of gadopentetate dimeglumine-enhanced T1-weighted images. AJR Am J Roentgenol 1992;158:1043–1050

18. Zawin M, McCarthy S, Scoutt L et al. Monitoring therapy with a gonadotropin-releasing hormone analog: utility of MR imaging. Radiology 1990;175:503–506

19. Zawin M, McCarthy S, Scoutt L. High-field MRI and US evaluation of the pelvis in women with leiomyomas. Magn Reson Imaging 1990;8:371–376

20. Dudiak CM, Turner DA, Patel SK et al. Uterine leiomyomas in the infertile patient: preoperative localization with MR imaging versus US and hysterosalpingography. Radiology 1988;167: 627–630

21. Balen F, Hall-Craggs M, Allen C, Lees R. Comparison of MR imaging with US contrast-enhanced hysterography for the delineation of submucosal fibroids. Radiology 1993;189:206

22. Weinreb JC, Brown CE, Lowe TW et al. Pelvic masses in pregnant patients: MR and US imaging. Radiology 1986;159: 717–724

23. Weinreb JC, Barkoff ND, Megibow A, Demopoulos R. The value of MR imaging in distinguishing leiomyomas from other solid pelvic masses when sonography is indeterminate. AJR Am J Roentgenol 1990;154:295–299

24. Curtis M, Hopkins MP, Zarlingo T et al. Magnetic resonance imaging to avoid laparotomy in pregnancy. Obstet Gynecol 1993;82:833–866

25. Kier R, McCarthy SM, Scoutt LM et al. Pelvic masses in pregnancy: MR imaging. Radiology 1990;176:709–713

26. Aubel S, Wozney P, Edwards RP. MRI of female uterine and juxta-uterine masses: clinical application in 25 patients. Magn Reson Imaging 1991;9:485–491

27. Rotter AJ, Lundell CJ. MR of intravenous leiomyomatosis of the uterus extending into the inferior vena cava. J Comput Assist Tomor 1991;15:690–693

28. Kawakami S, Sagoh T, Kumada H et al. Intravenous leiomyomatosis of uterus: MR appearance. J Comput Assist Tomogr 1991;15:686–689

29. Kaszar-Seibert DJ, Gauvin GP, Rogoff PA et al. Intracardiac extension of intravenous leiomyomatosis. Radiology 1988;168: 409–410

30. Shida T, Yoshimura M, Chihara H, Nakamura K. Intravenous leiomyomatosis of the pelvis with re-extension into the heart. Ann Thorac Surg 1986;42:104–106

31. Martin E. Leiomyomatous lung lesions: a proposed classification. AJR Am J Roentgenol 1983;141:269–272

32. Brumback RA, Brown BS, Sobie P et al. Leiomyomatosis peritonealis disseminata. Surgery 1985;97:707–713

33. Goldberg MF, Hurt WG, Frable WJ. Leiomyomatosis peritonealis disseminata: report of a case and review of the literature. Obstet Gynecol 1977;49:46–52

34. Pearce PH. Leiomyomatosis peritonealis disseminata. Am J Obstet Gynecol 1982;144:133–134

35. Renigers SA, Michael AS, Bardawil WA et al. Sonographic findings in leiomyomatosis peritonealis disseminata: a case report and literature view. J Ultrasound Med 1985;4:497–500

36. Dodd GD, Budzik RF. Lipomatous tumors of the pelvis in women: spectrum of imaging findings. AJR Am J Roentgenol 1990;155:317–322

37. Villanueva AJ, Martinez-Noguera A, Perez C et al. Uterine myolipoma: CT and US. Abdom Imaging 1993;18:402–403

38. Jacobs JE, Markowitz SK. CT diagnosis of uterine lipoma. AJR Am J Roentgenol 1988;150:1335–1336

39. Stevens SK, Hricak H, Campos Z. Teratomas versus cystic hemorrhagic adnexal lesions: differentiation with proton-selective fat-saturation MR imaging. Radiology 1993;86:481–488

40. Guinet C, Buy JN, Ghossain MA et al. Fat suppression techniques in MR imaging of mature ovarian teratomas: comparison with CT Eur J Radiol 1993;17:117–121

41. Togashi K, Nishimura K, Itoh K et al. Adenomyosis: diagnosis with MR imaging. Radiology 1988;166:111–114

42. Togashi K, Ozasa H, Konishi I et al. Enlarged uterus: differentiation between adenomyosis and leiomyoma with MR imaging. Radiology 1989;174:531–534

43. Reinhold C, McCarthy S, Bret PM et al. Diffuse adenomyosis comparison of endovaginal US and MR imaging with histopathologic correlation. Radiology 1996;199:151–158

44. Tavassoli FA, Norris HJ. Mesenchymal tumours of the uterus. VII. A clinicopathological study of 60 endometrial stromal nodules. Histopathology 1981;5:1–10

45. Baggish MS. Mesenchymal tumors of the uterus. Clin Obstet Gynecol 1974;17:51–85

46. Weissman A, Talmon R, Jakobi P. Cavernous hemangioma of the uterus in a pregnant woman. Obstet Gynecol 1993;81: 825–827

47. Weigman A, Talmon R, Jakobi P et al. Cavernous hemangioma of the uterus in a pregnant woman. Obstet Gynecol 1993; 81:825–827

48. Hawes DR, Hemann LS, Cornell AE, Yuh WTC. Hemangioma of the uterine cervix: sonographic and MR diagnosis. J Comput Assist Tomogr 1991;15:152–154

49. Salazar OM, Bonfiglio TA, Patten SF. Uterine sarcomas: natural history, treatment, and prognosis. Cancer 1978;42:1152–1160

50. Platz CE, Benda JA. Female genital tract cancer. Cancer 1995;75:270–294

51. Bitterman P, Chun B, Kurman RJ. The significance of epithelial differentiation in mixed mesodermal tumors of the uterus: a clinicopathologic and immunohistochemical study. Am J Surg Pathol 1990;14:317–328

52. Shapeero LG, Hricak H. Mixed müllerian sarcoma of the uterus: MR imaging findings. AJR Am J Roentgenol 1989;153:317–319

53. McLeod AJ, Zornoza J, Shirkhoda A. Leiomyosarcoma: computed tomographic findings. Radiology 1984;152:133–136

54. Takemori M, Nishimura R, Sugimura K. Magnetic resonance imaging of uterine leiomyosarcoma. Arch Gynecol Obstet 1992;251:215–218

55. Rose PG, Piver MS, Tsukada Y, Lau T. Patterns of metastasis in uterine sarcoma: an autopsy study. Cancer 1989;63:935–938

56. Choi BI, Lee WJ, Chi JG, Han JK. CT manifestations of peritoneal leiomyosarcomatosis. AJR Am J Roentgenol 1990; 155:799–801

57. Janus C, White M, Dottino P et al. Uterine leiomyosarcoma: magnetic resonance imaging. Gynecol Oncol 1989;32:79–81

58. Pattani SJ, Kier R, Deal R, Luchansky E. MRI of uterine leiomyosarcoma. Magn Reson Imaging 1995;13:331–333

59. Chang KL, Crabtree GS, Lim-Tan SK et al. Primary uterine endometrial stromal neoplasms: a clinicopathologic study of 117 cases. Am J Surg Pathol 1990;14:415–438

60. Togashi K. Normal Pelvic Structures. MRI of the Female Pelvis. Igaku-Shoin, Tokyo, 1993, pp 29–33

61. Outwater EK. MR imaging of the pelvis. In: Haaga J, Lanzieri C, Sartoris D, Zerhouni E, Eds. Computed Tomography and Mag-

netic Resonance Imaging of the Whole Body (vol. 2). CV Mosby, St. Louis, 1994, pp 1393–1404

62. Szolar DH, Ranner G, Lax S, Preidler K. MRI appearance of gestational choriocarcinoma within the myometrium. Eur J Radiol 1994;18:61–63

63. Sanders C, Rubin E. Malignant gestational trophoblastic disease: CT findings. AJR Am J Roentgenol 1987;148:165–168

64. Hricak H, Demas BE, Braga CA et al. Gestational trophoblastic neoplasm of the uterus: MR assessment. Radiology 1986;161:11–16

65. Mirich DR, Hall JT, Kraft WL et al. Case report: metastatic adnexal trophoblastic neoplasm: contribution of MR imaging. J Comput Assist Tomogr 1988;12:1061–1067

66. Outwater EK, Schiebler ML. Pelvic fistulas: findings on MR images. AJR Am J Roentgenol 1993;160:327–330

67. Hricak H. Postoperative and postradiation changes in the pelvis. Magn Reson Q 1990;6:276–297

68. Goldman SM, Fishman EK, Gatewood OMB et al. CT in the diagnosis of enterovesicle fistulae. AJR Am J Roentgenol 1985;144:1229–1233

69. Mayer DP, Shipilov V. Ultrasonography and magnetic resonance imaging of uterine fibroids. Obstet Gynecol Clin North Am 1995;22:667–725

70. Outwater EK, Schiebler ML. Magnetic resonance imaging of the vary. MRI Clin North Am 1994;2:245–274

18

Hysterosalpingography of the Myometrium

JACQUES S. ABRAMOWICZ

VIVIAN LEWIS

Besides congenital abnormalities, the two conditions that mostly affect the myometrium are adenomyosis and leioymomata.

ADENOMYOSIS

Adenomyosis is a common disease of perimenopausal women. It is due to the presence of endometrial glands and stroma within the myometrium. The origin is the endometrial basal layers, and, thus, adenomyosis does not undergo significant cyclic changes secondary to variations in hormone levels as opposed to endometriosis, although bleeding sometimes occurs. Adenomyosis may be focal and appear to have a pseudocapsule forming a nodule or adenomyoma. It usually is more generally diffuse, in the anterior and more particularly the posterior wall of the uterus. In diffuse adenomyosis, there is often general enlargement of the uterus mostly due to thickening of the posterior wall secondary to local smooth muscle hyperplasia. The major clinical symptoms are menorrhagia and dysmenorrhea, but these are rare and most women are asymptomatic.

The typical appearance on hysterosalpingography (HSG) is due to penetration of contrast into the myometrial muscle layer. This produces delicate, small, diverticula-like projections from the cavity into the uterine wall (Fig. 18.1). Delayed films show a honeycomb appearance. Other methods, however, such as magnetic resonance imaging[1] or ultrasonography[2] are more effective (Fig. 18.2).

LEIOMYOMATA

Leiomyomata are nonencapsulated but well-circumscribed benign tumors of immature smooth muscle cell origin. Various amounts of connective and/or fibrous tissue may be present. They are the most frequent solid pelvic tumour and can be found in 25% to 50% of women. Classification is according to location: submucus, intramural, and subserous. Submucous leiomyomata tend to be symptomatic earlier and more frequently than the others: abnormal (usually heavy) uterine bleeding is the most common complaint. Other symptoms may include pelvic pain, infertility, dysmenorrhea, and complications of pregnancy. Growth of the tumor is often disproportionate to its blood supply. Secondary degeneration can occur. Hyaline degeneration is the most common, but calcification, myxomatous, and red (or carneous) degeneration also occur. Malignant degeneration is rare.

Leiomyomata can often be diagnosed by HSG[3] (Fig. 18.3), but this is generally not the method of choice. Submucous or intramural leiomyomas may disturb the uterine cavity and, thus, sometimes require greater volumes of dye. They will usually appear as filling defects (Fig. 18.4). When the leiomyoma is fundal and bulges within the cavity, the uterus may appear bicornuate or even have a pseudo-T-shape (Fig. 18.5). Polyps can have a similar appearance but do not usually cause alterations in the uterine cavity. Ultrasonography is usually more sensitive in demonstrating leiomyomas. In one study of surgical specimens, ultrasonography had an 87% prediction rate and HSG only 31%.[4] The better prediction rate of ultrasound is not unexpected, as HSG generally shows only the leiomyomas that distort the uterine cavity. This distortion is sometimes an indication for surgery for patients with infertility or recurrent pregnancy loss.

LEIOMYOMA VARIANTS

Several variants can be characterized by histology (bizarre, cellular, epithelioid lipoleiomyoma) or by growth patterns (metastasizing leiomyoma, intravenous leiomyomatosis, and diffuse peritoneal leiomyomatosis). HSG is of no use in differentiating these variants from other "ordinary" leiomyomata.

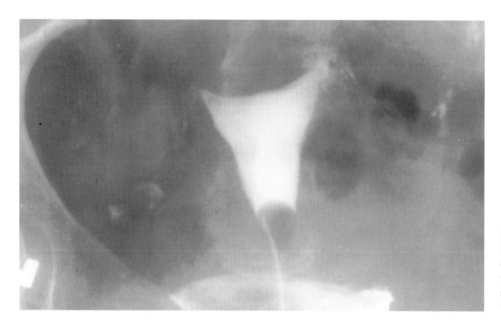

Figure 18.1 This 42-year-old nulligravida had long-standing dysmenorrhea and infertility. Adenomyosis was found histologically. The HSG shows typical projections of dye into the right cornual area.

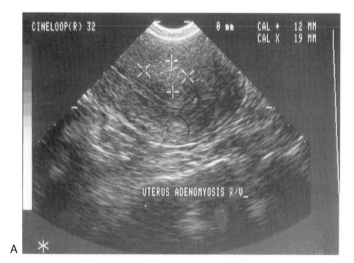

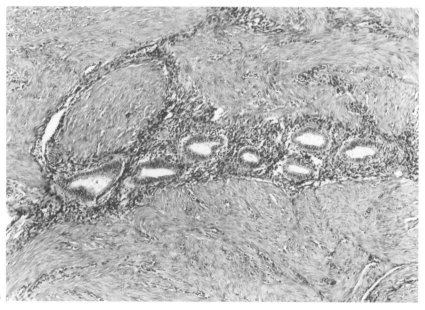

Figure 18.2 (A) Transvaginal ultrasonography shows two distinct hyperechoic areas within the myometrium. This patient underwent hysterectomy because of intractable pelvic pain. (B) Adenomyosis is shown in this slide, taken from the anterior wall of the uterus. There are well-developed islands of endometrial glands within the myometrium. (Courtesy of Dr. Eric Buffong, Jacksonville, NC.)

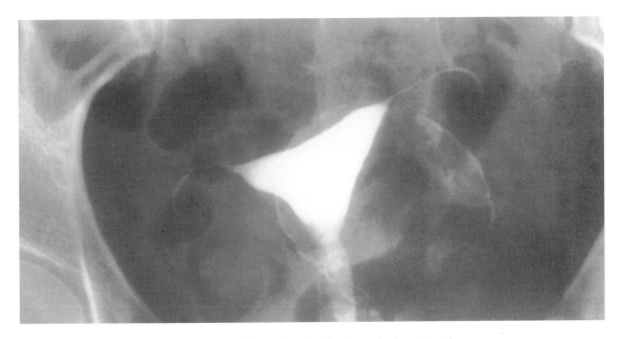

Figure 18.3 This patient was a 34-year-old nulligravida with infertility and pelvic discomfort. The HSG shows a normal uterine cavity and tubes. There is also a large, round calcification behind the uterus due to a calcified, pedunculated myoma.

Histologic Variants

Bizarre (Symplastic or Pleomorphic) Leiomyomas

A particular form of benign degenerative change involves giant cells. These have very large nuclei (single or multiple) but do not have other signs of malignancy. Patients are usually young, and this histology is often found in oral contraceptive users or after pregnancy.[5]

Cellular Leiomyoma

Cellular leiomyoma is a benign smooth tumor. Cellularity is greatly increased in comparison to surrounding tissue. No mitotic activity is present.

Epithelioid Leiomyoma

Smooth muscle cells undergo changes that lead to morphology similar to epithelial, plexiform, clear cell, or atypical histology with somewhat unclear malignant potential. Leiomyoblastoma is another rare variant with large nuclei and strongly eosinophilic cytoplasm.

Lipoleiomyoma

Lipoleiomyoma are characterized by foci of adipose tissue seeded among the smooth muscle fibers.

Variants by Growth Patterns

Benign Metastasizing Leiomyomas

The typical cellular pattern of leiomyomas can be demonstrated in pulmonary tumors or lymph nodes usually after hysterectomy for leiomyomata.

Intravenous Leiomyomatosis

Smooth muscle tissue grows as worm-like masses into the broad ligament vascular spaces or into veins of the pelvis and

Figure 18.4 A 39-year-old woman with infertility and prolonged, heavy menstrual flow. The uterine cavity shows a large filling defect. After hysteroscopic resection of her myoma, the patient had a term pregnancy.

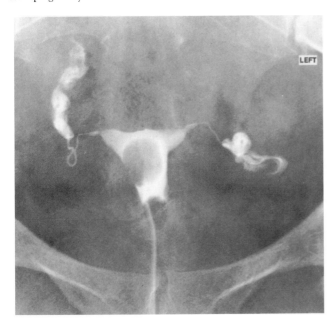

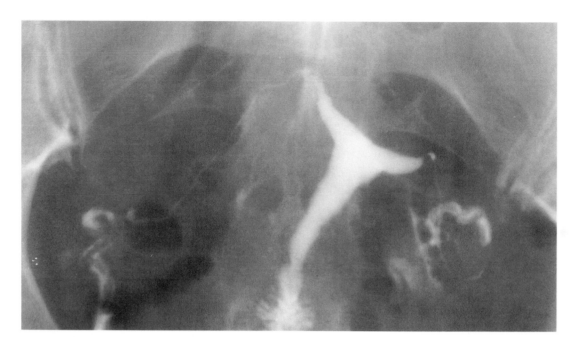

Figure 18.5 This 41-year-old woman had infertility and menorrhagia. HSG showed a pseudo-T-configuration of the uterine cavity due to intramural myomas.

has been known to reach the vena cava or even the right atrium. No atypia is present.

Disseminated Peritoneal Leiomyomatosis

Multiple small myomas are seeded over the surface of the lower abdomen and/or pelvis. This is usually, but not always, associated with pregnancy and regresses postpartum.

VASCULAR TUMORS

Vascular tumors are rare, usually congenital, but do not cause clinical disturbances until 40 to 60 years, when they produce abnormal menstrual patterns. They comprise hemangiomata (which, like leiomyomas, can be subserous, pedunculated or intramural) and the even rarer lymphangiomata.

ADENOMATOID TUMORS

Usually small and asymptomatic, adenomatoid tumors are rare and mostly found by chance, near the serosal surface. They lack atypia, mitotic activity, and myometrial invasion.

MALIGNANT CONDITIONS

Sarcomas are rare, comprising 5% or less of uterine malignancies. They consist of leiomyosarcoma (and epithelioid and

myxoid variants), endometrial stromal tumors, and heterologous sarcomas and mixed epithelial–nonepithelial tumors. No characteristic HSG patterns have been described.

POSTOPERATIVE APPEARANCE

With the increase in the number of infertility patients, the cost-containment issues, and the desire to preserve fertility, conservative or minimally invasive surgery for leiomyoma will become more common. There is limited experience on the use of HSG before and after myomectomy.[6,7] Scarring can occur after removal of fibroids (Fig. 18.6). Lev-Toaff et al.[7] describe their findings on HSG after myomectomy in 32 patients. They consisted of normalization of the uterine cavity shape and/or dimensions, including resolution of cavity asymmetry, particularly in the cornual region, patency of previously obstructed fallopian tubes, and disappearance of filling defects. In 4 of 32 patients, distortion of the uterine cavity persisted after surgery: filling defects as signs of residual leiomyomata or postoperative synechiae. HSG can, therefore, be very useful as a preoperative assessment to evaluate cavity distortion as well as tubal distortion or compression and to assist in the localization of leiomyomata that might, otherwise, be missed.[8]

Other causes of uterine scarring include caesarean section and perforation. Scar from a previous cesarean section may appear on HSG as a jagged defect in the normally smooth lower segment.[9] Depending on the healing process after surgery, the defect may be small or very large and appear as an outpouching. Uterine perforation secondary to a dilatation

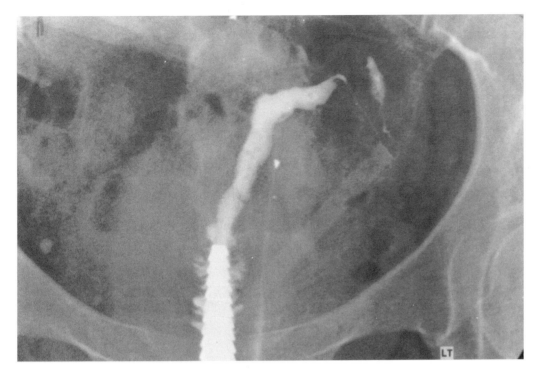

Figure 18.6 HSG after removal of multiple myomas from the patient in Fig. 18.4. Resection of the fundal myoma resulted in scarring of the right cornual portion of the uterus.

and curettage, even if followed by laparotomy for repair, will not usually leave a scar large enough to be recognizable by HSG.

Another rare pathology is diverticulum of the uterus. This may be secondary to a surgical procedure or due to a congenital weakness of the uterine cavity. Diagnosis is by HSG, which demonstrates a typical bulging of the uterine cavity.[10]

REFERENCES

1. Brosens JJ, DeSouza NM, Barker FG et al. Endovaginal ultrasonography in the diagnosis of adenomyosis uteri: identifying the predictive characteristics. Br J Obstet Gynaecol 1995;102:471–474

2. Togashi K, Ozasa H, Konishi I et al. Enlarged uterus: differentiation between adenomyosis and leiomyomas with MR imaging. Radiology 1989;171:531–534

3. Karasick S, Lev-Toaff AS, Toaff ME. Imaging of uterine leiomyomas. AJR Am J Roentgenol 1992;158:799–805

4. Dudiak C, Turner DA, Patel SK et al. Uterine leiomyomas in the infertile patient: preoperative localization with MR imaging versus US and hysterosalpingography. Radiology 1988; 167:627–630

5. Evans HL, Chawla SP, Simpson C, Finn KP. Smooth muscle neoplasms of the uterus other than ordinary leiomyoma. A study of 46 cases, with emphasis on diagnostic criteria and prognostic factors. Cancer 1988;62:2239–2247

6. Weinstein D, Aviad Y, Polishuk AZ. Hysterography before and after myomectomy. AJR Am J Roentgenol 1977;129:899–902

7. Lev-Toaff AS, Karasick S, Toaff ME. Hysterosalpingography before and after myomectomy: clinical value and imaging findings. AJR Am J Roentgenol 1993;160:803–807

8. Ramon Garcia C, Pfeifer SM. Myomectomy. In: Nichols DH, Ed. Gynecology and Obstetric Surgery. CV Mosby, St. Louis, 1993, pp 606–623

9. Schwimmer M, Heiken JP, McClennan BL, Friedrich ER. Postoperative hysterosalpingrogram: radiographic–surgical correlation. Radiology 1985;157:313–317

10. Buell JI, Perkins MB. Diverticulum of the uterus. Am J Obst Gynecol 1962;84:244–243

19

Ultrasonography and Sonosalpingography of the Fallopian Tube

GAUTAM N. ALLAHBADIA

SADHANA K. DESAI

The earliest accurate description of the fallopian tube was provided by Gabriellus Fallopius in his *Observationes Anatomicae* in 1561:

This seminal duct originates from the cornua uteri, it is thin, very narrow, of white colour, and looks like a nerve. After a short distance, it begins to broaden and to coil like a tendril, winding its folds almost up to the end. There, having become very broad, it shows an extremitas of the nature of skin and colour of flesh, the utmost end being very ragged and crushed like the fringe of worn out clothes. Further, it has a great hole which is held closed by the fimbriae which lap over each other. However, if they spread out and dilate, they create a kind of opening which looks like a flaring bell of a brazen tube. Because the course of the seminal duct, from its origin up to its end, resembles the shape of this classical instrument—anyhow, whether the curves are existing or not, I named it the tuba uteri.

This century has marked the development of diagnostic procedures for tubal pathology with the introduction of hysterosalpingography (HSG), ultrasonography, magnetic resonance imaging, radionuclide HSG, and laparoscopy.

Tubal disease causes infertility in one of three infertile couples. The most common etiology of tubal occlusion is previous salpingitis, which may be clinical or subclinical. Inflammation may completely resolve, or it may damage the mucosa of the endosalpinx, or cause agglutination of the fimbria, with distal or proximal obstruction.[1] HSG is usually the first tool used to assess tubal disease, as it is simple and cost-effective. Diagnostic laparoscopy also plays a role, and both procedures complement one another, as each provides information about one or more segments of the tube.

Transvaginal sonography can be used to demonstrate dilated fallopian tubes and establish their relationship to the ovary. Visualization of normal nondistended tubes remains a challenge, and only rarely can they be recognized. The proximal end of the tube can sometimes be followed for about 1 to 2 cm after it leaves the cornua.

DEVELOPMENTAL ANOMALIES

Structural congenital anomalies of the fallopian tube are rare. Tubes associated with uterine abnormalities such as a rudimentary horn or bicornuate uterus may be hypoplastic or partially atretic.[2,3] Bilateral absence of the ampullary muscularis has been reported.[4] Infertility patients who were exposed in utero to diethylstilbestrol may have shortened, sacculated, and convoluted fallopian tubes with the fimbria being described as constricted and the os as pinpoint.[5] Apparent congenital absence of a segment of the tube, tubal duplication, and accessory tubes have been reported.[6]

BENIGN CONDITIONS

Salpingitis Isthmica Nodosa

Salpingitis isthmica nodosa (SIN) results from the formation of diverticula from the main lumen of the tube, which can become so complex that they replace the normal anatomy. They consist of hard, distended, rosary-like lesions in the isthmus of the fallopian tubes. The etiology of SIN is presumably infective. It cannot be diagnosed on ultrasound and requires HSG.

Adenomatoid Tumors

Benign adenomatoid tumors are the most common benign tumor They are usually small, circumscribed tumors (1 to 2 cm in diameter) and confined to the smooth muscle wall of the tube.

Lipoma

Lipomas have manifested themselves as adnexal masses,[7] and there is a report of an angiomyolipoma of the fallopian tube.[8] An ultrasound diagnosis is usually impossible, and clinicians take refuge in other diagnostic modalities. A case of lipoma of the mesosalpinx, which presented as an adnexal mass, was

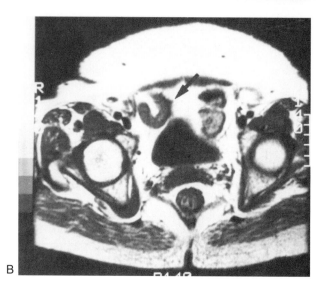

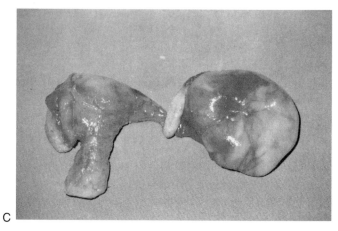

Figure 19.1 Lipoma of the mesosalpinx. (**A**) Transabdominal ultrasound showing a hypoechoic adnexal mass (arrow). There are no characteristic features. (**B**) Computed tomography scan showing the sausage-shaped solid adnexal mass (arrow). (**C**) Hysterectomy specimen showing the mesosalpingeal lipoma.

suspected on computed tomography scan and confirmed on histopathology (Fig. 19.1).

MALIGNANT CONDITIONS

Fallopian Tube Carcinoma

Adenocarcinoma is the most common primary malignancy of the fallopian tube and accounts for 0.3% of all gynecologic cancers.[9-12] The fallopian tubes are often involved secondarily from lesions arising in adjacent sites such as ovaries, endometrium, gastrointestinal tract, as well as from the breast.

Ultrasound appearances of fallopian tube carcinoma can be complex, similar to that of a pyosalpinx or a fluid-filled tube with adjacent solid components that are not part of the ovary, cervix, or uterus. There may also be "sausage-like" cystic masses with papillary projections similar to hydrops tubae profluens.[13] Color Doppler imaging may show a highly vascular adnexal mass and low resistance flow on pulsed Doppler suggesting malignancy.

INFLAMMATORY CONDITIONS

Pelvic inflammatory disease (PID) is an acute or chronic process caused by ascending infection. It is commonly sexually transmitted but can also occur by direct spread from pelvic surgery, diverticulitis, ruptured appendiceal abscess, or post-partum sepsis, and it can cause permanent damage to the upper reproductive tract.

Chlamydia trachomatis has evolved as the most serious and common pathogen of PID and results in extensive and irreversible tubal damage that develops slowly over a long time. A complicated immunologic process is thought to be responsible for the scar tissue formation in patients affected by this bacterium.[14] The degree of tubal damage varies, and obstructive consequences are generally accepted to be the principal cause of infertility.[15] The extent of peritubal and periovarian adhesions is the primary determinant of tubal blockage, and intratubal pathology is of secondary importance. The diagnosis of PID is often based on laparoscopy.[16]

The three stages of PID are hyperemia, frank salpingitis, and tubo-ovarian abscess.[17]

Hysterosalpingo-contrast sonography (HyCoSy) can be useful in the treatment of patients with PID. Doxycycline solution is used instead of contrast material to avoid the possibility of exacerbating the infectious process.

In chlamydial salpingitis, low viscous material may accumulate near the fimbriated ends. Some of this tubal exudate can be safely and successfully removed with antibiotic lavage. A 2-mm balloon catheter is inserted into the uterine cavity and inflated. Doxycyline solution is then instilled, and the flow through the tubes is monitored with transvaginal color Doppler. Clinical symptoms resolve more quickly, and the distended tube regains its normal appearance and shrinks back to its original caliber.[18]

Acute PID

Acute PID is usually not evident on ultrasound. Intraluminal fluid will accumulate later after the tube becomes blocked. Hyperemia, swelling, tortuosity, and purulent exudate from the lumen and the serosal surfaces of the tubes are the main characteristics of acute PID. Blood vessels in the tubal wall can be identified by color Doppler in the early phase of the disease. The ovaries are enlarged and globular, and they may contain multiple cysts (infected follicles) and have indistinct margins.[19]

Chronic PID

Hydrosalpinx, Pyosalpinx

The obstruction of the fimbriated end results in fluid collection in the tube, producing a hydrosalpinx. This appears as a tubular anechoic structure with thickened mucosal folds and nodular projections into the lumen on ultrasound. The absence of blood flow on color Doppler helps differentiate the hydrosalpinx from a large blood vessel. The appearance of internal echoes in the distended lumen with the absence of blood flow suggests pyosalpinx. On transverse sections, the dilated tube appears as a cystic structure with internal mural indentations.

Damage from salpingitis to the distal portions of the fallopian tubes include hydrosalpinx, pyosalpinx, partial fimbrial obstruction without hydrosalpinx formation, and interstitial salpingitis. Involvement of proximal segments of the tube may result in isthmic and cornual stenosis or blockage. Finally, the whole tube may become involved, resulting in proximally blocked tubes with distal hydrosalpinges.

Two classically recognized appearances of hydrosalpinx are hydrosalpinx simplex and hydrosalpinx follicularis. In hydrosalpinx simplex, the tube is dilated, the lumen is single, and there are no adhesions between the mucosal folds. Ultrasound will show a tubular anechoic structure (Fig. 19.2). In hydrosalpinx follicularis, the tubal lumen is divided transversely into locules by mucosal folds that have agglutinated together, forming compartments or pseudoglandular spaces.

At operation, a hydrosalpinx is seen to have either thin or thick walls. In thin-walled hydrosalpinx, the fallopian tube is grossly distended by copious straw-colored fluid, which makes it appear translucent. In thick-walled hydrosalpinx, the wall is fibrous, and the lumen is smaller and contains little fluid. In both types, the terminal part of the tube is completely

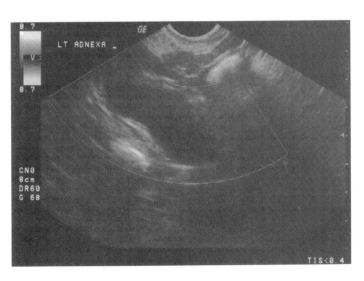

Figure 19.2 Hydrosalpinx simplex. A convoluted tubular liquid filled mass is seen in the left adnexa.

blocked, and the fimbriae are obscured. The distinction between thin-walled and thick-walled hydrosalpinx is important; not only do their morphologic and histologic features differ, but also the pregnancy rate after tubal microsurgery is much lower for thick-walled than for thin-walled hydrosalpinx.[20]

Tubo-ovarian Abscess

Tubo-ovarian abscess is the most severe form of an acute infection. The continuous spillage of purulent material from the tube reaches the neighboring structures (ovary, bowel, and omentum). The ultrasound appearance will show a complex dense hypoechoic mass with internal septa. Acoustic enhancement and absence of blood flow will confirm the presence of fluid. The outer margins of the abscess are irregular and indistinct, and identification of tube and ovary may be difficult.

Ultrasound findings suggestive of PID include thickened, fluid-filled tubes alone or a thickened tube adjacent to an ovary forming a tubo-ovarian abscess.[21] The tube usually "embraces" the ovary, which loses its typical structure of stroma and follicles. Some of the ovarian follicles may still be recognized, thus enabling localization of the "ovarian" part of the tubo-ovarian abscess. The tube may be dilated and partially filled with fluid, as shown by fluid-debris levels. The cul-de-sac may contain echogenic pus. As the abscess develops, there is loss of anatomic landmarks (Fig. 19.3).

Figure 19.3 Tubo-ovarian abscess. The patient was 32 years old and had been on an in vitro fertilization program because of tubal disease and endometriosis. She became febrile after an ovum pickup and developed lower abdominal pain. She ran a protracted course, despite the exhibition of antibiotics, and this scan was taken 42 days after ovum pick up. The ovary and tube could not be distinguished from this complex mass (arrows), which is mostly solid. After 6 months, the mass became more complex as omentum and bowel became agglutinated. This caused so much chronic pain that a salpingoopherectomy was performed. (Courtesy of Dr. Warwick Birrell, Sydney, Australia.)

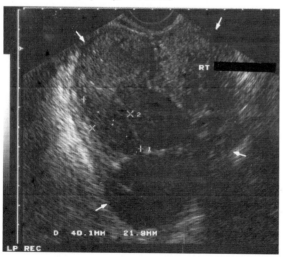

Actinomycosis

Actinomycotic infection of the tube is uncommon and is usually a complication of an intrauterine contraceptive device (IUCD).[22,23] Almost 85% of cases have occurred in women who have had an IUCD in place for more than 3 years,[24] the infection being more common with use of plastic rather than copper IUCDs.[25]

Actinomycosis can result in the formation of destructive,[26] often multiple, abscesses involving the ovary and fallopian tube. In one study, almost 90% of patients with actinomyces were found to have a tubo-ovarian abscess.[27] The mass may appear to be a dilated tube or to be more inflammatory, being bound down to pelvic structures with adhesions or fistula formation. Pus is present in the shaggy-walled cavities within the tube.[28]

Tuberculosis

Genital tuberculosis varies with the population studied and their geographic location. It is uncommon in developed countries. The fallopian tubes are the most common site of initial infection in genital tuberculosis, and infection of the endometrium, myometrium, cervix, and vagina is probably due to spread from a focus in the tubes. The disease rarely produces symptoms in the early stages and is usually detected during the investigation of infertility, the first signs being seen on HSG (Figs. 19.4 and 19.5)

Tuberculosis occurs most often in the ampulla of the tube. Infection of the intramural and isthmic segments is uncommon. Sonographic appearances of tuberculosis may show a collection of infected fluid in the pouch of Douglas. The fluid will have diffuse low-level echogenicity, and floating particulate matter will be evident within the fluid if the gain is increased.

At laparotomy, the tube feels rigid on palpation and the ampulla may be dilated, but the fimbriae usually appear normal and the ostium is open. Adhesions between the tube and ovary may develop and either close the fimbrial end and cause complete distal occlusion or cause constriction of the proximal end of the dilated ampulla, resulting in a characteristic "tobacco pouch" appearance at HSG.[29] The general appearance is similar to that of nontuberculous chronic salpingitis, except in those rare cases that are secondary to peritoneal tuberculosis when there are foci on the serosal surface. The infection is usually limited to the mucosa, but caseating granulomata may extend into the tubal wall, resulting in focal calcification. In tuberculous pyosalpinx, there is a necrotic, cheesy exudate in the lumen of the tube.

ISCHEMIA AND ISCHEMIC NECROSIS

Adnexal Torsion

Torsion is the most common anatomic displacement of the tube and is often associated with ovarian cysts or tumor.[30,31] Tubal enlargement secondary to hydrosalpinx or pyosalpinx[31] or previous sterilization[32] are additional causes, but torsion may occur in the absence of adnexal disease.

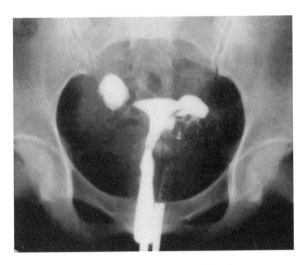

Figure 19.4 HSG showing bilateral hydrosalpinges in a patient with proven genital tuberculosis.

Typically, the patient is of reproductive age with 12% to 18% of adnexal torsion occurring during pregnancy[33] and becoming a gynecologic emergency. Venous outflow is compromised early, and the resulting congestion may lead to arterial compression. The adnexa are often swollen and edematous, with hemorrhagic infarction and gangrene. Ultrasonography will show an absence of color Doppler signals on the ipsilateral side. Unilateral absence of color flow indicates complete adnexal torsion. If an early diagnosis can be made, infarction can be prevented by simply unwinding the adnexa without resection.[34] Isolated torsion of the fallopian tube is a rare condition.[35]

Torsion of Accessory Fallopian Tube

Torsion of an accessory tube is rare. The ultrasound findings of two cases of fallopian tube duplication in premenarchal girls, both of whom had undergone torsion, were reported by Thonell et al.[36] Complex cystic structures were found at surgery, and pathologic examination confirmed the torsion of accessory fallopian tubes.

SONOGRAPHIC DIAGNOSIS OF TUBAL OCCLUSION

Sonosalpingography

Sonosalpingography using color Doppler flow mapping[37] is an accurate and safe method of evaluating tubal patency. There is no exposure to ionizing radiation or to potentially allergic iodinated contrast agents.[38]

The Doppler effect uses ultrasound to detect the flow of sterile saline as it passes transcervically through the uterine cavity into the fallopian tubes and subsequently spills in the pouch of Douglas. Color seen passing through the fallopian tubes and into the cul-de-sac is defined as patent; no color

flow is defined as occlusion. Obstruction can be observed at any point along the course of the tube.[39]

Ultrasound Contrast Agents

The evaluation of tubal patency by direct imaging of the tubal passage using a contrast agent was reported in 1988 and 1989 by Deichert et al.[40,41] Several ultrasonographic contrast agents have been developed to enhance imaging of the anatomic structures and allow better definition. These include Albunex (human albumin encapsulated in microbubbles), Echovist (stabilizing microbubbles with microparticles of physiologic saccharide galactose), and SH U 454 (chemically identical to Echovist with a minor galenic modification of the microparticles).[42]

Hysterosalpingo-Contrast Sonography

It is possible to examine both the uterine cavity and the fallopian tubes with HyCoSy. An echogenic contrast for ultrasound is administered via a transcervical balloon catheter (Fig. 19.6). The contrast is injected slowly (1 to 2 ml) every 5–10 seconds. The flow of multiple fractions of the contrast through each fallopian tube is seen in real-time using a transvaginal probe with either two dimensional or color Doppler. A tube is regarded as patent if intratubal flow can be seen for at least 5 to 10 seconds.

The supplementary use of Doppler techniques (duplex, color Doppler, pulsed Doppler) provides additional information in cases of suspected tubal occlusion and assists with diagnostic accuracy. The demonstration of a pulsed waveform from the tube is diagnostic of tubal patency.

SUMMARY

Ultrasonography, whether abdominal or transvaginal, cannot demonstrate the normal fallopian tubes. Normal fallopian tubes can only be identified if they contain a contrast mate-

Figure 19.5 HSG in a patient with genital tuberculosis showing intrauterine adhesions with fixed beaded tubes.

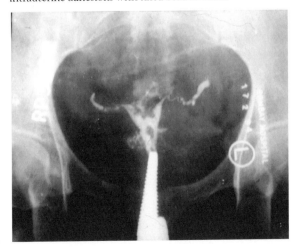

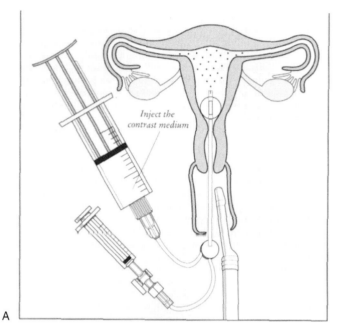

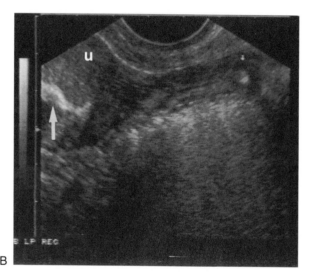

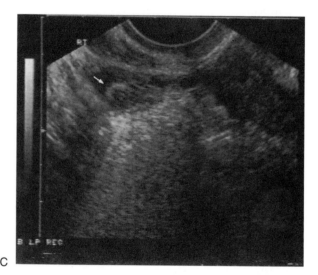

Figure 19.6 HyCoSy. **(A)** The transcervical balloon catheter is positioned inside the uterine cavity. The balloon is then inflated to fix the catheter in position. The covered transvaginal ultrasound probe is inserted into the vagina and, the echo-contrast medium (1 to 2 ml) is slowly injected into the uterus via the catheter. (From Schering Health Care Ltd, West Sussex, UK, with permission.) **(B)** This transvaginal scan in the coronal plane through the left uterine angle (u) shows contrast medium (large arrow) in the uterine cavity and in the midportion of the visible fallopian tube (small arrow) The ampulla is not on the plane of view. **(C)** On the right side, the contrast medium (arrow) can be seen curving down into the ampullary portion of the tube. The procedure is easier to demonstrate on real-time, as the flow is observed for only 5 to 10 seconds.

rial. The tubes become distended and fluid filled as part of an infectious process, forming a hydrosalpinx or pyosalpinx, and then they can also be seen.

ACKNOWLEDGMENTS

The principal author thanks Master Medical Equipment Pvt. Ltd., Delhi and Bombay (Sony Thermal Printer, Japan), and Kody Elcot Ltd. (Fukuda Denshii FF Sonic 4500, Japan) for their support for this project.

REFERENCES

1. Fortier KJ, Haney AF. The pathologic spectrum of uterotubal junction obstruction. Obstet Gynecol 1985;65:93–99

2. Farber M, Mitchell GW, Jr. Bicornuate uterus and partial atresia of the fallopian tube. Am J Obstet Gynecol 1979;134:881–884

3. Knab DR, Blanco LJ. Mullerian duct agenesis with unilateral functioning segment of the rudimentary uterine horn. Am J Obstet Gyneol 1978;132:222–224

4. Tulusan AH. Complete absence of the muscular layer of the ampullary part of the fallopian tubes. Arch Gynecol 1984;234:279

5. De Cherney AH, Cholst I, Naftolin F. Structure and function of the fallopian tubes following exposure to diethylstilbestrol (DES) during gestation. Fertil Steril 1981;36:741–745

6. Silverman AY, Greenberg EI. Absence of segment of the proximal portion of a fallopian tube. Obstet Gynecol 1983;62:90S–91S

7. Winer-Muram HT, Muram D. Retroperitoneal lipoma manifested as an adnexal mass. J Tenn Med Assoc 1988;81:225–226

8. Katz DA, Thom D, Bogard P, Dermer MS. Angiomyolipoma of the fallopian tube. Am J Obstet Gynecol 1984;148:341–343

9. Eddy GL, Copeland LJ, Gershenson DM et al. Fallopian tube carcinoma. Obstet Gynecol 1984;64:546

10. Hu CY, Taymor ML, Hertig AT. Primary carcinoma of the fallopian tube. Am J Obstet Gynecol 1950;50:58

11. Roberts JA, Lifshitz S. Primary adenocarcinoma of the fallopian tube. Gynecol Oncol 1982;13:301

12. Sieck UV. Primary adenocarcinoma of the fallopian tube. Aust NZ J Obstet Gynecol 1978;18:147

13. Ajjimakorn S, Bhamarapravati Y, Israngura N. Ultrasound appearance of fallopian tube carcinoma. J Clin Ultrasound 1988;16:516–518

14. Morrison RP et al. Immunology of Chlamydia trachomatis infection: immunoprotective and immunopathogenic responses. Adv Host Defense Mech 1992;8:57–84

15. Woodruff JD, Pauerstein CJ, Eds. The Fallopian Tube: Structure, Function, Pathology and Management. Williams & Wilkins, Baltimore, 1969, pp 342–346

16. Jacobsen L, Westrom L. Objectivised diagnosis of acute PID. Am J Obstet Gynecol 1969;105:1088–1098

17. Birnholz JC. Endometriosis and inflammatory disease. Semin Ultrasound 1983;4:184.

18. Toth M, Chervenak FA. Clinical and ultrasound dimensions of infections of the ovary and Fallopian tube. In: Kurjak A, Ed. Ultrasound and the Ovary. Parthenon Publishing, London, 1994, p 175

19. Toth M, Chervenak FA. Transvaginal color Doppler ultrasound in pelvic inflammatory disease. In Bourne TH, Jauniaux E, Jurkovic D, Eds. Transvaginal Colour Doppler. Berlin, Springer-Verlag, 1995, p 151

20. Brosens IA, Gordon AG. The abnormal Fallopian tube. In: Tubal Infertility Brosen IA, Gordon AG, eds. JB Lippincott, Philadelphia, 1989, pp 26–29

21. Timor-Tritsch IE, Rottem S, Lewit N. The fallopian tubes. In Timor-Tritsch IE, Rottem S, Eds. Transvaginal Sonography (2nd ed.). Elsevier Science Publishing, New York, 1991, p 139

22. Dische FE, Burt JM, Davison NJH, Puntambekar S. Tuboovarian actinomycosis associated with intrauterine contraceptive devices. J Obstet Gynecol Br Commonw 1974;81:724–729

23. Surur F. Actinomycosis of the female genital tract. NY State J Med 1974;74:408–411

24. Schmidt WA. IUD's, inflammation, and infection: assessment after 2 decades of use. Hum Pathol 1982;13:878–881

25. Keebler C, Chatwani A, Schwartz R. Actinomycosis infection associated with intrauterine contraceptive devices. Am J Obstet Gynecol 1983;145:596

26. Chapin DS, Sullinger JC. A 43 year old woman with left buttock pain and a presacral mass. N Engl J Med 1990;323:183

27. Burkman R, Schlesselman S, McCaffret L et al. The relationship of genital tract actinomycetes and the development of pelvic inflammatory disease. Am J Obstet Gynecol 1982;143:585–589

28. Wheeler JE. Disease of the fallopian tube. In: Kurman RJ, Ed. Blaustein's Pathology of the Female Genital Tract (4th ed.). Springer-Verlag, New York, 1994, p 539

29. Elkin M. Urogenital tuberculosis. In: Pollack HM, Ed. Clinical Urography. WB Saunders, Philadelphia, 1990, pp 985–986

30. Demopoulos RI, Bigelow B, Vasa U. Infarcted uterine adnexa: associated pathology. NY State J Med 1978;78:2027–2029

31. Lee RA, Welch JS. Torsion of the uterine adnexa. Am J Obstet Gynecol 1967;97:974–977

32. Bernardus RE, Van der Slikke JW, Roex AJM et al. Torsion of the fallopian tube: Some considerations on its aetiology. Obstet Gynecol 1984;64:675

33. Isager-Sally L, Weber T. Torsion of the fallopian tube during pregnancy. Acta Obstet Gynecol Scand 1985;64:349–351

34. Ben-Rafael Z, Bider D, Mashiach S. Unwinding of ischaemic haemorrhagic adnexum via laparoscopy. Fertil Steril 1990;53:569–571

35. Kurzbart E, Mares AJ, Cohen Z et al. Isolated torsion of the fallopian tube in premenarcheal girls. J Pediatr Surg 1994;29:1384–1385

36. Thonell SH, Kam A, Resnick G. Torsion of accessory fallopian tube: ultrasound findings in two premenarchal girls. Australas Radiol 1993;37:393–395

37. Peters AJ, Coulam CB. Hysterosalpingography using colour Doppler sonography. Am J Obstet Gynecol 1991;164:1530–1534

38. Yarali H, Gurgan T, Erden A, Kisnisci HA. Colour Doppler hysterosalpingosonography: a simple and potentially useful method to evaluate fallopian tubal patency. Hum Reprod 1994;9:64–66

39. Peters AJ, Stern JJ, Coulam CB. Hysterosalpingography using color Doppler sonography. J Ultrasound Med 1991;10:537–558

40. Deichert U, van de Sandt M, Lauth G, Daume E. Transvaginal contrast hysterosonography. A new diagnostic procedure for the differentiation of intrauterine and myometrial findings. Geburtshilfe Frauenheilkd 1988;48:835–844

41. Deichert U, Schlief R, Van de Sandt M, Juhnke I. Transvaginal hysterosalpingo-contrast-sonography (HyCoSy) compared with conventional tubal diagnostics. Hum Reprod 1989;4:418–424

42. Stern JJ, Coulam CB. Color Doppler hysterosalpingography. In: Jaffe R, Pierson RA, Abramowicz JS, Eds. Imaging in Infertility and Reproductive Endocrinology. JB Lipincott, Philadelphia, 1994, p 339

Computed Tomography and Magnetic Resonance Imaging of the Fallopian Tube

SATOSHI KAWAKAMI

The fallopian tubes are predisposed to infection when the pelvis is affected by inflammatory disease, and they are usually involved when traumatic events overtake the ovaries. Malignant change of the tubes is rare, but when it does occur, it usually involves the ovaries. Imaging of the tubes, then, is an integral part of imaging the entire female pelvis. Ultrasound is the method of choice, but computed tomography (CT) and magnetic resonance imaging (MRI) can be helpful, especially in difficult cases.

DEVELOPMENTAL ANOMALIES

Fusion Defects

Müllerian duct anomalies of the fallopian tube may be hypoplastic, partially atretic, or distended with blood. Menstrual blood accumulates in the noncommunicating horn or vagina and forms a hematometra or hematocolpos.[1–6] Sometimes the blood collects in the fallopian tube, forming a hematosalpinx, appearing on CT or MRI as a cystic mass.[1,2,4–6] The hematosalpinx is not highly attenuating like fresh blood but has low attenuation on noncontrast CT.[5] On MRI, the hematosalpinx is often hyperintense on T1-weighted images, as is a hematocolpos in the chronic stage (Fig. 20.1). In addition to pelvic CT or MRI, upper abdominal examination may be useful because müllerian duct anomalies are often associated with renal anomalies. The most common anomaly is renal agenesis ipsilateral to the noncommunicating uterine horn, and the second most common is an ipsilateral pelvic kidney.[5]

INFLAMMATORY CONDITIONS

Acute Salpingitis

Acute salpingitis is more common in users of intrauterine contraceptive devices (IUCDs) and in women with multiple sexual partners.[7] CT and MRI changes in the acute stage may be subtle. Pelvic peritonitis is suggested by inflammatory exudate, which has a signal intensity equal to or greater than that of simple liquid on both T1- and T2-weighted images, along the uterine or adnexal surfaces, and in the pouch of Douglas.[8,9] Changes in the fat planes, the indistinct borders of pelvic organs, and accentuated fascial lines can also be seen[8] (Fig. 20.2).

The CT of a tubo-ovarian abscess shows a thick-walled, liquid, dense, tubular or spheric mass[10,11] (Fig. 20.3A). Internal septa are common[10] (Figs. 20.3 and 20.4). On MRI, the liquid content commonly has a signal intensity identical to or slightly greater than that of simple liquid on T1- and T2-weighted images (Figs. 20.3 and 20.4), but signal characteristics similar to that of blood may be seen. The inner layer of the cyst wall occasionally is faintly hyperintense on T1-weighted images and hypointense on T2-weighted images, suggesting blood[8] (Fig. 20.3B & C).

Differentiation between inflammatory masses and adnexal neoplasms is occasionally difficult if the mass enhances due to granulation (Fig. 20.3E). Although gas is the most specific sign of abscess, it is unusual in tubo-ovarian abscess.[10] Compared with neoplasms, inflammatory masses have an indistinct border because of the inflammatory extension to the surrounding fat and the loss of the fat planes between the mass and the uterus.[11] Posterior extension may cause thickening of the uterosacral ligaments and effacement of presacral and perirectal fat, resulting in increased density on CT and decreased or heterogeneous intensity on T1-weighted images of MRI. Luminal narrowing of bowel loops, infiltration of perirectal fat, and indistinct borders between the pelvic mass and the bowel suggest rectosigmoid involvement.[10] The pelvic ureters, which form the posterior boundary of the ovarian fossa, may be compressed, and unilateral hydronephrosis may be seen on CT or MRI. Inflammatory para-aortic lymphadenopathy can occur near the level of the renal hila in tubo-ovarian abscess; however, lymphadenopathy does not necessarily suggest a malignancy.[10]

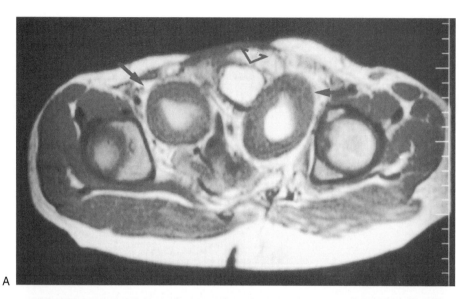

A

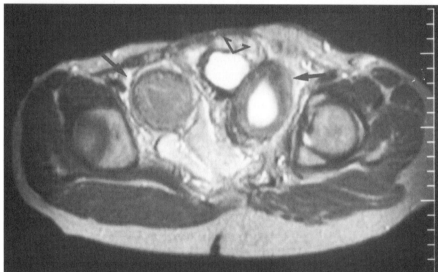

B

Figure 20.1 Hematosalpinx seen in a case of uterine duplication associated with vaginal agenesis. A 22-year-old woman with multiple congenital abnormalities caused by maldevelopment of the urogenital sinus. Because of an absence of the cervix and the vagina, both uterine horns have formed a hematometra (arrows). The blood in the left uterus is hyperintense on T1- and T2-weighted images, while the blood in the right uterus is hypointense on T2-weighted images. The round structure continuous with the left uterine horn, which is hyperintense on T1- and T2-weighted images (arrowheads), is probably a hematosalpinx. **(A)** Axial T1-weighted image (TR600/TE20). **(B)** Axial T2-weighted image (TR2,000/TE80).

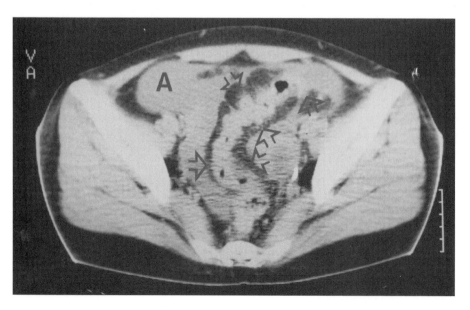

Figure 20.2 Acute salpingitis. Non-contrast-enhanced CT scan. A 30-year-old woman with abdominal pain and fever. CT showed the irregular margins of intestinal loops (arrowheads) and increased attenuation in the fat planes, and ascites (A). These suggest pelvic peritonitis, although this amount of liquid is unusual in pelvic inflammatory disease. Acute salpingitis is among the differential diagnosis, but pelvic peritonitis due to acute appendicitis, for instance, could not be distinguished on CT alone, because there was no obvious adnexal mass.

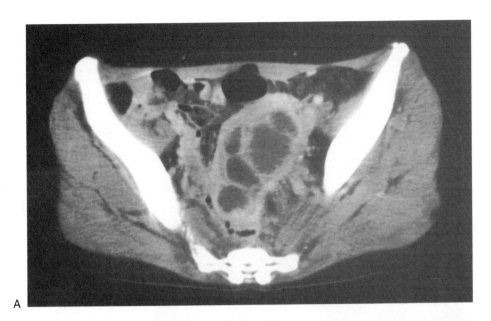

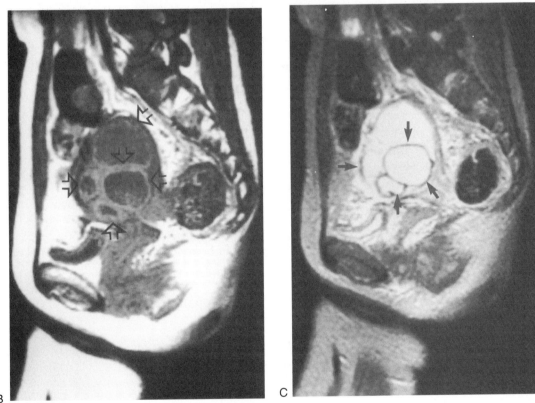

Figure 20.3 Tubo-ovarian abscess. A 41-year-old woman after vaginal hysterectomy. Left ovarian inflammation was suspected clinically. On CT, a thick-walled, liquid mass with septa was seen. On MRI, the inner layer of the cyst wall had linear hyperintense signals on T1-weighted images (Fig. B, arrowheads) and hypointense signals on T2-weighted images (Fig. C, arrows). With contrast, the cyst walls were enhanced and very thick. Well-enhanced tissue was also observed within the lesion (Figure E, arrow). If a clinical history was not available, it would be difficult to distinguish this lesion from ovarian cancer. Left salpingo-oophorectomy established the diagnosis of tubo-ovarian abscess. **(A)** Contrast-enhanced CT scan. **(B)** Sagittal T1-weighted image (TR600/TE20). **(C)** Sagittal T2-weighted image (TR2,000/TE80). (*Figure continues.*)

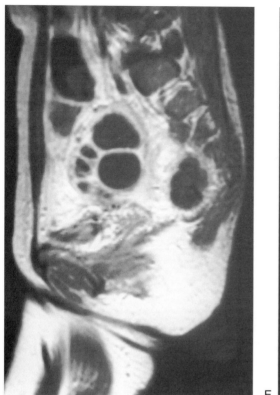
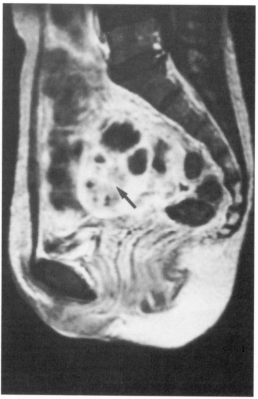

D   E

Figure 20-3. (*Continued*). (**D & E**) Sagittal T1-weighted image with contrast (TR600/TE20).

Differentiation from an inflammatory mass arising from other organs, such as an appendiceal or diverticular abscess, is another problem. Anterior displacement of the mesosalpinx suggests an ovarian or tubal origin. Endometriomas have a variable signal intensity on T1- and T2-weighted images.[12] In the absence of gas, a tubo-ovarian abscess may be radiologically indistinguishable from an endometrioma.[10]

Chronic Salpingitis

Hydrosalpinx and Pyosalpinx

Small tubal carcinomas may present as a hydrosalpinx.[13] On CT, it usually has an attenuation equal to that of water, with a slight enhancement of the wall[14] (Fig. 20.5). The signal intensity on MRI is nonspecific.[8] Typically, hydrosalpinx has a signal intensity of simple liquid, is hypointense on T1-weighted images, and is hyperintense on T2-weighted images (Fig. 20.6); occasionally, however, it may have a signal intensity greater than that of simple liquid on T1-weighted images.[8] Pyosalpinx also tends to have a greater intensity than that of simple liquid on T1-weighted images, and it is difficult to distinguish between hydrosalpinx and pyosalpinx on intensity alone. Hydrosalpinx can be associated with tubal carcinoma, and contrast-enhanced images are needed to detect an enclosed small solid tumor[8,15] (Fig. 20.7).

A hydrosalpinx or pyosalpinx can form a large mass, and differentiation from an ovarian mass is sometimes necessary

(Fig. 20.8). The clue to the diagnosis of a hydrosalpinx is its tubular or retort shape.[13–16] Bowel loops can also appear as a tubular cyst, but they can be excluded because of continuity with adjacent loops.[17] The rare intravenous leiomyomatosis can also be tubular in shape and may mimic a hydrosalpinx on T2-weighted images. Contrast helps to differentiate them, because leiomyomatosis markedly enhance.[18]

Granulomatous Salpingitis

Actinomycosis

Actinomyces is an opportunistic pathogen that is usually seen after trauma or surgery or in patients with neoplasms or foreign bodies. Actinomycosis is a chronic suppurative, granulomatous, fibrosing process that spreads by direct extension, forming abscesses, fistulas, and sinuses.[7] Proteolytic enzymes made by the microbe enable direct extension of infection, accounting for the spread into the abdominal wall.[19] The fallopian tube can be subject to actinomycosis, producing a large fibrous mass often including the ovary.[7] Although definitive diagnosis requires anaerobic cultures, awareness of its existence is important because it is potentially lethal but curable.[19]

The radiologic signs of pelvic actinomycosis are nonspecific, but CT and MRI can show the extent and character of the disease.[19,20] Pelvic actinomycosis usually (70%) forms a large pelvic mass that is mostly solid with focal low-attenuation areas on CT (Fig. 20.9), but mostly cystic masses with

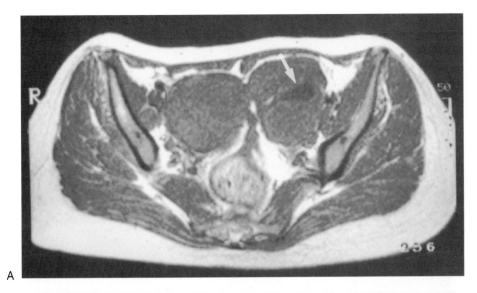

A

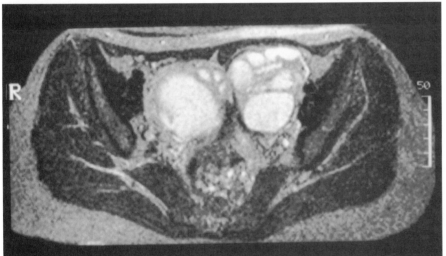

B

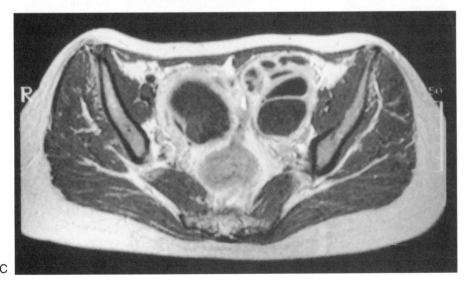

C

Figure 20.4 Tubo-ovarian abscess. A 40-year-old woman with abdominal pain and fever. On T1-weighted images, the lesion predominantly has a slightly greater signal than that of pure liquid. A small component with a signal intensity equal to that of pure liquid is also present (arrow). On T2-weighted images, the liquid content is hyperintense. The thick wall of the lesion is relatively hypointense. After contrast, the thick walls and internal septa are strongly enhanced. **(A)** Axial T1-weighted image (TR600/TE13). **(B)** Axial T2-weighted image (TR2,000/TE80). **(C)** Axial T1-weighted image with contrast (TR600/TE13).

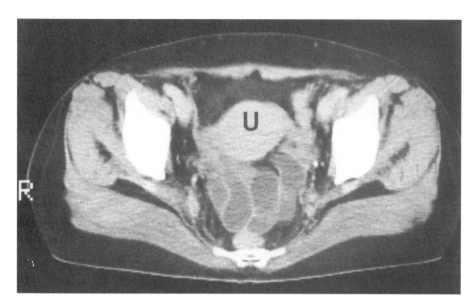

Figure 20.5 Contrast-enhanced CT scan of a hydrosalpinx (after tubal ligation). A 46-year-old woman presented with severe right lower abdominal pain, which began with menstruation. She had a tubal ligation 17 years before. CT showed well-defined, folded tubular structures behind the uterus (U). Surgery revealed bilateral simple hydrosalpinges following tubal ligation.

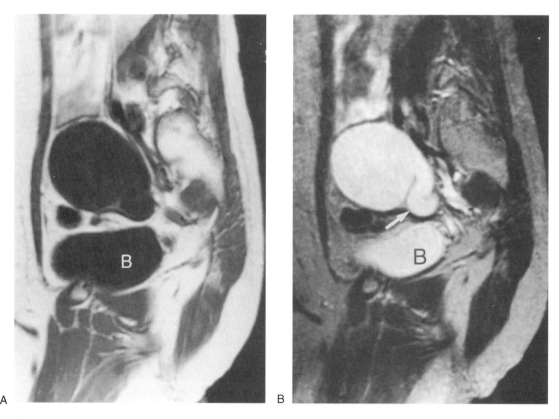

Figure 20.6 MRIs of hydrosalpinx. A 37-year-old woman was referred because of an adnexal mass. The lesion is homogeneous and hypointense on T1-weighted images and hyperintense on T2-weighted images. The typical retort shape of the lesion (arrow) was sufficient to make a diagnosis of hydrosalpinx confirmed at surgery (B = urinary bladder). **(A)** Sagittal T1-weighted image (TR600/TE20). **(B)** Sagittal T2-weighted image (TR2,000/TE80).

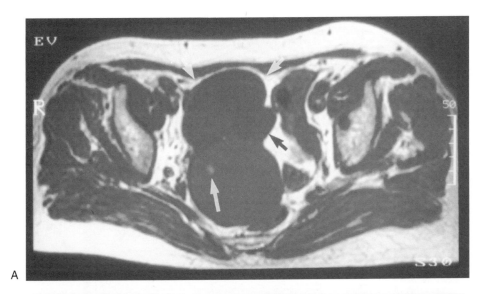

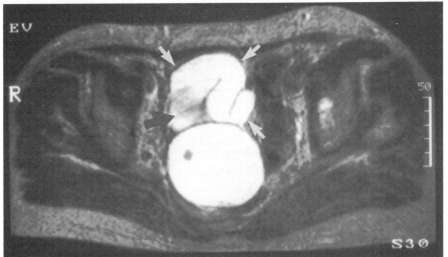

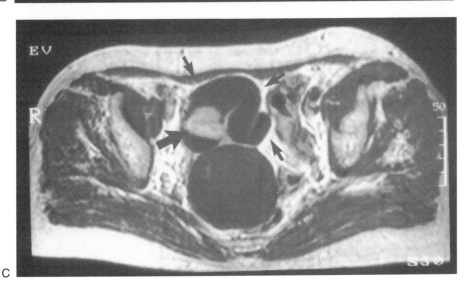

Figure 20.7 Small tubal carcinoma within hydrosalpinx. A 68-year-old woman with lower abdominal pain. A cystic mass in the pelvis is serpentine in shape (smallest arrows), which would be sufficient to make a diagnosis of hydrosalpinx. On T1-weighted images, solid tumor within the hydrosalpinx is not identified. **(A)** A small hemorrhagic hyperintense area is noted (lowest white arrow). **(B)** On T2-weighted images, solid tumor with a relatively hypointense signal may be noted within the hyperintense hydrosalpinx (black arrow) but is not so clear. **(C)** With contrast, solid tumor is strongly enhanced and is easily identified (large black arrow). **(A)** Axial T1-weighted image (TR600/TE13). **(B)** Axial T2-weighted image (TR4,500/TE100). **(C)** Axial T1-weighted image with contrast (TR600/TE13).

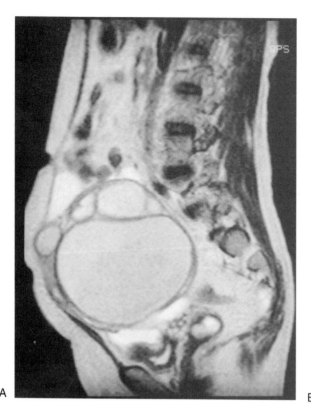

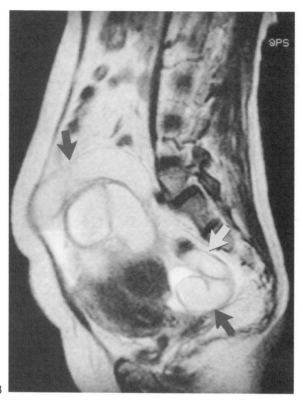

Figure 20.8 Chronic pyosalpinx presenting as a large cystic mass. A 44-year-old woman presented with a lower abdominal mass. Because clinical symptoms, such as abdominal pain, fever, and leukocytosis were absent, the provisional diagnosis before MRI was ovarian cystadenoma or cystadenocarcinoma. **(A & B)** Sagittal T2-weighted images (TR3500/TE80). **(A)** MRI showed a large cystic mass with multiple septa, mimicking ovarian cystadenoma at the central part of the lesion. **(B)** However, at the periphery of the lesion, tubular structures characteristic of distended fallopian tubes were seen (arrows). MRI diagnosis was hydrosalpinx or chronic pyosalpinx, confirmed at surgery. (Courtesy of Dr. Kohichi Kawakami, Hyogo, Japan.)

thickened walls, due to abscess formation, have also been reported. Solid components consist of granulation tissue.[20] On MRI, the inflammatory tissue is of mixed signal intensity both on T1- and T2-weighted images, while the abscess shows hypointensity on T1-weighted images and hyperintensity on T2-weighted images.[19] Dense contrast enhancement in the walls or solid components may be seen, which is a sign of acutely inflamed tissues or dense fibrosis (Fig. 20.9B).[20] Narrowing of the colon (Fig. 20.9C) or hydronephrosis may be seen as a result of extension to the adjacent organs with fibrosis.[19,20] In actinomycosis, regional lymphadenopathy is uncommon.[20]

The prevalence of pelvic actinomycosis increases in women using IUCDs.[19–21] In radiologic descriptions of pelvic actinomycosis, the prevalence of use of IUCDs is between 75% and 100%.[19,20] On CT and MRI, an IUCD appears as a linear low density or intensity, depending on the composition of the IUCD (Fig. 20.9D). Actinomycosis should be considered when a mainly solid pelvic mass is seen in a patient with long-term use of an IUCD. *Actinomyces* tends to invade across tissue planes and boundaries with involvement of colon, small

intestine, greater omentum, and abdominal wall, which is rare in neoplastic conditions.[20] This and the lack of regional lymphadenopathy relative to the size of the mass suggest actinomycosis rather than malignancy. Specific diagnosis of actinomycosis by imaging alone is impossible, and if actinomycosis is suspected histology is needed to make the diagnosis. Treatment for actinomycosis requires removal of the IUCD and intravenous penicillin with drainage of abscesses.[20]

Tuberculosis

Tuberculosis has been the predominant cause of granulomatous salpingitis, accounting for approximately 5% of all cases of salpingitis in many areas of the world.[22] Sexual transmission is extremely rare. Secondary spread from a primary infection is the usual route.[7] Sterility and amenorrhea are the most common symptoms.[7] CT and MRI cannot specifically diagnose pelvic tuberculosis, but some findings are suggestive. CT often shows calcified pelvic and abdominal nodes, a sequela of healed pelvic tuberculosis. Bilateral, predominantly solid adnexal masses, containing scattered small calcifications are

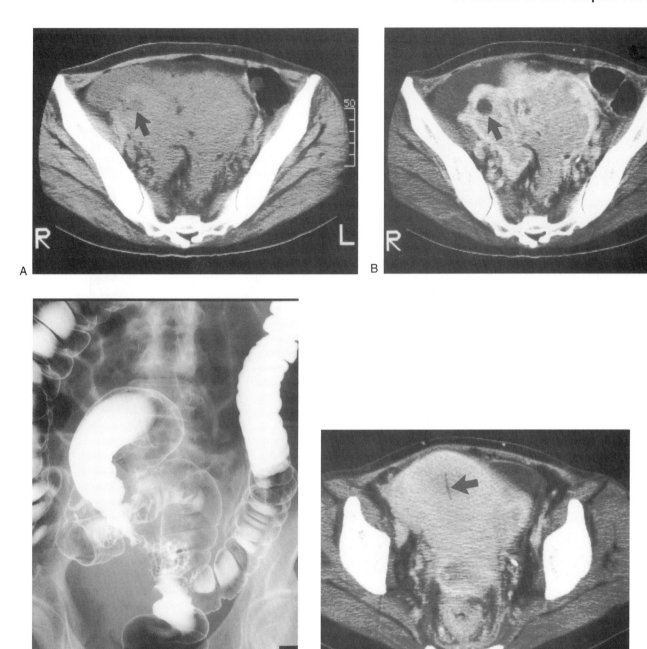

Figure 20.9 Actinomycosis. A 37-year-old woman presented with lower abdominal distension. (**A & B**) On CT, there was a solid pelvic mass with a small cystic component (arrows) around the uterus. The solid part was well enhanced, especially at the periphery. Narrowing of the rectosigmoid and sigmoid colons was also noted on barium enema. A malignant ovarian tumor was suspected, but actinomycosis was found at laparotomy. (**D**) Retrospectively, an IUCD (arrow), within the uterus, was a clue to the diagnosis. (**A**) CT before contrast. (**B**) Contrast-enhanced CT scan. (**C**) Barium enema. (**D**) Contrast-enhanced CT scan.

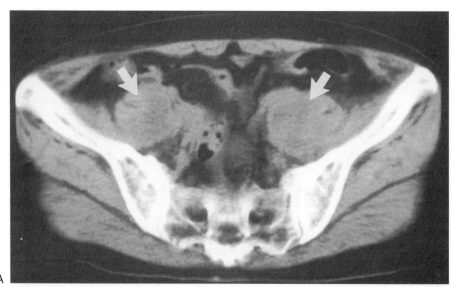

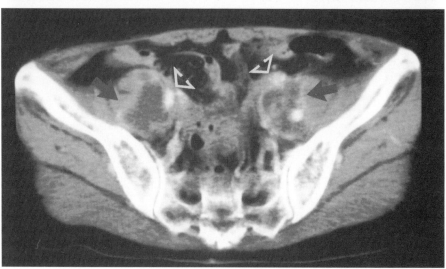

Figure 20.10 Pelvic tuberculosis (lymphadenitis). A 73-year-old woman with diabetes mellitus presented with fever. CT showed bilateral masses along the iliopsoas muscles (arrows). They had slightly higher attenuation than that of pure liquid on precontrast CT. With contrast, the lesions were cystic masses with thick, strongly enhanced walls. They were lateral to the iliac vessels (arrowheads) and were thought to be iliac lymph nodes. Because of their marked cystic necrosis and coalescent nature, tuberculous lymphadenitis was suspected. Ultrasound-guided needle aspiration confirmed the diagnosis. **(A)** CT without contrast. **(B)** CT with contrast.

suggestive of tuberculous involvement.[23] CT is preferred to MRI to make the diagnosis because of the superiority in detecting these calcified lesions, and sometimes multiple cystic lymph nodes with a tendency to conglomerate are also seen (Fig. 20.10).

Parasitic Salpingitis and Other Miscellaneous Conditions

The pinworm, *Enterobius vermicularis*, can migrate up the genital tract and embed in the tube. A tubo-ovarian or fibrous nodular mass may be present. The ova are released, provoking a granulomatous reaction and disseminating in the peritoneum, simulating metastatic carcinoma.[24] Schistosomiasis is one of the most common causes of granulomatous salpingitis. In Africa, tubal infections occur in as many as 20% of unselected women at autopsy. Grossly, fibrosis surrounds the ova, producing a nodular or fibrotic tube. Hydatid disease due to *Echinococcus granulosus* can also cause a complex mass in the pelvis.[7]

Sarcoidosis of the tube is rarely reported but can accompany disseminated disease. Tubal distension, tubo-ovarian adhesions, an ovarian abscess, or multiple serosal nodules may be seen. Crohn's disease may involve the tube and the ovary to produce a granulomatous salpingo-oophoritis.[25,26] Fistulas from bowel to tube may also occur. Foreign matter, which may be introduced into the tube in the course of gynecologic investigations, especially hysterosalpingography, can cause a lipoid or granulomatous salpingitis.[7]

On CT or MRI, it is difficult to diagnose these conditions from their appearance alone. Findings from other organs, such as mediastinal lymphadenopathy in sarcoidosis or thickening of the bowel wall in Crohn's disease, may help. Clinical and pathologic information including specific culture and stains are necessary to exclude bacterial or other granulomatous diseases.

MALIGNANT CONDITIONS

Primary Tubal Carcinoma

Primary carcinoma of the fallopian tube is one of the most rare malignancies. It usually affects older women.[27] The striking difference between tubal and ovarian carcinoma is the early manifestation of symptoms such as abnormal bleeding and vaginal discharge in tubal carcinoma.[27] Tubal carcinoma has a tendency to produce copious amounts of thin serous liquid. Although these patients may seek medical help at an earlier stage than patients with ovarian carcinoma, it is extremely difficult to make a correct diagnosis because of the rarity of the disease and the small size of the lesion.[28] The low 5-year survival is attributable to delayed diagnosis rather than to high malignancy.[29]

An associated hydrosalpinx affects the CT and MRI appearance of tubal carcinoma. When hydrosalpinx is absent, tubal carcinoma is a small, solid lobulated adnexal mass. The tube, filled with tumor and distended to a fusiform shape, accounts for the lobulation on CT and MRI. The lesion is attenuated to that of a nonspecific soft tissue mass on CT[15] (Fig. 20.11). The signal intensi-

ties on MRI are homogeneously hypointense on T1-weighted images and relatively hyperintense on T2-weighted images[15] (Figs. 20.7 and 20.12 to 20.14). With contrast, the lesion is homogeneously enhanced (Figs. 20.7 and 20.13). Small cystic components caused by necrosis or hemorrhage are sometimes seen at the periphery of the mass.[15] Peripheral cysts are usually hypointense on T1-weighted images unless hemorrhage is present (Fig. 20.13). It may be difficult to distinguish it from surrounding bowel loops on CT because of the lobulation (Fig. 20.12).[15] Oral contrast should be used to detect tubal carcinoma on CT.

When there is an associated hydrosalpinx, the entire lesion appears as a large cystic adnexal mass with a small solid component, which is a tubal carcinoma (Fig. 20.14). The cystic component is an associated hydrosalpinx, and it exhibits a characteristic tubular shape.[15] A contrast study is necessary to identify the solid tumor within, because a small carcinoma may appear as a hydrosalpinx[8,13] (see Fig. 20.7).

Associated findings in tubal carcinoma are intrauterine liquid collection (Fig. 20.12B), peritumoral ascites (Figs. 20.12 and 20.13), and hydrosalpinx[15] (Figs. 20.7 and 20.14). Peritumoral ascites is markedly hyperintense on T2-weighted images and distinguishes the border of the tumor[8] (Figs. 20.12C and 20.13C). On physical and ultrasound examination, tubal carcinoma can be confused with a uterine leiomyoma.[15] Uterine leiomyomas are of low signal intensity with or without speckling on T2-weighted images, while tubal carcinoma is hyperintense[15,30,31] (Fig. 20.13). Tubal carcinoma can be misinterpreted as an ovarian cystadenocarcinoma if there is an associated hydrosalpinx.[15] The shape of the hydrosalpinx may be a clue to the diagnosis of tubal carcinoma[15] (Fig. 20.14).

Figure 20.11 Tubal carcinoma. Contrast-enhanced CT. A 58-year-old woman presented with bleeding. A relatively small, solid adnexal mass was seen on CT (arrow).

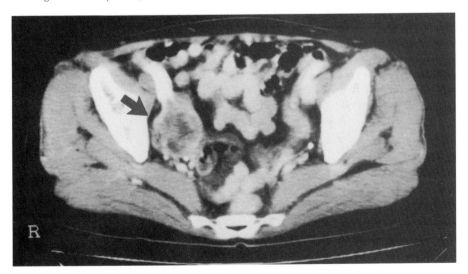

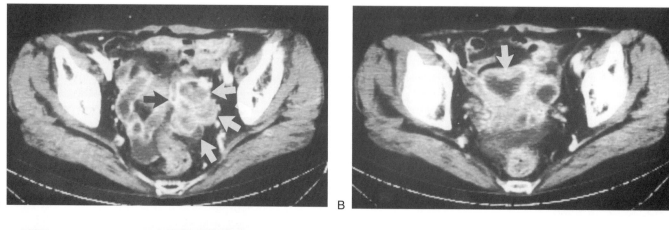

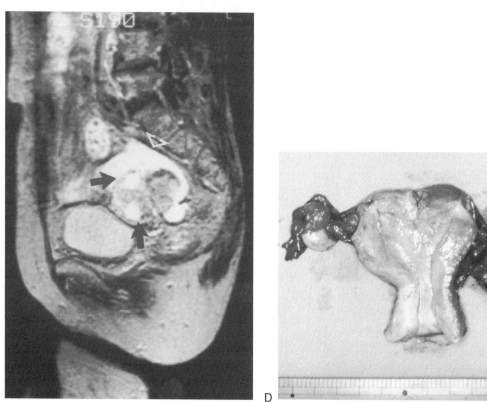

Figure 20.12 Tubal carcinoma mimicking intestinal loops on CT. A 56-year-old woman presented with bleeding. An adnexal tumor was suspected on physical examination and ultrasound. **(A)** On CT, the lesion (arrows) was lobulated and resembled bowel loops which were not opacified with oral contrast material. **(B)** On CT at the uterine corpus, intrauterine liquid was seen as a wide central area of low attenuation (arrow). **(C)** On T2-weighted MRI, the tumor was homogeneous and relatively hyperintense. Peritumoral ascites (arrowhead) was markedly hyperintense and helped demarcate the lesion. Distinct hyperintense cysts, were noted at the periphery (arrows). **(D)** In the gross specimen, a tumor of the fallopian tube was noted. **(A & B)** CT with contrast. **(C)** Sagittal T2-weighted image (TR2,000/TE80). **(D)** Gross specimen.

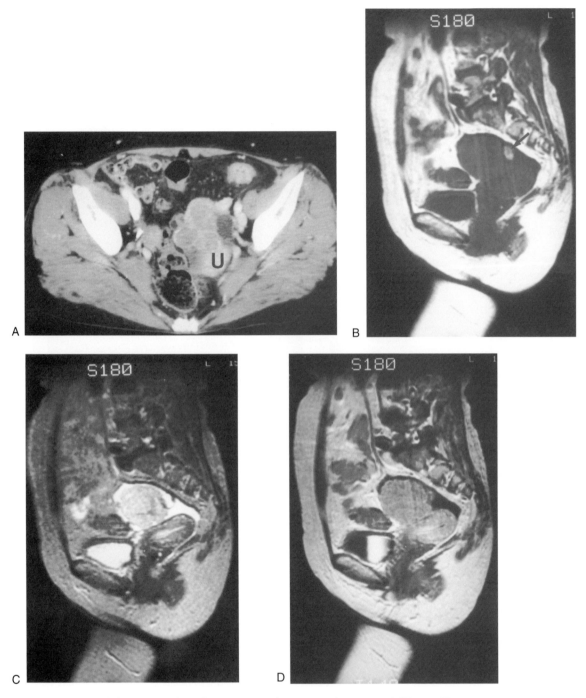

Figure 20.13 Tubal carcinoma clinically misinterpreted as a uterine leiomyoma. A 57-year-old woman presented with bleeding. A uterine leiomyoma was suspected by physical examination and ultrasound because of its contiguous position. CT was not thought to be adequate to make the diagnosis of adnexal tumor (U, uterus). Retrospectively, however, the lobulation and thin enhancing rim of the lesion and the presence of the peripheral cyst suggest a solid adnexal tumor. On T1-weighted MRI, the lesion was homogeneous and hypointense and was not separable from the uterus and peritumoral ascites. The peripheral cyst had a hyperintense signal on T1-weighted images, in this case (Fig. B) (arrow) due to hemorrhage. On T2-weighted MRI, the lesion was separate from the uterus and peritumoral ascites. The relative hyperintensity of the tumor helps to exclude the diagnosis of uterine leiomyoma. With contrast, the tumor was homogeneously enhanced. **(A)** Contrast-enhanced CT scan. **(B)** Sagittal T1-weighted image (TR600/TE20). **(C)** Sagittal T2-weighted image (TR2,000/TE80). **(D)** Sagittal T1-weighted image with contrast enhancement (TR600/TE20).

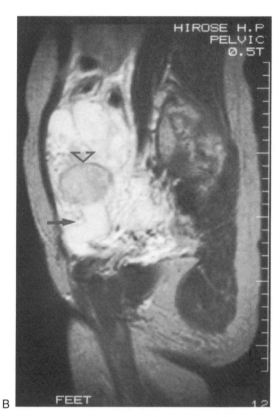

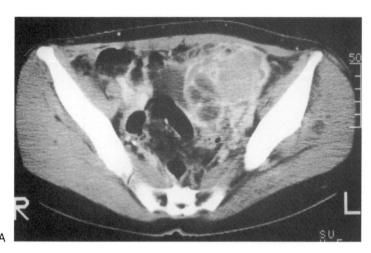

Figure 20.14 Tubal carcinoma with hydrosalpinx. A 46-year-old woman with lower abdominal distension and abnormal genital bleeding. On CT, the mass has mixed solid and cystic components, mimicking ovarian cystadenocarcinoma. On MRI, a hyperintense solid part is the true tumor (arrowhead). The cystic part is serpentine, which indicates a hydrosalpinx (arrow). This shape of a hydrosalpinx suggests a tubal carcinoma rather than an ovarian cystadenoma or carcinoma. **(A)** CT with contrast. **(B)** Sagittal T2-weighted image (TR2,000/TE80).

ISCHEMIA

Adnexal Torsion

Adnexal torsion is a rare but important cause of abdominal pain.[32] The usual predisposing factor is cystic enlargement of the ipsilateral ovary.[7] A benign ovarian cyst or tumor is present in 65% to 80% of patients, and a malignant ovarian tumor is present in 5% to 15%.[7,33] Paraovarian cysts are also associated with torsion.[7] Exceptionally, torsion may occur in the absence of an apparent adnexal mass, usually in children, because normal adnexa in this age group are especially mobile, allowing torsion at the mesosalpinx with changes in position or intra-abdominal pressure.[7,34] There is right-sided predominance of adnexal torsion, with an approximately 3:2 ratio, and the incidence increases in pregnancy.[32] It is thought that this is due to the decreased space on the left side of the lower abdomen and pelvis, which is occupied by the sigmoid colon or to the differences in venous drainage of the two ovaries.[32]

The symptoms include gradual or sudden onset of pain indistinguishable from other causes of acute abdominal pain.[35] Although adnexal torsion is often considered as an acute event, a subacute form does occur and makes the diagnosis still more difficult.[36] Ultrasound is the most widely used imaging modality for the diagnosis of torsion,[37,38] and the role of CT or MRI is limited. Subacute torsion may unexpectedly be seen at CT or MRI examinations performed for suspected malignancy.[36] Any delay in surgery results in complete gangrenous change of the ovary.

There are two types of torsion of the fallopian tube: torsion of both the fallopian tube and the ovary and isolated tubal torsion. Torsion of both the fallopian tube and the ovary occurs more often than that of either alone, since the broad ligament acts as a fulcrum.[32] Isolated tubal torsion may be related to hydrosalpinx, tubal neoplasm, and previous sterilization[39] however, torsion with no apparent underlying pathology has also been reported.[37,40]

CT and MRI of adnexal torsion will differ if the torsion is complete or incomplete,[36] as there are no specific CT or MRI signs for incomplete torsion.[36] In contrast, complete torsion with hemorrhagic infarction has specific CT and MRI signs. When the torsion is complete, the blood supply is obstructed, and gangrenous and hemorrhagic necrosis results.[36] Internal hemorrhage is not always present (20% to 50%), but if so, it can be identified by high attenuation on precontrast CT or by hyperintensity on T1-weighted MRI[36,41] (Fig. 20.15). A swollen pedicle and absent enhancement are diagnostic.[36] A "beaked" or serpentine protrusion is frequently discovered at the periphery of a mass after complete torsion. Because the protrusion extends from the lesion to the uterus, it has an edematous pedicle due to obstructed venous drainage.[36] The lack of enhancement indicates absent flow[36] (Fig. 20.16). Prominently engorged blood vessels appear as enhancing vessels surrounding the mass on dynamic CT scanning or linear flow voids on MRI[36,42] (Fig. 20.16).

In addition to the appearance of the ovarian mass, the appearance of the fallopian tube is important in diagnosing torsion of both ovary and the tube.[41] A swollen tube can be identified on CT as a tubular structure extending from the uterus and partly covering the adnexal mass.[41] In a series of 10 cases, an adnexal mass was present in all 10, the fallopian tube was thickened in 8, there was hemorrhage in 6, and heterogeneous contrast uptake in 5. These signs suggest torsion even when the changes in the ovary or mass are not obvious.[41]

Isolated tubal torsion is rare. The tube is an elongated, convoluted cystic mass, tapering as it nears the uterus.[37] Internal hemorrhage may be seen on CT or MRI as increased attenuation or signal intensity within the lesion (Fig. 20.17). Demonstration of the ipsilateral ovary strongly suggests isolated tubal torsion.[37]

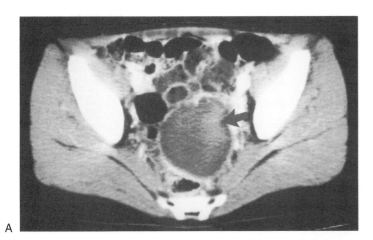

A

Figure 20.15 Complete torsion with hemorrhagic infarction. A 10-year-old presented with insidious onset of lower abdominal pain, which became severe 10 days previously. CT showed a cystic mass with an enclosed area of high attenuation due to blood (arrow). On MRI, the periphery of the lesion was hyperintense on T1- and T2-weighted images, which was consistent with subacute hematoma. At surgery, there was an ovarian cyst that had undergone torsion. (**A**) CT with contrast. (**B**) Sagittal T1-weighted image (TR600/TE20). (**C**) Sagittal T2-weighted image (TR2,000/TE80).

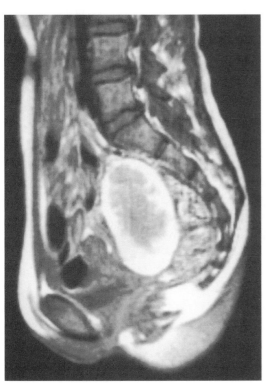

B

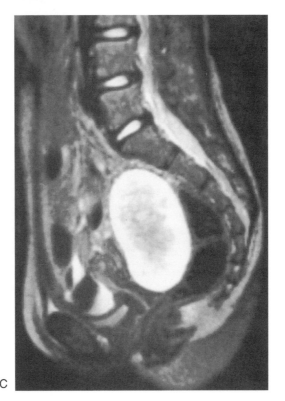

C

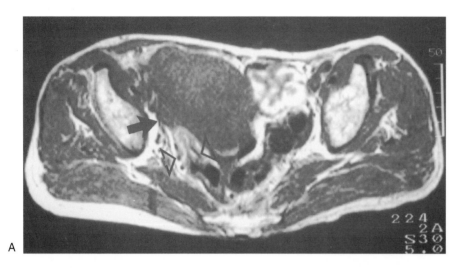

A

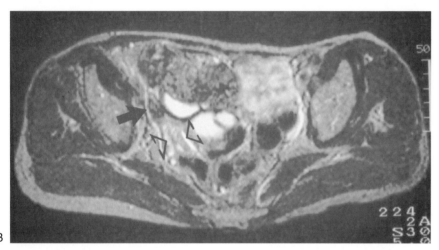

B

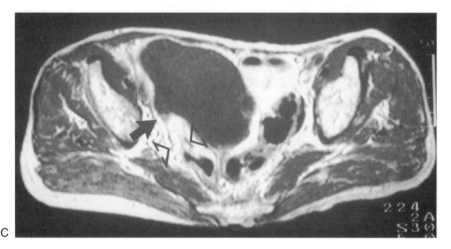

C

Figure 20.16 Complete torsion with hemorrhagic infarction. A 72-year-old woman presented with abdominal pain for 4 days. A right adnexal mass has a beaked protrusion (arrows), to which engorged vessels are converging (arrowheads). The wall, minute septa, and protrusions completely fail to enhance, indicating interruption to blood flow. At surgery there was complete torsion of a mucinous cystadenoma. **(A)** Axial T1-weighted image (TR600/TE20). **(B)** Axial T2-weighted image (TR2,000/TE80). **(C)** Axial T1-weighted image with contrast (TR600/TE20).

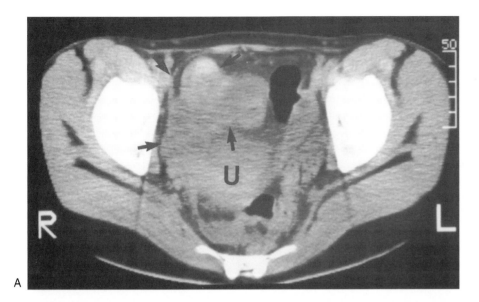

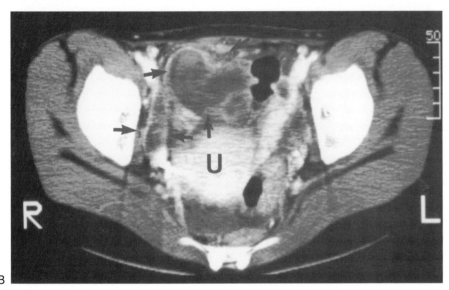

Figure 20.17 Torsion of hydrosalpinx caused by tubal ligation. A 28-year-old woman presented with an acute onset of abdominal pain. Tubal ligation had been performed 4 years before. **(A)** Pre-contrast CT showed a right adnexal mass of high attenuation indicating blood. (arrows). **(B)** After contrast, a tubular cystic mass was more clearly identified (arrows). Torsion of hydrosalpinx was confirmed by surgery. U, uterus.

POSTOPERATIVE APPEARANCE

Post Tubal Ligation

Tubal ligation increases the risk of hydrosalpinx.[14,16,39] Pelvic inflammation or surgery may cause scarring of the fimbriated end of the tube. Surgical ligation of the other end may thus cause hydrosalpinx formation.[16] When a tubular cyst is seen on CT or MRI in patients who have had a tubal ligation, a hydrosalpinx is a possibility (Figs. 20.5 and 20.18). When a hemorrhagic adnexal mass is identified on CT or MRI in a patient with a history of tubal ligation and com-

plaining of acute abdominal pain, torsion with gangrene of a hydrosalpinx should be considered (Fig. 20.17).

SUMMARY

CT and MRI are important in the assessment of pathology of the fallopian tubes, particularly for the diagnosis of malignancy and chronic inflammation. While ultrasound is the usual method of imaging the pelvis, it is important to recognize the appearances of the tubes on CT and MRI, as tubal

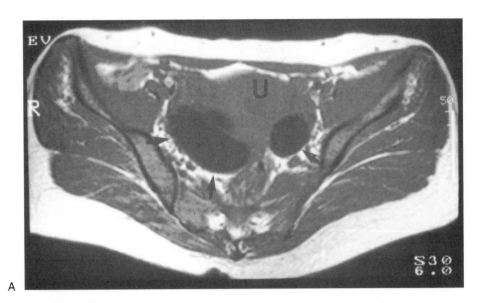

A

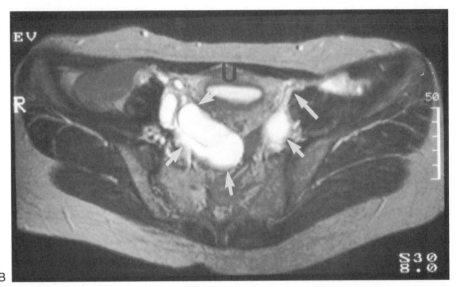

B

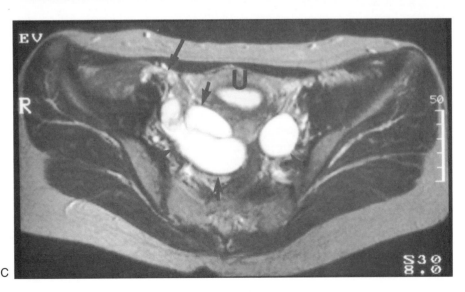

C

Figure 20.18 Hydrosalpinx after tubal ligation. A 34-year-old woman with a history of tubal ligation 5 years before. She had no symptoms. Screening ultrasound revealed bilateral cystic adnexal masses (arrows). They were homogeneous and hypointense on T1-weighted images and hyperintense on T2-weighted images. They were tubular and folded. The continuity of the lesions with the uterine cornua was clearly demonstrated (Figures B and C, arrows). (A) Axial T1-weighted image (TR600/TE20). (B) Axial T2-weighted image (TR4,500/TE100). (C) Axial T2-weighted image 1 cm caudal to Figure B. U, uterus.

pathology will be seen in patients undergoing pelvic examinations for other reasons.

REFERENCES

1. Carrington BM, Hricak H, Nuruddin RN et al. Müllerian duct anomalies: MR imaging evaluation. Radiology 1990;176:715–720
2. Knab DR, Blanco LJ. Müllerian duct agenesis with a unilateral functioning segment of the rudimentary uterine horn. Am J Obstet Gynecol 1978;132:222–224
3. Farber M, Mitchell GW. Bicornuate uterus and partial atresia of the fallopian tube. Am J Obstet Gynecol 1979;134:881–884
4. Berman L, Stringer DA, Stonge O et al. Case report: unilateral haematocolpos in uterine duplication associated with renal agenesis. Clin Radiol 1987;38:545–547
5. Silber CG, Magness RL, Farber M. Duplication of the uterus with a non-communicating functioning uterine horn. Mt Sinai J Med 1990;57:374–377
6. Yoder IC, Pfister R. Unilateral hematocolpos and ipsilateral renal agenesis: report of two cases and review of the literature. AJR Am J Roentgenol 1976;127:303–308
7. Wheeler JE. Diseases of the fallopian tube. In: Kaufman RJ, Ed. Blaustein's Pathology of the Female Genital Tract (3rd ed.) Springer-Verlag, New York, 1987, pp 409–436
8. Togashi K. Other pelvic organs. In: Togashi K, Ed. MRI of the Female Pelvis. Igaku-shoin, Tokyo, 1993, pp 281–306
9. Lupetin AR, Dash N, Schapiro RL et al. MR evaluation of the female pelvis with a 0.5 Tesla superconducting magnet. Presented at the Radiological Society of North America Meeting, Washington DC, 1984
10. Wilbur AC, Aizenstein RI, Napp TE. CT findings in tuboovarian abscess. AJR Am J Roentgenol 1992;158:575–579
11. Ellis JH, Francis IR, Rhodes M et al. CT findings in tuboovarian abscess. J Comput Assist Tomogr 1991;15:589–592
12. Togashi K. Endometriosis. In: Togashi K, Ed. MRI of the Female Pelvis. Igaku-shoin, Tokyo, 1993, pp 203–225
13. Shamam OM, Bennett WF, Teteris NJ, Finer RM. Primary fallopian tube adenocarcinoma presenting as a hydrosalpinx: CT appearance. J Comput Assist Tomogr 1988;12:674–675
14. Togashi K, Nishimura K, Itoh K et al. Computed tomography of hydrosalpinx following tubal ligation. J Comput Assist Tomogr 1986;10:78–80
15. Kawakami S, Togashi K, Kimura I et al. Primary malignant tumor of the fallopian tube: appearance at CT and MR imaging. Radiology 1993;186:503–508
16. Russin LD. Hydrosalpinx and tubal torsion: a late complication of tubal ligation. Radiology 1986;159:115–116
17. Tessler FN, Perella RR, Fleischer AC, Grant EG. Endovaginal sonographic diagnosis of dilated fallopian tubes. AJR Am J Roentgenol 1989;153:523–525
18. Kawakami S, Sagoh T, Kumada H et al. Intravenous leiomyomatosis of uterus: MR appearance. J Comput Assist Tomogr 1991;15:686–689
19. O'Connor KFO, Bagg MN, Croley MR, Schabel SI. Pelvic actinomycosis associated with intrauterine devices. Radiology 1989;170:559–560
20. Ha HK, Lee HJ, Kim H et al. Abdominal actinomycosis: CT findings in 10 patients. AJR Am J Roentgenol 1993;161:791–794
21. Maloney J, Cho SR. Pelvic actinomyocosis. Radiology 1983;148:388
22. Anderson JR. Genital tuberculosis. In: Novak ER, Woodfuff JD, Eds. Novak's Gynecologic and Obstetric Pathology with Clinical and Endocrine Relations (8th ed). WB Saunders, Philadelphia, 1979, 557–559
23. Walzer A, Koenigsberg M. Ultrasonographic demonstration of pelvic tuberculosis. J Ultrasound Med 1983;2:139–140
24. Fitzgerald TB, Mainwarning AR, Ahmed A. Pelvic peritoneal oxyuriasis simulating metastatic carcinoma. J Obstet Gynecol Br Commonw 1974;81:248
25. Brooks JJ, Wheeler JE. Granulomatous salpingitis secondary to Crohn's disease. Obstet Gynecol 1977;49:31s
26. Wlodarski FM, Trainer TD. Granulomatous oophoritis and salpingitis associated with Crohn's disease. Am J Obstet Gynecol 1975;122:527
27. Raju KS, Barker GH, Wiltshaw E. Primary carcinoma of the fallopian tube. Br J Obstet Gynaecol 1981;88:1124–1129
28. Diasia PJ. Tumors of the fallopian tube. In: Scott JR, Disaia PJ, Hammond CB, Spellacy WN, Eds. Danforth's Obstetrics and Gynecology (6th ed.) JB Lippincott, Philadelphia, 1990, pp 1055–1065
29. Novak ER, Woodruff JD. Tumor of the tube, paraovarium, and uterine ligaments. In: Novak ER, Woodfuff JD, Eds. Novak's Gynecologic and Obstetric Pathology with Clinical and Endocrine Relations (8th ed). WB Saunders Philadelphia, 1979, pp 334–342
30. Hricak H, Tsholakoff D, Heinrichs L et al. Uterine leiomyomas: correlation of MR, histopathologic findings, and symptoms. Radiology 1986;158:385–391
31. Weinreb JC, Barkoff ND, Megibow A, Demopoulos RD. The value of MR imaging in distinguishing leiomyomas from other solid pelvic masses when sonography is indeterminate. AJR Am J Roentgenol 1990;154:295–299
32. Warner MA, Fleischer AC, Edell SL et al. Uterine adnexal torsion: sonographic findings. Radiology 1985;154:773–775
33. Lee RA, Welch JS. Torsion of the uterine adnexa. Am J Obstet Gynecol 1967;97:974
34. Schultz LR, Newton WA, Clatworthy HW, Jr. Torsion of previously normal tube and ovary in children. N Engl J Med 1963;268:343–346
35. DiSaia PJ. Ovarian disorders. In: Scott JR, Disaia PJ, Hammond CB, Spellacy WN, Eds. Danforth's Obstetrics and Gynecology (6th ed.). JB Lippincott, Philadelphia, 1990, pp 1067–1120
36. Kimura I, Togashi K, Kawakami S et al. Ovarian torsion: CT and MR imaging appearances. Radiology 1994;190:337–341
37. Elcahlal U, Capsi B, Schachter M, Borenstein R. Isolated tubal torsion: clinical and ultrasonographic correlation. J Ultrasound Med 1993;2:115–117
38. Rosado WM Jr, Trambert MA, Gosink BB, Pretorius DH. Adnexal torsion: diagnosis by using color doppler sonography. AJR Am J Roentgenol 1992;159:1251–1253
39. Bernardus RE, Van der Silkke JW, Roex AJM et al. Torsion of the fallopian tube: some considerations on its etiology. Obstet Gynecol 1984;64:675–678
40. Chambers JT, Thiagarajah S, Kitchin JD. Torsion of the normal fallopian tube in pregnancy. Obstet Gynecol 1979;54:487–489
41. Ghossain MA, Buy JN, Bazot M et al. CT in adnexal torsion with emphasis on tubal fidings: correlation with ultrasound. J Comput Assist Tomogr 1994;18:619–625
42. Bellah RD, Griscom NT. Torsion of normal uterine adnexa before menarche: CT appearance. AJR Am J Roentgenol 1989;152:123–124

21

Hysterosalpingography of the Fallopian Tube

VIVIAN LEWIS

JACQUES S. ABRAMOWICZ

HISTORY

Burns, in the 19th-century edition of *Principles of Midwifery*, was the first to recognize that diseased fallopian tubes are an important cause of infertility, but tests of tubal patency were not developed until about 100 years later.[1] The first observation of the uterine cavity by intravenous injection of a bismuth paste and roentgenography came from Rindfleish in 1910.[2] The term *hysterosalpingogram* to indicate images of both the uterus (*hyster*, in Greek) and the fallopian tubes (*salpinx*, in Latin) originated a few years later, with the first reports describing injection of different contrast media through the cervix.[3] Rubin[4,5] went on to develop and popularize his insufflation technique, which involved injection of gas into the cervix and checking for free gas by x-ray, auscultation, patient symptoms, or changes in insufflation pressure, eventually reporting over 80,000 cases. The high false-negative rate of insufflation and greater amount of information gained through imaging techniques have completely superseded his test. Subsequently, many modifications in contrast media, techniques, instruments, and indications have been introduced.[1,6,7]

TECHNIQUE

Hysterosalpingography (HSG) is well tolerated in an outpatient setting. It is usually scheduled during the follicular phase of the cycle. Premedication generally consists of either acetaminophen or a nonsteroidal anti-inflammatory drug. The patient empties her bladder and is placed in the supine position. Bimanual pelvic examination is performed to assess uterine position and exclude tenderness, and a speculum is placed to allow cleansing of the vagina and cervix. Paracervical block can be used but is usually not necessary. The cannula used for dye injection is generally one of three types: cone shaped (such as Kidde or Jarcho), balloon type (such as

Sholoff or Harris), or suction cup-like apparatus (such as Malmstrom). After placement of an appropriate cannula in the cervix, contrast is injected slowly until the uterine cavity and fallopian tubes are outlined. Films are obtained to document uterine and tubal anatomy with a view toward minimizing radiation. Sometimes a scout film is taken before injection of contrast, to look for calcification or soft tissue masses. An early film of the uterus should be taken to look for filling defects, followed by one or two films to document tubal patency and another to show dispersion of dye through the pelvis. Oblique films are sometimes useful in imaging different planes of the uterus and in determining location of tubal patency when dye from one tube spreads rapidly through the pelvis.[8–10]

Contrast material is basically of two types: oil or water based (Table 21.1), and each has its proponents. Those who support oil-based contrast claim a higher spontaneous pregnancy rate in the months after HSG, especially in women with unexplained infertility. One randomized controlled trial comparing oil- with water-based media showed an overall odds ratio of pregnancy of 1.89 (95% confidence interval =1.33 to 2.68).[11] The proponents of water-based media point to a higher complication rate with oil, which has caused granuloma formation in the peritoneum and tubes[9,12] and a case of coma due to cerebral embolization from intravascular oil form an HSG.[13] Additionally, there is evidence of a lower chance of pregnancy in patients with tubal factor infertility after oil-based HSG.[11]

INDICATIONS

Infertility, especially when tubal abnormalities are suspected, is the most common indication for HSG.[8,14] It is principally used for screening but is also often employed in conjunction with tubal surgery (both pre and postoperatively) and as a therapeutic technique (Fig. 21.1). Uterine abnormalities can also be diagnosed.

Table 21.1 Comparison of Oil- and Water-Soluble Medium

	Oil	Water Soluble
Viscosity	High	Low to moderate
Radiopacity	Good	Moderate to good
Absorption	Very slow (up to several months)	Very prompt (excretion through kidneys in 20–60 min)
Toxicity	None observed	Rare
Allergic reaction	None observed	Occasional
Peritoneal reaction	Only with large amounts	Transient
Pain	Mild–moderate	Mild–moderate
Pregnancy rate (controlled trials)	19–54%	11–40%
Dangers	Intravasation, pulmonary embolism, granuloma formation	None
Iodine content	>400 mg/ml	280–350 mg/ml
Convenience	24-hr delayed film required	

(Modified from Abramowicz and Lewis,[10] with permission.)

CONTRAINDICATIONS

Pregnancy is the most obvious contraindication to HSG. The risks in terms of instrumentation and radiation are minimal.[9,15] Nonetheless, it is customary to schedule the study just after menstruation (day 5 to 12 of the cycle). In anovulatory patients, a pregnancy test may be advisable before the procedure.

The procedure should be avoided when there is active uterine bleeding. This is particularly true after intrauterine manipulation, such as curettage, when venous intravasation of contrast is almost certain. A small amount of bleeding, at the end of the menses or secondary to a submucous fibroid is not an absolute contraindication. When interpreting the films, it should be remembered that blood clot could be the cause of a filling defect, rather than intrauterine pathology.[10]

Acute pelvic inflammatory disease (PID) is an absolute contraindication to HSG. Peritonitis after HSG was the cause of death in 6 of the 11 fatalities reported in the world literature.[9] In patients who have previously had acute PID, cervical cultures should be obtained. DNA probes for *Neisseria gonorrhea* and *Chlamydia trachomatis* offer lower false-negative rates and ease of specimen handling.[16] If abnormal, antibiotics are prescribed and the procedure is rescheduled 1 to 2 months after therapy.[17] Often, the organism is anaerobic and difficult to eradicate. Some believe that HSG is contraindicated when there is clear evidence of previous acute PID, in which case, laparoscopy may be preferable to establish tubal patency.

COMPLICATIONS

The principal complications are lower abdominal pain, febrile morbidity and pelvic infection, vascular intravasation with risks of pulmonary embolism if an oil-soluble dye is used, the risks of ovarian radiation, uterine perforation, and dye allergy.[6,8,9,17,18] Pain is a common complaint during and after HSG. The initial manipulation of the cervix, with tenaculum application and catheter insertion, is the first component. This can be minimized by the use of a catheter that does not require use of a tenaculum or by injection of a local anesthetic into the anterior lip of the cervix before grasping it. Cramping because of uterine distension with contrast medium introduces another painful component. This is particularly problematic when tubal obstruction prevents spillage of dye into the peritoneal cavity. In those cases, the pain usually worsens as more medium is injected. Premedication with analgesics such as prostaglandin synthesis inhibitors is often helpful.[19,20] Slow injection and limited dye volume also reduce the pain.

Acute PID is one of the most feared complications of HSG, as it may further reduce fertility. The frequency in large series lies between 0.3% and 6.0%, depending on the population and the diagnostic criteria.[7,9,12] Patients who have had previous pelvic infection, or who have had pelvic surgery for infection, or those with previous adnexal tenderness are at greater risk.[21] No laboratory test can predict the risk of subsequent pelvic infection. However, since *C. trachomatis* has most often been cited as the culprit in postprocedure infection, some authors advocate checking for serum antibodies to this organism.[22,23] In one series, there was good correlation between antibodies and tubal occlusion; although two of the five women who developed infectious complications after HSG did not have antibodies.[23] Cervical cultures are also limited in that there is sometimes residual infection in the endometrium or tubes, despite negative cervical studies.[24,25] Doxycycline is the agent of choice for prophylaxis,[17] but in a low-risk group it is not indicated. Oil-soluble media may be associated with less inflammation than water-soluble media.[18] Abdominal pain or temperature that persists more than 1 to 2 days after HSG suggests inflammation (Fig. 21.2).

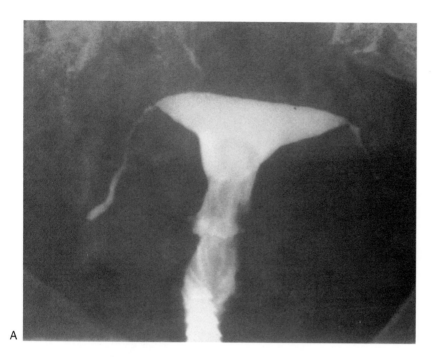

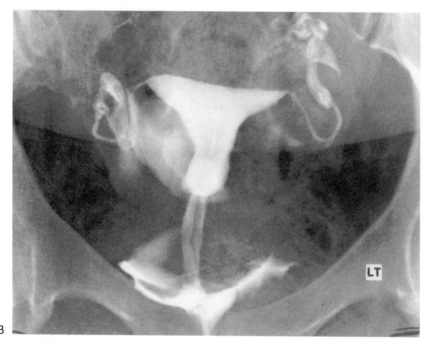

Figure 21.1 A 34-year-old gravida 2, para 2 had a postpartum tubal ligation. She presented 6 months later for tubal reanastomosis. (**A**) The preoperative HSG shows a normal uterine cavity and patent proximal tubal segments. (**B**) Postoperative HSG shows free intraperitoneal spill of dye.

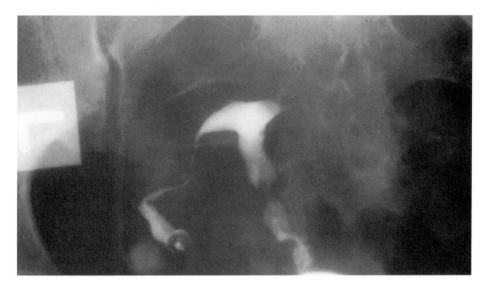

Figure 21.2 A 28-year-old gravida 0, para 0 with infertility whose HSG shows left distal tubal occlusion and right proximal occlusion. The patient presented 12 hours after the HSG with abdominal pain, tenderness, and fever. She was hospitalized with a diagnosis of salpingitis and treated with parenteral antibiotics.

Vascular or lymphatic intravasation occurs when the contrast penetrates the uterine musculature, blood vessels, or lymphatics.[26] This has been described in as many as 6% of cases.[27] The theoretical danger is embolism, but, with the use of water-soluble media, this hazard is almost nonexistent.[8] The most common cause of this complication is inadvertent insertion of the cannula into the myometrium and excessive injection pressure.[7] Predisposing factors for intravasation are recent uterine surgery, endometrial scarring, fibrosis, and ulcerations[8,9] (Fig. 21.3). If intravasation is suspected during the examination, the procedure should be immediately interrupted and the patient closely observed.

Embolism of contrast medium is a rare event that is usually not serious but that has been fatal in several cases.[28–31] The consequences depend on the type of intravasation and the type of dye used. Vascular intravasation allows access of con-

Figure 21.3 This 35-year-old woman was exposed to diethylstilbestrol (DES) in utero, which apparently resulted in distortion and scarring of the endometrial cavity. Excessive injection pressure resulted in marked intravasation of dye. The patient was asymptomatic except for pelvic cramping.

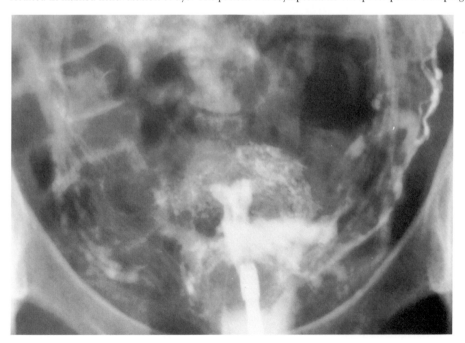

trast medium to other organs, particularly the lungs, heart, kidneys, and brain. Most of the fatalities occurred with the vascular intravasation of oil-soluble medium.[32] Although there was a report of a fatal embolus in 1959 after the use of water-soluble media, this medium contained methylcellulose, and to the best of our knowledge, it is no longer in use.[12] With the use of modern water-soluble media, vascular intravasation is probably dissipated rapidly, without consequence.[8,9] Lymphatic intravasation seems inconsequential.[28]

The amount of radiation to pelvic and abdominal organs during HSG varies depending on the technique, instruments, and experience of the examiner. Gonadal exposure has been estimated at 75 to 1,053 mrad, depending largely on duration of fluoroscopy.[9] Two studies showed no deleterious effects of HSG in undiagnosed early gestations.[33,34] Nevertheless, it is wise to follow the 10-day rule: All diagnostic x-ray examinations should be performed during the first 10 days of the menstrual cycle.[35]

Some rarer complications of HSG have been described. Allergic reactions can range from simple malaise to anaphylactic shock.[36,37] It is possible to perforate the uterus or create a false passage in the cervix.[6] Heavy postoperative bleeding has also been described.[6] There are cases of prolonged retention of the contrast, particularly when oil-soluble medium is used.[38,39] Last, there are rare instances of deranged thyroid function tests resulting from absorption of iodine contained in the medium.[40]

ANATOMY

Normal fallopian tubes are about 6 to 15 cm in length and can be divided into the interstitial, isthmic, ampullary, and infundibular segments.[9] The interstitial portion has a narrow lumen and arises at an oblique angle from the corners of the uterine cavity (cornua). The uterotubal junction consists of thick concentric smooth muscle layers. At this location, the endothelium is ciliated and normally forms villi. The isthmus is lateral to this; it also has a very thin lumen and thick muscular layer. This muscular layer becomes thinner and the mucosal layer more prominent, moving into the distal, ampullary region and eventually the fimbria[9] (Fig. 21.4).

DEVELOPMENTAL ABNORMALITIES

Defects of the müllerian and paramesonephric system are common gynecologic and obstetric findings. It is impossible to know how common they are because these abnormalities are often asymptomatic. The American Society for Reproductive Medicine describes seven classes of abnormalities, based on the uterine configuration.[41] The tubal anomalies may be related to these major uterine anomalies; nevertheless, there are cases of isolated tubal problems, which are apparently congenital. There are no formal classification systems

for tubal anomalies, but they can be thought of as abnormalities of complete tubal absence, partial absence, duplication (partial or complete), and diverticulae.

Unilateral absence of a tube is a common finding in cases of unicornuate uterus.[41] Fertility is generally normal in these women, although there may be obstetric risks such as premature labor. There are also cases where the ipsilateral ovary is absent[42–44] and cases of contralateral gonadal agenesis in which the ovary was surgically transposed.[42] It is unknown whether this represents a developmental failure or in utero adnexal torsion and necrosis. There are also reports of segmental tubal atresia. The midsegment may be absent, with preservation of the proximal and distal segments (Fig. 21.5). Rarely, the distal segment may be absent, as in one case reported of laparoscopic salpingostomy and subsequent pregnancy.[45]

Duplication of part or all of the fallopian tube has also been reported. Series of HSGs or laparoscopies in patients with infertility suggest an incidence between 4% and 10%.[46,47] It is much less common in normally fertile women.[47,48] Accessory tubes are sometimes seen at surgery for elective sterilization[43] or ectopic pregnancy.[46] The pathogenesis is not understood, but these anomalies may result from simultaneous invagination of coelomic epithelium in embryonic life.[43]

Tubal polyps are thought by some authors to be a developmental anomaly wherein there has been partial duplication of the tubal endothelium. They most often occur in the proximal portion of the tube and may be seen in 1% to 3% of HSGs.[49,50] Tubal polyps can arise in the uterus or tube and may sometimes be confused with redundant mucosa. Their significance in the infertile patient is controversial. Microsurgical resection with tubal implantation or reanastomosis has yielded variable results.[49,50]

TUBAL CANCER

The incidence of carcinoma of the fallopian tubes is approximately 0.3% to 1.1% of all gynecologic malignancies.[51] Most cases occur in postmenopausal women, although it has been reported in a patient in her teens. The symptoms are nonspecific and insidious and may include vaginal discharge, abdominal distension, and pelvic pain, usually colicky. Abnormal vaginal bleeding is present in over 50% of patients. There is usually a palpable adnexal mass, which appears on ultrasound or CT as a hydrosalpinx.[52] Abnormalities of the HSG have been reported; usually, there is a hydrosalpinx with irregular borders and internal debris, giving a cloudy or muddy appearance.[53] This is not the best way to make the diagnosis, because of the possibility of spreading malignant cells into the peritoneum.[53] At surgery, the tube usually appears cystically dilated. Adenocarcinoma is by far the most common pathologic finding, although squamous cell, endometrioid, and mixed müllerian tumors have also been reported.[51] Treatment is abdominal hysterectomy and bilateral salpingo-oophorectomy, with adjuvant chemotherapy. Prognosis is

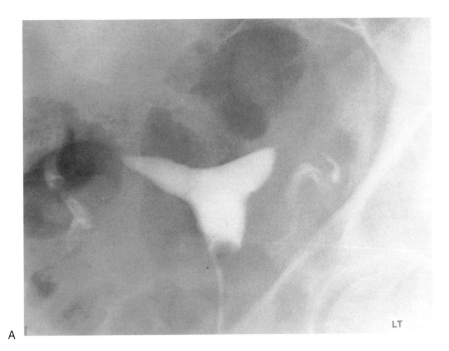

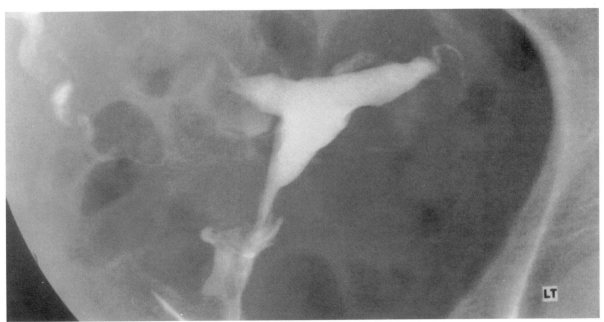

Figure 21.4 This gravida 1, para 1 presented with a 2-year history of infertility and a normal workup. **(A)** Dye in both tubes and a normal rugal pattern. **(B)** Free dispersal of dye through the pelvis.

poor because the tumors are often discovered at an advanced stage.[52]

HYDATID DISEASE

Hydatid cysts are found rarely in the broad ligament or ovary.[54,55] This infection is usually acquired during childhood but only becomes symptomatic 5 to 20 years later, as a result of growth and dissemination of the cysts. Hepatic cysts are often visible as diffuse radiolucent areas on plain x ray. Ultrasound may show fluid-filled masses with internal echoes due to calcification.[56] The reproductive tract is rarely the primary site.

FALLOPIAN TUBE ABNORMALITIES IN INFERTILE PATIENTS

HSG remains the least invasive and most cost-effective means of showing tubal patency. It can also show intraluminal disease not evident at laparoscopy; however, a disadvantage of HSG is that it provides only limited information about peritubal adhesions and none about endometriosis.[57] While some causes of pathology are common to all portions of the tube, there are considerations particular to each segment.

PROXIMAL TUBAL OCCLUSION

Obstruction of the isthmic part of the tube is fairly common. Studies have shown that the incidence ranges from 5% to 20%.[58,59] In this portion of the tube, infertility can be related to fibrosis after infection or endometriosis. The latter occurs in about 10% of proximally occluded tubes and is often present without other pelvic endometriosis.[60] Salpingitis isthmica nodosa (SIN) is commonly seen in this area of the tube.[61] HSG cannot resolve the cause (Fig. 21.6).

SIN is a pathologic entity in which there are nodular areas in the tube, characteristically seen in the proximal or midtubal segments (Fig. 21.7). Histologically, pockets of endosalpinx, or necrotic debris and macrophages, are seen within the muscularis of the tube.[60] The etiology is unknown, but SIN is thought to result from chronic inflammation. The radiographic appearance is quite characteristic, with a webbed pattern of dye around the lumen resulting from the multiple outpouchings into the myosalpinx.[58] A small series of salpingoscopies in these patients showed a 19% incidence of intraluminal abnormalities.[62] Clinically, there is an increased incidence of tubal occlusion and ectopic pregnancy.

The intramural portion of the tube cannot be distinguished from the isthmic portion. Consequently, lesions originating in the uterus such as synechiae, polyps, or fibroids can easily occlude the lumen.[63] Furthermore, the narrow caliber

of the lumen makes it particularly susceptible to obstruction by mucous plugs or amorphous material.

The anatomy here makes it a common location for muscle spasm. The tube arises from two layers of thick smooth muscle, contiguous with the uterus, which sometimes undergo spasm as a result of distension from injection with media. This can be treated by injection of glucagon, a beta sympathomimetic, or a prostaglandin antagonist.[64,65] Some patients have unexplained occlusion. When resection and reanastomosis of obstructed proximal tube was the standard treatment, histopathology showed no abnormality in up to half of these cases.[60] Recent technology has allowed canalization of the tubes with excellent results, diagnostically and therapeutically. Failure to cannulate the tubes is highly suggestive of intrinsic pathology[66] (Fig. 21.8).

ROLE OF SELECTIVE CANNULATION

Hysteroscopic or fluoroscopic guidance is often used to correct tubal obstruction in infertile patients. Selective cannulation has also been used for sterilization, treatment of ectopic pregnancy, and placement of gametes or embryos in assisted reproduction. The latter are usually performed under sonographic guidance.[67] Technique depends upon patient history and available personnel and equipment.

Fluoroscopically guided tubal cannulation is scheduled in much the same manner as conventional HSG. Prophylactic antibiotics are used, and small doses of midazolam and fentanyl are commonly given during the procedure. A technique using a modified angioplasty balloon catheter, first described by Confino et al.,[68] probably allows for lysis of intratubal ad-

Figure 21.5 This HSG shows the right proximal tubal segment, which ends abruptly. At laparoscopy, the mid portion of the tube was absent. The fimbria appeared normal at laparoscopy.

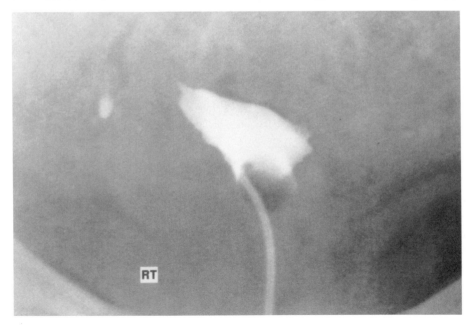

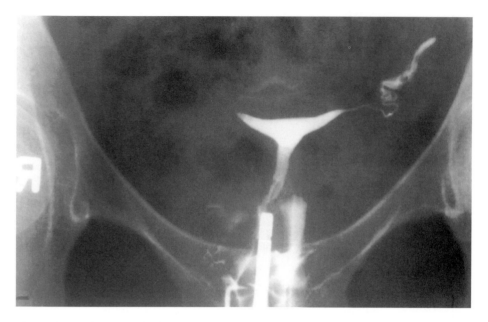

Figure 21.6 This woman had infertility and chronic pelvic pain. This HSG shows occlusion of the right proximal tube. Although fluoroscopically directed cannulation of the right tube was successful, the patient went to surgery 6 months later because of pain and continued infertility. There were endometrial adhesions from the proximal tube to the ovary.

Figure 21.7 This patient was infertile after partial salpingectomy for a right ectopic pregnancy. HSG shows typical SIN in the remaining right tubal segment. There was also subtle evidence of SIN in the left proximal tube, although it was clearly patent. IVF was suggested.

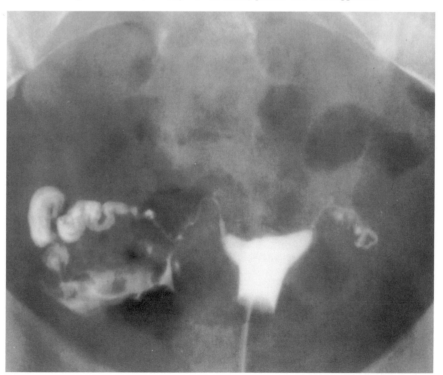

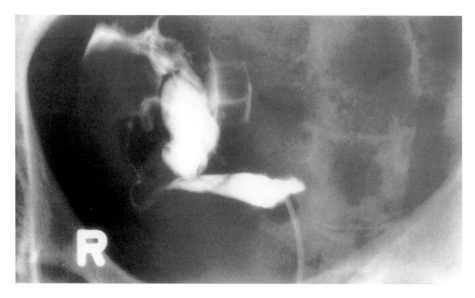

Figure 21.8 This 32-year-old woman had chronic anovulation and infertility. When HSG showed loculated spill of dye from the right tube and proximal occlusion of the left tube, hysteroscopic cannulation was recommended. Laparoscopy, performed concurrently, showed dense adhesions around the right tube and a nodular, convoluted left tube, suggestive of SIN. Hysteroscopic cannulation was not successful.

hesions and dilatation of the cornua and tubal isthmus. Another method developed by Thurmond et al.[69] used a system of coaxial catheters and guidewires to canalize the tube. Both methods result in successful cannulation in 85% to 90% of obstructed tubes.[8] Pregnancy rates with either method range between 7% and 39%. Ectopic pregnancies are reported in 5% to 13% of cases.[67–69] This may reflect underlying pathology, as well as damage from the procedure. Reocclusion rates are not known, but there is evidence that the balloon method may maintain patency for longer.[8] Complications are similar to those with HSG, except for a tubal perforation rate of 2% to 5%.[67] These injuries usually heal without any intervention.

Hysteroscopic tubal cannulation is usually performed in patients who also need laparoscopy. It is not recommended in an office setting, because of the difficulty in distinguishing relief of obstruction from tubal perforation.[70] Laparoscopy is carried out concurrently with operative hysteroscopy. A series of Teflon cannulas are introduced through the operating port of the hysteroscope, once the tubal ostium is visualized. Laparoscopic assistance with a blunt probe is sometimes helpful in straightening the angle of the uterotubal junction. Tubal patency rates and pregnancy rates are similar.

TUBAL OCCLUSION: MIDSEGMENT

Isolated midsegment occlusion is uncommon and may result from congenital atresia,[71] inflammation, or peritubal adhesions. Tuberculosis is an important infectious agent in this part of the tube.[72] Although genital tuberculosis is rare, its frequency recently has increased. There is often accompanying

evidence of Asherman Syndrome. The HSG findings are suggestive of SIN, isthmic diverticulosis, and adnexal or lymph node calcification.[8] The tubes may also contain segments of constriction alternating with dilatation. HSG is contraindicated in the presence of acute infection (Fig. 21.9).

Postoperative adhesions with tubal distortion can effect the midtubal segment. Surgery for infertility, myomectomy, and childhood inguinal herniorrhaphy are possibly causative.[72] Ectopic pregnancy is fairly common, and treatment may result in tubal occlusion (Fig. 21.10). There are also reports of untreated, arrested ectopic pregnancies that were found at surgery for midtubal obstruction. Endometriosis at this site is rare. Prognosis with surgery is fair, except for patients with tuberculosis.[73] As with other types of tubal surgery, the risk of subsequent ectopic pregnancy is high.[72]

DISTAL TUBAL OCCLUSION

The distal portion of the fallopian tube is the most common site of occlusive disease. Tubal infection can cause fibrosis, dilatation, and destruction of the normal ciliated epithelial cells that line the tube. Currently, C. trachomatis is the most common organism causing infection. The acute episode is unrecognized in 50% to 80% of women[74] because of its frequently subclinical course. It is also a difficult organism to culture, especially from the cervix. The availability of genetic technologies[16] has supplanted the use of cultures for the detection of the organism when cervical infection is suspected. In many patients with tubal damage, the organism is no longer present in the cervix. While many investigators have shown that C.

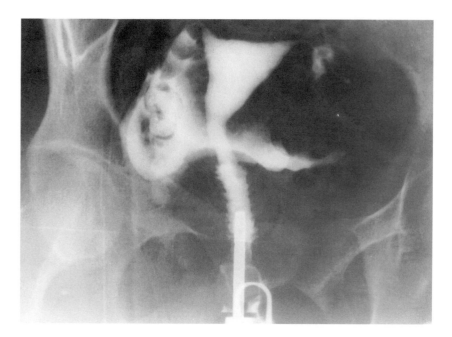

Figure 21.9 This 38-year-old nulligravida acquired genitourinary tuberculosis while living in India. HSG shows dilatation and occlusion of the left tube and loculated spill from the right tube.

trachomatis can reside in the upper genital tract (endometrium and tubes), the invasive methods necessary to do so make this clinically impractical.[24,25] Studies have shown a striking correlation between immunoglobulin G antibodies to *C. trachomatis* and tubal occlusion.[75] It has been suggested that immunoglobulin G antibodies should be used instead of HSG to

screen for tubal disease[76] because of lower cost and noninvasive nature.

Treatment for distal occlusion is either surgery or in vitro fertilization (IVF). Patients with preservation of tubal rugae and normal tubal caliber have a better prognosis at surgery (Figs. 21.11 and 21.12). Absence of peritubal adhesions is also

Figure 21.10 This 28-year-old infertile woman had undergone left midtubal salpingostomy for ectopic pregnancy 2 years before this HSG. In this view, the sharp angulation of the proximal tube and the shortened tubal length are suggestive of peritubal adhesions.

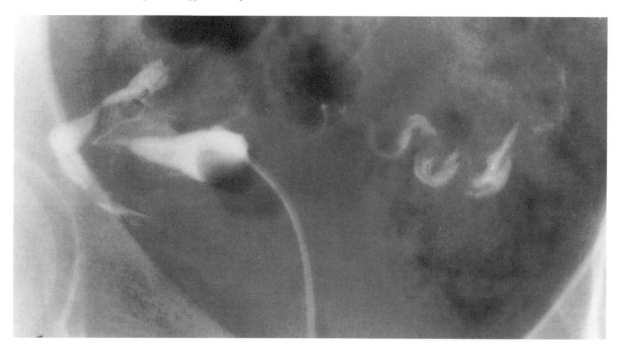

Table 21.2 The American Society for Reproductive Medicine Classification System of Distal Tubal Occlusion.

	<3 cm	3–5 cm	>5 cm
Distal ampullary diameter			
Left	1	4	6
Right	1	4	6
Tubal wall thickness	Normal/thin	Moderately thickened or edematous	Thick and Rigid
Left	1	4	6
Right	1	4	6
Mucosal folds at neostomy site	Normal/>75% preserved	35–75% preserved	<35% Preserved Adherent mucosal fold
Left	1	4	6
Right	1	4	6
Extent of adhesions	None/minimal/mild	Moderate	Extensive
Left	1	3	6
Right	1	3	6
Type of adhesions	None/filmy	Moderately dense (or vascular)	Dense
Left	1	2	4
Right	1	2	4

Prognostic Classification for Terminal salpingostomy (Salpingoneostomy)   Additional Findings _____

		LEFT	RIGHT	
A	Mild	_____ 1.3	_____	
B	Moderate	_____ 9–10	_____	
C	Severe	_____ >10	_____	

(From the American Fertility Society.[81] With permission of the American Society for Reproductive Medicine.)

Figure 21.11 This 32-year-old infertile nulligravida had no risk factors for sexually transmitted diseases. In this HSG, the dilated ampullary portion of the left tube shows some preservation of rugal folds.

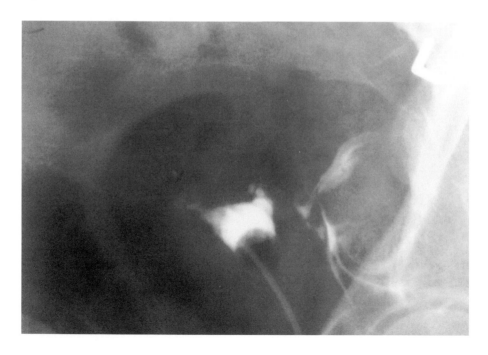

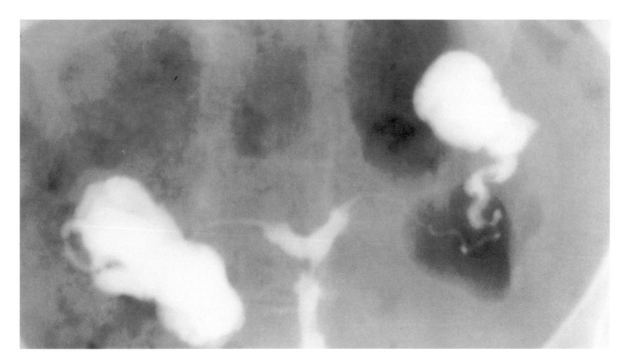

Figure 21.12 In contrast to the patient in Figure 23.10, this 29-year-old woman was exposed to DES in utero and had a right ectopic pregnancy, treated by salpingostomy, prior to this HSG. The configuration of the endometrial cavity and the dilated lower uterine segment are common among patients exposed to DES. This patient also has markedly dilated tubes with absent rugal folds. IVF was recommended.

Figure 21.13 This 27-year-old had a history of chlamydia cervicitis and presented with a 2-year history of infertility. In this view, both tubes are convoluted, and the ampullary segments are dilated. Spillage of dye was seen in subsequent films.

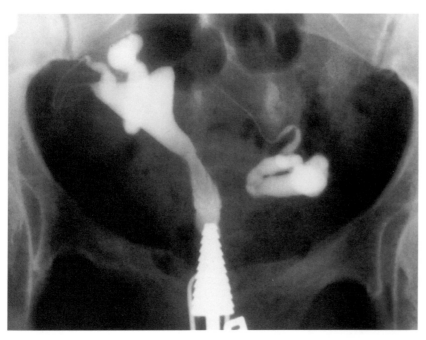

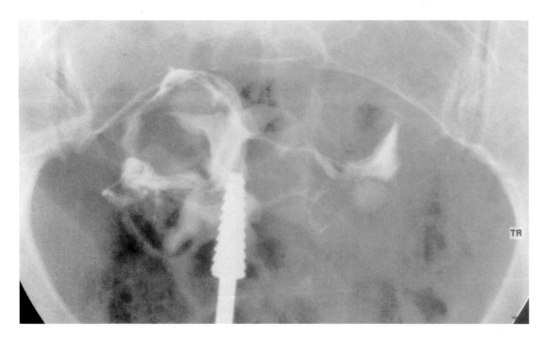

Figure 21.14 There is free spill of dye from the left tube. However, there is a sharply demarcated pool of dye at the right distal tube, which was the site of previous salpingostomy.

important in determining chance of pregnancy[77] (Table 21.2). The recent development of falloposcopy may help to refine radiographic prognostic signs.[78] Hydrosalpinx can also affect prognosis with IVF. It is thought that the tubal secretions somehow dilute the endometrial secretions that are important in embryo implantation.[79]

Peritubal adhesions often mimic distal tubal occlusion. HSG is suggestive in up to 75% of proven cases.[80] Previous infection, surgery, endometriosis, and inflammatory bowel disease are common causes. The HSG findings include tubal convolutions (particularly if fixed in nature), loculated spill of dye, vertical position of the tube, ampullary dilatation, and peritubal halo (double contour appearance of the tube due to pooling of dye around a patent hydrosalpinx) (Figs. 21.13 and 21.14). The latter is especially hard to distinguish from distal tubal occlusion.[80] Endometriosis sometimes causes contraction and scarring of the broad ligament, which causes the tube to appear convoluted. However, there is a high false-negative rate for HSG detection of tubal abnormalities, especially in the diagnosis of peritubal abnormalities.[57]

REFERENCES

1. Maguiness SD, Djahanbakhch O, Grudzinskas JG. Assessment of the fallopian tube. Obstet Gynecol Surv 1992;47:587–603
2. Rindfleisch W. Darstellung des cavum uteri (Imaging of the uterine cavity). Berl Klin Wochenschr 1910;17:780
3. Kaldor J. Achievements of uterosalpingography. Am J Surg 1930;8:1245–1249
4. Rubin IC. Nonoperative determination of patency of the fallopian tubes, by means of intrauterine inflation with oxygen and production of artificial pneumoperitoneum. JAMA 1920;75:661

5. Rubin IC. Uterotubal Insufflation. CV Mosby, St. Louis, 1947, pp 389–412
6. Siegler AM. Dangers of hysterosalpingography. Obstet Gynecol Surv 1967;22:284–308
7. Siegler AM. Hysterosalpingogram. Fertil Steril 1983;40:139–158
8. Yoder IC, Hall DA. Hysterosalpingography in the 1990's. AJR Am J Roentgenol 1991;157:675–683
9. Yoder IC. Techniques, normal anatomy and complications. In: Yoder IC, Ed. Hysterosalpingography and Pelvic Ultrasound. Little, Brown, Boston, 1988, pp 1–35
10. Abramowicz JS, Lewis V. Hysterosalpingography of the normal pelvis. In: Jaffe R, Pierson RA, Abramowicz JS, Eds. Imaging in Infertility and Reproductive Endocrinology. Lippincott, Philadelphia, 1994, pp 313–320
11. Watson A, Vandekerckhove P, Lilford R et al. A meta-analysis of the therapeutic role of oil soluble contrast media at hysterosalpingography: a surprising result? Fertil Steril 1994;61:470–477
12. Winfield AC. Techniques and complications of hysterosalpingography. In: Winfield AC, Wentz AC, Eds. Diagnostic Imaging in Infertility (2nd ed.). Williams & Wilkins, Baltimore, 1992, pp 13–28
13. Dan V, Ezra D, Oelsner G et al. Cerebral embolization and coma after hysterosalpingogram with oil-soluble contrast medium. Fertil Steril 1990;53:939–940
14. Pontifex G, Trichopouolos D, Karpathios S. Hysterosalpingography in the diagnosis of infertility (statistical analysis of 3437 cases). Fertil Steril 1972;23:829–833
15. Jacobson A, Conley JG. Estimation of fetal doses to patients undergoing diagnostic X-ray procedures Radiology 1976;120:683–685
16. Limberger RJ, Biega R, Evancoe A et al. Evaluation of culture and Gen-Probe PACE 2 assay for the detection of Neisseria gonorrhoea and Chlamydia trachomatis in endocervical specimens transported to a state health laboratory. J Clin Microbiol 1992;30:1162–1166

17. Pittaway DE, Winfield AC, Maxson W et al. Prevention of acute pelvic inflammatory disease after hysterosalpingogram: efficacy of doxycycline prophylaxis. Am J Obstet Gynecol 1983;147:623–626

18. Lindequist S, Justesen P, Larsen C, Rasmussen F. Diagnostic quality and complications of hysterosalpingography; oil- versus water-soluble contrast media—a randomized prospective study. Radiology 1991;179:69–74

19. Owens OM, Schiff I, Kaul AF et al. Reduction of pain following hysterosalpingogram by prior analgesic administration. Fertil Steril 1985;43:146–148

20. Lorino CO, Prough SG, Aksel S et al. Pain relief in hysterosalpingography. A comparison of analgesics. J Reprod Med 1990;35:533–536

21. Stumpf PG, March CM. Febrile morbidity following hysterosalpingography: identification of risk factors and recommendations for prophylaxis. Fertil Steril 1980;33:487–492

22. Moller BR, Allen J, Toft B et al. Pelvic inflammatory disease after hysterosalpingography associated with Chlamydia trachomatis and Mycoplasma hominis. Br J Obstet Gynaecol 1984;91:1181–1187

23. Forsey JP, Caul EO, Paul ID, Hull MG. Chlamydia trachomatis, tubal disease and the incidence of symptomatic and asymptomatic infection following hysterosalpingography. Hum Reprod 1990;5:444–447

24. Campbell LA, Patton DL, Moore DE et al. Detection of Chlamydia trachomatis deoxyribonucleic acid in women with tubal infertility. Fertil Steril 1993;59:45–50

25. Shepard MK, Jones RB. Recovery of Chlamydia trachomatis from endometrial and fallopian tube biopsies in women with infertility of tubal origin. Fertil Steril 1989;52:232–238

26. Drukman A, Rozin S. Uterovenous and utero-lymphatic intravasation in HSG. J Obstet Gynaecol Br Emp 1951;58:73–78

27. Norris S. The hysterogram in the study of sterility. Can Med Assoc J 1956;75:1016–1020

28. Zachariae F. Venous and lymphatic intravasation in hysterosalpingography. Acta Obstet Gynecol Scand 1955;34:131–149

29. Levinson JM. Pulmonary oil embolism following hysterosalpingography. Fertil Steril 1963;14:21–27

30. Breitlander K, Hinrich S. Pulmonary embolism following hysterosalpingography with Iodopin (Lungenembolie nach Hysterosalpingographie mittels Jodipin-Reaktionsloser). Zentralbl Gynakol 1941;65:124–129

31. Gajzago E. Ein im Anschluss an Hysterographie durch Olembolie verursachter Todestall. Zentralbl Gynakol 1931;55:543–544

32. Nunley WC, Jr, Bateman BG, Kitchin JD, Pope TL. Intravasation during hysterosalpingography using oil-base contrast medium—a second look. Obstet Gynecol 1987;70:309–312

33. Sternberg J. Irradiation and radiocontamination during pregnancy. Am J Obstet Gynecol 1970;108:490–513

34. Goldenberg RL, White R, Magendantz HG. Pregnancy during the hysterogram cycle. Fertil Steril 1976;27:1274–1276

35. Warrick CK. Radiology now: the "10-day rule." Br J Radiol 1973;46:933–934

36. Capdeville R, Remy J. Un accident majeur d'hysterosalpingographie (A major complication of hysterosalpingography). J Radiol 1983;64:561–562

37. Schuitemaker NW, Helmerhorst FM, Tjon A et al. Late anaphylactic shock after hysterosalpingography. Fertil Steril 1990;54:535–536

38. Malter IJ, Fox RM. Prolonged oviduct retention of iodized contrast medium. Obstet Gynecol 1972;40:221–224

39. Eisenberg AD, Winfield AC, Page DL et al. Peritoneal reaction resulting from iodinated contrast material: comparative study. Radiology 1989;172:149–151

40. Slater S, Paz-Carranza J, Solomons E, Perlmutter M. Effects of HSG on assay of thyroid function. Fertil Steril 1959;10:144–149

41. The American Fertility Society. The AFS classification of adnexal adhesions, distal tubal occlusion, tubal occlusion secondary to tubal ligation, tubal pregnancies, muellerian anomalies, and intrauterine adhesions. Fertil Steril 1988;49:944–955

42. Kim SJ, Cho DJ, Song CH. Ovarian transposition with subsequent intrauterine pregnancy. Fertil Steril 1993;59:468–469

43. Venyo AKG. Supernumerary fallopian tubes. Br J Obstet Gynaecol 1993;100:183–188

44. Sirsenia LA. Unexplained absence of an ovary and uterine tube. Postgrad Med J 1978;54:443–444

45. McBean JH, Brumstead JR. Pregnancy after laparoscopic neosalpingostomy in a patient with atresia of the distal fallopian tubes. Fertil Steril 1994;61:1163–1164

46. Beyth Y, Koplovic J. Accessory tubes: a possible contributing factor in infertility. Fertil Steril 1982;38:382–383

47. Yablonski M, Sarge T, Wild RA. Subtle variations in tubal anatomy in infertile women. Fertil Steril 1990;54:455–458

48. Coddington CC, Chandler PE, Smith GW. Accessory fallopian tube. A case report. J Reprod Med 1990;35:420–421

49. Gordts S, Boeckx W, Vasquez G, Brosens I. Microsurgical resection of intramural tubal polyps. Fertil Steril 1983;40:258–259

50. Stangell JJ, Chervenak FA, Mouradian-Davidian M. Microsurgical resection of bilateral tube polyps. Fertil Steril 1981;35:580–582

51. Cheung AN, So KF, Ngan HY, Wong LC. Primary squamous cell carcinoma of fallopian tubes. Int J Gynaecol Pathol 1994;13:92–95

52. DiSaia PJ, Creasman WT. Carcinoma of the fallopian tube. In: DiSaia PJ, Creasman WT, Eds. Clinical Gynecologic Oncology (4th ed.). Mosby Year Book, St. Louis, 1993, pp 458–466

53. Robey M, Goiran JP, Robey F, Salleron A. L'adenocarcinome de la trompe de Fallope. J Gynecol Obstet Biol Reprod (Paris) 1972;1:581–590

54. Khan JS, Steele RJC, Stewart D. Enterobius infestation of the female genital tract causing generalized peritonitis. Br J Obstet Gynaecol 1981;88:681–683

55. McMahon JN, Connolly CE, Long SV, Meehan FP. Enterobius granulomas of the uterus, ovary and pelvic peritoneum. Two case reports. Br J Obstet Gynaecol 1984;91:289–290

56. Kammerer WS, Schantz PM. Echinococcal disease. Infect Dis Clin North Am 1993;7:605–618

57. Johnson WK, Ott DJ, Chen MY et al. Efficacy of hysterosalpingography in evaluating endometriosis. Abdom Imaging 1994;19:278–280

58. Yoder IC. Diseases of the fallopian tube. In: Yoder IC, Ed. Hysterosalpingography and Pelvic Ultrasound. Little, Brown, Boston, 1988, pp 37–82

59. Thurmond AS, Novy M, Rosch J. Terbutaline in diagnosis of interstitial fallopian tube obstruction. Invest Radiol 1988;23:209–210

60. Sulak PJ, Letterie GS, Coddington CC et al. Histology of proximal tubal occlusion. Fertil Steril 1987;48:437–440

61. Clent PB. Diseases of the peritoneum. In: Kurman RJ, Ed.

Blaustein's Pathology of the Female Genital Tract (4th ed.). Springer-Verlag, New York, 1994, pp 647–703

62. Gurgan T, Urman B, Yarali H et al. Salpingoscopic findings in women with occlusive and nonocclusive salpingitis isthmica nodosa. Fertil Steril 1994;61:461–463

63. Lewis V, Abramowicz JS. Hysterosalpingography of the abnormal pelvis. In: Jaffe R, Pierson RA, Abramowicz JS, Eds. Imaging in Infertility and Reproductive Endocrinology. Philadelphia, JB Lippincott, 1994, pp 321–333

64. Winfield AC, Pittaway D, Maxson W et al. Apparent cornual occlusion in HSG: reversal by glucagon. AJR Am J Roentgenol 1982;139:525–527

65. Lang EK. Organic vs functional obstruction of the fallopian tubes: differentiation with prostaglandin antagonist- and beta 2-agonist-mediated hysterosalpingography and selective ostial salpingography. AJR Am J Roentgenol 1991;157:77–80

66. Letterie G, Sakas EL. Histology of proximal tubal obstruction in cases of unsuccessful canalization. Fertil Steril 1991;56:831–835

67. Jansen RPS, Anderson JC, Sutherland P. Non-operative embryo transfer to the fallopian tubes. N Engl J Med 1988;319:288–291

68. Confino E, Friberg J, Gleicher N. Transcervical balloon tuboplasty. Fertil Steril 1986;46:963–966

69. Thurmond AS, Novy M, Uchida BT, Rosch J. Fallopian tube obstruction: selective salpingography and recanalization. Radiology 1987;163:511–514

70. Thurmond AS, Novy MJ. Transcervical fallopian tube catheterization for management of proximal tube obstruction. In: Winfield AS, Wantz AC, eds. Diagnostic Imaging and Infertility. Williams & Wilkins, Baltimore, 1992, pp 192–207

71. Richardson DA, Evans MI, Talerman A, Maroulis GB. Segmental absence of the fallopian tube. Fertil Steril 1982;37:577–579

72. Urman G, Gomel V, McComb P, Lee N. Midtubal occlusion: etiology, management and outcome. Fertil Steril 1992;57:747–750

73. Saracoglu OF, Mungan T, Tanzer F. Pelvic tuberculosis. Int J Gynaecol Obstet 1992;37:115–120

74. Thejls H, Rahm VA, Rosen G, Gnarpe H. Correlation between chlamydia infection and clinical evaluation, vaginal wet smears and cervical swab test in female adolescents. Am J Obstet Gynecol 1987;157:974–976

75. Minassian SS, Wu CH. Chlamydia antibody by enzyme-linked immunosorbent assay and associated severity of tubal factor infertility. Fertil Steril 1992;58:1245–1247

76. Dabekausen YA, Evers JL, Land JA, Stals FS. Chlamydia trachomatis antibody testing is more accurate than hysterosalpingography in predicting tubal factor infertility. Fertil Steril 1994;61:833–837

77. Donnez J, Nisolle M, Casanas-Roux F et al. Carbon dioxide laser laparoscopic surgery: adhesiolysis, salpingostomy and fimbrioplasty. In: Donnez J, Nisolle M, Eds. An Atlas of Laser Operative Laparoscopy and Hysteroscopy. Parthenon, New York, 1994, pp 97–113

78. Kerin J, Daykhovsky L, Segalowitz J et al. Falloposcopy: a microendoscopic technique for visual exploration of the human fallopian tube from the uterotubal ostium to the fimbria using a transvaginal approach. Fertil Steril 1990;54:390–400

79. Anderson AN, Yue Z, Meng FJ, Petersen K. Low implantation rate after in-vitro fertilization in patients with hydrosalpinges diagnosed by ultrasonography. Hum Reprod 1994;9:1935–1938

80. Karasick S, Goldfarb AF. Peritubal adhesions in infertile women: diagnosis with hysterosalpingography. AJR Am J Roentgenol 1989;152:777–779

81. The American Fertility Society. The American Society for Reproductive Medicine classification systems of distal tubal occlusion. Fertil Steril 1988;49:944–955

22

Ultrasonography of the Ovary

ANIL TAILOR

ELISABETH HACKET

THOMAS BOURNE

It has never been easier to study the ovary. The recent development of relatively noninvasive imaging techniques such as ultrasound and laparoscopy and the development of ovarian hormone assays have enabled great progress to be made in the study of ovarian pathophysiology. The ovaries have previously been misunderstood because of their inaccessability. For example, in 400 BC, Hippocrates thought that the ovaries were the female equivalents of testes, with the right ovary producing male offspring and the left ovary producing females. Aristotle was even further from the truth in believing that the female had no seed. Following these early observations, it was almost 2,000 years before Versalius described the follicle in his famous work *De Fabrica* in 1543. In later editions, he was probably referring to the corpus luteum when he described a structure within the ovary as being "like a rather large pea full of a yellow fluid." Niels Stenson in 1667 in his *Myologiae* finally made the observation that the human ovary contains eggs, confirming that their function may be similar to that of the ovaria in birds. The first pathologic ovary was described by Matthew Braille in 1789 (a benign teratoma), and the first oophorectomy was reported in 1809 by Ephraim McDowell. A formal study of ovarian pathology using ultrasound was first reported by Donald and colleagues in 1958.[1] Transvaginal ultrasound has since been developed to give high-resolution images of the ovary and a better understanding of the ovarian cycle. An ultrasound image does not provide a histologic diagnosis; it can only give an indication of the risk of the particular pathology being present. Ultrasound findings must be considered in relation to the clinical picture and may well alter the patient's management, particularly with the option of minimal access surgical techniques. Depending on the risk of malignancy as judged by the ultrasonologist, the appropriate management could be laparotomy by a gynecologic oncologist, laparoscopic surgery by a gynecologist, or simply observation. Accurate assessment of the ovarian cyst found incidentally in an asymptomatic woman is necessary to avoid unnecessary surgical intervention. An examination of the ovary using ultrasound can clearly only be of value if it changes the management of the patient and leads to an improved clinical outcome.

This chapter concentrates on the ultrasound criteria of benign and malignant lesions and the evaluation of the relative risk of any ovarian mass harboring a malignancy. It then focuses on some specific examples of ovarian pathophysiology.

GRAY SCALE IMAGING OF THE ABNORMAL OVARY

Transabdominal sonography (TAS) is useful for the evaluation of large tumors extending beyond the range of a vaginal probe, but the limited resolution does not provide accurate morphologic information. For this, we rely on high-resolution transvaginal sonography (TVS).

The appearance of any adnexal mass can be described in terms of the following: the size or volume of the lesion; the number of cysts (monocystic or multicystic); the number of locules for a given cyst (unilocular or multilocular) (Fig. 22.1); echogenicity (hyperechoic, hypoechoic or anechoic); cyst outline (regular or irregular); papillary projections (presence or absence) (Fig. 22.2); wall thickness; septal thickness; echo-dense foci (presence or absence); acoustic shadowing; mobility of the lesion; and finally, the presence or absence of ascites. The presence of hydronephrosis, intrahepatic lesions, or other intra-abdominal masses is clearly relevant.

The Size of a Lesion

Ovarian size can be measured in three perpendicular planes and the volume calculated according to the formula for a prolate ellipsoid ($\pi/6 \times D_1 \times D_2 \times D_3$). In clinical practice, the largest diameter is usually used as the most convenient index; furthermore, it is associated with little interobserver variability. The risk of malignancy rises with increasing tumor size. Granberg and colleagues[2] reported the macroscopic naked eye appearances of a series of ovarian tumors that had been removed from both pre- and postmenopausal women. They described 1,017 tumors, of which 789 (77.6%) were benign, 25 (2.5%) were borderline, and 203 (20.0%) were malignant.

319

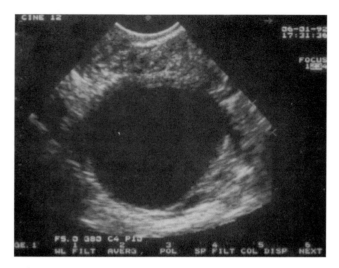

Figure 22.1 A persistent simple anechoic unilocular cystic lesion of less than 5.0 cm in diameter in a postmenopausal women. The risk of malignancy is very low. Histology for this lesion was shown to be a serous cystadenoma. Although surgery was performed, it might be argued that in view of the ultrasound appearances it was not necessary.

The tumors were divided into three categories based on their maximum diameters: less than 5 cm, 5 to 10 cm, and greater than 10 cm. Ninety four percent of the tumors less than 5 cm were benign, 8 (2.2%) were borderline, and 14 (3.8%) were malignant. When lesions are measured using ultrasonography, similar results are obtained. Granberg et al.[3] performed preoperative TVS on 180 masses in both pre- and post-menopausal women. One hundred and forty one (78%) were benign, and 39 (21%) were malignant. Of the 54 tumors that measured less than 5 cm, only 1 was malignant. Similar findings have been reported by Sassone et al.[4] who found that

Figure 22.2 A persistent cystic lesion of less than 5.0 cm in a postmenopausal woman. There is a large papillary projection present in the cavity. This is an ominous morphologic sign. Histology revealed a cystadenocarcinoma.

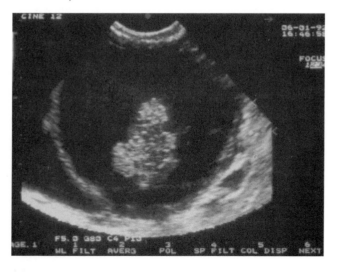

97% of masses less than 5 cm were benign, irrespective of menopausal status.

The survey of ovarian cyst histology by Granberg et al.[2] also demonstrated how the risk of malignancy rises with increasing cyst size. This study shows a positive predictive value for malignancy of 5.9% for cysts less than 5 cm, 21.3% from 5 to 10 cm, and 43.6% if over 10 cm. On the basis of these data, it seems unwise to apply morphologic or Doppler criteria for malignancy for swellings greater than 10 cm in diameter and possibly also for those between 5 and 10 cm. The data derived from ultrasonography are more variable. Granberg et al.[3] reported that the risk of malignancy for lesions over 10 cm was as high as 71.8%, but the data of Sassone et al.[4] suggest that the risk is of the order of 12.5%. This discrepancy can be largely explained by the different prevalence of malignancy in the two series: 21.7% in the former and 5% in the latter. Others have stratified their data according to menopausal status.[5,6] Their findings reflect the prevalence of malignancy seen in the postmenopausal population (Table 22.1). Notwithstanding these limitations, the probability of malignancy associated with tumors over 10 cm is too high for conservative management, irrespective of the morphologic or color Doppler appearances. Furthermore, tumors of this size are unsuitable for morphologic or evaluation, as they extend beyond the depth of penetration of most vaginal ultrasound probes. When the lesion is less than 5.0 cm, the risk of malignancy is relatively low, and other gray scale features or Doppler information can be used to clarify the situation. Between 5 and 10 cm, the management is controversial. If the entire cyst structure can be visualized by TVS, then a morphologic or Doppler evaluation may be a reasonable strategy. If not, the risk of malignancy must be of concern. For these reasons, morphologic and Doppler assessment are only relevant to ovarian lesions under 5.0 cm. For larger lesions, more detailed ultrasound findings are unlikely to alter the management of the patient.

The management of the special but common case of an absolutely simple cyst in a woman of reproductive age is controversial when considering whether to monitor sonographically, aspirate under ultrasound guidance, or excise via a laparotomy. When these cysts are large (>10 cm in diameter), it can be difficult to be certain that the entire cyst wall is thin and regular, especially when some regions may be beyond the focal region of the ultrasound probe for an adequate examination. For cysts less than 10 cm, aspiration may be successful in dealing with a proportion of them,[7–9] however, caution is required in interpreting these data. The "gold standard" for assuming that all these cysts were benign relies upon the finding that none of these women developed a malignancy in the ovary treated by aspiration after 1 or 2 years[7] follow-up. It is also reassuring that the cytology of the aspirated fluid was benign. Given the paucity of knowledge of the natural history of ovarian cancer and the observation that ovarian cyst fluid cytology does not correlate well with histology, this clinical problem will continue to vex clinicians. Similar but smaller (< 5 cm) cysts in postmenopausal women also present difficulties in manage-

Table 22.1 Positive Predictive Value of Size in Differentiating Benign From Malignant Ovarian Tumors

Author	Population	N	Prevalence of Malignancy (%)	Positive Predictive Value		
				<5 cm	5–10 cm	>10 cm
Granberg et al 1989[2]	All ages	1,017	22.4	5.9	21.3	43.6
Granberg et al 1990[3]	All ages	180	21.7	1.9	11.5	71.8
Sassone et al 1991[4]	All ages	200	5.0	3.3	7.2	12.5
Moyle et al 1983[103]	All ages	106	30.1	22.2[a]	14.6[b]	42.9
Luxman et al 1991[5]	Postmenopausal	102	28.4	13.9	35.6	38.1
Rulin and Preston,[6] 1987	Postmenopausal	150	31.3	3.1	10.9	63.5
Rulin and Preston[6] and Luxman et al[5] (combined)	Postmenopausal	257	30.0	8.7	22.0	57.1
Bourne et al 1993[18]	Familial ovarian cancer (all ages)	61	9.8	9.8	—	—

[a] <4 cm

[b] 4–10 cm

ment. Little is known about the natural history of these cysts in this population who are more likely to harbor a malignancy by virtue of their age. Kroon and Andolf[10] studied 32 postmenopausal women with these small simple cysts followed up for a period ranging from 1 to 9 years. The authors reported that 12 of these cysts disappeared completely, 1 increased in size, and none had been diagnosed with a malignancy in the intervening period. It was concluded that stationary lesions could be monitored sonographically and that surgery should be reserved for those who are symptomatic or have a past or family history of ovarian, breast, or colon cancer (Table 22.1).

Locules and Septa

A loculated cyst is one that is divided into compartments by septa. It may be difficult to distinguish a loculated cyst from a multicystic ovary, which contains a number of separate cysts. The commonly used term of *simple cyst* refers to a unilocular cyst with no irregular features (Fig. 22.3). In contrast, the term *complex cyst* refers to a cyst that has all or a combination of features such as multicysts, multiloculations, and/or the presence of papillary projections. Published data show that multilocular lesions are more likely to be malignant and were initially reported in 69 patients.[11] Unilocular cysts were present in 42 (61%) and multilocular lesions in 27 (39%). Two (5%) of the unilocular cysts and 16 (59%) of the multilocular cysts were subsequently shown to be malignant. TAS was used, so the results must be interpreted with caution. Complex cysts are more likely to be malignant, as shown by Granberg et al.[2] This study included 499 (49%) unilocular, 438 (43%) multilocular, and 80 (8%) solid tumors. Only 5 of the unilocular cysts harbored malignant or borderline pathology (1%), compared to 191 (44%) of those described as multilocular. Of the 80 solid tumors, 32 (39%) were malignant or borderline. The data show the tendency toward malignancy with increasing morphologic complexity, but with much

overlap. Attempts to produce weighted morphology scoring systems must therefore carry an inherent risk of missing cancer. The study by Granberg et al.[3] of 180 tumors examined by TVS confirmed these findings. Two earlier studies using TAS that classified lesions as unilocular or complex cysts also showed the relatively low risk of malignancy associated with unilocular cysts (1.8% to 2.6%).[12,13] With complex cysts, however, 24.2% were malignant in one study[13] and 72.7% in another.[13] The data from these are summarized in Table 22.2.

If size of the lesion is included as a variable as well as the presence or absence of solid papillary projections, more useful information can be extracted. In both (histology and ultrasonography-based) studies by Granberg et al.[2,3] that have been discussed, none of the unilocular lesions less than 5 cm

Figure 22.3 A simple, anechoic, unilocular ovarian cyst. The lesion measures less than 3.0 cm in its largest diameter. As long as the entire cyst wall has been surveyed, the risk of cancer in such a persistent lesion is low.

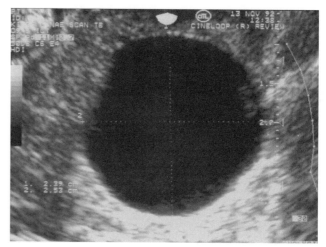

Table 22.2 Positive Predictive Value of Locularity in Differentiating Benign From Malignant Ovarian Tumors

Author	Year	Population	N	Prevalence of Malignancy (%)	Positive Predictive Value (%)		
					Unilocular	Multilocular	Solid
Granberg et al[2]	1989	All ages	1,017	22.4	1.0	40.3	39.2
Granberg et al[3]	1990	All ages	180	21.7	1.8	37.4	12.5
Valentin et al[14]	1994	All ages	149	18.8	5.8	17.9	57.9
Meire et al[11]	1978	All ages	69	26.1	4.8	59.3	—
					Unilocular	Complex	
Hermann et al[12]	1987	All ages	206	18.0	1.8	24.2	
Deland et al[13]	1979	All ages	60	28.3	2.6	72.7	
Luxman et al[5]	1991	Postmenopausal	102	28.4	6.1	39.1	
Bourne et al[18]	1993	Familial ovarian cancer (all ages)	61	9.8	0	15.4	

were malignant (Table 22.3). Table 22.2 shows that while the overall positive predictive value toward malignancy for a multilocular lesion with any size is 37.4%, if it is 10 cm or more, the risk of malignancy exceeds 90% (Table 22.3).

The data suggest that the only lesion that is associated with a very low risk of malignancy is one that is simple, unilocular, and less than 5.0 cm in size. Any variation in size or morphology is associated with an increased risk of malignancy.

Papillary Projections

Papillary projections from the cyst wall into the lumen are the result of localized overgrowth of epithelium (Fig. 22.4). Histology usually reveals stroma of variable density covered by tall columnar epithelium. The entire cyst wall must be examined to exclude papillary projections. Subtle irregularities of the wall of a cyst may be difficult to identify.

The significance of papillary projections has always been recognized, even with the rudimentary ultrasound equipment available in the early 1970s, and is the feature most strongly associated with malignancy. Returning to the data of Granberg et al.[2] 152 of 1,017 tumors showed macroscopic evidence of papillary projections. Of these, 81 (53%) were ei-

ther malignant or borderline. In their subsequent study, ultrasound tended to overdiagnose the presence of papillary projections. These were reported in 51 tumors by ultrasonography compared to 43 on macroscopic examination of removed tissues. The associated risk of malignancy in these 43 cases was 67%.[3] With TAS, Meire et al.[11] found that 83% of the tumors with solid projections in their series were cancers, and Valentin et al.[14] also showed the high risk of malignancy associated with papillary projections demonstrable with TVS (Table 22.4). The likelihood of malignancy increases with the number of such irregularities present,[3] but a persistent

Figure 22.4 A magnified view of the wall of a lesion that was found to be a stage 1 mucinous cystadenocarcinoma. Note the scale on the left, this projection is only 3.0 mm across, but is irregular. This underlines the importance of fully assessing the entirety of a cyst wall. If the lesion is obscured or out of range of the probe being used, morphology must not be used to characterize a lesion.

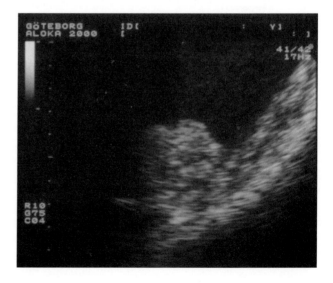

Table 22.3 Positive Predictive Value of Size and Locularity in Differentiating Benign From Malignant Ovarian Tumors

Size	Probability of Malignancy (%)		
	Unilocular	Multilocular	Solid
<5 cm	0	7.7	0
5–10 cm	0	17.3	9.1
>10 cm	11.1	92.3	75.0

(From Granberg et al.,[3] with permission.)

Table 22.4 Positive and Negative Predictive Values of the Presence of Papillary Projections in Differentiating Benign From Malignant Ovarian Tumors

Author	Year	N	Number With Papillary Projections	Percentage of Cystic Tumors With Papillary Projections	Positive Predictive Value	Negative Predictive Value
Granberg et al[2]	1989	1,017	152	16.2	53.3	85.4
Granberg et al[3]	1990	180	43	29.7	67.4	94.1
Meire et al[11]	1978	69	18	26.1	83.3	94.1
Valentin et al[14]	1994	149	42	32.3	40.5	89.7

cyst with even one papillary projection should be removed because of the risk of malignancy.

Wall and Septal Thickness

It is difficult to standardize the measurements of cyst wall and septal wall thickness and to recognize these structures consistently. Benign ovarian cysts are more likely to have thin and smooth septa compared to the thick irregular septa associated with malignancy.[15] A thick septum has been arbitrarily defined as one greater than 3.0 mm (Fig. 22.5). Using this cutoff, Meire and colleagues[11] found that, of 27 multilocular lesions, 19 had thin septa and 8 thick septa. Nine (47%) of those with thin septa and seven (88%) with thick septa were malignant.[11] Sassone *et al.*[4] incorporated these features into a morphologic scoring system but with limited success. False-positives arose with benign teratomas and endometriomas. Of the 24 benign teratomas, over 50% had thick walls. This led the same group to another scoring system that retained a score for septal thickness but excluded wall thickness.[16]

Overall, the current data do not support the use of septal thickness as a variable. This is understandable, given that cancer does not develop in a linear fashion. If we overempha-

size these measurements, it may be that the earliest, "simplest looking" cancers will be missed when they are most curable.

Echo-Dense Foci and Acoustic Shadowing

Echo-dense foci are areas within the lesion that appear almost white on the gray scale image because they are highly reflective. They may represent dystrophic calcification near necrotic areas or calcific densities such as teeth within a dermoid cyst (benign teratoma). These foci usually cause acoustic shadowing that is suggestive of a benign teratoma. Gas within bowel is also highly reflective and casts an acoustic shadow and can be mistaken for a dermoid. Lerner and colleagues[16] introduced this feature in their new morphology scoring system, weighting it so that lesions scored lower if they had shadowing. This was intended to offset the high scores of benign teratomas with mixed echogenicity, irregular cyst outline, and thick walls.[4] Their results showed that, although 86.2% of the teratomas had shadowing, 28.6% of malignant and borderline tumours also shadowed, so calcifications cannot be seen as entirely reassuring.[16]

This shows the difficulty of rigidly adhering to objective scoring systems. Most teratomas would be diagnosed by sub-

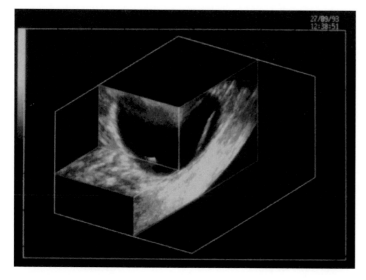

Figure 22.5 Three-dimensional ultrasound image showing a small septum. Very occasionally a small morphologic defect such as this will be more easily detected using this new technology. This lesion was a serous cystadenoma. The septum is thin, but it is not possible to be categoric about the size of a particular septum and the risk of carcinoma.

jective assessment, without need to resort to morphologic scoring systems.

Echogenicity of the Lesion

Serous fluid within an ovarian cyst is virtually anechoic and appears black on ultrasound (Fig. 22.3). In contrast, cysts containing mucinous fluid may have a faint homogeneous gray appearance due to low-level echoes and yet still appear less echoic than the surrounding stromal element of the ovary. A collection of blood or pus tends also to be homogeneously hypoechoic and is often described as having a "ground-glass" appearance, a feature common to endometriomas. There is often acoustic enhancement posteriorly because the lesion contains fluid. Solid elements in an enlarged ovary will tend to have a heterogeneous hyperechoic appearance and have shadowing or no effect posteriorly.

The relative echogenicity of an ovarian lesion is important in almost all scoring systems, with completely anechoic lesions scoring low and heterogeneously hyperechoic lesions scoring high. Moyle and colleagues[17] reported a retrospective study of 106 ovarian neoplasms scanned transabdominally. Six percent of anechoic lesions were found to be malignant compared to 35% of those with mixed hypoechoic and hyperechoic areas. Echogenicity is a helpful indicator for predicting malignancy, but like many of the other morphologic characteristics described above, it cannot be used alone.

Persistence of the Lesion

The most important second-stage test is a repeat scan to determine whether a lesion is persistent or not. This is particularly so in women of reproductive age when functional cysts may mimic malignancy but then resolve with time. An example of this is in the familial cancer screening study performed by Bourne et al.[18] Of 1,601 women screened, only 692 (43%) underwent just one scan; the remainder had serial scans. Sixty one (3.8%) finally underwent surgery, as the cysts resolved in many of the remainder. A repeat scan should always be performed even in postmenopausal women, as transient bowel masses can be confused with ovarian masses, but they do not persist. Some women undergoing surgery for pelvic masses may benefit from a preoperative scan.

MORPHOLOGY SCORING SYSTEMS

It should be possible to decide whether a cyst is simple, unilocular, anechoic, and lacking septa and papillary projections. Provided the whole lesion has been visible and is within the focal range of the vaginal probe, it is most unlikely to be malignant. If any atypical morphologic features are present, the risk of malignancy increases. Attempts have been made to allocate scores to morphologic features and correlate the total score with the risk of malignancy. Such an approach must be of concern, given the lack of understanding of the natural history of ovarian pathology. It is not known whether a thin septum grows thick, or an irregular wall becomes a papillary projection and if so, over what time scale.

The morphology index is calculated by adding scores given for various features. The inclusion of continuous variables such as wall thickness means that ranges of values have to be assigned scores, on the assumption that the progression from benign to malignant disease is continuous for that variable.

One of the first attempts to give ultrasound appearances a numeric score was reported by Finkler and colleagues.[19] It was not a true scoring system, in that the numeric index was not calculated by adding individual scores of the characteristics, but rather on the basis of "pattern recognition." A specified score was given to a combination of characteristics; for example, a clear cyst with slightly irregular outline was given a score of 2, and a multilocular or irregular cystic mass with papillary projections was given a score of 8. They chose 7 as a cutoff to indicate malignancy. Of their 37 malignant tumors in 102 patients, this scoring system correctly identified only 23 (62%) of the malignant and 62 (95%) of the benign tumors in the series. Instead of a score, the adnexal masses could have been directly labeled as either malignant or benign according to the same predefined characteristics.

Sassone and colleagues[4] suggested a true scoring system that incorporated four variables: inner wall structure, wall thickness, septal thickness, and echogenicity. After a retrospective analysis of 143 patients with adnexal masses, a cutoff value of 9 was selected in order to achieve 100% sensitivity for the detection of malignancy. This was associated with a relatively high false-positive rate of 17%. Many of the false-positive diagnoses arose from benign teratomas. The scoring system was then applied prospectively to 94 adnexal masses including 16 malignancies.[20] The detection rate for cancer was 94%, the specificity 87%, and positive predictive value 60%. This system was applied to a further series of 36 benign and 27 malignant tumors.[21] Four cancers were missed (a detection rate of 85.2%), and there were 11 false-positive test results for cancer, which reduced the specificity to 69.4% and positive predictive value to 67.6%.

Another version of this scoring system was proposed by Lerner and colleagues[16] with three important differences. The variable called *wall thickness* was replaced by another described as *acoustic shadowing*, the number of categories for each variable was reduced to a maximum of three, and the individual score for each category was reduced. A mass with acoustic shadowing was given a lower score to indicate a reduced probability of malignancy. This was designed to reduce the index score of benign teratomas. They evaluated their new system on 350 masses, of which 31 were malignant. Using a numeric cutoff value of 3, the detection rate for malignancy was 97%. The false-positive rate was 23% and the positive predictive value only 29.4%. Furthermore, in view of the relatively low prevalence of malignant disease in the study population, the data should be interpreted with caution. The surgical stage of the cancers evaluated is another important variable. In the literature, most cancers assessed by scoring systems (and color Doppler) are either at a late stage or the stages are not stated. Little is still known about the morphologic appearances of very early cancers.

Lerner et al.[16] included age as a variable by adding a tenth of the patient's age to the overall score. This reduced the number of false-positive test results and improved the specificity and positive predictive values to 81% and 33.3%, respectively. The mean ages of patients with benign and malignant lesions were 43 and 60 years, respectively, which is consistent with the expected distribution of the disease in the population.

The menopausal status of the patient is a consideration at the time of any scan. This is illustrated clearly in the study by Valentin et al.[14] In their study of 149 women examined preoperatively, 42% were postmenopausal and yet 75% of all the malignant tumors in their series were in this menopausal group.[14]

Perhaps the most clear indication of the performance of the prospective application of morphologic assessments and color Doppler imaging of persistent ovarian masses can be derived from the familial ovarian cancer screening study published by Bourne et al. in 1993.[18] The morphologic scoring system in this study is shown in Table 22.5. It was applied to persistent ovarian masses of less than 5.0 cm maximum diameter. A positive result was defined as a score of 5 or more.

In this study, 1,601 women with a family history of ovarian cancer underwent ovarian cancer screening using TVS.[18] Sixty-one women had a persistent ovarian mass. Six of these were primary ovarian cancers, of which five were FIGO (International Federation of Gynecology and Obstetrics) stage Ia. Therefore, the odds of finding cancer at surgery for women with a positive screen result were about 1:9. After applying the morphology score, the number of false-positive test results was reduced by 89% from 55 to 6. As a result, the odds of finding cancer at surgery for a woman with a positive screen result would have been 1:1. This improvement was gained at the expense of missing a cancer, and the detection rate fell to 83%. If the lesions had just been described as being simple and unilocular or complex as a basis for referral for surgery, the number of false-positive results would have fallen by 40% from 55 to 33. Thus, the odds of finding cancer at surgery would have been 1:6. The performance of different second-stage tests in the Kings College Hospital ovarian cancer screening program are seen in Table 22.6. Another factor regarding this study is the prevalence effect. In a study of a group at risk of developing the disease, the chance of finding cancer at surgery is, by definition, increased, simply because the disease is more common in the group of women studied.

The presence or absence of certain morphologic features may be useful when trying to discriminate between benign and malignant ovarian masses. The use of morphologic scor-

Table 22.5 Morphology Scoring System Used in the Kings College Familial Ovarian Cancer Screening Program

	0	1	2
Number of cysts	—	Monocystic	Multicystic
Number of locules	Unilocular	Multilocular	—
Papillary projections	Absent	—	Present
Cyst outline	Regular	—	Irregular
Echogenicity	Anechoic	Mixed or random	Uniform

(From Bourne et al.,[18] with permission.)

Table 22.6 The Performance of Different Second-Stage Tests in an Ovarian Cancer Screening Program

	Detection Rate	No. of False Positives	Odds[a]
No second-stage test	100%	55 [13]	1:9
Unilocular or complex	100%	33 [nd]	1:6
Morphology score (MS ≥ 5)	83%	6 [1]	1:1
Low PI (≤ 1.0)	80%	13 [0]	1:3
Low PI or MS ≥ 5	100%	15 [1]	2:5

[a] Odds ratio of finding cancer at surgery.

Brackets denote the figures for postmenopausal women.

nd, no data available for postmenopausal women.

(From Bourne et al.,[18] with permission.)

ing systems is associated with a reduction in the detection rate for cancer. The chance of a simple unilocular cyst of less than 5.0 cm diameter being malignant, particularly in a younger woman, appears to be very low indeed (<1.0%). A simple division into simple cysts, which can be treated conservatively, and complex cysts, that cannot, will reduce the false-positive rate for cancer, and be more likely to maintain the detection rate. Extensive use of scoring systems will be associated with missed opportunities to diagnose cancer. Teratomas and endometriomas have such specific morphologic features that they can be characterized on the basis of subjective "pattern recognition." and conservative management is justified.

It was hoped that the addition of color Doppler would assist morphology scoring. Clinically, color Doppler would be useful if it allowed conservative management of complex lesions or, conversely, if it indicated surgery on simple cysts. In our experience, the use of color Doppler has had neither of these effects, despite claims to the contrary.

COLOR DOPPLER IMAGING OF THE ABNORMAL OVARY

Early in the development of ovarian cancer, there are changes in tissue vascularity, induced by angiogenic factors. Studies of transgenic mice have shown that, for at least one type of cancer, angiogenesis occurs during the transition from hyperplasia to neoplasia.[22] In another study, there was a strong correlation between ovarian cancer and the expression of messenger RNA for platelet-derived endothelial growth factor (thymidine phosphorylase).[23]

Doppler techniques have been used in animal models to identify areas of altered vascularization within tumors as small as 50 mg.[24] Vascular morphology was further evaluated by digital angiography, which demonstrated correlation between the site of high velocity, low impedance signals, and the presence of arteriovenous anastomoses.[25]

In humans, too, malignant lesions have high diastolic flow, probably reflecting low impedance distal to the point of sampling. This may be because new vessels associated with a rapidly growing tumor have little vascular tone due to the absence of the tunica media and, as a result, form low impedance shunts. The attempt to characterize benign and malignant lesions on the basis of vascularity arose along with widespread use of transvaginal color Doppler.[26]

One of the first reports on the use of transvaginal color Doppler to discriminate between benign and malignant ovarian lesions was published by Bourne et al. in 1989.[27] Thirty women with no apparent pelvic pathology and 18 women with ovarian tumors were examined. All seven cases of invasive cancer showed evidence of neovascularization with low impedance blood flow. One serous cystadenoma of borderline malignancy did not demonstrate an abnormal blood flow pattern, and there was one false-positive (a benign teratoma). Two of the invasive cancers were at stage Ia, suggesting that Doppler can detect ovarian cancer when it is still confined within the capsule. In this report, a pulsatility index (PI) of less than 1.0 was used as a cutoff to indicate the presence of low impedance vessels suggestive of neovascularization. The fact that this early report contained both one false-positive and one false-negative suggests that the technique was never destined to answer the problem of classifying persistent ovarian lesions. Indeed, this paper has one or two other surprising features. The mean PI for premenopausal ovaries was found to be 4.9. Subsequently, it has been shown that low impedance flow is a common finding through much of the menstrual cycle.[28,29] It seems likely that using equipment with relatively low sensitivity, the authors recorded waveforms from just outside the ovary, rather than the ovary itself. Of the premenopausal women with benign tumors in the study, 20% showed low impedance blood flow.

Since this report,[27] there have been a number of studies of benign and malignant masses using transvaginal color Doppler. Aspects of tumor vascularity that have been described include qualitative features such as a simple assessment of the presence or absence of vascularity, the site of vascularization, and the presence of a notch in the flow velocity waveform. Quantitative data generated from such flow-velocity waveforms have been based on the PI, resistance index, peak systolic velocity, and time-averaged maximum velocity (mean velocity). A summary of some of these studies is presented in Tables 22.7 to 22.9.

The Presence or Absence of Blood Flow

The presence or absence of blood flow is a crude indicator of the likelihood of malignancy and is highly dependent on the sensitivity of the equipment used. Normal high-resistance vascularity is pulsatile with color Doppler. It often disappears in diastole, and the velocity according to the color bar is low. In contrast, vascularity associated with malignancy tends to be disordered and branching in nature, with continuous flow in diastole and high velocities (see Plates 22.1 and 22.2). The difference between presence and absence of flow may be subtle and almost a "feeling" for the presence or absence of cancer. The results of studies that report presence or absence of blood flow are shown in Table 22.7.

The findings are not surprising. Color Doppler detects flow in over 95% of malignant masses as well as from 35% to 90% of benign tumors. The absence of flow seems associated with a low risk of malignancy, but a test with a false-positive rate of over 80% is unacceptable. It is difficult to interpret data that have not been stratified for menopausal status or the stage of the cancers. Another cause of false-positives is the coincidental presence of functional cysts, many of which normally have low-resistance flow. In Plate 22.1, there is a ring of intense vascularity next to a dermoid cyst, and low impedance signals were recorded; however this was because of a coexistent corpus luteum, not the dermoid. Similarly, Plate 22.1 shows a

Table 22.7 Percentage of Ovarian Tumors With Detectable Flow on Color Doppler Examination

Author	Year	N	Prevalence of Malignancy (%)	Percentage with Detectable Flow (%) Benign	Malignant	Positive Predictive Value (%)	Negative Predictive Value (%)
Tekay et al[30]	1992	72	15.3%	44.3	81.8	28.9	94.4
Timor-Tritsch et al[20]	1993	115	13.9%	78.8	100	17.0	100
Wu et al[104]	1994	410	25.1%	34.9	96.1	43.4	97.8
Zanetta et al[31]	1994	80	41.3%	66.0	100	51.6	100
Prompeler et al[41]	1994	83	49.4%	83.3	97.6	53.3	87.5
Valentin et al[14]	1994	149	18.8%	87.6	96.4	20.3	93.8
Chou et al[32]	1994	108	23.1%	59.0	100	42.4	100
Stein et al[33]	1995	170	29.2%	87.0	97.9	30.1	94.1
Tailor et al[107]	1995	47	17.0%	74.3	100	21.6	100

Table 22.8 Use of PI for Differentiating Benign From Malignant Ovarian Tumors

Author	Year	N	Prevalence of Malignancy (%)	Cutoff (PI)	Sensitivity (%)	Specificity (%)	Positive Predictive Value (%)	Negative Predictive Value (%)
Bourne et al[27]	1989	20	40.0	1.0	87.5	91.7	87.5	91.7
Fleischer et al[105]	1991	26	19.2	1.0	100	90.5	71.4	100
Tekay and Joupilla[30]	1992	72	15.3	1.0	100	29.6	32.1	100
Weiner et al[95]	1992	53	32.1	1.0	94.1	97.2	94.1	97.2
Fleischer et al[105]	1993	96	27.1	1.0	88.9	91.3	80.0	95.5
Hamper et al[106]	1993	31	19.4	1.0	66.7	76.0	40.0	90.5
Timor-Tritsch et al[20]	1993	115	13.9	0.62	87.5	97.4	87.5	97.4
Zanetta et al[31]	1994	80	41.3	1.0	97.0	91.5	88.9	97.7
Prompeler et al[41]	1994	83	49.4	0.80	82.9	25.7	79.1	78.8
Kawai et al[35]	1994	109	36.7	1.25	70.0	88.4	77.8	83.6
Stein et al[33]	1995	170	27.6	1.0	67.4	66.4	46.3	82.6
Tailor et al[107]	1995	47	17.0	0.90	87.5	59.0	30.4	95.8

corpus luteum within the wall of a simple ovarian cyst. The corpus luteum had low impedance signals, and the cyst was not malignant.

Color Doppler information must be interpreted with an understanding of the clinical picture as well as the gray scale images. Color Doppler information should be quantified, although a fairly accurate estimate of the likely impedance and peak systolic velocity of an area of flow can be made from the character of the colored area. Normal ovaries are perfused, so the presence of blood flow is nonspecific.

Site of Vascularization

The location of flow within ovarian lesions has been classified as being either central, peripheral, or within a septum or papillary projection. It is said that blood flow in solid projections is particularly ominous, followed by septal flow, with capsular flow more likely in benign cysts. The presence of a papillary projection or septum increases the risk of malignancy, irrespective of the color Doppler findings, and such a mass would warrant surgery irrespective of the Doppler characteristics.

Table 22.9 Use of Resistance Index for Differentiating Benign From Malignant Ovarian Tumors

Author	Year	N	Prevalence of Malignancy (%)	Cutoff (Resistance Index)	Sensitivity (%)	Specificity (%)	Positive Predictive Value (%)	Negative Predictive Value (%)
Kurjak et al[39]	1991	680	8.2	0.4	98.2	99.8	98.2	99.8
Tekay and Joupilla[30]	1992	72	15.3	0.5	45.5	90.1	41.7	91.4
Hata et al[21]	1992	63	42.9	0.72	92.6	52.8	59.5	90.5
Hamper et al[106]	1993	31	19.4	0.5	33.3	80.0	28.6	83.3
Timor-Tritsch et al[20]	1993	115	13.9	0.46	93.8	98.7	93.8	98.7
Wu et al[104]	1994	410	25.1	0.4	68.0	97.4	89.7	90.1
Zanetta et al[31]	1994	80	41.3	0.56	84.8	91.5	87.5	89.6
Prompeler et al[41]	1994	83	49.4	0.5	85.0	77.1	81.0	81.8
Bromley et al[108]	1994	33	36.4	0.6	66.7	81.0	66.7	81.0
Chou et al[32]	1994	108	23.1	0.5	88.0	91.8	84.6	93.8
Stein et al.[33]	1995	170	27.6	0.5	50.0	79.4	51.1	78.7
Tailor et al[107]	1995	47	17.0	0.6	87.5	53.8	28.0	95.5

The significance of flow within septa or papillary projections is not clear. It is common to observe low-velocity flow within a septum even in the absence of cancer (see Plates 22.3 and 22.4). In Plate 22.3, low-velocity flow is seen within the septa of a benign lesion. This contrasts with the high-velocity flow from a septum within a cancer in Plate 22.4. The color bar shows the relative velocities in the lesions.

Many studies have examined the presence or absence of blood flow from the center of ovarian masses; reports show that, for cancers where flow is detectable, 75% to 100% will have central flow, whereas the corresponding figure for benign tumors is from 5% to 40%.[30–35] Relevance of data must be seen in relation to the morphology of the ovarian lesions, because malignant lesions are more likely to have a stromal central component where vascularity could be found.

Peripheral vascularity must be interpreted with caution, as it may arise from outside the ovary or be compounded by movement artifact from the adjacent iliac vessels.

The Presence of a Notch in the Flow-Velocity Waveform

The diastolic notch is a trough that may occur in the flow-velocity waveform at the end of systole and beginning of diastole. A notch is thought to indicate the presence of a smooth muscle media in the vessel wall and high impedance distally, suggesting normal vascularity. Efforts have been made to standardize this feature by suggesting that the difference between the maximum flow at the beginning of diastole and the minimum flow at the end of systole should be at least 10% of the peak systolic velocity (PSV).[14]

A notch is seen in the waveforms of 15% to 90% of benign tumors but in few malignant ones.[14,34,36] The likely explanation for this is that, in the majority of benign tumors, blood flow will be located peripherally and that a pelvic vessel from outside the ovary could be sampled inadvertently. These vessels would be expected to have a notch in the waveform.

Indices of Blood Flow

Pulsatility Index

The relative merits of PI for discriminating benign from malignant ovarian tumors have been reported in several studies and consistently show that the PI is lower in malignant than benign tumors. The overlap between the values is such that discrimination is not perfect. Some benign tumors will exhibit neovascularization to sustain continued growth. Similarly, in malignant tumors, the blood vessels may be invaded by cancerous cells and cause tumor emboli, which in turn may increase the impedance to flow.

The cut off for PI that has been used most commonly is 1.0. Table 22.8 shows parameters of test performance derived from some of these reports. Wide ranges in the detection rate for cancer have been reported, ranging from 67% to 100%. In contrast, the specificity ranges from 26% to 97%. Using the PI

to make a diagnosis must be associated with missing some cancers and wrongly diagnosing some benign tumors as malignant. This emphasizes the point that Doppler information must be considered in combination with the morphologic appearance.

Resistance Index

The difficulties in using the resistance index (RI) for discriminating the benign from the malignant have been similar to those encountered with the use of the PI. While the RI is lower in malignant tumors, considerable overlap has been observed in the ranges for both benign and malignant tumors. Hence, both the sensitivity and specificity are compromised. Most reports have calculated a different cutoff for the RI in order to select the best specificity for a given sensitivity (see Table 22.9). This table shows that the cutoffs have ranged from 0.4 to 0.72.

It is clear from Tables 22.8 and 22.9 that the results obtained using indices of blood flow to discriminate between benign and malignant tumors are far from uniform. The data of Hata et al.[37] suggest that the appropriate cutoff values for indices of impedance to determine normal and abnormal blood flow within the ovary have yet to be determined. In eight cases of ovarian cancer, the mean RI value was 0.503 +/− 0.122. This group was unable to discriminate between the blood flow of a corpus luteum cyst, an endometrioid ovarian cyst, and carcinoma. In one case, internal iliac blood flow was mistaken for blood flow within the ovary. Data from our own clinic (Table 22.10) also demonstrate a clear overlap between the blood flow within normal physiologic ovarian cystic lesions and carcinoma.[38] The use of an arbitrary cutoff value of 0.40 seems likely to result in a number of both false-positive and false-negative results. Kurjak et al.[39] have presented data on color Doppler findings in 624 benign and 56 malignant ovarian masses. Presumed neovascularization was demonstrated in 6 of 7 stage I primary ovarian cancers, and in 48 of 49 of the other malignant lesions in the study. In all of the cases where neovascularization was seen, the RI was again less than 0.40. In our series of 8 cases of stage I ovarian carcinomas, neovascularization was seen in all invasive carcinomas; the details of each case as well as their RI values are seen in Table 22.11.[40] From these data, it can be seen that using a cutoff value of 0.40 would have led to a number of false-negative diagnoses of cancer. In this context, the work of Tekay and Joupilla[30] is of some interest. Their data suggest that the use of arbitrary discriminatory cutoff values of RI and PI does not discriminate between benign and malignant tumors.[30] According to these results, classifying an ovarian tumor on the basis of an RI value of less than 0.4 would detect less than 40% of malignancies. It is difficult to explain the huge discrepancies between studies, especially when the data of Tekay and Joupilla[30] are contrasted with the data of Kurjak et al.[39] covering 14, 317 symptomatic and asymptomatic women. Of the 8,620 asymptomatic women recruited to this study, 7, 495 were premenopausal, yet only one false-positive test result and two false-negative test results were recorded. Given the

Table 22.10 Range of Values for Indices of Intraovarian Blood Flow

Variable	Follicle (Post-Luteinizing Hormone) (n = 12)		Corpora Lutea (n = 30)		Early Invasive Ovarian Cancer (n = 7)	
	Mean	Range	Mean	Range	Mean	Range
RI	0.48	0.36–0.58	0.43	0.28–0.54	0.46	0.33–0.78
PI	0.62	0.39–0.99	0.56	0.30–0.73	0.61	0.40–0.96
Velocity (cm/sec)	26.1	14.3–45.2	43.2	16.1–73.4	44.0	35.2–57.5[a]

[a] n = 3

Kings College Hospital Ovarian Cancer Screening Clinic, 1991

(From Bourne,[26] with permission.)

overlap demonstrated in Table 22.10 between follicles, corpora lutea, and cancer, it is difficult to explain these data which no other group has been able to replicate (Tables 22.10 and 22.11).

PSV and Time-Averaged Maximum Velocity

PSV and time-averaged maximum velocity (TAMXV) are both angle-dependent. When interrogating intratumoral blood vessels, it is not possible to determine the angle of insonation, and hence a correction cannot be achieved. Few data refer to the use of velocity. Fleischer and colleagues[36] found no difference between the PSVs in benign and malignant tumors. Prompeler and colleagues[41] found a difference, with malignant lesions having a PSV of 30 cm/sec or more, with a sensitivity and specificity of 76% and 79%, respectively. Valentin and colleagues[14] also found a significant difference in the peak systolic velocities, and using a cutoff of 12

cm/sec, they were able to achieve a sensitivity and specificity of approximately 93% and 54%, respectively.

TAMXV is a synonym of the mean velocity during one cycle of systole and diastole. Evaluation of TAMXVs has also shown significant differences between benign and malignant tumors. Using a cutoff of 15 cm/sec, Prompeler and colleagues[41] achieved a sensitivity and specificity of 88% and 83%, respectively. While Valentin and colleagues[14] used a cutoff of 8.5 cm/sec and achieved values of approximately 86% and 65%, respectively. Data from our unit suggest that these indices of flow velocity may improve discrimination between benign and malignant.[42] When combined with impedance, for a given detection rate, the number of false-positive test results is reduced. These results are summarized in Table 22.12 and are derived from an ongoing study in which 47 adnexal tumors have been examined preoperatively. Eight were subsequently found to be malignant. Table

Table 22.11 Early Stage Ovarian Cancers Examined by Transvaginal Color Doppler Showing Intraovarian Indices of Impedance to Blood Flow

Case No.	Age	Menopausal Status	Histologic Classification	FIGO Stage	RI	PI	Peak Systolic Velocity
1	63	Post	Serous cystadenocarcinoma (borderline)	Ia	0.96	5.50	—
2	54	Pre	Endometrioid cystadenocarcinoma	Ia	0.64	0.96	—
3	46	Pre	Endometrioid cystadenocarcinoma (borderline)	Ia	0.34	0.56	57
4	52	Post	Serous cystadenocarcinoma	Ia	0.39	0.57	70
5	52	Post	Serous cystadenocarcinoma	Ib	0.38	0.44	35
6	53	Post	Endometrioid cystadenocarcinoma	Ic	0.58	0.80	26
7	30	Pre	Serous cystadenocarcinoma (borderline)	Ia	0.43	0.59	15
8	37	Pre	Serous cystadenocarcinoma	Ic	0.33	0.49	40
9	38	Pre	Serous cystadenocarcinoma	IIa	0.41	0.56	32

(From Bourne,[26] with permission.)

Table 22.12 Sensitivities and Specificities Obtained With Different Doppler Indices

Criteria for Malignancy	Sensitivity (%)	Specificity (%)
PI ≤ 0.90	87.5	59.0
RI ≤ 0.60	87.5	53.8
PSV ≥ 15 cm/sec	87.5	66.7
TAMXV ≥ 12 cm/sec	87.5	76.9
PI ≤ 0.90 and PSV ≥ 15 cm/sec	87.5	76.9
RI ≤ 0.65 and PSV ≥ 15 cm/sec	87.5	74.4
PI ≤ 1.0 and TAMXV ≥ 12 cm/sec	87.5	84.6
RI ≤ 0.65 and TAMXV ≥ 12 cm/sec	87.5	82.1

(n = 47, benign = 39, malignant = 8)
(From Tailor et al.,[107] with permission.)

22.12 shows that, when only one criterion is used to diagnose malignancy, a TAMXV equal to or greater than 12 cm/sec and PI less than or equal to 1.0 gives optimal test performance. However, these data are still preliminary. An argument against the use of velocity indices to discriminate between benign and malignant has been that it suffers from interobserver variability. This problem was recently addressed by Sladkevicius and Valentin,[43] who concluded that, although there was some degree of variability in the absolute values when two observers measured PSV and TAMXV, there was generally interobserver agreement in classifying tumors based on cutoff limits. They concluded that, in terms of reproducibility, it would be possible to use Doppler measurements of TAMXV and PSV to characterize adnexal masses (see Plate 22.5 and Table 22.12).

BENIGN OVARIAN CONDITIONS

Non-neoplastic Cysts

Follicular Cysts

Developing ovarian follicles normally reach a diameter of 20 to 25 mm, and then they rupture at ovulation (Plate 22.6 and Fig. 22.6). At this stage, they are simply called *follicles* and are lined by granulosa cells. If they fail to ovulate and continue to grow, the cyst can reach huge proportions. Regardless of size, they are seen as simple cysts with thin walls, sharply defined regular borders, and echolucent fluid within. In most cases, these cysts are an incidental finding in an asymptomatic woman who may give a history of menstrual irregularity. These cysts are usually small and transient, and a follow-up scan at an interval of 6 weeks will in most cases show that they have disappeared. Hormonal therapy has been advocated for them, but it is likely that the cysts that respond to hormone therapy would have resolved anyway with time. Occasionally,

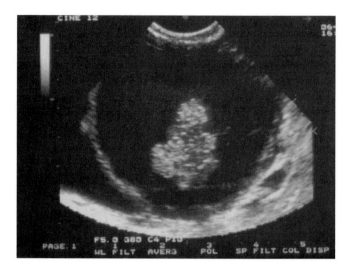

Figure 22.6 A hemorrhagic cyst. Note the web-like echogenic area filling the cyst and the region on the right where the clot has retracted leaving a gap between it and the wall of the cyst. This was asymptomatic and relatively small. A repeat scan 3 weeks later showed that the area had resolved.

they cause pain if hemorrhage into the cyst cavity occurs (Fig. 22.7), and ultrasound-guided transvaginal puncture of the cyst should relieve symptoms.

Corpus Luteal Cysts

The morphology, volume, and vascularity of the corpus luteum undergo profound changes during the ovarian cycle. Following ovulation, the corpus luteum may be barely discernible; however, with time, the center of the corpus luteum may appear anechoic and cystic or hemorrhagic (Plate 22.7).

Figure 22.7 In this follicle, hemorrhage is just starting to occur. Although difficult to see, the contents of the follicle are no longer completely anechoic, and the appearance of some "web-like" strands are just becoming discernible.

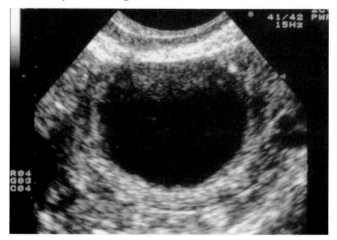

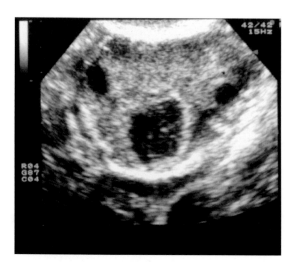

Figure 22.8 A typical cystic mature corpus luteum. Note the echogenic wall and the debris within its central area.

and Fig. 22.8). Changes in corpus luteum volume and blood flow that occur are of interest, as they mirror function.[28] These changes in volume and PSV in relation to the time of a positive urinary luteinizing hormone self-test and the first day of menses of the next cycle are shown (Figs. 22.9 and 22.10). PSV declines rapidly from about the ninth or tenth day after a positive urinary dipstick, and it can be hypothesized that this is associated with the onset of innervation of the vasculature of the corpus luteum. This might facilitate the action of prostaglandins on the vasculature of the corpus luteum, leading to a decrease in PSV and the onset of functional luteolysis. The highly vascular appearances of a mature corpus luteum are shown in Plate 22.8. This is a result of angiogenesis, leading to invasion of the theca interna and the zona granulosa by a network of proliferating capillaries extending from the theca externa.

Corpora lutea cysts may grow to a size of 5 to 10 cm in diameter. They have thin walls, but unlike follicular cysts, they can often have an irregular outline and are likely to have hemorrhagic contents. They usually resolve with time. Occasionally, the cyst cavity will persist with regression of the vasculature and hormone production, the so-called "corpus albicans" cyst.

Hemorrhage is common with corpus luteum cysts. It may have a fine "web-like" appearance, form a "jelly-like" area across the cyst, or have a ground-glass appearance like an endometrioma, depending on how organized the blood in the cyst cavity has become. One study on the ultrasonographic characteristics of 76 hemorrhagic cysts found a mean diameter of 5 cm, with a range from 2.5 cm to 16 cm.[44] A small proportion of these cysts were also accompanied by free fluid in the pouch of Douglas.

The management of hemorrhagic cysts in young women is conservative, as most will regress. Aspiration under ultrasound guidance will relieve symptoms in some cases, but the fluid may be too viscous to remove. Laparoscopic surgery will deal with the remaining few that persist or when the symptoms are too severe for the patient to wait for spontaneous resolution.

Theca Lutein Cysts

Hyperreactio luteinalis is the term used to describe the cystic ovarian enlargement that can be associated with gestational trophoblastic disease. Theca lutein cysts relate to the same condition. Similar changes can be observed in the ovaries of some women receiving drugs such as clomiphene citrate or human menopausal gonadotropin for the treatment of infertility (Fig. 22.11). Hyperreactio luteinalis has been reported in both normal singleton[45–47] and twin pregnancies[48] as well as in pregnancies affected by nonimmune hydrops fetalis.[49,50] One study reported the incidence of hyperreactio luteinalis in a series of untreated hydatidiform moles as 25%, with a mean cyst diameter of 7 cm (ranging 3 to 20 cm);[51] hence the ab-

Figure 22.9 Changes in corpus luteum volume and PSV and serum progesterone in relation to onset of menses. (From Bourne et al.[28] With permission of the American Society for Reproductive Medicine.)

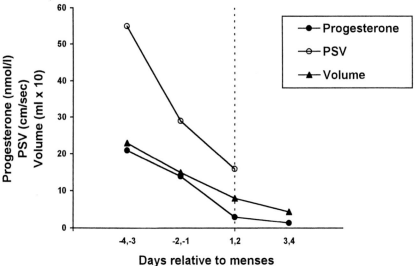

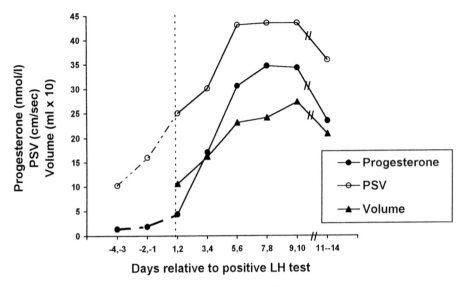

Days relative to positive LH test

Figure 22.10 Changes in corpus luteum volume and PSV and serum progesterone in relation to positive urinary luteinizing hormone (LH surge). (From Bourne et al.[28] With permission of the American Society for Reproductive Medicine.)

sence of these cysts does not make the diagnosis of gestational trophoblastic disease less likely.

In practical terms, the ultrasound picture often consists of the typical cystic appearance within the uterus accompanied by large hypoechoic ovarian cysts extending beyond the depth of penetration of the vaginal probe. In some cases, only one ovary is affected.[51] The presence of these lesions indicates an increased risk for the development of postmolar trophoblastic disease; this risk is further increased if the cysts are bilateral.[51] The cysts may cause abdominal pain, but in many women, the condition is asymptomatic, and many are only recognized at the time of a routine scan during pregnancy or at cesarean section.[52]

Figure 22.11 The typical appearances of a stimulated ovary following oocyte retrieval; the scan was performed on the day of embryo transfer. Note the multiple follicles, some showing evidence of hemorrhage and debris within them.

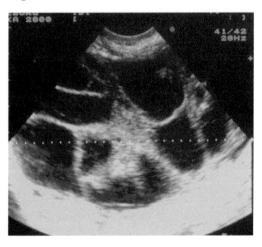

Serous Inclusion Cysts

Serous inclusion cysts are most often found in postmenopausal women, although they can occur in premenopausal women, being incorrectly diagnosed as follicles. These cysts arise as a result of cortical invagination of the surface germinal epithelium. They are typically small (1 to 3 cm), thin walled, unilocular, regular in outline, and anechoic. Color Doppler usually fails to reveal any vascularization in association with the cyst. They are frequently seen in postmenopausal women attending familial ovarian cancer screening and are in most cases managed by repeating the scan about 8 to 12 weeks later. In the majority of cases, they are seen to persist, and as long as they do not enlarge or develop complex morphologic or Doppler features, they are monitored annually.

Endometriomata and Endometriosis

Discrete small deposits of functioning endometrial tissue on peritoneal surfaces cannot be demonstrated with ultrasound. If pelvic endometriosis develops into hemorrhagic tumors when the cyclically discharging ectopic endometrium cannot empty itself, these endometriomata can be well seen. Endometriotic cysts probably account for about 15% to 20% of all adnexal masses that undergo surgery. Although many reports describe them as having typical ultrasound features,[53–55] they are a common source of false-positive diagnoses of cancer. Ovarian endometriomata are well-circumscribed thin or thick-walled cysts that contain homogeneously echogenic fluid. This so called "ground-glass" appearance (Fig. 22.12) is due to altered blood. Furthermore, internal septa have been described in about 10% to 30% of all endometriotic cysts seen.[53,54] The fluid may be hypoechoic, so in some cases it is necessary to increase the gain setting to detect the low-level echogenicity. There may be a fluid–fluid level (Fig. 22.13).

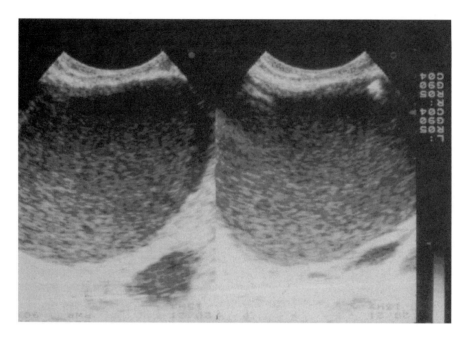

Figure 22.12 A split-screen view of an endometrioma. The "ground-glass" appearance of the contents is the classic but not specific sign of these lesions. Note that the wall is slightly irregular, and there is the suggestion of a small solid projection and septa in the left-and right-hand images, respectively. Endometriomas invariably score highly in any morphologic scoring system designed to detect malignancy.

Diagnostic accuracy is superior transvaginally;[55] however, the appearances are not always classic. The hemorrhagic contents may have a trabecular pattern that looks complex, so mucinous epithelial and endometrioid tumors may be part of the differential diagnosis along with hemorrhagic cysts and dermoids. The role of color Doppler imaging in the diagnosis of endometriomata is not clear. In many cases, the impedance is low, with high diastolic flow especially during the menstrual phase but with an RI invariably above 0.40.[56] Given the fact that low impedance flow can be seen at virtually any phase of the menstrual cycle, such a simple analysis seems unlikely to be useful. The majority of endometriomata have characteristic features and a clinical history to support the diagnosis.

Ovarian Remnant Syndrome

The ovarian remnant syndrome is the development of symptoms, usually pain, due to the development of cysts in residual ovarian tissue that was inadvertently left after bilateral oophorectomy. Often, the original surgery was difficult due to the presence of endometriosis or pelvic inflammatory disease (PID), and ultrasonography is likely to be more successful at demonstrating the remnant than laparoscopy, as it is likely to be buried under adhesions.[57] A mass may be palpable in some cases.[57,58] In one case, ultrasonography revealed a 5-cm well-circumscribed heterogeneously hyperechoic pelvic mass that was a hemorrhagic corpus luteum. A tubular fluid-filled structure posterior to it was found to be the obstructed ureter.[59] A

cyst may not be obvious, so it may be helpful to give a 10-day course of clomiphene citrate to stimulate follicular development, which may be easier to identify on ultrasound.[60] A low level of circulating follicle stimulating hormone (FSH) is also a good indicator of the presence of functioning ovarian tissue; furthermore, even if the patient is on hormone replacement therapy, the FSH level may not be suppressed, so a high level would indicate no functioning residual tissue. If the patient's

Figure 22.13 A 5-cm unilocular cyst with a regular outline and a definite fluid level between the anechoic contents and the homogeneously isoechogenic "ground-glass" contents of the cyst. Laparoscopy revealed an endometrioma.

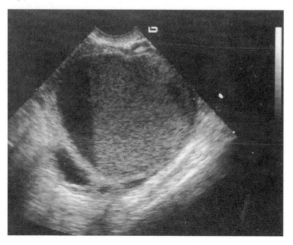

symptoms are relieved with a trial of gonadotropin releasing hormone analogs,[61] it is likely that surgical removal of the remnant will be successful.

The management of ovarian remnant syndrome is not simple. Surgical removal may be difficult, as they are often fixed to the pelvic side wall. Furthermore, the presence of an ovarian remnant is not a guarantee that it is causing the pain, and this is a real concern, given the risks of surgery associated with such cases.[62] Preoperative ultrasonic localization may be of value.

Differential Diagnosis of Non-neoplastic Cysts

Pelvic Inflammatory Disease

PID refers to the infection of the female upper genital tract. In its acute phase, PID can present with a pyosalpinx or tubo-ovarian abscess, and in its chronic form, it can exist as hydrosalpinx. In the early stages of infection, the only sonographic signs that may be visible are endometrial cavity fluid and free fluid in the pouch of Douglas. The fallopian tubes may still be indistinct from the surrounding structures unless there is a considerable amount of pelvic fluid. As acute PID progresses, a fluid collection may be identified inside one or both of the tubes within 72 hours of the onset of symptoms.[63] This collection is seen in the ampullary portion of the tube, which is also the area most commonly damaged and the frequent site of ectopic pregnancies. The spillage of this purulent material into the pelvis in severe cases will lead to the formation of the tubo-ovarian abscess. Sonographically, this appears as a complex cystic mass with thick irregular walls, septa, and heterogeneous echogenicity. These appearances, along with the clinical picture of severe tenderness, fever, and leukocytosis, will usually lead to the correct diagnosis. In the chronic phase of this condition, the pus is replaced by clear fluid trapped by the obstruction of the fimbriated end of the tube, giving the appearances of a hydrosalpinx. Sonographically, an "elongated" cystic structure with "incomplete" septa representing thickened mucosal folds are seen. Nodular structures almost like small papillary projections protruding into the lumen are also characteristic signs. A normal ovary adjacent to the structure will usually betray the cystic structure as a hydrosalpinx.

Ultrasonography has also been of some use in the treatment of both the pyosalpinx and tubo-ovarian abscess. Toth and Chervenak[63] have successfully carried out antibiotic lavage of the tubal contents in the acute phase of the condition. They monitored the flow of antibiotic solution through the tubes and into the abdominal cavity using ultrasound. This resulted in a shortened recovery period and preservation of tubal patency confirmed by hysterosalpingography. Similarly, sonography has also been applied successfully for the treatment of tubo-ovarian abscess. In a prospective study, 40 women with tubo-ovarian abscesses were randomized to have either conventional medical therapy with antibiotics or the latter in combination with early ultrasound-guided transvaginal drainage[64] and were shown to have a faster recovery and lower rate of surgical morbidity.

Paratubal Cysts

Paratubal or paraovarian cysts occur mostly in premenopausal women and are responsible for about 10% of all adnexal masses.[65] The prevalence of these lesions in the population is not known due to the lack of data on normal women. They occur mainly in the broad ligament but may be seen associated with the terminal portion of the fallopian tube. They are usually derived from the mesothelial covering of the peritoneum or remnants of paramesonephric and mesonephric origin, so histologically, they are covered by a single layer of ciliated columnar or flattened epithelium.[65] These simple cysts can be complicated by torsion, hemorrhage, or rupture. Malignant change has also been reported to occur in about 2% to 3%,[66,67] and it should be suspected if there are papillary projections. As the true prevalence of these cysts is not known, it is difficult to ascertain the true rate of malignant change. These cysts are usually thin-walled, simple, and anechoic. The diagnosis depends on identifying the ipsilateral ovary separate from it (Fig. 22.14). If the ovary cannot be clearly seen separate from the cyst, or sliding independently when transducer pressure is applied, the cyst is probably ovarian in origin.

In asymptomatic women in whom the cyst is small and simple, no further action is necessary. For symptomatic women or those who have large or complex-looking cysts, surgery may be indicated if a follow-up scan after 2 or 3 months shows no resolution.

Figure 22.14 A small thin-walled unilocular cyst can be clearly seen here to be separate from the normal ovary adjacent to it. This is a paraovarian cyst. When the lesion was pushed by the transducer, it could be seen to move separately—the "sliding organ" sign.

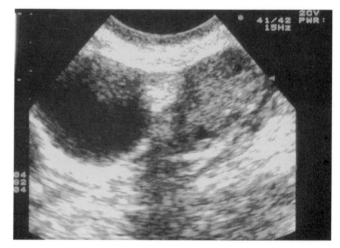

Ultrasound of Surgical Emergencies Related to the Ovary

Adnexal Torsion

Adnexal torsion a rare but important cause of abdominal pain. Early diagnosis is essential to prevent its sequelae of ischemic injury necessitating salpingo-oophorectomy. It can occur throughout life from the neonatal to postmenopausal periods but is most common in the first three decades of life. There is an increased incidence in early pregnancy and in some series has accounted for 12% to 26% of the patients with adnexal torsion.[68,69] Some have reported a predominance of this condition on the right side,[70,71] said to be due to the relatively decreased space on the opposite side because of the sigmoid colon. This adds to the difficulties in making a correct clinical diagnosis, because it is commonly mistaken for appendicitis. It presents with unilateral pelvic pain associated with nausea, vomiting, and leukocytosis. Some have a history of intermittent pain, which represents spontaneously resolving subacute torsion. In most reported series, the duration of the symptoms before diagnosis is approximately 2 to 3 days.

The prior presence of an adnexal mass either as a cystic ovarian enlargement or as a hydrosalpinx is commonly a precipitating feature of this condition, and in a majority of these cases, an adnexal mass is seen sonographically. In some cases, the enlargement may develop following the torsion as congestion and edema occurs (see massive ovarian edema below). The mass appears relatively echogenic, possibly due to edema and hemorrhage. In one reported series of 13 cases scanned transabdominally and confirmed to have torsion operatively, all had an adnexal mass ranging from 4 to 10 cm.[71] They were located in the midline in 70% and appeared solid in 30% and cystic in 40% Recently, color Doppler imaging has been reported to give signs to facilitate the diagnosis of this condition.[72,73] The Doppler findings may range from high resistance, low-velocity arterial flow and absent venous return[72] to complete absence of intraovarian flow.[73]

Massive Ovarian Edema

Massive ovarian edema is a rare condition most commonly associated with young menarcheal women with some cases reported in prepubertal girls.[74,75] The most common presenting complaints are intermittent lower abdominal pain, menstrual irregularity, and more rarely virilization.[76] Most cases are unilateral.[77] The pathogenesis is not certain, but some believe that it may be due to repeated partial torsion of the ovary. This may account for the intermittent pain and discovery of an ovary with partial torsion at laparotomy.[78,79] The other possibility is that it is a variant of polycystic ovarian syndrome.[78,80]

Macroscopically, the affected ovary is usually uniformly enlarged to a size of approximately 8 to 10 cm with a smooth white outer surface with no capsular thickening. On incision of this capsule, copious amount of clear fluid exudes from the edematous stroma. Histologically, the key feature is diffuse interstitial edema with luteinization of theca and stromal cells in cases complicated by virilization.[81]

The ultrasound appearances are of an enlarged ovary, and while the echogenicity may be normal, the internal architecture of the ovary will seem blurred. The management of this is surgical, with oophorectomy usually necessary, but some patients have responded to wedge resection to diagnose the condition followed by fixation of the ovary to the uterus to prevent further torsion.[75,82] Interestingly, in one reported case of bilateral ovarian edema and unilateral partial torsion, the removal of the torsed ovary led to resolution of edema in the other ovary after therapy with oral contraceptives.[79]

Ultrasound in Ovarian-Related Endocrine Disorders

Polycystic Ovarian Syndrome

Polycystic ovarian syndrome (PCOS) is a condition first described by Stein and Leventhal[83] as having a classic triad of chronic oligomenorrhea, hirsutism, and obesity. It is now increasingly realized that these features are not universally present. Many of the patients are diagnosed to have this condition during investigation for infertility. Classically, it has been diagnosed mainly on the basis of abnormal serum hormone profile and confirmed by laparoscopy, which reveals mildly enlarged ovaries bilaterally having a smooth and thickened white or grayish capsule. Under this capsule, some of the small cysts may be visible. Sonography has an important role in the noninvasive management of this condition, as it can also exclude other uterine and adnexal causes of oligomenorrhea, especially when an increased incidence of ovarian tumors has been reported in association with PCOS.[84] Because many of the women are being investigated for infertility, the initial and subsequent sonographic examinations provide useful information regarding the response to therapy with ovulation induction. The morphologic appearances sonographically can range from the completely normal-looking ovary to one that is mildly enlarged with an increased number of follicles. The latter are usually located peripherally and appear to be smaller. Also commonly found is an increase in stromal echogenecity, presumably as a result of numerous tissue–fluid interfaces (Fig. 22.15). A recent study comparing the sonographic appearances in normal women and those with this condition reported the mean size of follicles, number of follicles, and total ovarian volume in the two groups.[85] The mean size, number of follicles, and the total ovarian volume in the group with PCOS were 3.8 mm, 9.8, and 9.8 cm,[3] respectively. This contrasted with 5.1 mm, 5, and 5.9 cm,[3] respectively, for the normal group.[85] The investigators also found an increased stromal echogenecity in 94% of the women with PCOS compared with 10% in the normal group. They reported that normal and PCOS ovaries could be discriminated sonographically with a sensitivity of 92% and specificity of

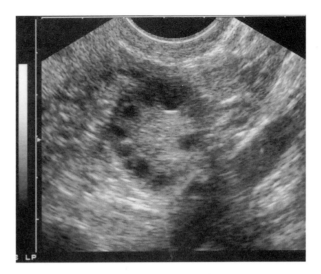

Figure 22.15 Ultrasound of a polycystic ovary. There is slight enlargement of the ovary with numerous small follicles around the periphery with an associated increase in stromal echogenicity because of the tissue–fluid interfaces

97% on the basis of follicular size and ovarian volume. Considerable overlap was seen in these parameters between the two groups. This illustrates the important point that the typical appearances of a polycystic ovary are not always present in women confirmed to have this condition on the basis of clinical features and abnormal hormone profiles. Conversely, it also illustrates the fact that some women who have normal cycles and none of the symptoms of PCOS described above may have ovaries that may appear polycystic sonographically. Since PCOS is essentially a condition diagnosed on the basis of an abnormal hormone profile, the temptation to diagnose PCOS on the basis of sonographic appearances must be resisted.

The changes in vascularity in patients with PCOS have been investigated with Doppler sonography. It appears that intraovarian vascularity is increased, giving reduced impedance and a paradoxic increase in impedance in the uterine arteries,[86] the latter postulated to be due to the vasoconstrictive effects of the increased androgens. It is unlikely that Doppler sonography on its own will allow discrimination of the normal and PCOS ovaries, but it may have a complementary role with gray scale studies in achieving this goal.

Luteoma of Pregnancy

Luteoma of pregnancy is thought to be the solid counterpart to theca lutein cysts described above. Though rare, they occur with normal pregnancies rather than gestational trophoblastic disease and are more commonly unilateral. They cause virilization of the mother in about 30% of cases, and about 50% of female infants from these patients will also be virilized.[87] Microscopically, hyperplasia of the luteinized theca interna is seen,[47] and there may be numerous mitoses.[88] Macroscopically, there is solid enlargement of the ovary to 6 to 10 cm in

diameter, but lesions of up to 25 cm in size have been reported.[89] They may be an incidental finding at cesarean section. The ultrasound appearances are of an ovary with moderate diffuse solid enlargement.[90]

Stromal luteomas have histologic characteristics and endocrine consequences similar to those of pregnancy luteomas,[88] but they are usually found in postmenopausal women who present with vaginal bleeding due to the endometrial hyperplasia associated with excessive ovarian hormone production. They, too, appear as solid enlargement of the ovary.

Ultrasound of Benign Ovarian Tumors

Mature Teratoma (Dermoid)

Dermoid cysts are common ovarian masses in women of reproductive age. In 10% of cases, they are bilateral, and because of the totipotent nature of the germ cells from which they grow, they usually contain a bizarre mixture of tissues from different origins. About 30% have teeth, and many more have elements such as hair and apocrine glands producing sebum. Malignant change is rare but is almost always squamous cell carcinoma arising from the skin elements. They are usually complex and cystic, and most measure between 5 to 10 cm at the time of presentation.[91,92]

On ultrasonography, no other ovarian condition has such a variable appearance. They may be simple and anechoic or complex with mixed echogenicity and multiloculations. The presence of hair and sebum often gives a homogeneous hyperechoic appearance that is well circumscribed (Fig. 22.16).

Figure 22.16 A 3.5-cm dermoid cyst. Although echogenic, these lesions are often isoechogenic with surrounding bowel. This can be seen in this case when the cyst contents are compared to the bowel that can be seen in the far field. Often, a dermoid will appear simply as a space-occupying area that does not move with the rest of the bowel. It is not difficult to persuade oneself that a lesion felt on bimanual examination is not present, because it cannot be seen on ultrasound.

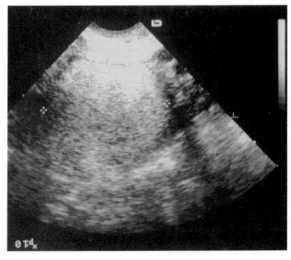

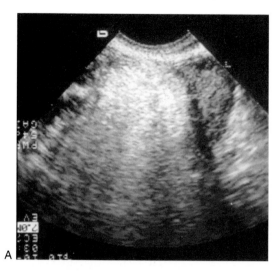
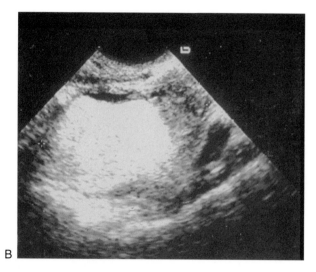

Figure 22.17 Echogenic areas in the pelvis similar to a dermoid cyst. They are not the same. **(A)** An area of bowel overlying the ovary, and two normal ovaries were identified separate from it. **(B)** A true dermoid cyst within the ovary. Perhaps paradoxically, the shadowing due to bowel appears more sharp compared to the way the hyperechogenicity of the dermoid tends to have a more diffuse margin with the normal ovarian stroma.

This hyperechogenicity is similar in appearance to stool-filled large bowel and may cause confusion (Fig. 22.17). On occasion, all that can be discerned is a space-occupying effect. Close examination as well as manipulation during the scan will show that bowel around the area of interest is moving, while the area in question remains static. Great care must be taken to avoid missing a large dermoid when an ovarian mass is suspected in a young women. The presence of teeth causes echo-dense foci with acoustic shadowing.

Most morphologic scoring systems would score these lesions as "malignant," but the characteristic features of brightly echogenic sebum, teeth, or hair allow accurate diagnosis by the subjective approach. Using color Doppler imaging, few dermoid cysts appear to have detectable flow,[30–32] however, the functional ovarian tissue beside it may.

Benign Epithelial Tumors

Serous and mucinous cystadenoma are classified in the broad category of common epithelial tumors. The latter account for 70% of all ovarian neoplasms and 90% of all malignant tumors.[93] They arise from the germinal epithelium covering the ovary or occasionally from a focus of endometriosis. Histologically, there are five major subtypes, namely, serous, endometrioid, mucinous, clear cell, and Brenner tumors. Subtyping is not an exact science, even on histology. Variability occurs in diagnosis not only when two pathologists are shown the same tumor but also when one pathologist is asked to report on tissue obtained from the same tumor.[94] The reported intraobserver and interobserver variability were 64% and 52%, respectively. Therefore, when this "gold standard" cannot be exact, sonography can hardly be expected to perform

any better. The most sonography can be expected to achieve is to enable the differentiation between benign and malignant, but as is noted in the section on morphology assessment of the ovary, there has been only limited success.

SEROUS CYSTADENOMA

Thirty percent of all ovarian neoplasms are serous epithelial tumors, and 60% of these are benign, 30% are malignant, and 10% are borderline. Ten percent of serous cystadenomas are bilateral.[93] They are usually about 5 to 10 cm in size but can range from 1 to 20 cm. Most serous cystadenomata are unilocular or bilocular, and the septa in loculated cysts are usually thin and often diaphanous to undulate when gently nudged with the transducer. The cyst fluid is serous, which imparts an anechoic appearance on sonography (Fig. 22.18). These cystadenomas usually lack papillary projections, but if present, the risk of the cyst being borderline or malignant increases with the number present. On color Doppler imaging, many benign serous tumors do not have detectable flow,[30,31] but when present, it is usually high impedance flow.[31,95]

MUCINOUS CYSTADENOMA

Twenty percent of all ovarian neoplasms are mucinous epithelial tumors, and 85% of these are benign, 10% are malignant, and 5% are borderline. Five percent of these benign mucinous cystadenomata are bilateral.[93] Unlike serous lesions, mucinous tumors are most often multilocular and are frequently larger. These cystadenomata generally are 15 to 30 cm when discovered. Their septa and cyst walls are thin and regular. The mucinous fluid can either be thick and viscous or thin and watery but usually has low-level echogenicity on

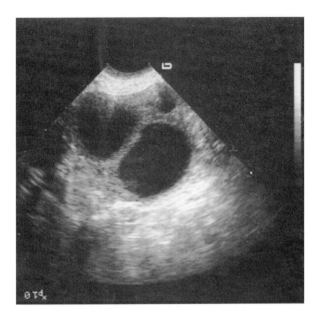

Figure 22.18 A small serous cystadenoma with regular cyst outlines and anechoic cyst contents. Two of the cystic compartments are seen to be separated by a thin band of tissue, which could represent a septum.

sonography (Fig. 22.19). Like their serous counterparts, the number of papillary projections varies and is related to an extent on the histology.

Brenner Tumors

Three percent of all ovarian neoplasms are Brenner tumors. They are mostly benign, and only less than 2% show borderline or malignant change. They are frequently small, with

Figure 22.19 A larger mucinous cystadenoma with a regular cyst outline and a thin septum. The contents are homogeneously hypoechoic. In some cases, the gain setting on the gray scale has to be increased to visualize the hypoechogenicity.

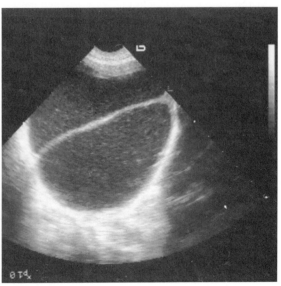

60% being under 2 cm across and 90% to 95% being discovered incidentally when the ovaries are removed for other reasons.[96] Less than 10% are bilateral. Most are solid and well circumscribed with foci of calcification. Infrequently, the tumor is multicystic with papillary projections, which are suggestive of malignancy.[93] On sonography, they appear similar to other solid ovarian neoplasms such as fibrothecomata, which are seen as hypoechoic lesions with calcifications and acoustic shadowing. They can easily be mistaken for pedunculated fibroids. These tumors are known to be associated with endometrial hyperplasia,[97] and in about 4% to 14% the endometrium will be thickened.

Fibroma and Fibrothecoma

Pathologically, fibroma and fibrothecoma are a spectrum of tumors with varying proportions of stromal and thecal elements called fibromata and fibrothecomas at the two extremes. With few exceptions they are benign and account for about 4% of all ovarian neoplasms. Between 3% and 10% are bilateral, and their size can range from 1 to 20 cm.[93] Thecomas, but not fibromas, are hormone producing and secrete estrogen or rarely androgens when the thecal cells are luteinized. The former will therefore cause a thickened endometrium and may lead to an endometrial carcinoma in 20%.[93] Fifteen percent of fibromata cause ascites, and about 1% also develop a pleural effusion (Meig syndrome), which is more commonly on the right.[93]

The classic ultrasound appearance of a fibrothecoma is the unusual combination of a uniformly hypoechoic mass with intense posterior acoustic shadowing.[98,99] In fibromata, but not thecomas, calcification is also seen. A separate ipsilateral ovary is not seen. The differential diagnosis in these cases includes both pedunculated and broad ligament fibroids, but a separate ipsilateral ovary should be seen. With fibroids, the identification of a pedicle and blood supply from the uterus also confirms the diagnosis (Plate 22.9). On color Doppler imaging, when flow is detected, the impedance is usually high.[31,32]

MALIGNANT OVARIAN TUMORS

Granulosa Cell Tumors

Almost all granulosa cell tumors are considered malignant, and they account for about 10% of all ovarian cancers. Five percent of them occur before puberty, and the rest are evenly distributed over the reproductive and postmenopausal years. About 5% are bilateral.[93] The ultrasonographic appearances are variable, with some of the smaller solid tumors appearing hyperechoic, with calcifications similar to uterine fibroids (Fig. 22.20). The larger complex cystic tumors may be indistinguishable from the epithelial malignancies. Most of these tumors are functional and produce estrogen, and so in postmenopausal women, this may lead to an increase in endometrial thickness, due to endometrial hyperplasia in some and

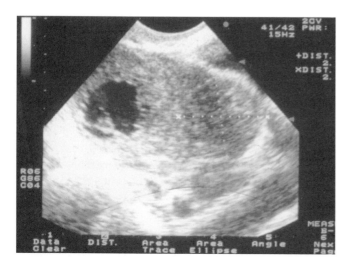

Figure 22.20 A granulosa cell tumor in a 32-year-old woman. The cystic area on the left is a mature corpus luteum. On the right, delineated by the calipers is a small 2.5-cm solid lesion within the ovary. It has mixed echogenicity suggesting a degree of calcification. Color Doppler showed two separate areas of vascularity within this ovary, one around the corpus luteum and another around this lesion. Repeat scans showed this area to be persistent morphology and vascularity. Surgery confirmed the diagnosis.

endometrial carcinoma in about 5% Few data relate to the use of color Doppler in the diagnosis of these tumors. Our experience is that it can be valuable for recognition of small solid tumors within the ovary. Granulosa tumors are invariably vascular, and so the presence of flow may give an indication of the presence of an isoechogenic solid lesion that might be difficult to recognize using gray scale alone. A recent case report on the diagnosis of a small solid Sertoli-Leydig tumor illustrated the use of color Doppler in this context.[100]

Cystadenocarcinomas

Cystadenocarcinomas account for 90% of all primary malignant ovarian tumors.[93] About 50% of serous and 25% of mu-

cinous cystadenocarcinomas are bilateral.[93] Serous cystadenocarcinomas are usually larger than their benign counterparts, with more than 95% being greater than 5 cm and more than 50% greater than 15 cm. They are usually multiloculated, with numerous papillary projections, and the septa are often thickened and nodular (Fig. 22.21). These cystadenocarcinomata are said to have psammoma bodies in about 30% of the cases. Histologically, these are calcified laminated spheroids about 50 μm in diameter and may be seen at sonography as speckles of calcification associated with acoustic shadowing. In approximately half of all cases of serous cystadenocarcinomas, ascites is seen as free fluid in the pouch of Douglas. They also almost always have detectable flow, which is generally of low impedance quality.[32,95]

Mucinous adenocarcinomata are generally larger than the malignant serous tumors and can range from 5 to 50 cm across. Apart from the size, the consequences of the other characteristics such as septal thickness and regularity, solid elements, and flow analysis on color Doppler imaging are similar to their serous counterparts.[31,32,95] Mucinous tumors rarely have psammoma bodies and as such tend not to have calcification as often.

CLINICAL OPINIONS

1. A simple unilocular cyst 5.0 cm or less in diameter is unlikely to be malignant, particularly in a premenopausal woman. Unless there is a risk factor for cancer in the history, such cysts do not warrant surgical intervention.

2. Functional ovarian cysts resolve with time. Before any elective surgery, a repeat scan should be performed in 6 to 8 weeks to allow time for spontaneous resolution and thus assess its persistence.

3. The more complex a tumor, the more likely it is to be malignant. The presence of papillary projections is a particu-

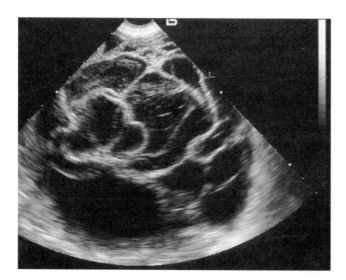

Figure 22.21 Cystadenocarcinoma. A large complex cyst with multiple haphazard septa. The septa are not of uniform thickness or echogenecity. Some of the locules are seen to contain debris, and although this section of the ovary does not contain any obvious vegetations arising from the cyst wall, these were present in other sections. This appearance in a postmenopausal woman in conjunction with free fluid is indicative of a malignant lesion.

larly ominous sign. The application of any current morphology scoring system to evaluate a tumor will compromise the detection rate for early cancer.

4. Some tumors such as benign teratomas (dermoids) and endometriomata often have gray scale ultrasound appearances that allow them to be characterized purely on the basis of pattern recognition.

5. In women with an increased risk of ovarian cancer, there is a prevalence effect, which means that the odds of finding cancer at surgery for a persistent ovarian mass are high, irrespective of the gray-scale or Doppler findings.

6. Color Doppler has serious limitations in women of reproductive age. Impedance indices obtained from the follicle and corpus luteum can be similar to those seen in early cancer. In postmenopausal women, the finding of low impedance, high-velocity blood flow is more predictive of carcinoma.

7. Ultrasound findings must be interpreted in light of the patient's clinical history, menopausal status, day of cycle, and drug therapy, in order to know if the findings are appropriate.

8. Ultrasound findings can only give an indication of risk of any given pathology being present. The histologic examination of removed tissues is the standard by which we are regularly judged.

SUMMARY

Color Doppler information can be used to improve diagnostic confidence, but the limitations of the technique must be remembered. In postmenopausal women, there are no physiologic events occurring within the ovary that alter vascularity. In our ovarian cancer screening program, there have been very few false-positive results from postmenopausal women.[18] In premenopausal women, this is not the case. Angiogenesis and low impedance indices are normally seen in the corpus luteum and the preovulatory follicle. Vascular information derived from the ovary must be viewed critically and related to normal physiologic events in the patient's ovarian cycle, and any abnormal findings must be subjected to a repeat scan. For the purposes of ovarian cancer screening, we book repeat scans on premenopausal patients between days 3 and 11 of their cycle, to avoid the majority of functional cysts. It seems likely that low impedance blood flow will be obtained from the majority of premenopausal ovaries at some time or other, due to the dynamic nature of the ovaries in terms of both their vasculature and morphology. So, though it is claimed that transvaginal color Doppler can be used to detect ovarian cancer before it is otherwise discernible, and that it should be utilized to characterize the nature of cystic ovarian lesions in pregnancy,[101] little data support the former statement and support the latter. These problems have been discussed elsewhere.[102]

The relative merits of transvaginal color Doppler are very well illustrated by the prospective ovarian cancer screening study by Bourne et al.[18] Data derived from this study are shown in Table 22.6. As already stated, 61 of 1,601 women were found to have persistent ovarian masses and referred to surgery. Six of these were found to have primary ovarian cancer. In the initial stages of the program, Doppler equipment was not available, and the first cancer was detected without its use. If the cutoff had been set at 1.0 for the PI, the number of false-positives would have been reduced from 55 to 13, but one cancer would have been missed. The odds of finding cancer at surgery for women with a positive result would have been 1:3. In this large prospective screening study, a morphology scoring system performed better than color Doppler in terms of reducing the false-positive rate. The evaluation of a cyst as morphologically simple or complex maintained a better sensitivity. The best screening algorithm defined a positive test result as either having a high morphology score or low impedance flow. This seems a reasonable approach to the problem.

With high-resolution TVS, we can obtain excellent images of the ovary in most women. It is the interpretation of these images that is the current challenge. The ovary is a dynamic organ in which cyst formation is a normal, cyclic phenomenon. The findings must be interpreted in the context of the clinical picture, the patient's age and menopausal status, and the phase of her cycle. Even with this, the reliable classification of persistent ovarian masses can still be problematic. Ultrasound does not give us histologic information, yet this is what the clinician seeks. We have only indirect methods of discriminating between benign and malignant ovarian lesions, and these methods are limited by our lack of understanding of the natural history of ovarian cancer.

ACKNOWLEDGMENTS

We are grateful to Keymed Ltd. (Southend, UK), Berner Medicinteknik (Sweden), and the ALOKA Co. Ltd. (Tokyo, Japan) for the use of their ultrasound equipment both at Kings College Hospital, London, and Sahlgrenska University Hospital, Göteborg, Sweden. Financial support for A.T. and the ovarian cancer screening clinic is provided by the Linbury Trust. T.B. is supported by the Swedish Medical Research Council grant number 2873.

REFERENCES

1. Donald I, MacVicar J, Brown TG. Investigation of abdominal masses by pulsed ultrasound. Lancet 1958;1:1188–1195
2. Granberg S, Wikland M, Jansson I. Macroscopic characterization of ovarian tumors and the relation to the histological diagnosis: criteria to be used for ultrasound evaluation. Gynecol Oncol 1989;35:139–144

3. Granberg S, Norstrom A, Wikland M. Tumors in the lower pelvis as imaged by vaginal sonography. Gynecol Oncol 1990;37:224–229

4. Sassone AM, Timor-Tritsch IE, Artner A et al. Transvaginal sonographic characterization of ovarian disease: evaluation of a new scoring system to predict ovarian malignancy. Obstet Gynecol 1991;78:70–76

5. Luxman D, Bergman A, Sagi J, David MP. The post-menopausal adnexal mass: correlation between ultrasonic and pathologic findings. Obstet Gynecol 1991;77:726–728

6. Rulin MC, Preston AL. Adnexal masses in postmenopausal women. Obstet Gynecol 1987;70:578–581

7. Khaw KT, Walker WJ. Ultrasound guided fine needle aspiration of ovarian cysts: diagnosis and treatment in pregnant and non-pregnant women. Clin Radiol 1990;41:105–108

8. De Crespigny LC, Robinson HP, Davoren RAM, Fortune D. The "simple" ovarian cyst: aspirate or operate? Br J Obstet Gynaecol 1989;96:1035–1039

9. Granberg S, Crona N, Enk L et al. Ultrasound-guided puncture of cystic tumors in the lower pelvis of young women. J Clin Ultrasound 1989;17:107–111

10. Kroon E, Andolf E. Diagnosis and follow-up of simple ovarian cysts by ultrasound in postmenopausal women. Obstet Gynecol 1995;85:211–214

11. Meire HB, Farrant P, Guha T. Distinction of benign from malignant ovarian cysts by ultrasound. Br J Obstet Gynaecol 1978;85:893–899

12. Hermann UJ, Locher GW, Goldhirsch A. Sonographic patterns of ovarian tumors: prediction of malignancy. Obstet Gynecol 1987;69:777–781

13. DeLand M, Fried A, van Nagell JR, Donaldson ES. Ultrasonography in the diagnosis of tumors of the ovary. Surg Gynecol Obstet 1979;148:346–348

14. Valentin L, Sladkevicius P, Marsal K. Limited contribution of Doppler velocimetry to the differential diagnosis of extrauterine pelvic tumours. Obstet Gynecol 1994;83:425–433

15. Morley P, Barnett E. The use of ultrasound in the diagnosis of pelvic masses. Br J Radiol 1970;43:602–616

16. Lerner JP, Timor-Tritsch IE, Federman A, Abramovich G. Transvaginal ultrasonographic characterization of ovarian masses with an improved, weighted scoring system. Am J Obstet Gynecol 1994;170:81–85

17. Moyle JW, Rochester D, Sider L et al. Sonography of ovarian tumors: predictability of tumor type. AJR Am J Roentgenol 1983;141:985–991

18. Bourne TH, Campbell S, Reynolds KM et al. Screening for early familial ovarian cancer with transvaginal ultrasonography and colour blood flow imaging. Br Med J 1993;306:1025–1029

19. Finkler NJ, Benacerraf B, Lavin PT et al. Comparison of serum CA 125, clinical impression, and ultrasound in the preoperative evaluation of ovarian masses. Obstet Gynecol 1988;72:659–664

20. Timor-Tritsch LE, Lerner JP, Monteagudo A, Santos R. Transvaginal ultrasonographic characterization of ovarian masses by means of color flow-directed Doppler measurements and a morphologic scoring system. Am J Obstet Gynecol 1993;168:909–913

21. Hata K, Hata T, Manabe A et al. A critical evaluation of transvaginal Doppler studies, transvaginal sonography, magnetic resonance imaging, and CA 125 in detecting ovarian cancer. Obstet Gynecol 1992;80:922–926

22. Folkman J, Watson K, Ingber D, Hanahan D. Induction of angiogenesis during the transition from hyperplasia to neoplasia. Nature 1989;339:58–61

23. Reynolds K, Farzaneh F, Collins WP et al. Association of ovarian malignancy with expression of platelet-derived endothelial cell growth factor. J Natl Cancer Inst 1994;86:1234–1238

24. Ramos I, Fernandez LA, Morse SS et al. Detection of neovascular signals in a 3 day Walker 256 rat carcinoma by CW Doppler ultrasound. Ultrasound Med Biol 1988;14:123–126

25. Shimamoto K, Sakuma S, Ishigaki T, Makino N. Intratumoral blood flow: evaluation with color Doppler echography. Radiology 1987;165:683–685

26. Bourne TH. Transvaginal color Doppler in gynecology (review). Ultrasound Obstet Gynecol 1991;1:359–373

27. Bourne TH, Campbell S, Steer C et al. Transvaginal colour flow imaging: a possible new screening technique for ovarian cancer. Br Med J 1989;299:1367–1370

28. Bourne TH, Hagstrom HG, Hahlin M et al. Ultrasound studies of vascular and morphological changes in the corpus luteum during the menstrual cycle. Fertil Steril 1996;65:753–758

29. Campbell S, Bourne TH, Waterstone J et al. Transvaginal color blood flow imaging of the periovulatory follicle. Fertil Steril 1993;60:433–438

30. Tekay A, Joupilla P. Validity of pulsatility and resistance indices in classification of adnexal tumors with transvaginal color Doppler ultrasound. Ultrasound Obstet Gynecol 1992;2:338–344

31. Zanetta G, Vergani P, Lissoni A. Color Doppler ultrasound in the preoperative assessment of adnexal masses. Acta Obstet Gynecol Scand 1994;73:637–641

32. Chou C, Chang CH, Yao B, Kuo H. Color Doppler ultrasonography and serum CA 125 in the differentiation of benign and malignant ovarian tumours. J Clin Ultrasound 1994;22:491–496

33. Stein SM, Leifer-Narin S, Johnson MB et al. Differentiation of benign and malignant adnexal masses: Relative value of grayscale, color Doppler, and spectral Doppler sonography. Am J Roentgenol AJR 1995;164:381–386

34. Maly Z, Riss P, Deutinger J. Localization of blood vessels and qualitative assessment of blood flow in ovarian tumors. Obstet Gynecol 1995;85:33–36

35. Kawai M, Kikkawa F, Ishikawa H et al. Differential diagnosis of ovarian tumors by transvaginal color-pulse Doppler sonography. Gynecol Oncol 1994;54:209–214

36. Fleischer AC, Rodgers WH, Kepple DM et al. Color Doppler sonography of ovarian masses: a multiparameter analysis. J Ultrasound Med 1993;12:41–48

37. Hata K, Makihara K, Hata T et al. Transvaginal color Doppler imaging for hemodynamic assessment of reproductive tract tumors. Int J Gynecol Obstet 1991;36:301–308

38. Bourne TH, Jurkovic D, Waterstone J et al. Intra-follicular blood flow during human ovulation. Ultrasound Obstet Gynecol 1991;1:63–69

39. Kurjak A, Zalud I, Alfirevic Z. Evaluation of adnexal masses with transvaginal color ultrasound. J Ultrasound Med 1991;10:295–297

40. Bourne T, Reynolds K, Campbell S. Ovarian cancer screening. [Review.] Eur J Cancer 1991;27:655–659

41. Prompeler HJ, Madjar H, Sauerbrei W et al. Quantitative flow measurements for classification of ovarian tumors by transvaginal color Doppler sonography in postmenopausal patients. Ultrasound Obstet Gynecol 1994;4:406–413

42. Tailor A, Jurkovic D, Bourne TH et al. A comparison of intra-tumoural indices of blood flow velocity and impedance for the diagnosis of ovarian cancer. Ultrasound Med Biol 1996;22:837–843

43. Sladkevicius P, Valentin L. Interobserver agreement in the results of Doppler examinations of extrauterine pelvic tumours. Ultrasound Obstet Gynecol 1995;6:91–96

44. Baltarowich OH, Kurtz AB, Pasto ME et al. The spectrum of sonographic findings in hemorrhagic ovarian cysts. AJR Am J Roentgenol 1987;148:901–905

45. Bradshaw KD, Santos-Ramos R, Rawlins SC et al. Endocrine studies in a pregnancy complicated by ovarian theca lutein cysts and hyperreactio luteinalis. Obstet Gynecol 1986;67:66S–69S

46. Okadome M, Kaku T, Tsukamoto N et al. Hyperreactio luteinalis in normal singleton pregnancy. Int J Gynecol Obstet 1989;29:365–371

47. Wajda KJ, Lucas JG, Marsh WL, Jr. Hyperreactio luteinalis. Benign disorder masquerading as an ovarian neoplasm. [Review.] Arch Pathol Lab Med 1989;113:921–925

48. Lindow SW, Munoz WP. Spontaneous regression of large theca lutein cysts in a twin pregnancy. A case report. S Afr Med J 1985;67:185–186

49. Hatjis CG. Nonimmunologic fetal hydrops associated with hyperreactio luteinalis. Obstet Gynecol 1985;65:11S–13S

50. Reubinoff BE, Mor-Yosef S, Shushan A et al. Hyperreactio luteinalis associated with non-immune hydrops fetalis—the role of pituitary hormones. Eur J Obstet Gynecol Reprod Biol 1994;53:144–146

51. Montz FJ, Schlaerth JB, Morrow CP. The natural history of theca lutein cysts. Obstet Gynecol 1988;72:247–251

52. Barad DH, Gimovsky ML, Petrie RH, Bowe ET. Diagnosis and management of bilateral theca lutein cysts in a normal term pregnancy. Diagn Gynecol Obstet 1981;3:27–30

53. Athey PA, Diment DD. The spectrum of sonographic findings in endometriomas. J Ultrasound Med 1989;8:487–491

54. Kupfer MC, Schwimer SR, Lebovic J. Transvaginal sonographic appearance of endometriomata: spectrum of findings. J Ultrasound Med 1992;11:129–133

55. Volpi E, Grandis TD, Zuccaro G et al. Role of transvaginal sonography in the detection of endometriomata. J Clin Ultrasound 1995;23:163–167

56. Kurjak A, Kupesic S. Scoring system for prerdiction of ovarian endometriosis based on transvaginal color and pulsed Doppler sonography. Fertil Steril 1994;62:81–88

57. Pettit PD, Lee RA. Ovarian remnant syndrome: diagnostic dilemma and surgical challenge. Obstet Gynecol 1988;71:580–583

58. Webb MJ. Ovarian remnant syndrome. Aust N Z J Obstet Gynaecol 1989;29:433–435

59. Phillips HE, McGahan JP. Ovarian remnant syndrome. Radiology 1982;142:487–488

60. Siddall-Allum J, Rae T, Rogers V et al. Chronic pelvic pain caused by residual ovaries and ovarian remnants. Br J Obstet Gynaecol 1994;101:979–985

61. Koch MO, Coussens D, Burnett L. The ovarian remnant syndrome and ureteral obstruction: medical management. J Urol 1994;152:158–160

62. Elkins TE, Stocker RJ, Key D et al. Surgery for ovarian remnant syndrome. Lessons learned from difficult cases. J Reprod Med 1994;39:446–448

63. Toth M, Chervenak FA: Transvaginal color Doppler ultrasound in pelvic inflammatory disease In: Bourne TH, Jauniaux E, Jurkovic D, Eds. Transvaginal Colour Doppler: The Scientific Basis and Practical Application of Colour Doppler in Gynaecology (1st ed). Springer -Verlag Berlin, 1995, pp146–152

64. Perez-Medina T, Huertas MA, Bajo M. Early ultrasound-guided transvaginal drainage of tubo-ovarian abesses: a randomised study. Ultrasound Obset Gynecol 1996;7:435–438

65. Athey PA, Cooper NB. Sonographic features of paraovarian cysts. Am J Roentgenol AJR 1985;144:83–86

66. Genadry R, Parmley T, Woodruff JD. The origin and clinical behaviour of the paraovarian tumor. Am J Obstet Gynecol 1977;129:873–880

67. Stein AL, Koonings PP, Schlaerth JB et al. Relative frequency of malignant parovarian tumors: should parovarian tumors be aspirated? Obstet Gynecol 1990;75:1029–1031

68. Nichols DH, Julian PJ. Torsion of the adnexa. Clin Obstet Gynecol 1985;28:375–380

69. Graif M, Shalev J, Strauss S et al. Torsion of the ovary: sonographic features. AJR Am J Roentgenol 1984;143:1331–1334

70. Warner MA, Fleischer AC, Edell SL et al. Uterine adnexal torsion: sonographic findings. Radiology 1985;154:773–775

71. Helvie MA, Silver TM. Ovarian torsion: sonographic evaluation. J Clin Ultrasound 1989;17:327–332

72. Fleischer AC, Williams LL, Jones HW. Transabdominal and transvaginal color Doppler sonography of ovarian masses. In: Fleischer AC, Jones HW, Eds. Early Detection of Ovarian Carcinoma with Transvaginal sonography—Potentials and Limitations (1st Ed). Raven Press, New York 1993, pp 85–144

73. Desai SK, Allahbadia GN, Dalal AK. Ovarian torsion: diagnosis by color Doppler ultrasonography. Obstet Gynecol 1994;84:699–701

74. Roth LM, Deaton LM, Sternberg WH. Massive ovarian oedema. A clinicopathologic study of five cases including ultrastructural observations and review of the literature. Am J Surg Pathol 1979;3:11–21

75. Chervenak FA, Castadot MJ, Wiederman J, Sedlis A. Massive ovarian edema: review of world literature and report of two cases. Obstet Gynecol Surv 1980;35:677–684

76. Patty JR, Galle PC, McRae MA. Massive ovarian edema in a woman receiving clomiphene citrate. A case report. [Review.] J Reprod Med 1993;38:475–479

77. VanWingen T, Upton RT, Cloherty MG et al. Bilateral massive ovarian edema. A case report. J Reprod Med 1984;29:875–877

78. Sageshima M, Masuda H, Kawamura K, Shozawa T. Massive ovarian edema associated with polycystic ovary. Acta Pathol Jpn 1990;40:73–78

79. Hubbell GP, Punch MR, Elkins TE, Abrams GD. Conservative management of bilateral massive edema of the ovary. A case report. J Reprod Med 1993;38:61–64

80. Roth LM. Massive ovarian edema with stromal luteinisation: a newly recognised virilising syndrome apparently related to partial torsion of the mesovarium. Am J Clin Pathol 1971;55:757–760

81. van den Brule F, Bourque J, Gaspard UJ, Hustin JF. Massive ovarian edema with androgen secretion. A pathological and endocrine study with review of the literature. [Review.] Horm Res 1994;41:209–214

82. Kleiner GK, Solomon L, Greston WM, Lev-Gur M. Wedge resection in massive edema of the ovary. Am J Obstet Gynecol 1978;132:107–108

83. Stein IF, Leventhal ML. Amenorrhoea associated with bilateral polycystic ovaries. Am J Obstet Gynecol 1935;29:181–191

84. Babaknia A, Calfopoulos P, Jones HW. The Stein-Leventhal syndrome and coincidental ovarian tumors. Obstet Gynecol 1976;47:223–224

85. Pache TD, Wladimiroff JW, Hop WC, Fauser BC. How to discriminate between normal and polycystic ovaries: transvaginal US study. Radiology 1992;183:421–423

86. Battaglia C, Artini PG, D'Ambrogio G et al. The role of color Doppler imaging in the diagnosis of polycystic ovary syndrome. Am J Obstet Gynecol 1995; 172:108–113

87. Cronje HS. Luteoma of pregnancy. S Afr Med J 1984;66:59–60

88. Kraus FT: Female genitalia. In: Kissane JM, Anderson WAD, Eds. Anderson's Pathology (8th ed., vol. 2) CV Mosby, St. Louis 1985, pp1451–1545

89. Garcia-Bunuel R, Berek JS, Woodruff JD. Luteomas of pregnancy. Obstet Gynecol 1975;45:407–414

90. Illingworth PJ, Johnstone FD, Steel J, Seth J. Luteoma of pregnancy: masculinisation of a female fetus prevented by placental aromatisation. Br J Obstet Gynaecol 1992;99:1019–1020

91. Sisler CL, Siegel MJ. Ovarian teratomas: a comparison of the sonographic appearance in prepubertal and postpubertal girls. AJR Am J Roentgenol 1990;154:139–141

92. Sandler MA, Silver TM, Karo JJ. Gray-scale ultrasonic features of ovarian teratomas. Radiology 1979;131:705–709

93. Ritchie AC. Female reproductive system. In: Ritchie AC, Ed. Boyd's Textbook of Pathology (9th ed., vol. 2). Lea & Febiger, London, 1990, pp 1294–1384

94. Cramer SF, Roth LM, Ulbright TM et al. Evaluation of reproducibility of the World Health Organisation classification of common ovarian tumours. Arch Pathol Lab Med 1987;111:819

95. Weiner Z, Thaler I, Beck D et al. Differentiating malignant from benign ovarian tumors with transvaginal color flow imaging. Obstet Gynecol 1992;79:159–162

96. Balasa RW, Adcock LL, Prem KA et al. The Brenner tumour: a clinicopathologic review. Obstet Gynecol 1977;50:120–128

97. Yoonessi M, Abell MR. Brenner tumours of the ovary. Obstet Gynecol 1979;54:90–96

98. Yaghoobian J, Pinck RL. Ultrasound findings in thecoma of the ovary. J Clin Ultrasound 1983;11:91–93

99. Diakoumakis E, Vieux U, Seife B. Sonographic demonstration of thecoma: report of two cases. Am J Obstet Gynecol 1984;150:787–788

100. Yanushpolsky EH, Brown DL, Smith BL. Localisation of small ovarian Steroli-Leydig cell tumors by transvaginal sonography with color Doppler. Ultrasound Obstet Gynecol 1995; 5:133–135

101. Anonymous. First catch your deer. [Editorial.] Lancet 1990;336:147

102. Campbell S, Bourne TH, Collins WP. Detection of early ovarian cancer. [Letter.] Lancet 1990;336:436

103. Moyle JW, Rochester D, Sider L et al. Sonography of ovarian tumors: predictability of tumor type. Am J Roentgenol 1983; 141:985–991

104. Wu CC, Lee CN, Chen TM et al. Factors contributing to the accuracy in diagnosing ovarian malignancy by color Doppler ultrasound. Obstet Gynecol 1994;84:605–608

105. Fleischer AC, Rodgers WH, Rao BK et al. Transvaginal color Doppler sonography of ovarian masses with pathological correlation. Ultrasound Obstet Gynecol 1991;1:275–278

106. Hamper UM, Sheth S, Abbas FM et al. Transvaginal color Doppler sonography of adnexal masses: differences in blood flow impedance in benign and malignant lesions. Am J Roentgenol 1993;160:1225–1228

107. Tailor A, Natucci M, Bourne TH et al. Comparative assessment of adnexal masses using colour and power Doppler imaging [abstract]. Ultrasound Obstet Gynecol 1995;5:25

108. Bromley B, Goodman H, Bencerraf BR. Comparison between sonographic morphology and Doppler waveform for the diagnosis of ovarian malignancy. Obstet Gynecol 1994;83:434–437

Computed Tomography and Magnetic Resonance Imaging of the Ovary

KATHRYN A. OCCHIPINTI

Recent advances in magnetic resonance imaging (MRI) sequences and surface coils (fast T2-weighted sequences and pelvic phased array coil) have improved resolution and contrast in MRI of the ovary. MRI is now the method of choice when ultrasound is indeterminate in evaluation of the ovary and adnexal masses, such as cysts, endometriomas, and pelvic inflammatory disease (PID). MRI can also be used to diagnose more uncommon conditions, such as peritoneal pseudocysts, adnexal torsion, massive ovarian edema, and rare forms of ectopic pregnancy.

Many processes that involve the ovary can be imaged with computed tomography (CT). CT is less desirable than MRI for imaging the ovary, however, due to the necessity of exposing the patient to ionizing radiation, lack of multiplanar imaging capability, and poor soft tissue contrast when compared with both ultrasound and MRI.

The use of intravenous contrast for MRI (gadopentetate dimeglumine) is essential for the MRI evaluation of internal architecture of ovarian masses. Both contrast-enhanced MRI and CT can be used in the preoperative evaluation and preliminary staging of women with suspected ovarian carcinoma.

Although controversial, cross-sectional imaging with MRI or CT has also been suggested as an alternative to routine second-look laparotomy after initial treatment for ovarian carcinoma.

MRI OF BENIGN OVARIAN DISORDERS

Non-neoplastic Cysts

The ovary is a dynamic organ in which follicles and functional cysts develop throughout life.[1-3] Ultrasound is preferred for the evaluation of follicular development and ovarian cysts, as it is noninvasive, readily available, and inexpensive when compared with MRI, but ovarian follicles and cysts are well visualized on MRIs as well (Fig. 23.1).

Follicular Cyst

Ovarian follicles as small as several millimeters can be clearly seen with MRI. A follicular cyst is defined as a persistent follicle 3 cm or larger.[4] On MRI, follicular cysts usually have the high signal intensity of simple fluid (low signal intensity on T1-weighted images, high signal intensity on T2-weighted images). High signal intensity will be present on both T1- and T2-weighted sequences if the cyst becomes hemorrhagic (Fig. 23.2). The wall of a follicular cyst is thin and enhances with intravenous contrast, while the center of the cyst does not enhance and remains low signal intensity.

A corpus luteum normally forms during the second half of the menstrual cycle and undergoes hemorrhagic involution if pregnancy does not occur. Exaggeration of the normal involutional process may cause the corpus luteum to enlarge to the size of a cyst.[5] A corpus luteum cyst with internal hemorrhage will appear as a high signal intensity, round lesion on both T1- and T2-weighted images (Fig. 23.2).

Theca Lutein Cysts

Theca lutein cysts are ovarian cysts that histologically are surrounded by luteinized theca cells and develop in response to high levels of endogenous hormones. Theca lutein cysts are commonly found in patients with hydatidiform moles, but they may also develop after overstimulation of the ovaries by clomiphene or gonadotropins and in cases of multiple, or even rarely, singleton pregnancies. Theca lutein cysts are almost always multiple and bilateral and cause gross enlargement of the ovary, to 10 or 20 cm in diameter. The MRI appearance of bilateral, multiple, large cysts with signal intensity of simple fluid is characteristic.

Serous Inclusion Cysts

Serous inclusion cysts are nonfunctional cysts found on the surface of the ovary in postmenopausal women. These cysts are the result of repeated ovulation with infolding of the surface epithelium and retention of serous or bloody fluid.[6] They are usually asymptomatic and may appear and disappear without consequence throughout postmenopausal life.[3] The MRI diagnosis of a serous inclusion cyst can be suggested if a round lesion with thin walls and central signal intensity of fluid is visualized. Follow-up examination is necessary in the postmenopausal woman to differentiate a simple cyst from a serous cystadenoma or cystadenocarcinoma, which can have a similar appearance.

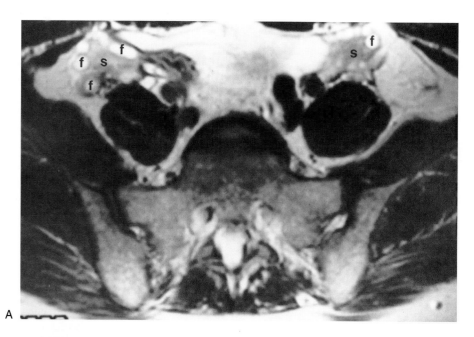

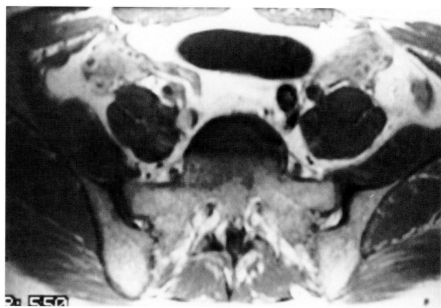

Figure 23.1 Normal ovary. **(A)** Axial T2-weighted image of the ovaries in a reproductive-age woman obtained with a phased-array coil. The central ovarian stroma (s) is low signal intensity, surrounded by high signal intensity follicles (f). **(B)** Contrast-enhanced axial T1-weighted image obtained with a phased-array coil in the same woman demonstrates enhancement of ovarian stroma. Follicles do not enhance, and they remain low signal intensity.

Differential Diagnosis of Non-neoplastic Cysts

Endometriosis

The diagnosis of endometriosis is often made at laparoscopy, as no currently available imaging modality is able to detect the small peritoneal implants and adhesions found in early stage disease.[7] In the diagnosis of ovarian endometriomata, MRI is more sensitive than ultrasound or CT, with sensitivity varying from 68% to 90% and specificity from 83% to 96%.[8,9] The most useful application

of MRI is in the diagnosis of extraperitoneal lesions that are difficult to visualize at surgery in the rectovaginal septum, presacral region, urinary bladder wall, abdominal wall, and sciatic nerve.[10]

Endometrial implants have been described as intermediate signal intensity on T1-weighted images. On T2-weighted images, both high signal intensity (like normal endometrial tissue) and low signal intensity (from fibrosis) have been described.[11,12] Endometriomas are of variable signal intensity due to superimposed acute and chronic hemorrhage but most commonly demonstrate high signal intensity on both T1- and T2-weighted

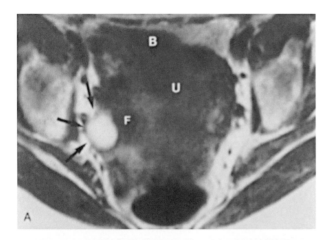

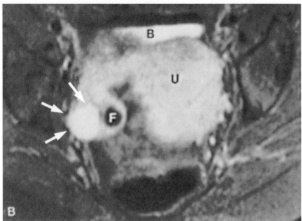

Figure 23.2 Ovary with two follicle cysts. **(A)** Axial T1-weighted image of the right ovary demonstrates a low signal intensity follicle cyst (F) and an adjacent high signal intensity ovarian cyst (arrows). U, uterus; B, bladder. **(B)** After intravenous contrast enhancement with gadolinium-DTPA, fat-saturated axial T1-weighted images demonstrate enhancement of the ovarian stroma. A low signal intensity follicle cyst (F) is well delineated against the enhancing stroma. The second ovarian cyst remains of high-signal intensity (arrows), verifying the presence of hemorrhage. U, uterus; B, bladder. (From Occhipinti et al.,[27] with permission.)

images, with regions of low signal intensity from hemosiderin (shading) on T2-weighted images (Fig. 23.3). A fluid–fluid level may also be visualized. Fat saturation images are useful for identifying small lesions and for verifying the presence of hemorrhage[13] (Fig. 23.3). A fibrotic wall often develops around the endometrioma and appears as a low signal intensity rim on T1- and T2-weighted images. After administration of intravenous contrast, the wall of an endometrioma may enhance, and loculations may be seen. Ovarian endometriomata cannot be reliably differentiated from functional hemorrhagic ovarian cysts by MRI, as both will have similar location and signal intensity.

Pelvic Inflammatory Disease

Clinical history and physical examination can establish a diagnosis of PID. Early PID may not be demonstrated by ultrasound. If hydrosalpinges, pyosalpinges, or a tubo-ovarian ab-

scess develop, these abnormalities can be visualized sonographically. When the diagnosis is not clear on ultrasound, MRI can be used to distinguish between a dilated fallopian tube and a cystic ovarian mass. A tortuous fallopian tube folded on itself can usually be identified in at least one plane on axial, sagittal, or coronal images. Serous fluid within the tube is of similar signal intensity to water (low intensity on T1-weighted images and high intensity on T2-weighted images); pyosalpinx or hemorrhagic fluid will appear as high-signal intensity and will be noted on both T1- and T2-weighted sequences.[14] In the patient with PID, the walls of the fallopian tubes, which are not usually demonstrated by MRI, can be visualized and can enhance with intravenous contrast.

Paratubal Cysts

Occasionally, adnexal cysts are not ovarian in origin. Remnants of the wolffian duct system include the hydatid cysts of Morgagni, which are found along the course of the fallopian tubes, and paratubal cysts, which are located in the broad ligament. These remnants are often seen as persistent simple cysts, separate from the ovary. Hydatid cysts of Morgagni are usually under 1 cm in diameter, while paratubal cysts are usually greater than 1 cm. Both are usually thin-walled with no solid elements and contain simple serous fluid. They are usually asymptomatic but when located close to the ovary, they may be difficult to differentiate from functional ovarian cysts.[15]

Peritoneal Pseudocysts

Peritoneal pseudocysts (or mesenteric inclusion cysts) are formed within the pelvis when normal peritoneal fluid (fluid that is released from the ovary during normal ovulation) becomes trapped in the pelvis by adhesions that have resulted from previous PID or endometriosis. Pseudocysts have an irregular shape because the outer surface is not a true wall but is composed of the adjacent ovary, uterus, and pelvic sidewall. Septa within the pseudocyst and distortion of pelvic anatomy may make differentiation from cystic tumor difficult by ultrasound.[16] MRI can demonstrate the extent of the pseudocyst and the septa within it. MRI signal intensity characteristics of the uterus and ovary (on T2-weighted and contrast-enhanced T1-weighted images) can also be used to identify the location of these pelvic organs around the cystic fluid collection. Signal intensity within the cyst is most often that of simple fluid (low on T1-weighted images and high on T2-weighted images) but has also been reported to be high on T1-weighted images due to hemorrhage, with layering of hemosiderin seen as low-signal intensity on T2-weighted sequences. If endometriosis is the cause of the adhesions in patients who develop peritoneal pseudocysts, ovarian endometriomata may be a concurrent finding.

CT OF BENIGN OVARIAN DISORDERS
Non-neoplastic Cysts

CT images may vaguely demonstrate normal ovarian follicles (Fig. 23.4). Functional ovarian cysts appear as round masses with thin walls and enclosed fluid with the attenuation value of water[17] (Fig. 23.5). The walls will enhance after administration of

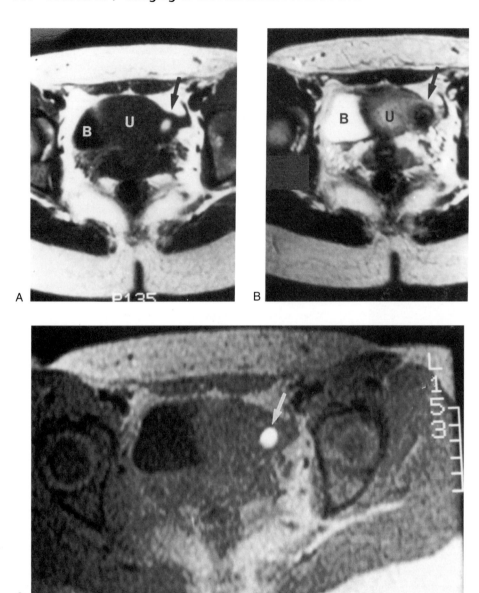

Figure 23.3 Endometriosis. **(A)** Axial T1-weighted sequence demonstrates a high-signal intensity focus in the left adnexa (arrow). U uterus; B, bladder. **(B)** Axial T2-weighted sequence
demonstrates an intermediate and low-signal intensity lesion in the left adnexa (arrow), with a
low-signal intensity rim (due to fibrosis), consistent with an endometrial implant/endometrioma.
U, uterus; B, bladder. **(C)** Fat-saturation axial T1-weighted sequence verifies the lesion is hemorrhagic, as it remains high signal intensity (arrow).

intravenous contrast. If internal septa are present, they will also
enhance (Fig. 23.5). Hemorrhagic cysts can be identified by the
high attenuation value of subacute hemorrhage, and a fluid–fluid
level may be present within a functional cyst on CT.[18]

Endometriosis

Peritoneal endometrial implants and adhesions in mild endometriosis are not evident on CT images. Endometriomas have
a nonspecific appearance on CT images and can have attenuation values of soft tissue or cystic masses.[19] As with functional
cysts, subacute hemorrhage can be detected in endometriomas
by the high attenuation value on CT.[20] MRI with fat saturation

is more sensitive than CT, however, and is preferable if cross-
sectional imaging is requested before staging laparoscopy.

MRI OF SURGICAL EMERGENCIES RELATED
TO THE OVARY

Adnexal Torsion and Massive
Ovarian Edema

Adnexal torsion is defined as rotation of the ovary and fallopian tube around the broad ligament. Rarely, the ovary alone
may undergo torsion around the mesovarium. Torsion may oc-

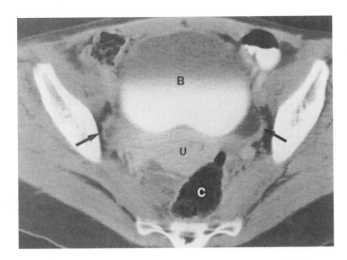

Figure 23.4 Contrast-enhanced CT section through normal uterus and adnexa in a reproductive-age woman. Although the ovaries are not clearly delineated, low attenuation regions that represent follicles can be visualized (arrows). U, uterus; B, bladder; C, sigmoid colon. (From Occhipinti et al.,[27] with permission.)

cur at all ages. In both children and adults, some cases will occur with normal ovaries, but often, an underlying ovarian mass predisposes to torsion by enlarging the ovary and lifting it out of the pelvis.[21] The most common ovarian mass associated with torsion is the dermoid cyst. A cystadenoma, functional ovarian cyst, or rarely, a malignant tumor may also occur. With ovarian torsion, restriction of the venous supply will occur first and result in hemorrhagic venous infarction; arterial flow will be compromised later. The clinical presentation usually suggests a surgical emergency, with severe pelvic pain that must be differentiated from ectopic pregnancy or appendicitis.

MRI will show the ovarian mass associated with an enlarged, edematous ovary and dilated fallopian tube on T1- and T2-weighted images (Fig. 23.6). With hemorrhagic infarction of the associated ovarian mass, a high signal intensity rim can be seen on the T1-weighted image.[22]

Massive edema of the ovary is believed to be the result of intermittent ovarian torsion and usually occurs in women 20 to 30 years of age, often in a normal ovary. Compromise of venous and lymphatic drainage results in marked enlargement of the ovary from edema that collects in the central ovarian stroma. Ascites and Meig syndrome can be associated. MRIs of the ovary show the high signal intensity fluid within the enlarged ovary on the T2-weighted images.[23]

MRI OF OVARIAN-RELATED ENDOCRINE DISORDERS

Ovarian Disorders Associated With Increased Androgen Production

Polycystic Ovaries

Polycystic ovaries are characterized by an increase in the amount of central stroma and multiple, small, 8- to 10-mm im-

mature follicles in the periphery of the ovary. Transvaginal ultrasound can detect the small follicles and hypertrophied central stroma in women with polycystic ovaries.[24] MRI findings have been reported from images obtained with a body coil and include low signal intensity of the central stroma on T2-weighted images, along with multiple small peripheral follicles of similar size.[25] Decrease in the signal intensity of normal ovarian stroma is also present on MRIs of the normal ovary obtained with fast spin echo (FSE) weighting, and the diagnosis of polycystic ovaries therefore remains a clinical one.

Stromal Hyerplasia and Stromal Hyperthecosis

Mild hyperplasia of the medullary and cortical stroma is a common pathologic finding in postmenopausal women, but when the histologic distinction between the medulla and cortex is obscured, stromal hyperplasia is diagnosed.[26] The clinical findings are secondary to excessive androgen production from the excess stroma and can be associated with diabetes, hypertension, and obesity.

Stromal hyperthecosis is a combination of stromal hyperplasia and luteinized theca cells, which occurs in women of reproductive age. This entity is clinically similar to polycystic ovarian syndrome, with menstrual irregularity and obesity. Virilization is often more severe and progressive with stromal hyperthecosis and does not respond to medical therapy, as do polycystic ovaries. Bilateral oophorectomy may be necessary to halt the virilization process in severe cases.

MRI findings in stromal hyperthecosis include bilateral enlargement of the ovaries with multiple cysts of various sizes.[27]

Tumors Associated With Excess Androgen Production

The most common ovarian tumor to cause virilization is the Sertoli-Leydig cell tumor (androblastoma). Brenner tumors and the rare lipid cell tumor also secrete androgens. The granulosa cell tumor and the thecoma, which usually produce es-

Figure 23.5 Contrast-enhanced CT section of a benign folliculer cyst of the right ovary with a single septum (arrows) in a reproductive-age woman. U, uterus; B, bladder; C, sigmoid colon. (From Occhipinti et al.,[27] with permission.)

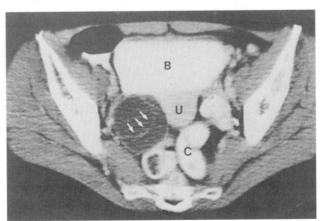

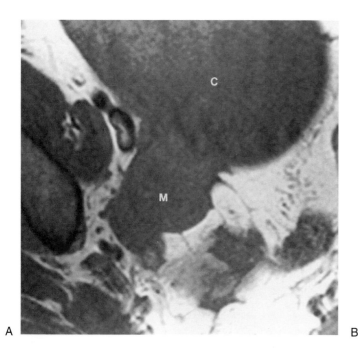

A

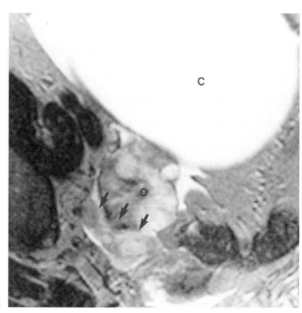

B

Figure 23.6 Ovarian torsion. **(A)** Axial T1-weighted image performed with a phased-array coil shows an adnexal mass (M) and adjacent large, low signal intensity cyst (C). **(B)** Axial T2-weighted fast spin echo (FSE) image demonstrated the adnexal "mass," which actually represents an enlarged, markedly edematous ovary (o) and a coiled, edematous tube posteriorly (arrows). The cyst (C) has characteristic high signal intensity. At pathology, ovarian torsion was found with a hemorrhagic, infarcted ovary and a large simple cyst. (Figure **B** from Outwater and Schiebler,[12] with permission.)

trogen, have rarely been reported to produce androgens. Patients with virilizing ovarian tumors usually have higher levels of serum testosterone (>150 nl/dl) than those with polycystic ovaries or stromal hyperthecosis.

MRI finding of Sertoli-Leyding tumors, lipid cell, and Brenner tumors have not been described in the literature but would be expected to have signal characteristics of predominantly solid tumors. Lipid cell tumors contain varying amount of lipid histologically, which in theory might be detected by MRI. Rare virilizing granulosa cell tumors have been described as predominantly cystic histologically, while thecomas are predominantly solid.[28]

Tumors Associated With Excess Estrogen Production

Granulosa cell tumors and thecomas commonly produce estrogen. Clinical manifestations of the granulosa cell tumor include pseudoprecocious puberty, amenorrhea, abnormal uterine bleeding in the reproductive years, and uterine bleeding after the menopause. Sexual precocity is rarely associated with the thecoma, but symptoms are otherwise the same. Granulosa cell tumours are prone to rupture and may recur 20 to 30 years after treatment.[29] Granulosa cell tumors may be solid, cystic, or both, and are of low-grade malignancy. Thecomas are often difficult to separate from fibromas histologically but both are solid, benign tumors.

The MRI appearance of the granulosa cell tumor is most often a multicystic mass with solid components (Fig. 23.7).

Figure 23.7 Juvenile granulosa cell tumor in a pregnant patient. Axial T2-weighted image shows the gravid uterus and fetus (curved arrows) and a left-sided unilocular mass (M). The presence of a papillary excrescence (straight arrow) is noted within the mass. Juvenile granulosa cell tumor was removed at surgery. (From Outwater and Schiebler,[12] with permission.)

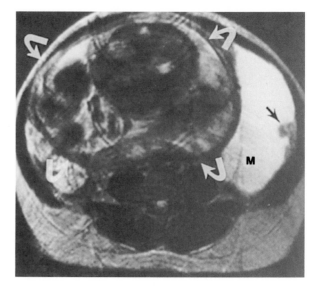

The cystic component can contain serous fluid or clotted blood.[29] Although MRI characteristics of a pure thecoma have not been described, fibro thecomas would be expected to have similar signal intensity characteristics and very low signal intensity on T2-weighted images.[30]

MRI DIFFERENTIATION OF BENIGN AND MALIGNANT OVARIAN MASSES.

As a women advances in age, the over-all chance that an ovarian tumor will be malignant increases, from 1 in 15 in the second decade to 1 in 3 by 45 years of age.[31] As a result, much MRI research has focused on developing criteria that can be used to differentiate benign from malignant masses.

The dermoid cyst, the most common benign ovarian tumor in younger women, can be reliably diagnosed by MRI if fat can be identified within the tumor. The largest group of ovarian tumors, the serous and mucinous cystic tumors, have an appearance more difficult to consign to the definitely benign category by cross-sectional imaging. This is due to the histologic appearance of these tumors, which is on a continuum from the benign to the malignant forms. Benign lesions generally lack solid components (except for the less common cases of serous or mucinous papillary cystadenomas, which can have a few soft tissue protrusions, or papillary projections). Papillary projections are a common finding in borderline and malignant tumors, and if they are present on cross-sectional images, malignancy must be considered. Other signs of malignancy commonly found in high-grade malignant tumors include a predominantly solid component, often with necrosis, and thick irregular walls.

MRI features that suggest that an adnexal mass is benign include

1. Size less than 4 cm
2. Entirely cystic components
3. Wall thickness less than 3 mm
4. Lack of internal structure
5. Absence of ascites
6. Absence of invasive characteristics, such as peritoneal disease or adenopathy.[32]

These criteria were developed in conjunction with the use of intravenous contrast, which visualizes the internal structure of an ovarian mass.[33] The wall of the lesion, internal septa, papillary projections, and solid components will enhance after administration of intravenous contrast (Fig. 23.8). Using the above criteria, preoperative characterization of ovarian lesions by MRI is reported to be as high as 95%.[34]

MRI VS. CT DIFFERENTIATION OF BENIGN AND MALIGNANT OVARIAN MASSES

Due to its multiplanar imaging capability, MRI is superior to ultrasound or CT in the differentiation of adnexal and uterine masses.[7,35] MRI is also invaluable in the investigation of the

Figure 23.8 Borderline serous cystadenocarcinoma with papillary projections. **(A)** Axial T2-weighted FSE image of a right ovarian mass in a 24-year-old that is predominantly cystic with low signal intensity papillary projections (arrows). The uterus (U), with normal zonal anatomy, is well-visualized adjacent to the mass. **(B)** Pathologic specimen with interior of the opened cyst shows granular papillary projections. Histologic diagnosis was a borderline malignancy. Peritoneal washings obtained at surgery were negative for malignant cells. (From Outwater and Schiebler,[12] with permission.)

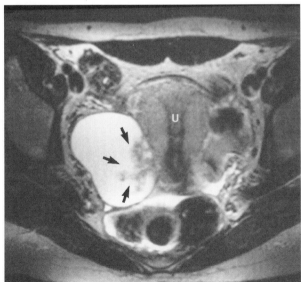

A

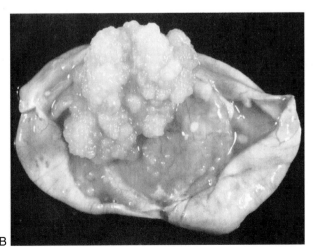

B

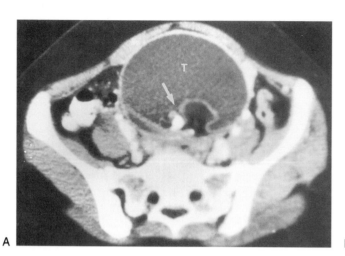
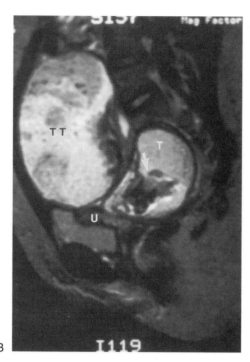

A   B

Figure 23.9 Benign teratoma. **(A)** CT image demonstrates a large cystic lesion (T) with a Rokitansky protruberance (arrow) containing chunks of calcification. CT findings are characteristic of a teratoma. **(B)** Sagittal T2-weighted MRI in the same patient again demonstrates the teratoma (T) noted on CT, with low-signal intensity calcification in the Rokitansky protruberance (arrow). A second, larger teratoma (TT) can also be visualized adjacent to the first, due to the large field of view offered by MRI. The relationship of both teratomas to the uterus (U) is easily seen on one image.

pregnant patient with an indeterminate adnexal mass on ultrasound due to its lack of ionizing radiation, large field of view, and superior soft tissue characterization (Fig. 23.7).[36] A prospective comparison of MRI, transvaginal sonography with Doppler, and carcinoembryonic antigen (CEA) 125 found MRI to have the highest rate of accuracy in differentiating benign from malignant ovarian lesion.[37] One study directly compared CT and non-contrast-enhanced MRI and found them to be similar in classification of ovarian tumors, although MRI was found superior in the over all classification of adnexal lesions.[38]

MRI OF BENIGN OVARIAN TUMORS

In women over 45 years, benign epithelial ovarian tumors (serous and mucinous cystadenomas) are the most common ovarian tumors, accounting for 80% of all benign neoplasms.[39] Fibromas and fibrothecomas are more rare tumors of stromal origin, which occur in a small percentage of patients both before and after menopause.

Mature Teratoma (Dermoid Cyst)

The mature teratoma (dermoid cyst) is the most common benign ovarian tumor found in women under 45 years. These teratomas are composed of mature tissue from two or more embryonic germ cell layers. Most consist primarily of a cystic component that resembles the epidermis and contains sebaceous material, hair, calcification or teeth, and possibly a soft tissue mass that a projects into the lumen called a *Rokitansky protuberance*. Less common forms of mature teratomas are the monodermal types and include the struma ovarii (mature thyroid tissue predominates) and carcinoid tumors. Both of these tumors contain primarily solid tissue.

MRI with fat saturation will demonstrate high signal intensity fat on T1-weighted images, which will become low signal intensity with the application of fat saturation. These MRI findings can be used to diagnose a dermoid cyst. Chemical shift artifact, if present, is diagnostic of fat within the tumor as well. Chemical shift artifact is not always present and is limited by tumor shape, field of view, and orientation of the lipid–water interface in the plane of section.[40,41] The dermoid plug can often be visualized as a solid component, but calcification, which most commonly appears as low signal intensity on both T1- and T2-weighted images, is not as easily identified by MRI as it is with CT (Fig. 23.9). MRI characteristics of the rare struma ovarii type of teratoma are that of a nonspecific solid mass with cystic components.[42]

Serous and Mucinous Cystadenoma

The serous cystadenoma is a thin-walled, unilocular, or multilocular tumor that is filled with serous fluid. The mucinous cystadenoma is less common, almost always multilocular, and often very large (15 to 30 cm in diameter).[43] Each locule in a mucinous cystadenoma is filled with watery or thick mucinous fluid. Hemorrhage and papillary projections may be found histologically in benign forms but are much more common in borderline and malignant forms.

Both serous and mucinous cystadenomas are well demonstrated on MRI. The tumor can be visualized arising from the ovary on T2-weighted images and on contrast-enhanced T1-weighted images (Fig. 23.10). The cystic locules of serous cystadenomas follow signal intensity of simple fluid (low on T1-weighted images, high on T2-weighted images), while the cystic locules of mucinous cystadenomas are of varying signal intensity, depending on the ratio of water and mucin in each (either high or low signal intensity on T1 and T2-weighted images). After intravenous contrast administration, the wall of these cystic lesions, as well as any internal septa, will enhance on T1-weighted images (Fig. 23.10).

Fibroma and Fibrothecoma

Benign ovarian fibromas are solid ovarian tumors that arise from the ovarian stromal cells. The histology of the fibrothecoma often blends imperceptibly with the fibroma. When the tumor enlarges over 10 cm, Meig syndrome (ascites and hydrothorax associated with a benign tumor) may be present. Ovarian fibromas are multiple, bilateral, and calcified in patients with the basal cell nevus syndrome.[44] The MRI appearance is that of a well-circumscribed, low signal intensity tumor on both T1 and T2-weighted images. The multiplanar imaging capability provided by MRI can allow differentiation from a uterine leiomyoma, which has similar signal intensity.

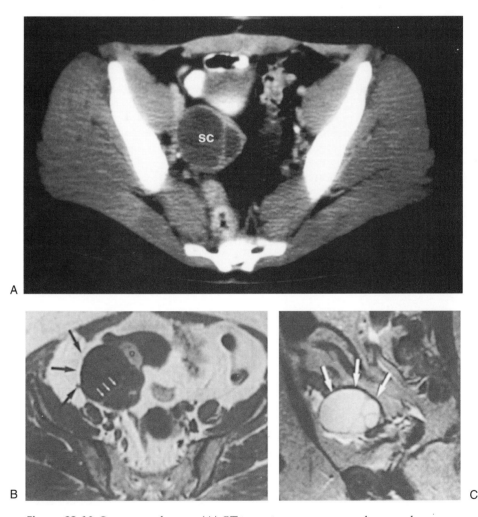

Figure 23.10 Serous cystadenoma. **(A)** CT image in a postmenopausal woman demonstrates a cystic lesion with enhancing walls and a septum (sc). Surgical resection confirmed a serous cystadenoma. **(B)** Axial contrast-enhanced T1-weighted image demonstrates a serous cystadenoma (black arrows) arising from the right ovary (o). Enhancing ovarian stroma and tumour septa (white arrows) are well-visualized against the low signal intensity serous fluid within the lesion. **(C)** Sagittal T2-weighted image demonstrates high signal intensity fluid within the serous cystadenoma (arrows). Septa are now low signal intensity. (B & C from Occhipinti et al.,[27] with permission.)

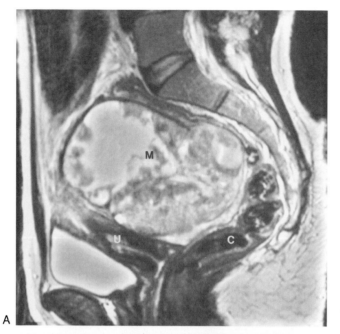

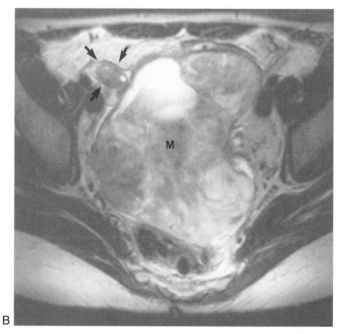

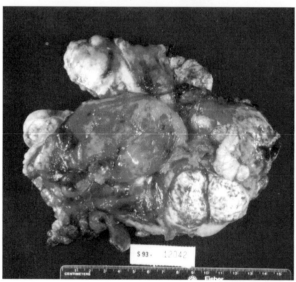

Figure 23.11 Endometroid carcinoma. **(A)** Sagittal T2-weighted FSE image obtained with a multicoil shows a large cystic and solid mass (M) located above the uterus and anterior to the sigmoid colon (C). U, uterus. **(B)** Axial T2-weighted FSE image demonstrates the extensive solid components of the mass (M). The right ovary (arrows) shows no evidence of tumor excrescences in the lining of the cystic portion of the mass. **(C)** Gross appearance of the mass. Histology showed a poorly differentiated endometroid adenocarcinoma of the left ovary. (From Outwater and Schiebler,[12] with permission.)

CT OF BENIGN OVARIAN TUMORS

Mature Teratoma (Dermoid Cyst)

The dermoid cyst appears as a well-circumscribed ovarian mass by CT scan. The sebaceous contents measure fat attenuation,[45] and a fat–fluid level may be present, often with a hair ball floating at the interface; foci of calcification or teeth are well demonstrated as high attenuation foci within the Rokitansky nodule[46] (Fig. 23.9). Torsion of the tumor has been reported as thickening of the cyst wall and dilatation of the ipsilateral fallopian tube on CT images.[47] Fat attenuation on CT is diagnostic of a teratoma.

Serous and Mucinous Cystadenoma; Fibroma and Fibrothecoma

Serous and mucinous cystadenomas appear as cystic masses with thin walls on CT images (Fig. 23.10). Fluid within the locules would be expected to be close to that of water attenuation in serous cystadenomas, or of slightly higher attenuation, consistent with protein in mucinous cystadenomas.[48] The thin walls of these cystic tumors enhance after intravenous contrast administration (Fig. 23.10). The CT appearance of an ovarian fibroma is that of a nonspecific, solid adnexal lesion. Ovarian fibromas cannot be easily differentiated from an exophytic leiomyoma or other soft tissue mass within the pelvis by CT.

CT AND MRI OF OVARIAN CARCINOMA

Ovarian carcinoma is the most common cause of death from a malignancy of the female reproductive tract; most women present late with stage III disease, and over all survival is only 41%.[49] The current method for staging of ovarian carcinoma is surgical exploration, with hysterectomy, bilateral oophorectomy, omentectomy, and peritoneal washings. Cryoreduction is also performed at the initial surgery and is considered optimal if any tumor fragments left behind are less than 2 cm in diameter. The role of CT and MRI in staging of ovarian carcinoma is controversial but has gained renewed importance with the realization that surgical understaging and suboptimal cryoreduction can be found in 30 to 40% of cases at initial surgery.[50] The stage at presentation directly affects prognosis of ovarian carcinoma, and adequate cryoreduction has been directly related to improved survival by enhancing the effect of chemotherapy.[51] As a result, cross-sectional imaging for preoperative assessment was recommended at the 1995 National Institutes of Health (NIH) Consensus Conference in order to assess lesions preoperatively that may be difficult to visualize at surgery and therefore avoid surgical understaging as well as to optimize cryoreduction.[52]

CT and MRI have been found to perform similarly in the staging of ovarian carcinoma in two prospective comparative studies, with over all accuracy from the larger series 77% for CT and 78% for MRI.[53,54] Both modalities are limited in the detection of small, 5 to 8 mm peritoneal implants, which are consistently missed when located within the mesentery and small bowel. Peritoneal implants have been reported as a limiting factor in the staging of ovarian carcinoma on several other reports of CT and MRI staging.[55,56] In two reports prediction of cancer resectability was found to be excellent, with 100% achieved with CT and 91% with MRI,[57,58] and either modality can fulfill the NIH criteria for prediction of optimal cryoreduction. In a report that assessed only CT findings of ovarian carcinoma referable to the abdomen, CT was found to predict the success of primary debulking surgery successfully.[59]

CT AND MRI OF MALIGNANT OVARIAN TUMORS

Ovarian carcinoma is classified by cell type, and the most common cell type of origin is the ovarian epithelium. Serous cystadenocarcinoma accounts for 40% of all ovarian malignancies, followed by endometroid carcinoma (15% to 25%), mucinous cystadenocarcinoma (10%), and the rare clear cell carcinoma.[60]

MRI and CT findings suggestive of a malignant ovarian tumor include a thick, irregular wall, thick septa, papillary projections, and a large soft tissue component with necrosis. Both MRI and CT demonstrate enhancement of the soft tissue components of the lesions after administration of intravenous contrast; necrotic and cystic portions of the tumor will not enhance and become more visible (Fig. 23.11). MRI signal intensity characteristics help in the diagnosis of cystic regions and in determining cyst contents (simple vs. mucinous or hemorrhagic), as previously described.

CT AND MRI STAGING OF OVARIAN CARCINOMA

CT and MRI staging criteria have been developed to correspond to the FIGO (International Federation of Gynecology and Obstetrics) classification followed at surgical staging (Table 23.1). Both modalities must be able to detect tumor limited to one or both ovaries for stage I disease, detect a small amount of ascites and extension of the ovarian mass into the pelvic organs for stage II disease, and demonstrate peritoneal implants and omental involvement for stage III disease. Hepatic or distant metastases is a stage IV diagnosis.

CT and MRI appearance of pelvic extension to the uterus appears as localized distortion of the uterine contour or irregular tumor–myometrial interface. An additional feature of MRI is disruption of the normal uterine zonal anatomy on T2-weighted images and on contrast-enhanced T1-weighted images (Fig. 23.12). Sigmoid colon invasion can be diagnosed by both modalities as loss of tissue planes between the tumor and sigmoid colon or direct encasement by tumor.

Table 23.1 CT/MRI Modified Staging of Ovarian Carcinoma[a]

Stage	Criteria
I	Tumor limited to ovaries
Ia	Limited to one ovary; no ascites (intact capsule/no tumor external surface of capsule)
Ib	Limited to both ovaries, no ascites (+)
Ic	Stage Ia or Ib with ascites (or with tumor on surface; capsule ruptured, peritoneal washings positive for malignant cells)
II	Growth involving one or both ovaries; pelvic extension
IIa	Extension and/or metastases to the uterus and/or fallopian tubes
IIb	Extension to other pelvic tissues
IIc	Tumor either stage IIa or IIb with ascites (+ +)
III	Tumor involving one or both ovaries; peritoneal implants outside the pelvis and/or retroperitoneal or inguinal nodes including superficial liver metastases (histologically proven malignant extension to small bowel or omentum)
IIIa	Tumor grossly limited to the true pelvis (includes microscopic seeding of abdominal peritoneal)
IIIb	<2-cm implants of abdominal peritoneal surfaces
IIIc	>2-cm implants of abdominal peritoneal surface and/or retroperitoneal or inguinal nodes
IV	Growth involving one or both ovaries; distant metastases; parenchymal liver metastases

[a] Additional staging criteria used in pathologic and surgical staging are in parentheses.

(+), same as in Ia; (+ +), same as in Ic.

(From Forstner et al.,[54] with permission.)

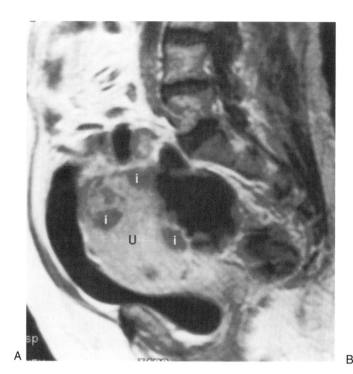
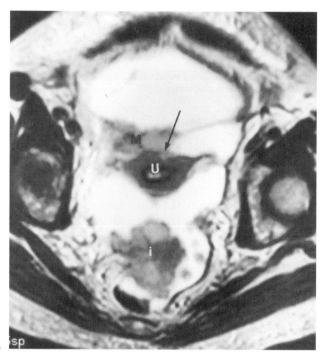

Figure 23.12 MRI appearance of uterine invasion and peritoneal implants. **(A)** Sagittal contrast-enhanced T1-weighted image demonstrates the enhancing uterus (U) with multiple, low signal intensity, enhancing implants (i) involving the uterine myometrium. **(B)** Axial T2-weighted image demonstrates the uterus (U) with ovarian mass (M) directly anterior. The solid portion of the mass disrupts the superficial myometrium (arrow), but preservation of overall zonal anatomy is otherwise noted. Peritoneal implants (i) are visualized in the cul-de-sac and are of variable signal intensity. Implants are well-delineated against the high-signal intensity ascites.

The appearance of tumor extension outside the pelvis is similar on both CT and MRI. Omental cake appears as a feathery or nodular infiltration with thickening of the omentum in both CT and MRI (Fig. 23.13). On MRI, signal intensity of omental fat is also decreased on T1 and T2-weighted images. Enhancement of tumor in the omentum is present with both CT and MRI.

Peritoneal implants appear as nodular or plaque-like lesions that project from the peritoneal surfaces in the pelvis and abdomen and enhance with contrast. The MRI signal intensity of peritoneal implants is usually intermediate to low on T1-weighted images and variable on T2-weighted images. When implants are low signal intensity on T2-weighted sequences, the appearance of peritoneal implants in the cul-de-sac is particularly striking against high signal intensity ascites (Fig. 23.12). Calcification within peritoneal implants can make small implants visible on CT images.[61]

CT AND MRI IN EVALUATION OF RECURRENT OVARIAN CARCINOMA

Second-look laparotomy has been performed in the past on a routine basis to evaluate patients with ovarian carcinoma after initial treatment. However, recent reports have deter-

mined that surgical cryoreduction performed at second-look laparotomy is not superior to chemotherapy for most patients, and routine debulking does not have a significant impact on patient survival.[62] At a recent NIH consensus conference, second-look laparotomy was no longer recommended on a routine basis.[63]

Both CT and MRI can be of value in assessing patients with recurrent ovarian carcinoma in order to determine which patients may not benefit from surgical re-evaluation. CT findings in implants greater than 2 cm on the diaphragm or liver surface, suprarenal adenopathy, and pleural or hepatic parenchymal disease were evaluated in one study as representing unresectable disease. CT was found to be 92.3% sensitive and 79.3% specific in predicting surgical outcome and determined to be an accurate measurement for prediction of successful surgical cryoreduction.[64]

MRI can also be used as a cross-sectional imaging modality to detect ovarian cancer recurrence and determine which patients may not be suitable for second-look laparotomy.[65] MRI findings of recurrent disease are similar to those in CT. Tumor detection is improved with even small amounts of ascites on MRI. Tumors that are best detected by MRI are those in the cul-de-sac of the pelvis, in the vaginal cuff, or on the liver surface. Detection is limited for peritoneal lesions in the pelvis, abdomen, and mesentery. With MRI, accuracy of 82% is re-

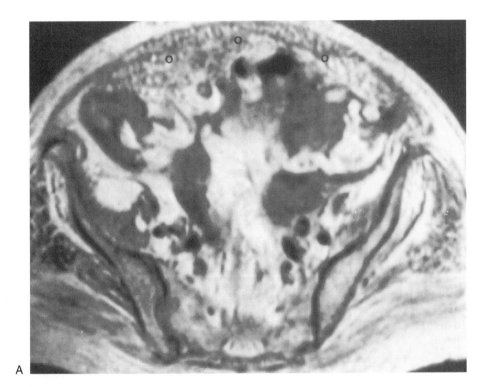

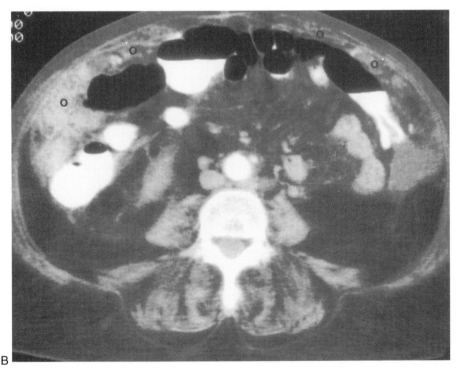

Figure 23.13 MRI and CT appearance of omental cake. **(A)** Axial T2-weighted image of the abdomen demonstrates the feathery appearance of low-signal intensity omental cake (o). **(B)** CT scan in the same patient demonstrates infiltration of the normal fatty omentum by soft-tissue omental cake (o).

ported for tumors with diameter of greater than 2 cm, which can be used to detect significant disease. This was found even in the absence of elevated CEA levels.[65]

SUMMARY

Due to its lack of ionizing radiation, multiplanar capability, and superb soft tissue resolution, MRI can play an integral role in evaluation of the ovary. Although ultrasound is the screening procedure of choice, MRI can be performed if ultrasound is indeterminate in evaluation of adnexal masses, including simple cysts, complex cysts, endometriosis, or PID. MRI can also perform an integral role in evaluation of more rare ovarian entities such as paratubal cysts or peritoneal pseudocysts, and in surgical emergencies.

MRI with administration of intravenous contrast can be used to evaluate ovarian masses, stage ovarian carcinoma, and evaluate patients for recurrent disease prior to second-look laparotomy.

REFERENCES

1. Cohen HL, Eisenberg P, Mandel F, Haller JO. Ovarian cysts are common in premenarchal girls: a sonographic study of 101 children 2-12 years old. AJR Am J Roentgenol 1992;159:89–91
2. Cohen HL, Shapiro MA, Mandel FS, Shapiro ML. Normal ovaries in neonates and infants: a sonographic study of 77 patients 1 day to 24 months old. AJR Am J Roentgenol 1993;160:583–586
3. Levine D, Gosink BB, Wolf SI et al. Simple adnexal cysts: the natural history in postmenopausal women. Radiology 1992;184:653–659
4. Morrow CP, Townsend DE. Tumour-like conditions of the ovary. In: Morrow CP, Townsend DE, Eds. Synopsis of Gynecologic Oncology (3rd ed.). Churchill Livingstone, New York 1987, p 339
5. Kurman RJ. Non-neoplastic lesions of the ovary. In: Kurman RJ, Ed. Blaustein's Pathology of the Female Genital Tract (3rd ed.). Springer-Verlag, New York, 1987, p 486
6. Disaia PJ. Ovarian disorders. In: Scott JR, Disaia PJ, Hammond CB, Spelacy WN, Eds. Danforth's Obstetrics and Gynecology (6th ed.). Lippincott, Philadelphia, 1990, p 1071
7. Dooms GC, Hricak H, Tscholakoff D. Adnexal structures: MR imaging. Radiology 1986;158:639–646
8. Togashi K, Nishimura K, Kimura I et al. Endometrial cysts: diagnosis with MR imaging. Radiology 1991;180:73–78
9. Outwater E, Scheibler ML, Owen RS, Schnall MD. Characterization of hemorrhagic adnexal lesions with MR imaging: blinded reader study. Radiology 1993;186:489–494
10. Binkovitz LA, King BF, Ehman RL. Sciatic endometriosis: MR appearance. J Comput Assist Tomogr 1991;15:508–510
11. Arrive L, Hricak H, Martin MC. Pelvic endometriosis: MR imaging. Radiology 1989;171:687–692
12. Outwater EK, Schiebler ML. Magnetic resonance imaging of the ovary. In: Mexrick R, Weinreb JC, Eds. Magnetic Resonance Imaging Clinics of North America. The Female Pelvis. WB Saunders, Philadelphia, 1994, p 257
13. Ha HK, Lim YT, Kim HS et al. Diagnosis of pelvic endometriosis: fat suppressed T1-weighted vs. conventional MR images. AJR Am J Roentgenol 1994;163:127–131
14. Occhipinti KA. Magnetic resonance imaging of abnormal pelvic anatomy. In: Jaffe R, Pierson RA, Abramowicz JS, Eds. Imaging in Infertility and Reproductive Endocrinology. JB Lippincott, Philadelphia, 1994, pp 264–266
15. Kimm JJ, Woo SK, Suh SJ, Morettin LB. Sonographic diagnosis of paraovarian cysts: value of detecting a separate ipsilateral ovary. AJR Am J Roentgenol 1995;164:1441–1444
16. Kurachi H, Murakami T, Nakamura H et al. Imaging of peritoneal pseudocysts: value of MR imaging compared with sonography and CT. AJR Am J Roentgenol 1993;161:589–591
17. Sawyer RW, Vick CW, Walsh JW, McClure PH. Computed tomography of benign ovarian masses. J Comput Assist Tomogr 1985;9:784–789
18. Scoutt LM, McCarthy SM, Moss A. Computed tomography and magnetic resonance imaging of the pelvis. In: Moss AA, Gamsu G, Genant H, Eds. Computed Tomography of the Body With Magnetic Resonance Imaging (2nd ed.). WB Saunders, Philadelphia, 1983, p 1215
19. Fishman EK, Scatarige JC, Saksouk F et al. Computed tomography of endometriosis. J Comput Assist Tomogr 1983;7:257–264
20. Buy JN, Ghossain MA, Mark AS et al. Focal hyperdense areas in endometriomas: a characteristic finding on CT. AJR Am J Roentgenol 1992;159:769–771
21. Russell P, Bannatyne P. Surgical Pathology of the Ovaries. Churchill Livingstone, New York, 1989, p 125
22. Kawakami K, Murata K, Kawaguchi N et al. Hemorrhagic infarction of the diseased ovary: a common MR finding in two cases. Magn Reson Imaging 1993;11:595–597
23. Lee AR, Kim KH, Lee BH, Chin SY. Massive edema of the ovary: imaging findings. AJR Am J Roentgenol 1993;161:343–344
24. Ardaens Y, Robert Y, Lemaitre L et al. Polycystic ovarian disease: contribution of vaginal endosonography and reassessment of ultrasonic diagnosis. Fertil Steril 1991;55:1062–1068
25. Mitchell DG, Gefter WB, Spritzer CE et al. Polycystic ovaries, MR imaging. Radiology 1986;160:425–429
26. Russell P, Bannatyne P. Surgical Pathology of the Ovaries. Churchill Livingstone, New York, 1989 p 113
27. Occhipinti KA, Frankel SD, Hricak H. The ovary, computed tomography and magnetic resonance imaging. In: Gooding GAW, Higgins CB, Eds. The Radiological Clinics of North America, Endocrine Radiology. WB Saunders, Philadelphia, 1993, pp 1122–1123
28. Morrow CP, Townsend DE. Sex-chord stromal neoplasms. In: Morrow CP, Townsend DE, Eds. Synopsis of Gynecologic Oncology (3rd ed.). Churchill Livingstone, New York, 1987, p 339
29. Scully RE. Granulosa-stromal cell tumours. In: Hartmass WH, Ed. Tumours of the Ovary and Maldeveloped Gonads, Atlas of Tumour Pathology (2nd series, fascicle 16) Armed Forces Institute of Pathology, Washington DC 1979, p 154–168
30. Carrington BM. The adnexae. In: Hricak H, Carrington BM, Eds. MRI of the Pelvis, Text Atlas. Martin Dunitz, London, 1991, p 190
31. Scully RE. General aspects of ovarian tumours. In: Hartmass WH, Ed. Tumours of the Ovary and Maldeveloped Gonads, Atlas of Tumour Pathology. (2nd series, Fascicle 16). Armed Forces Institute of Pathology, Washington, DC, 1979, p 31

32. Sica GT, Stevens SK, Hricak H et al. Comparison of unenhanced and contrast enhanced MR images in the evaluation of ovarian lesions. Presented at the 78th Scientific Assembly and Annual Meeting of the Radiological Society of North America, Chicago, 1992

33. Thurnher S, Hodler J, Baer S et al. Gadolinium-DOTA enhanced MR imaging of adnexal tumours. J Comput Assist Tomogr 1990;14:939–949

34. Stevens SK, Hricak H, Stern JL. Ovarian lesions: detection and characterization with gadolinium-enhanced MR images at 1.5T. Radiology 1991;181:481–488

35. Mitchell DG, Mintz MC, Spritzer CE et al. Adnexal masses: MR imaging observations at 1.5T, with US and CT correlation. Radiology 1987;162:319–324

36. Weinreb JC, Brown CE, Lowe TW et al. Pelvic masses in pregnant patients: MR and US imaging. Radiology 1986;159:717–724

37. Hata K, Hata T, Manabe A et al. A critical evaluation of transvaginal Doppler studies, transvaginal sonography, magnetic resonance imaging, and CA 125 in detecting ovarian cancer. Obstet Gynecol 1992;80:922–926

38. Ghossain MA, Buy JN, Ligneres C et al. Epithelial tumours of the ovary: comparison of MR and CT findings. Radiology 1991;181:863–870

39. Morrow CP, Townsend DE. Neoplasms derived from coelonic epithelium. In: Morrow CP, Townsend DE, Eds. Synopsis of Gynecologic Oncology (3rd ed.). Churchill Livingstone, New York, 1987, p 257

40. Togashi K, Nishimura K, Itoh K et al. Ovarian cystic teratomas: MR imaging. Radiology 1987;162:669–673

41. Smith RC, Lange RC, McCarthy SM. Chemical shift artifact: dependence on shape and orientation of the lipid–water interface. Radiology 1991;181:225–229

42. Outwater EK, Schiebler ML. Magnetic resonance imaging of the ovary. In: Mexrich R, Weinreb JC, Eds. Magnetic Resonance Imaging Clinics of North America. The Female Pelvis. WB Saunders, Philadelphia, 1994, pp 250–254

43. Scully RE. Mucinous tumours. In: Hartmass WH, Ed. Tumours of the Ovary and Maldeveloped Gonads, Atlas of Tumour Pathology (2nd series, fascicle 16). Armed Forces Institute of Pathology, Washington, DC, 1979, p 75.

44. Scully RE. Tumours in the thecoma-fibroma group. In: Hartmass WH, Ed. Tumours of the Ovary and Maldeveloped Gonads, Atlas of Tumour Pathology (2nd series, fascicle 16). Armed Forces Institute of Pathology, Washington, DC, 1979, p 182.

45. Friedman AC, Pyatt RS, Hartman DS et al. CT of benign cystic teratomas. AJR Am J Roentgenol 1982;138:659–665

46. Feldberg MA, vanWaes PF, Hendriks MJ. Direct multiplanar CT findings in cystic teratoma of the ovary. J Comput Assist Tomogr 1984;8:1131–1135

47. Buy JL, Ghossain MA, Moss AA et al. Cystic teratoma of the ovary: CT detection. Radiology 1989;171:697–701

48. Buy JL, Ghossain MA, Sciot C et al. Epithelial tumours of the ovary: CT findings and correlation with ultrasound. Radiology 1991;178:811–818

49. Cancer facts and figures—1994. American Cancer Society, New York, 1994, p 15

50. Young RC, Perez CA, Hoskins W. Cancer of the Ovary. In: DeVita VT, Hellman S, Rosenberg SA, eds. Cancer. Principles and Practice of Oncology (4th ed.). Lippincott, Philadelphia, 1993, pp 1226–1263

51. Smith JP, Day TG. Review of ovarian cancer at the University of Texas Medical Center, M.D. Anderson Hospital and Tumour Institute. Am J Obstet Gynecol 1979;153:984–993

52. NIH Consensus Conference. Ovarian cancer: Screening, treatment, and follow-up. JAMA 1995;273:491–497

53. Semelka RC, Lawrence PH, Shoenut JP et al. Primary ovarian cancer: prospective comparison of contrast-enhanced CT and pre and post contrast fat-suppressed MR imaging, with histologic correlation. J Magn Reson Imaging 1993;3:99–106

54. Forstner R, Hricak H, Occhipinti K et al. Value of CT and MR in the staging of ovarian cancer. Presented at the 80th Scientific Assembly and Annual Meeting of the Radiological Society of North America, Chicago, 1994

55. Jacquet P, Jelinek JS, Steves MA, Sugarbaker PH. Evaluation of computed tomography in patient with peritoneal carcinomatosis. Cancer 1993;72:1631–1636

56. Low RN, Sigeti JS. MR imaging of peritoneal disease: comparison of contrast-enhanced fast multiplanar spoiled gradient-recalled and spin-echo imaging. AJR Am J Roentgenol 1994; 163:1131–1140

57. Forstner R, Hricak H, Occhipinti K et al. Ovarian cancer: staging with CT and MR imaging Radiology 1995;197:619–626

58. Nelson BE, Rosenfield AT, Schwartz PE. Preoperative abdominopelvic computed tomographic prediction of optimal cytoreduction in epithelial ovarian carcinoma. J Clin Oncol 1993;11:166–172

59. Meyer JI, Kennedy AW, Fiedman R et al. Ovarian carcinoma: value of CT in predicting the success of debulking surgery. AJR Am J Roentgenol 1995;165:875–878

60. Scully RE. Serous tumours. In: Hartmass WH, Ed. Tumours of the Ovary and Maldeveloped Gonads, Atlas of Tumour Pathology (2nd series, fascicle 16). Armed Forces Institute of Pathology, Washington, DC, 1979, p 55

61. Mitchell DG, Hill MC, Hill S, Zaloudek C. Serous carcinoma of the ovary: CT identification of metastatic calcified implants. Radiology 1986;158:649–652

62. Podratz KC, Kinney WK. Second look operation in ovarian cancer. Cancer 1993;71 (suppl 4):1551–1558

63. NIH Consensus Development Panel on Ovarian Cancer. Screening, treatment and follow-up. JAMA 1995;273: 491–496

64. Nelson BE, Rosenfield AT, Schwartz PE. Preoperative abdominopelvic computed tomographic prediction of optimal cryoreduction in epithelial ovarian carcinoma. J Clin Oncol 1993;11:166–172

65. Forstner R, Hricak H, Powell CB et al. Ovarian cancer recurrence: value of MR imaging. Radiology 1995;196:715–720

Computed Tomography, Magnetic Resonance Imaging, and Ultrasonography of Nongynecologic Pelvic Masses

ZÉLIA M.S. CAMPOS

CLÁUDIO CAMPI DE CASTRO

MARIA HELENA S. CAMPOS

GIOVANNI GUIDO CERRI

This chapter describes the computed tomography (CT), magnetic resonance imaging (MRI), and ultrasound appearances of pelvic masses that do not arise from the female genital tract.

GASTROINTESTINAL TRACT MASSES

Inflammatory Diseases

Appendicitis

CT is said to be more accurate than ultrasound in the diagnosis of acute appendicitis, with a sensitivity of 96%, a specificity of 89%, and an accuracy of 94%.[1] Noncontrast scans may be used, although thin patients may require oral and intravenous contrast, due to difficulty identifying fat planes.

The normal appendix often appears as a small tubular or ringlike structure in the right lower quadrant. It may be collapsed or slightly filled with fluid or air, with a thin wall and surrounded by the homogeneous fat density of the normal mesentery. Appendicoliths may be seen as ringlike or homogeneous calcium-density structures, and their presence has no clinical significance unless accompanied by appendix wall thickening or periappendiceal inflammation.[2]

The CT signs of appendicitis depend on its evolution and severity. Acute appendicitis is characterized by an abnormal appendix or periappendiceal inflammatory process. The inflamed appendix is a tubular, fluid-filled structure measuring more than 5 mm in diameter, with a thickened wall, which

may enhance after an intravenous bolus injection of contrast.[1–3]

Periappendiceal inflammation is seen as blurring of periappendiceal fat, fascial thickening, fluid collections, or ill-defined soft tissue densities, when a phlegmon is present. Pericecal inflammation in association with an appendicolith is also diagnostic of appendicitis, when the appendix is not seen.

The ultrasound diagnosis of appendicitis is based on detection of a noncompressible fluid-filled distended appendix without peristalsis with a diameter of 7 mm or greater, in front of the psoas or in a retrocecal position. Pericecal inflammation (phlegmon) or abscess without visualization of the abnormal appendix are suggestive but not diagnostic of appendicitis.[1,4] The examination is positive if an appendicolith is identified as a discrete echogenic focus with an acoustic shadow and if the appendix is dilated and edematous[4] (Fig. 24.1).

Diverticulitis

Diverticulitis results when obstruction of the orifice of a diverticulum leads to localized inflammation. Bowel wall thickening, spasm, and obstruction can occur, and diverticula may perforate with abscess formation, causing peritonitis and fistulas.[5] Clinical findings include local pain, fever, nausea, vomiting, constipation and diarrhea, local tenderness, and a palpable mass. CT and contrast enema are the imaging methods of choice, but ultrasound may help in patients with pelvic pain and confusing symptoms.[5]

CT is the best initial test to evaluate diverticulitis because

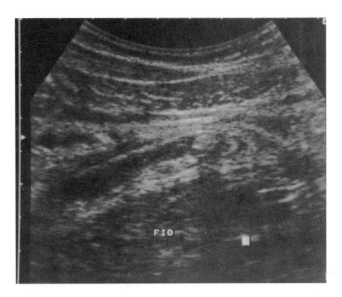

Figure 24.1 Transabdominal ultrasound of a 25-year-old woman with appendicitis. Note the dilated and inflamed appendix with an echogenic appendicolith with acoustic shadow.

it can define the extent of the disease better than a barium enema and has the ability to evaluate the whole abdomen and pelvis.[6] Pericolic inflammation will be found in 98% of cases and mural thickening in 70%. When it is over 1 to 3 cm, differentiation from bowel neoplasm may be difficult.[7] Fluid at the root of the mesentery and vascular engorgement is more common in sigmoid diverticulitis, distinguishing it from carcinoma.[8]

The most common sonographic feature of diverticulitis is an abnormal colonic segment at the point of maximum tenderness, seen as mural thickening over 4 mm, involving a segment 5 cm or longer. Inflamed diverticula are seen in up to 85% of cases, as shadowing outpouchings of the thickened bowel[5,9] (Fig. 24.2). In the early stages, ultrasound can show the image of the inflamed diverticulum. More severe cases may not be detected by ultrasound, presumably because the diverticulum is incorporated in the inflammatory process, and a CT should then be performed.[10]

Crohn's Disease

Two distinct phases of Crohn's disease are observed, acute and chronic. The acute phase is characterized by enlarged lymphoid follicles and aphthoid ulcerations. These mucosal changes are better evaluated by barium studies (Fig. 24.3A) and colonoscopy, and CT may be normal.[11,12] Pseudopolyps are sometimes seen. Bowel wall thickening is well documented by CT, with a double-halo or target appearance. The mucosa appears as a ring of soft tissue density, surrounded by a ring of attenuation of water (submucosal edema) or fat (fat infiltration), which is surrounded by a higher density ring, the muscularis propria. Mucosa and serosa show various degrees of enhancement following intravenous contrast, according to the clinical activity of the disease. This heterogeneous aspect of the bowel wall indicates absence of fibrosis, and the disease

is reversible with treatment. In the chronic phase, fibrosis predominates, the alterations are irreversible, and the thickened bowel wall shows homogeneous attenuation.[11,13]

The most common sonographic findings are "target lesions," where an echogenic center (luminal residues and air) is surrounded by a hypoechoic rim (thickening of submucosa and muscular areas). This is the pattern most commonly seen in Crohn's disease, representing segmental or diffuse bowel wall thickening[14-17] (Fig. 24.3B). Crohn's disease is a transluminal disease leading to fibrosis. This fibrosis is responsible for the formation of an echo-poor halo surrounding a central echogenic zone. In the earlier stages, with transmural edema and inflammation, the halo assumes a "ground-glass" appearance.[18]

Ulcerative Colitis

Acute, subacute, and chronic phases of ulcerative colitis are distinguished. In the acute phase, initial inflammatory mucosal changes are not detected by CT. With progressive disease, severe mucosal ulceration denudes portions of the colon wall, generating pseudopolyps, which may be seen on CT when sufficiently large. Mural thinning, perforations, and pneumatosis may be detected on CT scans in patients with toxic megacolon.[7,11] In subacute and chronic phases, mural thickening and luminal narrowing are demonstrated by CT. The muscularis mucosa is markedly hypertrophied, causing diffuse or segmental narrowing of the lumen and shortening of the colon. The submucosa is thickened because of edema in acute and subacute cases and because of fat deposition in chronic cases. CT shows a target or halo pattern in these phases, where the lumen is surrounded by a ring of soft tissue density (mucosa, lamina propria, and hypertrophied muscularis mucosae), which is surrounded by a low-density ring (fatty infiltration of the submucosa), which in turn is surrounded by a ring of soft-tissue density (muscularis propria).

On ultrasound, the mucosa and submucosa initially become thickened and hypoechoic as a result of edema, with colonic motility being maintained. Haustrations are lost with progressive disease. The typical wall stratification is maintained[19] (Fig. 24.4). Hydrocolonic sonography (sonography with water enema) shows the normal sonographic stratified appearance of the colonic wall in patients with acute ulcerative colitis.[20] Later, there is absence of peristalsis. If extensive pseudopolyposis occurs, the wall thickness increases, often accompanied by loss of wall stratification.[19] Mural thickening, however, is less intense than in Crohn's disease.[15] Intramural high-amplitude echoes with acoustic shadowing may be observed in ulcerative colitis associated with pneumatosis intestinalis.[21]

Neoplasms

Small Bowel

Small bowel malignant lesions are characterized by eccentric or asymmetric mural thickening, a lobulated inner and outer

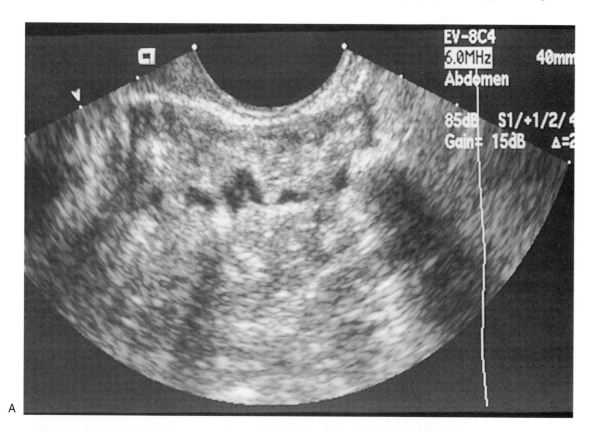

A

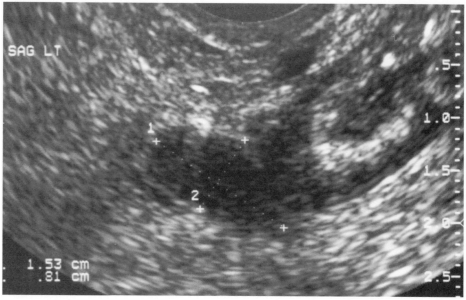

B

Figure 24.2 Diverticulitis: transvaginal ultrasound. **(A)** Longitudinal images of a colonic segment with thick wall and diverticula, seen as hyperechoic outpouchings with acoustic shadow. (Courtesy of Dr. Rita Secaf, São Paulo, Brazil.) **(B)** Axial image of a segment of colon with a 1.53 × 0.8 cm diverticulum. (Courtesy of Dr. Deborah Levine, Boston, Massachusetts.)

contour, and/or a focal tissue mass exceeding 2 cm from the lumen to the serosal surface. Narrowing of the lumen, a spiculated outer contour of the mass, and an abrupt transition between normal and abnormal intestinal wall may be seen. Local or distant metastases, regional lymphadenopathy, and ascites suggest neoplasm. Leiomyomas and leiomyosarcomas are bulky, eccentrically grown images, sometimes calcified, and may have a low-attenuation center when larger than 4 cm. Adenocarcinomas are generally single soft tissue density masses causing lumen narrowing and obstruction. Carcinoids

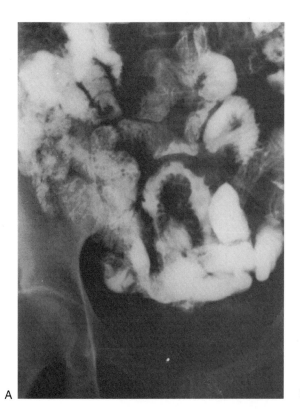

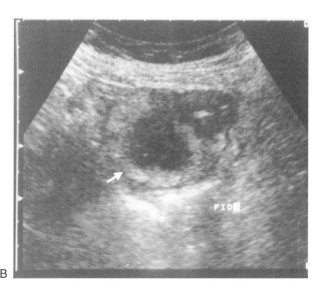

A

B

Figure 24.3 Crohn's disease in a 43-year-old woman. **(A)** Small bowel enema shows an ileal loop with irregular contours and thin lumen. **(B)** Axial images, where a thickened bowel loop is seen with a hyperechoic center and hypoechoic wall, contiguous to an abscess with thickened wall and fluid contents (arrow). (Courtesy of Dr. Denise P. Vezozzo, São Paulo, Brazil.)

Figure 24.4 Ulcerative colitis. Axial image, with better demonstration of air trapped inside an ulceration. The bowel wall is thickened but not as intensely as in Crohn's disease.

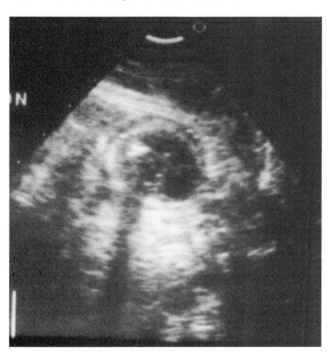

present with radiating soft tissue strands in the mesentery with displacement of small bowel loops and a small mesenteric mass in the right lower quadrant.[22] Calcification may be seen in carcinoid tumors, and the triad of a calcified mesenteric mass, radiating strands, and adjacent bowel wall thickening, associated with retroperitoneal lymphadenopathy, should be considered suggestive.[23–25]

MRI has limitations in evaluating small bowel neoplasms, due to long acquisition times leading to low spatial resolution and lack of a good intraluminal contrast agent for the small bowel.[22]

Most intrinsic neoplasms of the small bowel, such as adenocarcinoma, leiomyosarcoma, and carcinoids, have a "target-like" appearance on ultrasound. The wall thickening is more intense, asymmetric, and irregular, when compared with inflammatory bowel disease, with loss of normal wall stratification.[22] Benign leiomyomas are common small bowel tumors, seen as sharply demarcated spheric masses (Fig. 24.5). Carcinoids appear as hypoechoic, homogeneous, predominantly intraluminal masses with a smooth intraluminal contour, attached to the wall by a broad base with interruption of the submucosa and thickening of the muscularis propria.

The small intestine and mesentery may be involved by metastases and other masses arising in the peritoneum, retroperitoneum, and lymph nodes. Small bowel lymphoma appears as markedly hypoechoic thickened bowel wall with

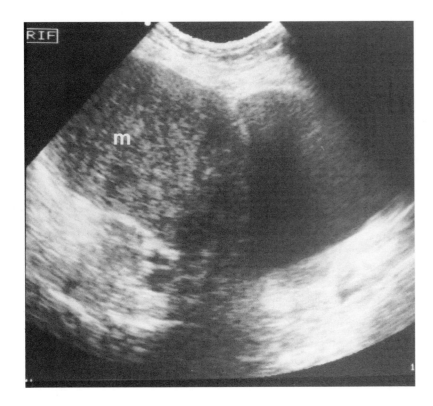

Figure 24.5 A 60-year-old woman with a small bowel leiomyoma. The leiomyoma is seen as a well-circumscribed oval solid mass (M).

hypoechoic lymph nodes and dilatation of the involved intestine.[22,26] The main sonographic patterns are circumferential involvement of the bowel wall, bulky tumors, and nodular extraluminal spread.[27] The adjacent mesenteric nodes may be involved, making a "sandwich" or mesenteric "cake" sign, consisting of an echogenic band containing the subperitoneal fat and connective tissue of the small bowel mesentery encased by multiple lobulated, hypoechoic masses.[22]

Colon and Rectum

Colorectal carcinoma is one of the most common cancers, with approximately one half of the cancers found in the rectum and sigmoid, and the rest scattered throughout the proximal colon. The peak incidence is about 70 years of age.[28,29]

CT shows a soft tissue density mass or focal thickening within the rectum or colon wall (Fig. 24.6). When the lesion is restricted to the intestinal wall, the outer contour is generally smooth. Irregular outer contour or soft tissue density strands in the perirectal or pericolonic adipose tissue indicates extension beyond the intestinal wall. Extracolonic tumor spread is suggested by loss of tissue fat planes between the large bowel and surrounding muscles.

Due to the relatively fixed position of the rectosigmoid, MRI is more accurate in staging cancer than CT. Colorectal tumors are seen as masses or focal wall thickening, with similar or slightly higher signal than muscle on T1-weighted images (Fig. 24.7). T1-weighted images are better than T2-weighted images in demonstrating intramural lesions and also extracolonic tumor extension. T2-weighted images show bet-

ter contrast between muscle and tumors, particularly when uterine or pelvic sidewall invasion is suspected.[28]

Endorectal surface coil MRI provides increased detail of the rectal wall with better delineation of the different layers

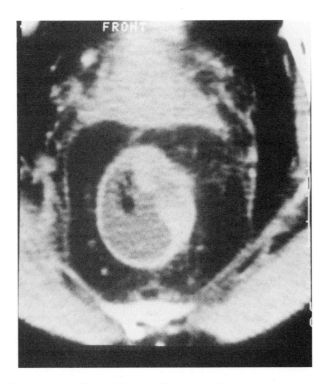

Figure 24.6 CT in a 34-year-old woman with a rectal carcinoma. Note focal thickening of laterosuperior rectal wall.

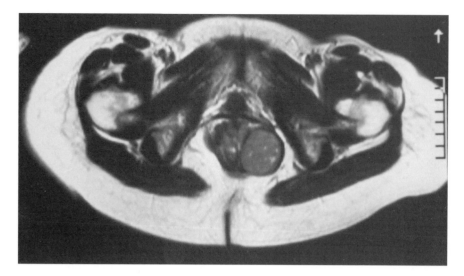

Figure 24.7 MRI axial T2-weighted image of a rectal carcinoma in a 60-year-old woman.

than with other MRI techniques. The results equal those of transrectal ultrasound for staging small tumors in the rectal wall. In more advanced cases, MRI with double surface coil gives additional information about tumor spread and local lymph node evaluation.[30]

Transabdominal ultrasound may detect large colorectal tumors, but its main use is in evaluating abdominal metastasis

and ascites. Transrectal sonography (including endoscopic sonography) is preferred to evaluate local extension and local nodal metastasis of colorectal carcinomas. It is a useful, precise, and reliable diagnostic tool for staging purposes of rectal carcinoma.[29,31–33]

Transrectal ultrasonography can show the various layers of the colon wall, enabling determination of depth of tumor

Figure 24.8 A 70-year-old woman with a rectal carcinoma. Transrectal ultrasound shows a mass with irregular contours.

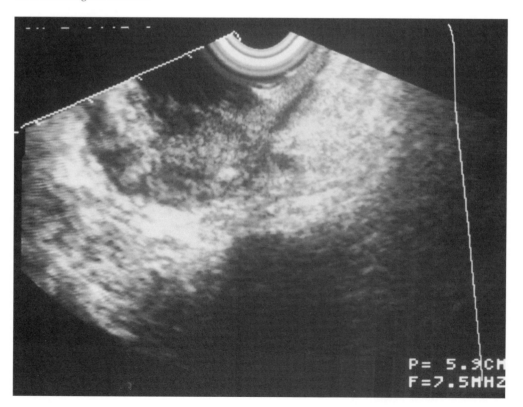

penetration into the wall.[28,33] A colon tumor appears as a hypoechoic mass whose margins can be outlined and related to the layers in the colon or rectal wall (Fig. 24.8). The depth of infiltration can be assessed from evidence of disruption of the different segments of the colon or rectal wall. The intraluminal component can be seen as a polypoid or exophytic mass. Pericolonic or perirectal abnormalities can be seen. Peritumoral inflammation or radiation changes, also hypoechoic, may simulate tumor. Colorectal carcinoma in adolescent females is frequently associated with ovarian metastases. In adolescents, a smaller proportion of colorectal ovarian metastases are multicystic when compared to adults. These lesions are frequently large and may be complex, multicystic, or solid.[34]

VASCULAR PELVIC MASSES

Varices

Pelvic varices are frequently seen in patients with unexplained chronic pelvic pain,[35] and may simulate adnexal masses[36] or hydrosalpinx.[37] Transabdominal or transvaginal ultrasonography (TAS or TVS) may be used to identify pelvic varices,[35] which appear as multiple dilated vessels lying within the broad ligament.[38] The presence of circular or linear anechoic structures with a diameter greater than 5 mm, which are found in transverse and oblique sections of the lateral fornices, are indicative of pelvic varices. The vascular nature of these structures is confirmed with the Valsalva maneuvre and in the upright position,[39] which is important if no abnormal vessels are seen during supine scanning, as filling of these vessels is gravity dependent.[35] Transvaginal color Doppler may differentiate pelvic varices from other adnexal masses.[36,40] Doppler shows a venous signal of varying amplitude, similar to that seen in other dilated venous systems.[38] Giant pararectal varices may also be found in patients with portal hypertension.[41] Doppler examination demonstrates venous flow, confirming the presence of varices.[42]

On CT, pelvic varices are seen as multiple tubular soft tissue density parauterine structures with enhancement following intravenous contrast. Giant pararectal varices may be found in patients with portal hypertension. CT scans show multiple tubular lesions of soft tissue attenuation, surrounding the sigmoid colon and rectum. Venous contrast shows early homogeneous enhancement, confirming the diagnosis of varices.

Aneurysms

Aneurysms of the aorta and iliac arteries are potentially lethal and often clinically silent. The most important type of aneurysm affecting the abdominal aorta or iliac arteries is the atherosclerotic aneurysm due to weakening of the arterial wall.[43] Males are more susceptible to aortic aneurysms than females.[43,44] There is a tendency for aneurysms to occur in the distal aorta and proximal iliac arteries, with most iliac artery

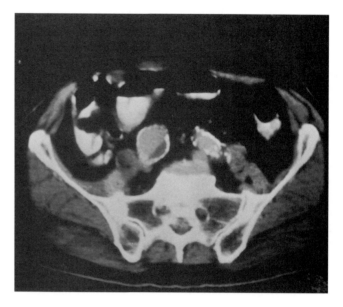

Figure 24.9 CT of a 72-year-old woman shows a right common iliac artery aneurysm, with mural thrombus and a calcified wall.

aneurysms being associated with aortic aneurysms. Isolated iliac aneurysms are less common but more dangerous, as they are usually large by the time of diagnosis. Ruptured iliac aneurysms may be accompanied by nonspecific pelvic pain, delaying diagnosis until shock occurs. The aorta is considered aneurysmal if the diameter is greater than 3 cm.[43]

The symptoms of an iliac artery aneurysm are often those of compression of the intrapelvic structures, including neurologic symptoms or those due to rupture or decreased venous flow. The diagnosis is based on ultrasound, conventional or helical CT, and angiography for the definition of laterality and extension.[45–47] CT angiography, performed with helical CT, may replace digital subtraction angiography in the diagnosis of iliac artery aneurysms.[48] The location, size, and extent of the aneurysm, as well as wall calcification and intra-aneurysmal thrombus are well demonstrated by helical CT[49] (Fig. 24.9). MRI, including MRI angiography, may be used to evaluate intrapelvic aneurysms, with or without intravenous contrast.[50–52]

Ultrasound is used to demonstrate the shape and any focal increase in the caliber of the affected vessel and the presence of thrombi, dissection, rupture, and wall calcification.

MASSES OF NEURAL ORIGIN

Pheochromocytoma

Pheochromocytoma is a catecholamine-secreting tumor that arises from the chromaffin cells of the sympathoadrenal system.[53] Lesions may be found at any point in the paraganglionic system, which extends from the carotid body to the floor of the pelvis.[54] Approximately 18% to 22% of pheochromocytomas are found at extra-adrenal locations.[55] Extra-adrenal pheochromocytomas (also called paragangliomas) are found intra-abdominally, originating from the sympathetic chains or from the organs of Zuckerkandl.[53] They are often multicentric (15% to 24%)[55] and have been found in the bladder, distal ureter, sacrococcygeal area, anus, broad ligament of the uterus, ovary, and vaginal wall.[53,55] Extra-adrenal pheochromocytomas are more likely to be malignant than those found in the adrenal gland.[55]

Nonfunctioning tumors are usually large when diagnosed, with symptoms of abdominal or back pain or palpable mass. Functioning tumors are generally small when detected due to paroxysmal symptoms (such as palpitations, headache, sweating, and pallor), hypertension, and midline mass. The classic triad of headache, palpitations, and sweating is common in functioning tumors, and is related to excessive norepinephrine secretion.[55]

Pheochromocytomas of the bladder are mostly located on the dome or in the trigone of the bladder. The female/male ratio is 3:2, with an average of 41 years.[54] Pheochromocytoma of the bladder may be accompanied by headache, fainting, palpitations, blurred vision, sweating or hypertension related to urination, bladder distention, abdominal palpation, defecation or sexual intercourse, as well as hematuria.[54–58] Biochemical diagnosis is based on increased urinary or plasma catecholamines (epinephrine and norepinephrine).[55]

CT is favored for the localization of extra-adrenal pheochromocytomas, after metaiodobenzylguanidine (MIBG) scan.[53,55] Evaluation of the lesions may be limited in patients with paucity of retroperitoneal fat,[56] and bladder lesions may be missed if scans are obtained only after contract[55] and the urine has opacified. On MRI, pheochromocytomas are typically hypointense on T1-weighted images and hyperintense on T2-weighted images allowing differentiation from other tumors.[55,59–61]

Ultrasonography is less expensive than CT and can demonstrate adrenal and retroperitoneal pheochromocytomas, but it does not show tumors measuring less than 2 cm and does not permit visualization of retroperitoneal areas obscured by bowel gas.[53,59] Bladder pheochromocytomas may be well demonstrated by ultrasound.[57] Sonographically, a bladder pheochromocytoma appears as a sharply demarcated soft tissue mass. The lesion may be solid or may contain foci of hemorrhage and necrosis. Hypoechoic areas have been attributed to old hemorrhage and necrosis, and hyperechoic areas have been attributed to acute hemorrhage. Doppler sonography shows low-impedance flow with little systolic–diastolic variation, reflecting low resistance to blood flow within the highly vascularized fibrous trabeculae and sinusoids characteristic of pheochromocytomas.[61]

Peripheral Nerve Sheath Tumors

Benign nerve sheath tumors are schwannoma (neurilemoma) and neurofibroma. Malignant nerve sheath tumors are usually referred to as malignant schwannoma.[62]

Schwannoma

The schwannomas or neurinomas are usually isolated benign tumors, except when associated with von Recklinghausen's disease, when they are multiple and potentially malignant.[63] Schwannomas are most commonly found in the retroperitoneum but may appear anywhere in the pelvis. Benign schwannoma, also known as neurilemoma, neurinoma, and perineural fibroblastoma, is an encapsulated tumor that arises from neural sheaths of peripheral nerves. Women are affected twice as often as men.[64] Schwannomas can be solitary, arising at various anatomic sites or associated with von Recklinghausen neurofibromatosis. In the pelvis, they may simulate ovarian tumors.[63,65] (Fig. 24.10). Ultrasound will show the cystic or solid nature of the lesions.[63] MRI findings of neurilemomas include masses of low signal intensity on T1-weighted images and of high signal intensity on T2-weighted images because of the long T1 and long T2 relaxation times of the tumor tissue.[64]

Neurofibroma

Pelvic neurofibromatosis is rare. Neurofibromas originate from Schwann cells and may occur in any location, although they are predominantly found in the skin. They can also involve other organs. Neurofibromas may originate from the pelvic autonomic plexus and lead to upper and lower urinary tract obstruction because of their anatomic location. Plexiform neurofibromatosis is a form of generalized dysplasia of neuroectodermal and mesodermal tissue characterized by multiple, bilateral neurofibromas involving the spinal and paraspinal nerves.[66] Pelvic neurofibromas, as part of neurofi-

Figure 24.10 Benign schwannoma in a 23-year-old woman with sacral pain, irradiating to right thigh and leg and dyspareunia. The CT shows a heterogeneous mass, exiting the sacral neural foramen.

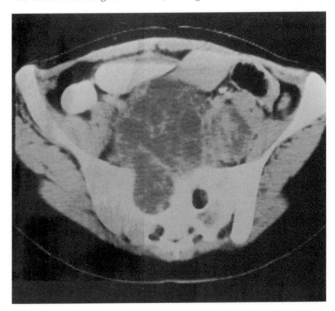

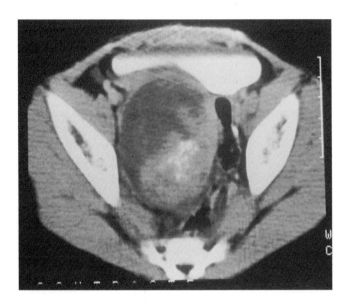

Figure 24.11 Ganglioneuroma in a 6-year-old girl. CT shows a heterogeneous mass with hypoattenuating areas and calcifications, compressing the posterior wall of the bladder.

bromatosis, can be located anywhere along the urogenital tract. The most frequently affected pelvic organ is the urinary bladder. Other less frequent locations are the cervix, perineum, pelvic floor, and ovary.[67] Plexiform neurofibromas can become very large and involve local structures.[68]

CT generally shows a homogeneous mass with attenuation values of 20 to 30 Hounsfield units (HU) that may show contrast enhancement.[68] Cystic or hemorrhagic changes are usually not seen.[64] The lower attenuation results from a high content of fat or Schwann cells within the tumor. On MRI, neurofibromas are slightly hyperintense in relation to muscle, with hyperintense septa, secondary to myelinated axons. These septa appear hypointense on T2-weighted images due to collagen fibers. Following gadolinium administration, neurofibromas enhance similarly to intracranial neuromas.[68]

Ultrasound may show hypoechoic lesions behind the bladder, adjacent to neural foramina. Neurofibromas may have a fat component, so the presence of pelvic sidewall masses of high echogenicity in the absence of acoustic shadowing should suggest a fat-containing tumor.[69] Anterior sacral meningoceles, associated with neurofibromatosis, are seen on CT as cystic masses that enhance after intrathecal contrast anterior to the sacrum.[70] MRI shows a communicating stalk in the sagittal plane.[70] Ultrasound shows a cystic mass adjacent to the sacrum.[70]

Ganglioneuroma

Ganglioneuromas are typically benign slow-growing tumors, found mainly in children and young adults. Diagnosis may be delayed, according to their location. Pelvic retroperitoneal location is rare.[71,72] Ganglioneuroma, the benign counterpart of neuroblastoma, may occur spontaneously or after chemotherapy or radiation therapy for neuroblastoma[73] (Fig. 24.11).

URINARY TRACT MASSES

Kidney

Pelvic Kidney

The most common form of simple renal ectopy is a pelvic kidney in the true pelvis or adjacent to the sacrum (sacral kidney). Bilateral renal ectopy is rare, occurring in 10% of patients with renal ectopia.[74,75] If the kidney lies at the level of the iliac crest, this is called abdominal ectopy. Pelvic kidney may be associated with other malformations. Symptoms are usually due to an associated condition, such as pain from obstruction or infection associated with reflux.[74] The pelvic kidney is often palpable and may be misinterpreted as a pelvic tumor. Ultrasound assists in identifying the ectopic renal tissue with a characteristic pattern of renal parenchyma, collecting systems, and renal sinus echoes anterior to the iliac vessels[74,75] (Fig. 24.12) and also confirms the empty ipsilateral renal fossa.[75] Pelvic kidney resembles a normal kidney on CT and should not be misdiagnosed as a pelvic mass. On CT and MRI, a functioning mass of renal parenchyma can usually be identified (Figs. 24.13 and 24.14).

Horseshoe Kidney

Horseshoe kidney is the most common anomaly of renal form, occurring in approximately 1:400 births, with a 2:1 male predominance. The two kidneys on either side of the midline are connected by an isthmus, preventing normal rotation. The isthmus is usually located in front of the aorta and inferior vena cava.[74] The horseshoe kidney is usually abdominal with its inferior pole extending into the pelvis. Horseshoe kidneys are generally asymptomatic, unless obstruction or infection occurs.

Ultrasound diagnosis of horseshoe kidneys depends on the demonstration of an isthmus or band of renal tissue across the midline of abdomen connecting the lower poles of the kidneys.[76] The CT appearances of horseshoe kidney are the same as normal kidney, with the exception of a centrally located isthmus joining the lower poles of the kidneys. CT helps in defining the relationship of the kidney to the major vessels[74] (Fig. 24.15).

Transplantation

Transplanted kidneys are most commonly situated in the pelvis and have the same appearance as normal kidneys, differentiating them from pelvic masses. Ultrasound can assess the vitality of the transplanted kidney and also detect any complications such as lymphoceles, urinomas, hematomas, and abscesses, which may mimic pelvic masses (Figs. 24.16 and 24.17).

Lymphoceles are the most common peritransplant fluid collections, occurring in 1% to 15% of patients.[77,78] Persistent leakage of lymph from interrupted pelvic lymphatics results in collection of lymph within an epithelialized cavity.[78]

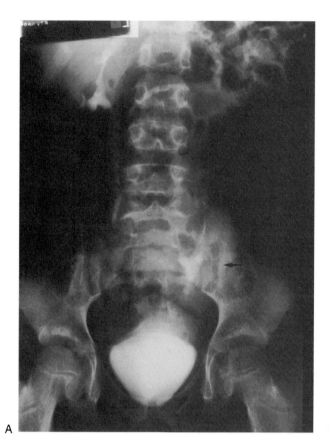

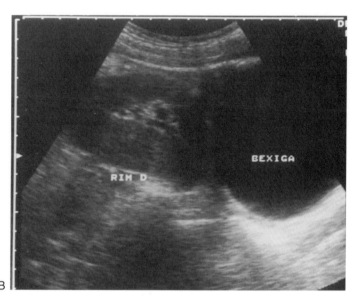

Figure 24.12 A 19-year-old woman. Uterine and ovarian agenesis (not shown). **(A)** Urography demonstrates a pelvic left kidney (arrow). **(B)** Transabdominal ultrasound shows a pelvic kidney. RIM D, right kidney; BEXIGA, urinary bladder. (Courtesy of Dr. Denise P. Vezozzo, São Paulo, Brazil.)

Figure 24.13 Right pelvic kidney in a 32-year-old woman. CT without intravenous contrast administration

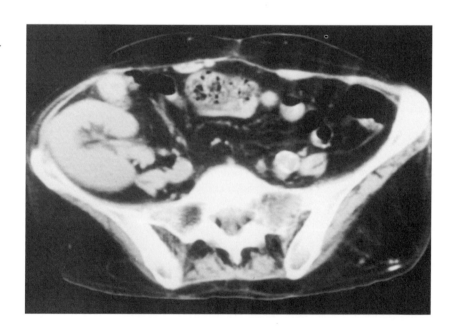

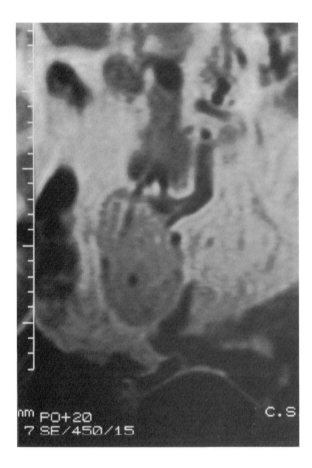

Figure 24.14 This coronal T1-weighted postcontrast image in a 29-year-old woman shows the right pelvic kidney.

Figure 24.15 An axial proton-density weighted MRI in a 36-year-old woman demonstrates horseshoe kidneys, anterior to aorta and inferior vena cava.

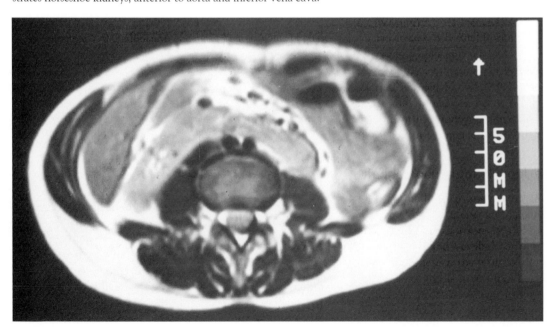

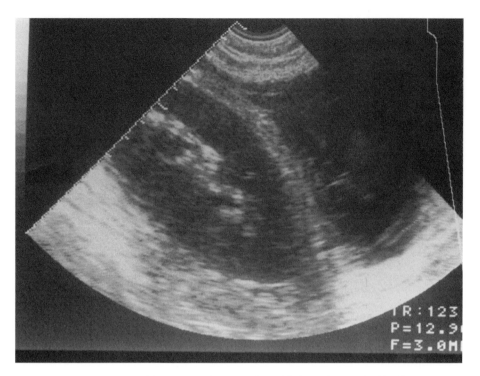

Figure 24.16 A 33-year-old woman with a transplanted kidney close to the bladder.

Lymphorrhea from the hilar lymphatics of the donor kidney may also cause post-transplant lymphoceles. Ultrasound shows fluid-filled structures that often contain fine septa, which may be difficult to distinguish from urinomas. They are usually seen between the kidney and the bladder.[79] The well-defined sonolucent pelvic mass may displace the bladder.[77] Infected lymphoceles may show internal complex echoes.[80]

Urinomas are frequently detected in the early postoperative period and can result from leaks from the renal pelvis,

Figure 24.17 CT shows a left iliac fossa transplanted kidney and an infected hematoma in the right iliac fossa following appendectomy in a 42-year-old woman.

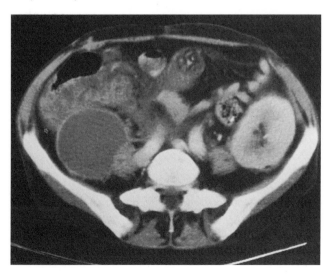

ureteroneocystostomy, or bladder. They are commonly situated near the lower pole of the transplant or near the bladder. On ultrasound, they do not have a distinctive appearance, and aspiration may be necessary to make the diagnosis. Abscesses are relatively common peritransplant fluid collections, and the ultrasonographic appearance is nonspecific, with the location in relation to the graft being variable. Septa and internal echogenicity may be seen. Hematomas tend to be sonographically complex in nature.[81]

On CT, the morphology, attenuation, and contrast enhancement are the same as normal kidneys. On CT, lymphoceles are seen as round or oval collections with sharp borders and CT values between 0 and 20 HU. On non-contrast-enhanced scans, lymphoceles are difficult to distinguish from urinomas. Following contrast, many urinomas opacify, while lymphoceles do not.[79]

Ureter

Ureteric Dilatation

Congenital megaloureter is caused by deficiency and derangement of the ureteric smooth muscle fibers with associated fibrosis, resulting in a failure of normal peristalsis in the affected segment and subsequent functional obstruction. This obstruction occurs approximately 2 cm above the ureteral orifice, and this segment is of normal caliber.[74] Ultrasound appearances are dilatation of the distal ureter, often disproportionate to the appearance of the upper collecting system; lower ureteral hyperperistalsis; and a sharply tapered, incurving, distal adynamic segment, 1 to 3 cm long.[82] A tortuous di-

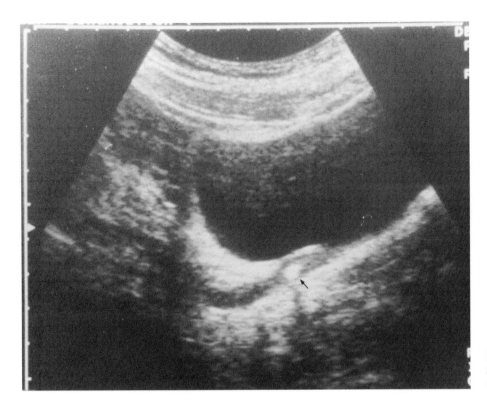

Figure 24.18 Transabdominal ultrasound. A hyperechoic calculus is seen in the dilated terminal ureter (arrow).

lated ureter may simulate a cystic pelvic mass. Obstructive distal ureteral calculi may lead to ureteral dilatation and appear as a hypoechoic persistent tubular structure close to the bladder. Calculi are hyperechoic structures in the distal ureter, with acoustic shadowing[83] (Fig. 24.18). Transperineal, transrectal, and transvaginal sonography are useful to detect distal ureteric calculi.[84–86]

Although hydronephrosis can usually be diagnosed by urography, pyelography, or ultrasound, the etiology of the obstruction may not be apparent. CT usually helps by identifying the cause of ureteric obstruction, such as tumors, inflammatory processes, and radiation fibrosis.[87] Noncontrast helical CT is a rapid and accurate method for demonstrating ureteric calculi causing renal colic. The reformatted views produce images similar in appearance to excretory urograms; however, the quality of reformatted images may be suboptimal when there is little retroperitoneal fat.[88]

MRI is useful to evaluate megaloureter and hydronephrosis using a techinique called RARE-MR urography in the presence of contraindications to intravenous urography or failure to locate the level of obstruction by ultrasound or for patients in renal failure.[89]

Ureterocele

A ureterocele is a focal dilatation of the submucosal portion of the distal ureter. It may be simple or ectopic. A simple ureterocele, also known as adult-type ureterocele, is associated with a single collecting system and occurs in the normal position on the trigone.[74] Ectopic ureteroceles are usually associated with the ureter from the upper pole of a duplicate

collecting system. This dilatation may extend to the bladder neck or even into the posterior urethra.[74] Ureteroceles produce the classic ultrasound sign of a "cyst within a cyst," that is, a cystic structure within the bladder.[90] Simple ureteroceles are easily identified on the posteroinferior bladder wall (Fig. 24.19). Ectopic and simple ureteroceles are dynamic structures, changing in shape and size according to intravesical pressure. Small ureteroceles are seen on dynamic scans filling and emptying several times per minute.[91,92]

During excretory urography, the orthotopic (simple) ureterocele, is seen as the classic "cobra head" deformity of the distal ureter protruding into the bladder lumen in the region of the trigone. If the ureter is opacified with contrast, the central portion of the ureterocele also is opacified in continuity with the remainder of the ureter but is surrounded by a lucent rim, representing the bladder mucosa around the ureterocele.

CT shows a nonopacified ureterocele[74] as a round or fusiform filling defect in the bladder. When opacified, the ureterocele shows a soft tissue linear contour separating the lumen of the ureterocele and urine inside the bladder. MRI may demonstrate the ureterocele as a thin, hypointense, linear, round structure inside the bladder, without the need for contrast.

Bladder

Diverticulum

A congenital bladder diverticulum, called a Hutch diverticulum, is in close relationship with the ureteral orifice, typically opening just above and lateral to it and often with associated reflux.[93]

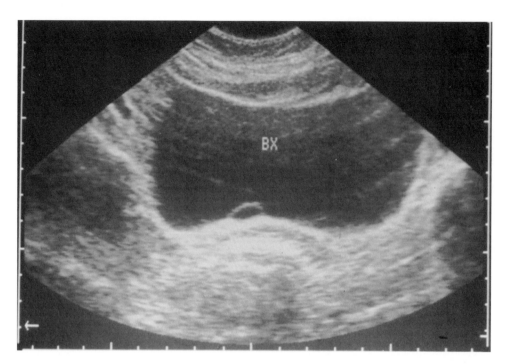

Figure 24.19 A ureterocele is seen adjacent to the bladder wall.

Acquired bladder diverticula due to outlet obstruction are rare in women. A large bladder diverticulum may be larger than the bladder and displace it to the opposite side.[93] The diverticulum is seen with a thin wall and the bladder with its thickened wall. A large lateral wall diverticulum tends to deviate the ipsilateral distal ureter medially. There is a higher incidence of tumor inside bladder diverticula than inside the bladder itself.[93] Ultrasound is useful to evaluate bladder diverticula. Echo-free outpouchings from the bladder are readily seen, and filling defects such as stones or tumor within a diverticulum can be seen[93] (Fig. 24.20).

CT is also suitable for evaluation of bladder diverticula. Stones inside diverticula are seen in noncontrast CT scans as hyperdense structures, and tumors present as soft tissue masses arising from the diverticular wall and protruding into the contrast-filled diverticulum (Fig. 24.20). MRI can also be used to evaluate tumors inside bladder diverticula.[93,94]

Post Radiotherapy

Radiation cystitis is associated with edema and hemorrhage in the acute phase. It may resolve completely, or it may progress to mucosal ulceration, fibrosis, small capacity bladder, and, rarely, calcification.[93] Diffuse fibrotic thickening of the bladder wall following radiotherapy may be impossible to distinguish from tumor[96] (Figs. 24.21 and 24.22).

Tumors

Benign bladder tumors are rare. Leiomyoma is the most common, found in women from 30 to 50 years of age. It is usually seen in the trigone or lateral walls as a smooth mural mass protruding into the bladder lumen. If there is a large extravesical component, the bladder will be compressed or displaced. Extravesical leiomyomas may be difficult to differentiate from a uterine leiomyoma.[93]

The most common malignant bladder tumor is the transitional cell carcinoma, accounting for approximately 90% of all bladder tumors. Involvement of pelvic lymph nodes is common, and hematogenous spread is most frequent to liver and lungs and less frequently to bones, producing lytic lesions. The most common clinical finding is painless hematuria, which can be microscopic or gross.[95]

Bladder tumors appear on ultrasound as echogenic masses projecting into the bladder lumen (Fig. 24.23). The bladder wall has a more intense echo pattern than tumor tissue, which permits distinction of early superficial lesions from those invading the deeper layers of the bladder wall. The disadvantage of TAS is its inability to assess lymph node status, unless the nodes are grossly enlarged.[96] Less common malignant bladder tumors are squamous cell carcinoma, adenocarcinoma, and lymphoma,[93] which also cause focal thickening of bladder wall or focal masses.

CT and MRI are useful in differentiating between tumor limited to the bladder wall and more extensive disease[95,96] but not in the detection of superficial bladder tumors. Cystoscopy with biopsy is the definative method of diagnosing bladder cancer and should be used in all patients who have unexplained hematuria. CT is more effective than ultrasound in staging bladder cancer by allowing better assessment of tumor invasion through the wall into perivesical fat and surrounding

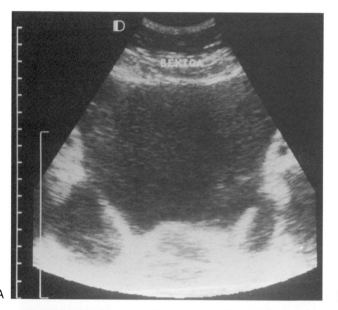

A

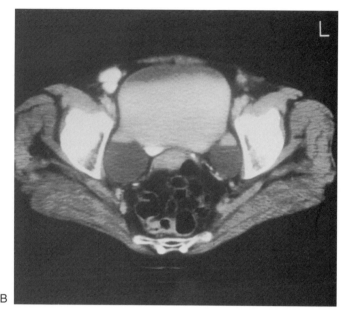

B

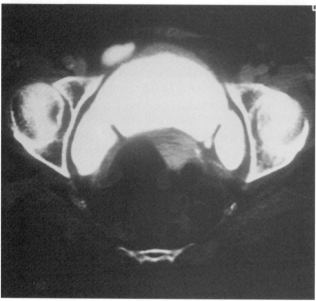

C

Figure 24.20 Bladder diverticula in a 74-year-old woman. (A) Pelvic ultrasound shows hypoechoic structures communicating with bladder lumen. (B) CT after intravenous contrast. Two posterior bladder diverticula are partially opacified. (C) After intravesical contrast, the communication between the diverticula and bladder is well demonstrated. (Courtesy of Dr. Renato A. Sernik, São Paulo, Brazil.)

structures and evaluation of lymph node enlargement.[93,95,96] On MRI, bladder tumors are hyperintense on T2-weighted images, in contrast to low-signal normal bladder wall (Fig. 24.24). Transmural invasion presents as an area of lower intensity in the perivesical fat. Gadolinium-DTPA causes enhancement of the tumor and increases contrast between tumor and adjacent muscle and allows improved assessment of extent of bladder wall invasion by transitional cell carcinoma.[93,95–98] MRI cannot differentiate between enlarged lymph nodes due to tumor and those enlarged due to reactive hyperplasia or other benign conditions.[96]

Urachus

The allantois attaches the bladder dome to the umbilicus. In fetal life, the bladder is an abdominal organ, and later de-

scends to the pelvis. As this happens, the bladder dome narrows to form the urachus, which elongates with bladder descent. Normally, the urachus becomes completely obliterated, forming a fibrous cord called the *umbilical ligament*.[93,99] Patent urachus or complete persistence of the urachus extends from the bladder dome to the umbilicus. A patent portion of the urachus communicating with the umbilicus is called a *urachal sinus*.[100] Segmental failure of closure of the urachus at the bladder attachment results in a urachocele, or urachal diverticulum in the dome of the bladder. Failure of closure of a portion of the urachus between the umbilicus and the bladder forms a urachal cyst.[93,100] Urachal sinus and patent urachus, due to their small diameter, are better evaluated by high-resolution ultrasound or fistulography than by CT.[100]

Urachal cysts are generally silent, except when there is associated infection.[93] They are seen by ultrasound as a midline

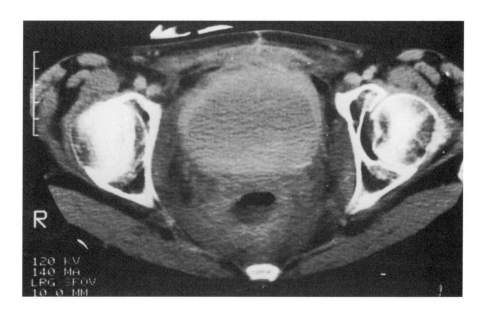

Figure 24.21 CT shows thickening of bladder and rectum following radiotherapy in a 55-year-old woman.

unilocular clear cystic structure, above the bladder, often extending to the umbilicus.[101–104] Mucous content may give the appearance of a complex echogenic cystic mass.[102] Internal echoes and wall thickening or irregularity in a urachal cyst denote a complication such as infection, carcinoma, or post-traumatic hematoma.[103] Infected urachal cysts (pyourachus) account for 23% of symptomatic urachal anomalies.[100] Pyourachus may present acutely, particularly if intraperitoneal

perforation has occurred, or as an abdominal-pelvic mass.[100] It can mimic urinary tract infection, inflammatory bowel disease, pelvic inflammatory disease, appendicitis, or Meckel's diverticulum.[101]

Most malignant urachal neoplasms are adenocarcinomas, and they are usually asymptomatic until the bladder is invaded and hematuria occurs, with a poor prognosis (Fig. 24.25). Other symptoms include dysuria, frequent urination, and umbilical discharge.[103,105–107] Ultrasound may show a supravesical complex mass, which may have foci of calcification.[93,106]

CT is valuable in diagnosing urachal carcinomas by showing the extravesical location of the tumor. The demonstration of a calcified mass above or anterior to the bladder, in contact with the anterior abdominal wall, is highly suggestive of urachal carcinoma. The mass may invade the bladder, extend anterosuperiorly to the umbilicus, or both.[93,104,108,109] Irregu-

Figure 24.22 A sagittal T1-weighted image in a 49-year-old woman 10 years after hysterectomy, demonstrating bladder wall thickening following radiotherapy.

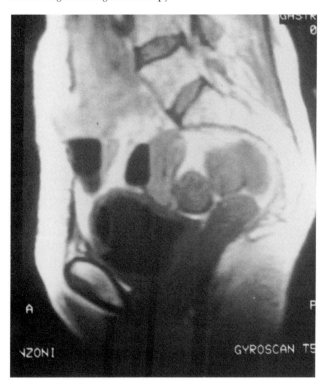

Figure 24.23 Bladder tumor (transitional cell carcinoma), shown as a solid mass with irregular margins on the bladder floor.

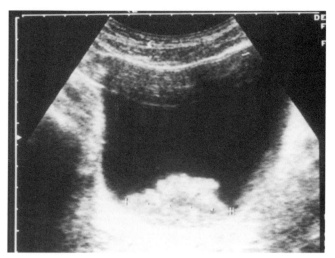

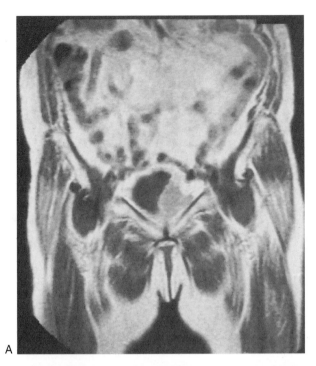

A

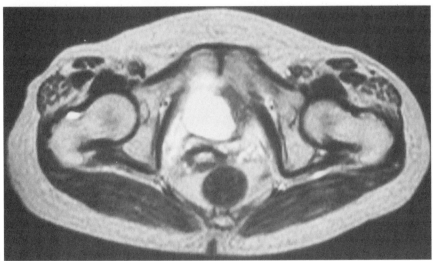

B

Figure 24.24 MRI of transitional cell carcinoma in a 38-year-old woman. **(A)** Coronal T1-weighted, postcontrast image demonstrating thickening of left lateral bladder wall, with contrast enhancement. **(B)** Axial T2 weighted image showing the lesion with lower signal than urine and perivesical fat.

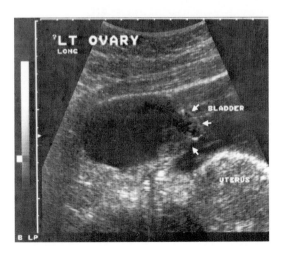

Figure 24.25 A sagittal transabdominal scan of a 46-year-old woman who presented with painless hematuria. The urinary bladder is seen on the right with a urachal cyst on the left and an adenocarcinoma invading the bladder wall (arrows). The cyst on the left of the image was not the left ovary.

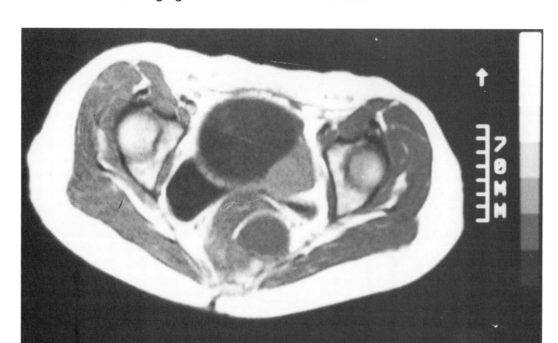

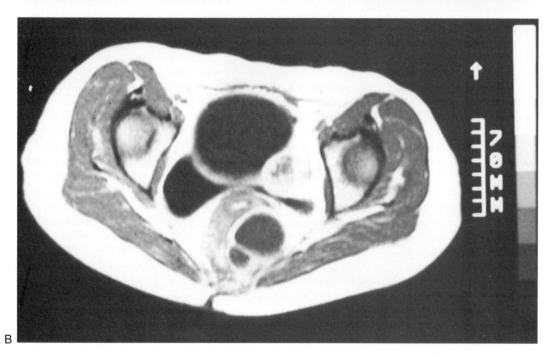

Figure 24.26 MRI of urachus carcinoma in a 48-year-old woman. **(A)** Axial T1-weighted precontrast image. **(B)** Axial T1-weighted postcontrast images. A cystic mass is seen anterior to the bladder, with a solid component that enhances following contrast.

larity or wall thickening of a urachal cyst should suggest the possibility of carcinoma.[103]

MRI may allow improved staging of carcinoma of the urachus by its multiple imaging planes[102] (Fig. 24.26). Sagittal MRI shows the shape of the tumor and the urachal ligament extending toward the umbilicus.[110] A carcinoma should be suspected when a mass is present in the dome of the bladder associated with mostly extravesical extension in the midline and calcification.

MISCELLANEOUS SOFT TISSUE MASSES

Postsurgery, Post-traumatic, and Inflammatory Lesions

Hematoma

CT appearance of a hematoma of the rectus abdominis muscle and sheath is usually an ovoid or spindle-shaped superficial hyperdense mass of the anterior abdominal wall. Large rectus sheath hemorrhages may extend into the pelvis, compressing the viscera. Fluid levels may be seen in acute hematomas.[111] CT attenuation of the hematoma depends on its age. Acutely extravasated blood is the same density as circulating blood. Blood density increases with clot formation and clot retraction, remaining elevated for several days and reabsorption taking weeks or months. Hematomas may be homogeneous or heterogeneous. They may have density similar to other pelvic structures, and intravenous contrast must be used to differentiate them.[112]

On MRI, intra-abdominal or intrapelvic hematomas may show a characteristic concentric-ring configuration after 3 weeks, with a thin, dark peripheral rim on all pulse sequences and a bright inner ring most distinctive on T1-weighted images, indicating a maturing hematoma.[113] Acute hematomas may be isointense to muscle on T1-weighted images, becoming more intense with time; inhomogeneous streaks are present by the end of the first week. Both abscesses and solid tumors can mimic hematomas at this stage. Fluid levels of sedimented blood may be confounded with hematomas.[113] Subacute and chronic hematomas have areas of high signal intensity on both T1- and T2-weighted images.[114]

The ultrasound appearance will depend on the organization and duration and may be cystic or complex with internal heterogeneous, low-level echoes.[115] They may be rounded, oblong, or irregular, with walls of varying thickness and regularity. Large collections may be mistaken for the bladder and need aspiration for differentiation.[116]

Abscess

The typical CT appearance of an abscess is a low-attenuation, fluid-filled, encapsulated, well-defined mass with no central enhancement after contrast. The density of the mass is typically 2 to 29 HU, and rim enhancement may be seen. In solid organs, the mass is usually oval, and when extraparenchymal,

the mass conforms to, or may displace, adjacent structures. Gas inside the lesion is highly indicative of an abscess and is seen in 50% of all cases.[112,117] A gas–liquid level inside an abscess may indicate the presence of a fistulous communication to the gastrointestinal tract.[118] The CT appearance of an abscess may be nonspecific and indistinguishable from normal unopacified bladder and bowel or noninfected fluid collections such as urinoma, mesenteric cyst, necrotic tumor, loculated sterile ascites, and liquified hematoma.[112]

On ultrasound, pelvic abscess formation appears as fluid collections displacing adjacent structures, sometimes multiloculated, with debris, tiny septa, thick walls, and variable size and echogenicity. Posterior acoustic enhancement may help to characterize a fluid lesion, and debris may be seen within. Gas appears as an image with a "dirty shadow" (an acoustic shadow with multiple low-level internal echoes). There may also be a gas–liquid level and debris–fluid level within the lesion.[115,117]

Lymphocele (Lymphocyst)

Lymphoceles, also called *lymphocysts*, can occur after kidney transplantation, radical hysterectomy, and pelvic lymph node dissection for cervical or endometrial malignancy.[119–124] Lymphadenectomy is the only reliable method for the assessment of lymphatic spread in gynecologic oncology. One potential complication is pelvic lymphocele, a lymph-filled extraperitoneal space with no epithelial lining. Large lymphoceles may cause abdominal or pelvic pain, tenesmus, urinary frequency, hydronephrosis, leg edema, and/or deep venous thrombosis.[124–127] Pelvic lymphocysts following lymphadenectomy in gynecologic malignancy have a reported incidence of 1% to 3%. Eighty to 90% occur within the first 3 weeks after radical pelvic surgery, and they can be bilateral. They must be differentiated from other postoperative complications such as abscess or ureteric injury.[128]

On CT, lymphoceles are smooth and thin-walled, low-attenuation cystic collections, sharply demarcated from surrounding structures.[121,128–130]

Peritoneal Inclusion Cyst

Peritoneal inclusion cysts are also called benign cystic mesotheliomas, mesothelial cysts of the peritoneum, and loose cysts of the peritoneal cavity[131–133] and usually occur postpartum or following pelvic surgery, endometriosis, or pelvic inflammatory disease (PID).[131,132,134–137] Occasionally, one or more cysts may occur in various locations throughout the peritoneal cavity distant from the ovary.[131,132,137,138]

They develop from diminished peritoneal absorption of fluid and normally functioning ovaries and are caused by secretion of fluid by the ovary trapped in surrounding scarred peritoneum in patients with extensive pelvic adhesions. The peritoneal lining that forms the wall of a peritoneal inclusion cyst has been altered by inflammation, fibrosis, and mesothelial proliferation, and does not have the absorptive capacity of the normal peritoneum.[131,136,138]

The cysts are uni- or multilocular, with or without septa, and are usually densely adherent to, but do not replace, the ovary, thus indicating their nonovarian origin. The ovarian parenchyma is usually normal. The fibrous wall is smooth and may be up to 5 mm in thickness. An ovary surrounded by septa and fluid is the most common finding on ultrasound. Doppler examination shows low resistive flow in the septa.[135] Transvaginal ultrasound may be used to guide drainage or injection of sclerosing agents. There is a high recurrence rate of peritoneal inclusion cysts after aspiration or surgical treatment.[139]

MRI will show a multilocular cystic mass with thin septa in the pelvic cavity, showing hypointensity of the cyst contents on T1 images and variable hyperintense signals on T2 images.[140]

Necrotizing Fasciitis of the Pelvis

Infections of the abdominal wall are usually divided into necrotizing fasciitis if localized to the subcutaneous fat and superficial fascia and pyomyositis if they involve the muscles alone.[141]

Necrotizing fasciitis is a life-threatening infection that usually is secondary to a polymicrobial infection that may develop spontaneously after vaginal, vulvar, or abdominal surgery, blunt or penetrating trauma, venous stasis, or decubitus ulcers.[142-145] Most infections occur in the perineum and genitalia.[145] Necrotizing fasciitis may complicate percutaneous drainage of intra-abdominal abscesses guided by ultrasound or CT.[146]

The clinical presentation is that of a rapidly progressing inflammatory process, initially appearing as mild cellulitis or edema with inflammation, causing extensive necrosis of fascia and subcutaneous tissue with initial sparing of muscle.[142,143] Fever, pain, swelling, and bullae may be seen.[145] Severe septicemia with multiple organ failure can develop early in the course of the disease.[143] Toxic shock syndrome may be associated with necrotizing fasciitis.[147] Delay in diagnosis carries a high mortality rate.[142,143,145] Radiography may show soft tissue gas.[144,145] Ultrasound is of limited use, unless fluid or pus collections are present or superficial structures are involved. Gas in the superficial soft tissues may hinder imaging of deeper structures. Abscesses within the anterior abdominal wall can appear anechoic, weakly echogenic, or occasionally highly echogenic, depending upon the amount of necrotic tissue debris and gas they contain.[148,149]

The main CT features of necrotizing fasciitis are gas within the superficial fascia, gas distributed in a linear fashion corresponding to the superficial fascia, and predominance of fascial involvement. Lesser involvement of muscle occasionally occurs. There is frequent associated inflammation of the subcutaneous fat and skin.[150] Abscesses can involve the subcutaneous fat, the muscle layers or both, and may appear on CT as fluid-filled lesions or a solid "plaque-like" thickening of the abdominal wall.[149]

MRI is useful for separating cellulitis from deeper, necrotizing soft tissue infections that require surgical intervention.

In the former, abnormal signal intensity is confined to the subcutaneous fat, whereas a necrotizing infection displays increased signal intensity on T2-weighted images within muscles and extending along fascial planes, which may be accompanied by peripheral enhancement on T1-weighted images following intravenous gadolinium.[151,152] MRI can be particularly useful in delineating a collection of inflammatory fluid at the interface of muscle and fascia in areas of necrosis.[153]

Fatty Tumors

Lipomatous tumors are commonly found in women. The majority are benign cystic ovarian teratomas; however, malignant degeneration of benign cystic teratomas, nonteratomatous lipomatous ovarian tumors, and lipomatous uterine tumors should be excluded. Nongynecologic fatty tumors of the pelvis are lipomas and liposarcomas.[154]

Lipoma

Benign pelvic lipomas are uncommon retroperitoneal masses composed of mature lipocytes and minimal fibrous tissue. They are usually well-defined, encapsulated masses that produce a mass effect rather than invade adjacent structures and appear hyperechoic on ultrasound.[154]

CT appearances of pelvic lipomas are generally of homogeneous fat density, except for a few thin low-density septa.[154,155] They are usually sharply marginated, showing less attenuation than the patient's normal fat, and unless a capsule is seen, lipomas cannot be distinguished from localized fat collections.[155-157]

Liposarcoma

Liposarcomas represent approximately 25% of soft tissue sarcomas and 10% to 20% of all primary retroperitoneal tumors.[158,159] Calcium may be found in liposarcomas.[154] Liposarcomas should be suspected when a fatty mass displays one or more of the following characteristics: inhomogeneity, infiltration or poor margination, and/or CT attenuation values greater than the patient's normal fat or contrast enhancement.[156,157,160] (Fig. 24.27). Three patterns of attenuation may be observed: solid tissue, mixed fat and solid tissue, and pseudocystic. They can be sharply marginated and have a pseudocapsule.[156] Well-differentiated liposarcomas have imaging characteristics of lipomas. Liposarcomas with a low grade of differentiation may present variable degrees of necrosis, giving them imaging characteristic of nonspecific masses.[155] MRI shows well-differentiated liposarcomas with fat signal intensity; other types of liposarcomas may be hypointense on T1-weighted images and hyperintense on T2-weighted images.[160] Ultrasound shows a heterogeneous, predominantly hyperechoic, retroperitoneal mass.[161-162]

Pelvic Lipomatosis

Pelvic lipomatosis is a benign condition characterized by increased deposition of normal fat in the pelvis, and at times is

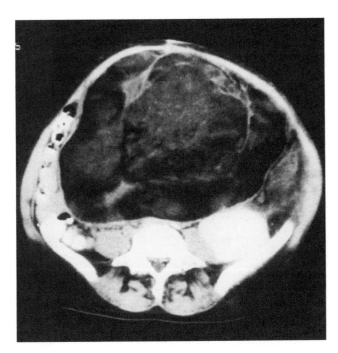

Figure 24.27 CT of myxoid liposarcoma in a 49-year-old woman. A large hypoattenuating abdominopelvic mass with internal septa and some areas of soft-tissue attenuation. Courtesy of Dr. Elvira Carvalhal, São Paulo, Brazil.

associated with a fibrous tissue response. It is more common in males than in females and is usually confined to the pelvis, although retroperitoneal involvement may occur. Deformity of the bladder and extrinsic compression of rectosigmoid may be seen.[163,164] Ultrasound may show the bladder compressed by a hyperechoic mass; however, the fatty mass may be easily missed.[155,164]

CT is preferred for evaluation of pelvic lipomatosis because of the highly negative attenuation of fat.[155] In pelvic lipomatosis, the pelvic cavity is infiltrated by a fat density tissue; the CT numbers are generally equal to or more negative than the patient's normal fat. The abnormal fat is usually evenly distributed throughout the pelvis.[156,164] MRI shows high amounts of hyperintense fat surrounding the bladder[165] or rectosigmoid.

Fibrous Tumors

Desmoid (Aggressive Fibromatosis)

The desmoid tumor is the most common neoplasm of the rectus abdominis muscle and sheath. It arises in the musculoaponeurotic structures of the abdominal wall, especially below the level of the umbilicus. It is a completely encapsulated fibroma and is so hard that it creaks when it is cut. Eighty percent of cases are in women who have had children. They occasionally occur in scars of old hernial or other abdominal operations. Consequently, trauma, stretching of the muscle fibers during pregnancy, or possibly a small hematoma of the abdominal wall appear to be a predisposing factor. Metastasis and sarcomatous changes do not occur, although they have a strong tendency toward local recurrence and focal invasion.[166,167]

On ultrasound, desmoid tumors are generally well-defined hypoechoic formations, but they may have a cystic, solid, or even heterogeneous appearance (Fig. 24.28). Treatment usually consists of wide excision, otherwise recurrence commonly takes place.[168]

Intra-abdominal desmoids appear as soft tissue masses that generally do not enhance on CT[167,169] (Fig. 24.28B). MRI may show desmoids as masses that are hypointense to muscle on T1-weighted images, and hypo- or slightly hyperintense on T2-weighted images, without enhancement following intravenous gadolinium injection. Sagittal and coronal images may be obtained with MRI, allowing a better delineation of extension of the lesion.[167]

Fibroma

Fibromas, or leiomyomas, are benign tumors usually found in the uterus; however, rarely they occur in the ovaries and nongynecologic sites such as in the round ligament, peritoneum, and retroperitoneum.

Round ligament fibromas are rare. They are usually single, unilateral, and they are clinically silent, although there may be a traction-like sensation in the inguinal region as the mass is moved during pelvic examination. Their size may vary from small masses to enormous ones. Ultrasonography shows a heterogeneous mass. The location of the tumor may not be precisely determined by ultrasound.[170]

Leiomyomatosis peritonealis disseminata is a rare benign disorder, characterized by multiple benign nodules composed of smooth muscle, myofibroblasts, and fibroblasts[171] varying in size from a few millimeters to 10 cm in diameter in the submesothelial mesenchyma of the abdominal cavity and pelvis. The nodules occur on the surfaces of abdominal and pelvic organs, the omentum, mesentery, parietal peritoneum, and in round or broad ligaments. The disease is usually not symptomatic; patients may complain of nonspecific pelvic pain, or the nodules may be found incidentally. The tumors are vascular, and ultrasound shows pelvic tumors with solid and cystic components, separate from the uterus.[172]

Retroperitoneal leiomyomas are seen on CT as soft tissue density masses[173] or as irregularly marginated masses with central cyst formation, related to necrosis or hemorrhage, and no calcification. Peritoneal leiomyosarcomatosis is seen on CT as soft tissue density of peritoneal or mesenteric masses, with low attenuation central areas and absence of lymph node enlargement and occasionally associated ascites.[174]

Malignant Fibrous Histiocytoma

Malignant fibrous histiocytoma is a pleomorphic sarcoma and is the most common soft tissue sarcoma of late adult life, although it can be seen at any age.[176,177] It can be found in the abdominal cavity or retroperitoneum and in the mesentery.[175,177,178] Extraretroperitoneal sites of tumor include the

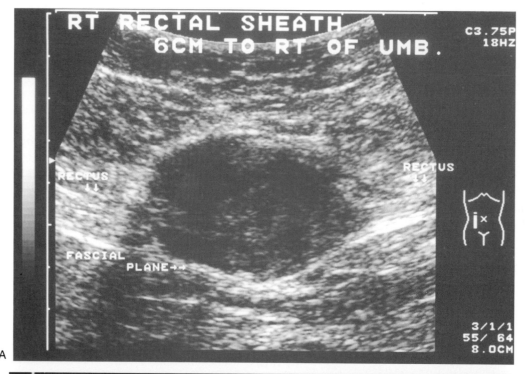

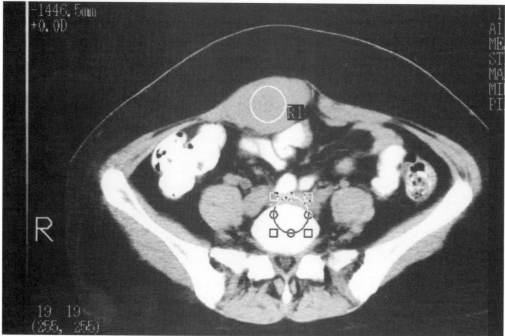

Figure 24.28 A 32-year-old who presented 9 months after cesarean section with a firm right-sided lower abdominal wall mass. **(A)** Ultrasound shows a well delineated mass of low echogenicity. **(B)** Corresponding CT shows a homogeneous mass to the right of the midline (circle). Although confirmed on needle biopsy the patient refused operation and 2 years later no evidence could be seen of the swelling, either clinically or on imaging.

small intestine, colon and rectum, appendix, peritoneal cavity, liver, spleen, and stomach.[176]

Retroperitoneal fibrous histiocytomas may cause fever, malaise and weight loss, leukocytosis, and anemia.[175,178] Abdominal distension and hernias due to increasing abdominal pressure, ascites caused by liver metastases, and local infiltration of major vessels as well as ileus symptoms may be present. Local recurrence and metastases are frequent. Metastases most frequently occur in lung and regional lymph nodes.[178–180] Bone, muscle, or bowel invasion is rare, and commonly extrinsic pressure and displacement of adjacent structures are seen.[175]

Ultrasound shows the tumors to be well circumscribed, generally hypoechoic (the most frequent pattern) with internal echoes. Necrotic and cystic areas with thick septa[175,176,181] and calcification may be seen. Differential diagnosis includes circumscribed mesotheliomas, other forms of sarcomas, metastases of carcinomas, pseudomyxoma, and tuberculosis.[176,178]

Precontrast CT shows large, solid lesions (40 to 60 HU), with areas of necrosis and/or hemorrhage represented by scattered areas of lower density (30 to -10 HU), with occasional calcifications (Fig. 24.29). Postcontrast scans may show heterogeneous hypervascularity, which is persistent and located peripherally in cases of necrosis. Infiltration or encasement of adjacent organs such the psoas, aorta, or iliac arteries can be demonstrated.[175,176]

Primary retroperitoneal tumor can be suspected when a mass is identified extraperitoneally without invasion of any adjacent organs. It is impossible to differentiate a primary

Figure 24.29 CT of a malignant fibrohystiocytoma in a 1-year-old girl. A heterogeneous mass is seen with contrast enhancement, and internal calcification is surrounded by low density material.

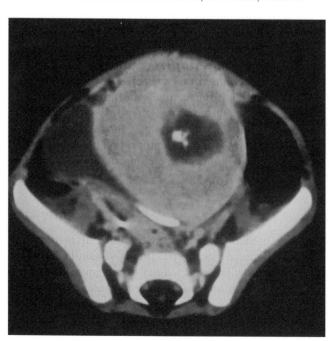

retroperitoneal mass from a tumor arising in the affected organ when visceral invasion or encasement is present. Fibrous histiocytoma cannot be differentiated from other nonfatty mesenchymal or germ cell tumors or from neurogenic tumors by imaging alone. It should be considered in the differential diagnosis of retroperitoneal primary tumors, since it is one of the most common soft tissue sarcomas of adult life and is commonly found in the retroperitoneum.[175]

On MRI, soft tissue malignant fibrous histiocytomas may show poor margin definition, internal low signal septa, and heterogeneous high signal intensity on T2-weighted images.[182]

TUMORS OF LYMPHATIC ORIGIN

Lymphangioma

Lymphangiomatosis is a congenital maldevelopment of the lymphatic system.[183] There are three basic forms:

1. Capillary lymphangioma, a focal tumefaction with ill-defined borders, composed of dilated lymphatic vessels with a rich cellular stroma of connective tissue
2. Cavernous lymphangioma, consisting of dilated lymphatic sinuses generally filled with a chylous fluid
3. Cystic lymphangioma, a thin-walled cystic structure, lined with endothelium[184]

The natural history of lymphangioma includes progressive growth with compression and infiltration of adjacent structures. They cross fascial planes, infiltrate viscera, and extend along neurovascular bundles. Lymphedema, lymphorrhea, lymphatic effusions, and infections are common, and spontaneous involution is rare.[183] The most commonly affected sites are the face and neck; pelvic and mesenteric lymphangiomas are rare.[185,186]

Ultrasound shows fluid-filled structures with well-defined walls[185] and fine septa in cystic lymphangiomas[183,184] and allows differentiation of the ovaries, which may be engorged by chylous fluid, from adjacent small bowel loops and lymphatic pools.[183]

CT shows the lesions and their relation to adjacent structures with enhancement of the lymphatic vessels following injection of contrast and in guiding needle and catheter placement for sclerosing therapy.[183]

CT appearances of lymphangiomas and lymphangiomatosis are variable. The mesenteric and retroperitoneal lymphangiomas are round, thin-walled tumors, with homogeneous attenuation, with fatty density zones (less than 0 HU), sometimes with slight peripheral enhancement. They may cause displacement without invasion of adjacent structures. Less common and nonspecific presentations are of soft tissue density infiltrative tumors, without cystic areas. Calcification and fluid–fluid levels may be present, in cases of hemorrhage or superinfection.[184–186] MRI shows abnormal lymphatic pools and channels, as well as diffuse pelvic lymphedema.[183]

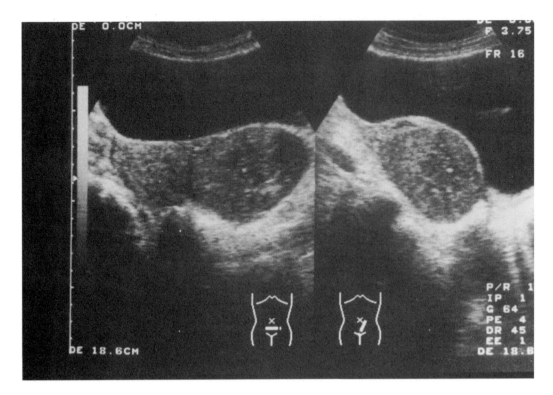

Figure 24.30 A 27-year-old woman with a pelvic lymphoma. Oval heterogeneous parauterine masses, simulating ovarian tumor. (Courtesy of Dr. Ayrton Pastore, São Paulo, Brazil.)

Figure 24.31 A T1-weighted image following intravenous contrast administration demonstrates right internal iliac lymphadenopathy in a 67-year-old woman.

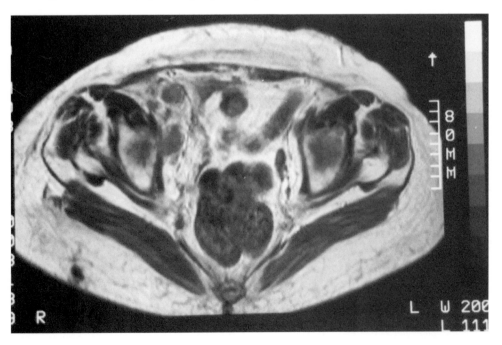

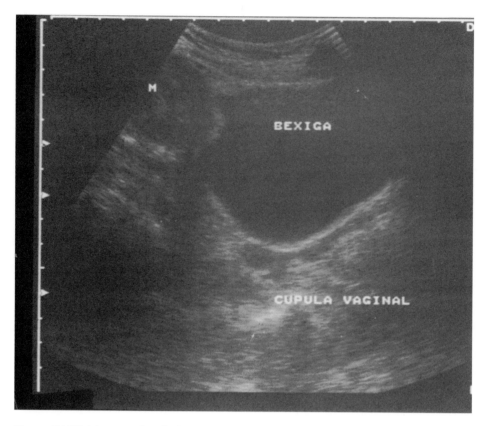

Figure 24.32 Metastatic lymphadenopathy shown as a solid paravesical mass (M) in 60-year-old woman with a previous hysterectomy. Bexiga, bladder; cupula vaginal, vagina. (Courtesy Dr. Denise P. Vezozzo, São Paulo, Brazil.)

Lymphadenopathy

Lymphoma, leukemia, tuberculosis, inflammatory conditions, and metastatic malignancy of genital, intestinal, or urinary tract origin may cause enlargement of the lymph nodes (lymphadenopathy), generally seen as hypoechoic nodules or confluent masses (Fig. 24.30).

MRI can detect para-aortic, paracaval, iliac, and inguinal lymphadenopathies[187] (Fig. 24.31). In comparison with noncontrast CT, MRI gives higher image contrast between enlarged lymph nodes, vessels, and muscles.[188] Enlarged pelvic lymph nodes are equally well seen by MRI, CT, and ultrasound[188,189] (Fig. 24.32).

PERITONEAL LESIONS

Mesothelioma

Approximately 33% of mesotheliomas are found in the abdomen and are formed by cystic mesothelioma, benign adenomatoid tumor, and the malignant mesothelioma.[190]

Cystic mesothelioma of the peritoneum is a rare benign form that occurs predominantly in middle-aged women and tends to recur locally.[190–195] The pathogenesis is unknown, although peritoneal irritation and previous laparotomy may contribute.[192,196] Local recurrence rate between 3 months to 22 years postresection is 27% to 75%.[190] Multiple thick- and thin-walled cystic areas are seen distributed throughout the abdomen and pelvis,[192,193] and rarely, free-floating pelvic cysts are seen.[196] Circumscribed cystic lesions encase loops of bowel and can compress intraperitoneal organs.[193] They do not invade adjacent organs or omentum, nor are they metastatic.[190,193,194]

The differential diagnosis includes pseudomyxoma peritonei, lymphangioma, mesenteric cysts, enteric duplication cysts, and cystadenoma or cystadenocarcinoma of the ovary.[190,192,196] Ultrasonography usually shows a heterogeneous mass.[194]

Malignant mesothelioma is an uncommon neoplasm arising from the serosal surfaces of the peritoneum. Ultrasound shows sheetlike or nodular peritoneal thickening, soft tissue hypoechoic masses, fixation of the intestinal loops, mesenteric thickening, and ascites, which is disproportionate to the degree of tumor dissemination.[193,197–200]

Malignant peritoneal mesothelioma can be divided into two basic groups: one with a predominant, usually upper abdominal, mass and scattered intra-abdominal nodules, and the other with a diffuse intraperitoneal solid desmoplastic effect, which tends to envelop the bowel viscera[191] (Fig. 24.33).

Metastatic

Pseudomyxoma Peritonei

Pseudomyxoma peritonei may be benign or malignant and is defined as intraperitoneal accumulation of a mucoid substance. It is caused by mucus-secreting implants throughout the abdominal cavity, that is, ruptured mucinous adenocarcinoma of the ovary or the appendix or mucocele of the appendix.[193,201–204] The most common clinical findings are ascites, mass, distension, and abdominal pain.[201,202,204] Serum carcinoembryonic antigen (CEA) is commonly abnormally high.[201,204]

The characteristic CT findings of pseudomyxoma peritonei are massive ascites or loculated fluid collections causing hepatic and mesenteric scalloping[204–205] (Fig. 24.34). These cystic and low-attenuation tumor masses appear without lymphadenopathy in the presence of intrinsically normal viscera.[205] Mucinous ascites is generally heterogeneous and of fat density with attenuation values greater than those of water. Fluid ascites may be homogeneous with attenuation values greater than water. Hepatic, splenic, and mesenteric scalloping, ascitic septa, and loculi may be demonstrated by CT. Low-attenuation soft tissue masses with internal mottled densities and scattered curvilinear peripheral calcifications may be seen. Curvilinear calcifications, which are rare, omental thickening, and multiple septate cystic lesions are suggestive of pseudomyxoma peritonei. A characteristic central displacement of bowel loops and compression of abdominal viscera may be seen.[201,202,206,207]

Figure 24.33 CT of peritoneal mesothelioma shows soft tissue density masses encasing bowel loops in a 67-year-old woman.

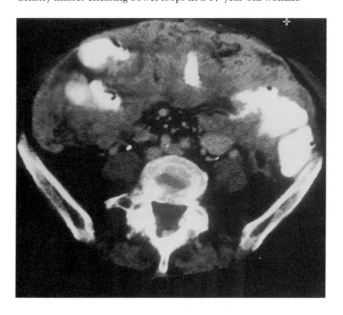

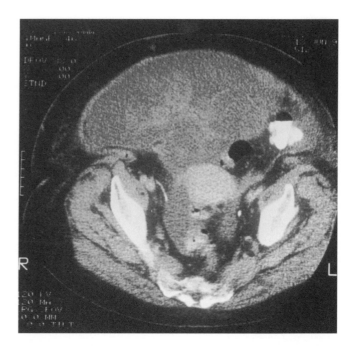

Figure 24.34 Peritoneal pseudomyxoma in a 70-year-old woman 1 year after resection of colon carcinoma. Hypo-attenuating material is seen in the peritoneal cavity and surrounding the uterus.

MRI helps in the differential diagnosis of ascites.[205] MRI shows the myxomatous material with low signal intensity on T1-weighted images and high signal intensity on T2-weighted images, indicating long T1 and T2 values, which are, however, shorter than those of ascites, pseudocysts, and water-like fluid.[208] Both implants and mucoid ascites are hypointense on T1-weighted images, with signal intensity approaching that of muscle. On T2-weighted images, however, there is general hyperintensity of signals, which is more pronounced in mucoid ascites than in implants, and which approaches signal intensities of water.[209] T2-weighted images accentuate the differences between mucinous ascites and fluid ascites better than T1-weighted images do. The signal intensity of the adjacent peritoneal implants is slightly higher than that of fat.[206] Mucin in the cysts will produce an increased signal intensity on T1-weighted and T2-weighted images.[190]

Ultrasound features of pseudomyxoma peritonei are of an echogenic mantle with echogenic loculated ascites, multiple intraperitoneal cysts, and multiple bowel indentations.[207] The ascites can sometimes seem "solid," with the transducer not deforming the ascites but compressing the adjacent bowel loops.[201,206] It may also have numerous "suspended" echoes that do not mobilize as the patient changes position.[206] The internal echoes represent semi-solid gelatinous masses or the walls of tiny highly echogenic mucinous cysts.[204] A cystic mass may be seen, generally in the right iliac fossa, with or without peripheral calcifications.[202] Ultrasound is a helpful tool to guide paracentesis,[206] and the diagnosis can be confirmed, but local recurrence is common.[203,204]

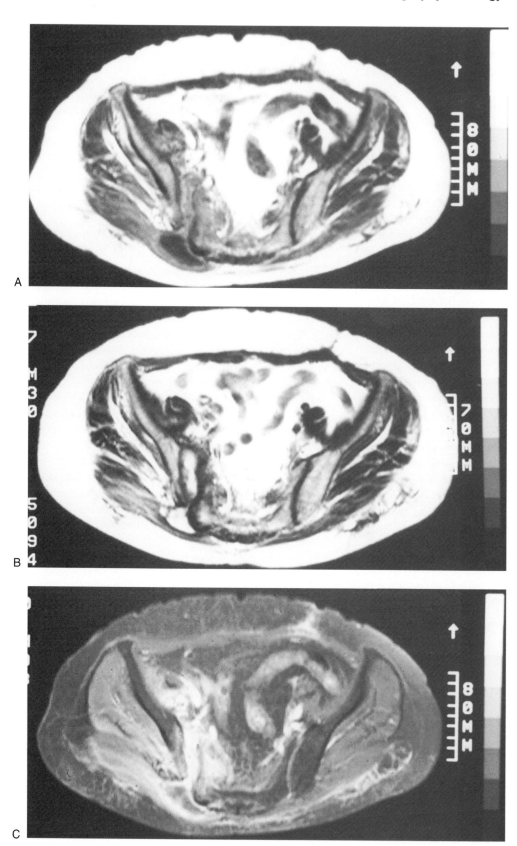

Figure 24.35 MRI of pyoarthritis with right iliac osteomyelitis in a 66-year-old woman. **(A)** Axial T1-weighted postcontrast image. **(B)** Axial T2-weighted image. **(C)** Axial T1-weighted fat-suppressed postcontrast image. A right iliac hyperintense area is seen on the T2-weighted image, and fluid collection with peripheral enhancement is seen in the right sacroiliac joint, extending to the gluteus muscle posteriorly.

Peritoneal Carcinomatosis

Peritoneal carcinomatosis can also diffusely infiltrate the abdominal wall and mesentery, thicken the bowel wall, and show cystic components and ascites.[193] Common sources are adenocarcinomas of the ovary, colon, and stomach.[193,210] On ultrasound and CT, secondary tumor is usually diffuse and consists of small nodules that can give a large nodular appearance.[193] Ascites is seen in 75% of patients, sometimes with debris, and 50% of these patients can have loculated ascites.[193] Peritoneal carcinomatosis can diffusely infiltrate the abdominal wall and mesentery, thicken the bowel wall, and show cystic components and ascites.[193] Omental involvement may be seen by ultrasound as nodular, cake-like thickening, and infiltration of fat. Small nodular implants on the surface of the omentum, peritoneum, or bowel serosa may also be detected. Another ultrasound feature of peritoneal carcinomatosis is the interruption of the anterior hyperechoic peritoneal line, corresponding to a tumoral involvement of the peritoneum prior to nodule formation.[211]

CT will show peritoneal implants, ascites, mesenteric implants, and omental involvement.[210] Another CT sign of peritoneal carcinomatosis is a discrete linear peritoneal thickening detected more easily in the presence of ascites.[211]

MRI findings in peritoneal carcinomatosis include ascites, seedings along small intestine and colon, stellate pattern of the mesentery, linear or tiny nodular infiltrations of the omentum, and subperitoneal fat (ligamentous, mesenteric, and mesocolic), focal or segmental wall thickenings, loss of unilateral colonic haustration with sacculation on the contralateral side, and nodular soft tissue masses along different locations of the peritoneal surfaces.[212,213]

MUSCULOSKELETAL TUMORS

Osteomyelitis

Osteomyelitis of pelvic bones is generally secondary to extension of a pelvic abscess to the pelvic bones or extension from a decubitus ulcer. The most common agents are anaerobic bacteria. Clinically, it may simulate other pelvic conditions such as appendicitis and septic arthritis of the hip joint.[214]

CT helps to differentiate cortical or periosteal involvement from intramedullary disease and to detect complicating abscesses and the need for surgery. CT features of pelvic osteomyelitis include an increase in intramedullary density due to the accumulation of infected debris within the bone marrow and intra-osseous or intra-articular gas. Fistulous tracts may be seen with the gastrointestinal and central nervous systems.[214] Early osteomyelitis is seen as a radiolucent area in the intramedullary bone. In early sacro-iliac arthritis, indistinct joint margins are seen, followed by irregularity of the margins. The CT signs of retroperitoneal, retrofascial, or gluteal abscesses are an abnormal hypodense mass, displacement of adjacent structures, obliteration of surrounding tissue planes, gas collections, and peripheral enhancement.[215]

MRI may be a helpful diagnostic tool to evaluate early changes of infection in the sacroiliac area. It is very sensitive for detecting bone marrow abnormalities, but it is nonspecific and cannot distinguish osteomyelitis from sacroiliitis[216] (Fig. 24.35).

Ultrasound may help to detect pelvic abscesses related to pelvic osteomyelitis, evaluating the solid or cystic nature of the lesion, but CT is preferred to determine the intraperitoneal or extraperitoneal location of the mass.[215]

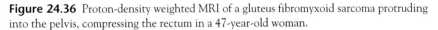

Figure 24.36 Proton-density weighted MRI of a gluteus fibromyxoid sarcoma protruding into the pelvis, compressing the rectum in a 47-year-old woman.

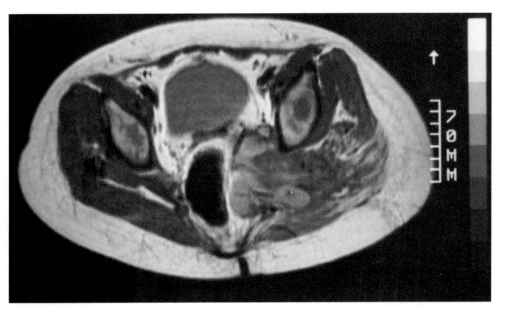

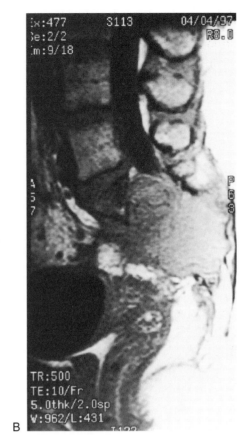

Figure 24.37 Recurrence of sacral giant cell tumor in a 50-year-old woman. (A) CT showing sacral lytic mass with soft tissue component protruding into the pelvis. (B) Sagittal T1-weighted images showing the sacral mass with intrapelvic extension.

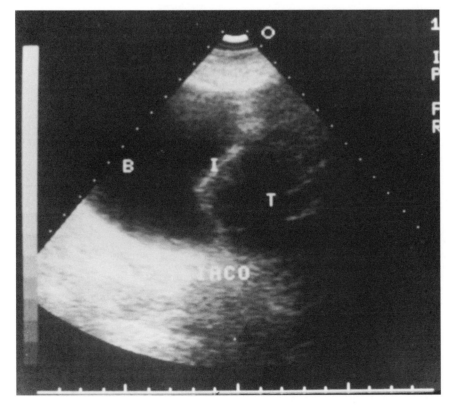

Figure 24.38 Pelvic ultrasound of a rhabdomyosarcoma (T), compressing the urinary bladder (B). (Courtesy of Dr. Ayrton Pastore São Paulo, Brazil.)

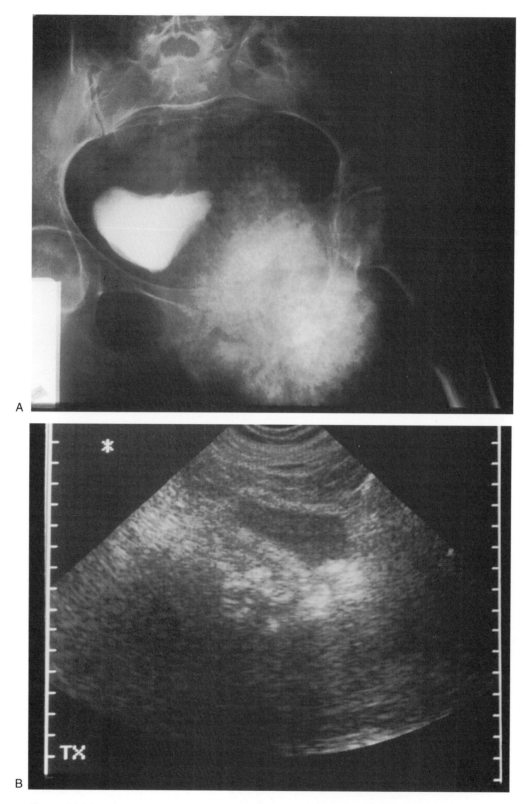

Figure 24.39 Pubic osteosarcoma in a 31-year-old woman. **(A)** Urography demonstrates a calcified mass dislocating the bladder. **(B)** Pelvic ultrasound shows the urinary bladder and the tumor calcifications, seen as hyperechoic zones.

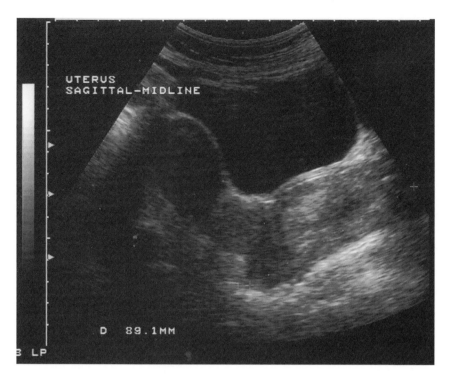

Figure 24.40 A 24-year-old woman who presented with dyspareunia. A firm smooth mass was palpable in the rectovaginal septum on bimanual examination. It was removed surgically and proved to be a benign rhabdomyoma. (Courtesy of Dr. Kenneth Atkinson, Sydney, Australia.)

Tumors

CT and MRI are the most appropriate methods to evaluate musculoskeletal tumors of the pelvis. The interior of the mass and the relationship between the mass and pelvic organs, as well as between neural and other musculoskeletal structures of pelvic wall, can be well defined (Figs. 24.36 and 24.37).

The use of ultrasound on the evaluation of musculoskeletal masses is limited. As the majority of musculoskeletal pelvic masses are situated on or close to the pelvic walls, only a study of the surface of the lesion can be performed. Ultrasound may help to disclose the relationship between the mass and other pelvic organs (Figs. 24.38 and 24.39). Figure 24.40 shows a rare rhabdomyoma of the rectovaginal septum which caused dyspareunia.

REFERENCES

1. Balthazar EJ, Birnbaum BA, Yee J et al. Acute appendicitis: CT and US correlation in 100 patients. Radiology 1994; 190:31–35
2. Birnbaum BA, Balthazar EJ. CT of appendicitis and diverticulitis. Radiol Clin North Am 1994;32:885–898
3. Curtin KR, Fitzgerald SW, Nemcek Jr AA et al. CT diagnosis of acute appendicitis: imaging findings. AJR Am J Roentgenol 1995;164:905–909
4. Jeffrey RB, Jain KA, Nghiem HV. Sonographic diagnosis of acute appendicits: interpretive pitfalls. AJR Am J Roentgenol 1994;162:55–59
5. Yacoe ME, Jeffrey RB, Jr. Sonography of appendicitis and diverticulitis. Radiol Clin North Am 1994;32:899–912
6. Trenkner S, Thompson WM. In patients with left lower quadrant pain, should barium enema or CT be used for initial evaluation? AJR Am J Roentgenol 1995;165:733
7. Jacobs JE, Birnbaum BA. CT of inflammatory disease of the colon. Semin Ultrasound CT MR 1995;16:91–101
8. Padidar AM, Jeffrey RB, Jr, Mindelzun RE, Dolph JF. Differentiating sigmoid diverticulitis from carcinoma on CT scans: mesenteric inflammation suggests diverticulitis. AJR Am J Roentgenol 1994;163:81–83
9. Alonso Sánchez JM, Acebo García M, Matas Gómez V. Ultrasonography of acute diverticulitis of the colon. Rev Esp Enferm Dig 1994;86:835–837
10. Ide C, Van Beers B, Pauls C, Pringot J. Diagnosis of acute colonic diverticulitis: comparison with echography and tomodensitometry. J Belge Radiol 1994;77:262–267
11. Gore RM, Balthazar EJ, Ghahremani GG, Miller FH. CT features of ulcerative colitis and Crohn's disease. AJR Am J Roentgenol 1996;167:3–15
12. Pompili GG, Damiani G, Mariani P et al. Computerized tomography in the diagnosis of Crohn disease. Radiol Med 1994;88:44–48
13. Klein HM, Wein B, Adam G et al. The computed tomographic morphology of Crohn's disease and ulcerative colitis. Rofo Fortschr Geb Rontgenstr Neuen Bildgeb Verfahr 1995; 163:9–15
14. Solvig J, Ekberg O, Lindgren S et al. Ultrasound examination of the small bowel: comparison with enteroclysis in patients with Crohn disease. Abdom Imaging 1995;20:323–326
15. Lim JH, Ko YT, Lee DH et al. Sonography of inflammatory bowel disease: findings and value in differential diagnosis. AJR Am J Roentgenol 1994;163:343–347
16. Khaw KT, Yeoman LJ, Saverymuttu SH et al. Ultrasonic patterns in inflammatory bowel disease. Clin Radiol 1991; 43:171–175
17. Gore RM. Cross-sectional imaging of inflammatory bowel disease. Radiol Clin North Am 1987;25:115–131

18. Joseph AE. Ultrasound scanning. Scand J Gastroenterol Suppl 1994;203:24–27
19. Gore RM, Laufer I. Ulcerative colitis and granulomatous colitis: idiopathic inflammatory bowel disease. In: Gore RM, Levine MS, Laufer I, Eds. Textbook of Gastrointestinal Radiology. WB Saunders, Philadelphia, 1994, pp. 1098–1141
20. Limberg B. Diagnosis of colonic tumors and chronic inflammatory colonic diseases by hydrocolonic sonography. Radiologe 1993;33:407–411
21. Vernacchia FS, Jeffrey RB, Laing FC, Wing VW. Sonographic recognition of pneumatosis intestinalis. AJR Am J Roentgenol 1985;145:51–52
22. Vecchioli A, De Franco A, Maresca G, Gore RM. Small bowel. Cross-sectional imaging. In: Gore RM, Levine MS, Laufer I, Eds. Textbook of Gastrointestinal Radiology WB Saunders, Philadelphia 1994, pp. 789–801
23. Pantongrag-Brown L, Buetow PC, Carr NJ et al. Calcification and fibrosis in mesenteric carcinoid tumor: CT findings and pathologic correlation. AJR Am J Roentgenol 1995;164: 387–391
24. Woodard PK, Feldman JM, Paine SS, Baker ME. Midgut carcinoid tumors: CT findings and biochemical profiles. J Comput Assist Tomogr 1995;19:400–405
25. Sugimoto E, Lörelius LE, Eriksson B, Öberg K. Midgut carcinoid tumors—CT appearance. Acta Radiologica 1995;36: 367–371
26. Watanabe Y, Takahiro I, Horibe K et al. Advanced primary non-Hodgkin's lymphoma of the small intestine in childhood: report of four cases. Jpn J Surg 1994;24:1023–1027
27. Goerg C, Schwerk WB, Goerg K. Gastrointestinal lymphoma: sonographic findings in 54 patients. AJR Am J Roentgenol 1990;155:795–798
28. Thoeni RF, Laufer I. Colon. Polyps and cancer. In: Gore RM, Levine MS, Laufer I, eds. Textbook of Gastrointestinal Radiology. WB Saunders, Philadelphia, 1994, pp. 1160–1199
29. Thompson WM, Trenkner SW. Staging colorectal carcinoma. Radiol Clin North Am 1994;32:25–37
30. Masi A, Olmastroni M, Lascialfari L et al. Magnetic resonance with endorectal coil in the locoregional staging of rectal carcinoma. Radiol Med 1995;90:431–437
31. Isern AM, Fernández C, Salamanca M et al. Transrectal ultrasonography in the preoperative staging of rectal adenocarcinoma. Cross-sectional study 1991–1994. GEN (Venezuela) 1995;49:104–110
32. Fedyaev EB, Volkova EA, Kuznetsova EE. Transrectal and transvaginal ultrasonography in the preoperative staging of rectal carcinoma. Eur J Radiol 1995;20:35–38
33. Wojtowycz AR, Spirt BA, Kaplan DS, Roy AK. Endoscopic US of the gastrointestinal tract with endoscopic, radiographic, and pathologic correlation. Radiographics 1995;15:735–753
34. Kauffman WM, Jenkins JJ 3rd, Helton K et al. Imaging features of ovarian metastases from colonic adenocarcinoma in adolescents. Pediatr Radiol 1995;25:286–288
35. Kennedy A, Hemingway A. Radiology of ovarian varices. Br J Hosp Med 1990;44:38–43
36. Juhász B, Kurjak A, Lampé LG. Pelvic varices simulating bilateral adnexal masses: differential diagnosis by transvaginal color Doppler. J Clin Ultrasound 1992;20:81–84
37. Jain KA, Jeffrey RB, Jr, Sommer FG. Gynecologic vascular abnormalities diagnosis with Doppler US. Radiology 1991;178:549–551
38. Hodgson TJ, Reed MWR, Peck RJ, Hemingway AP. Case report: the ultrasound and Doppler appearances of pelvic varices. Clin Radiol 1991;44:208–209
39. Giacchetto C, Cotroneo GB, Marincolo F et al. Ovarian varicocele: ultrasonic and phlebographic evaluation. J Clin Ultrasound 1990;18:551–555
40. Thibault PK, Lewis WA. Recurrent varicose veins. Part 1: evaluation utilizing duplex venous imaging. J Dermatol Surg Oncol 1992;18:618–624
41. Walsh G, Williams MP. Case report: giant pararectal varices—computed tomographic appearances. Br J Radiol 1995; 68:203–204
42. Berger RB, Taylor KJW, Rosenfield AT. Pelvic varices simulating cystic ovaries: differentiation by pulsed Doppler. J Clin Ultrasound 1982;10:186–189
43. Zwiebel WJ. Aortic and iliac aneurysms. In. Zwiebel WJ, Ed. Introduction to Vascular Ultrasonography (3rd ed.). WB Saunders, Philadelphia, 1992, pp. 351–366
44. Gillum RF. Epidemiology of aortic aneurysm in the United States. J Clin Epidemiol 1995;48:1289–1298
45. Morbidelli A, Caron R, Caldana G et al. Aneurysm of the iliac artery. Minerva Chir 1995;50:767–771
46. Lozano P, Julià J, Corominas C, Gomez F. Ruptured aneurysms of the internal iliac artery. Report of two cases. J Cardiovasc Surg (Torino) 1995;36:591–594
47. Raptopoulos V, Rosen MP, Kent KC et al. Sequential helical CT angiography of aortoiliac disease. AJR Am J Roentgenol 1996;166:1347–1354
48. Rieker O, Düber C, Schmiedt W et al. CT angiography versus intra-arterial DSA in abdominal aortic aneurysms. Rofo Fortschr Geb Rontgenstr Neuen Bildgeb Verfahr 1996; 165:17–23
49. Gomes MN, Davros WJ, Zeman RK. Preoperative assessment of abdominal aortic aneurysm: the value of helical and three-dimensional computed tomography. J Vasc Surg 1994; 20:367–375
50. Prince MR. Gadolinium-enhanced MR aortography. Radiology 1994;191:155–164
51. Kaufman JA, Geller SC, Petersen MJ et al. MR imaging (including MR angiography) of abdominal aortic aneurysms: comparison with conventional angiography. AJR Am J Roentgenol 1994;163:203–210
52. Sardelic F, Fletcher JP, Ho D, Simmons K. Assessment of abdominal aortic aneurysm with magnetic resonance imaging. Australas Radiol 1995;39:107–111
53. Samaan NA, Hickey RC, Shutts PE. Diagnosis, localization, and management of pheochromocytoma. Pitfalls and follow-up in 41 patients. Cancer 1988;62:2451–2460
54. Hansen LU, Jess P, Hermansen K, Lorentzen M. Phaeochromocytoma—an unusual cause of haematuria. Scand J Urol Nephrol 1992;26:319–321
55. Whalen RK, Althausen AF, Daniels GH. Extra-adrenal pheochromocytoma. J Urol 1992;147:1–10
56. Goldfarb DA, Novick AC, Bravo EL et al. Experience with extra-adrenal pheochromocytoma. J Urol 1989;142:931–936
57. Caissel J, Ghaddar Y, Léandri P et al. Multiple pheochromocytomas revealed by a hemorrhagic tumor of the bladder. Ann Urol 1986;20:209–212
58. Dial P, Marks C, Bolton J. Current management of paragangliomas. Surg Gynecol Obstet 1982;155:187–192
59. van Gils APG, van Erkel AR, Falke THM, Pauwels EKJ. Mag-

netic resonance imaging or metaiodobenzylguanidine scintigraphy for the demonstration of paragangliomas? Eur J Nuc Med 1994;21:239–253

60. Schmedtje JF, Sax S, Pool JL et al. Localization of ectopic pheochromocytomas by magnetic resonance imaging. Am J Med 1987;83:770–772

61. Crecelius SA, Bellah R. Pheochromocytoma of the bladder in an adolescent: sonographic and MR imaging findings. AJR Am J Roentgenol 1995;165:101–103

62. Agarwal M, Azzopardi A, Mufti GR. Giant pre-sacral neurofibroma. Postgrad Med J 1992;68:55–56

63. Fauchery A, de Meeûs JB, Turc I et al. Benign pelvic schwannoma. A case report. J Gynecol Obstet Biol Reprod 1994;23:279–282

64. Kim SH, Choi BI, Han MC, Kim YI. Retroperitoneal neurilemoma: CT and MR findings. AJR Am J Roentgenol 1992;159:1023–1026

65. Khatib RA, Khalil AM, Saba MI et al. Case report. A pelvic retroperitoneal schwannoma presenting as an adnexal mass. Gynecol Oncol 1994;53:242–244

66. Gierada DS, Erickson SJ. MR imaging of the sacral plexus: abnormal findings AJR Am J Roentgenol 1993;160:1067–1071

67. Blickstein I, Lurie S. The gynaecological problems of neurofibromatosis. Aust NZ J Obstet Gynaecol 1990;30:380–382

68. Niku SD, Mattrey RF, Kalota SJ, Schmidt JD. MRI of pelvic neurofibromatosis. Abdom Imaging 1995;20:176–178

69. Geake TMS. Case of the month. A pain in the pelvis. Br J Radiol 1986;59:943–944

70. Green WJ, Green AE, Jr. Large pelvic mass in a patient with neurofibromatosis. Invest Radiol 1988;23:772–774

71. Pastore C, Marchiori G, D'Annibale A et al. Retroperitoneal ganglioneuroma. A case report and review of the literature. Minerva Chir (Italy) 1994;49:1129–1132

72. Kurzel RB, Durso N. Pelvic ganglioneuroma during pregnancy. A case report. J Reprod Med 1990;35:286–288

73. Hayes FA, Green AA, Rao BN. Clinical manifestations of ganglioneuroma. Cancer 1989;63:1211–1214

74. Dunnick NR, Sandler CM, Amis ES, Jr, Newhouse JH. Congenital anomalies. In: Textbook of Uroradiology (2nd ed.). Williams & Wilkins, Baltimore, 1997, pp 15–43

75. Sherer DM, Rideout J. Transvaginal sonography of pelvic kidney. J Clin Ultrasound 1994;22:214–215

76. Banerjee B, Brett I. Ultrasound diagnosis of horseshoe kidney. Br J Radiol 1991;64:898–900

77. Burgos FJ, Teruel JL, Mayayo T et al. Diagnosis and management of lymphoceles after renal transplantation. Br J Urol 1988;61:289–293

78. Gill IS, Hodge EE, Munch LC et al. Transperitoneal marsupialization of lymphoceles: a comparison of laparoscopic and open techniques. J Urol 1995;153:706–711

79. Dunnick NR, Sandler CM, Amis ES, Jr, Newhouse JH. Renal transplantation. In: Textbook of Uroradiology (2nd ed.). Williams & Wilkins, Baltimore, 1997, pp 236–253

80. Ridge JA, Manco-Johnson ML, Weil R, III. Ultrasonographic diagnosis of infected lymphocele after kidney trasnplantation. Eur Urol 1987;13:31–34

81. Letourneau JG, Day DL, Feinberg SB. Ultrasound and computed tomographic evaluation of renal transplantation. Radiol Clin North Am 1987;25:267–279

82. Wood BP, Ben-Ami T, Teele RL, Rabinowitz R. Ureterovesical obstruction and megaloureter: diagnosis by real-time US. Radiology 1985;156:79–81

83. Saita H, Matsukawa M, Fukushima H et al. Ultrasound diagnosis of ureteral stones: its usefulness with subsequent excretory urography. J Urology 1988;140:28–31

84. Hertzberg BS, Kliewer MA, Paulson EK, Carroll BA. Distal ureteral calculi: detection with transperineal sonography. AJR Am J Roentgenol 1994;163:1151–1153

85. Laing FC, Benson CB, DiSalvo DN et al. Distal ureteral calculi: detection with vaginal US. Radiology 1994;192:545–548

86. Lerner RM, Rubens D. Distal ureteral calculi: diagnosis by transrectal sonography. AJR Am J Roentgenol 1986; 147:1189–1191

87. Bosniak MA, Megibow AJ, Ambos MA et al. Computed tomography of ureteral obstruction. AJR Am J Roentgenol 1982;138:1107–1113

88. Sommer FG, Jeffrey RB, Jr, Rubin GD et al. Detection of ureteral calculi in patients with suspected renal colic: value of reformatted noncontrast helical CT. AJR Am J Roentgenol 1995;165:509–513

89. Roy C, Saussine C, Jahn C et al. Evaluation of RARE-MR urography in the assessment of ureterohydronephrosis. J Comput Assist Tomogr 1994;18:601–608

90. Griffin J, Jennings C, MacErlean D. Ultrasonic evaluation of simple and ectopic ureteroceles. Clin Radiol 1983;34:55–57

91. Nussbaum AR, Dorst JP, Jeffs RD et al. Ectopic ureter and ureterocele: their varied sonographic manifestations. Radiology 1986;159:227–235

92. Andrew WK, Thomas RG, Aitken FG. Simple ureteroceles—ultrasonographic recognition and diagnosis of complications. S Afr Med J 1985;67:20–22

93. Dunnick NR, Sandler CM, Amis ES, Jr, Newhouse JH. The urinary bladder. In: Textbook of Uroradiology (2nd ed.). Williams & Wilkins, Baltimore, 1997, pp 396–439

94. Dondalski M, White EM, Ghahremani GG, Patel SK. Carcinoma arising in urinary bladder diverticula: imaging findings in six patients. AJR Am J Roentgenol 1993;161:817–820

95. Klein L, Pollack HM. Computed tomography and magnetic resonance imaging of the female lower urinary tract. Radiol Clin North Am 1992;30:843–860

96. Husband JE. Staging bladder cancer. Clin Radiol 1992;46:153–159

97. Tanimoto A, Yuasa Y, Imai Y et al. Bladder tumor staging: comparison of conventional and gadolinium-enhanced dynamic MR imaging and CT. Radiology 1992;185:741–747

98. Kim B, Semelka RC, Ascher SM et al. Bladder tumor staging: comparison of contrast-enhanced CT, T1- and T2-weighted MR imaging, dynamic gadolinium-enhanced imaging and late gadolinium-enhanced imaging. Radiology 1994;193:239–245

99. Collins GN, Sunderland GT, Crossling FT. Urachal cyst: an unusual cause of hydronephrosis. Br J Urol 1990;65:305–306

100. Herman TE, Shackelford GD. Pyourachus: CT manifestations. J Comput Assist Tomogr 1995;19:440–443

101. Awwad J, Azar G, Soubra M. Sonographic diagnosis of a urachal cyst in utero. Acta Obstet Gynecol Scand 1994; 73:156–157

102. Al-Hindawi MK, Aman S. Benign non-infected urachal cyst in an adult: review of the literature and a case report. Br J Radiol 1992;65:313–316

103. Lapin J. Adenocarcinoma of a urachal cyst. Can Assoc Radiol J 1992;43:230–231

104. Nagasaki A, Sumitomo K, Iwanaga M et al. Remnants of urachus in infants and children—the problems of diagnosis and treatment. Jpn J Surg 1991;21:167–171

105. Vergos M, Messina MH, Lhomme Desages B, Chapuis O. Cancer of the middle umbilical fold a rare form of bladder tumor. J Chir (Paris) 1992;129:165–168

106. Ravi R, Shrivastava BR, Chandrasekhar GM et al. Adenocarcinoma or the urachus. J Surg Oncol 1992;50:201–203

107. Irwin PP, Weston PMT, Sheridan W, Matthews PN. Transitional cell carcinoma arising in a urachal cyst. Br J Urol 1991;67:103–104

108. Brick SH, Friedman AC, Pollack HM et al. Urachal carcinoma: CT findings. Radiology 1988;169:377–381

109. Korobkin M, Cambier L, Drake J. Computed tomography of urachal carcinoma. J Comput Assist Tomogr 1988;12:981–987

110. Maeda H, Kinukawa T, Kuhara H et al. MR findings in urachal carcinoma. AJR Am J Roentgenol 1992;158:1171

111. Pastakia B, Horvath K, Kurtz D et al. Giant rectus sheath hematomas of the pelvis complicating anticoagulant therapy: CT findings. J Comput Assist Tomogr 1984;8:1120–1123

112. Churchill RJ. CT of intra-abdominal fluid collections. Radiol Clin North Am 1989;27:653–666

113. Hahn PF, Saini S, Stark DD et al. Intraabdominal hematoma: the concentric-ring sign in MR imaging. AJR Am J Roentgenol 1987;148:115–119

114. Unger EC, Glazer HS, Lee JKT, Ling D. MRI of extracranial hematomas: preliminary observations. AJR Am J Roentgenol 1986;146:403–407

115. Levot J, Gisserot D, Boyer B et al. Non-gynecologic liquid images of pelvis. Echographic study. J Radiol (Paris) 1987;68:293–303

116. Rifkin MD, Needleman L, Kurtz AB et al. Sonography of nongynecologic cystic masses of the pelvis. AJR Am J Roentgenol 1984;142:1169–1174

117. Gagliardi PD, Hoffer PB, Rosenfield AT. Correlative imaging in abdominal infection: an algorithmic approach using nuclear medicine, ultrasound, and computed tomography. Semin Nucl Med 1988;18:320–334

118. Fukuya T, Hawes DR, Lu CC, Barloon TJ. CT of abdominal abscess with fistulous communication to the gastrointestinal tract. J Comput Assist Tomogr 1991;15:445–449

119. Lopes AD, Hall JR, Monaghan JM. Drainage following radical hysterectomy and pelvic lymphadenectomy: dogma or need? Obstet Gynecol 1995;86:960–963

120. Paul MTS, Brémond A, Rochet Y. Avoiding peritonization after pelvic surgery for cancer. The results from 157 cases. J Gynecol Obstetr Biol Reprod 1991;20:957–960

121. Petru E, Tamussino K, Lahousen M et al. Pelvic and para-aortic lymphocysts after radical surgery because of cervical and ovarian cancer. Am J Obstet Gynecol 1989;161:937–941

122. Terada KY, Roberts JA. Lymphoceles following second-look laparotomy for ovarian cancer. Gynecol Oncol 1988;29:382–384

123. Pennehouat G, Mosseri V, Durand JC et al. Lymphocysts and peritonealisation after lymphadenectomy for cancers of the uterus. J Gynecol Obstet Biol Reprod 1988;17:373–378

124. Aronowitz J, Kaplan AL. The management of a pelvic lymphocele by the use of a percutaneous indwelling catheter inserted with ultrasound guidance. Gynecol Oncol 1983;16:292–295

125. Conte M, Panici PB, Guariglia L et al. Pelvic lymphocele following radical para-aortic and pelvic lymphadenectomy for cervical carcinoma: incidence rate and percutaneous management. Obstet Gynecol 1990;76:268–271

126. La Fianza A, Campani R, Dore R et al. CT in the diagnosis and treatment of lymphoceles following gynecologic cancer surgery. Radiol Med 1993;86:106–115

127. Gilliland JD, Spies JB, Brown SB et al. Lymphoceles: percutaneous treatment with povidone-iodine sclerosis. Radiology 1989;171:227–229

128. Perrin LC, Goh J, Crandon AJ. The treatment of recurrent pelvic lymphocysts with marsupialization and functioning omental flap. Aust NZ J Obstet Gynaecol 1995;35:195–197

129. Mann WJ, Vogel F, Patsner B, Chalas E. Management of lymphocysts after radical gynecologic surgery. Gynecol Oncol 1989;33:248–250

130. Chow CC, Daly BD, Burney TL et al. Complications after laparoscopic pelvic lymphadenectomy: CT diagnosis. AJR Am J Roentgenol 1994;163:353–356

131. Moran RE, Older RA, De Angelis GA et al. Genitourinary case of the day. Peritoneal inclusion cyst in a patient with a history of prior pelvic surgery. AJR Am J Roentgenol 1996;167:247,250

132. González Carro PS, Monés Xiol J, Vidal Alvarez P et al. Multilocular peritoneal inclusion cysts in puerperium. Rev Esp Enferm Dig 1991;80:127–129

133. McFadden DE, Clement PB. Peritoneal inclusion cysts with mural mesothelial proliferation. A clinicopathological analysis of six cases. Am J Surg Pathol 1986;10:844–854

134. Ross MJ, Welch WR, Scully RE. Multilocular peritoneal inclusion cysts (so-called cystic mesotheliomas). Cancer 1989;64:1336–1346

135. Sohaey R, Gardner TL, Woodward PJ, Peterson CM. Sonographic diagnosis of peritoneal inclusion cysts. J Ultrasound Med 1995;14:913–917

136. Hoffer FA, Kozakewich H, Colodny A, Goldstein DP. Peritoneal inclusion cysts: ovarian fluid in peritoneal adhesions. Radiology 1988;169:189–191

137. Cancelmo RP. Sonographic demonstration of multilocular peritoneal inclusion. Case Report. J Clin Ultrasound 1983;11:334–335

138. Hederström E, Forsberg L. Entrapped ovarian cyst. An unusual case of persistent abdominal pain. Acta Radiol 1990;31:285–286

139. Lipitz S, Seidman DS, Schiff E et al. Treatment of pelvic peritoneal cysts by drainage and ethanol instillation. Obstet Gynecol 1995;86:297–299

140. Yaegashi N, Yajima A. Multilocular peritoneal inclusion cysts (benign cystic mesothelioma): a case report. J Obstet Gynaecol Res 1996;22:129–132

141. Sharif HS, Clark DC, Aabed MY et al. MR imaging of thoracic and abdominal wall infections: comparison with other imaging procedures. AJR Am J Roentgenol 1990;154:989–995

142. Wilkinson EJ. Benign diseases of the vulva. In: Kurman RJ, Ed. Blaustein's Pathology of the Female Genital Tract (4th ed). Springer-Verlag, New York, 1994, p 55

143. Gauperaa T, Sundsfjord A, Andersen BM. Necrotising fasciitis and ishiorectal abscess. Eur J Surg 1995;161:211–212

144. Marn CS. Anterior abdominal wall. In: Gore RM, Levine MS, Laufer, Eds. Textbook of Gastrointestinal Radiology. Philadelphia, WB Saunders, 1994, p 2407

145. Resnick D, Niwayama G. Osteomyelitis, septic arthritis, and soft tissue infection: mechanisms and situations. In: Resnick D, Ed. Diagnosis of Bone and Joint Disorders. WB Saunders, Philadelphia, 1995, p 2386

146. Holley DT, McGrath PC, Sloan DA. Necrotizing fasciitis as a complication of percutaneous catheter drainage of an intra-abdominal abscess. Am Surg 1994;60:197–199

147. Farley DE, Katz VL, Dotters DJ. Toxic shock syndrome associated with vulvar necrotizing fasciitis. Obstet Gynecol 1993;82:660–662

148. Razi-syed S, Jafri SZH. Necrotizing fasciitis and myositis: a case report. Comput Med Imaging Graph 1994;18:213–216

149. Walshaw CF, Deans H. CT findings in necrotising fasciitis—a report of four cases. Clin Radiol 1996;51:429–432

150. Beauchamp NJ, Jr, Scott WW, Jr, Gottlieb LM, Fishman EK. CT evaluation of soft tissue and muscle infection and inflammation: a systematic compartment approach. Skeletal Radiol 1995;24:317–324

151. Anderson MW. Muscles. In: Higgins CB, Hricak H, Helms CA, Eds. Magnetic Resonance Imaging of the Body (3rd ed.). Lippincott-Raven Press, New York, 1997, p 1331

152. Rahmouni A, Chosidow O, Mathieu D et al. MR imaging in acute infectious cellulitis. Radiology 1994;192:493–496

153. Kaufman JL. Clinical problem-solving: necrotizing fasciitis. N Engl J Med 1994;331:279

154. Dodd GD, III, Budzik RF, Jr. Lipomatous tumors of the pelvis in women: spectrum of imaging findings. AJR Am J Roentgenol 1990;155:317–322

155. Le Vot J, Solacroup JC, Muyard B et al. Adipose tissue in imaging of the pelvis. Ann Radiol 1990;33:23–30

156. Friedman AC, Hartman DS, Sherman J et al. Computed tomography of abdominal fatty masses. Radiology 1981; 139:415–429

157. Berens BM, Azarvan A. Bladder outlet obstruction due to pelvic lipoma: computerized tomography, magnetic resonance imaging and radiographic evaluation. J Urol 1991;145:138–139

158. Long Pretz P, Detry R, Kestens PJ, Haot J. Liposarcoma of the left fossa ischiorectalis. Acta Chir Bel, 1988;88:151–154

159. Ulusoy E, Adsan Ö, Beyribey S et al. Primary retroperitoneal liposarcoma: a case report and review of the literature. Int Urol Nephrol 1995;27:691–695

160. Lachachi F, Antarieu S, Valleix D, Descottes B. Bulky retroperitoneal liposarcoma. One case report. J Chir (Paris) 1995;132:309–313

161. Lopes Filho GJ, Carvalho SMT, Scalabrini M et al. Abdominal liposarcomas. Rev Assoc Med Bras 1995;41:219–226

162. Kutta A, Engelmann U, Schmidt U, Senge T. Primary retroperitoneal tumors. Urol Int 1992;48:353–357

163. Hold M, Olbert F, Schlegl A et al. Pelvic lipomatosis—its appearance on radiography and computed tomography. Radiologe 1981;21:300–302

164. Calès P, Blanc H, Bories P et al. Pelvic lipomatosis: value of computerised axial tomography; a case report. Ann Med Interne 1984;135:533–536

165. Allen FJ, De Kock MLS. Pelvic lipomatosis: the nuclear magnetic resonance appearance and associated vesicoureteral reflux. J Urol 1987;138:1228–1230

166. Lappas JC. Benign tumors. In: Gore RM, Levine MS, Laufer I, Eds. Textbook of Gastrointestinal Radiology. WB Saunders, Philadelphia, 1994 p 898

167. Greget M, Veillon F, Meyer C et al. Desmoid tumor in Gardner's syndrome. Case report. J Radiol 1994;75:199–202

168. Rains AJH, Capper WM, Eds. Bailey and Love's Short Practice of Surgery (15th ed.). HK Lewis, London, 1971, p 1050

169. Lambroza A, Tighe MK, DeCosse JJ, Dannenberg AJ. Disorders of the rectus abdominis muscle and sheath: a 22-year experience. Am J Gastroenterol 1995;90:1313–1317

170. Combes B, Ledoux A, Provendier B. A huge fibroma of the round ligament developing as an abdominal extra-peritoneal mass. J Gynecol Obstet Biol Reprod (Paris) 1988;17:347–349

171. Zaloudek C, Norris HJ. Mesenchymal tumors of the uterus. In: Kurman RJ, Ed. Blaustein's Pathology of the Female Genital Tract (4th ed.). Springer-Verlag, New York, 1995, pp 487–528

172. Abulafia O, Angel C, Sherer DM et al. Computed tomography of leiomyomatosis peritonealis disseminata with malignant transformation. Am J Obstet Gynecol 1993;169:52–54

173. Hayasaka K, Yamada T, Saitoh Y et al. CT evaluation of primary benign retroperitoneal tumor. Radiat Med 1994;12:115–120

174. Villanueva A, Pérez C, Sabaté JM et al. CT manifestations of the peritoneal leiomyosarcomatosis. Eur J Radiol 1993;17:166–169

175. Goldman SM, Hartman DS, Weiss SW. The varied radiographic manifestations retroperitoneal malignant fibrous histiocytoma revealed through 27 cases. J Urol 1986;135:33–38

176. Bruneton JN, Drouillard J, Rogopoulos A et al. Extraretroperitoneal abdominal malignant fibrous histiocytoma. Gastrointest Radiol 1988;13:299–305

177. Faragher IG, Bennett TM, Cass AJ. Primary malignant fibrous histiocytoma of the retroperitoneum. Aust N Z J Surg 1988;58:915–917

178. Hauser H, Beham A, Uranüs S et al. Malignant fibrous histiocytoma of the mesentery—a rare cause of abdominal pain. Case report with a review of literature. Gastroenterology 1993;31:735–738

179. Stever MR, Hernandez E, Sakas EL. Malignant fibrous histiocytoma of the pelvis. Gynecol Oncol 1988;30:285–290

180. Raney RB, Jr, Allen A, O'Neill J et al. Malignant fibrous histiocytoma of soft tissue in childhood. Cancer 1986; 57:2198–2201

181. Duchat A, Landel JF, Villand J et al. Mesenteric malignant fibrous istiocytoma. Ultrasonic and computed tomographic findings. Report on one case. Radiology 1985;66:241–244

182. Miller TT, Hermann G, Abdelwahab IF et al. MRI of malignant fibrous histiocytoma of soft tissue: analysis of 13 cases with pathologic correlation. Skeletal Radiol 1994;23:271–275

183. Molitch HI, Unger EC, Witte CL, vanSonnenberg E. Percutaneous sclerotherapy of lymphangiomas. Radiology 1995; 194:343–347

184. Azais O, Drouineau J, Vandermarcq P et al. Pelvic cystic lymphangioma. Report on one adult case. J Radiol 1989; 70:209–212

185. Cyna-Gorse F, Frija J, Yana C et al. From lymphangioma to lymphangiomatosis. A report on 10 cases. J Radiol 1989; 70:381–387

186. Hoeffel JC, Winants D, Marchal AL et al. Right pelvic cystic lymphangioma. Chir Pediatr 1988;29:219–221

187. Greco A, Jelliffe AM, Maher EJ, Leung AWL. MR imaging of lymphomas: impact on therapy. J Comput Assist Tomogr 1988;12:785–791

188. Nyman R, Rehn S, Glimelius B et al. Magnetic resonance imaging, chest radiography, computed tomography and ultrasonography in malignant lymphoma. Acta Radiol 1987; 28:253–262

189. Williams MP, Olliff JFC. Magnetic resonance imaging in extranodal pelvic lymphoma. Clin Radiol 1990;42:264–268

190. Romero JA, Kim EE, Kudelka AP et al. MRI of recurrent cystic mesothelioma: differential diagnosis of cystic pelvic masses. Gynecol Oncol 1994;54:377–380

191. Smith TR. Malignant peritoneal mesothelioma: marked variability of CT findings. Abdom Imaging 1994;19:27–29

192. Takenouchi Y, Oda K, Takahara O et al. Report of a case of benign cystic mesothelioma. Am J Gastroenterol 1995; 90:1165–1167

193. Preidler KW, Steiner H, Szolar D, Kern R. Cystic appearance of a malignant peritoneal mesothelioma by ultrasonography and computed tomography: a case report. Eur J Radiol 1994;18:137–139

194. Hasan AKH, Sinclair DJ. Case report: calcification in benign cystic peritoneal mesothelioma. Clin Radiol 1993;48:66–67

195. O'Neil JD, Ros PR, Storm BL et al. Cystic mesothelioma of the peritoneum. Radiology 1989;170:333–337

196. Bhandarkar DS, Smith VJ, Evans DA, Taylor TV. Benign cystic peritoneal mesothelioma. J Clin Pathol 1993;46:867–868

197. Akhan O, Kalyoncu F, Özmen MN et al. Peritoneal mesothelioma: sonographic findings in nine cases. Abdom Imaging 1993;18:280–282

198. Cozzi G, Bellomi M, Frigerio LF et al. Double contrast barium enema combined with non-invasive imaging in peritoneal mesothelioma. Acta Radiol 1989;30:21–24

199. Gupta S, Gupta RK, Gujral RB et al. Peritoneal mesothelioma simulating pseudomyxoma peritonei on CT and sonography. Gastrointest Radiol 1992;17:129–131

200. Yeh HC, Chahinian AP. Ultrasonography and computed tomography of peritoneal mesothelioma. Radiology 1980; 135:705–712

201. Delinière F, Arnaud JP, Casa C et al. Pseudomyxoma peritonei. Report on 19 cases. J Chir (Paris) 1993;130:141–145

202. Khoda J, Sebbag G, Lantzberg L et al. Cystadenocarcinoma with peritoneal involvement (pseudomyxoma peritonei). Is surgical resection alone sufficient? Ann Chir 1992;46:636–641

203. Marin Pérez-Tabernero A, Alvarado Alvarez E, Munoz de la Espada J et al. Pseudomyxoma peritonei. J Chir (Paris) 1994; 131:51–52

204. Landen S, Bertrand C, Maddern GJ et al. Appendiceal mucoceles and pseudomyxoma peritonei. Surg Gynecol Obstet 1992;175:401–404

205. Matsuoka Y, Ohtomo K, Itai Y et al. Pseudomyxoma peritonei with progressive calcifications: CT findings. Gastrointest Radiol 1992;17:16–18

206. Walensky RP, Venbrux AC, Prescott CA, Osterman FA, Jr. Pseudomyxoma peritonei. AJR Am J Roentgenol 1996; 167:471–474

207. Lee HH, Agha FP, Weatherbee L, Boland CR. Pseudomyxoma peritonei. Radiologic features. J Clin Gastroenterol 1986; 8:312–316

208. Weigert F, Lindner P, Rohde U. Computed tomography and magnetic resonance of pseudomyxoma peritonei. J Comput Assist Tomogr 1985;9:1120–1122

209. Buy JN, Malbec L, Ghossain MA et al. Magnetic resonance imaging of pseudomyxoma peritonei. Eur J Radiol 1989; 9:115–118

210. Villanueva A, Pérez C, Sabaté JM et al. Peritoneal carcinomatosis. Review of CT findings in 107 cases. Rev Esp Enferm Dig 1995;87:707–714

211. Rioux M, Michaud C. Sonographic detection of peritoneal carcinomatosis: a prospective study of 37 cases. Abdom Imaging 1995;20:47–51

212. Chou CK, Liu GC, Su JH et al. MRI demonstration of peritoneal implants. Abdom Imaging 1994;19:95–101

213. Chou CK, Liu GC, Chen LT, Jaw TS. MRI manifestations of peritoneal carcinomatosis. Gastrointest Radiol 1992; 17:336–338

214. Merine D, Fishman EK, Magid D. CT detection of sacral osteomyelitis associated with pelvic abscesses. J Comput Assist Tomogr 1988;12:118–121

215. Simons GW, Sty JR, Starshak RJ. Retroperitoneal and retrofascial abscesses. J Bone Joint Surg Am 1983;65:1041–1058

216. Haliloglu M, Kleiman MB, Siddiqui AR, Cohen MD. Osteomyelitis and pyogenic infection of the sacroiliac joint. MRI findings and review. Pediatr Radiol 1994;24:333–335

Ultrasonography of the Pediatric and Adolescent Pelvis

LORI L. BARR

HARRIS L. COHEN

Sonography is often the only modality necessary for the investigation of problems of the reproductive system in girls. The clinical presentation varies with age. A neonate may present with ambiguous genitalia. A palpable abdominal mass may occur at any age. A child may present with premature breast bud development or vaginal bleeding. In an adolescent, lower abdominal pain is a common presenting symptom. Failure of onset of menses is another cause for imaging of the reproductive organs in older girls.

SONOGRAPHIC TECHNIQUES

Most pediatric pelvic sonograms use a transabdominal approach with a partially or fully filled bladder. Mostly, the bladder is filled by having the patient drink before the examination. In infants where frequent voiding occurs, an off-midline approach with slight compression may be helpful in maximizing the use of the bladder to visualize the contralateral pelvis. Occasionally, it may be necessary to fill the bladder by catheterization of the bladder to visualize the uterine fundus or a mass arising from the pelvis. Sterile water instilled into the rectum with a small bore catheter can help to move air and stool out of the rectosigmoid and to demonstrate the more anterior pelvic organs.

In general, the highest frequency possible is used for pelvic sonograms, attempting to balance the near field resolution of higher frequency transducers with the penetration of lower frequency transducers. In infants, a 7.5-MHz or broad-bandwidth transducer in the range from 5 to 10 MHz is appropriate. As the child grows, a lower frequency transducer may be needed to allow greater penetration. In most children older than infants, a 5-MHz transducer provides the best resolution of the reproductive organs.

Transvaginal sonography is usually reserved for children who are sexually active or, in rare cases, where the information to be obtained is considered of critical importance and both the parents and the child consent. Transvaginal scanning under a general anesthetic can provide additional information about the reproductive system. Transperineal scanning is useful in the workup of vaginal atresia and distension of the vagina and the size of its distal obstruction. Transperineal scanning can be used in the virginal patient and has been used to evaluate some cases of imperforate anus.

NORMAL ANATOMY

The uterus, fallopian tubes, and upper two-thirds of the vagina begin forming at 6 weeks gestational age from fusion of right- and left-sided müllerian ducts. The shape and size of the uterus and ovaries change during pediatric life. In the first months of life, under the influence of high gonadotropins, the cervical length is twice that of the fundus (Fig. 25.1).[1] The mean uterine length in the newborn is 3.4 cm.[2] This decreases as gonadotropin levels decrease (4 to 12 months), resulting in a mean length of 3.0 cm.[2] An endometrial echo is seen in half of girls under 6 months of age.[3] After the first year of life, the uterus is usually tube shaped with the anteroposterior measurement of the cervix equal to that of the fundus (Fig. 25.2).[1] The length gradually decreases until age 4 and then steadily increases[3] with a mean premenarchal measurement of 4.3 cm.[4,5] Reference curves for uterine lengths and fundal/cervical ratios versus age are presented in Figures 25.3 and 25.4, respectively.[3] After puberty, the uterus measures 5 to 8 cm in length and no longer maintains a neutral position. It may be anteverted or retroverted (Fig. 25.5). The change from tube shaped to postmenarcheal pear shaped is a function of patient age and size as well as estradiol levels.[5]

The ovaries can appear anywhere along their embryologic course from the inferior border of the kidney. Normally, they are alongside the uterus and best seen on ultrasound on transverse images. The ovaries can be seen at all ages, although it is more difficult to see them in the very young. The volume and configuration vary with age and gonadotropin levels. In infants, the mean volume is 0.6 +/- 1.03 cc, but volumes can

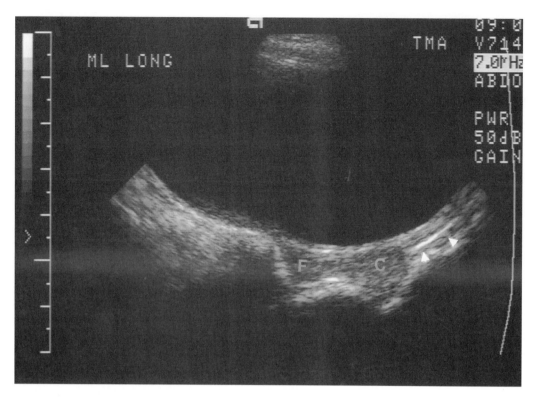

Figure 25.1 Longitudinal midline sonogram through the fully distended bladder of a 1-year-old demonstrating a spade-shaped uterus. Note that both the anteroposterior measurement and the length of the cervix (C) are longer than that of the fundus (F). The vagina appears as an echogenic stripe distal to the cervix (C) (arrowheads).

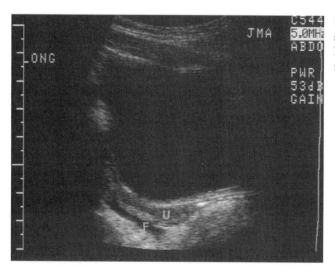

Figure 25.2 A 7-year-old girl with right lower quadrant pain shows a normal tube-shaped uterus (U), common before puberty. Note the tiny amount of free fluid in the cul-de-sac (F) which is a normal finding during childhood.

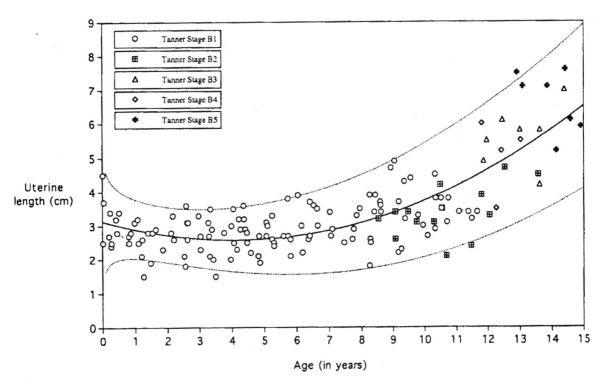

Figure 25.3 Uterine lengths versus age and for various stages of puberty. (From Griffin et al.,[3] with permission.)

Figure 25.4 Uterine fundus virgule cervix ratios versus age and for various stages of puberty. (From Griffin et al.,[3] with permission.)

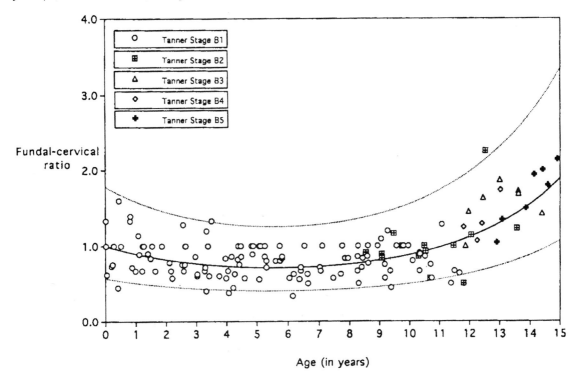

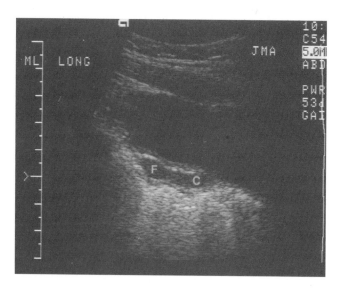

Figure 25.5 This 12-year-old girl has a normal, early, pear-shaped uterus with enlargement of the fundus (F) compared to the cervix (C) and slight anteversion consistent with the onset of menarche.

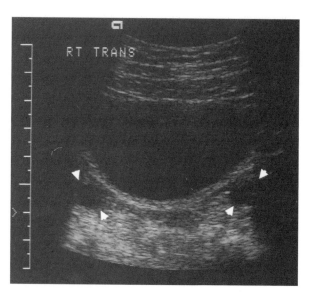

Figure 25.7 Transverse sonogram through the full bladder of a 6-month-old demonstrates the macrocysts in both ovaries (arrowheads).

be as great as 3.5 cc.[6] Two appearances of the pediatric ovary have been described. One is a homogeneous pattern of echogenicity without cysts (Fig. 25.6),[2,5,7] and the other (more common) pattern is heterogeneous with enclosed follicles. Ovarian follicles are commonly seen throughout childhood (Fig. 25.7),[6,8] but cysts larger than 9 mm in diameter are only occasionally seen.[8] The mean normal volume in the second decade is 7.8 cc (range from 1.7 to 18.5 cc).[9]

The vagina appears as an echogenic stripe distal to the cervix. Infants commonly reflux urine into the vagina. Small amounts of vaginal fluid seen should not

Figure 25.6 Note the homogeneous appearance of the ovaries (arrowheads) on the transverse sonogram obtained through a full bladder of a 2-year-old.

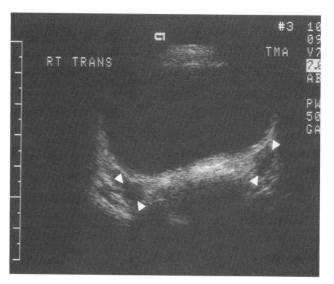

alarm the imager. A small amount of fluid in the cul-du-sac is another normal finding in children.

CLINICAL PRESENTATIONS

Ambiguous Genitalia

When ambiguous genitalia are discovered in the newborn, the identification of the reproductive organs is paramount in the decision on how to rear the child. Anomalies range from aplasia to duplication and ectopia, and the investigation often includes a contrast fistulogram or vaginogram as well as a sonogram. Imaging is correlated with sex chromosome studies, hormone assays, gonadal biopsy, and surgical exploration. The role of ultrasound is to identify the uterus.[4,10–12]

During the sixth week of fetal life, müllerian ducts develop lateral to the wolffian ducts. In males, the testes secrete müllerian inhibiting factor (which causes the adjacent müllerian duct to involute) and testosterone (which differentiates the wolffian duct into epididymis, seminal vesicles, and vas deferens).[10,13] Testosterone also causes formation of male genitalia from the urogenital sinus tract.

Formation of the upper vagina, uterus, and fallopian tubes occurs by 11 weeks of fetal life as long as there are no testes or high levels of androgens. The lower one-third of the vagina develops by elongation of the primitive vaginal plate into a core of tissue where the müllerian system joins the urogenital sinus. The core canalizes by week 20. In normal females, the wolffian system degenerates.[4,10,14]

Patients with nonconcordant genital, gonadal, and chromosomal sex fall into three groups: female intersex, true hermaphrodites, and male intersex.[14] Female intersex is most often due to virilization of karyotypically normal females because of congenital adrenal hyperplasia. It is sometimes due to a masculinizing ovarian tumor in the mother during pregnancy or to the administration of androgens. The external genitalia are masculinized with clitoral hypertrophy, labial fusion, and elongation of the urethra. On ultrasound, the internal anatomy is normal. If genital reconstruction and correct sex assignment are successful, patients are potentially fertile.[4,15] Differential considerations include male infants with hypospadias and bifid scrotum. Ultrasound is helpful in identifying homogeneously echogenic testes in these patients.[16]

The true hermaphrodite is rare and has an array of genital appearances. A 46, XX karyotype is typical, and the patient may have combined or separate ovarian and testicular tissue. Gonadal biopsy is usually required for diagnosis. Case reports have shown that the ovarian portion of an ovotestis can be identified by the presence of follicles.[17]

Male intersex is usually due to inadequate fetal androgen production after the time of maximal sexual structure sensitivity. This leads to incomplete production of müllerian inhibition factor and partially masculinized genitalia.[10,13] Absent or incomplete fusion of the müllerian system leads to uterine anomalies (Fig. 25.8). The incidence is 0.1% to 0.5% of all women.[18,19] The kidneys should be scanned when a reproductive organ anomaly is found because of the close relationship and proximity of the developing metanephric and müllerian systems in fetal life.[13] There is a higher incidence of pregnancy complications among these patients. Müllerian dysgenesis results in absent or rudimentary female reproductive organs. When associated with renal and skeletal anomalies, one should consider Mayer-Rokitansky-Kuster-Hauser

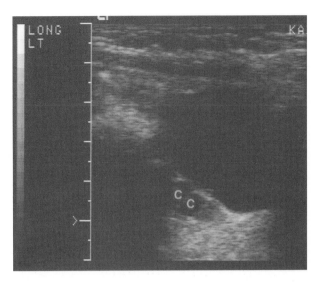

Figure 25.9 Longitudinal sonogram of the left ovary of a 1-year-old with normal macrocysts (C).

syndrome. These patients are karyotypically and phenotypically normal.[20]

Palpable Mass

A mass may be detected in the abdomen during prenatal sonography or by palpation on neonatal examination, prompting a pelvic sonogram. Maternal hormones/neonatal gonadotropin levels stimulate the development of benign ovarian cysts of varying size throughout childhood (Fig. 25.9). Many surgeons treat simple ovarian cysts conservatively even when relatively large in size.[21] Compression of adjacent structures and rupture or torsion have been reported to produce symptoms in the infant.[22] If sonographic evaluation shows torsion, then concern is greater. The most common mass of the ovary in all ages is the ovarian follicle. The diagnosis of ovarian cyst is complicated by hemorrhage in the older child. The ultrasound features of hemorrhage depend upon the age of the hemorrhage (Figs. 25.10 and 25.11). A homogeneous area of increased echogenicity with good through-transmission may be seen. In others, as the hemorrhage liquifies, fluid/debris levels are present. Follow-up demonstrates a decrease in size and a change in echogenicity, confirming the diagnosis of hemorrhagic cyst and excluding more significant masses. If symptoms deteriorate or if there is an increase in volume on follow-up, surgery is indicated.[23]

Simulators of ovarian cysts include enteric duplication cysts, intrapelvic ureteroceles, mesenteric cysts (Fig. 25.12), cysts from a multicystic dysplastic kidney, a distended utricle (müllerian duct remnant), a Gartner's duct cyst (wolffian duct remnant), a dilated ureter from reflux or obstruction, or an anterior meningocele. If a hypoechoic muscular rim is identified subjacent to the echogenic lining of the cyst, then the diagnosis of an enteric duplication may be made with cer-

Figure 25.8 Transverse sonogram through the bladder of a 16-year-old showing two uteri (arrowheads). This patient was known to have uterus didelphys from the combination of the ultrasound findings and the clinical finding of two vaginas.

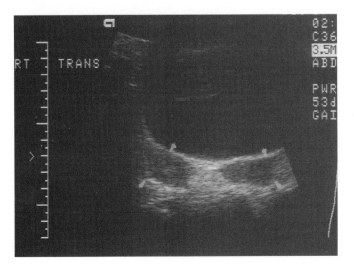

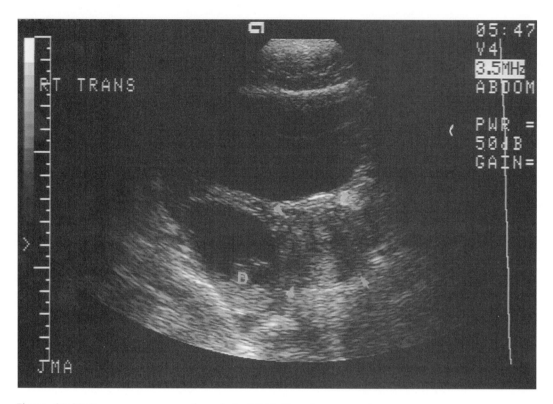

Figure 25.10 Transverse sonogram through the full bladder of a teenager demonstrates dependent debris (D) in the 5-cm right ovarian cyst complicated by hemorrhage. The uterus (arrowheads) has a normal echogenic endometrium.

Figure 25.11 Longitudinal sonogram of the left ovary in a 15-year-old with an inhomogeneous mass, which has increased through transmission consistent with subacute hemorrhage in an ovarian cyst (arrowheads). The uterus (U) is anterior to the left ovary.

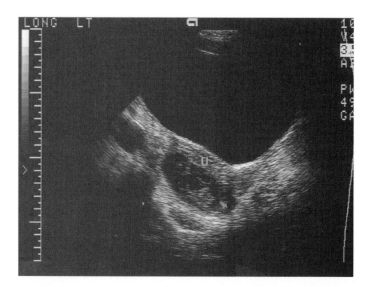

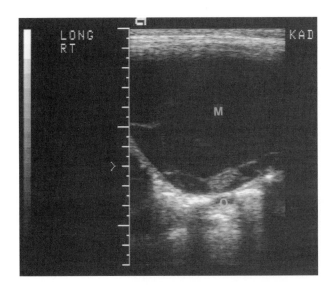

Figure 25.12 Longitudinal sonogram of 4-month-old's right lower quadrant demonstrates a septate mesenteric cyst (M) separate from the ovary (O).

tainty.[23] In patients with ventriculoperitoneal shunts, cerebrospinal fluid pseudocyst formation is also a consideration. The search for the shunt tip is easier if a recent abdominal x-ray demonstrates the position of the tube.

Fifteen percent of neonatal pelvic masses are due to congenital vaginal obstruction and resulting hydrocolpos or hydrometrocolpos.[13] Symptoms occur in the newborn and again at puberty. If vaginal obstruction is not discovered neonatally, the diagnosis will not be made until the menarche, when the patient will complain of cyclic pelvic pain and primary amenorrhea and may be found to have a palpable abdominal mass. Hydrometrocolpos may be associated with malformations of the cloacal or urogenital sinus and imperforate anus.[24] The cause of congenital vaginal obstruction in the absence of cloacal or urogenital sinus malformations is usually an obstructing membrane in close proximity to, and often inseparable from, the imperforate hymen.[25,26] Vaginal stenosis and atresia consist of a thick transverse septum occluding the upper one-third of the vagina at the site of fusion of the müllerian and sinus derivatives. Vaginal stenosis and atresia are associated with cardiac, gastrointestinal, genitourinary, and skeletal anomalies.[13] Sonography is useful in demonstrating the vaginal distension, which is thin-walled, from distension of the uterus, which has a thicker (muscular) wall. A sonographically complex appearance of the fluid usually indicates blood (hematometrocolpos). When the genitourinary system communicates with the vagina, the hydrometrocolpos may be less echoic (Fig. 25.13).[27] Transperineal ultrasound helps to define the width of the vaginal septum.[28]

Isolated hematometra suggests cervical obstruction either due to dysgenesis or to obstruction of the horn of a bicornuate system. These anomalies are associated with other genitourinary tract anomalies such as renal agenesis (Fig. 25.14).

Precocious Puberty

The development of secondary sex characteristics before age 8 is termed *precocious puberty*. Symptoms include breast bud development, axillary and pubic hair growth, gonadal enlargement, and ovulation. Most cases are idiopathic with premature activation of the hypothalamic-pituitary-gonadal axis.[29,30] Intracranial tumors and other causes of increased intracranial pressure may result in precocious puberty. Sonography helps to differentiate precocious puberty from pseudoprecocious puberty, the latter being due to secondary activation of gonadal tissue. Sonographically, true isosexual precocious puberty has an enlarged uterus and symmetrically enlarged ovaries. In one study, the mean ovarian volume in patients with true isosexual precocity was 2.47 cc compared to an ovarian volume of 2.09 cc in pseudoprecocious puberty.[31] More notable was the difference in uterine volumes (4.38 cc in true isosexual precocity vs. 2.96 cc in pseudoprecocious puberty).[31] Marked asymmetric enlargement of the ovaries is suggestive of pseudoprecocious puberty caused by either an ovarian mass (cyst or tumor) or a feminizing adrenal tumor. The most common ovarian lesion implicated is the granulosa-theca cell tumor, although simple cysts, dysgerminomas, choriocarcinomas, theca-lutein cysts, and teratomas have also caused hormonal stimulation.[32] Granulosa-theca cell tumors are the most common tumors to arise from the sex cord.

Vaginal Bleeding

While vaginal bleeding may precede the onset of menses, clinical considerations in the first decade include tumor, sexual abuse, and foreign bodies such as toilet tissue. Sonography of the vagina is helpful in demonstrating tumors. Malignant tumors of the vagina are more common in children than benign ones. The most common malignant tumor of the vulvovaginal region is embryonal rhabdomyosarcoma.[33] These tumors present early in infancy along the anterior wall of the vagina close to the cervix. When carcinoma of the vagina occurs in childhood, it is usually clear cell adenocarcinoma. These are usually diagnosed in patients over 13 years of age. One predisposing factor is antenatal diethylstilbestrol (DES) exposure. Both rhabdomyosarcomas and carcinomas of the vagina have a similar sonographic appearance of an inhomogeneous mass with mixed echogenicity, with or without extension to the cervix and uterus (Fig. 25.15).

Pelvic Pain

The differential diagnosis of childhood pelvic pain includes ovarian torsion, cysts, tumors, pelvic inflammatory disease, and acute appendicitis. Ovarian torsion describes rotation of the ovary on its pedicle. It is often associated with the acute onset of sharp ipsilateral pain. Torsion is said to be more common on the right and in ovaries of greater volume (postmenarchal or enlarged by a mass).[34,35] Small degrees of torsion may lead to edema and venostasis, which eventually

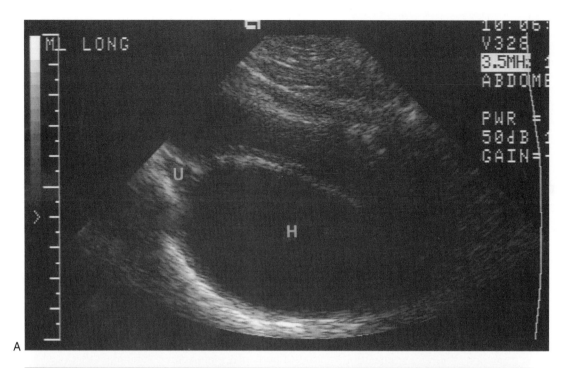

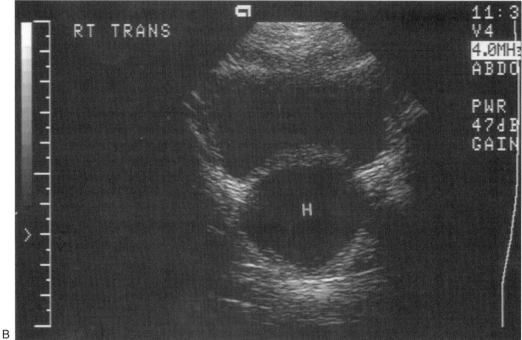

Figure 25.13 (**A**) Longitudinal midline sonogram of an 8-year-old with a urinary tract infection with distension of the vagina due to anechoic fluid, hydrocolpos (H). The uterus (U) is seen above the vagina. (**B**) Transverse sonogram of the same patient showing the midline location of the hydrocolpos (H). While the thin wall discounts the possibility of hydrometra, other differential considerations include ectopic ureterocele and vaginal reflux of urine.

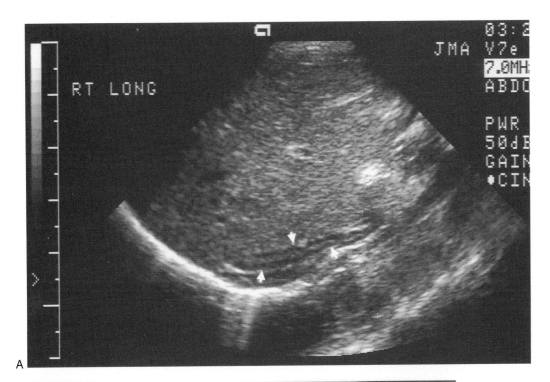

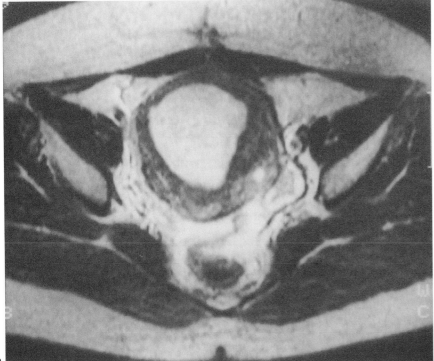

Figure 25.14 **(A)** Longitudinal sonogram of the right renal fossa of a 1-year-old with no right kidney seen on prenatal sonography. An elongated adrenal gland (arrowheads) suggesting nonascent of the right kidney. Scanning of the abdomen and pelvis revealed right renal agenesis, normal left kidney, and incidental macrocysts of the right ovary. **(B)** Transverse sonogram of the same patient through the bladder demonstrates uterus bicornis bicollis with isolated hematometra of the right uterine horn (arrows). Note the fluid in the endometrial cavity of the small right horn surrounded by prominent endometrial echoes due to maternal hormonal stimulation in the newborn. The left uterine horn is more normal in size (arrowheads).

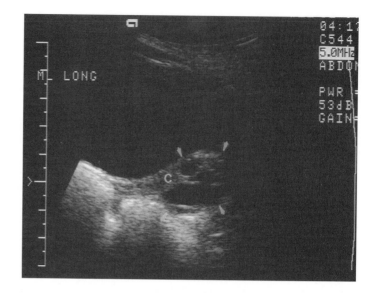

Figure 25.15 Longitudinal sonogram through the bladder of a 6-year-old with vaginal bleeding shows a multi cystic mass (arrowheads) filling the proximal vagina and pouch of Douglas. It is inseparable from the cervix (C). At surgery this was a clear cell adenocarcinoma.

causes arterial compromise and infarction. The sonographic appearance of ovarian torsion is variable. The most specific picture is that of a unilaterally enlarged solid ovary with multiple peripheral follicles (Fig. 25.16). This appearance is different when a cyst or neoplasm is present. Sonographic variability is also related to the degrees of internal hemorrhage and stromal edema. Doppler detection of moving blood in the center of the ovary helps to direct the diagnosis away from torsion, especially if flow is also seen in the asymptomatic ovary. Technical differences are probably responsible for the not uncommon failure to obtain a Doppler signal even from normal ovaries. Unhappily, some cases of ovarian torsion have been reported with central flow on color Doppler.[36]

Ovarian masses are more common than uterine masses and are usually cysts. Cysts may also arise in paraovarian locations. Ovarian neoplasms are rare in childhood but more common than uterine neoplasms. The classification of ovarian neoplasms is the same as that in adults. The cells of origin are the germ cell, surface epithelium, sex cord, and secondary invasion due to metastasis. Unlike adults, among whom epithelial cell tumors are most common, the germ cell is the most likely cell of origin in pediatric ovarian tumors. They represent 60% of all pediatric ovarian neoplasms. About 60% of the germ cell neoplasms of children are benign.[37] Germ cell tumors are complex adnexal masses on ultrasound examination (Fig. 25.17). The presence of a mural nodule, echogenic focus with

Figure 25.16 (A) Longitudinal sonogram of the left ovary of a 12-year-old with lower left quadrant pain demonstrates an inhomogeneous, hyperechoic appearance to the ovarian parenchyma with peripheral microcysts. Note the size of the ovary marked by electronic markers. (B) Longitudinal sonogram of the normal right ovary (markers) in the same patient.

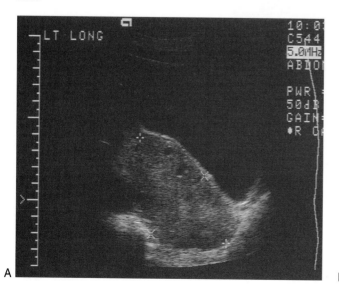

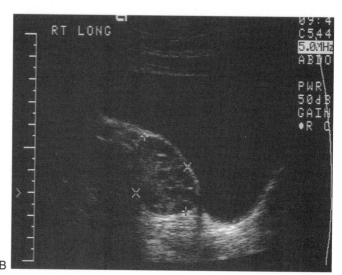

A   B

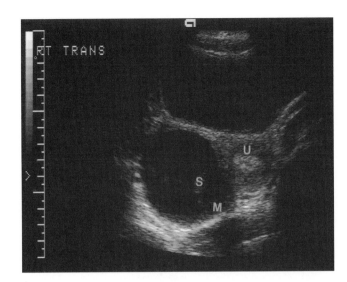

Figure 25.17 Transverse sonogram of a teenager with a urinary tract infection shows a predominantly cystic mass of the right ovary containing a septum (S) and a mural nodule (M). This was a dermoid cyst.

posterior shadowing, or a fat–fluid level is most suggestive of the diagnosis of benign teratoma. The teratoma is the most common of the germ cell tumors, with approximately one-third being malignant.[38] The germinoma is the next most common germ cell tumor arising from the ovary.

Tumors arising from the surface epithelium are responsible for 20% of childhood ovarian tumors.[39] These include cystadenoma, mucinous cystadenoma, cystadenofibroma, and cystadenocarcinoma. Serous cystadenoma is the most frequent of the epithelial tumors in children, but they rarely occur before puberty. Sonographically, they are predominantly cystic and can become quite large. Septa and low-level internal echoes are common.

Sex cord tumors account for 12% of childhood ovarian neoplasms, with the granulosa-theca cell tumor being the most common. This tumor is unique, in that affected girls usually present with precocious puberty rather than pelvic pain. The second most common sex cord tumor is the fibroma. These may be associated with ascites and pleural effusion in Meig syndrome. Bilateral fibromas are associated with Gorlin syndrome.

Metastases to the ovary are exceedingly rare and account for only 1% of pediatric ovarian tumors. Leukemia and lymphoma are the most common causes. Other primary sites include breast, endometrium, stomach, rhabdomyosarcoma, and neuroblastoma. The ovarian metastases of colorectal carcinoma in childhood can become quite large and difficult to differentiate from cystadenomas.[40] Metastatic involvement is often bilateral. Bilateral multicystic ovaries may also occur in benign conditions such as juvenile hypothyroidism. In general, ovarian neoplasms can have any appearance apart from a simple unilocular cyst. Solid or papillary projections, capsular invasion, or pelvic fixation are suggestive of malignancy.

Care needs to be taken when interpreting the appearances of the ovary. Air in the colon can produce an image that mimics that of a solid or dense tumor. Air causes a "dirty" shadow on ultrasound examination (Fig. 25.18). If in doubt, the physician should examine the patient again after the patient has had a bowel action. The ovaries may also become obscured by large pelvic neoplasms arising from outside the reproductive system. Burkitt's lymphoma commonly arises in the ileocecal region and may obscure the right ovary (Fig. 25.19).

Pelvic pain in the sexually active girl may be caused by ectopic or other pregnancy-related complication.[41] The imaging features are no different from adults. Pelvic pain may also be due to pelvic inflammatory disease, which has an annual incidence of 2% among 15 to 29-year-olds.[41] *Neisseria gonorrhea* and *Chlamydia trachomatis* are the most likely causes, and cervical excitation and vaginal discharge are usually present. Although salpingitis cannot be seen sonographically, salpingoophoritis may be demonstrated by adherent ovaries with increased mean adenexal volumes of greater than 11 cc.[42] A tuboovarian abscess (Fig. 25.20) appears as a complex adnexal mass replacing apparently normal ovarian tissue. It is difficult to differentiate from an endometrioma and hemorrhagic ovarian cyst without appropriate clinical information.

Delayed Menarche

Failure of onset of menses may be the result of an imperforate hymen and the subsequent development of hematometrocol-

Figure 25.18 Transverse sonogram of a teenager with a sharply circumscribed mass adjacent to the uterus (U) with highly echogenic material centrally. The right adnexa was not clearly identified. At surgery, no pathology was found. Attention to the hypomuscular rim subjacent to the echogenic mucosa (arrowheads) identifies this "mass" as a loop of colon containing air. Note the "dirty" shadowing of the air. If the muscular rim is identified surrounding a simple cyst, it identifies the cyst as an enteric duplication.

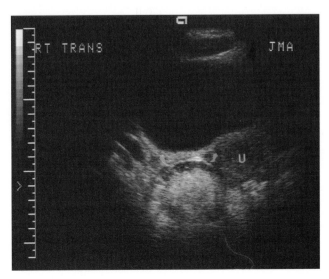

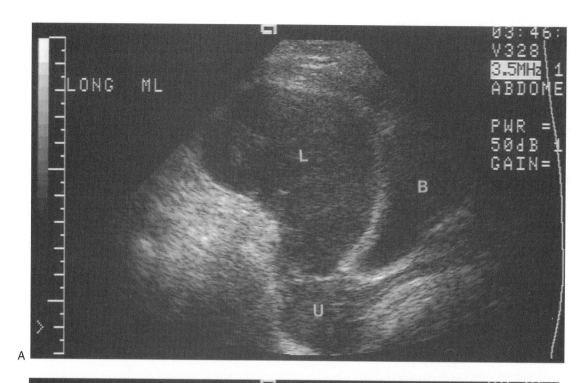

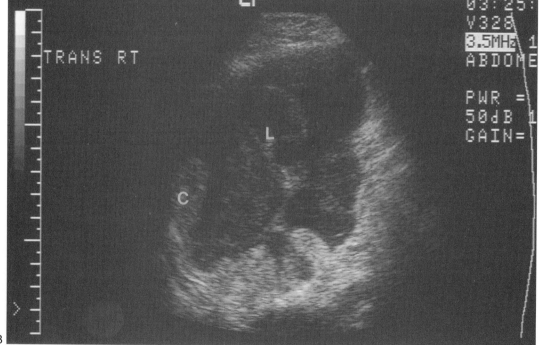

Figure 25.19 **(A)** Longitudinal midline sonogram showing displacement of the uterus (U) by a large hypoechoic mass representing Burkitt's lymphoma (L), which compresses the bladder (B). **(B)** Transverse sonogram of the right lower quadrant shows the close relationship of the lymphoma (L) to the compressed cecum (C).

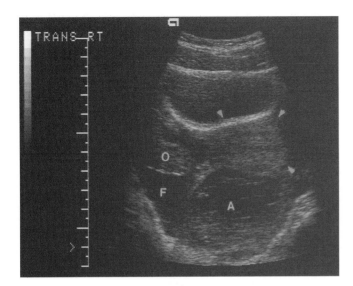

Figure 25.20 Transverse sonogram of a teenager with pelvic inflammatory disease. Note the indistinct appearance of the uterus (arrowheads). The right ovary (O) floats in free intrapelvic fluid (F). An ill-defined cystic mass with low-level internal echoes represents an abscess. The appearance of the abscess is nonspecific and is difficult to differentiate from endometrioma or hemorrhagic ovarian cyst.

pos. Another consideration is gonadal dysgenesis secondary to Turner syndrome. In pure gonadal dysgenesis (45, X0), streak ovaries are present. In mosaic states, the ovaries can approach normal size, but a small uterus is usually present. A T-shaped uterus and vaginal atresia are associated with intrauterine exposure to DES. Adenosis and clear cell adenocarcinoma of the vagina are also associated with DES exposure.[43] The most common cause of hypoplasia of the uterus is the lack of estrogen produced at the pituitary, hypothalamic, or ovarian level.

SUMMARY

With the exception of the evaluation of complex uterine anomalies and the staging of large, potentially malignant tumors, sonography is the modality of choice for evaluation of the pediatric pelvis.

REFERENCES

1. Nussbaum AR, Sanders RC, Jones MD. Neonatal uterine morphology as seen on real-time US. Radiology 1986;160:641–643
2. Hingsbergen EA, Barr LL. Normal ultrasound measurements of infant uterus and ovaries. IPR 1991, Stockholm, Sweden, 1991, p 80
3. Griffin IJ, Cole TJ, Duncan KA et al. Pelvic ultrasound measurements in normal girls. Acta Paediatr 1995;84:536–543
4. Eisenberg P, Cohen H, Mandel F et al. US analysis of premenarchal gynecological structures. J Ultrasound Med 1991;10:S30
5. Salardi S, Orsini LF, Cacciari E et al. Pelvic ultrasonography in premenarchal girls: relation to puberty and sex hormone concentrations. Arch Dis Child 1985;60:120–125
6. Cohen HL, Shapiro MA, Mandel FS, Shapiro ML. Normal ovaries in neonates and infants: a sonographic study of 77 patients 1 day to 24 months old. AJR Am J Roentgenol 1993;160:583–586
7. Orsini L, Salardi S, Pilu G et al. Pelvic organs in premenarchal girls: real-time ultrasonography. Radiology 1984;153:113–116
8. Cohen HL, Eisenberg P, Mandel F, Haller JO. Ovarian cysts are common in premenarchal girls: a sonographic study of 101 children 2–12 years old. AJR Am J Roentgenol 1992; 159:89–91
9. Cohen HL, Tice HM, Mandel FS. Ovarian volumes measured by US: bigger than we think. Radiology 1990;177:189–192
10. Grimes CK, Rosenbaum DM, Kirkpatrick JA, Jr. Paediatric gynecologic radiology. Semin Roentgenol 1982;17:284–301
11. Cremin BJ. Intersex states in young children: the importance of radiology in making a correct diagnosis. Clin Radiol 1974;25: 63–73
12. Haller J, Bass I, Nardi P, Novogroder M. A problem-oriented approach to the imaging of pediatric endocrine disorders. Semin Ultrasound 1985;6:321
13. Cohen HL, Haller JO. Pediatric and adolescent genital abnormalities. Clin Diagn Ultrasound 1989;24:187–215
14. Goldman H, Eaton D. Pediatric uroradiology. In: Elkin M, Ed. Radiology of the Urinary System. Little Brown, Boston, 1980, p 1034
15. Moore KL, Ed. Urogenital system. Intersexuality. In: Before We Are Born, Basic Embryology and Birth Defects (3rd ed.). WB Saunders, Philadelphia, 1989 pp 195–197
16. Cohen HL, Bober SE, Bow SN. Imaging of the pediatric pelvis: the normal and abnormal genital tract and simulators of its diseases. Urol Radiol 1992;14:273–283
17. Eberenz W, Rosenberg HK, Moshang T et al. True hermaphroditism: sonographic demonstration of ovotestes. Radiology 1991;179:429–431
18. Wiersma AF, Peterson LF, Justema EJ. Uterine anomalies associated with unilateral renal agenesis. Obstet Gynecol 1976;47:654–657
19. Woolf RB, Allen WM. Concomitant malformations: the frequent simultaneous occurrence of congenital malformations of the reproductive and urinary tracts. Obstet Gynecol 1953;2: 236–265
20. Rosenberg HK, Sherman NH, Tarry WF et al. Mayer-Rokitansky-Kuster-Hauser Syndrome: US aid to diagnosis. Radiology 1986;161:815–819
21. Amodio J, Abramson S, Berdon W et al. Postnatal resolution of large ovarian cysts detected in utero. Report of two cases. Pediatr Radiol 1987;17:467–469
22. Sherer D, Shah Y, Egers P, Woods J. Prenatal sonographic diagnosis and subsequent management of fetal adnexal torsion. J Ultrasound Med 1990;9:161–163
23. Warner BW, Kuhn JC, Barr LL. Conservative management of large ovarian cysts in children: the value of serial pelvic ultrasonography. Surgery 1992;112:749–755
24. Barr LL, Hayden CK, Jr, Stansberry SD, Swischuk LE. Enteric duplication cyst in children: are their ultrasonographic wall characteristics diagnostic? Pediatr Radiol 1990;20:326–328

25. Reed MH, Griscom NT. Hydrometrocolpos in infancy. Am J Roentgenol Radium Ther Nucl Med 1973;118:1–13

26. Dewhurst J. Genital tract obstruction. Pediatr Clin North Am 1981;28:331–344

27. Nussbaum-Blask A, Sanders R, Gearhart J. Obstructed uterovaginal anomalies: demonstration with sonography. Part 1. Neonates and infants. Radiology 1991;179:79–83

28. Scanlan KA, Pozniak M, Fagerholm M, Shapiro S. Value of transperineal sonography in the assessment of vaginal atresia. AJR Am J Roentgenol 1990;154:545–548

29. Grimes CK, Rosenbaum DM, Kirkpatrick JA, Jr. Pediatric gynecologic radiology. Semin Roentgenol 1982;17:284–301

30. Haller JO, Friedman AP, Shaffer R, Lebensart DP. The normal and abnormal ovary in childhood and adolescence. Semin Ultrasound 1983;4:206–225

31. Paesano PL, Vanzulli A, Fasolato V et al. Sonographic evaluation of premature puberty. [Abstract.] Radiology 1993;189 (suppl P):125

32. Eberlein WR, Bongiovanni AM, Jones IT, Yakovac WC. (no article name). J Pediatr 1960;57:484–497

33. Breen JL, Bonamo JF, Maxson WS. Genital tumors in children. Pediatr Clin North Am 1981;28:355–368

34. Little H, Crawford D, Meister K. Hematocolpos: diagnosis made by ultrasound. J Clin Ultrasound 1978;6:341–342

35. Nussbaum-Blask A, Sanders R, Rock J. Obstructed Utero-vaginal anomalies demonstrated with sonography. Part II, Teenagers. Radiology 1991;179:84–88

36. Quillin SP, Siegel MJ. Transabdominal color Doppler ultrasonography of the painful adolescent ovary. J Ultrasound Med 1994;13:549–555

37. Kurman RJ, Norris HJ. Germ cell tumors of the ovary. Pathol Annu 1978;13:291

38. Creasman WT, Fetter BF, Hammond CB, Parker RT. Germ cell malignancies of the ovary. Obstet Gynecol 1979;53:226–230

39. Breen JL, Maxson WS. Ovarian tumors in children and adolescents. Clin Obstet Gynecol 1977;20:607–623

40. Kauffman WM, Jenkins JJ, 3rd, Helton K et al. Imaging features of ovarian metastases from colonic adenocarcinoma. Pediatr Radiol 1995;25:286–288

41. Weckstein LN. Current perspective on ectopic pregnancy. Obstet Gynecol Surv 1985;40:259–272

42. Golden N, Cohen HL, Gennari G, Neuhoff S. The use of pelvic ultrasonography in the evaluation of adolescents with pelvic inflammatory disease. Am J Dis Child 1987;141:1235–1238

43. Ostergard DR. DES-related vaginal lesions. Clin Obstet Gynecol 1981;24:379–394

Computed Tomography and Magnetic Resonance Imaging of the Pediatric and Adolescent Pelvis

MARILYN J. SIEGEL

Sonography remains the initial study of choice for the assessment of suspected ovarian and uterine lesions.[1,2] Computed tomography (CT) and magnetic resonance imaging (MRI) are helpful to establish the origin of a mass when the results of sonography are equivocal, to determine the full extent of neoplastic or inflammatory lesions, and to characterize further the morphology of complex congenital uterine and vaginal malformations.[3,4] This chapter reviews the CT and MRI findings of gynecologic abnormalities in children.

TECHNIQUE

Sedation

Sedation is needed for the CT and MRI evaluation of pediatric patients 5 years of age and younger to minimize motion artifacts. Children over 5 years of age usually will cooperate after verbal reassurance and explanation of the procedure and will not require sedation. Oral chloral hydrate, 50 to 100 mg/kg, with a maximum dosage of 2,000 mg, is preferred for children younger than 18 months, while intravenous pentobarbital sodium, 6 mg/kg with a maximum dose of 200 mg, is used in children older than 18 months.[5,6] Other methods of sedation include intramuscular or rectal barbiturate and a combination of meperidine, chlorpromazine, and promethazine, commonly referred to as a "cardiac cocktail." Because intravenous barbiturate sedation results in fewer failures and has a shorter mean time of duration than these other analgesics, it is preferred by many pediatric radiologists. Regardless of the choice of drug, the use of parenteral sedation requires the facility and ability to resuscitate and maintain adequate cardiorespiratory support during and after the examination.

After being sedated, the infant or child is placed on a blanket on the CT or MRI table, and the arms are extended above the head to provide an easily accessible route for intravenous injection. When necessary, the upper arms can be restrained with sandbags, adhesive tape, or Velcro straps.

Patients who are to undergo parenteral sedation should have no liquids by mouth for 3 hours and no solid foods for 6 hours prior to examination. Patients who do not require sedation, but who are to receive intravenous contrast, should receive nothing per mouth for 3 hours to minimize the possibility of nausea or vomiting with aspiration during administration of contrast medium.

CT: TECHNICAL CONSIDERATIONS

Intravenous Contrast Material

Differentiation of pelvic vessels and lymph nodes is facilitated by the use of intravenous contrast material. An intravenous line should be in place when the child arrives in the radiology department in order to reduce patient agitation that might otherwise occur with venipuncture performed for administration of contrast material. The largest gauge butterfly needle or plastic cannula that can be placed is recommended. Either low-osmolar or high-osmolar contrast media can be used and administered by hand injection or via a mechanical injector. The latter type of administration is preferred if a 22-gauge or larger needle can be placed in an antecubital vein. A flow rate of 1.5 ml/s is desirable for 22-gauge needles, while a 2.0 ml/s rate is recommended for 20-gauge needles. A hand injection is preferred for smaller caliber needles in the antecubital region and for needles positioned in the hand. The recommended dose of contrast is 2 ml/kg, not to exceed a total of 4 ml/kg or 100 ml.

CT scanning may be performed with either a dynamic incremental or a spiral (helical) technique. With either technique, scanning is begun after 100% of the contrast medium has been administered.

The advantage of spiral scanning over conventional dynamic imaging is improved vascular enhancement, which allows confident differentiation of vessels from lymph nodes. However, the spiral CT survey study is often completed before

411

a significant amount of contrast material has reached the bladder. Delayed scanning can allow contrast medium to accumulate in the bladder, facilitating recognition of pelvic fluid collections.

Oral Contrast Material

Oral contrast material is routinely given for pelvic CT examinations, to prevent bowel loops being mistaken for a mass or abnormal fluid collection. Optimal bowel opacification can be achieved using a dilute (1% to 2%) solution of barium or water-soluble, iodine-based contrast agent given by mouth or through a nasogastric tube. To increase patient acceptance, the contrast agent can be mixed with fruit juice. Complete opacification of the stomach, small bowel, and proximal colon is usually possible if the oral contrast agent is given 60 minutes before scanning. The volume varies with patient age (Table 26.1). The descending and rectosigmoid colon, even if unopacified, can be recognized by their location and fecal contents, but if opacification of these segments is needed, a contrast enema can be administered.

Imaging Techniques

CT examinations should be performed with scan times of 1 second or less. Contiguous, 8-mm collimated sections at 8-mm intervals are adequate for most pelvic CT studies in children over 5 years of age. Decreased collimation (4 mm) and reduced scanning intervals (4 mm) are used in infants and children under 5 years of age and in evaluating the extent of pelvic neoplasms.

CT sections are obtained with breath holding at suspended inspiration if the patient is cooperative and at resting lung volume if the patient is sedated. With the spiral technique, an excellent quality study can be obtained even if the patient is quietly breathing.

Table 26.1 Age vs. Oral Contrast

Age	Dose Given 60 Min Before Study
Less than 1 mo	2–3 oz (60–90 ml)
1 mo to 1 yr	4–8 oz (120–240 ml)
1–5 yr	8–12 oz (240–360 ml)
6–12 yr	12–16 oz (360–480 ml)
13–15 yr	16–20 oz (480–600 ml)
16–18 yr	24 oz (720 ml)

MRI: TECHNICAL CONSIDERATIONS

Coil Selection

MRI examinations should be performed with the smallest coil that fits tightly around the body part being studied.[7] A head coil usually is adequate in infants and small children, while a whole-body coil or phased-array surface coil is needed for larger children and adolescents.

Pulse Sequences

Both T1- and T2-weighted sequences are needed to allow lesion detection and characterization. T1-weighted sequences are acquired with a conventional spin echo technique (TR 300 to 500 ms, TE as short as possible). The advantages of the T1-weighted image are improved contrast between soft tissue structures and fat and images without respiratory-related artifacts, resulting in increased lesion detection. T1-weighted images also are useful to characterize hemorrhagic and fatty components of masses.

T2-weighted sequences (TR > 2,000 ms, TE > 70 ms) provide excellent contrast between tumor and adjacent soft tissues and are superior to T1-weighted images for tissue characterization. The T2-weighted sequences can be acquired with conventional or fast spin echo (also known as turbo spin echo) techniques. Fast spin echo sequences allow a substantial reduction in imaging time, although they may result in some loss of contrast between fat and other similarly intense fluid and tissues.

Fat suppression can be done with either short T1 inversion recovery or fat saturation techniques. Fat suppressed T1- and T2-weighted sequences increase the contrast range of non-fatty tissues and improve lesion conspicuity. Gadolinium administration, especially in combination with fat suppression, is useful for further defining cystic and solid elements of neoplasms and the relationship of neoplasm to adjacent pelvic structures.[8]

The gradient echo technique results in a high signal in flowing blood and is used to evaluate the patency of vessels and to differentiate vessels and lymph nodes.[9,10] The evaluation of blood flow with the gradient echo sequence requires the use of technical parameters (TR/TE of 25 to 40/8 to 10, flip angle of 30 to 40 degrees) that are tailored for vascular imaging. A two-dimensional sequential mode is used for routine MRI angiography, while a three-dimensional mode is useful for multiplanar reconstructions.

Transaxial images with 4- to 8-mm slice thickness at 5- to 10-mm intervals generally suffice in children 5 years of age and older. In younger children, 4-mm sections at 5-mm intervals are obtained. Transaxial images are particularly useful to show the relationship of the uterus to the adnexa and to assess tumor extension to the pelvic sidewalls and lymph nodes. They are also best to display vaginal anatomy. Transaxial views are supplemented by images in either the coronal or sagittal plane. Coronal images are a useful adjunct to define further the relationship of the uterus to the ovaries, parametrium, and pelvic floor, and they are valuable in delineating lateral extension of tumor and lymphadenopathy. Sagittal images display the relationship of the uterus to the urinary bladder and the rectum. A 128-to-192 matrix and one or two signal acquisitions are useful to shorten the imaging time. Oral contrast agents are not widely used in MRI of the pediatric pelvis.

NORMAL PELVIS

Ovaries

The ovaries lie on either side of the uterus within the mesoovarium of the broad ligament with their axes parallelling the iliac vessels. Based on sonographic criteria, the neonatal ovary is approximately 15 mm long, 3 mm wide, and 2.5 mm thick, with a volume less than 0.7 cm.[1,2,11–14] A gradual age-related increase in ovarian volume begins about 6 years of age. At puberty, the ovaries reach their adult size, measuring approximately 2.5 to 5 cm in length, 1.5 to 3 cm in width, and 0.6 to 1.5 cm in thickness, with a volume between 1.8 and 5.7 cm.[1,2,14,15]

Multiple cystic structures, representing follicles, are typically visible in the cortex of the ovary. During the follicular phase (days 1 to 14), primordial follicles mature, with appearance of the dominant follicle by day 5 to 7 of the cycle. Following ovulation, the empty follicle fills with blood, lipid, and lutein to form a corpus luteum, which persists for 14 days. After that time, the corpus luteum degenerates unless fertilization has occurred. Eventually, this structure is replaced with fibrous tissue, forming the corpus albicans. Follicular or corpus luteum cysts have an upper diameter of 3 cm.

The ovaries of pubertal girls are more likely to be seen on CT and MRI than are the ovaries of prepubertal girls. On CT, the ovaries appear as avoid structures, posterolateral to the body of the uterus. They may be of homogeneous soft tissue density, but more often they are of low attenuation, reflecting the presence of small follicles (Fig. 26.1).[16] Individual follicles often cannot be identified on CT. On T1-weighted MRIs, the ovaries have a low to medium signal intensity, are isointense or slightly hyperintense to muscle. On T2-weighted images, the periphery of the ovary, containing multiple follicles, increases in signal intensity and is hyperintense to fat, while the central stroma becomes isointense to fat (Fig. 26.2).[17,18] Individual follicles are more likely to be seen on MRI than on CT.

Uterus and Vagina

The uterus, similar to the ovary, changes in size and morphology with age. The neonatal uterus is a tubular structure with a cervix and corpus of equal size. Based on established

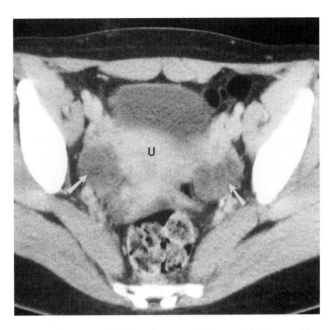

Figure 26.1 Normal pubertal ovaries, CT scan of a 15-year-old girl. The ovaries (arrows) are of low attenuation reflecting the presence of multiple follicles. U = uterus.

sonographic criteria, uterine length in the neonate ranges between 2.3 and 4.6 cm, while the anteroposterior diameter is between 0.8 and 2.2 cm.[1,13,14] The neonatal uterus is relatively large because of in utero stimulation by maternal hormones. As the level of exogenous hormones declines during the first month of life, the uterus decreases in size. From infancy to about 7 years of age, uterine size remains stable, measuring between 2.5 and 3.3 cm in length and 0.4 and 1.0 cm in anteroposterior diameter.[1,13,14] The corpus and cervix remain similar in size. Following puberty, the uterus increases in size, with the corpus enlarging more than the cervix, producing the adult pear-shaped uterus. In the pubertal girl, uterine length ranges between 5 to 8 cm and anteroposterior diameter varies between 1.5 and 3 cm.[12,14]

Identification of the uterus on CT and MRI may be difficult in very young prepubertal girls. As puberty approaches, the uterus increases in size and is easily identifiable behind the bladder. On CT, it appears as an oval soft tissue mass. With intravenous contrast administration, the myometrium and endometrium show intense enhancement, particularly in adolescent girls. The endometrial canal may have a lower attenuation, reflecting secretions or blood (Fig. 26.3).[16] Differentiation of the uterus and cervix is difficult on CT scanning.

The premenarcheal uterus, cervix, and vagina have low-to-medium signal intensity and indistinct zonal anatomy. The signal intensity increases slightly on T2-weighted images. In pubertal girls, the uterus has a homogeneous medium signal intensity on T1-weighted images.[19,20] It exhibits a characteristic zonal anatomy on T2-weighted images.[19,20] The central high signal intensity zone represents endometrium, the adja-

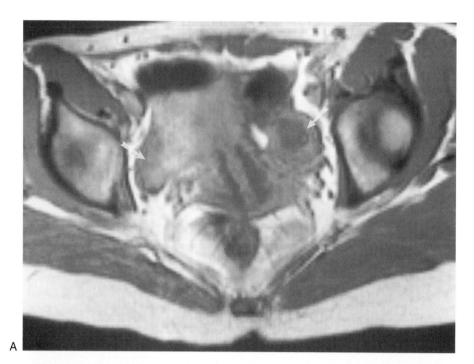

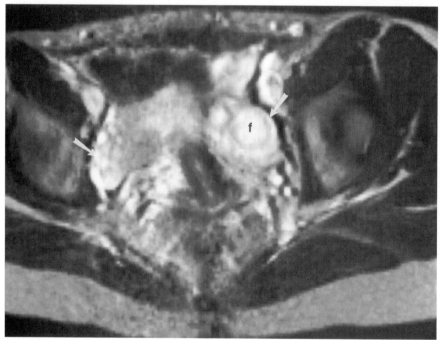

Figure 26.2 Normal ovaries, MRI of a 15-year-old girl. **(A)** Coronal T1-weighted image (TE 600/TR15) demonstrates relatively homogeneous, medium signal intensity ovaries (arrows). **(B)** On T2-weighted transaxial image (TE3,500/TR90), the ovaries (arrows) demonstrate high signal intensity. The left ovary contains a 2.5-cm dominant follicle (f).

cent low-intensity layer corresponds to inner myometrium, and the peripheral intermediate signal intensity layer corresponds to the outer myometrium (Fig. 26.4). Endometrial width varies throughout the menstrual cycle.[21–23]

The endometrium is thinnest (1 mm) immediately after menstruation and increases in width during the follicular and

secretory phases. The width is significantly larger in the secretory phase (mean, 5 mm) than in the follicular phase (mean, 3.1 mm).[23] In pubertal girls taking oral contraceptives, endometrial width is markedly reduced in both phases (mean, 1.1 mm).[23]

The cervix and vagina also have homogeneous low-to-

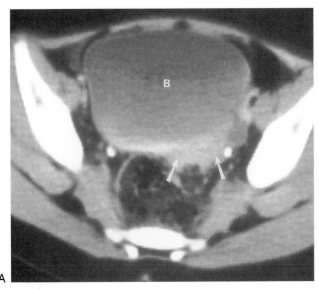

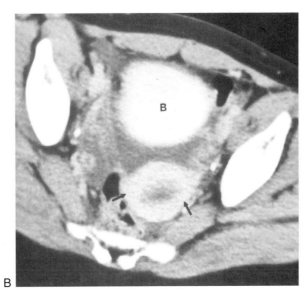

Figure 26.3 Normal uterus, CT. **(A)** Three-year-old girl. The uterus (arrows) is seen as a homogeneous oval soft tissue mass located behind the bladder (B). **(B)** Postpubertal 13-year-old-girl, menstrual phase. The uterus (arrows) is larger in size and has a low attenuation center surrounded by enhancing myometrium. B, = bladder.

medium signal intensity on T1-weighted images. On T2-weighted images, the normal cervix frequently displays a central stripe of high signal intensity, reflecting cervical mucosa and secretions in the canal. The periphery of the cervix has two signal intensities: an inner low-intensity layer, corre-

Figure 26.4 Normal pubertal uterus and vagina, MRI of a 16-year-old girl. Sagittal MRI (TR 3,500/TE90) shows the characteristic uterine anatomy: a high signal endometrial (e) cavity, a low signal inner myometrium (arrowhead), and an intermediate signal outer myometrium (m). The vagina has two zones of different signal intensities: a high signal intensity canal (c) and a lower signal intensity wall (arrows).

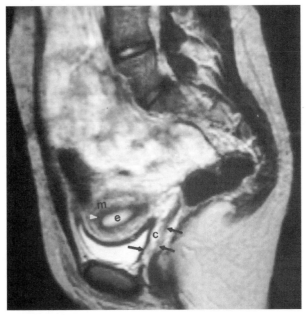

sponding to fibrous stroma, and an outer, medium intensity layer, representing muscle.[19] The paracervical tissue has a homogeneous medium signal intensity on T1-weighted images, and it increases in signal intensity on T2-weighted images. In contrast to the uterus and the cervix, the vagina has two layers: a high signal intensity center and a subadjacent low signal intensity wall.[19] As does the uterus, the vaginal endometrium varies in thickness with changes in hormonal status.

CONGENITAL ABNORMALITIES

Ultrasonography and MRI have both been shown to be useful methods for evaluating patients with congenital uterine or vaginal anomalies.[14,24-31] CT can detect and differentiate congenital anomalies, but it is not performed routinely, because it utilizes ionising radiation[32] and has suboptimal soft tissue contrast compared with MRI.

Uterine Agenesis or Hypoplasia

Uterine malformations occur in 0.1% to 0.5% of all women.[19,24] The uterus and upper two-thirds of the vagina arise from fused portions of the müllerian ducts, while the lower vagina and vestibule arise from the urogenital sinus. Uterine agenesis is the result of nondevelopment of the müllerian ducts and is most often associated with the testicular feminization or the Mayer-Rokitansky-Kuster-Hauser syndromes. Affected patients present with primary amenorrhea. Testicular feminization is characterized by a male (46,XY) karyotype, female external genitalia, a blind-ending vagina, and absent uterus. The gonads are testes that produce normal

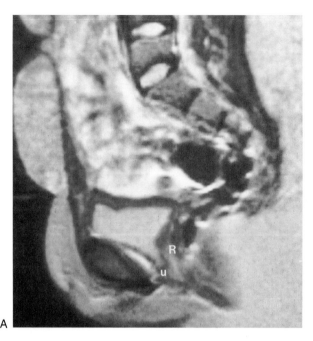
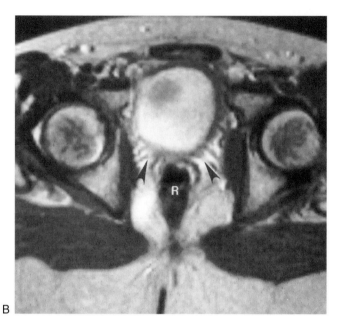

Figure 26.5 Vaginal atresia, 16-year-old girl with absent menses. **(A)** Sagittal MRI.
(B) Transaxial T2-weighted images (TR2,000/TE60) demonstrate absence of the uterus,
cervix, and vagina. Fatty tissue (arrowheads) fills the space normally occupied by the vaginal fornices on the transaxial image. R, rectum, u, urethra.

male levels of testosterone, but there is end-organ insensitivity to androgens. Mayer-Rokitansky-Kuster-Hauser syndrome
is characterized by a normal female karyotype, the presence of
normal ovaries, and the absence of both the uterus and
vagina.[26] Müllerian remnants may be present in place of the
uterus. Associated renal and skeletal anomalies occur in 50%
and 12% of patients, respectively.[14]

Uterine hypoplasia can be an isolated finding, but more
frequently it is associated with Turner syndrome. In Turner
syndrome, ovarian size varies with karyotype. In patients with
45,XO karyotype, the ovaries are either absent or are fibrous
streaks. Uterine size remains prepubertal with increasing age.
Patients with chromosomal mosaicism (XO/XX) have a spectrum of findings ranging from streak ovaries and an infantile
uterus to normal size gonads and uterus. Uterine agenesis or
hypoplasia is best displayed on T2-weighted sagittal images,
while vaginal agenesis is best shown on transaxial scans (Fig.
26.5). In addition to a small uterus, patients with uterine hypoplasia have poor zonal differentiation and reduced endometrial and myometrial widths.[24]

Uterine Duplication

Uterine duplication results from complete or partial nonfusion of the müllerian ducts.[33] The spectrum includes uterus
didelphys (two vaginas, two cervices, and two uterine corpora); uterus bicornis, either bicollis uterus (single vagina,
two cervices and two uterine corpora) or unicollis uterus (one
vagina, one cervix, and two uterine corpora); and uterus sep-

tus (single uterus, cervix and vagina, with a septum dividing
the uterus into two compartments) (Fig. 26.6). Neonates usually present with a pelvic mass, while adolescent girls present
with hematocolpos or hematometra. Occasionally, duplication anomalies are detected incidentally during obstetric
sonography.

On CT or MRI, uterus didelphys and uterus bicornis have
a bilobed shape with concave outer walls in contrast to the
normal fundal convexity (Fig. 26.7). The two cornua usually
are separated by myometrium, which exhibits a medium signal intensity on T1-weighted images and a higher signal intensity on T2-weighted images. The MRI appearance of septate uterus is that of a single uterine fundus with a convex
fundal contour and a central septum dividing the endometrium into two cavities (Fig. 26.8).[24,29] The septum typically
has a low signal intensity on both T1- and T2-weighted images, consistent with fibrous tissue.[24,29] Occasionally, however,
a bicornuate uterus displays a low signal intensity band between the two fundi.[24,30] In these cases, fundal contour can help
to separate a bicornuate from a septate uterus. The accuracy
of MRI for diagnosing uterine anomalies has been reported to
be 100% versus an accuracy of approximately 90% for endovaginal sonography and 55% for hysterosalpingography.[30,34]

Congenital Vaginal Obstruction

Congenital vaginal obstruction can be encountered in the
neonatal period or at the time of menarche. In the neonate,
vaginal obstruction may be the result of vaginal atresia or
stenosis, a transverse septum, or a cloacal malformation. In

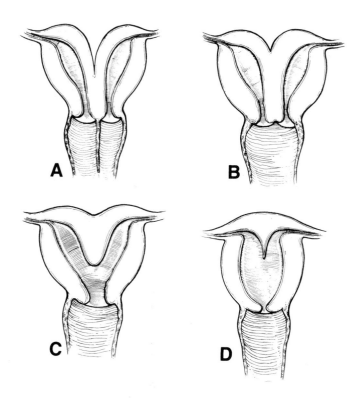

Figure 26.6 Uterine duplication anomalies. Diagrammatic representation of common anomalies. (A) Uterus didelphys. Two uteri, two cervices, two vaginas. (B) Uterus duplex bicollis. Two uteri, two cervices, one vagina. (C) Uterus duplex unicollis. Two uteri, one cervix, one vagina. (D) Uterus septus. Single uterus divided by a septum, one vagina (From Cooperberg and Kidney,[33] with permission.)

Figure 26.7 Didelphys uterus, 17-year-old girl with periodic pelvic pain. (A) Coronal T2-weighted image (TR 2,100/TE90) shows two widely separate uterine fundi (u). (B) More anterior coronal image shows two separate endocervical canals (c) and vaginal fornices (arrowheads).

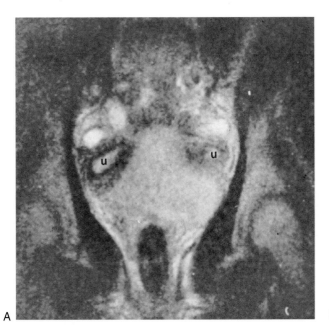

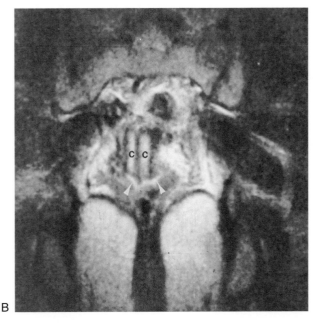

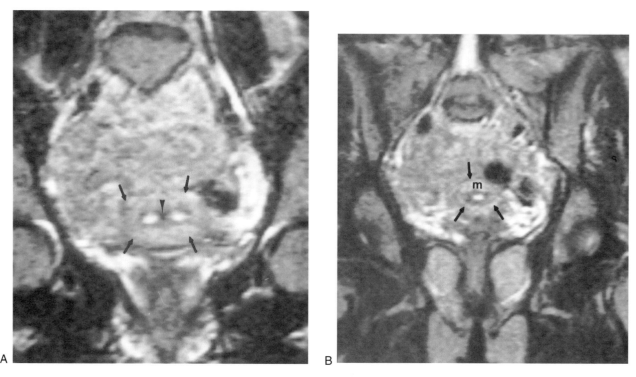

Figure 26.8 Septate uterus, 16-year-old girl. **(A)** Coronal T2-weighted image (TR2, 100/TE90) shows a single uterine fundus (arrows) with two high signal endometrial cavities separated by a low intensity septum (arrowhead). **(B)** At a more posterior level, the two fundi have fused to form a single body (arrows) with normal zonal anatomy. m, myometrium. (From Siegel,[4] with permission.)

Figure 26.9 Hydrocolpos in a 13-year-old girl with amenorrhea and recurrent pelvic pain. CT scan through the pelvis demonstrates a dilated fluid-filled vagina (V). An imperforate membrane was found at operation. B, bladder; R, rectum.

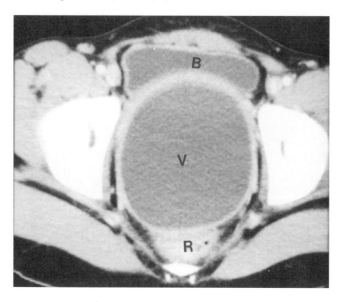

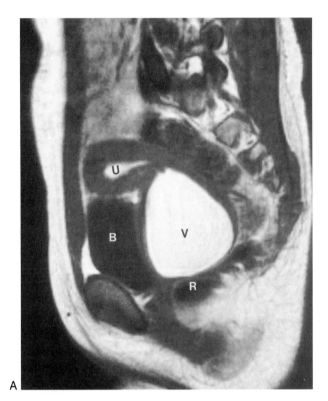
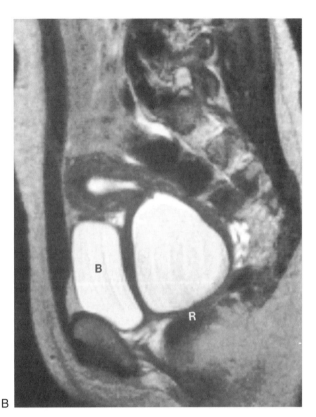

A   B

Figure 26.10 Hematocolpos and hematometra in a 1-month-old girl with vaginal atresia and a cloacal anomaly. **(A)** T1-weighted (TR600/TE15) sagittal image shows a dilated vagina (V) and uterine cavity (U). The high signal intensity of the fluid within the vaginal and uterine cavities is compatible with blood. **(B)** On a T2-weighted (TR4,200/TE90) image, the signal intensity in the vaginal and uterine cavities remains high. Note the indistinct uterine zonal anatomy, typical of the premenarcheal uterus. R, rectum; B, bladder. At operation, the point of atresia was in the distal third of the vagina.

adolescent girls, it is most often the result of a simple imperforate membrane. Affected neonates present with a palpable pelvic or abdominal mass resulting from the production and excessive accumulation of vaginal and/or uterine secretions in utero secondary to maternal hormone stimulation. In addition to secretions, urine may be found within the vagina or uterus of patients with cloacal anomalies. Adolescent patients present with cyclic lower abdominal pain or a mass caused by acute hematometra and a history of absent menses. There is an increased association of congenital anomalies (e.g., imperforate anus, esophageal or duodenal atresia, congenital heart disease, and renal abnormalities) in neonates with vaginal atresia.

On CT, the dilated vagina and uterus appear as midline, near-water density masses (Fig. 26.9).[32] The distended vagina has a thin, almost imperceptible wall, while the uterus has a thicker muscular wall. Wall enhancement may be seen after administration of intravenous contrast. The signal intensity of the luminal fluid is variable on MRI. Serous fluid or urine has a low signal intensity on T1-weighted images and a high signal intensity on T2-weighted images (Fig. 26.10).[31] The signal intensity increases on T1-weighted images if the con-

tents are hemorrhagic.[28] Intra-abdominal extension or hydronephrosis, caused by ureteral compression, can be seen in long-standing obstruction.

PELVIC MASSES

Sonography remains the primary imaging study to evaluate patients with suspected gynecologic pathology because of its absence of ionizing radiation, widespread availability, ease of performance, and lower cost. Ultrasonography can reliably differentiate ovarian from uterine masses and cystic from solid lesions. CT or MRI is useful when sonography is technically suboptimal because of patient obesity or abundant bowel gas, both of which attenuate the sound beam, or when the results of sonography are equivocal.[35,36] Both CT and MRI can delineate the size and character of a mass and its relationship to adjacent pelvic viscera. They have similar ability to differentiate fluid, fat, and soft tissue. CT is more sensitive than MRI in detecting small gas bubbles and calcifications. MRI is superior to CT in allowing a topographic display of anatomy because of its capability to provide direct multiplanar images. With rare exceptions, such as ovarian teratomas, neither CT nor MRI are capable of providing a definitive histologic diagnosis.

OVARIAN CYSTS

Functional Cysts

Benign functional cysts account for most ovarian masses in childhood. Neonatal ovarian cysts result from exaggeration of normal follicular development due to in utero stimulation by maternal hormones. The end result is a palpable pelvic or abdominal mass. Functional cysts occur in pubertal girls when a follicular cyst or corpus luteum fails to involute and continues to enlarge secondary to hormonal stimulation. They range between 3 and 10 cm in diameter. While usually asymptomatic, functional cysts may cause symptoms of pain due to torsion, hemorrhage, or rupture. The CT and MRI appearance of ovarian cysts is similar to cysts elsewhere in the body. On CT, functional cysts appear as water-density, round or ovoid structures with imperceptible walls that do not enhance after in-

travenous contrast administration (Fig. 26.11). When they contain clear serous fluid, they have a low signal intensity on T1-weighted images and high signal intensity on T2-weighted sequences (Fig. 26.12).[17,35,36] A fluid–debris level or septa may be seen if torsion occurs. If the cyst is very large, it can extend into the upper abdomen and may be confused with a mesenteric or omental cyst.

Hemorrhagic Cysts

When blood vessels within a follicular or corpus luteal cyst rupture, a hemorrhagic cyst develops. These cysts typically are found in pubertal girls who present with acute pelvic pain. On CT, acute hemorrhage has a high attenuation value; old blood has an attenuation value nearer water density. The signal intensity is variable on T1-and T2-weighted images, depending on whether the blood is acute or chronic (Fig. 26.13).[17,36] The differential diagnosis of a hemorrhagic cyst is a cystic neoplasm. Sequential imaging, usually with sonography, can be useful to exclude neoplasm. Hemorrhagic ovarian cysts decrease in size over time, while cystic tumors remain unchanged or increase in size.

Figure 26.11 Nonhemorrhagic functional cyst. CT of a 14-year-old girl with pelvic pain and a mass. A large left ovarian cyst (C) displaces the urine-filled bladder (B) to the right. The cyst is well circumscribed, has a thin wall, and is of near-water density. A simple follicular cyst was confirmed at operation.

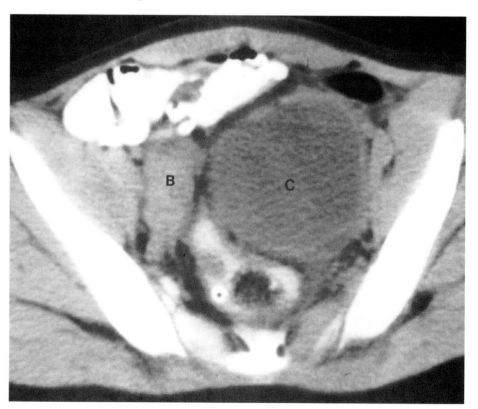

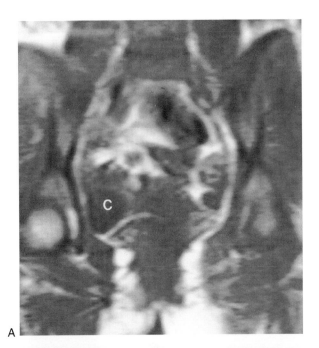

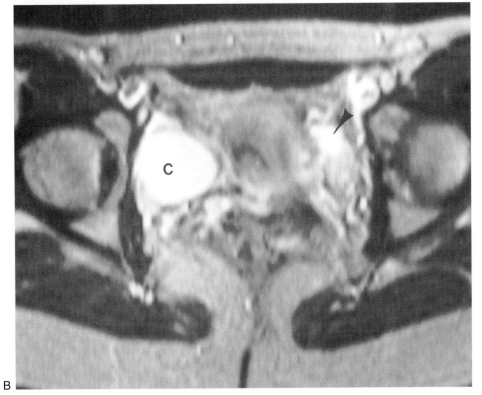

Figure 26.12 Nonhemorrhagic functional cyst, discovered incidentally on MRI performed for chronic hip pain. **(A)**Coronal T1-weighted MRI (TR500/TE17) show a 4-cm round, low-intensity cyst (C) arising in the right ovary. **(B)** On the T2-weighted image (TR3,000/TE90), the cyst (C) has a signal intensity higher than subcutaneous fat. A normal physiologic follicle (arrowhead) is noted in the left ovary. (From Siegel,[4] with permission.)

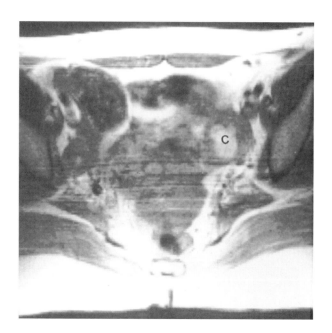

Figure 26.13 Hemorrhagic ovarian cyst, discovered incidentally. Transaxial T1-weighted (TR700/TE20) MRI shows a slightly hyperintense cyst (C) in the left ovary. The signal intensity is consistent with subacute blood. (From Siegel,[4] [Courtesy of Dr. George Bissett III, Durham, North Carolina], with permission.)

Figure 26.14 Polycystic ovary disease, 15-year-old girl with Stein-Leventhal syndrome. **(A)** T1-weighted images (TR700/TE20) shows low signal intensity ovaries (O). **(B)** T2-weighted image (TR2,500/TE80) shows multiple, small, high signal intensity cysts with surrounding low signal intensity stroma. (From Siegel,[4] [Courtesy of Dr. George Bissett III, Durham, North Carolina], with permission.)

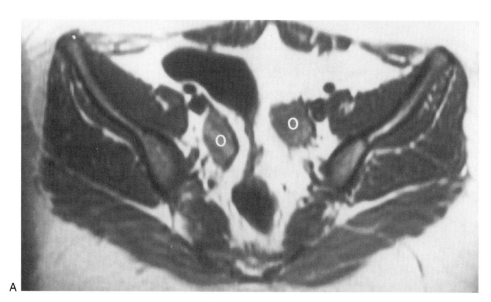

A

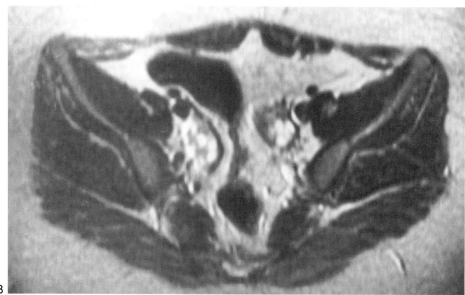

B

Polycystic Ovary Disease

Polycystic ovary disease (Stein-Leventhal syndrome) is a syndrome characterized by amenorrhea, obesity, and hirsutism. Both ovaries are enlarged in approximately 70% of patients (mean volume of 14 ml) and contain multiple small cysts.[37,38] Ovarian size and morphology are normal in the remaining patients. On CT, the ovaries demonstrate low attenuation. The MRI appearance is that of multiple, small, peripheral cysts with low signal intensity on T1-weighted sequences and high signal intensity on T2-weighted sequences (Fig. 26.14). The parenchyma exhibits low-signal intensity on T1-and T2-weighted images, corresponding to cellular stroma.[39]

OVARIAN TUMORS

Benign Tumors

Teratomas, the most common true pediatric ovarian neoplasms, may be subdivided into mature, immature (containing embryonic neural elements), and malignant types.[40–42] The first group accounts for more than 90% of ovarian germ cell tumors. Affected patients usually present with a pelvic or abdominal mass, although they may present with pain if the tumor undergoes torsion, rupture, or hemorrhage. Teratomas usually range in diameter from 5 to 10 cm and are bilateral in 25% of cases.

A specific diagnosis of an ovarian teratoma is possible on CT or MRI when fatty elements are identified within an ovar-

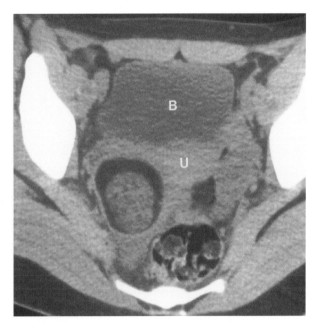

Figure 26.16 Benign ovarian teratoma, 15-year-old girl with a solid pelvic mass on sonography. CT scan shows a complex mass containing soft tissue and fat lying to the right of the uterus (U). On pathologic section, the teratoma contained fat primarily and a small amount of hair. Even in the absence of calcific elements, the fatty tissue is reliable enough to suggest a diagnosis of teratoma. B, bladder.

ian tumor.[43–45] In one series of 43 cystic teratomas (41 benign and 2 malignant) imaged by CT, fat was noted in 93%, Rokitansky protuberances in 81%, teeth or calcific elements in 56%, and a fat–fluid level in 12% of lesions.[43] Calcific elements and fat are most often located in the Rokitansky protuberance or dermoid plug arising from the cyst wall (Figs. 26.15 and 26.16). Occasionally, the intracystic fat is mobile and shifts position.[44] Benign cystic teratomas contain some soft tissue elements, but the presence of large amounts of soft tissue (> 50% volume) should increase the suspicion of malignant transformation.[43,45]

Benign teratomas have varying signal intensities, depending on their tissue composition.[35,36,46,47] On T1-weighted images, fat appears as an area of high signal intensity, while serous fluid and calcifications have low signal intensity. On T2-weighted images, both fat and serous fluid are of high signal intensity (Fig. 26.17). Calcifications, teeth, bone, hair, and fibrous tissue have low signal intensity on both pulse sequences. Gradient echo and fat suppression techniques are especially useful for demonstrating small amounts of fatty tissue.[47–49] Other MRI findings of cystic teratomas include mural protrusions or nodules, fat–fluid levels, and gravity-dependent or floating debris.[46]

Malignant Neoplasms

Malignant ovarian masses comprise 2% of all pediatric malignancies. Germ cell tumors (dysgerminoma, immature or malignant teratoma, endodermal sinus tumor, embryonal carcinoma,

Figure 26.15 Cystic ovarian teratoma, 10-year-old girl with complex pelvic mass on sonography. A CT scan through the mid pelvis shows a large near-water density mass containing peripheral fat (arrows) and calcifications. A mature teratoma was found at operation.

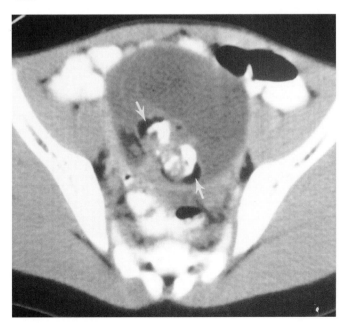

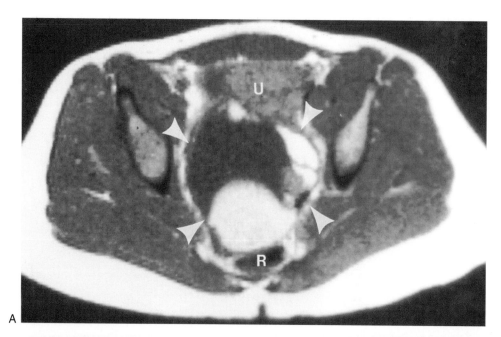

A

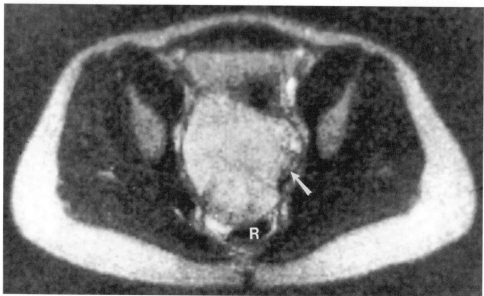

B

Figure 26.17 Cystic ovarian teratoma, young woman with a palpable mass. **(A)** Transaxial T1-weighted (TR500/TE30) image shows a large mass (arrowheads) posterolateral to the uterus (U). The anterior aspect of the mass has a relatively low signal intensity, while the posterior and left lateral aspects of the mass have a high signal intensity equal to that of fat. **(B)** On a T2-weighted image, (TR1,500/TE90) the signal intensity of the anterior portions of mass is higher than that of subcutaneous fat, while the intensity of the posterior component is equal to subcutaneous fat. The low signal intensity focus laterally (arrow) corresponded to calcification and hair on pathologic specimen. R, rectum. (From Siegel,[4] with permission.)

choriocarcinoma) account for 60% to 90% of malignant neoplasms; stromal tumors (Sertoli-Leydig cell, granulosa-theca cell, and undifferentiated neoplasms) have a 10% to 13% incidence; and epithelial carcinomas account for 5% to 11% of malignant ovarian lesions.[41,50] Malignant tumors tend to occur in pubertal girls and are usually larger than 10 cm in diameter at presentation. CT features suggesting malignancy include a solid or complex mass with ill-defined or irregular borders and cen-

tral necrosis, thick septa, or papillary projections (Figs. 26.18 and 26.19). Ascites, lymphadenopathy, peritoneal or omental implants, and hepatic metastases are associated findings (Fig. 26.20). On MRI, malignant ovarian neoplasms appear as heterogeneous masses with low-to-intermediate signal intensity on T1-weighted images and intermediate or high signal intensity masses on T2-weighted images. Other findings include a thickened irregular wall or septa and ascites.[51]

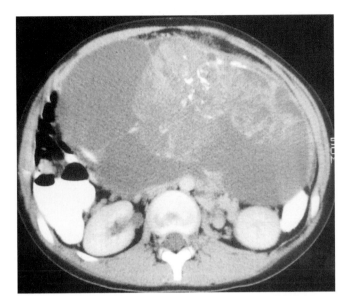

Figure 26.18 Immature teratoma containing glial elements, 13-year-old girl with a large pelvoabdominal mass. CT shows a complex mass with a large central soft tissue plug containing calcification. The solid enhancing elements of the teratoma were shown histologically to contain neuroepithelium.

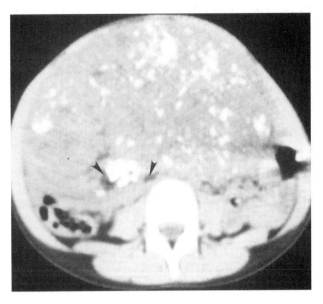

Figure 26.19 Malignant ovarian teratoma, 11-year-old girl with a palpable abdominal mass. Noncontrast CT image shows a solid mass with large amounts of calcification and scattered areas of fat (arrowheads).

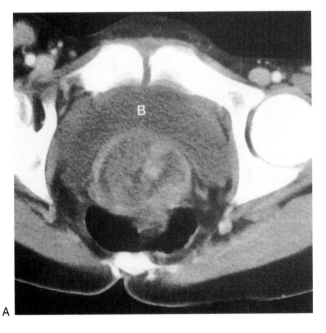

Figure 26.20 Mucinous ovarian carcinoma with omental implants, 14-year-old girl with abdominal distension and weight loss. **(A)** CT scan through the pelvis shows a complex mass with cystic and solid components behind the bladder (B). (*Figure continues.*)

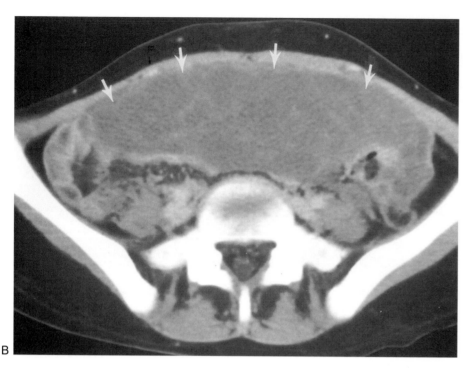

Figure 26.20 (*Continued*). (**B**) CT scan through the upper abdomen demonstrates diffuse omental involvement (omental cake) (arrows) anterior to bowel loops.

Malignant ovarian neoplasms spread by direct extension or via hematogeneous or lymphatic dissemination. They also may spread by implanting on peritoneal or omental surfaces. Intraperitoneal seeding occurs predominantly in epithelial cancers having mucinous components. Peritoneal tumor implants appear as soft tissue nodules on the lateral peritoneal surfaces of the abdomen on CT and as medium signal intensity nodules on MRI.[51] Omental implants, also termed an "omental cake," appear as discrete nodules or as conglomerate soft tissue masses beneath the anterior abdominal wall on CT (Fig. 26.20) and as medium signal intensity masses on MRI. Peritoneal and omental implants often enhance after administration of gadolinium diethylenetriamine-penta-acetic acid.

UTERINE AND VAGINAL MASSES

Rhabdomyosarcoma

Rhabdomyosarcoma is the most common malignant tumor of the vagina and uterus in children, usually presenting as a pelvic mass or vaginal discharge or bleeding.[52] CT or MRI are warranted for staging, especially to evaluate hematogeneous or lymphatic spread to liver, lymph nodes, or lung. On CT, rhabdomyosarcoma appears as a soft tissue mass with an attenuation value approximating that of muscle (Fig. 26.21). Necrosis or calcification also may be present, along with variable enhancement after intravenous administration of con-

trast material. Metastases to pelvic lymph nodes can be seen if the involved nodes are enlarged. Rhabdomyosarcoma has a low signal intensity on T1-weighted and a high signal intensity on T2-weighted MRIs (Fig. 26.22).[53] T1-weighted images are best for depicting the primary tumor, lymphadenopathy, and invasion of perivesical fat. Contrast enhancement also may improve tumor detection. A less frequent vaginal malignancy is clear cell adenocarcinoma. It should be considered in adolescents with a history of in utero exposure to diethylstilbestrol. The imaging features are similar to those of rhabdomyosarcoma.

Gestational Trophoblastic Diseases

Gestational trophoblastic disease is a rare cause of a uterine mass in an adolescent girl. It represents a spectrum of tumors varying from the relatively benign hydatidiform mole to the malignant invasive mole or choriocarcinoma. The diagnosis of molar pregnancy is based on clinical findings and the demonstration of elevated serum levels of human chorionic gonadotropins. Sonography is the initial study for the diagnosis of trophoblastic disease, but it is not as useful as CT or MRI in detecting the full extent of tumor in patients with invasive mole or choriocarcinoma. The CT findings of gestational trophoblastic disease are (1) a normal-size uterus with heterogeneous enhancement; (2) a uniformly enlarged uterus with low-density areas; or (3) a lobular uterus with focal uter-

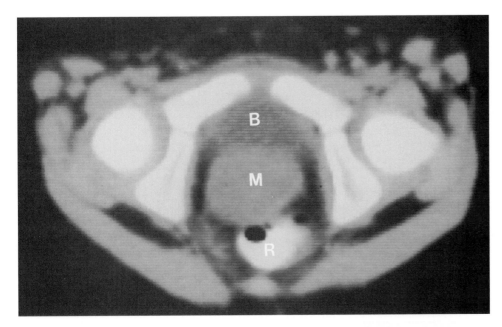

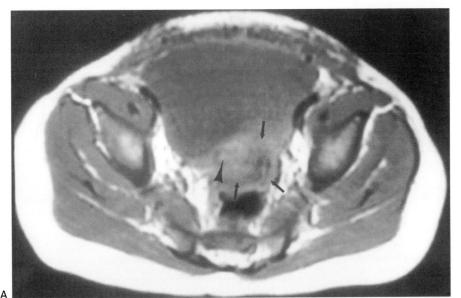

A

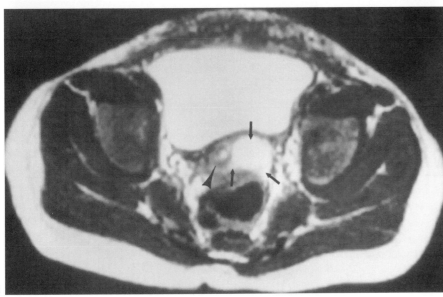

B

Figure 26.21 Vaginal rhabdomyosarcoma in a 2-year-old girl with vaginal bleeding. CT. CT scan of the pelvis shows a soft tissue mass (M) between the bladder (B) and rectum (R). The soft tissues in the right pelvic wall posterolaterally are thickened secondary to prior biopsy. (From Siegel,[4] with permission.)

Figure 26.22 Vaginal rhabdomyosarcoma, MRI. (A)Transaxial MRI (TR2, 500/TE90) shows an intermediate signal intensity mass (arrows) arising from the left vaginal fornix. (B)On T2-weighted image, the signal intensity of the mass increases and is equal to that of bladder (B). The interface between the bladder and rectum is well demarcated. Arrowhead, uterus. (From Siegel,[4] with permission.)

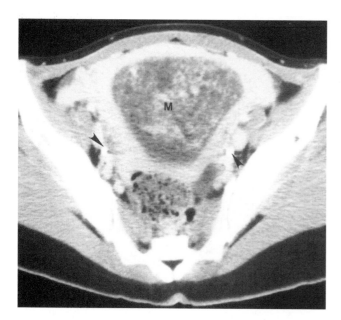

Figure 26.23 Gestational trophoblastic disease. On CT, the uterus shows heterogeneous enhancement with a large mass (M), containing cystic and solid components, filling the uterine cavity. The uterine wall is thick, and the ureters (arrowheads) are dilated because of compression by the dilated uterus. Engorged pelvic vessels are also seen in the parametrial fat. Histologic examination showed a hydatidiform mole without local invasion.

ine or cervical enlargement with or without hypodense areas (Fig. 26.23).[54,55] Occasionally, a gestational sac with a small fetal pole can be noted within the endometrial cavity. On MRI, gestational trophoblastic disease appears as heterogeneous, hypervascular masses within an enlarged uterus. Zonal anatomy is indistinct.[56] This tumor is hypervascular, and dilated vessels can be noted within the tumor or in the adjacent adnexa on both CT and MRI. The ovaries are frequently enlarged and contain multiple theca lutein cysts. Distant metastases to the liver or the lung also may be present.

PELVIC PAIN

Adnexal Torsion

Adnexal torsion should be considered in young girls with acute or recurrent pelvic pain. Torsion results from rotation of the ovary or fallopian tube on its vascular pedicle, causing compromise of lymphatics and venous, arterial flow, and ultimately infarction. Torsion can occur in the presence of normal adnexa, or it can occur in association with an underlying mass, usually a teratoma or ovarian cyst. CT and MRI are useful when ultrasonography is indeterminate. On both CT and MRI, the edematous and possibly hemorrhagic ovary is en-

larged and may contain multiple, peripheral dilated follicles (Fig. 26.24).[57] Associated findings include engorged blood vessels on the affected side, ascites, obliteration of pelvic fat planes, and an underlying cyst or tumor (Fig. 26.25).[58,59]

Inflammatory Disease

Pelvic inflammatory disease affects girls of reproductive age and is usually due to *Neisseria gonorrheae* or *Chlamydia trachomatis*.[60] The inflammatory process begins in the vagina and cervix and then ascends to the endometrium and fallopian tubes. From the fallopian tubes, the infection can spread to the ovaries, parametrium, and peritoneal cavity. The diagnosis is usually made clinically, based on symptoms of pelvic pain, vaginal discharge, fever, and cervical motion tenderness. Sonography is useful for identifying complications such as pyosalpinx, tubo-ovarian abscess, and cul-de-sac abscess, and for assessing the response to treatment. CT plays an important role in evaluating the extent of adnexal and peritoneal abcesses. The CT appearance of a tubo-ovarian abscess, and also a pyosalpinx, is that of a low-attenuation pelvic mass with thick walls and with loss of fat planes between the mass and the adjacent pelvic organs (Fig. 26.26).[61,62] Internal septa, air or an air–liquid level also may be noted (Fig. 26.27). Thickening of the uterosacral ligaments and bowel wall, increased density in the pelvic fat, narrowing or irregularity of the rectosigmoid colon, hydronephrosis and hydroureter, and inflammatory lymphadenopathy are other common findings.

Figure 26.24 Adnexal torsion, 14-year-old girl with solid mass on sonography and acute pelvic pain. **(A)** CT shows an enlarged left ovary (O) lying behind the bladder. U, uterus. (*Figure continues.*)

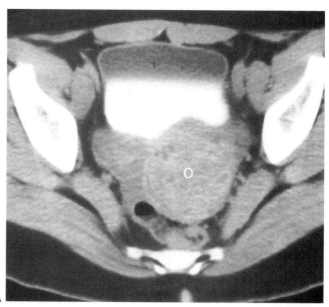

A

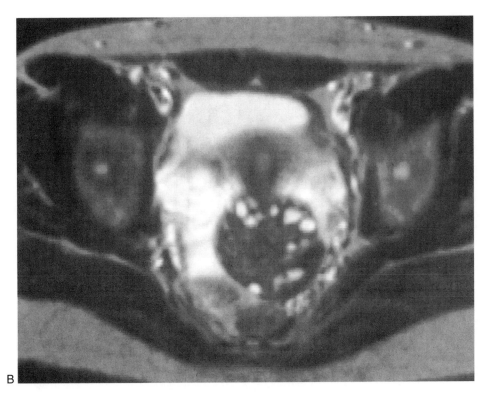

Figure 26.24 (*Continued*). **(B)** Transaxial T2-weighted image (TR2,500/TE90) demonstrates multiple high signal intensity peripheral cysts within an enlarged low signal intensity ovary. Note that the ovary lies behind the uterus, rather than in its usual position lateral to the uterus. Pathologic examination revealed an infarcted ovary. (From Surratt and Siegel,[2] with permission.)

Figure 26.25 Adnexal torsion secondary to an ovarian cyst in a 14-year-old girl with 1-day history of acute pelvic pain. CT scan shows a well-circumscribed cyst (C) with thick walls lying anterior to the uterus (U). Surgery revealed a twisted, infarcted right ovary with a follicular cyst.

Figure 26.26 Pyosalpinx. CT scan shows near-water density masses (asterisk) with enhancing walls behind the bladder **(B)**. The adjacent soft tissues are thickened, and there is loss of the pelvic fat planes due to inflammation.

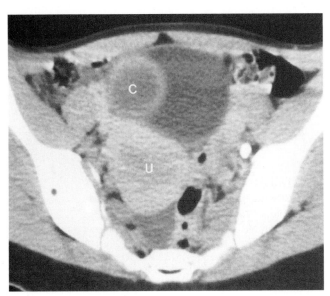

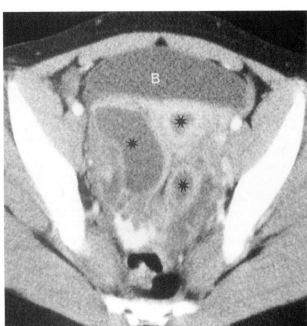

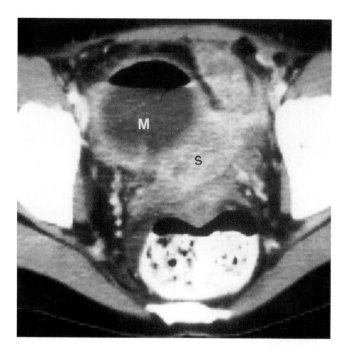

Figure 26.27 Tubo-ovarian abscess in a 16-year-old girl with fever and severe pelvic pain. CT scan shows a well-circumscribed mass (M) with a thick enhancing wall and air–fluid level in the right adnexa. Also noted are inflammatory changes in the adjacent sigmoid colon (s).

REFERENCES

1. Siegel MJ, Surratt JT. Pediatric gynecologic imaging. Obstet Gynecol Clin North Am 1992;19:103–127

2. Surratt JT, Siegel MJ. Imaging of pediatric ovarian masses. Radiographics 1991;11:533–548.

3. Dietrich RB, Kangarloo H. Pelvic abnormalities in children: assessment with MR imaging. Radiology 1987;163:367–372

4. Siegel MJ. Magnetic resonance imaging of the pediatric pelvis. Semin Ultrasound CT MR 1991;12:475–505

5. Bisset GS, 3rd, Ball WS, Jr. Preparation, sedation and monitoring of the pediatric patient in the magnetic resonance suite. Semin Ultrasound CR MR 1991;12:376–378

6. Siegel MJ. Pediatric applications. In: Lee KTL, Sagel SS, Stanley RJ, Eds. Computed Body Tomography with MRI Correlation (2nd ed.). Raven Press, New York, 1989, pp 1063–1099

7. Siegel MJ. MR imaging of the pediatric abdomen. Magn Res Imaging Clin N Am 1995;3:161–182

8. Semelka RC, Lawrence PH, Shoenut JP et al. Primary ovarian cancer: prospective comparison of contrast-enhanced CT and pre-and postcontrast, fat-suppressed MR imaging, with histologic correlation. J Magn Reson Imaging 1993;3:99–106.

9. Bradley WG, Jr, Waluch V, Lai KS et al. The appearance of rapidly flowing blood on magnetic resonance images. AJR Am J Roentgenol 1984;143:1167–1174

10. Shady KL, Siegel MJ, Brown JJ. Preoperative evaluation of intraabdominal tumors in children: gradient-recalled echo vs spin-echo MR imaging. AJR Am J Roentgenol 1993;161:843–847

11. Cohen HL, Tice HM, Mandel FS. Ovarian volumes measured by US: bigger than we think. Radiology 1990;177:189–192

12. Ivarsson SA, Nilsson KO, Persson PH. Ultrasonography of the pelvic organs in prepubertal and postpubertal girls. Arch Dis Child 1983;58:352–354

13. Orsini LF, Salardi S, Pilu G et al. Pelvic organs in premenarchal girls: real-time ultrasonography. Radiology 1984;153:113–116.

14. Siegel MJ. Female pelvis. In: Siegel MJ, Ed. Pediatric Sonography. Raven Press, New York, 1995, pp 437–477

15. Sample WF, Lippe BM, Gyepes MT. Gray-scale ultrasonography of the normal female pelvis. Radiology 1977;125:477–483

16. Rigsby CK, Siegel MJ. CT appearance of pediatric ovaries and uterus. J Comput Assist Tomogr 1994;18:72–76

17. Dooms GC, Hricak H, Tscholakoff D. Adnexal structures: MR imaging. Radiology 1986;58:639–646

18. Stevens SK. The adnexa. In: Higgins CB, Hricak H, Helms CA, Eds. Magnetic Resonance Imaging of the Body (2nd Ed.). Raven Press, New York, 1992, pp 865–889

19. Hricak H, Popovich MJ. The uterus and vagina. In: Higgins CB, Hricak H, Helms CA, Eds. Magnetic Resonance Imaging of the Body (2nd ed.). Raven Press, New York, 1992, pp 817–863

20. McCarthy S, Scott G, Majumdar S et al. Uterine junctional zone: MR study of water content and relaxation properties. Radiology 1989;171:241–243

21. Demas BE, Hricak H, Jaffe RB. Uterine MR imaging: effects of hormonal stimulation. Radiology 1986;159:123–126

22. Haynor DR, Mack LA, Soules MR et al. Changing appearance of the normal uterus during the menstrual cycle: MR studies. Radiology 1986;161:459–462

23. McCarthy S, Tauber C, Gore J. Female pelvic anatomy: MR assessment of variations during the menstrual cycle and with use of oral contraceptives. Radiology 1986;160:119–123

24. Carrington BM, Hricak H, Nuruddin RN et al. Müllerian duct anomalies: MR imaging evaluation. Radiology 1990;176:715–720

25. Fedele L, Dorta M, Brioschi D et al. Magnetic resonance evaluation of double uteri. Obstet Gynecol 1989;74:844–847

26. Fedele L, Dorta M, Brioschi D et al. Magnetic resonance imaging in Mayer-Rokitasky-Küster-Hauser syndrome. Obstet Gynecol 1990;76:593–596

27. Hamlin DJ, Pettersson H, Ramey SL, Moazam F. Magnetic resonance imaging of bicornuate uterus with unilateral hematometrosalpinx and ipsilateral renal agenesis. Urol Radiol 1986;8:52–55

28. Hricak H, Chang YC, Thurnher S. Vagina: evaluation with MR imaging. Part I. Normal anatomy and congenital anomalies. Radiology 1988;169:169–174

29. Mintz MC, Thickman DI, Gussman D, Kressel HY. MR evaluation of uterine anomalies. AJR Am J Roentgenol 1987;148:287–290

30. Pellerito JS, McCarthy SM, Doyle MB et al. Diagnosis of uterine anomalies: relative accuracy of MR imaging, endovaginal sonography, and hysterosalpingography. Radiology 1992;183:795–800

31. Togashi K, Nishimura K, Itoh K et al. Vaginal agenesis: classification by MR imaging. Radiology 1987;162:675–677

32. Fields SI, Katz S, Beyth Y. Computed tomography of unilateral hematometrocolpos. J Comput Assist Tomogr 1988;12:530–531

33. Cooperberg PL, Kidney MR. Ultrasound evaluation of the uterus. In: Callen PW, Ed. Ultrasonography in Obstetrics and Gynecology. WB Saunders Philadelphia 1988, pp 393–411

34. Reuter KL, Daly DC, Cohen SM. Septate versus bicornuate uteri: errors in imaging diagnosis. Radiology 1989;172:749–752

35. Mitchell DG, Mintz MC, Spritzer CE et al. Adnexal masses: MR imaging observations at 1.5 T, with US and CT correlations. Radiology 1987;162:319–324

36. Mitchell DG, Outwater EK. Benign gynecologic disease: applications of magnetic resonance imaging. Top Magn Reson Imag 1995;7:26–43

37. Hann LE, Hall DA, McArdle CR, Seibel M. Polycystic ovarian disease: sonographic spectrum. Radiology 1984;150:531–534

38. Yeh HC, Futterweit W, Thornton JC. Polycystic ovarian disease: US features in 104 patients. Radiology 1987;163:111–116

39. Mitchell DG, Gefter WB, Spritzer CE et al. Polycystic ovaries: MR imaging. Radiology 1986;160:425–429

40. Ablin A, Issacs H, Jr. Germ cell tumors. In: Pizzo PA, Poplack DG, Eds. Pediatric Oncology. JB Lippincott, Philadelphia, 1989, pp 713–731

41. Breen JL, Bonamo JF, Maxson WS. Genital Tract Tumors in Children. Pediatr Clin North Am 1981;28:355–367

42. Castleberry RP, Kelly DR, Joseph DB, Cain WS. Gonadal and extragonadal germ cell tumors. In: Fernbach DJ, Vietti TJ, Eds. Clinical Pediatric Oncology. Mosby Year Book, St. Louis, 1991, pp 577–594

43. Buy JN, Ghossain MA, Moss AA et al. Cystic teratoma of the ovary: CT detection. Radiology 1989;171:697–701

44. Muramatsu Y, Moriyama N, Takayasu K et al. CT and MR imaging of cystic ovarian teratoma with intracystic fat balls. J Comput Assist Tomogr 1991;15:528–529

45. Quillin SP, Siegel MJ. CT features of benign and malignant teratomas in children. J Comput Assist Tomogr 1992;16:722–726

46. Togashi K, Nishimura K, Itoh K et al. Ovarian cystic teratomas: MR imaging. Radiology 1987;162:669–673

47. Yamashita Y, Hatanaka Y, Torashima M et al. Mature cystic teratomas of the ovary without fat in the cystic cavity: MR features in 12 cases. AJR Am J Roentgenol 1994;163:613–616

48. Kier R, Smith RC, McCarthy SM. Value of lipid-and water-suppression MR images in distinguishing between blood and lipid within ovarian masses. AJR Am J Roentgenol 1992;158:321–325

49. Yamashita Y, Torashima M, Hatanaka Y et al. Value of phase-shift gradient-echo MR imaging in the differentiation of pelvic lesions with high signal intensity at T1-weighted imaging. Radiology 1994;191:759–764

50. Altman AJ, Schwartz AD. Tumors of the sexual organs. In: Altman AJ, Schwartz AD, Eds. Malignant Diseases of Infancy, Childhood and Adolescence (2nd ed.). WB Saunders, Philadelphia, 1983, pp 84–509

51. Ghossain MA, Buy NJ, Ligneres C et al. Epithelial tumors of the ovary: comparison of MR and CT findings. Radiology 1991;181:863–870

52. Cohen MD. Tumors involving multiple tissues or organs. In: Cohen MD, Ed. Imaging of Children with Cancer. Mosby Year Book, St. Louis, 1992, pp 308–369

53. Fletcher BD, Kaste SC. Magnetic resonance imaging for diagnosis and follow-up of genitourinary, pelvic, and perineal rhabdomyosarcoma. Urol Radiol 1992;14:263–272

54. Davis WK, McCarthy S, Moss AA, Braga C. Computed tomography of gestational trophoblastic disease. J Comput Assist Tomogr 1984;8:1136–1139

55. Sanders C, Rubin E. Malignant gestational trophoblastic disease: CT findings. AJR Am J Roentgenol 1987;148:165–168

56. Hricak H, Demas BE, Braga CA et al. Gestational trophoblastic neoplasm of the uterus: MR assessment. Radiology 1986;161:11–16

57. Bellah RD, Griscom NT. Torsion of normal uterine adnexa before menarche: CT appearance. AJR Am J Roentgenol 1989;152:123–124

58. Kimura I, Togashi K, Kawakami S et al. Ovarian torsion: CT and MR imaging appearances. Radiology 1994;190:337–341

59. Kawakami K, Murata K, Kawaguchi K et al. Hemorrhagic infarction of the diseased ovary: a common MR finding in two cases. Magn Reson Imaging 1993;11:595–597

60. Shafer MA, Sweet RL. Pelvic inflammatory disease in adolescent females. Epidemiology, pathogenesis, diagnosis, treatment, and sequelae. Pediatr Clin North Am 1989;36:513–532

61. Ellis JH, Francis IR, Rhodes M et al. CT findings in tuboovarian abscess. J Comput Assist Tomogr 1991;15:589–592

62. Wilbur AC, Aizenstein RI, Napp TE. CT findings in tuboovarian abscess. AJR Am J Roentgenol 1992;158:575–579

Ultrasonography of Pathologic Pregnancy Conditions

JOHN C. ANDERSON

JONATHAN CARTER

There have been few fields of medicine in which a new technology has been embraced as has ultrasound in obstetrics. The ability of ultrasound to image soft tissues allows the contents of the uterus to be seen as never before. The diagnosis of abortion, ectopic pregnancy, and gestational trophoblastic disease is now only as far away as the nearest ultrasound machine. This has completely changed obstetric care, including the first trimester, when patients no longer languish in a hospital bed for days waiting for a threatened miscarriage to declare itself. Now the diagnosis is made rapidly, allowing definitive treatment and resumption of a normal life.

ABORTION

There is no difference in the meaning of the words *abortion* or *miscarriage*, although laypersons often use the former when they mean that a pregnancy was terminated intentionally and the latter when they mean that the pregnancy terminated spontaneously. The conceptus is technically an embryo until 8 weeks after fertilization (10 menstrual weeks). Death of the embryo during the first few weeks is common, with only a small proportion recognized as spontaneous abortions. Many early pregnancy failures cause only a slightly late or unusually heavy period.

The principal cause of early pregnancy failure is a chromosomal abnormality, with at least 50% of all first-trimester abortions associated with changes in the number or structure of the chromosomal complement[1,2] (Fig. 27.1).

Other causes of first-trimester spontaneous abortion include certain viral syndromes, underlying maternal diseases, congenital abnormalities of the reproductive system, or the presence of an intrauterine contraceptive device (IUCD).

Threatened Abortion

An abortion is said to be *threatened* if vaginal bleeding occurs without pain during the first 20 weeks of pregnancy. The cervix is closed on visual examination. An ultrasound scan may show a normal pregnancy, or it may show an area of extramembranous hemorrhage. The prognosis for these pregnancies is good.

Complete and Incomplete

Abortion is said to be *complete* if all the products of conception are expelled. This can happen whether fetal heart motion is present or not. Usually, the products of conception are incompletely expelled in the first trimester, and trophoblast remains in the uterus, causing bleeding, pain, and potentially, infection. In a complete abortion, the uterus will be empty.

Inevitable

Inevitable abortion is due to cervical dilatation secondary to uterine contractions. It presents with vaginal bleeding and cramping lower abdominal pain. This results from prostaglandin release as the placenta and membranes separate from the uterine site. Once the internal os is dilated to 1 or 2 cm and products of conception occupy the cervical canal, the pregnancy will abort, either completely or incompletely. The diagnosis is usually clinical, and made by inspection of the external cervical os. Ultrasound may show a gestation sac with enclosed fetus and dilated cervical os, occasionally with membranes bulging through the os into the vagina. In the absence of pain and bleeding (i.e., if the condition is due to an incompetent cervix), it is occasionally possible to prevent a miscarriage by suturing the cervix closed.

Missed Abortion

A *missed abortion* refers to a nonviable pregnancy where the products of conception are retained in the uterine cavity 4 or more weeks after death. The symptoms of pregnancy subside, but there is maternal failure to recognize that the pregnancy is not ongoing, and there is no bleeding, and the products of conception are not expelled (Fig. 27.2).

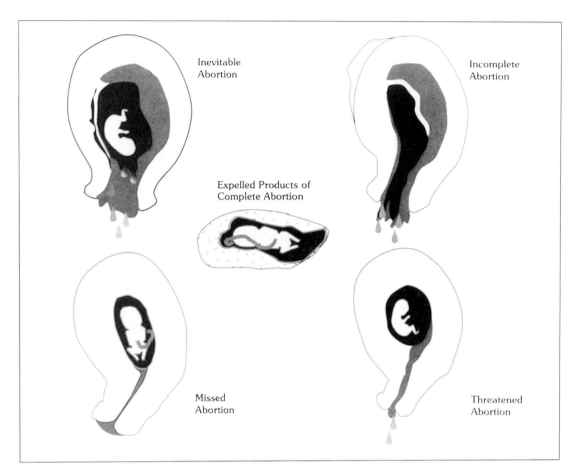

Figure 27.1 Diagrammatic illustrations demonstrating differences between threatened, inevitable, complete, incomplete, and missed abortions. (From Carter,[43] with permission.)

Figure 27.2 Missed abortion. Transvaginal echogram of an intrauterine gestation sac with enclosed fetus whose crown rump length equalled 9 weeks and 5 days. A previous scan and period of amenorrhea dated the pregnancy at 11 weeks and 3 days. Fetal heart movement was not present on real-time or M-mode. The pregnancy could be described as a missed abortion or early intrauterine fetal death.

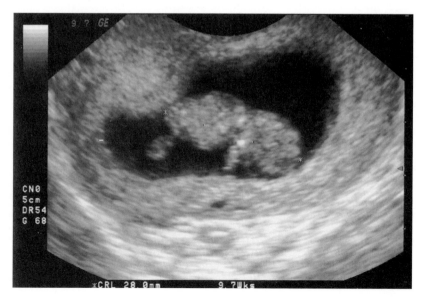

Blighted Ovum

In an elegant experiment in 1978 with manufactured hexa-parental mice, Markert and Petters[3] showed that, in the 64-celled mouse blastocyst, three cells, and probably only three, are the source of all adult tissue. Twelve cells become yolk sac, allantois, and amnion, and the remaining 49 become tropho-blast.

It seems reasonable to assume, therefore, that if an adverse event in embryogenesis results in the death of these three cells a pregnancy could continue for a time without a co-existent fetus. A gestation sac over 15 mm without fetal pole should be considered *anembryonic*. Otherwise it may be called a blighted ovum. Most anembryonic pregnancies are those where there has been early embryonic or fetal death. Transvaginal sonography (TVS) shows a gestation sac that is often larger than expected for the stated period of amenorrhea, and that usually becomes irregular in shape as time passes. In addition, the decidual reaction around the sac loses its bright echogenicity, and no fetus can be found (Fig. 27.3).

ECTOPIC GESTATION

Ectopic pregnancy can be defined as the implantation of a fertilized ovum outside the uterine cavity. The reported incidence is 1:90 pregnancies. Of these, 95% are tubal (ampullary, isthmic, fimbrial, or in the interstitial portion of the tube).[4] Ovarian, abdominal, and cervical ectopics are less common. Other rare sites of implantation include vaginal[5] and intraligamentous sites[6] (Fig. 27.4). A remarkable case of an intramyometrial ectopic pregnancy in a previous cesarean section scar is shown in Figure 27.5. This patient required an emergency hysterectomy to secure hemostasis.

There is an association between infertility and ectopic pregnancy. The increased incidence of multiple pregnancy with ovulation induction and in vitro fertilization further increases the risk for both ectopic and heterotopic (coexistent intrauterine and ectopic) gestation, with data suggesting the rate is 1 in 7,000 pregnancies[7,8] The hydrostatic forces generated during embryo transfer may also contribute to the increased risk.

Factors increasing the risk of ectopic pregnancy:

1. Any tubal abnormality that may prevent passage of the zygote or result in delayed transit
2. Infertility and patients undergoing ovulation induction or in vitro fertilization
3. Previous pelvic surgery
4. Previous tubal pregnancy
5. History of tubal reconstructive surgery or unsuccessful tubal ligation
6. Pelvic inflammatory disease or pelvic infection resulting in peritubal adhesions
7. IUCD usage
8. Salpingitis and damage to the tubal mucosa

The ectopic pregnancy undergoes hemorrhage, then detachment from the tube, followed by absorption or extrusion out of the tubal ostium, or rupture through the tubal wall. Pregnancy hormone production results in uterine enlargement and decidual reaction in the endometrium. Ectopic pregnancy presents with pain, abnormal vaginal bleeding, and a palpable adnexal mass,[9] and/or adnexal tenderness and usually a period of amenorrhea.

In cases of ectopic pregnancy, transvaginal ultrasound confirms the absence of an intrauterine gestation sac. Early identification of an adnexal mass and free fluid in the pelvis and the measurement of endometrial thickness increase the accu-

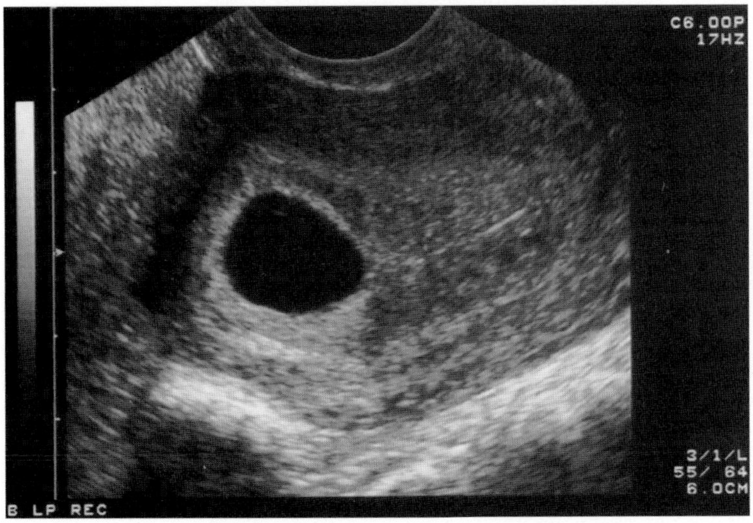

Figure 27.3 Blighted ovum. Transvaginal scan showing an enlarged uterus containing an empty gestation sac.

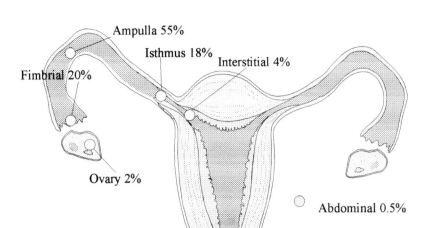

Figure 27.4 Relative frequency of sites of implantation of ectopic pregnancies.

racy of diagnosis. Correlation with serum β-human chorionic gonadotropin (β-hCG) (>25 IU/L) contributes to the diagnosis when the sonographic findings are nonspecific. An absolute diagnosis of ectopic pregnancy without surgery requires the demonstration of an extrauterine fetal heart. It is sometimes difficult to distinguish an ectopic pregnancy without a pseudogestation sac from an early normal or failed intrauterine pregnancy where no gestation sac can be seen. A pseudogestation sac results from fluid within the uterus producing a saclike appearance, resembling a gestation sac.

Scanning should include the uterus, the cavity, the endometrium, the cornual and cervical areas of the uterus, the adnexa, and the pouch of Douglas. Note should be taken of any transducer tenderness.

Ultrasound Findings

The ultrasound demonstration of a live embryo in the adnexa is specific for ectopic pregnancy (Fig. 27.6). Early pregnancy located outside the uterine cavity but developing normally

Figure 27.5 (A) Ectopic pregnancy in a cesarean section scar. A transabdominal sagittal scan through the distended bladder shows the gestation sac with enclosed living fetus below and in front of the empty uterine cavity. The patient required an emergency hysterectomy to control massive bleeding. (Courtesy of Dr. Glenn McNally, Sydney, Australia.) **(B)** Operative photograph of the gestation sac just before hysterectomy. (Courtesy of Dr. Mark Beale, Sydney, Australia.)

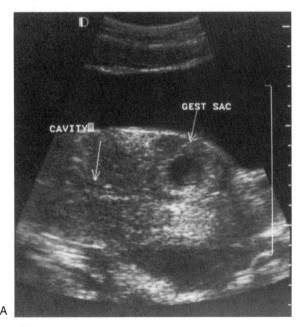

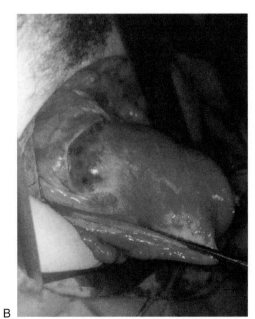

will resemble a normal intrauterine pregnancy. A nonruptured tubal ectopic pregnancy will be on the same side as the corpus luteum in 85% of cases. A comparison should be made of the tubal ring and the corpus luteum after both structures are examined separately.

The decidual-chorionic lines (double-decidual sign) are used to identify an intrauterine pregnancy before the visualization of the yolk sac or embryo, but in certain cases, these are unreliable. The double-decidual sign is to be distinguished from the decidual cast or pseudogestion sac of ectopic pregnancy.[10] A decidual cast is an intrauterine fluid collection surrounded by a single decidual layer as opposed to the two concentric rings of the double-decidual sign.

Color flow Doppler may also provide additional differentiation between a true intrauterine pregnancy and the pseudogestation sac of an ectopic pregnancy.[11] An abundant blood supply around the trophoblast will be demonstrated with an ectopic pregnancy. An ectopic tubal ring may be present, consisting of a hyperechoic trophoblastic decidual ring around the hypoechoic chorionic cavity. The fallopian tube may be visualized as a distended, fusiform structure, containing echogenic fluid (blood).

The presence of echogenic free fluid (hemoperitoneum) or blood in the pouch of Douglas suggests a ruptured or leaking ectopic pregnancy in patients without sonographic evidence of an intrauterine pregnancy. Fluid in the pouch of Douglas is found in between 10% and 30% of cases.[12–16]

Sonography of a cornual/interstitial pregnancy will show a bulge in the cornual area of the uterus where an extremely thin myometrial mantle surrounds the hyperechoic trophoblastic ring of a more advanced gestation sac.[17]

Cervical pregnancy is rarely seen. The cervix will contain a chorionic sac with enclosed fetal or embryonic heartbeats. Sonographically, the intact sac will be seen passing through the cervix. Color Doppler sonography will detect the uterine artery containing the chorionic sac at the level of the cervix.[18] The uterine cavity will be empty. These pregnancies can result in heavy bleeding, which is difficult to control, as the cervix is poor at contracting, because it contains few muscle fibers. Methotrexate by ultrasound-guided injection is sometimes used to stop development of the pregnancy and allow regression of the sac, reducing the risk of bleeding from subsequent curettage.

Ovarian pregnancy is rare and may be difficult to diagnose. On ultrasound, when the ovary contains the hyperechoic trophoblastic ring and the ovary can be independently displaced, an ovarian ectopic pregnancy should be considered.

Ultrasound is valuable for localizing abdominal pregnancy. The diagnosis is suggested if the empty uterus is seen separate from the fetus, there is no uterine mantle around the pregnancy or fetus, the placenta is an unusual location, or fetal structures are "crowded" due to extreme oligohydramnios.[19] In any case of an unusual abdominal mass in the reproductive years, one should keep in mind the possibility of an abdominal pregnancy. A search for fetal heart movement may give the clue to an unusual diagnosis.

GESTATIONAL TROPHOBLASTIC NEOPLASIA

Incidence

Approximately 85% of patients with a hydatidiform mole will follow a benign course after evacuation, while 15% will subsequently develop locally invasive disease, and 5% eventually prove to have metastatic lesions. Risk factors for the development of persistent or recurrent disease includes age greater than 40 years, a uterus large for dates, a high initial hCG titer, marked trophoblast proliferation, and a blood group of AB or B.

Symptoms

Presenting symptoms of persistence or recurrence include irregular vaginal bleeding; theca-lutein cysts; uterine subinvolution or asymmetric enlargement, and most importantly, persistently elevated or abnormally regressing serum hCG titers. Trophoblast may perforate the myometrium, causing intraperitoneal bleeding, or erode into uterine vessels, causing vaginal bleeding. Bulky necrotic tumor may involve the uterine wall and serve as a nidus for infection, leading to pelvic pain and vaginal discharge.

Partial hydatidiform moles can also have malignant sequelae, but in contrast to complete moles, no cases of choriocarcinoma have been documented after partial hydatidiform mole. When metastases occur, they are generally found in the lungs, vagina, vulva, and broad ligament;[20–24] however, they may also appear in the brain, liver, and heart.

Diagnosis

The diagnosis of persistent or recurrent disease is confirmed by an abnormal regression of the hCG titer. A metastatic survey is then performed to document disease extent, and then a

Figure 27.6 Ectopic pregnancy. The gestation sac is seen outside the uterus. A yolk sac and fetal heart movement are seen within the gestational sac, confirming the diagnosis.

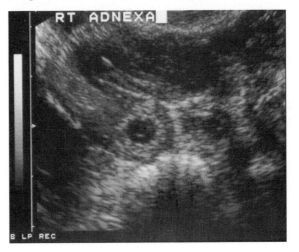

stage or prognostic scoring level is assigned. The classic ultrasound appearance of a hydatidiform mole will result in multiple small sonolucent areas, which correspond to the "grape-like" vesicles seen on gross inspection. These changes are usually seen after 10 weeks' gestation because the trophoblastic proliferation and hydropic changes are not present earlier. Early detection by TVS has resulted in the reduced incidence of molar pregnancy, as the products of conception are evacuated before they undergo further hydropic change and proliferation.[25]

With TVS, the diagnosis of invasive or recurrent gestational trophoblastic disease can be documented by demonstrating lesions invading the myometrium[17] (Figs. 27.7 and 27.8). Transabdominal sonography and computed tomography are suboptimal and may miss these lesions. The trophoblastic implants can be monitored throughout therapy. Figure 27.9 shows the correlation between lesion size and β-hCG titer in such a patient. As the β-hCG titer regresses, there appears to be an initial lag in the regression of the tumor implant. There is an inverse relationship between the β-hCG titer, tumor size, and the pulsatility index (PI).

Residual trophoblastic tissue within the uterine cavity is easily diagnosed by TVS (Plate 27.1), and this may be the only indication for a repeat curettage. When the only residual disease is in the myometrium and the uterus is empty, a repeat curette is unhelpful. While β-hCG titers remain the main determinant of treatment of gestational trophoblastic disease, we have been able to demonstrate that TVS with color flow Doppler is a useful adjunct in the following:

1. Determining the site of the persistent focus of trophoblast in gestational trophoblastic disease.

2. Monitoring its response to therapy.

3. Assessing adnexal pathology.

4. Allowing treatment response to be assessed while awaiting results of the β-hCG titer because uterine artery and intratumoral PI correlate with β-hCG titer.

Tumor Markers

hCG is a glycoprotein hormone composed of α and β-subunits and is similar to the other glycoprotein hormones produced by the pituitary. The α-subunits are essentially identical, while the β-subunits, although structurally similar, differ to an extent that confers specific biologic sensitivity on the intact hormone. The antigenic properties of glycoprotein hormones paved the way for development of radioimmunoassay (RIA) procedures to quantify hormone concentrations in small amounts of body fluid. In the case of hCG, RIA-enhanced hormone sensitivity is approximately 100-fold over that of bioassays, making it the method of choice for monitoring gestational trophoblastic disease.[19]

β-subunit assays allow hCG to be measured selectively in concentrations as low as 5 mIU/ml. Until recently, the measurement of free β-subunit has received little attention because of the difficulties encountered in trying to discriminate between the free subunit and intact hCG. Antibodies against the β-subunit usually recognize the intact hormone (the basis for the β-subunit RIA), and separation of the β-subunit from hCG was difficult. Nonetheless, evidence suggests that free β-subunit accounts for as much as 15% of the total β-subunit immunoactivity present in sera from patients with choriocarcinoma.[25] Khazaeli et al.[26] found a high ratio of free β-subunit to total hCG in patients who went on to develop persistent disease, a finding that holds promise for using this assay in the early identification of high-risk patients.

Figure 27.7 An isoechoic, well-circumscribed lesion within the myometrium.

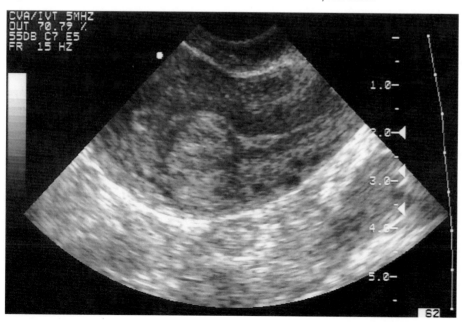

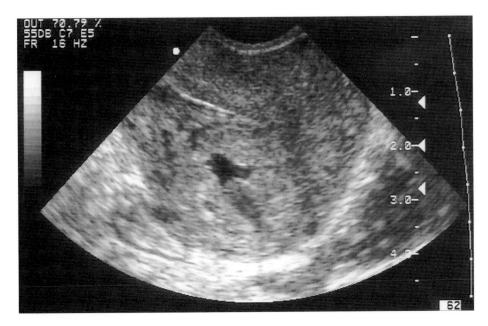

Figure 27.8 An isoechoic lesion with cystic component within the myometrium with extension through to the uterine serosa.

Treatment

Repeat Uterine Curettage

The long-standing practice of routinely recuretting patients after a hydatidiform mole to remove residual tissue is of little value and may be harmful, at least if the initial evacuation has been accomplished by suction curettage.[27]

Hysterectomy

If metastatic disease is excluded, then a hysterectomy may be indicated to remove the focus of resistant tumor in older patients who have completed their childbearing. It should be performed under a chemotherapy "window" to provide an extra safeguard against potential metastatic spread.

Chemotherapy

The main indication for chemotherapy is an abnormal serum hCG regression. Brewer et al,[28] studying hCG regression, found 15% patients with elevated titers at 60 days after evacuation. Of these patients, half had choriocarcinoma and the other half had invasive moles. In the United States, there is a more liberal attitude toward treatment. Serum β-hCG values rising for 2 weeks (3 weekly titers) or values on a plateau ($\pm$ 10%) for 3 weeks or more, or the presence of metastasis are all indications for chemotherapy.

In general, patients assigned to a low-risk prognostic scoring group may be adequately treated with methotrexate alone, while patients in the (high-risk) treatment failure group are given combination, multiagent chemotherapy, and the currently advocated regimen is the EMA/CO (etoposide-methotrexate-actinomycin-D-cytoxan-oncovin) regimen

Figure 27.9 Graph showing tumor size, PI, and Log β-hCG titers throughout therapy.

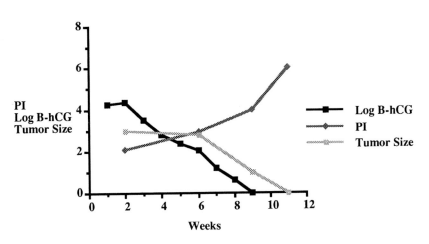

Choriocarcinoma

Choriocarcinoma, or invasive mole with metastasis, is a malignant form of gestational trophoblastic disease where there is abnormal proliferation of trophoblastic tissue following a gestational event. It is usually preceded by a molar pregnancy (50%), abortion (25%), normal pregnancy (22%), and after an ectopic pregnancy (3%).[29] The tumor tends to metastasize to the liver, lung, brain, gastrointestinal tract, and bone, where bleeding may ensue.

Ultrasound may show a large, irregular, echogenic mass occupying the uterine cavity. The disease involves local myometrial invasion with increased tissue proliferation. Irregular cystic areas within the mass may be visible as a result of internal hemorrhage.

Color Doppler is useful in the evaluation of low impedance values inside the richly vascularized tissue of the lesion.[30]

Placental Site Trophoblastic Tumor

Placental site trophoblastic tumor is a neoplasm composed predominantly of intermediate trophoblast. It is generally benign but may be highly malignant. It resembles the trophoblastic infiltration of the endometrium, and the myometrium of the placental bed is the rarest form of gestational trophoblastic disease.

Typically, patients are of reproductive years with either amenorrhea or abnormal bleeding, often with uterine enlargement, and a positive pregnancy test.

These tumors often invade through the myometrium to the serosa, causing perforation.[31] Invasion deep into the myometrium, broad ligament and the ovary has been reported.[32,33]

INFLAMMATORY CONDITIONS

Infection

Postoperative pelvic infection tends to arise in an area of devascularized, damaged tissue or in a hematoma.

Patients who become infected following induced abortion will present with abdominal pain, purulent vaginal discharge, and often, vaginal bleeding. The cervix may be open, and products of conception palpable. The uterus is often enlarged, boggy to palpation, and tender. Tender masses may be felt in the adnexa, and there may be evidence of trauma to the vagina or cervix.

PELVIC MASSES IN PREGNANCY

Uterine Fibroids

Uterine fibroids are commonly found in 0.3% to 2.6% of all pregnancies.[34] Large fibroids can complicate pregnancy by causing an increase in spontaneous abortions and ectopic pregnancies in early pregnancy, premature labor, placental abruption, fetal malpresentation, and soft tissue dystocia during labor.[35]

Ultrasound appearances will usually show an irregularly shaped uterine wall. There may be indistinct margins between uterus and fibroids because they have originated from the uterine wall (Fig. 27.10). Encapsulation and pedunculation of the fibroid occasionally occur, and these will appear separate from the uterus.

Fibroids have variable internal echo texture depending on the degree of degenerative change within. Solid fibrous connective tissue within a fibroid that has not undergone degeneration will have decreased echogenicity. Carneous degeneration caused by acute disruption of the blood supply and consequently necrosis and infarction will show increased echogenicity and the appearance of cystic areas.

Ovarian Tumors

The majority of ovarian tumors found in pregnancy are asymptomatic and benign and may be an incidental finding at any stage. Routine ultrasound examinations have shown an ovarian mass once in every 190 to 350 pregnancies, more common than are clinically detected. Ovarian tumors are commonly physiologic (corpora lutea); however, benign dermoid cysts and benign cystadenomas occur with decreasing frequency. Malignant neoplasms are rare and are found in less than 1% of ovarian neoplasms in pregnancy.[36,37]

The signs and symptoms produced by ovarian tumors in pregnancy need to be differentiated from other pathology. The ultrasound appearances of size, shape, and echogenicity assist in making a diagnosis.

Corpus luteum cysts are commonly found early in pregnancy.[38] They are typically unilocular, unilateral, less than 5 cm in size, and usually resolve spontaneously as the pregnancy progresses.[36] Theca-lutein cysts, which accompany 25% of hydatidiform moles, are bilateral, and the patient is likely to develop trophoblastic disease.[39]

Figure 27.10 Late first-trimester pregnancy with co-existing fibroid.

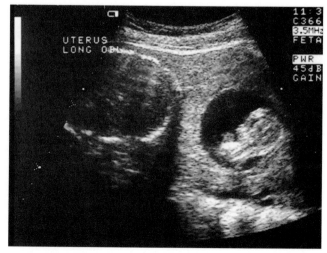

Aspiration of single unilocular cysts (5 to 10 cm in diameter) under ultrasound guidance can be performed safely and effectively. Laparotomy is usually required for cysts over 10 cm, multilocular cysts, cysts with solid components, and endometriomata, or if there is clinical evidence of rupture or torsion.[40]

Ultrasound appearances of malignant tumors usually show multilocular cysts with thick septa, solid areas within the tumor, invasion of the capsule, fixation, and free fluid in the abdomen. Color Doppler shows angiogenesis within the tumor.[41,42]

Intervention in a pregnancy that is complicated by ovarian tumor or pelvic mass is governed by the extent of clinical signs and symptoms and the stage of pregnancy.

SUMMARY

There are numerous uses of ultrasound in the investigation of the pathologic pregnancy and in the pregnancy complicated by other conditions. Future technical improvements can be expected to increase further the indications for ultrasound in pregnancy.

REFERENCES

1. Rushton D. Examination of products of conception from previable human pregnancies. J Clin Pathol 1981;34:819–835
2. Boue A, Boue J. Consequences of chromosome observations on the development of human conceptuses. In: Van Juhsingha EN, Tesh JM, Fara GM, Eds. Advances in the Detection of Congenital Malformations. European Teratology Society, Vienna, 1978, pp 33–49
3. Markert CL, Petters RM. Manufactured hexaparental mice show that adults are derived from three embryonic cells. Science 1978;202:56–58
4. Cartwright PS. Ectopic pregnancy. In: Jones HW III, Wentz AC, Burnett LC, eds. Novak's Textbook of Gynecology (11th ed.). Williams & Wilkins, Baltimore, 1988, pp 479–506
5. Duckman S, Suarez J, Spitaleri J. Vaginal pregnancy presenting as a suburethral cyst. Am J Obstet Gynecol 1984;149:572–573
6. Kobak AJ, Fields C, Pollack SL. Intraligamentary pregnancy: the extraperitoneal type of abdominal pregnancy. Am J Obstet Gynecol 1955;70:175–184
7. Hann LE, Bachman DM, McArdle CR. Coexistent intrauterine and ectopic pregnancy; a re-evaluation. Radiology 1984;152:151–154
8. Wong WSF, Mao K. Combined intrauterine and tubal ectopic pregnancy. Aust NZ J Obstet Gynecol 1989;29:76–77
9. Schwartz RO, Di Pietro DL. *b*-hCG as a diagnostic aid for suspected ectopic pregnancy. Obstet Gynecol 1980;56:197–203
10. Nelson PA, Bowie JD, Rosenberg ER. Early intrauterine pregnancy or decidual cast: An anatomic-sonographic approach. J Ultrasound Med 1983;2:543
11. Pellerito JS, Taylor KJW. Ectopic pregnancy. In: Copel JA, Reed KL, Eds. Doppler Ultrasound in Obstetrics and Gynecology. Raven Press, New York, 1994, p 41
12. Stiller RJ, de Regt RH, Blair E. Transvaginal ultrasonography in patients at risk for ectopic pregnancy. Am J Obstet Gynecol 1989;161:930–933
13. Fleischer AC, Pennell RG, McKee MS et al. Ectopic pregnancy: features at transvaginal ultrasonography. Radiology 1990;174:375–378
14. Rottem S, Thaler I, Timor-Trisch IE. Classification of tubal gestation by transvaginal ultrasonography. Ultrasound Obstet Gynecol 1991;1:197
15. Romero R, Copel JA, Kadar N et al. Value of culdocentesis in the diagnosis of ectopic pregnancy. Obstet Gynecol 1985;65:319–322
16. Timor-Trisch IE, Peisner DB, Monteagudo A. Transvaginal sonography in the diagnosis of ectopic pregnancy. In: Grunfeld L, ed. Ultrasonography in Reproductive Medicine. Infertil Reprod Clin North Am 1991;2:727–739
17. Jafri SZ, Loginsky SJ, Bouffard JA, Selis JE. Sonographic detection of interstitial pregnancy. J Clin Ultrasound 1987;15:253–257
18. Timor-Trisch IE, Monteagudo A, Mandeville EO et al. Successful management of viable cervical pregnancy by local injection of methotrexate guided by transvaginal sonography. Am J Obstet Gynecol 1994;170:737–739
19. Hertz RH, Timor-Trisch IE, Sokol RJ, Zador I. Diagnostic studies and fetal assessment in advanced extrauterine pregnancy. Obstet Gynecol 1977;50:63–65
20. Acosta-Sison H. Chorioadenoma destruens. A report of 41 cases. Am J Obstet Gynecol 1960;80:176
21. Hsu CT, Huang LC, Chen TY. Metastases in benign hydatidiform mole and chorioadenoma destruens. Am J Obstet Gynecol 1962;84:1412
22. Johnson TR, Comstock CH, Anderson DG. Benign gestational trophoblastic disease metastatic to pleura: unusual case of hemothorax. Obstet Gynecol 1979;53:509
23. Thiele RA, de Alvarez RR. Metastasizing benign trophoblastic tumors. Am J Obstet Gynecol 1962;84:1395
24. Wilson RB, Hunter JS, Jr, Dockerty MB. Chorioadenoma destruens. Am J Obstet Gynecol 1961;81:546–559
25. Jakob A, Jr, Overi L, Ditroi P et al. How does first trimester ultrasound influence the incidence of molar pregnancies? Ultrasound Obstet Gynecol 1994;4:50
26. Khazaeli MB, Hedayat, MM, Hatch KD et al. Radioimmunoassay of free beta-subunit of human chorionic gonadotropin as a prognostic test for persistent trophoblastic disease in molar pregnancy. Am J Obstet Gynecol 1986;155:320–324
27. Lao TT, Lee FH, Yeung SS. Repeat curettage after evacuation of hydatidiform nole. An appraisal. Acta Obstet Gynecol Scand 1987;66:305–307
28. Brewer JI, Eckman TR, Dolkart RE et al. Gestational trophoblastic disease. A comparative study of the results of therapy in patients with invasive mole and with choriocarcinoma. Am J Obstet Gynecol 1971;109:335–340
29. Callen PW. Ultrasound evaluation of gestational trophoblastic disease. In: Callen PW, Ed. Ultrasonography in Obstetrics and Gynecology (2nd ed.). WB Saunders, Philadelphia, 1988, pp 412–422
30. Kurjak A, Matijevic R, Kupesic S, Malda K. Gestational trophoblastic disease. In: Kurjak A, Ed. An Atlas of Transvaginal Color Doppler. Parthenon Publishing Group, London, 1994, p 125
31. Kurman RJ, Scully RE, Norris HJ. Trophoblastic pseudotumour

of the uterus. An exaggerated form of "syncytial endometritis" simulating a malignant tumour. Cancer 1976;38:1214–1226

32. Eckstein RP, Paradinas FJ, Bagshawe KD. Placental site trophoblastic tumour (trophoblastic pseudotumour): A study of four cases requiring hysterectomy, including one fatal case. Histopathology 1982;6:211–226

33. Kurman RJ, Scully RE, Norris HJ. Trophoblastic pseudotumour of the uterus. An exaggerated form of "syncytial endometritis" simulating a malignant tumour. Cancer 1976;38:1214–1226

34. Bezjin AA. Pelvic masses in pregnancy. Clin Obstet Gynecol 1984;27:402

35. Von Minsky LI. Sonographic study of uterine fibro-myomata in the non-pregnant state and during gestation. In: Sanders RC, James AE, eds. Ultrasonography in Obstetrics and Gynecology. Appleton-Century-Crofts, East Norwalk, CT, 1977, pp 297–328

36. Thornton JG, Wells M. Ovarian cyst in pregnancy: does ultrasound make traditional management inappropriate? Obstet Gynecol 1987;69:717–721

37. Hogston P, Lilford RJ. Ultrasound study of ovarian cysts in pregnancy: pregnancy: prevalence and significance. Br J Obstet Gynaecol 1986;93:625–628

38. Lavery JP, Koontz WL, Layman L et al. Sonographic evaluation of the adnexa during early pregnancy. Surg Gynecol Obstet 1986;163:319–323

39. Montz FJ, Schlaerth JB, Morrow CP. The natural history of theca lutein cysts. Obstet Gynecol 1988;72:247–251

40. Bider D, Ben-Rafael Z, Goldenberg M et al. Pregnancy outcome after unwinding of twisted ischaemic-haemorrhagic adnexa. Br J Obstet Gynecol 1989;96:428–430

41. Kurjak A, Zalud I, Jurkovic D et al. Transvaginal colour Doppler for the assessment of pelvic circulation. Acta Obstet Gynecol Scand 1989;68:131–135

42. Bourne T, Campbell S, Steer C et al. Transvaginal Color flow imaging; a possible new screening technique for ovarian cancer. Br Med J 1989;299:1367–1379

43. Carter J. An Atlas of Transvaginal Sonography. Lippincott Raven, Philadelphia, 1994, p III

Computed Tomography and Magnetic Resonance Imaging of Pathologic Conditions of Pregnancy

HYUN KWON HA

Ultrasound is usually the imaging method of choice for abortion, ectopic pregnancy, and gestational trophoblastic neoplasm, but magnetic resonance imaging (MRI) is sometimes used in equivocal cases or for staging of neoplasms. The value of MRI for specific diagnosis of pregnancy-related diseases is limited because most conditions appear as a nonspecific hemorrhagic mass on conventional T1- and T2-weighted images.[1,2]

INCOMPLETE ABORTION

The fetus and placenta are likely to be expelled together in abortions occurring before the 10th week, but separately thereafter.[3] When the placenta is retained in the uterus, ensuing bleeding is the principal sign of incomplete abortion. On T1- and T2-weighted images, a nonspecific heterogeneous or hemorrhagic mass is seen in the distended endometrial cavity. Without a clinical history, differentiating hemorrhagic masses from other conditions is impossible on conventional T1- and T2-weighted images. Contrast-enhanced MRI can demonstrate retained fetoplacental tissues because they are densely enhanced (Fig. 28.1).

ECTOPIC PREGNANCY

Ectopic pregnancy occurs when a fertilized ovum implants anywhere other than the uterine cavity. Although the most common location is the fallopian tube (90%), a zygote may implant in abdominal, ovarian, intraligamentous, cornual, intramural, or cervical sites. The diagnosis should be considered when uterine bleeding or pain in the lower abdomen occurs after the first 1 to 8 weeks after a missed menstrual period.[4] Rupture of the tube or uterus can be a catastrophic event because of massive hemorrhage and shock.

Tubal Form

Although many patients present with abdominal pain and shock, those patients with a clinically stable or "leaking" ectopic pregnancy pose a diagnostic challenge. MRI shows a pelvic fluid collection when an ectopic pregnancy is ruptured. The hemoperitoneum is hyperintense or isointense on T1-weighted images. An adnexal mass is seen in all patients and shows mixed or increased signal intensity on T1-weighted images and heterogeneity on T2-weighted images (Fig. 28.2). The heterogeneity may be associated with the repeated onset of hemorrhage, resulting in a mixture of blood of various ages. After contrast, adnexal masses often contain densely enhancing solid components of various sizes and consistencies (Fig. 28.2). These enhancing components, as with other forms of ectopic pregnancy, represent a remnant of fetoplacental tissues. A thin-walled theca-lutein cyst is often present.

The computed tomographic (CT) appearance of ruptured tubal ectopic pregnancy is very similar to the appearance on MRI. On contrast-enhanced CT, an adnexal mass is mostly cystic, with inhomogeneous attenuation due to the presence of hematoma (Fig. 28.3), and it contains densely enhancing solid components of fetoplacental tissue. The wall of an adnexal mass is sometimes thickened, and, if adhesions develop between the mass and adjacent small bowel loops, the walls of adjacent bowel loops are thickened. If a theca-lutein cyst is present on the same side as an ectopic pregnancy, it may simulate a multiseptate cystic mass. A hemoperitoneum can be diagnosed when a collection shows high attenuation compared to the surrounding muscles or shows a layering with higher attenuation in the dependent portion.

Uterine Ectopic

Compared with tubal pregnancy, uterine forms of ectopic pregnancy involving the cervix or the interstitial part of the tube are rare, but they can present a diagnostic problem in which MRI may be useful. The products of conception in

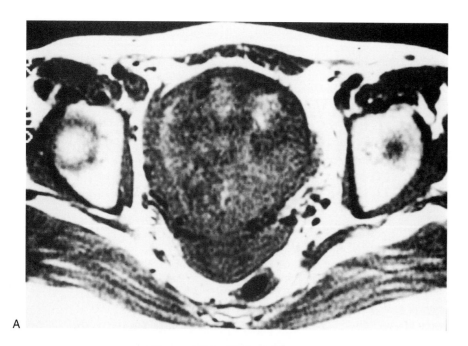

A

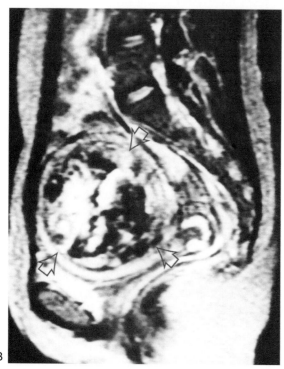

B

Figure 28.1 Incomplete abortion in a 37-year-old woman. **(A)** Axial T1-weighted image (TR400/TE15) shows a mass with scattered areas of hyperintensity in the enlarged uterus. **(B)** Sagittal T2-weighted image (TR800/TE80) shows a heterogeneous mass occupying and dilating the endometrial cavity (arrows). (*Figure continues.*)

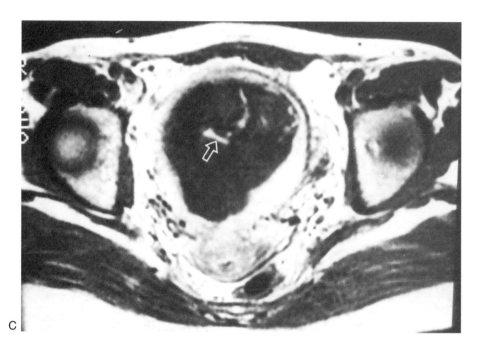

C

Figure 28.1 *(Continued).* **(C)** Axial contrast-enhanced image (TR400/TE15) shows densely enhancing fetoplacental tissues (arrow) within the mass in the endometrial cavity.

these patients cannot be completely removed, because the implantation site is inaccessible. Despite their uncommon occurrence, uterine forms of ectopic pregnancy have a higher mortality rate than tubal pregnancies.[5–8]

On MRI, an abnormal gestation sac appears as a well-defined, circumscribed uterine mass, sometimes hyperintense, isointense, or hypointense compared to the myometrium on T1-weighted images and heterogeneous on T2-weighted images (Fig. 28.4). The heterogeneity of this mass may be caused by the blood from hemorrhages occurring at various times before MRI. Using conventional T1- and T2-weighted images, distinguishing intrauterine forms of ectopic pregnancy from gestational trophoblastic tumors (especially choriocarcinoma) is impossible due to their similar morphologic and signal intensity patterns. However, a characteristic appearance of densely enhancing treelike solid components (Fig. 28.4) has been reported in these patients on contrast-enhanced MRI.[9] These proved to be fibrin strands and villous structures in a remnant of fetoplacental tissues. They are thought to be unique in cases of ectopic pregnancy and cannot be demonstrated by ultrasound.

Bader-Armstrong and colleagues[10] reported that T2-weighted images of a viable cervical pregnancy showed a homogeneously hyperintense gestation sac. MRI findings vary, because a dead fetus after 12 weeks may undergo fibrosis, skeletonization, saponification, mummification (Fig. 28.5), calcification, or adipous degeneration.[4,8]

Abdominal Pregnancy

Abdominal pregnancy is also one of the rare forms of ectopic pregnancy. The gestation sac is implanted on the abdominal peritoneum, and the diagnosis is difficult to make on ultrasound, as it is easy to miss the absence of myometrium around

the gestation sac. It is important to be aware that the condition exists and to think of it in unusual cases, or the diagnosis will not be made. These patients can reach term, and then require delivery abdominally (Fig. 28.6).

GESTATIONAL TROPHOBLASTIC NEOPLASIA

Gestational trophoblastic neoplasms (GTN) include hydatidiform mole, locally invasive mole, placental site trophoblastic tumor, and choriocarcinoma. Since the introduction of chemotherapeutic agents in 1956, the prognosis for GTN has improved dramatically. Even in the aggressive choriocarcinoma, which metastasizes to the lung, liver, and brain, multiagent chemotherapy achieves a complete remission in over 90% of patients.[11,12] Invasive mole can be treated with single-agent chemotherapy, and it is therefore important to make the correct diagnosis and avoid multiagent therapy with its associated severe toxicity.[11,12] Ultrasound is reliable and sensitive for the diagnosis of molar pregnancy, but MRI has become more useful for tumor detection and for staging trophoblastic diseases. CT is of limited value because of the difficulty obtaining multiplanar images and in making the distinction between endometrium and myometrium.

Hydatidiform Mole

Hydatidiform moles may be complete or partial. Complete moles do not have any fetal tissue, and the villi show generalized hydatidiform swelling and diffuse trophoblastic hyperplasia. The karyotype is 46, XX in 90% of cases,[13] and the chro-

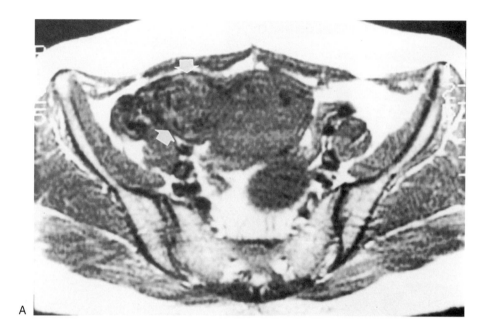

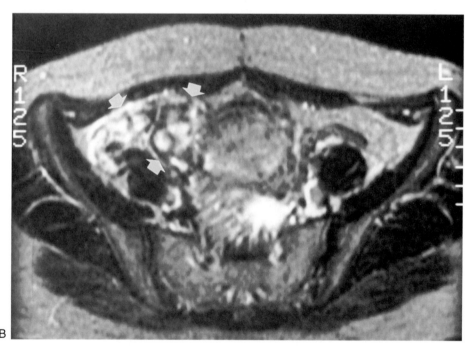

Figure 28.2 Ruptured tubal pregnancy in a 23-year-old woman. **(A)** Axial T1-weighted image (TR400/TE19) shows a heterogeneous mass (arrows) with focal areas of hyperintensity in the right adnexal region. **(B)** Axial T2-weighted image (TR2,000/TE80) shows a heterogeneous mass (arrows) in the right adnexa. (*Figure continues.*)

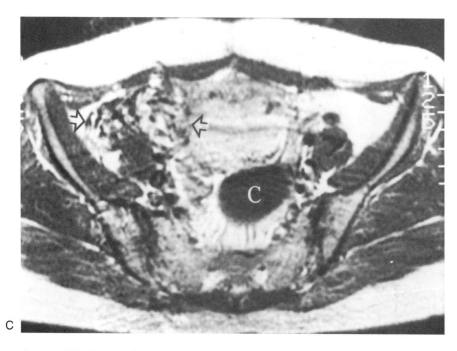

C

Figure 28.2 *(Continued)*. **(C)** Contrast-enhanced image (TR400/TE19) shows densely enhancing solid components in the right adnexal mass (arrows). A theca-lutein cyst (C) is also seen posterior to the uterus.

mosomes are almost always paternal in origin.[14] It is thought that complete moles follow fertilization of an ovum by a haploid sperm, which then duplicates its own chromosomes while the chromosomes from the ovum are lost or absent. In those moles with a 46,XY karyotype, the chromosomes have also been found to be paternal. Partial moles usually have identifiable fetal tissue and present with symptoms and signs of an incomplete or missed abortion. The ultrasound image is that of an incomplete or missed abortion, and the diagnosis is often made only after histologic examination of the curettings. They

Figure 28.3 Ruptured tubal pregnancy in a 30-year-old woman. Contrast-enhanced CT shows a mostly cystic mass with inhomogeneous attenuation of the fluid content and enhancing solid components in the right adnexal region.

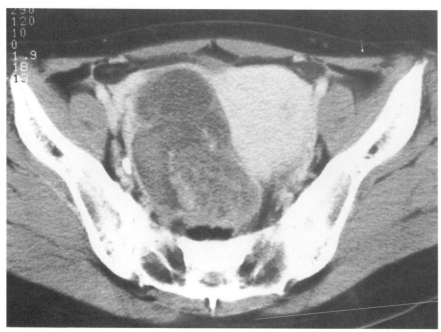

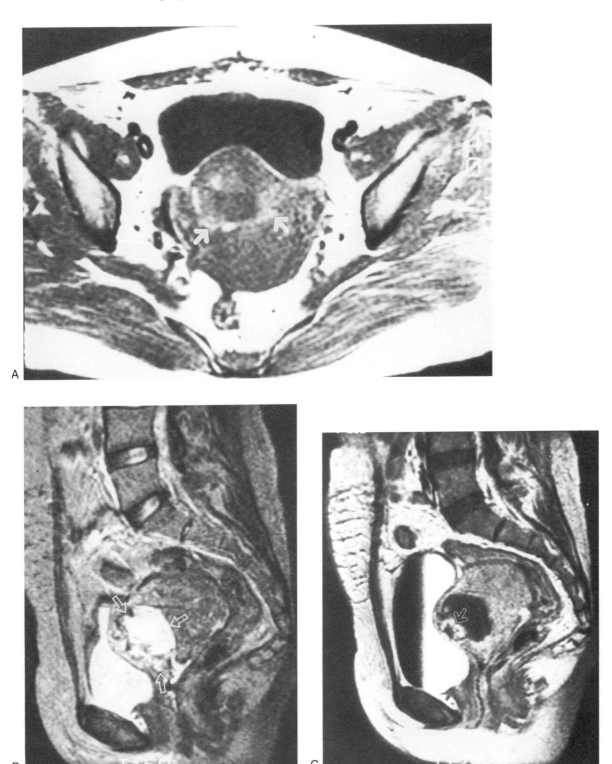

Figure 28.4 Interstitial pregnancy in a 32-year-old woman. **(A)** Axial T1-weighted image (TR600/TE11) shows a mass (arrows) with peripheral hyperintensity in the uterus. **(B)** Sagittal T2-weighted image (TR2000/TE80) shows a heterogeneous mass (arrows) in the isthmic portion of the tube. **(C)** Sagittal contrast-enhanced image (TR600/TE11) shows densely enhancing solid components (arrow) in the anterior aspect of the mass. (*Figure continues.*)

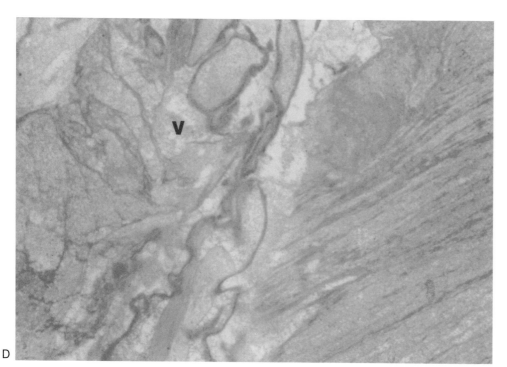

Figure 28.4 (*Continued*).
(**D**) Photomicrograph obtained from the densely enhancing solid components in Figure C show fibrin strands and villous structures (V) in the fetoplacental tissues (hematoxylin and eosin stain, ×400).

Figure 28.5 Mummified abdominal pregnancy with a lithopedion in a 56-year-old woman. (**A**) Plain abdominal radiograph shows a full-term fetus with calcified amniotic sac and twisted and calcified umbilical cord (C). (**B**) Unenhanced CT shows calcified amniotic sac and umbilical cord (arrow) with preservation of fetal skeletons.

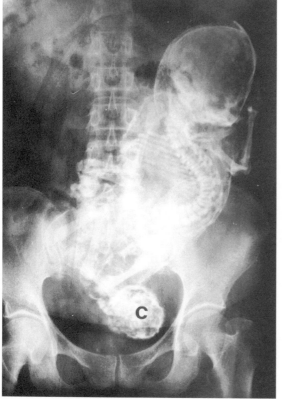

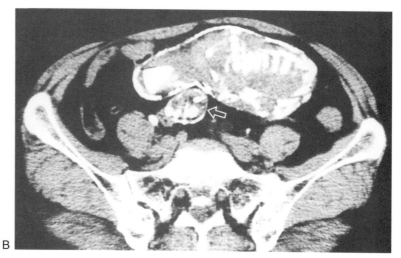

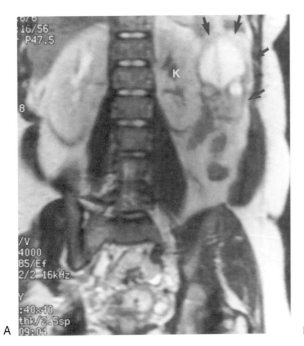 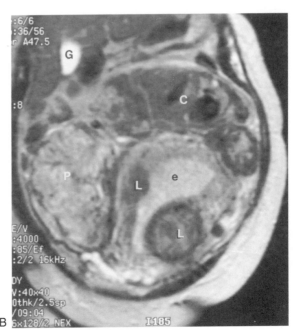

Figure 28.6 MRI of abdominal pregnancy. The patient underwent an exploratory laparotomy at 31 weeks' gestation. Both mother and baby did well postoperatively. **(A)** Coronal T2-weighted image demonstrates the head of a fetus (arrows) in the left upper quadrant of the abdomen, adjacent to the left kidney (K). **(B)** Coronal T2-weighted image more anteriorly demonstrates the empty endometrial cavity of the uterus (e) and leiomyomas scattered throughout the myometrium (L). The placenta (P) is located adjacent to the uterus, in the right lower quadrant of the abdomen. C, sigmoid colon; G, gallbladder. (Courtesy of Dr. Kathryn Occhipinti, Fort Lauderdale, Florida.)

usually have a triploid karyotype (69 chromosomes), with the extra set of haploid chromosomes originating from the father. When a living fetus is present, it usually is also triploid, and features of this may manifest themselves as intrauterine growth retardation. Presenting symptoms of complete and partial mole are shown in Table 28.1. The principal differences from an imaging viewpoint are the excessive uterine size, the large

theca-lutein cysts, and the characteristic "bunch of grapes" appearance in the group with complete mole.

On CT, complete hydatidiform moles appear as tiny densely enhancing cystic lesions, which distend the endometrial cavity (Fig. 28.7). These represent trophoblastic proliferations covering the wall of vesicular tissue.

Figure 28.7 Hydatidiform mole in a 32-year-old woman. Contrast-enhanced CT shows numerous molar tissues with densely enhancing wall, distending the endometrial cavity.

Table 28.1 Presenting Symptoms and Signs in Patients with Complete and Partial Molar Pregnancy*

Sign	Complete Mole N = 307 (%)	Partial Mole N = 81 (%)
Vaginal bleeding	97	73
Excessive uterine size	51	4
Prominent theca-lutein cysts	50	0
Toxemia	27	3
Hyperemesis	26	0
Hyperthyroidism	7	0
Trophoblastic emboli	2	0

* Adapted from Berkowicz RS et al. Pathobiol Annu 1981;11:391 and Obstet Gynecol 1985; 66:667, with permission.

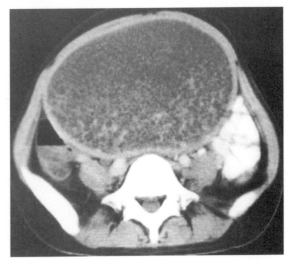

On MRI, a complete mole is hypointense on T1-weighted images and hyperintense on T2-weighted images, due to increased accumulation of stromal fluid. If vesicular molar tissue fills the whole uterine cavity, it appears as a large hyperintense mass on T2-weighted images. Contrast-enhanced MRI is useful for demonstrating the "bunch of grapes" appearance (Fig. 28.8) and for evaluating the degree of trophoblastic hyperplasia. This may be prognostic in predicting the development of malignancy.[15]

Invasive Mole

Locally invasive mole usually follows a molar pregnancy but can ensue after any gestational event, including normal pregnancy. The diagnosis is made by finding two or more elevated human chorionic gonadotropin (hCG) levels 8 weeks after evacuation of molar tissues.[16] Invasive GTN develops in 15% of patients who have had a mole evacuated.[17]

An invasive mole is clinically and pathologically benign.[12] It is defined as a molar gestation in which formed villous trophoblast penetrates the myometrium. The history frequently suggests the diagnosis. Typically, the story is of a patient who delivered a hydatidiform mole 4 to 12 weeks previously and who continued to bleed. MRI can be used to detect a mass in the myometrium when the hCG does not fall as expected after evacuation of a mole. If a mass is not demonstrated, early

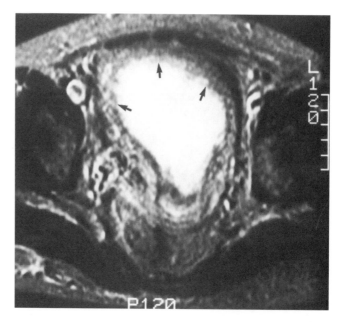

Figure 28.9 A 46-year-old woman with invasive mole. Because of persistence of elevated serum β-hCG titers after a molar evacuation, surgery was undertaken, confirming focal tumor invasion in the myometrium. Axial T2-weighted image (TR2,000/TE80) shows the endometrial cavity to be filled with hyperintense molar tissues. Disruption of the anterior half of the junctional zone in the myometrium (arrows) suggests an invasive mole.

Figure 28.8 Hydatidiform mole in a 45-year-old woman. Sagittal contrast-enhanced image (TR567/TE10) favorably shows the "bunch of grapes" appearance, and trophoblastic proliferations covering the wall of vesicular tissues are also densely enhanced.

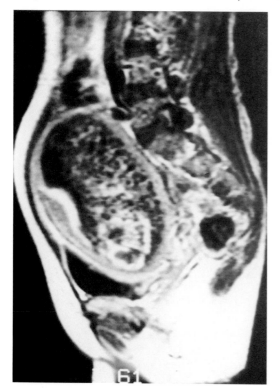

tumor detection is very difficult. Disruption of the junctional zone of the myometrium may be the only useful finding (Fig. 28.9).

On MRI, patients with an invasive mole usually have a poorly defined mass deeply invading the myometrium. This permeation of invasive mole is more easily seen on gross specimens than on MRI. It is caused by molar tissue invading the myometrium and blood vessels directly.[18] They sometimes appear as well-defined masses simulating a choriocarcinoma, especially in patients who have received chemotherapy before MRI. Therefore, the value of this external morphologic finding is limited.

On T1-weighted MRI, masses are usually heterogeneous with scattered areas of focal hyperintensity (Fig. 28.10) due to the presence of hemorrhagic areas.[19] On T2-weighted images, the masses are hyperintense or heterogeneous. After contrast, most masses have varying amounts of densely enhancing solid components that are confirmed as trophoblastic proliferation on pathology–MRI correlation.[19] In invasive moles, these components are present not only in the periphery but also in the center of the masses.

The detection of molar tissue-like structures within a mass is also of importance for the diagnosis of invasive mole. Usually, they appear as tiny cystic lesions within the densely enhancing zone of trophoblastic proliferation in a mass (Fig. 28.11). Differentiation from intratumoral vessels is difficult because of the small size of molar tissues (usually < 5 mm).

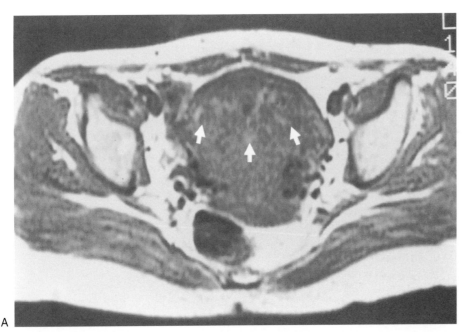

A

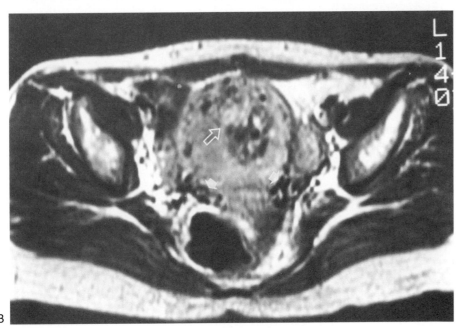

B

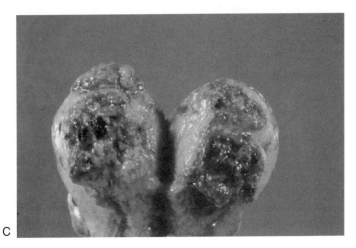

C

Figure 28.10 Invasive mole in a 48-year-old woman. **(A)** Axial T1-weighted image (TR600/TE11) shows a heterogeneous mass in the uterus with scattered areas of focal hyperintensity (arrows). **(B)** Axial contrast-enhanced image (TR550/TE11) shows densely enhancing solid components (open arrow) within the mass in association with increased intratumoral and adnexal (closed arrows) vascularity. **(C)** Cut gross pathologic section of the uterus shows a large permeative myometrial mass with villi and solid components of trophoblastic proliferation.

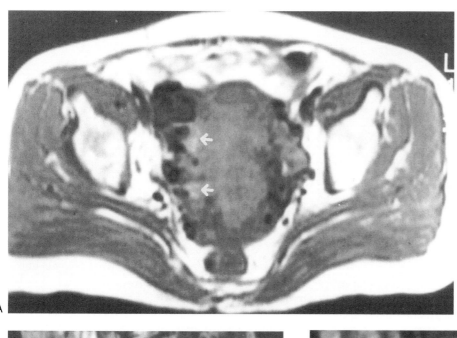

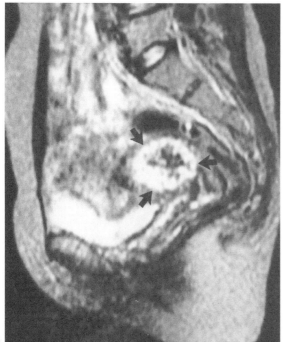

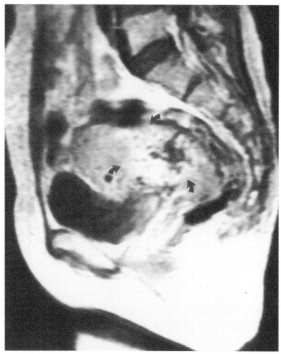

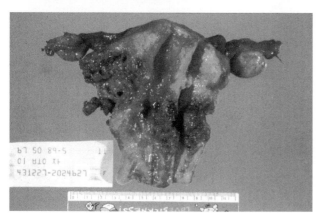

Figure 28.11 Invasive mole with uterine penetration in a 48-year-old woman. **(A)** Axial T1-weighted image (TR600/TE16) demonstrates increased adnexal and uterine vascularity associated with scattered areas of focal hyperintensity (arrows) along the right adnexa. **(B)** On sagittal T2-weighted image (TR2,000/TE90), a mass (arrows) is heterogeneous, the central hemorrhage is hypointense, and the peripheral zone with trophoblastic proliferation is hyperintense. **(C)** On sagittal contrast-enhanced, T1-weighted image (TR650/TE14), molar villi appear as tiny cystic lesions within the enhancing zone of the trophoblastic proliferation (arrows). **(D)** Surgical gross pathologic specimen of the uterus shows a permeative mass, deeply invading from the isthmus to the right cornual region and penetrating into the right adnexal region.

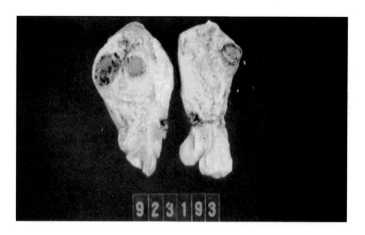

Figure 28.12 Choriocarcinoma in a 28-year-old woman. Cut gross pathologic specimen of the uterus shows well-defined masses with hemorrhage and necrosis.

The absence of signal void or the presence of unevenly thickened walls in the tiny cystic lesions is suggestive of molar tissue rather than of vessels. Due to the invasiveness of molar tissue, uterine penetration occasionally occurs (Fig. 28.11).

Most gestational tumors show increased uterine and adnexal vascularity.[20] On MRI, this is more commonly seen in cases of invasive mole rather than in choriocarcinoma. Therefore, on MRI, with the permeation of tumor into the myometrium, the invasive mole looks more aggressive than choriocarcinoma. Increased intratumoral vascularity is useful in distinguishing invasive mole from a choriocarcinoma.[19] In cases with prominent intramural vessels, a small myometrial mass may be missed.

Placental Site Trophoblastic Tumor

Placental site trophoblastic tumor is an uncommon variant of GTN that produces small amounts of hCG and human placental lactogen and that tends to remain confined to the uterus until late in its course. It is relatively insensitive to chemotherapy and requires surgical resection.

Choriocarcinoma

Choriocarcinoma (metastatic GTN) is a highly malignant tumor that follows in 4% of women who have had a hydatidiform mole evacuated.[17] Half of them are preceded by evacuation of a mole, but 20% are preceded by a spontaneous abortion, and 30% by a normal pregnancy. The gross appearance of choriocarcinoma is remarkably similar from case to case, and the tumor nodule shows severe central necrosis and hemorrhage due to lack of intrinsic tumoral vascularture.[18,21,22] In the uterus, the primary nodules may be single or multiple with a well-defined border (Fig. 28.12). Microscopically, choriocarcinoma is distinguished from invasive mole by the absence of formed chorionic villi.

In most cases of choriocarcinoma, MRI favorably demonstrates gross morphologic appearance. Characteristically, the tumor margins are nodular and well defined, as choriocarcinomas usually tend to invade the myometrium through the venous sinuses[18] (Fig. 28.13). Therefore, T1-weighted images are helpful in detecting these nodular types of hyperintense (hemorrhagic)

masses. On T2-weighted images, the masses are hyperintense, heterogeneous, or occasionally hypointense in signal intensity, depending upon the age of hemorrhage. Rarely, on T2-weighted images, a thin hemosiderin rim of hypointensity surrounds the mass, resulting from chronic hemorrhage (Fig. 28.14).

The tumor mass differs on contrast-enhanced MRI if the patient had a history of chemotherapy just before MRI. If the patient did not have pre-MRI chemotherapy, it appears as a mixed mass with central necrosis and irregularly enhancing solid peripheral components. A similar contrast enhancement was also described on a dynamic CT study in one case of choriocarcinoma.[23] After chemotherapy, these masses become nearly cystic due to increased tumoral necrosis. Intratumoral vascularity is minimal in most cases compared to those with invasive mole.[19]

Coagulative necrosis can develop within a mass as a result of sudden ischemia in patients treated with chemotherapy. It is isointense on T1-weighted images, hypointense on T2-weighted images, and mildly enhancing after administration of contrast (Fig. 28.15). Thus, because of variable tumor mass signal intensities after chemotherapy, a mass of less than 1.5 cm in diameter can be easily missed on conventional T1- and T2-weighted images. Therefore, a contrast-enhanced study is necessary as part of the workup for cases in which a small residual mass is suspected. Table 28.2 summarizes the MRI findings distinguishing choriocarcinoma from invasive mole.

Table 28.2 MR Characteristics of a Mass in Invasive Mole and Choriocarcinoma

	Choriocarcinoma	Invasive Mole
Tumor margin	Well-defined	Ill-defined
Hyperintense pattern on T1-weighted image	Nodular	Scattered
Intratumoral vascularity	Absent or minimal	Increased
Densely enhancing solid components	Peripheral	Diffuse
Molar tissue-like tiny cystic lesions	Absent	Present

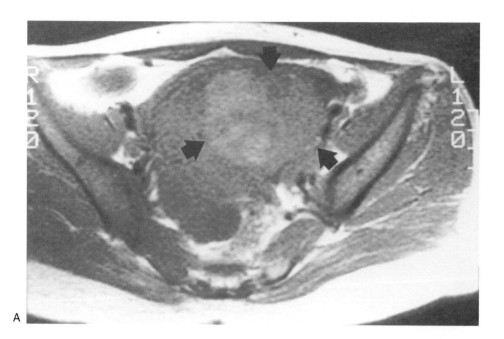

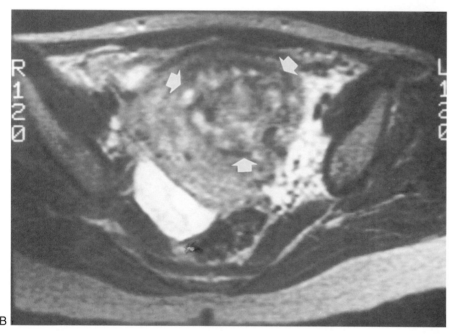

Figure 28.13 Choriocarcinoma in a 31-year-old woman. **(A)** Axial T1-weighted image (TR567/ TE11) shows a nodular hyperintense mass (arrows) in the uterus. **(B)** On axial T2-weighted image (TR2,000/TE80), the mass (arrows) appears to be heterogeneous. (*Figure continues.*)

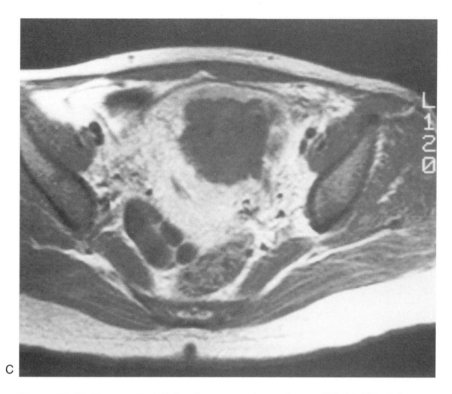

C

Figure 28.13 (*Continued*). **(C)** Axial contrast-enhanced image (TR567/TE11) demonstrates that the mass is almost completely necrotic.

Figure 28.14 Choriocarcinoma in a 31-year-old woman. **(A)** Axial T1-weighted image (TR566/TE11) shows a well-defined hyperintense mass in the uterus. (*Figure continues.*)

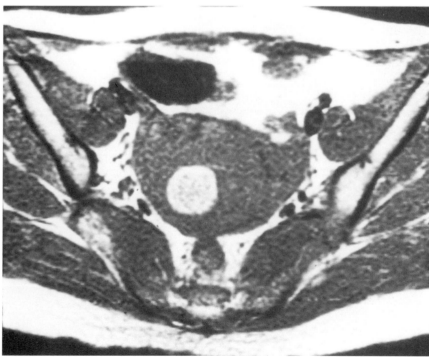

A

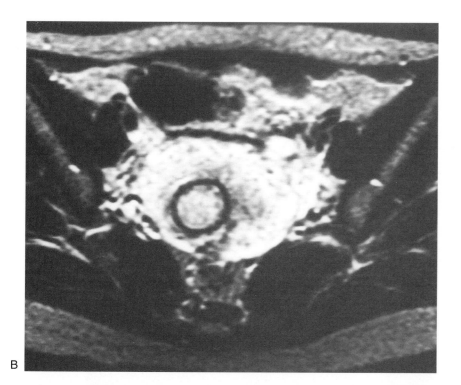

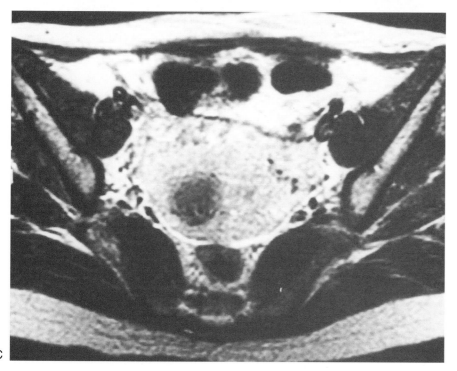

Figure 28.14 (*Continued*). **(B)** Axial T2-weighted image (TR2,200/TE80) shows a thin hypo-intense rim in the periphery of the mass due to hemosiderin deposition. **(C)** Axial contrast-enhanced image (TR566/TE11) favorably demonstrates severe central tumor necrosis.

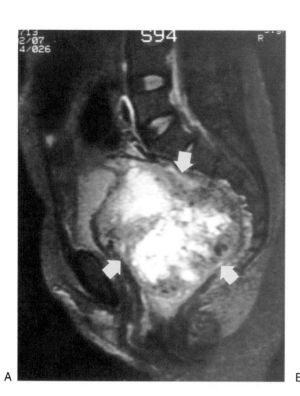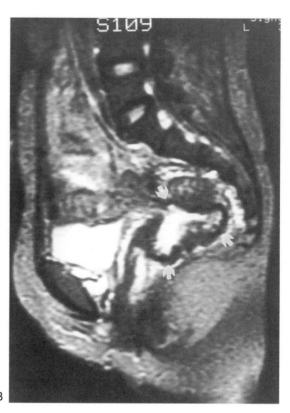

Figure 28.15 Recurrent choriocarcinoma in a 40-year-old woman who received five cycles of chemotherapy 1 year after hysterectomy. **(A)** Sagittal T2-weighted image (TR2,000/TE80) shows a large, heterogeneous mass (arrows) with central necrosis. Signal intensity in the solid area of the mass is nearly isointense relative to the adjacent muscle. **(B)** Repeated image of Figure A following three additional cycles of chemotherapy shows marked reduction in size of the mass (arrows). Previously isointense periphery of the mass (arrows) has become hypointense secondary to coagulation necrosis.

Theca-lutein cysts often develop in gestational trophoblastic neoplasms. The incidence varies from 15% to 50%. The frequency and size of theca-lutein cyst are not related to the hCG level.[24–26] These cysts can be unilateral or bilateral and have thin or thick walls. Morrow et al.[16] found that patients with theca-lutein cysts were at greater risk for persistent trophoblastic disease.

If serum hCG levels decrease after chemotherapy, the uterine volume and vascularity decrease to normal and the uterine zonal configuration becomes visible, indicating a favorable response.[27] For follow-up study in patients with gestational trophoblastic tumor during or after chemotherapy, ultrasound is preferred. However, it should be noted that a small mass can be missed or may appear to be smaller than its real size because the echogenicity of hemorrhagic tumor is similar to that of the uterus. Additionally, serum hCG levels were related to tumor detection on MRI, which was not useful in detecting disease in patients with a serum β-hCG level of 50 mIU/ml or less, but which could identify myometrial or extrauterine disease in about two-thirds of patients with a β-hCG level greater than 500 mIU/ml.[28]

SUMMARY

While ultrasound is firmly established as the imaging method of choice in the diagnosis of pathologic pregnancy conditions, CT and MRI both have a contribution to make when there is a diagnostic dilemma, especially in the case of gestational neoplastic diseases and unusual cases of ectopic pregnancy.

REFERENCES

1. Hricak H, Demas BE, Braga CA et al. Gestational trophoblastic neoplasm of the uterus: MR assessment. Radiology 1986;161: 11–16
2. Barton JW, McCarthy SM, Kohorn EI et al. Pelvic MR imaging findings in gestational trophoblastic disease, incomplete abortion, and ectopic pregnancy: are they specific? Radiology 1993;186:163–168
3. Cunningham FG, MacDonald PC, Gant NF, Eds. Williams Obstetrics (18th ed.). Prentice Hall, Upper Saddle River, NJ, 1989, pp 489–509

4. Benson RC. Current Obstetric and Gynecologic Diagnosis and Treatment. Lange Medical Publications, Los Altos, CA, 1976, pp 599–607

5. Jones HW, III, Wentz AC, Burnett LS. Novak's Textbook of Gynecology (11th ed.). Williams & Wilkins, Baltimore, 1988, pp 476–506

6. Iffy L, Kaminetzky HA. Principles and Practice of Obstetrics and Perinatology. Wiley, New York, 1981, pp 609–633

7. Quilligan EJ, Zuspan F. Douglas-Stromme Operative Obstetrics (4th ed.). Appleton-Century-Crofts, East Norwalk, CT, 1982, pp 219–252

8. Gompel C, Silverberg SG. Pathology in Gynecology and Obstetrics (3rd ed.). JB Lippincott, Philadelphia, 1985, pp 513–517

9. Ha HK, Jung JK, Kang SJ et al. MR imaging in the diagnosis of rare forms of ectopic pregnancy. AJR Am J Roentgenol 1993;160:1229–1232

10. Bader-Armstrong B, Shah Y, Rubens D. Use of ultrasound and magnetic resonance imaging in the diagnosis of cervical pregnancy. J Clin Ultrasound 1989;17:283–286

11. Hammond CB, Parker RT. Diagnosis and treatment of trophoblastic disease. Obstet Gynecol 1970;35:132–143

12. Lurain JR, Brewer JI. Invasive mole. Semin Oncol 1982; 9:174–180

13. Pattillo RA, Sasaki S, Katayama KP et al. Genesis of 46, XY hydatidiform mole. Am J Obstet Gynecol 1981;141:104

14. Kajii T, Ohama K. Androgenetic origin of hydatidiform mole. Nature 1977;268:633

15. Driscoll SG. Gestational trophoblastic neoplasms: morphological considerations. Hum Pathol 1977;8:529–539

16. Morrow CP, Kletzky OA, Disaia PJ et al. Clinical and laboratory correlates of molar pregnancy and trophoblastic disease. Am J Obstet Gynecol 1977;128:424–430

17. Berkowitz RS, Goldstein DP. Pathogenesis of gestational trophoblastic neoplasms. Pathobiol Annu 1981;11:391

18. Elston CW. Gestational trophoblastic disease. In Fox H, ed. Obstetrical and Gynecological Pathology (3rd ed.). Churchill Livingstone, Edinburgh, 1987, pp 1045–1078

19. Ha HK, Jung JK, Jee MK et al. MR imaging-pathologic correlation of gestational trophoblastic tumors. Gynecol Oncol 1995;57:340–350

20. de V Hendrickse JP, Cockshot WP, Evans KTE, Barton CJ. Pelvic angiography in the diagnosis of malignant trophoblastic disease. N Engl J Med 1964;17:859–866

21. Rosai J, Ed. Ackerman's Surgical Pathology. CV Mosby, St. Louis, 1989, pp 1179–1191

22. Silverberg SG, Ed. Principles and Practice of Surgical Pathology (2nd ed.). Wiley & Sons, New York, 1990, pp 1847–1856

23. Miyaska Y, Hachiya J, Furuya Y et al. CT evaluation of invasive trophoblastic disease. J Comput Assist Tomogr 1985;9:459–462

24. Baird AM, Beckly DE, Ross FGM. The ultrasound diagnosis of hydatidiform mole. Clin Radiol 1977;28:637–645

25. Cadkin AV, Sabbagha RE. Ultrasonic diagnosis of abnormal pregnancy. Clin Obstet Gynecol 1977;20:265–277

26. Requard CK, Mettler FA, Jr. The use of ultrasound in the evaluation of trophoblastic disease and its response to therapy. Radiology 1980;135:419–422

27. Hricak H, Demas BE, Braga CA et al. Gestational trophoblastic neoplasm of the uterus: MR assessment. Radiology 1986;161: 11–16

28. Barton JW, McCarthy SM, Kohorn EI et al. Pelvic MR imaging findings in gestational trophoblastic disease, incomplete abortion, and ectopic pregnancy: are they specific? Radiology 1993;186:163–168

Ultrasonography of the Postpartum Pelvis and Postabortal Pelvis

ANDREW McLENNAN

The *puerperium* refers to the postpartum period during which the body returns to its prepregnant state. It can also relate to the postabortal period. This is usually completed within 6 weeks and in the vast majority of patients is uncomplicated.

Ultrasound is not commonly performed in the postdelivery period but is useful in the evaluation of patients with uterine subinvolution, pain, blood loss, excessive vaginal discharge, and fever. The procedure is generally performed transabdominally after vaginal delivery, but transvaginal or transperineal approaches may be more useful after abortion or cesarean section.[1]

NORMAL POSTPARTUM UTERINE INVOLUTION

Immediately after normal delivery, the uterus weighs around 1,000 g and measures about 20 cm in the long axis. Serial ultrasound assessment of uterine involution is most accurately achieved using the long-axis measurement corrected for uterine angulation.[2] A sector transducer causes less distortion of the spongy early postpartum uterus than other transducers.

Involution is almost completed by the end of the first postpartum month with only a slight further decrease in length and volume over the second month. The mean dimensions reduce from 19.9 cm in the first 2 days to 11.2 cm at around 3 weeks and 8.7 cm at 6 to 8 weeks postpartum.[2] The uterine volume is reduced by approximately 40% in the first week, from 730 to 420 cc, and by 86% over 6 weeks, to about 100 cc.[3] This is achieved by a reduction in the size rather than the number of myometrial cells. The period of involution is prolonged in multipara compared with primipara (by up to 4 weeks)[2] and is reduced in breast-feeding women[3] and in preterm deliveries. The myometrium will appear heterogeneous on ultrasound due to the changes in uterine blood flow and reduction of tissue edema. Uterine fibroids, having achieved a steady state in the second and third trimesters, will also reduce in size but often remain larger than their prepregnant dimensions.

Within 2 or 3 days of delivery, the decidua remaining in the uterus becomes differentiated into two layers. The superficial layer becomes necrotic and is sloughed in the lochia. The basal layer contains endometrial glandular remnants, which proliferate, allowing rapid endometrial regeneration to occur everywhere, except at the placental site, by 10 days.[4] Within the uterine cavity, a small amount of fluid or brightly echoic air (incidentally introduced during the delivery process) are common findings in the immediate postpartum period and are of little clinical significance (Fig. 29.1). The endometrium usually returns to a homogeneous appearance of less than 1.0 cm diameter by the end of the second week.

As involution progresses, the uterine artery resistance index steadily increases, reaching nonpregnant levels by the end of the second month.[5] This reflects compression and hyaline obliteration of the new vessels formed within the uterus during pregnancy and reduction in caliber of the extrauterine vessels.

RETAINED PRODUCTS OF CONCEPTION

Post Delivery (> 20 Weeks)

Incomplete uterine evacuation following vaginal delivery or cesarean section usually presents within a few days of delivery with a secondary postpartum hemorrhage. This may be accompanied by painful uterine contractions and subinvolution. There is also an increased risk of endometritis.

Ultrasound usually reveals a uterus inappropriately large with uterine cavity distension.[6] The uterine cavity contents show mixed reflectivity with varying amounts of fluid, blood clot, membranes, and placental tissue. It can be difficult to distinguish blood clot (generally homogeneous in appearance) from placental tissue (generally echogenic).

In a study of 53 patients referred for possible retained products of conception, the most common finding in women with histologically proven retained placental tissue was an echogenic mass in the uterine cavity (Fig. 29.2).[7] Retained placental tissue was unlikely to be present where ultrasound revealed a normal endometrial stripe, endometrial fluid, or hyperechoic foci without an accompanying mass (a finding commonly associated with recent uterine instrumentation).[7]

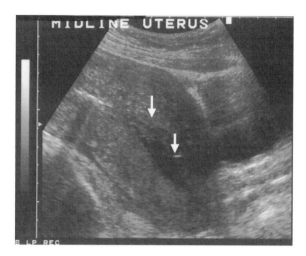

Figure 29.1 Blood (arrows) in the fundus 9 days postpartum. Part of the spectrum of normal uterine involution.

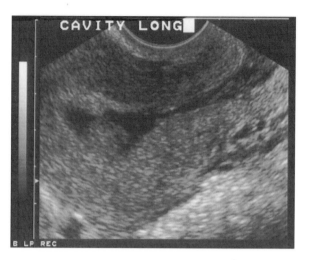

Figure 29.3 Retained products of conception 3 days after spontaneous abortion. Echogenic mass and blood clot extending to the cervix.

Expectant management, including the judicious use of antibiotics, may be appropriate when only small amounts of abnormal tissue, blood clot, or fluid are present in the uterine cavity. The presence of an echogenic mass or of a heterogeneous collection exceeding 15 mm in diameter in conjunction with troublesome bleeding warrants uterine curettage.

Post Spontaneous Abortion

Around 15% of all clinically apparent pregnancies will end in spontaneous abortion. Over 90% of these will occur in the first 12 weeks of amenorrhea. The risks increase with parity, maternal age (12% in women under 20 years of age and 28% in women over 40) and a smaller but similar increase with increased paternal age.[4]

Chromosomal abnormality is the causative factor in around 60% of first-trimester miscarriages. The majority of

Figure 29.2 Retained products of conception post delivery. Intrauterine echogenic mass 4 weeks after twin delivery.

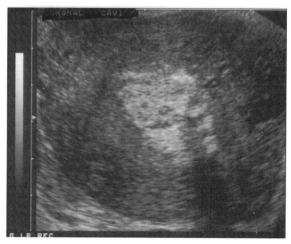

aneuploid miscarriages (autosomal trisomies, monosomy X, and triploidy) occur less than 8 weeks of amenorrhea. Euploid miscarriages that are caused by subtle genetic abnormalities[8] or maternal factors such as infection (*Listeria monocytogenes,* mumps, rubella), uterine anomalies, or immunologic conditions tend to peak at around 13 weeks of amenorrhea.

In one study, 501 of 17,369 first-trimester scans (2.8%) revealed asymptomatic early pregnancy failure (K. Nicolaides, personal communication, 1996). These comprised either missed abortion (demonstration of fetal parts in the absence of heart motion) or anembryonic pregnancy (a gestation sac of 25 mm diameter or greater with no fetal parts). Color Doppler in cases of missed abortion often shows large vascular lakes with high-velocity flows. These vascular lakes increase in size and number over time and eventually undermine the decidual layers, enabling detachment from the uterine wall.[9] Vaginal bleeding and abdominal pain in the presence of positive serum or urine β-human chorionic gonadotropin (β-hCG) is symptomatic of spontaneous (inevitable or incomplete) abortion.

Ultrasound is very sensitive in detection of products of conception (gestation sac, space-occupying collection or a thick (> 5 mm) endometrium of mixed echogenicity) but is less reliable in ruling out retained products of conception (Fig. 29.3).[10] An endometrial stripe of less than 2 mm predicted little likelihood of retained products of conception, while a moderately thick endometrium (2 to 5 mm) was not diagnostic.

Cervical dilatation and uterine curettage (D&C) has been the mainstay of treatment for over 50 years in both asymptomatic early pregnancy failure and symptomatic spontaneous abortion. The procedure makes up over half of all urgent gynecologic admissions and has complication rates between 4% and 10%.[11] Longitudinal studies of expectant[11] and medical[12] management of symptomatic spontaneous abortion have

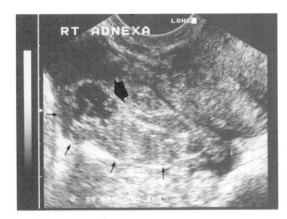

Figure 29.4 Heterotopic twin pregnancy. One month after a spontaneous miscarriage of an intrauterine pregnancy and D&C, this patient's pain persisted, and the β-human chorionic gonadotropin remained positive. A co-existent 5-cm right ectopic pregnancy mass (arrows) with gestation sac superiorly (large arrow) was subsequently found.

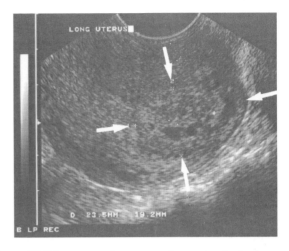

Figure 29.5 Invasive molar tissue at the uterine fundus (arrows) 3 weeks following evacuation of a hydatidiform mole (hCG 4,600 IU/ml). Transvaginal sagittal scan of the retroverted uterus.

shown lower complication rates, with no difference in number of days of bleeding or pain experienced or in hemoglobin levels when compared with patients managed by D&C. Those women with persistent heavy bleeding or ultrasound-measured retained products of 15 mm or more after 3 days should be referred for D&C.

One advantage of D&C is the histologic confirmation of normal chorionic villi to help exclude ectopic and molar pregnancies. Even if normal villi are obtained, persistence of low levels of β-hCG should trigger further sonographic evaluation for rare conditions such as heterotopic twin (ectopic) pregnancy (Fig. 29.4) or placental site trophoblastic tumor or invasive molar tissue (where color Doppler examination shows low impedance values within the richly vascularized tissue) (Fig. 29.5).[9]

Post Induced Abortion

Retained products of conception following termination of pregnancy show a range of sonographic features from a heterogeneous mix of blood and tissue (within days of the procedure) to echogenic masses (weeks to months after abortion) (Fig. 29.6). Perioperative ultrasound guidance of uterine curettage is valuable in the following situations:

- First-trimester termination failure due to uterine anomalies, and cervical stenosis.[13]
- Postabortal endomyometritis associated with retained products of conception[14] to ensure complete evacuation and prevent uterine perforation
- Second-trimester dilatation and evacuation to ensure complete removal of fetal parts

After induced abortion, there is no significant reduction in

Figure 29.6 Retained products of conception post induced abortion. **(A)** One week post abortion: heterogeneous mix of tissue and blood clot. **(B)** Four months post abortion: inspissated, echogenic retained placental fragments in the lower uterine cavity (arrows).

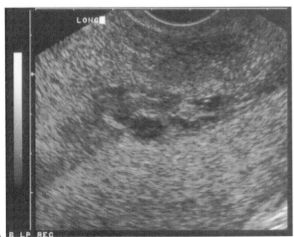

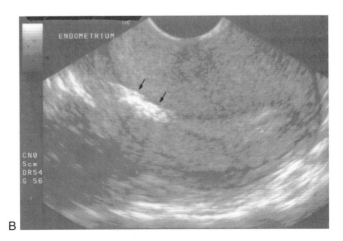

the rate of retained tissue, with or without the use of perioperative ultrasound.[15]

RETAINED PLACENTA

In most cases, the placenta separates spontaneously from the implantation site during the first few minutes after delivery. In approximately 1 per 2,500 deliveries, the placenta is unusually adherent to the implantation site. The decidua is scanty or absent, and the normal cleavage line through the spongy layer of the decidua is lacking.[4] This abnormality can result in one or more cotyledons attaching to (accreta) or penetrating (increta, percreta) the myometrium.

Predisposing factors include a history of uterine surgery, placenta previa, multiparity, or previous retained placenta. Antenatal ultrasonic features of placenta accreta include loss of the retroplacental hypoechoic zone, placental tissue contiguous with the myometrium, and multiple venous lakes occupying most of the thickness of the placenta displaying both laminar and pulsatile blood flow.[9,16] These findings are commonly associated with placenta previa and dilated vascular structures within nonplacental tissue.

Postpartum sonographic diagnosis of partial or complete placenta accreta has been less commonly described. This may be due to difficulty in distinguishing tissue boundaries in the postpartum uterus. The principal features noted are absence of the normal retroplacental hypoechoic zone (representing a defect in the decidua basalis and adjacent myometrium) and a marked thinning of the myometrial mantle beneath the placental bed.[17] Increased pulsatile blood flow in the adjacent myometrium has also been observed.[18]

Treatment of abnormally adherent placentae involves manual removal of the placenta, curettage with perioperative ultrasound, and uterine packing. Smaller areas of placenta accreta/increta may respond to (ultrasound-guided or systemic chemotherapy (methotrexate). In cases with persistent hemorrhage or sepsis, postpartum hysterectomy may be the only solution.

INFLAMMATORY CONDITIONS

Endo(myo)metritis

Puerperal infection is bacterial infection of the genital tract generally occurring 2 to 5 days after delivery or abortion. It complicates 2% to 3% of vaginal deliveries, 10% to 15% of cesareans (and over 40% in certain high-risk patients[19]) and up to 10% of abortion.[20] Infection (notably postabortal) remains an important cause of maternal mortality, contributing to 8% to 10% of deaths in recent surveys,[21,22] despite modern antibiotics and surgical practices. The clinical features include pyrexia (> 38°C), uterine and parametrial tenderness, abnormal bleeding, and offensive lochia. Postabor-

tal pelvic inflammatory disease (PID) can also produce tender adnexal masses.

Risk factors for puerperal infection include cesarean section after prolonged labor (particularly with rupture of membranes for greater than 6 hours), multiple vaginal examinations, and extensive vaginal lacerations.[19,23] Some studies have suggested that subclinical antenatal intrauterine infections might predispose to puerperal infection as well as to fetal morbidity.[24] Postabortal infection was more commonly seen in women harboring Chlamydia trachomatis (25%) and in those with a history of PID.[20]

The most common organisms responsible for infection are peptostreptococci, Bacteroides sp., streptococci, and coliforms.[25] Infection primarily involves the endometrium (decidua) and rapidly spreads to the adjacent myometrium and adnexa. Rarely, infection spreads via lymphatics to cause peritonitis or via pelvic circulation to cause septicemia.

Ultrasound generally has little role in the diagnosis and management of uncomplicated puerperal febrile morbidity other than exclusion of retained products of conception. Most patients respond to antibiotic therapy. In more severe cases of endomyometritis, the uterus may be inappropriately large and the myometrium relatively echo-poor with varying amounts of tissue, blood, or occasionally gas present within the uterine cavity.[6] There may be fluid in the pouch of Douglas.

Gas in the uterine cavity is diagnosed by hyperechoic foci with acoustic shadowing and/or reverberation artifact. This finding is seen in up to 21% of healthy women after normal vaginal delivery[26] and shows no difference from the reported incidence of 15% in women with proven endometritis.[27] Thus, endometritis cannot be inferred solely on the presence of endometrial gas.

Pelvic Abscess

Imaging has more utility in cases of puerperal febrile morbidity unresponsive to broad-spectrum antibiotic therapy. In a study of 31 such patients, 11 had hematomas, and 21 had endomyometritis (10 with ultrasound features), 13 of whom had other extrauterine abnormalities including abscess, hematoma, ovarian vein thrombosis, and vesicouterine fistula.[28] Ultrasound also has a pivotal role in guidance of drainage procedures and monitoring the progress of these abnormalities.

A pelvic abscess or infected hematoma can be either solid or cystic, depending on the degree of organization of the hematoma or whether it contains locules or pockets of pus.[29] An abscess will usually have a capsule. Differentiation of hematoma from abscess is often difficult, although the presence of bright echoes representing gas within the mass often indicates infection.[30]

Ovarian Vein Thrombosis

Ovarian vein thrombosis is a rare complication (1 in 5,800 uncomplicated vaginal deliveries[31]) and should be suspected when patients present with apparent late onset endometritis or pyelonephritis with unilateral pelvic and flank pain. Ultrasound usually reveals an adnexal mass that comprises a dilated, tortuous thrombosed ovarian vein with no Doppler signal. The enlarged vein is filled with echogenic thrombus anterior to the psoas muscle.[28] Treatment is with intravenous antibiotics and anticoagulants.

HEMORRHAGE

Primary Postpartum Hemorrhage

Primary postpartum hemorrhage is defined as loss of over 500 ml of blood within the first 24 hours of delivery. The incidence is approximately 5% of all deliveries and accounts for 28% to 33% of maternal deaths.[21,22] The common causes are uterine atony, retained placenta, or products of conception and local trauma to the genital tract.

Pelvic Hematoma

Genital tract damage does not always result in external hemorrhage. Complicated vaginal (notably rotational instrumental) deliveries can cause trauma to the paravaginal venous plexus, resulting in pelvic extraperitoneal hematoma formation (Fig. 29.7). They can be supralevator, extending into the broad ligament, or infralevator, extending to the vulva, perineum, or ischiorectal fossa.[32] They are rarely seen in the perivesical, vesicovaginal, or rectovaginal spaces due to dense fascial barriers. The hematomas can contain large blood volumes, which are occasionally sufficient to cause hemodynamic compromise.

Cesarean section delivery can also be associated with hematoma formation due to inadequate hemostasis. The potential sites are the anterior abdominal wall (subfascial),[1,29] bladder flap,[1,30] or laterally into the broad ligament and other retroperitoneal spaces.[32]

Figure 29.7 Left retroperitoneal hematoma (h) anterior to the psoas muscle 6 weeks after a normal vaginal delivery.

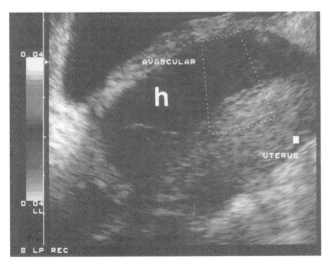

Uterine perforation is reported to complicate between 1 and 5 in every 1,000 first-trimester induced abortions. Most resultant bleeding is into the peritoneal cavity, but confined uterovesical fold hematomas can form after anterior uterine wall perforation, especially when the uterus is markedly retroverted.[33]

Pelvic hematomas often appear sonographically as large masses adjacent to the vagina or uterus,[6] which may distort neighboring pelvic organs. They are initially hypoechoic and smooth walled but become irregular and hyperechoic with progressive clotting and organization. Retroperitoneal hematomas are occasionally difficult to view with ultrasound, and computed tomography may be the preferred imaging modality.[28,32] Bladder flap hematomas (extraperitoneal hematoma between the anterior uterine wall and the posterior bladder wall) usually are seen as lenticular, solid, or complex echogenic masses between 2 and 10 cm. Masses of less than 2 cm probably represent normal wound healing.[1]

Subfascial Hematoma

Subfascial hematomas arise from extraperitoneal hemorrhage within the perivesical space posterior to the rectus muscles but anterior to the peritoneum. The ultrasound features are of a mostly cystic mass with occasional solid or gaseous elements depending on the degree of organization or infection.[29] They are commonly seen in association with bladder flap hematomas.

Uteroplacental Apoplexy

In more severe forms of placental abruption, widespread extravasation of blood into the myometrium and beneath the uterine serosa often occurs. This has been termed *uteroplacental apoplexy*, or *Couvelaire uterus*. Occasionally, these effusions are seen beneath the tubal serosa, in the broad ligament, and in the peritoneal cavity secondary to tubal passage of uterine blood.[4] These myometrial hematomas rarely interfere with uterine contraction sufficiently to produce severe postpartum hemorrhage. Ultrasound shows a thickened, generally hypoechoic myometrium, but the diagnosis is often made clinically at cesarean section due to the color and consistency of the uterus.

SUMMARY

Ultrasound has an important, if limited, role in the postpartum period. When complications develop after delivery or abortion, they are often effectively diagnosed and managed on clinical grounds alone.

Ultrasound is valuable in assessment of uterine involution and endometrial regeneration. Detection of retained placental fragments or products of conception is the most common indication for ultrasound use in the puerperium. In patients with puerperal febrile morbidity, especially those refractory to antibiotic therapy, ultrasound is able to show the cause in the majority of cases. Identification of paravaginal or pelvic collections can direct treatment and monitor progress.

REFERENCES

1. Hertzberg BS, Bowie JD, Kliewer MA. Complications of cesarean section: role of transperineal ultrasound. Radiology 1993;188:533–536

2. Wachsberg RH, Kurtz AB, Levine CD. Real-time ultrasound analysis of the normal postpartum uterus: technique, variability and measurements. J Ultrasound Med 1994;13:215–221

3. Galli D, Groce P, Chiapparini I, Dede A. Ultrasonic evaluation of the uterus in the puerperium (Italy) Minerva Ginecol 1993;45:473–478

4. Cunningham FG, MacDonald PC, Gant NF. Williams Obstetrics (18th ed.). East Norwalk, CT: Appleton & Lange, 1989 pp 245,461–476, 489, 507, 706

5. Reles A, Ertan AK, Kainer F, Dudenhausen JW. Doppler ultrasound images of the uterine artery and uterine involution in normal puerperium. Gynakol Geburtshilfliche Rundsch 1992;32(2):66–72

6. Andrew H. The post-partum uterus. In: Meire H, Cosgrove D, Dewbury K, Eds. Ultrasound in Obstetrics and Gynaecology. Churchill Livingstone, London, 1993, pp 506–508

7. Hertzberg BS, Bowie JD. Ultrasound of the postpartum uterus. Prediction of retained placental tissue. J Ultrasound Med 1991;10:451–456

8. Simpson JL. Genes, chromosomes and reproductive failure. Fertil Steril 1980;33:107–109

9. Timor-Tritsch IE. Colour Doppler ultrasound. In: Goldstein H, Timor-Tritsch IE, Eds. Ultrasound in Gynecology. Churchill Livingstone, New York, 1995, pp 245–247

10. Kurtz AB, Shlansky-Goldberg RD, Choi HY, Needleman L. Detection of retained products of conception following spontaneous abortion in the first trimester. J Ultrasound Med 1991;10:387–395

11. Nielsen S, Hahlin M. Expectant management of first-trimester spontaneous abortion. Lancet 1995;345:84–86

12. Henshaw RC, Cooper K, El-Rafaey H et al. Medical management of miscarriage: non-surgical uterine evacuation of incomplete or inevitable spontaneous abortion. BMJ 1993;306:894–895

13. Pennes DR, Bowerman RA, Silver TM, Smith SJ. Failed first trimester pregnancy termination: uterine anomaly as etiologic factor. J Clin Ultrasound 1987;15:165–170

14. Romero R, Copel JA, Jeanty P et al. Sonographic monitoring to guide the performance of postabortal uterine curettage. Am J Obstet Gynecol 1985;151:51–53

15. Mikkelsen AL, Felding C. The value of preoperative ultrasound examination in first trimester legally induced abortion. Clin Exp Obstet Gynecol 1994;21:150–152

16. Guy GP, Peisner DB, Timor-Tritsch IE. Ultrasound evaluation of uteroplacental blood flow patterns of abnormally located and adherent placentas. Am J Obstet Gynecol 1990;163:723–727

17. Shapiro JL, Sherer DM, Hurley JT et al. Postpartum ultrasonographic findings associated with placenta accreta. Am J Obstet Gynecol 1992;167:601–602

18. Polvi H, Pirhonen J, Makinen J et al. Postpartum diagnosis of placenta accreta with colour Doppler sonography. Ann Chir Gynaecol Suppl 1994;208:100–102

19. Gibbs RS. Clinical risk factors for puerperal infection. Obstet Gynecol 1980;55:178S–184S

20. Heisterberg L, Branebjerg PE, Bremmelgaard A et al. The role of vaginal secretory immunoglobulin A, Gardnerella vaginalis, anaerobes, and Chlamydia trachomatis in postabortal pelvic inflammatory disease. Acta Obstet Gynecol Scand 1987;66:99–102

21. Confidential enquiry into maternal mortality in England and Wales. 1985–7. HMSO, London, England

22. Report on maternal deaths in Australia, 1985–7. AGPS, Canberra, Australia

23. Gibbs RS. Maternal and Fetal Infections. In: Creasy RK, Resnik R, Eds. Maternal–Fetal Medicine. Principles and Practice. WB Saunders, Philadelphia, 1994, pp 622–627

24. Bergstrom S, Libombo A. Low birthweight and post partum endometritis-myometritis. Acta Obstet Gynecol Scand 1995;74:611–613

25. Gibbs RS, O'Dell TN, MacGregor RR. Puerperal endometritis: a prospective microbiologic study. Am J Obstet Gynecol 1975;121:919–925

26. Wachsberg RH, Kurtz AB. Gas within the endometrial cavity at postpartum ultrasound: a normal finding after spontaneous vaginal delivery. Radiology 1992;183:431–433

27. Madrazo BL. Postpartum sonography. In: Sanders RC James AE, Eds. The Principles and Practice of Ultrasonography in Obstetrics and Gynecology (3rd ed.). Appleton-Century-Crofts, East Norwalk, CT, 1985, p 454

28. Lev-Toaff AS, Baka JJ, Toaff ME et al. Diagnostic imaging in puerperal febrile morbidity. Obstet Gynecol 1991;78:50–55

29. Benacerraf BR. Pelvic sonography. In: Ryan KJ, Berkowitz R, Barbieri RL, Eds. Kistner's Gynaecology Principles and Practice (5th ed.). Year Book Medical Publishers, Chicago, 1990, p 690

30. Witlin AG, Sibai BM. Postpartum ovarian vein thrombosis after vaginal delivery: a report of 11 cases. Obstet Gynecol 1995;85:775–780

31. Yamashita Y, Torashima M, Harada M et al. Postpartum extraperitoneal pelvic hematoma: Imaging findings AJR Am J Roentgenol 1993;161:805–808

32. Baker ME, Bowie JD, Killam AP. Sonography of post-caesarean section bladder-flap haematoma. AJR Am J Roentgenol 1985;144:757–759

33. Elchalel U, Caspi B, Appelman Z, Manor Y. Ultrasound-directed diagnosis and treatment of pelvic hematoma after therapeutic abortion. J Clin Ultrasound 1993;21:55–57

Computed Tomography and Magnetic Resonance Imaging of the Postpartum Pelvis and Postabortal Pelvis

SEYED A. ROOHOLAMINI

ANH H. AU

RICHARD B. KURZEL

RAMESH C. VERMA

Although ultrasound should be considered first because it is cheaper, computed tomography (CT) is better at demonstrating some abnormalities in pregnancy-related conditions. Magnetic resonance imaging (MRI) usually confirms CT, but occasionally is superior in detection and characterization of soft tissue abnormalities. MRI also has multiplanar capability and does not use ionizing radiation but is time-consuming and expensive.

STRUCTURAL ABNORMALITIES

Uterine: Dehiscence and Rupture

The uterine wall can undergo scar dehiscence, uterine rupture, or perforation. Dehiscence is a discontinuity of the myometrium in a pre-existing scar. If it occurs in a healed cesarean section scar, it is usually asymptomatic and is an ongoing condition existing before the onset of labor. The defect does not penetrate the serosa, the fetal membranes remain intact, and there is no hemorrhage or extrusion of the fetus into the peritoneal cavity. Its incidence (2% to 4% of patients with a uterine scar) is 40 to 50 times higher than uterine rupture (1/2,200 deliveries)[1] and always occurs in a uterine scar. If it occurs in a healing scar, it can cause bleeding and can become infected.

Rupture of the uterus is an acute traumatic event that causes a defect in the uterine wall. If this is complete, there is direct communication with the peritoneal cavity.

If it is incomplete, the communication remains covered with visceral peritoneum or it opens into the broad ligament. Most ruptures (50% to 70%) occur in a scar, but the uterus can rupture if labor is obstructed, particularly in the patient of high gravidity. In the asymptomatic woman, dehiscence of the scar may be incidentally detected on postpartum ultrasonography.[2,3] CT is the most helpful modality to detect uterine dehiscence or rupture (Figs. 30.1 to 30.3) and can also show hematomas in the broad ligaments or adnexa.

Perforation is a traumatic event that usually results from the inadvertent puncturing of the wall of the uterus with a curette or other surgical instrument.

Skeletal: Pubic Symphyseal Rupture (Symphysitis or Separation)

Rupture of the joint of the symphysis pubis is rare and occurs usually during vaginal delivery, but it can occur in pregnancy. The cause is unknown, and the diagnosis is clinical.[4] There is tenderness over the symphysis, a palpable pubic diastasis, and pelvic pain associated with locomotor difficulty. Rupture of this joint causes the patient great distress and incapacity. Treatment consists of analgesics, use of an orthopedic walker, and a pelvic girdle (trochanteric belt) for support, while the pubic diastasis reduces.

A separation of 10 mm on plain radiography is diagnostic of symphyseal rupture.[5] MRI has been used to confirm symphyseal rupture[6] (Figs. 30.4 and 30.5).

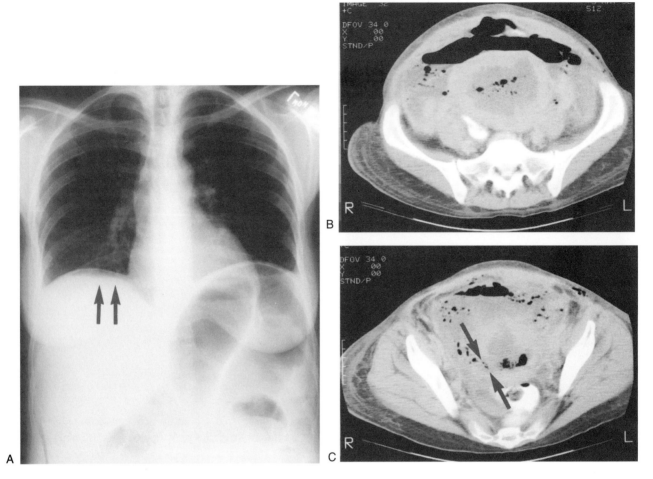

Figure 30.1 Uterine rupture or dehiscence. After cesarean section, this woman complained of pelvic pain and was tender over the uterus. There were ecchymoses under the umbilicus and a drop in hematocrit. **(A)** An erect abdominal radiograph 6 days after the cesarean section shows free gas (arrows) under the right hemidiaphragm. **(B & C)** CTs of the lower abdomen and pelvis 5 days later show liquid and gas in a markedly distended endometrial cavity. There is a discontinuity of the wall along the right posterolateral aspect of the uterus, consistent with uterine rupture or dehiscence of the sutures (arrows in Fig. C). Free liquid and gas are in the abdomen.

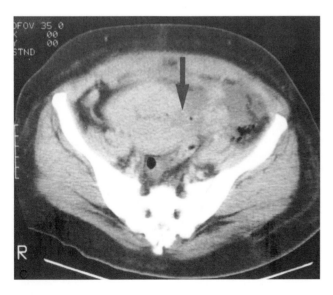

Figure 30.2 Uterine perforation. A 38-year-old gestational diabetic gravida 7, para 4 had a vaginal breech delivery. Retained products and postpartum hemorrhage necessitated curettage. CT shows a disruption of the lower segment of the uterine wall on the left, consistent with uterine perforation (arrow). The patient had a laparotomy with repair of the perforation.

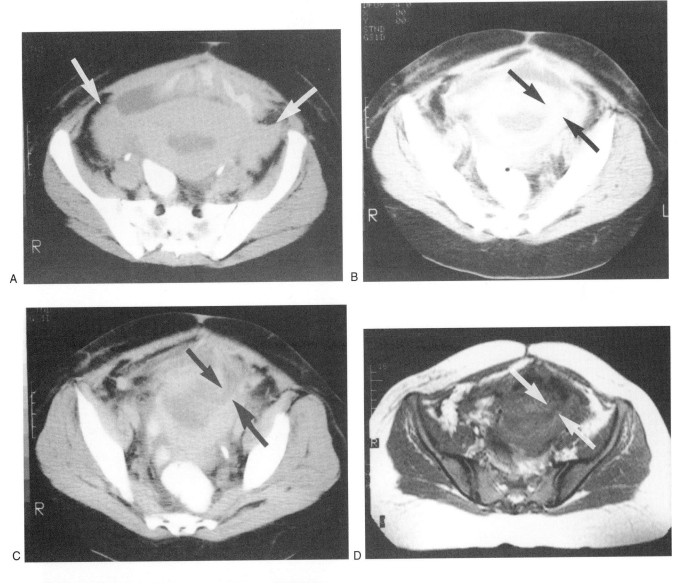

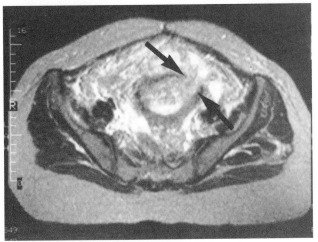

Figure 30.3 Uterine scar rupture. A 21-year-old gravida 3, para 2, with two previous cesarean sections, presented with fetal distress in second-stage labor. A forceps delivery was performed. Digital examination of the uterus, after delivery, suggested a uterine scar dehiscence. (A to C) CTs of the lower abdomen and pelvis show bilateral adnexal soft tissue densities, due to hematomas (arrows in Fig. A), and rupture of the left anterolateral aspect of the lower segment scar (arrows in Figs. B and C). (D) T1-weighted axial MRI of the lower abdomen and pelvis. (E) T2-weighted MRI confirms the uterine rupture (arrows in Figs. D and E). (Figs. B, C, and E from Rooholamini et al.,[8] with permission.)

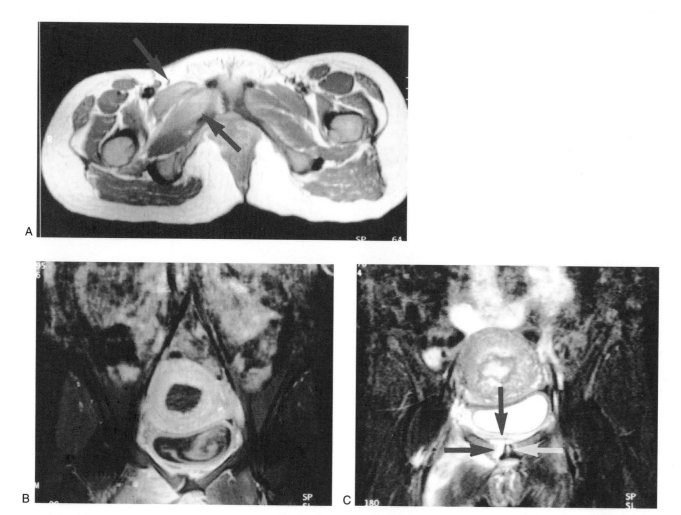

Figure 30.4 Symphyseal rupture. A 19-year-old gravida 1, para 0 was admitted at term in labor. She had a vacuum extraction because of a prolonged second stage. Immediately postpartum, she complained of pain in her symphysis pubis, groin, and perineum. A plain radiograph of the pelvis was unremarkable. **(A)** Axial T1-weighted MRI showed a 9-mm separation of the symphysis pubis: There was swelling of the right pectineus and external obturator muscles (arrows) with increased signal intensity. **(B)** Coronal T1-weighted images after gadolinium injection. **(C)** Coronal short-sterm inversion recovery (STIR) images show additional abnormal fluid collection signal intensities (arrows) along the mediosuperior and anterior aspects of the right pubic ramus and in the symphysis.

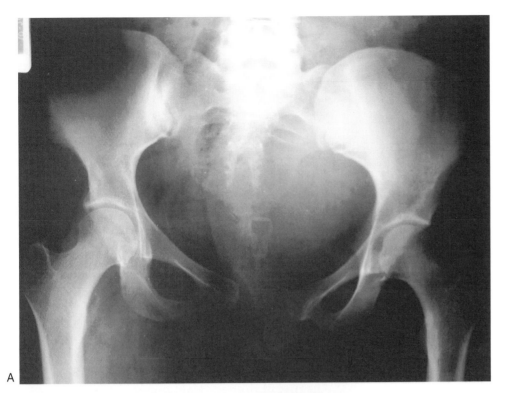

A

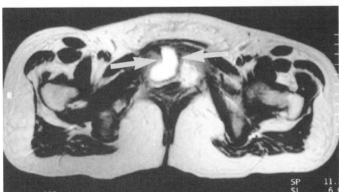

B

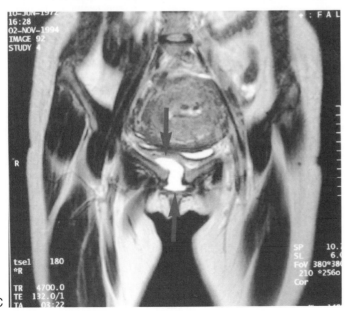

C

Figure 30.5 Symphyseal rupture. One day after a normal delivery, this patient complained of pain over the symphysis. A separation of the symphysis pubis was palpable. **(A)** Plain radiograph of the pelvis shows that it was 32 mm wide. **(B)** Axial fast spin echo (FSE, also known as turbo spin echo [TSE]) T2-weighted image 2 days later at the mid level of the symphysis shows separation of 21 mm. The abnormal fluid collection seen within the symphyseal cleft extends along the medial and posterior aspects of the pubic ramus on the right (arrows). **(C)** Coronal FSE T2-weighted image shows the separation of the symphysis with extension of the abnormal fluid collection along the medial, inferior, and superior borders of the right pubic ramus (arrows).

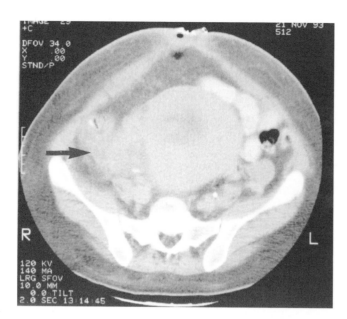

Figure 30.6 Broad ligament hematoma. A 28-year-old gravida 3, para 3 had a tubal ligation after a normal vaginal delivery. It was difficult to establish hemostasis. The patient developed a fever and low abdominal tenderness. CT showed that the endometrial cavity was distended and contained blood clot. There is a heterogeneous soft tissue density in the right adnexa and broad ligament, consistent with hematoma (arrow).

BLEEDING COMPLICATIONS

Uterine

Broad Ligament Hematoma

A hematoma within the broad ligament can occur during normal delivery but is generally a complication of cesarean section. Inadequate hemostasis will result in a drop in hematocrit and postoperative fever. If the hematocrit stabilizes and imaging shows no extension of the hematoma, treatment is expectant. Ultrasound and CT can both demonstrate hematomas in the broad ligaments (Fig. 30.6).

Intramural Uterine Hemorrhage (Couvelaire Uterus)

Placental abruption is premature separation of the placenta after 20 weeks of gestation. There is bleeding into the decidua basalis from small arterioles in the basal layer of the decidua, which are altered and prone to rupture. Resultant hemorrhage splits the decidua. Compression of the placenta leads to obliteration of the overlying intervillous space. Ultimately, there is destruction of the placental tissue in the involved area.

In more severe examples of abruptio placentae (especially when concealed), there are extensive hemorrhages in the substance of the muscular wall of the body of the uterus. In many cases, the uterus appears of a dark port wine color if seen at cesarean section or hysterectomy. This condition is known as *Couvelaire uterus*, or *uteroplacental apoplexy*.

These intramural hemorrhages do not interfere with uterine contractility and are not associated with postpartum hemorrhage. The condition is reversible and needs no treatment.

Retroperitoneal Hematoma

Intrapartum and postpartum formation of a retroperitoneal hematoma is rare. It is serious because of the potential size of the retroperitoneal space for blood loss. Retroperitoneal hematomata may be difficult to detect even with large blood loss. The patient may be hemodynamically unstable and may require transfusion and surgery. These hematomata may also become infected, and the patient can present with fever and leukocytosis. Ultrasound, CT, and MRI may be used to detect retroperitoneal hematomata, but the modality of choice is CT.[7] We have encountered one case of retroperitoneal hematoma as a complication of pudendal block (Fig. 30.7).

Wound Hematoma and Abscess

CT is an effective technique for detecting hematomas and abscesses. In a hematoma, CT shows a soft tissue density with or without areas of diminished attenuation depending upon its age. In an abscess, liquid, gas bubbles, fluid levels, and an enhancing rim may be present. Inflammatory strands surround the collection. Cases of incisional hematoma are seen in Figures 30.8 and 30.9.

Rectus Abdominis Hematoma

A hematoma within the rectus abdominis following cesarean section generally arises from rupture of a vessel within the belly of the muscle or slipping of a suture. The patient presents with pain and swelling in the incision.

The hematoma may be seen on ultrasound, CT, or MRI; however, CT is preferred (Fig. 30.10).

Figure 30.7 Retroperitoneal hemorrhage. A 17-year-old had a pudendal block in labor, and 15 cc of 1% lignocaine was injected on each side. Four days postpartum, she had a fever, rigors, diarrhea, and increasing abdominal pain radiating to the right lower quadrant and flank. There was mild abdominal distension, decreased bowel sounds, and tenderness on palpation in the right lower quadrant. Leukocytosis and low hematocrit were present. Heterogeneous fluid and soft tissue densities (arrows) in the right retroperitoneal space along the right iliacus and psoas muscles were seen on CT. These are consistent with retroperitoneal hemorrhage.

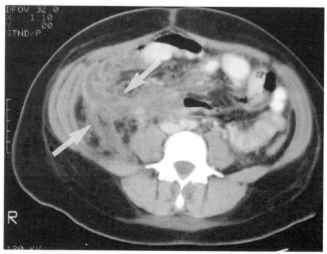

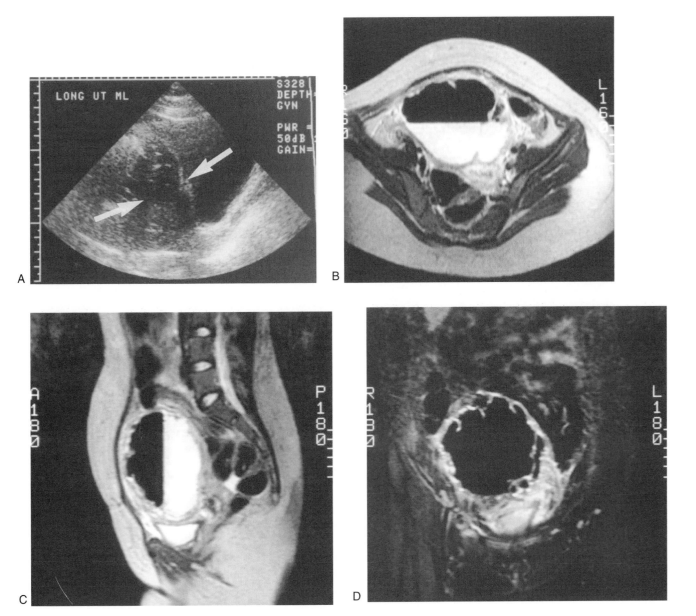

Figure 30.8 Infected intramural hematoma. A 25-year-old presented with fever and lower abdominal pain 3 weeks after cesarean section. **(A)** A longitudinal ultrasound of the pelvis shows an echogenic mass (arrows) behind the bladder. **(B)** Axial T2-weighted MRI. **(C)** Sagittal T2-weighted MRI shows the subserosal location of the collection. A fluid level is visible. **(D)** Coronal STIR MRI shows the upper part of the abscess containing gas. The margins of the abscess are irregular.

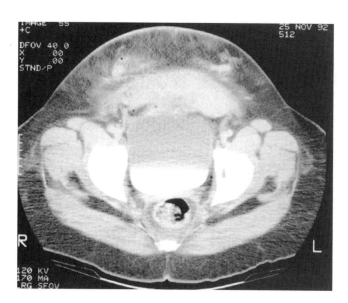

Figure 30.9 Infected incisional hematoma. Two days after cesarean section, a 32-year-old developed a fever. She did not respond to antibiotics. A CT 3 days later shows large heterogeneous soft tissue densities at the site of incision and in the underlying rectus abdominis muscle, consistent with hematoma and infection.

INFECTION

Postpartum Endometritis, Pyometra and Tubo-Ovarian Abscess

Pelvic ultrasound is not useful in making the diagnosis of postpartum pelvic cellulitis, because the image is normal. Pelvic collections such as abscesses and hematomas, on the other hand, can be seen on ultrasound, although it is usually not possible to

Figure 30.10 Rectus abdominis hematoma. CT image of the lower abdomen and pelvis in a 33-year-old woman following cesarean section. There is marked enlargement of the right rectus abdominis muscle (arrow) with a density similar to muscles, due to a hematoma. There is an area of diminished attenuation in the center due to breakdown of the blood clot. Thickened peritoneum, stranding of the pelvis, and areas of high density in the cul-de-sac represent hemoperitoneum.

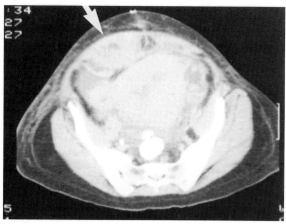

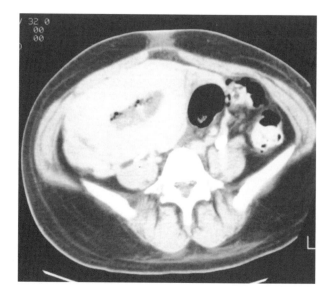

Figure 30.11 Puerperal endometritis. Five days after a normal vaginal delivery, a 26-year-old spiked a fever. A CT shows an endometrial cavity with heterogeneous density and containing gas bubbles, suggesting endometritis.

be sure whether the fluid is pus or blood on imaging features alone. The imaging features of endometritis, pyometra, and tubo-ovarian abscess are demonstrated in Figures 30.11 to 30.14.

Pelvic Thrombophlebitis and Ovarian Vein Thrombosis

CT is the modality of choice in visualizing a thrombus. A thrombosed vessel appears as a low-attenuation tubular

Figure 30.12 Pyometra. Three weeks after cesarean section, a 23-year-old presented with fever, abdominal pain, and heavy vaginal discharge of 1 weeks' duration. CT shows a fluid level in the endometrial cavity. The fluid is dense, consistent with pus. One liter of pus was drained from the uterus through the cervix.

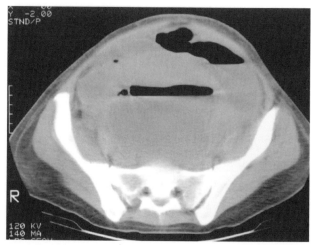

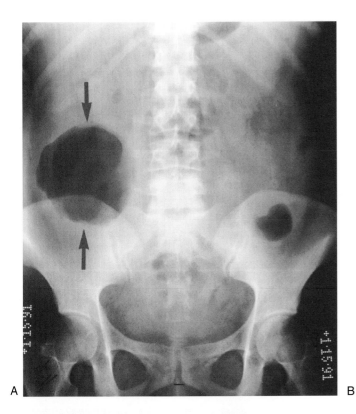

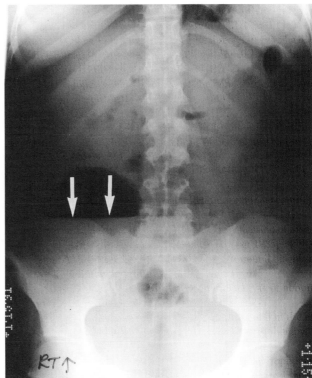

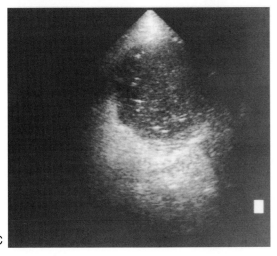

Figure 30.13 Tubo-ovarian abscess. A 22-year-old woman presented with right-sided abdominal pain, fever, and rigors 10 days after cesarean section. **(A)** Plain supine abdominal radiograph revealed gas (arrows). **(B)** Erect view revealed a fluid level (arrows) in the right lower quadrant. **(C)** Ultrasound of the right lower quadrant shows an echogenic mass with multiple internal echoes. A large right tubo-ovarian abscess was found at laparotomy.

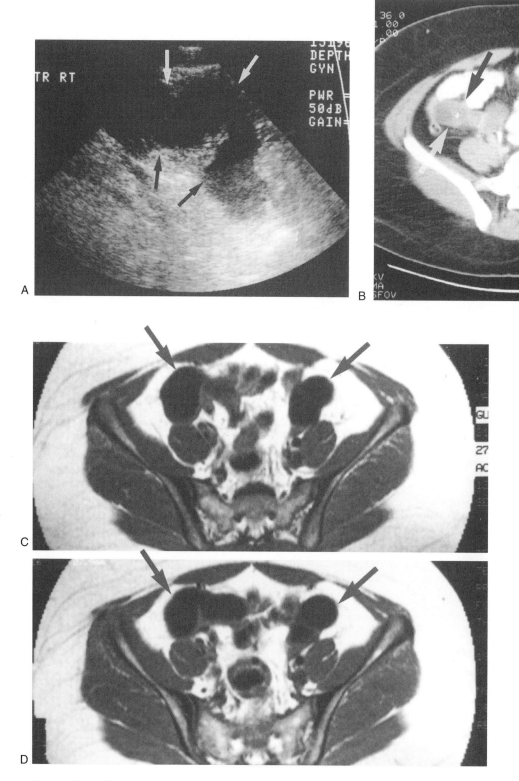

Figure 30.14 Hydrosalpinges. A 39-year-old gravida 2, para 1 presented with right lower quadrant pain, nausea, and vomiting. **(A)** Ultrasound revealed hydrosalpinges on both sides. The one on the right is shown (arrows). **(B)** CT showed a hydrosalpinx (arrows) with surrounding inflammatory strands, suggesting tubo-ovarian abscess. **(C & D)** Axial T1-weighted MRI showed marked dilatation of the fallopian tubes bilaterally (arrows) with diameters of 2 to 3 cm. The findings suggest bilateral pyosalpinges.

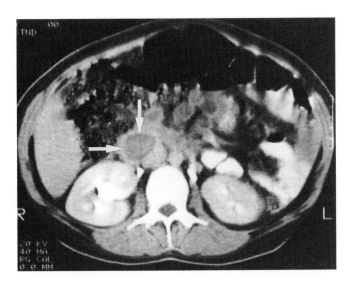

Figure 30.15 Thrombophlebitis of the ovarian vein. A 30-year-old, 1-week postpartum, complained of fever, lower abdominal and right flank pain. On CT there was a tubular structure (arrows) originating from the pelvis on the right side, lateral to the uterus and right ureter, and anterolateral to the right psoas, ascending cephalad. This had a center of low attenuation and an enhancing rim consistent with right ovarian vein thrombophlebitis. Surrounding inflammatory strands are present. The markedly dilated thrombotic right ovarian vein impinges upon the right lateral aspect of the inferior vena cava.

structure that can be followed on sequential images, to determine its extent. There is an enhancing rim. Inflammatory strands are present in the case of thrombophlebitis (Figs. 30.15 and 30.16). MRI also delineates the ovarian vein thrombosis as serpiginous structures with abnormal signal intensities, coursing along the retroperitoneum (Fig. 30.16). Thrombosed ovarian veins could be detected by ultrasonography, but CT is superior in determining their orientation, nature, and anatomic origin. CT also helps differentiate ovarian vein thrombosis from other clinically similar conditions such as appendicitis and appendiceal or pelvic abscesses.

Appendicitis

CT is the most helpful imaging technique to detect acute appendicitis with perforation and abscess formation. Ultrasound with graded compression is also helpful in making the diagnosis of acute appendicitis but is operator dependent. Appendicitis and appendiceal abscesses in the postpartum period are seen in Figures 30.17 and 30.18.

MISCELLANEOUS: FOREIGN BODIES

Surgical Sponge

Plain radiography will show the radiopaque marker in the surgical sponge, but the size of the granuloma or abscess formed around the foreign body can only be detected on CT or ultrasound. In addition, CT better evaluates the relationship of the granuloma mass or abscess to the bowel or other intra-abdominal structures. A retained surgical sponge following cesarean section is shown in Figure 30.19.

Intrauterine Contraceptive Device

At times, a patient will become pregnant in spite of having an intrauterine contraceptive device (IUCD) in place. The usual practice is to remove the IUCD early in the pregnancy, but as the pregnancy progresses, the IUCD with its strings will "migrate" up into the uterus, making it impossible to remove. If the pregnancy is allowed to go to term, the IUCD will be expelled, usually embedded in the placenta and amniotic membranes. If the IUCD is not retrieved, it may be embedded within the myometrium.

Occasionally, an IUCD may pass through the uterus into the peritoneal cavity. It will be seen in the pelvis on a plain radiograph, and ultrasound will show that it is not in the uterus. CT demonstrates the position of the IUCD in the adnexa (Fig. 30.20).

SUMMARY

The imaging workup of the postpartum and postabortal pelvis should commence with ultrasonography which can be performed at the bedside, lacks ionizing radiation, and is cost-effective. The usefulness of ultrasound is limited in the presence of obesity, gaseous distension, and an abdominal wound. CT is superior in detecting and delineating the extent of the abnormality, but it uses ionizing radiation and often requires intravenous contrast. MRI has the advantages of multiplanar capability, high soft tissue characterization, and lack of ionizing radiation, but it is more time-consuming, expensive, and its application is limited in patients with life-support appliances.

ACKNOWLEDGMENTS

The authors thank René Retana and Geoffrey Schieb for their secretarial and art work in the preparation of this chapter.

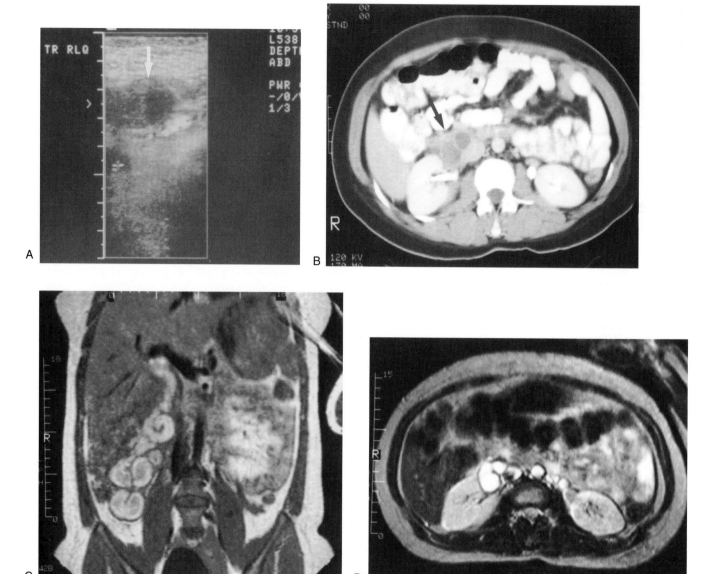

Figure 30.16 Ovarian vein thrombosis. Four days after confinement, a 32-year-old complained of nausea, vomiting, and diffuse abdominal pain, mostly in the right lower quadrant. She had a leukocytosis of 12,800/ml. **(A)** Transverse ultrasound image of the right lower quadrant shows a large mass (arrow) with internal echoes, due to a dilated right ovarian vein filled with thrombus. No flow was seen on color flow images. **(B)** CT of the pelvis and abdomen showed a large, tubular, low-attenuation structure originating from the pelvis on the right side (arrow) and extending cephalad retroperitoneally to the level of kidneys. This has a low-attenuation center and an enhancing rim and is surrounded by inflammatory strands. **(C)** Coronal T1-weighted MRI. **(D)** Axial T2-weighted MRI shows a tortuous structure originating from the pelvis and extending retroperitoneally to the level of the right kidney. Findings on CT and MRI are consistent with right ovarian vein thrombophlebitis. The patient recovered with antibiotic and anticoagulation therapy.

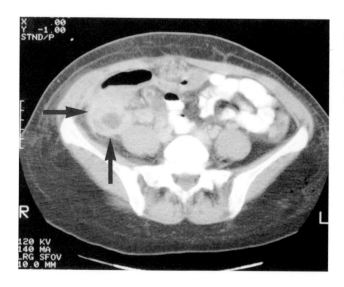

Figure 30.17 Appendiceal abscess. A 35-year-old woman, 2 weeks after cesarean section, complained of fever, anorexia, and right lower quadrant pain. CT shows a fluid collection in the right lower quadrant, due to an appendiceal abscess (arrows). Surrounding inflammatory strands are seen.

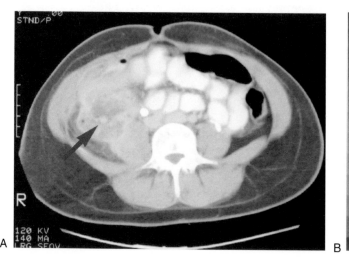
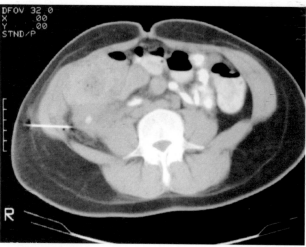

Figure 30.18 Appendiceal abscess. Six weeks after cesarean section, this patient complained of nausea, anorexia, fever, chills, and right lower quadrant pain radiating to her lower back. She had a leukocytosis of 13,000. A complex collection with indistinct margins was present in the right lower quadrant on an abdominal ultrasound. **(A)** CT showed an abnormal fluid collection with heterogeneous density, containing an appendicolith (arrow) and surrounded by inflammatory strands, diagnostic of a perforated retrocecal appendicitis with abscess formation. **(B)** The abscess was drained percutaneously.

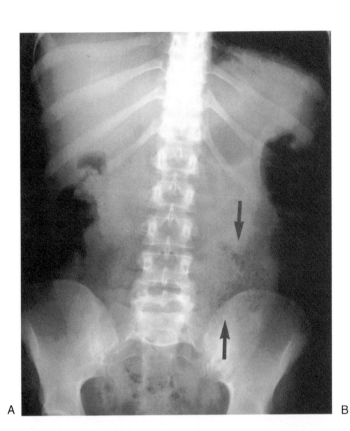

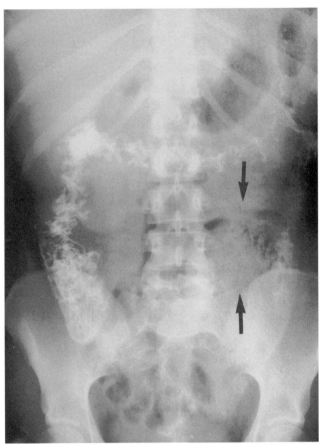

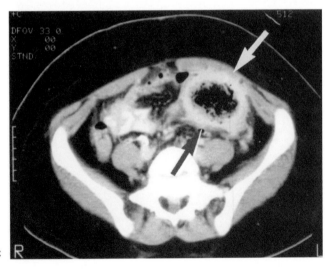

Figure 30.19 Surgical sponge. A 21-year-old woman presented with increasing left-sided lower abdominal pain, constipation, and vomiting for 3 weeks' duration. On physical examination, a 6 × 10-cm fixed and tender mass was palpable in the left lower quadrant. The patient had undergone a cesarean section 9 months previously in another country. **(A)** Plain abdominal radiograph shows gas and feces in the colon. There is an area of mottled opacity in the left lower quadrant with an appearance of feces (arrows). **(B)** Examination of the colon with barium showed that the area of mottled density (arrows) lies outside the colon. **(C)** CT shows a large mass (arrows) in the left lower quadrant. The mass is extraluminal and contains innumerable air bubbles in a honeycomb pattern. At laparotomy, a surgical sponge was found in the abdominal cavity with an inflammatory and fistulous communication with the small bowel. The densely enhanced circular periphery of the mass represents surrounding granulation tissue. In most countries, surgical sponges contain a radio-opaque thread that is visible on plain radiographs. (Figs. A and B from Rooholamini et al.,[8] with permission.)

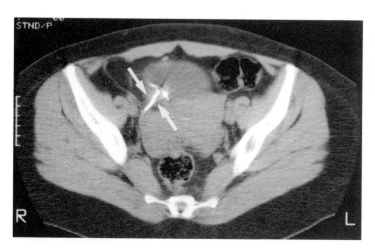

Figure 30.20 At the time of insertion of an IUCD, this patient had complained of lower abdominal pain for 3 months. The strings could not be seen on pelvic examination, and ultrasound showed that the IUCD was not in the uterine cavity. On CT, the IUCD (arrows) was seen in the right adnexa.

REFERENCES

1. Plauche WC. Rupture of the uterus. In: Nichols DH, Ed. Gynecologic and Obstetric Surgery. CV Mosby, St. Louis, 1993, pp 1135–1146
2. Acton CM. The ultrasonic appearance of a ruptured uterus. Austral Radiol 1978;22:254
3. Osmers R. Sonographic detection of a asymptomatic rupture of the uterus due to necrosis during the third trimester. Int J Gynecol Obstet 1988;26:279
4. Abramson D, Roberts SM, Wilson PD. Relaxation of the pubic joint in pregnancy. Surg Gynecol Obstet 1934;58:595–613
5. Lindsey RW, Leggon RE, Wright DG, Nolasco DR. Separation of the symphysis pubis in association with childbearing. A case report. J Bone Joint Surg [US] 1988;70:289–292
6. Kurzel RB, Au AH, Rooholamini SA, Smith W. Magnetic resonance imaging of the peripartum rupture of the symphysis pubis. Obstet Gynecol 1996;87:826–829
7. Korobkin M, Silverman PM, Quint LE, Francis IR. CT of the extraperitoneal space: normal anatomy and fluid collections. AJR Am J Roentgenol 1992;159:933–942
8. Rooholamini SA, Au AH, Hansen GC et al. Imaging of pregnancy-related complications. Radiographics 1993;13:753–770

31

Ultrasonography of the Postmenopausal Pelvis

DEBORAH LEVINE

In the United States, 35 million women (more than 25% of the female population) are postmenopausal. Because of their age, they are at increased risk for ovarian and endometrial cancers, which are two of the five most common causes of cancer deaths in women.[1] Clinical problems of postmenopausal women differ from those of premenopausal women. Vaginal bleeding, which is normal before the menopause, is worrisome for postmenopausal women. As the population grows and longevity increases, the number of postmenopausal women increases, and gynecologic cancers will become more common. It has been shown that the ovary and endometrium can be active after the menopause. A knowledge of the changes to be expected with aging is required to care for these women.

THE UTERUS

Myometrium

Fibroids

The normal postmenopausal uterus is atrophic (Fig. 31.1). After the menopause, the uterus decreases in size, with the most rapid decline occurring in the first 10 years.[2] Then there is a more gradual decline in size, frequently resulting in the uterus assuming a premenarchal configuration with the cervix being larger than the body of the uterus. This decrease in size is affected by parity. Uterine weight is greater in women of higher parity,[3] and in those with fibroids. Fibroids, like the uterus, decrease in size after menopause.

Fibroids, endometrial polyps, adenomyosis, or late endometrial cancer can enlarge the uterus. Calcification is often seen in patients with fibroids (Fig. 31.2). Calcification also occasionally occurs in the arcuate arteries. It may be seen in women with hypertension, diabetes, or renal failure (Fig. 31.3). It appears as small areas of hyperechogenicity with acoustic shadowing in the periphery of the myometrium along the course of the arcuate artery.[4] Calcification may cast dense shadows that limit visualization of the endometrium. Transvaginal sonography (TVS) is helpful in these patients,

since the higher frequency transducer allows visualization between or around areas of calcification.

Endometrium

Hormonal Replacement Therapy

If estrogen is given to postmenopausal women, it reduces the risk of osteoporosis, relieves atrophic vaginitis, and smooths the transition from high to low endogenous estrogen levels. Unfortunately, if given alone, there is a risk of causing endometrial cancer. The duration of estrogen use and the cumulative dose are major predictors of endometrial cancer.[5,6] For this reason, progesterone is usually given along with estrogen unless the woman has had a hysterectomy.

The progesterone induces endometrial atrophy, reducing the risk of cancer to that of postmenopausal women not receiving hormonal therapy.[7,8] Due to the side effects of progesterone (bloating, depression, and breast tenderness) and the increased risk of coronary artery disease with progestin,[5,7] minimal doses are used.

In the United States, estrogens are most frequently given from day 1 to day 25 of the month with progesterone added on day 13 to 16 and continued to day 25.[8] With this sequential regimen, withdrawal bleeding occurs in about 95% of patients under the age of 60. This proportion decreases with age, so that by age 65 only 60% will continue to experience light bleeding.[9] In order to decrease this bleeding, some patients take continuous daily estrogen and progesterone. This can lead to atrophy of the endometrium within 3 to 4 months.[10] Vaginal estrogen cream can be absorbed and have a trophic effect on the endometrium.[11]

Among women using hormonal replacement, the percentage of women with increased endometrial thickness varies with the regimen used.[12,13] Women not taking exogenous estrogens and those taking continuous combined estrogen and progesterone typically have atrophic endometria, with fewer than 15% having an endometrium greater than 8 mm.[12]

In contrast, approximately 50% of women using unopposed estrogen have an endometrial thickness greater than 8 mm in diameter.[12] This causes a diagnostic dilemma because

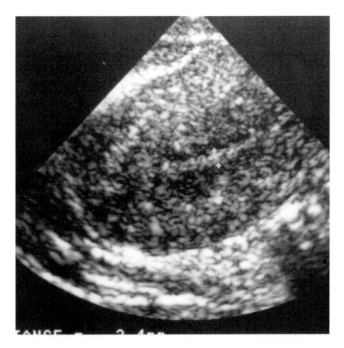

Figure 31.1 Sagittal TVS of a typical postmenopausal uterus with an atrophic endometrium measuring 2 mm (calipers).

of the increased incidence of endometrial hyperplasia, polyps, and carcinoma in women with an endometrial thickness greater than 8 mm. Women taking sequential hormone regimens also tend to have thick endometria. Since the endometria in these women can develop proliferative, secretory, and bleeding phases,[10] this thickness is likely to change with the phase of the hormone cycle. This change in endometrial thickness has been demonstrated in women in their sixth and seventh decade[13] (Fig. 31.4). These women may have a thick endometrium (up to 18 mm) in the middle of the hormone cycle. Thus, the sonographic appearance of the endometrium

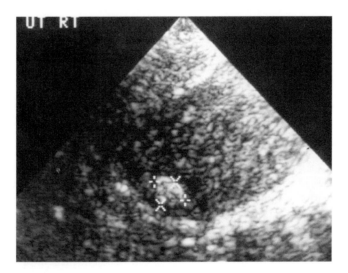

Figure 31.2 TVS of the uterus in a 60-year-old woman demonstrates a focal calcification (calipers) due to a degenerated fibroid.

is dependent upon the type of hormone regimen that the patient uses and, if she uses sequential hormones, the phase of the hormone cycle.

Therefore, if a thick endometrium is seen in a woman who is taking sequential hormones and who is in the middle of the hormone cycle, she should be rescanned after the completion of the progesterone phase of her cycle, or near the end of withdrawal bleeding, when the endometrium is theoretically at its thinnest. A persistently thick endometrium should be biopsied.

Tamoxifen

Tamoxifen is used in the treatment of breast cancer and as a preventive agent against the development of breast cancer in women with a hereditary risk. Although it is an estrogen antagonist in the breast, it acts as a mild estrogen agonist in the uterus and is therefore associated with increased risk of endometrial hyperplasia, polyps, and cancer. It causes a cystic appearance of the myometrium which may mimic endometrial thickening. This is thought to be due to reactivation of foci of adenomyosis within the inner layer of the myometrium[14,15] (Fig. 31.5). Therefore, in women who use tamoxifen and whose endometrium seems thick on ultrasound, biopsies frequently will show atrophy or insufficient tissue for diagnosis.[15,16] Sonohysterography may be helpful, since the endometrium can be seen to be thin and atrophic overlying a cystic appearing myometrium.[14] Women on tamoxifen with abnormal bleeding should undergo endometrial biopsy because of the risk of cancer.

A similar appearance of a thickened endometrium demonstrated by transvaginal scanning with atrophic tissue after biopsy has been reported in a breast cancer patient using megestrol acetate (an estrogen agonist).[17]

Endometrial bleeding

Bleeding may occur with normal atrophic endometrium, but it can also be due to hyperplasia, polyps, or cancer (all of which cause endometrial thickening). TVS is the method of choice to image the endometrium in women with postmenopausal bleeding and to screen women at risk for endometrial cancer (i.e., those women using unopposed estrogen and tamoxifen). It has been shown that ultrasound is more sensitive than endometrial biopsy in the detection of endometrial abnormalities. Shipley and colleagues[4] compared ultrasound and endometrial biopsy in the evaluation of asymptomatic postmenopausal women and found that endometrial biopsies were reported as an inadequate specimen or with some other nonspecific result in 70% of patients in whom either endometrial hyperplasia or polyps were subsequently proven. TVS had a sensitivity of 80% in the detection of endometrial abnormalities, compared to 30% sensitivity for endometrial biopsy. Van den Bosch et al.[18] evaluated symptomatic postmenopausal women, using 4 mm for endometrial thickness, and found a sensitivity of 82% for the detection of abnormal endometrial histology for TVS compared

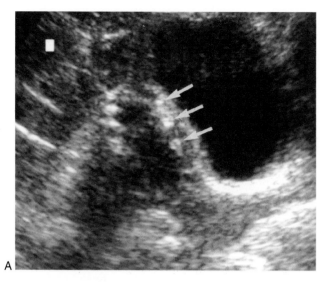

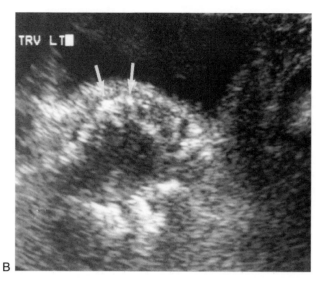

Figure 31.3 Arcuate artery calcifications in the uterus of an 80-year-old woman with hypertension demonstrate peripheral segmental calcifications (arrows). These calcifications are thought to be caused by cystic medial necrosis within the arcuate arteries. Visualization of the endometrium is limited by these calcifications on this transabdominal study **(A)** Sagittal view. **(B)** Transverse view.

to 45% for endometrial biopsy. These suggest that ultrasound, in addition to endometrial biopsy, is needed for the complete evaluation of symptomatic postmenopausal women.

The thickness of normal postmenopausal endometrium varies if there is bleeding or if hormones are in use. A clinically useful threshold for normal endometrial thickness in symptomatic women is 4 mm. A thickness of up to 8 mm is considered normal in asymptomatic women. A decision tree for endometrial thickness is shown in Figure 31.6.

Due to low estrogen levels, the endometrium of untreated postmenopausal women becomes atrophic. It appears as a thin echogenic line in the midline of the uterus. A hypoechoic halo may be seen surrounding the echogenic endometrium. This is commonly seen in premenopausal women, but is less obvious in most postmenopausal women. It has been shown that this hypoechoic area correlates histologically with the inner compact layer of the myometrium.[19] For this reason, it should not be included in endometrial measurements. Similarly, endometrial fluid, if present, should be excluded from the endometrial measurement (Fig. 31.7).

In postmenopausal women, the most frequent cause of bleeding is endometrial atrophy (due to the friable endometrium).[20,21] Sonography is a noninvasive method that can be used to minimize unnecessary biopsies. Many studies have shown that atrophic or benign endometria have a thickness of 4 mm or less.[22–27] Using a threshold of 5 mm, Granberg and co-workers[27] evaluated the endometrial thickness in 205 postmenopausal women with bleeding and found that 70% of curettages could have been avoided without missing any malignancies. Postmenopausal women with bleeding who have an endometrium greater than 4 mm should undergo a biopsy.

Endometrial Fluid

Endometrial fluid in the past has been thought to be an indicator of malignancy of the endometrium or cervix.[28] However, in the postmenopausal patient, endometrial fluid usually has a benign cause,[29,30] due to cervical stenosis from previous instrumentation or childbirth[30,31] (Fig. 31.8). Ultrasound often reveals tiny collections of fluid of less than 2 ml that are of no significance[12,13,31,32] (Fig. 31.7). The important sign is the thickness of the surrounding endometrium. A fluid collection surrounded by a thin endometrium, regardless of the amount of fluid, is likely to be benign[31] (Fig. 31.8). Fluid with any endometrial irregularity deserves a biopsy.

Tiny fluid collections can occasionally be detected within the myometrium of postmenopausal women. These are usually foci of adenomyosis. Adenomyosis is found in 15% to 20% of uteri postmortem.

Endometrial Hyperplasia

Endometrial hyperplasia is an abnormal proliferation of endometrial glands and stroma. This may result in histologic findings of cystically dilated glands to crowded glands with cellular atypia. Cystic hyperplasia is the most common and benign variant, with a low rate of progression to endometrial cancer.[33] Adenomatous and atypical forms of hyperplasia are precursors to endometrial carcinoma.

Endometrial hyperplasia is seen as thickening of the endometrium, which may be heterogeneous (Fig. 31.9). Hyperplasia usually is diffuse, but at times may be focal.[34] In cases of cystic hyperplasia, endometrial cysts may be visualized within an otherwise echogenic endometrium.

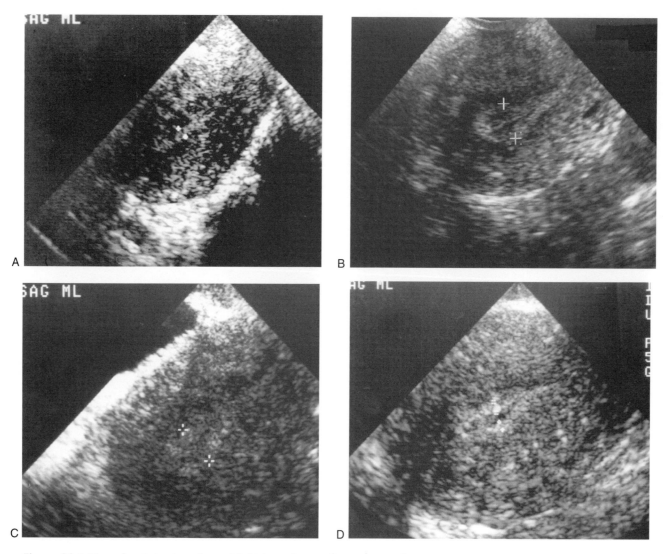

Figure 31.4 Normal variation in endometrial thickness from cyclic estrogen replacement in a 62-year-old woman. **(A)** Day 2, echogenic endometrium, 3 mm thick (calipers). **(B)** Day 9, three-layer endometrium, 10 mm thick. **(C)** Day 23, echogenic endometrium, 11 mm thick. **(D)** Day 27, echogenic endometrium with central debris, 5 mm thick. Women taking sequential hormones should be examined after the progesterone phase, when the endometrium is theoretically at it thinnest. (From Levine et al.,[13] with permission.)

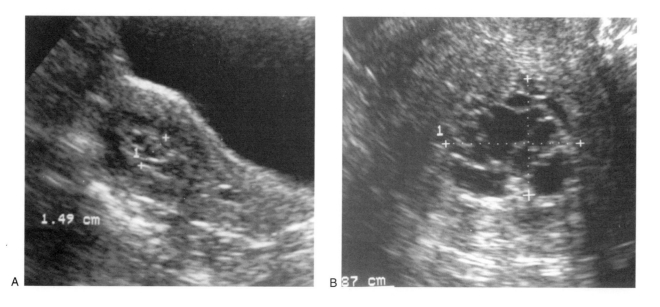

Endometrial Thickness (Double Layer)

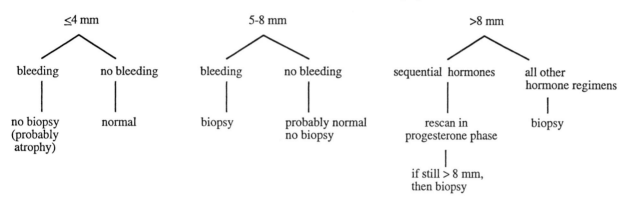

≤4 mm		5-8 mm		>8 mm	
bleeding	no bleeding	bleeding	no bleeding	sequential hormones	all other hormone regimens
no biopsy (probably atrophy)	normal	biopsy	probably normal no biopsy	rescan in progesterone phase	biopsy
				if still > 8 mm, then biopsy	

Figure 31.6 Decision tree for the evaluation of women with and without bleeding based on endometrial thickness and hormone use. (From Levine et al.,[13] with permission.)

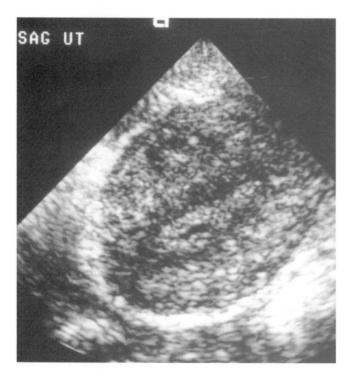

SAG UT

Figure 31.7 TVS shows a tiny endometrial fluid collection that did not change over a 1-year interval. Fluid should not be included in endometrial thickness measurements.

Figure 31.5 Cystic appearing endometria in two postmenopausal women taking tamoxifen. (A) Transabdominal view. (B) Transvaginal view. Both women had biopsies with unremarkable histology.

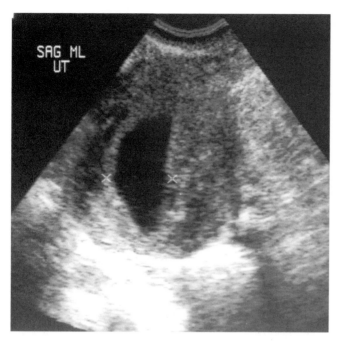

Figure 31.8 Sagittal view of the uterus in a 63-year-old asymptomatic woman placed on cyclic hormones demonstrates a large endometrial fluid collection. Her cervical stenosis was subsequently dilated, with drainage of the fluid. Endometrial biopsy was unremarkable.

Endometrial Polyps

Endometrial polyps often are difficult to distinguish from endometrial hyperplasia. However, if fluid is present within the endometrial cavity, it will outline a focal soft tissue mass, sometimes on a stalk (Fig. 31.10). Polyps can also be identified with color Doppler, when a single vessel is seen to enter

the middle of the mass. An important differentiation between polyps and submucosal fibroids is that polyps tend to have a homogeneous hyperechoic texture[35] (except for areas of cysts and vessels), whereas fibroids have a heterogeneous hypoechoic texture. Polyps do not distort the hypoechoic myometrial–endometrial interface, whereas submucosal fibroids frequently do cause distortion of this interface. Identification of polyps is important, since they are often missed with endometrial biopsies. The sonographic finding of a thick endometrium, in a patient in whom subsequent biopsy yields a report of "tissue insufficient for diagnosis" or "endometrial atrophy" raises suspicion that a polyp has been missed at biopsy.[13,29,36] These patients require a sonohysterogram or hysteroscopy.

Endometrial Cancer

Endometrial carcinoma is the most common gynecologic cancer, with 32,000 new cases reported in the United States in 1992[2] of whom 75% to 80% were postmenopausal. Risk factors include use of unopposed estrogen, obesity, and nulliparity. The disease is generally diagnosed at an early stage, usually because of uterine bleeding.

Endometrial carcinoma is suggested on ultrasound when the endometrium is heterogeneously echogenic with ill-defined hypoechoic areas and ill-defined margins between the endometrium and myometrium.[37] An ill-defined polypoid mass may be seen projecting within the endometrium[38] (Fig. 31.11). Advanced cases of endometrial cancer present with enlargement of the uterus, a lobular contour of the uterus, and mixed echogenicity of the myometrium[39] (Fig. 31.12). The depth of invasion can be demonstrated by transvaginal ultrasound[40,41] although magnetic resonance imaging (MRI) is more sensitive in this regard.[42] MRI also is useful in evalua-

Figure 31.9 Endometrial hyperplasia in a 63-year-old woman with a granulosa cell tumor (see Fig. 31.16). Sagittal view of the uterus demonstrates a 15-mm-thick endometrium (calipers) with a tiny cyst. The histology was endometrial hyperplasia, probably secondary to the estrogenic effect of the granulosa cell tumor.

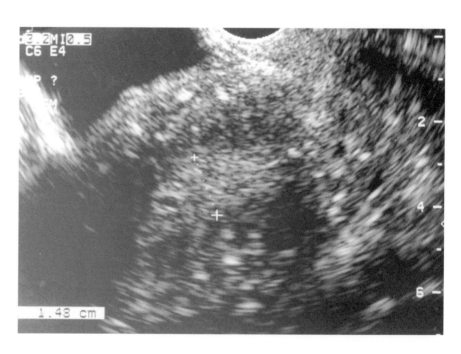

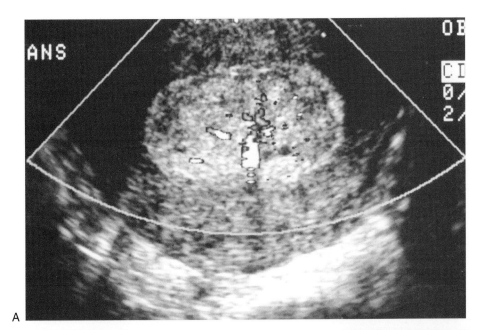

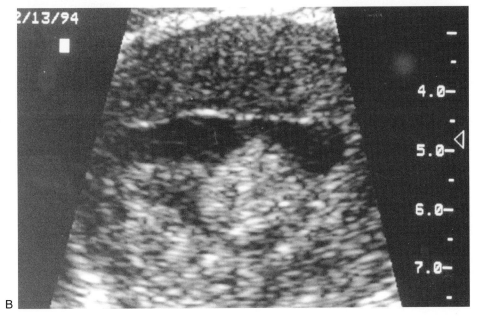

Figure 31.10 Endometrial polyps. **(A)** TVS in a 52-year-old woman demonstrates a thick echogenic endometrium (which measured 27 mm in the sagittal plane) with a single vessel entering centrally and branching, suggestive of a polyp. **(B)** TVS in a 51-year-old woman with fluid surrounding a pedunculated polyp.

tion of extrauterine extension and involvement of lymph nodes.

Doppler Evaluation of the Endometrium

There is disagreement in the literature regarding the utility of Doppler analysis of the endometrium, with calculation of the resistive index or pulsatility index, in the distinction between benign and malignant causes of endometrial thickening.[43–47] Since there is overlap in the resistive index findings in benign and malignant lesions, it is prudent to treat all cases of thickened endometrium as potentially malignant regardless of the blood-flow characteristics.

Sonohysterography

Sonohysterography is helpful in distinguishing polyps, submucosal fibroids, and endometrial hyperplasia in patients with postmenopausal bleeding. Sterile saline is instilled into the endometrial cavity through a pediatric feeding tube or a hysterosalpingography catheter. Scanning is performed transvaginally. In this manner, the discrimination between intracavitary, endometrial, and submucosal masses can be made.[48] Focal and diffuse processes can be distinguished. When focal areas of asymmetric endometrial thickening are identified, biopsy can be directed toward the site.[34,49] Because polyps and submucous fibroids can be distinguished from diffuse processes with sonohysterography, the technique can

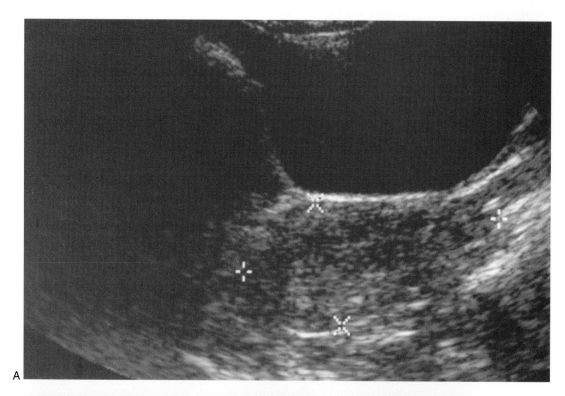

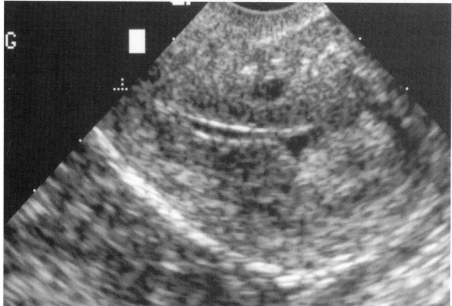

Figure 31.11 Endometrial carcinoma in a 62-year-old woman with abnormal bleeding. **(A)** Transabdominal sonography (TAS) of the uterus (calipers) shows an ill-defined endometrium. **(B)** TVS shows a focal area of endometrial thickening with invasion into the myometrium, consistent with endometrial carcinoma. Women with abnormal bleeding should be examined transvaginally in order to visualize the endometrium optimally.

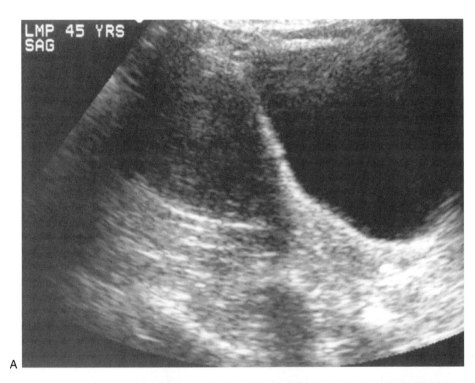

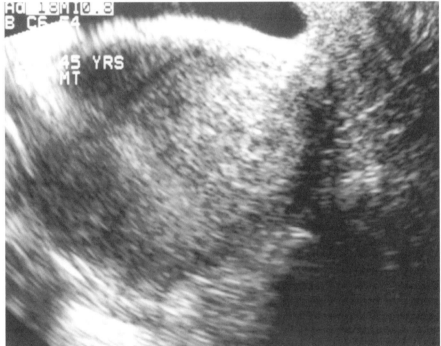

Figure 31.12 Endometrial carcinoma in a 90-year-old woman with vaginal bleeding. **(A)** TAS, midline view demonstrates an enlarged uterus. **(B)** TVS, sagittal view of the uterus demonstrates an ill-defined heterogeneous endometrium with invasion of the myometrium. This is the same patient as Figure 30.15. It is important to evaluate the adnexa in patients with endometrial abnormalities (and vice versa), since tumors of these organs are often synchronous.

help identify those patients who would benefit from hysteroscopy and a directed biopsy.[48]

THE OVARIES

Normal Ovaries

Ovarian size decreases after the menopause, with a rapid decline in ovarian volume in the first 5 to 10 years after menopause, and then a more gradual decrease in size.[50,51] Because of this, ovarian volumes in the first years after menopause should be interpreted with caution. This leads to difficulty in establishing a normal size for the postmenopausal ovary. Reports vary from 1.2 to 5.8 cm(Table 31.1). These values are probably high, since ovaries that were not visualized by ultrasound were excluded in the average size determination. Goswamy et al.[50] also reported that body weight, parity, and use of estrogens are associated with increased ovarian volume after the menopause. Given the variation in normal, a general guideline for ovarian size is that the ovarian volume should be less than 8 cc and should not be greater than twice the volume of the opposite side.[51,55,56]

The typical postmenopausal ovary is a hypoechoic, well-defined ovoid echo complex, usually measuring 2 cm or less in its greatest diameter (Fig. 31.13). Due to the absence of follicles, they are often difficult to identify. Visualization of normal postmenopausal ovaries varies from 20% to 99%[53,58,61,62] (Table 31.1). This variation is probably secondary to operator variations and patient population. Demonstration of the ovaries is known to decrease over the years after the menopause and also after hysterectomy.[62]

Ovarian Cysts

The previous contention that any palpable postmenopausal ovary should be removed[63] is no longer universally accepted. This is in a large part due to the ultrasound findings of benign-appearing cysts in the postmenopausal ovary. While in premenopausal women, most ovarian cysts result from cyclic hormonal stimulation, this stimulus is no longer present after menopause. Because 85% to 90% of malignancies are epithelial in origin[64–66] and the majority of these are cystic, the occurrence of any ovarian cyst in a postmenopausal woman has been considered potentially a cystic neoplasm and an indication for surgery. While in the past it was thought that any cyst within the postmenopausal ovary was abnormal, there is recent evidence that adnexal cysts are common in postmenopausal women. Small (< 5 cm), unilocular, anechoic postmenopausal cysts are unlikely to be malignant[41,62,66–74] (Fig. 31.14).

Wolf et al.[62] demonstrated that small anechoic cysts are seen in 15% of women on initial screen, with no association between cyst occurrence and patient age, length of time since

Table 31.1 Summary of the Current Literature on Postmenopausal Ovary Size

Author (Year)	No. of Patients	Age	Modality	Mean Volume (cm³)	Volume Range (cm³)	Ovaries Visualized (%)
Campbell et al[56] (1982)	31	50–59	TAS	4.3	1.5–10.4	84
Goswamy et al[52] (1983)	1,016	39–78	TAS	3.7	0.9–9.8	99
Hall et al[55] (1986)	30	51–80	TAS	—	<1.5–2.5	68
Granberg and Wikland[53] (1987)	11	—	TAS	1.2	—	71
	11	—	TVS	1.3	—	48
Goswamy et al[50] (1988)	2,221	44–79	TAS	3.6	1.0–14.0	99
Granberg et al[51] (1988)	36	—	TAS	1.4	—	87
Higgins et al[59] (1989)	260	41–86	TVS	2.9	0.4–7.8	87
Cohen et al[57] (1990)	50	>50[a]	TAS	5.8	1.2–14.1	48–75[a]
Schoenfeld et al[41] (1990)	17	50–76	TVS	1.3	—	—
Van Nagell et al[60] (1990)[b]	578	41–87	TVS	3.0	0.2–8.0	—
Wolf et al[62] (1991)	91	47–86	TAS	2.5	1.1–9.5	58[c]
	91	47–86	TVS	2.0	1.2–9.3	41[c]
Di Santis et al[58] (1993)	37	—	TVS	4.0	1.1–12.2	20

[a] Estimated from their data.

[b] Includes data from Higgins et al.[59]

[c] Values represent ovaries imaged in two planes. A much higher percentage was seen on one plane, 76% of ovaries were visualized in women who had not had a hysterectomy.

(From Levine,[93] with permission.)

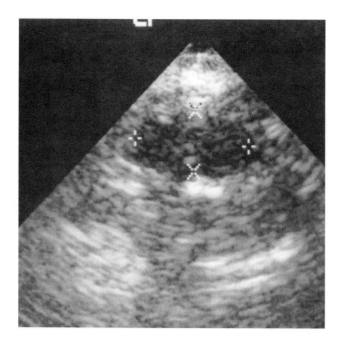

Figure 31.13 Transverse image of a normal postmenopausal ovary in a 54-year-old woman.

menopause, or hormone use. A follow-up study showed that cysts are seen in up to 23% of postmenopausal women over a 2-year interval and that these cysts can change in size.[75] Of 72 cysts observed over a period of 3 to 23 months, 38 (53%) disappeared completely, 20 (28%) were unchanged, 8 (11%) en-

larged by 3 mm or more, 2 (3%) decreased in size by 3 mm or more, and 4 (6%) both increased and decreased in size on repeated examination.[75] No association was found between changing cysts and length of time since menopause.

Other Ovarian Masses

Cystadenomas may appear as simple or complex cysts (Fig. 31.15). Other tumors found in postmenopausal women include granulosa cell tumors (Fig. 31.16), cystic teratomas (Fig. 31.17), and fibromas (Fig. 31.18).

Ovarian Cancer

Ovarian cancer is the leading cause of death from gynecologic malignancy in the United States. In 1994 approximately 24,000 new cases of ovarian cancer were diagnosed, with more than 13,600 women dying from the disease.[76] The lifetime incidence is 1 in 70 women. The high mortality rate is due to the disease presenting at a late stage, with greater than 70% of patients initially diagnosed having advanced disease (stage III and IV). Therefore, methods that improve the early detection should decrease mortality.

The risk of developing ovarian cancer increases with age. Women age 40 to 44 have an incidence of 16 cases/100,000 compared to women age 75 to 79 who have an incidence of 54/100,000.[77] Women at additional increased risk are those with a positive family history; history of endometrial, colon, or breast cancer; and increased ovulatory age (nulliparity and

Figure 31.14 Disappearing ovarian cyst. **(A)** Transverse view of the left ovary in a 68-year-old woman demonstrates a 4.7-cm anechoic cyst (C). **(B)** Follow-up examination 6 months later shows near complete resolution of the cyst, now 3 mm (calipers). Three months later, the cyst completely disappeared. (From Levine et al.,[75] with permission.)

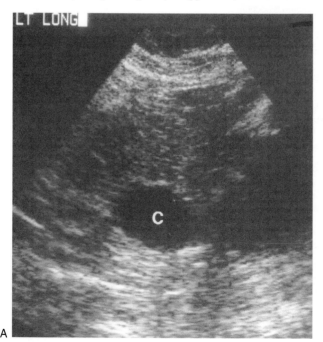

A

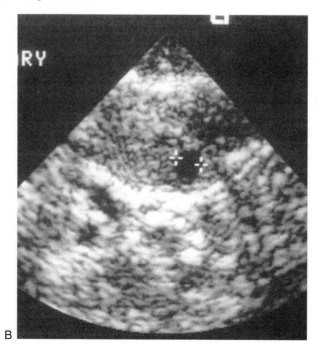

B

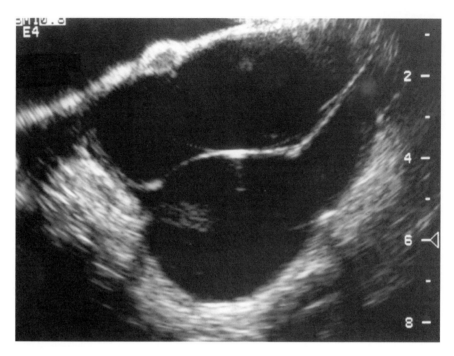

Figure 31.15 Transverse view of the left ovary in a 90-year-old woman showing a 6-cm cyst with a thin septum. Histologic examination revealed a serous cystadenoma. This is the same patient as Figure 30.12.

Figure 31.16 TAS of a 6-cm heterogeneous solid right adnexal mass in a patient with a thick endometrium (see Fig. 30.9). This was a granulosa cell tumor with associated endometrial hyperplasia.

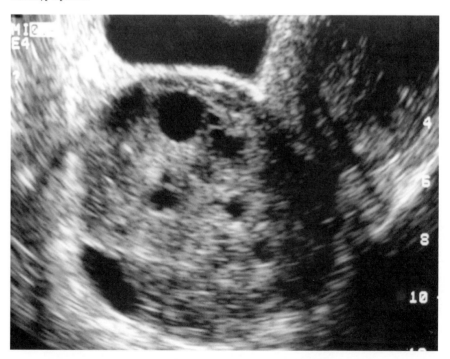

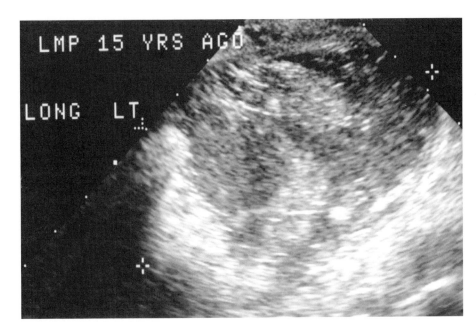

Figure 31.17 Dermoid in a 60-year-old woman. Longitudinal view of the left adnexa shows a 7-cm complex cystic mass with linear bright reflectors and echogenic material suggestive of a dermoid, confirmed at histology.

lack of oral contraceptive use).[76,78] Because ultrasound is sensitive in the detection of ovarian abnormalities, it has been advocated as a screening method for early ovarian cancer.[52,53,61,64,79–82]

When an ovarian abnormality is seen, some advocate the use of CA-125, a serum marker for ovarian cancer.[83] The CA-125 level has been shown to be elevated in over 80% of epithelial ovarian cancers.[84] CA-125 has been used to distinguish benign from malignant pelvic masses. In postmenopausal women, using a threshold of 35 U/ml, the positive predictive value is 87% to 98%, and the negative predictive value is 72% to 80%.[85,86] However, CA-125 has not

proved to be effective in screening for ovarian cancer, since only 50% of stage I ovarian malignancies have preoperative levels greater than 35 U/ml.[83]

Doppler Evaluation of the Ovaries

There have been numerous articles debating the value of color Doppler in identifying malignant masses. The consensus is that Doppler resistive index is not sensitive in distinguishing between benignancy and malignancy.[87–91] However, a low resistive index (< 0.4) is an unusual finding in a postmenopausal patient. Therefore, a cyst that appears morpho-

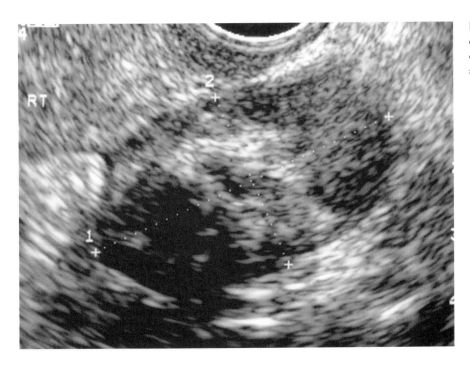

Figure 31.18 Fibrothecoma in a 68-year-old woman. Longitudinal view of the left ovary demonstrates a 5-cm heterogeneous solid mass.

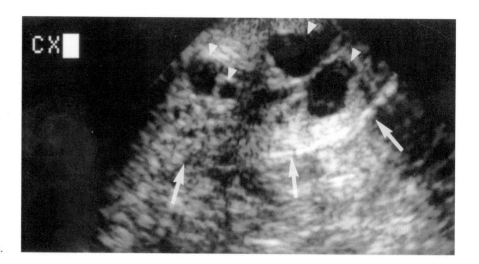

Figure 31.19 Sagittal view of the cervix demonstrates several small Nabothian cysts.

logically benign but which has a low resistive index should be regarded with suspicion after the menopause.[92] However, a morphologically suspicious lesion with a normal resistive index should still be treated with suspicion.

In the postmenopausal patient small (< 3 cm) anechoic cysts without suggestive morphology and with a normal resistive index do not require follow up. Larger cysts in this category may be treated conservatively but kept under observation.

THE CERVIX AND VAGINA

Nabothian cysts are common in the postmenopausal cervix. They are thought to be due to previous infection or inflam-

mation and are more common in older than in younger women. They typically communicate with the endocervical canal, are less than 2 cm in size, and may be multiple (Fig. 31.19). They are anechoic but may contain debris. The ovary may lie directly adjacent to the cervix, and it is important not to confuse them with ovarian lesions.

THE FALLOPIAN TUBES

Hydrosalpinx can occur in postmenopausal women (Fig. 31.20). It is seen as a dilated elongated cystic structure between the uterus and ovary. Color Doppler is helpful in distinguishing hydrosalpinx from adjacent vessels. Hydrosalpinx

Figure 31.20 A 50-year-old woman with a 5-cm hypoechoic multiseptated tubular adnexal mass, proved at surgery to be a hydrosalpinx.

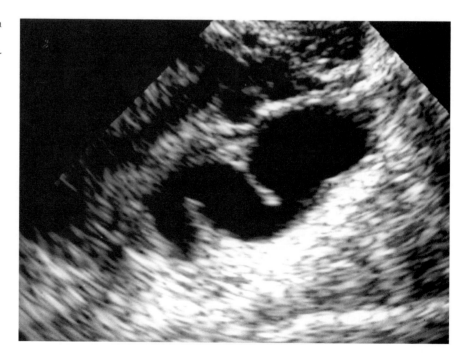

in the postmenopausal patient is often asymptomatic, and patients have usually had a hysterectomy or tubal ligation.

Tubo-ovarian abscess, while unusual in the postmenopausal patient, can occur. A history of vaginal discharge and fever can usually be elicited. If a cystic adnexal mass is seen in such a patient, a search of the uterus and ovaries should be carried out, as there is a close association between postmenopausal tubo-ovarian abscess and gynecologic malignancy.[15]

FREE FLUID

Small amounts of free fluid occasionally are seen in the cul-de-sac of asymptomatic postmenopausal women. A small amount of anechoic fluid is probably peritoneal and of no clinical concern. Larger amounts of fluid are not normal. Women with congestive cardiac failure may have increased fluid in the cul-de-sac. Free fluid with septa suggests malignancy, hemorrhage, or infection.

SUMMARY

Ultrasonography is a painless and inexpensive method of imaging the pelvis. In the postmenopausal woman, it is a useful way to demonstrate the endometrium of those women at risk for carcinoma. This applies particularly to those women on adjuvant hormone replacement therapy because of age, but also to those women on therapy for the prevention of recurrence of breast cancer. It also has applications in women at risk for cancer of the ovaries.

REFERENCES

1. Averette HE, Steren A, Nguyen H. Screening in gynecologic cancers. Cancer 1993;72:1043–1049.
2. American Cancer Society. Cancer Facts and Figures (vol. 5). American Cancer Society, Atlanta, 1992
3. Platt JF, Bree RL, Davidson D. Ultrasound of the normal nongravid uterus: correlation with gross and histopathology. J Clin Ultrasound 1990;18:15–19
4. Shipley CF, 3rd, Simmons CL, Nelson GH. Comparison of transvaginal sonography with endometrial biopsy in asymptomatic postmenopausal women. J Ultrasound Med 1994;13:99–104
5. Ernster VL, Bush TL, Huggins GR et al. Benefits and risks of menopausal estrogen and/or progestin hormone use. Prev Med 1988;17:201–223
6. Persson I, Adami HO, Bergkvist L et al. Risk of endometrial cancer after treatment with oestrogens alone or in conjunction with progestogens: results of a prospective study. Br Med J 1989;298:147–151
7. Wahl P, Walden C, Knopp R et al. Effect of estrogen/progesterone potency on lipid/lipoprotein cholesterol. N Engl J Med 1983;308:862–867
8. Whitehead M, Hillard TC, Crook D. The role and use of progestogens. Obstet Gynecol 1990;75:59S–76S
9. Gambrell RD, Jr. Prevention of endometrial cancer with progestogens. Maturitas 1986;8:159–168
10. Magos AL, Brincat M, Studd JW et al. Amenorrhea and endometrial atrophy with continuous oral estrogen and progestogen therapy in postmenopausal women. Obstet Gynecol 1985;65:496–499
11. Handa VL, Bachus KE, Johnston WW et al. Vaginal administration of low-dose conjugated estrogens: systemic absorption and effects on the endometrium. Obstet Gynecol 1994;84:215–218
12. Lin MC, Gosink BB, Wolf SI et al. Endometrial thickness after menopause: effect of hormone replacement. Radiology 1991;180:427–432
13. Levine D, Gosink B, Johnson L. Change in endometrial thickness in postmenopausal women on hormone replacement therapy. Radiology 1995;197:603–608
14. Goldstein SR. Unusual ultrasonographic appearance of the uterus in patient receiving tamoxifen. Am J Obstet Gynecol 1994;170:447–451
15. Cohen I, Rosen DJ, Shapira J et al. Endometrial changes in postmenopausal women treated with tamoxifen for breast cancer. Br J Obstet Gynaecol 1993;100:567–570
16. Cohen I, Rosen DJ, Tepper R et al. Ultrasonographic evaluation of the endometrium and correlation with endometrial sampling in postmenopausal patients treated with tamoxifen. J Ultrasound Med 1993;12:275–280
17. Lazebnik N, Hill LM, Robinson TM. Transvaginal sonography in a woman treated with megestrol acetate for breast cancer. J Ultrasound Med 1994;13:652–654
18. Van den Bosch T, Vandendael A, Van Schoubroeck D et al. Combining vaginal ultrasonography and office endometrial sampling in the diagnosis of endometrial disease in postmenopausal women. Obstet Gynecol 1995;85:349–352
19. Fleischer AC, Kalemeris GC, Machin JE et al. Sonographic depiction of normal and abnormal endometrium with histopathologic correlation. J Ultrasound Med 1986;5:445–452
20. Holst J, Koskela O, von Shoultz B. Endometrial findings following curettage in 2018 women according to age and indication. Ann Chir Gynaecol 1983;72:274–277
21. Kremer S, Kutcher R, Rosenblatt R et al. Postmenopausal tubo-ovarian abscess: sonographic consideration and clinical significance. J Ultrasound Med 1992;11:613–616
22. Karlsson B, Granberg S, Wikland M et al. Transvaginal ultrasonography of the endometrium in women with postmenopausal bleeding—a Nordic multicenter study. Am J Obstet Gynecol 1995;172:1488–1494
23. Nasri MN, Shepherd JH, Setchell ME et al. The role of vaginal scan in measurement of endometrial thickness in postmenopausal women. Br J Obstet Gynaecol 1991;98:470–475
24. Goldstein SR, Nachtigall M, Snyder JR, Nachtigall L. Endometrial assessment by vaginal ultrasonography before endometrial sampling in patients with postmenopausal bleeding. Am J Obstet Gynecol 1990;163(1 Pt 1):119–123
25. Varner RE, Sparks JM, Cameron CD et al. Transvaginal sonography of the endometrium in postmenopausal women. Obstet Gynecol 1991;78:195–199
26. Osmers R, Volksen M, Schauer A. Vaginosonography for early

detection of endometrial carcinoma? Lancet 1990;335:
1569–1571

27. Granberg S, Wikland M, Karlsson B et al. Endometrial thickness as measured by transvaginal ultrasonography for identifying endometrial abnormality. Am J Obstet Gynecol 1991;164:47–52

28. Breckenridge JW, Kurtz AB, Ritchie WGM, Macht ELJ. Postmenopausal uterine fluid collection: Indicator of carcinoma. AJR Am J Roentgenol 1982;139:529–534

29. Reid PC, Brown VA, Fothergill DJ. Outpatient investigation of postmenopausal bleeding. Br J Obstet Gynaecol 1993;100:498

30. McCarthy KA, Hall DA, Kopans DB, Swann CA. Postmenopausal endometrial fluid collections: always an indicator of malignancy? J Ultrasound Med 1986;5:647–649

31. Goldstein SR. Postmenopausal endometrial fluid collections revisited; look at the doughnut rather than the hole. Obstet Gynecol 1994;83:738–740

32. Lewit N, Thaler I, Rottem S. The uterus: a new look with transvaginal sonography. J Clin Ultrasound 1990;18:331–336

33. Woodruff JD, Pickar JH. Incidence of endometrial hyperplasia in postmenopausal women taking conjugated estrogens (Premarin) with medroxyprogesterone acetate or conjugated estrogen alone. The Menopause Study Group. Am J Obstet Gynecol 1994;170:1213–1223

34. Goldstein SR. Use of ultrasonohysterography for triage of perimenopausal patients with unexplained uterine bleeding. Am J Obstet Gynecol 1994;170:565–570

35. Kupfer MC, Schiller VL, Hansen GC, Tessler FN. Transvaginal sonographic evaluation of endometrial polyps. J Ultrasound Med 1994;13:535–539

36. Karlsson B, Granberg S, Hellberg P, Wikland M. Comparative study of transvaginal sonography and hysteroscopy for the detection of pathologic endometrial lesions in women with postmenopausal bleeding. J Ultrasound Med 1994;13:757–762

37. Sheth S, Hamper UM, Kurman RJ. Thickened endometrium in the postmenopausal woman: sonographic-pathologic correlation. Radiology 1993;187:135–139

38. Hulka CA, Hall DA, McCarthy K, Simeone JF. Endometrial polyps, hyperplasia, and carcinoma in postmenopausal women: differentiation with transvaginal sonography. Radiology 1994;191:755–758

39. Requard CK, Wicks JD, Mettler FA. Ultrasonography in the staging of endometrial adenocarcinoma. Radiology 1981;140:781–785

40. Fleischer AC, Gordon AN, Entman SS, Kepple DM. Transvaginal scanning of the endometrium. J Clin Ultrasound 1990;18(4):337–349

41. Schoenfeld A, Levavi H, Hirsch M et al. Transvaginal sonography in postmenopausal women. J Clin Ultrasound 1990;18:350–358

42. Yamashita Y, Mizutani H, Torashima M et al. Assessment of myometrial invasion by endometrial carcinoma: transvaginal sonography vs. contrast-enhanced MR imaging. AJR Am J Roentgenol 1993;161:595–599

43. Weiner Z, Beck D, Rottem S et al. Uterine artery flow velocity waveforms and color flow imaging in women with perimenopausal and postmenopausal bleeding. Correlation to endometrial histopathology. Acta Obstet Gynecol Scand 1993;72:162–166

44. Sheth S, Hamper UM, McCollum ME et al. Endometrial blood flow analysis in postmenopausal women: can it help differentiate benign from malignant causes of endometrial thickening? Radiology 1995;195:661–665

45. Carter J, Saltzman A, Hartenbach E et al. Flow characteristics in benign and malignant gynecologic tumors using transvaginal color flow Doppler. Obstet Gynecol 1994;83:125–130

46. Kurjak A, Shalan H, Sosic A et al. Endometrial carcinoma in postmenopausal women: evaluation by transvaginal color Doppler ultrasonography. Am J Obstet Gynecol 1993;169:1597–1603

47. Chan FY, Chau MT, Pun TC et al. Limitations of transvaginal sonography and color Doppler imaging in the differentiation of endometrial carcinoma from benign lesions. J Ultrasound Med 1994;13:623–628

48. Parsons AK, Lense JJ. Sonohysterography for endometrial abnormalities: preliminary results. J Clin Ultrasound 1993;21:87–95

49. Cullinan JA, Fleischer AC, Kepple DM, Arnold AL. Sonohysterography: a technique for endometrial evaluation. Radiographics 1995;15:501–514

50. Goswamy RK, Campbell S, Royston JP et al. Ovarian size in postmenopausal women. Br J Obstet Gynecol 1988;95:795–801

51. Granberg S, Wikland M. A comparison between ultrasound and gynecologic examination for detection of enlarged ovaries in a group of women at risk for ovarian carcinoma. J Ultrasound Med 1988;7:59–64

52. Goswamy RK, Campbell S, Whitehead MI. Screening for ovarian cancer. Clin Obstet Gynecol 1983;10:621–643

53. Granberg S, Wikland M. Comparison between transvaginal and transabdominal transducers for measuring ovarian volume. J Ultrasound Med 1987;6:649–653

54. Fleischer AC, McKee MS, Gordon AN et al. Transvaginal sonography of postmenopausal ovaries with pathologic correlation. J Ultrasound Med 1990;9:637–644

55. Hall DA, McCarthy KA, Kopans DB. Sonographic visualization of the normal postmenopausal ovary. J Ultrasound Med 1986;5:9–11

56. Campbell S, Goessens L, Goswamy R, Whitehead M. Real-time ultrasonography for determination of ovarian morphology and volume. A possible early screening test for ovarian cancer. Lancet 1982;1:425–426

57. Cohen HL, Tice HM, Mandel FS. Ovarian volumes measured by US: bigger than we think. Radiology 1990;177:189–192

58. Di Santis D, Scatarige J, Kemp G et al. A prospective evaluation of transvaginal sonography for detection of ovarian disease. AJR Am J Roentgenol 1993;161:91–94

59. Higgins RV, van Nagell JR, Jr, Donaldson ES et al. Transvaginal sonography as a screening method for ovarian cancer. Gynecol Oncol 1989;34:402–406

60. Van Nagell JR, Jr, Higgins RV, Donaldson ES et al. Transvaginal sonography as a screening method for ovarian cancer. A report of the first 1000 cases. Cancer 1990;65:573–577

61. Van Nagell JR, Jr, DePriest PD, Puls LE et al. Ovarian cancer screening in asymptomatic postmenopausal women by transvaginal sonography. Cancer 1991;68:458–462

62. Wolf SI, Gosink BB, Feldesman MR et al. Prevalence of simple adnexal cysts in postmenopausal women. Radiology 1991;180:65–71

63. Barber HRK, Graber EA. The PMPO Syndrome (postmenopausal palpable ovary syndrome). Obstet Gynecol 1971;38:921–923

64. Richardson GS, Scully RE, Nikrui N, Nelson JH, Jr. Common

epithelial cancer of the ovary (2). N Engl J Med 1985;312:474–483

65. Weiss NS, Homonchuk T, Young JLJ. Incidence of the histologic types of ovarian cancer: the U.S. third national cancer survey, 1969–1971. Gynecol Oncol 1977;5:161–167

66. Goldstein SR, Subramanyam B, Snyder JR et al. The postmenopausal cystic adnexal mass: the potential role of ultrasound in conservative management. Obstet Gynecol 1989;73:8–10

67. Andolf E, Jorgensen C. Cystic lesions in elderly women, diagnosed by ultrasound. Br J Obstet Gynaecol 1989;96:1076–1079

68. Hall DA, McCarthy KA. The significance of the postmenopausal simple adnexal cyst. J Ultrasound Med (US) 1986;5:503–505

69. Rulin MC, Preston AL. Adnexal masses in postmenopausal women. Obstet Gynecol 1987;70:578–581

70. Moyle JW, Rochester D, Sider L et al. Sonography of ovarian tumors: predictability of tumor type. AJR Am J Roentgenol 1983;141:985–991

71. Hurwitz A, Yagel S, Zion I et al. The management of persistent clear pelvic cysts diagnosed by ultrasonography. Obstet Gynecol 1988;72:320–322

72. Deland M, Fried A. Ultrasonography in the diagnosis of tumors of the ovary. Surg Gynecol Obstet 1979;148:346–348

73. Meire HB, Farrant P, Guha T. Distinction of benign from malignant ovarian cysts by ultrasound. Br J Obstet Gynaecol 1978;85:893–899

74. Granberg S, Wikland M, Jansson I. Macroscopic characterization of ovarian tumors and the relation to the histological diagnosis: criteria to be used for ultrasound evaluation. Gynecol Oncol 1989;35:139–144

75. Levine D, Gosink BB, Wolf SI et al. Simple adnexal cysts: the natural history in postmenopausal women. Radiology 1992;184:653–659

76. NIH consensus conference. Ovarian cancer. Screening, treatment, and follow-up NIH Consensus Development Panel on Ovarian Cancer. JAMA 1995;273:491–497

77. Yancik R, Ries LG, Yates JW. Ovarian cancer in the elderly: an analysis of Surveillance, Epidemiology and End Results Program data. Am J Obstet Gynecol 1986;154:639–647

78. Hartge P, Whittemore A, Itnyre J et al. Rates and risks of ovarian cancer in subgroups of white women in the United States. The Collaborative Ovarian Cancer Group. Obstet Gynecol 1994;84:760–764

79. Rodriguez MH, Platt LD, Medearis AL et al. The use of transvaginal sonography for evaluation of postmenopausal ovarian size and morphology. Am J Obstet Gynecol 1988;159:810–814

80. Andolf E, Svalenius E, Astedt B. Ultrasonography for early detection of ovarian carcinoma. Br J Obstet Gynaecol 1986;93:1286–1289

81. Campbell S, Bhan V, Royston P et al. Transabdominal ultrasound screening for early ovarian cancer. Br Med J 1989;299:1363–1366

82. Bhan V, Amso N, Whitehead MI et al. Characteristics of persistent ovarian masses in asymptomatic women. Br J Obstet Gynaecol 1989;96:1384–1391

83. Soper J, Hunter V, Kaly L et al. Preoperative serum tumor associated antigen levels in women with pelvic masses. Obstet Gynecol 1990;75:249–254

84. Jacobs I, Oram D. Potential screening tests for ovarian cancer. In: Sharp F, Mason W, Leake R, Eds. Ovarian Cancer: Biological and Therapeutic Challenges. WW Norton, London, 1990

85. Finkler NJ, Benacerraf B, Lavin PT et al. Comparison of serum CA 125, clinical impression, and ultrasound in the preoperative evaluation of ovarian masses. Obstet Gynecol 1988;72:659–664

86. Patsner B, Mann WJ. The value of preoperative serum CA-125 levels in patients with a pelvic mass. Am J Obstet Gynecol 1988;159:873–876

87. Carter JR, Lau M, Saltzman AK et al. Gray scale and color flow Doppler characterization of uterine tumors. J Ultrasound Med 1994;13:835–840

88. Levine D, Feldstein VA, Babcook CJ, Filly RA. Sonography of ovarian masses: poor sensitivity of resistive index for identifying malignant lesions. AJR Am J Roentgenol 1994;162:1355–1359

89. Salem S, White LM, Lai J. Doppler sonography of adnexal masses: the predictive value of the pulsatility index in benign and malignant disease. AJR Am J Roentgenol 1994;163(5):1147–1150

90. Hamper UM, Sheth S, Abbas FM et al. Transvaginal color Doppler sonography of adnexal masses: differences in blood flow impedance in benign and malignant lesions. AJR Am J Roentgenol 1993;160:1225–1228

91. Brown DL, Frates MC, Laing FC et al. Ovarian masses: can benign and malignant lesions be differentiated with color and pulsed Doppler US. Radiology 1994;190:333–336

92. Kurjak A, Shalan H, Matijevic R et al. Stage I ovarian cancer by transvaginal color Doppler sonography: A report of 18 cases. Ultrasound Obstet Gynecol 1993;3:195–198

93. Levine D. The postmenopausal pelvis. In: Nyberg DA, Hill LM, Bohm-Velez M et al. Eds. Transvaginal Ultrasound. Mosby Year Book, St. Louis, 1992, pp 233

32

Ultrasound Screening for Gynecologic Malignancy

JONATHAN CARTER

The aim of screening is to detect people with a particular disease from among the apparently healthy population. Screening tests are not diagnostic; they merely identify people who need further investigation.[1] A screening test is positive if it suggests the presence of the disease and negative if it does not.

The screening criteria have been formalized by the World Health Organization (WHO).[2] For a program to be effective, a disease should:

1. be a major cause of death or morbidity in the screened population.
2. have a preclinical phase during which screening could detect the disease while it is still curable.
3. have a reasonably high prevalence in the screened population.
4. be amenable to therapy.

Of the gynecologic tumors, cervical cancer most aptly fills these criteria, and the Papanicolaou cervical smear screening program has decreased the incidence of cervical cancer and its mortality.[3] Ultrasound is useful for imaging cervical pathology and blood flow, but it has no role in screening. Tumors of the uterine corpus are not suitable for screening, due to low prevalence rates, and those of the vulva and vagina are not suitable for screening, due to low mortality rates. The length of the preclinical phase of ovarian cancer is unknown, and its prevalence rate is low, but ovarian cancer fulfills the remainder of the WHO screening criteria, and screening programs are being developed in some centers.[4] Endometrial cancer has a high incidence in postmenopausal women, and with the increasing use of estrogen replacement therapy, a higher incidence is anticipated, so it is hoped that ultrasound can screen for early endometrial cancer. This chapter concentrates on the role of ultrasound in screening for ovarian and endometrial cancer.

OVARIAN CANCER

Incidence

Ovarian cancer has the dubious distinction of being the most deadly gynecologic cancer. More women die each year from ovarian cancer than from endometrial and cervical cancer combined. The death rate from ovarian cancer, unlike other cancers, is increasing.[5] Ovarian cancer will develop in 1:70 women (1.5%), and 1% of women will die from the disease.[6]

The etiology of ovarian cancer is unknown, but through epidemiologic studies, a number of factors have been incriminated. Ovarian cancer occurs most frequently in industrialized countries in the middle and upper socioeconomic groups. The prevalence of ovarian cancer is highest in women over 50 years (approximately 50 per 100,000).[7]

Women exposed in their infancy to perineal talc or asbestos, which were common components of older baby powders, appear to be at a modest risk of 1.5 (confidence interval [CI] 0.9 to 1.8) of developing ovarian cancer, possibly due to its ascent through the genital tract.[8] Ovaries in which ovulation has been suppressed by pregnancy, breast-feeding, or oral contraception are at lower risk of malignant change. The most important risk factor in the development of ovarian cancer is a family history, and in about 5% to 10%, there is another affected family member. A smaller group of affected women belong to one of the Familial Ovarian Cancer syndromes. In some, the familial risk is restricted to ovarian cancer. In others, the familial cancer risk extends to ovarian and breast cancer. The Cancer Family Syndrome is characterized by early onset of cancer of the colon and endometrium as well as a high risk of multiple other primary cancers including stomach, ovary, and kidney. Each of these syndromes is characterized by autosomal dominant transmission, an earlier age of onset (47.7 years compared to 59 years for epithelial ovarian cancer in the general population), and a predominance of the serous type of tumor with a trend toward more poorly differentiated adenocarcinomas and a high proportion of bilateral disease.[9,10]

Mother-to-daughter transmission is readily identifiable, but unaffected males may also be gene carriers in the ovarian cancer and breast–ovarian cancer syndromes, and they transmit the syndrome to half of their daughters. Half of their sons will be unaffected carriers of the gene.

Rationale for Screening

There is no doubt that ovarian cancer poses a major health and financial burden. The natural history of the disease is not understood, and evidence for a preclinical stage is circumstantial. Two large screening series from the United Kingdom confirmed that no individual screening test can achieve a specificity of 99%,[11,12] due to low prevalence of the disease and low overall sensitivity of the screening tests. Screening programs should screen entire populations, but due to the low background incidence of ovarian cancer, it has been suggested that attention initially be focused toward those at high risk, that is, those with a family history of ovarian cancer or other adenocarcinomas and possibly those over 50 years or with cancerophobia.

Currently, laparoscopy or laparotomy is required for patients with a positive ovarian cancer screening test. Therefore, the specificity of the test must be high, so that no more than 10 operations are needed to detect every case of ovarian cancer. That is, the positive predictive value (PPV) must be at least 10%. An annual screening test for ovarian cancer, even with 100% sensitivity, would require 99.6% specificity to achieve a positive predictive value of 10% (i.e., nine false-positive tests for each case of ovarian cancer identified).

Methods of Screening

Bimanual Pelvic Examination

Pelvic examination by a gynecologist was once thought to assess accurately the size and shape of the ovaries, but recent comparisons with transvaginal sonography (TVS), immediately before laparotomy have found that ultrasound is much more specific and sensitive than pelvic examination.[13,14] In a blind study performed at the University of Minnesota, findings at pelvic examination were compared to those at TVS. Overall, 22% of pelvic assessments (102 of a total of 472) did not agree with the ultrasound findings, and only 29% were consistent with the findings at laparotomy. This compares poorly with the 71% accuracy rate of ultrasound.[13]

Compared with transabdominal sonography (TAS), pelvic examination detects only 34% of adnexal masses and overreads 8%.[15] Macfarlane et al.[16] performed over 18,000 pelvic examinations in 1,300 women, detecting only 6 cancers. There is no evidence that case detection and survival from ovarian cancer have been improved by annual pelvic examinations, performed for other reasons, mainly cervical cancer screening. Pelvic examination is not a reliable way to detect early ovarian cancer.

Transabdominal Sonography

TAS has been the main imaging modality since the 1970s, and the image quality has steadily improved. In a series of 805 patients attending an outpatient clinic for a variety of reasons, Andolf et al.[15] detected abnormalities in 83, or 10.3%, of patients at an initial scan. Lesions detected in those subjected to laparotomy included five mucinous and serous cystadenocarcinomas, one serous cystadenocarcinoma, two borderline cancers, and one cecal cancer. None of the malignant and bor-

derline tumors were clinically detected before the ultrasound.[15] The remaining patients were found to have either normal or benign pathology.

In a much larger series by Campbell et al.,[12] TAS was used for ovarian cancer screening in 5,479 self-referred asymptomatic women. Abnormalities were detected by sonography in 326 subjects, or 5.9%, and surgically confirmed in all patients. In all, a total of five primary ovarian tumors and four metastatic ovarian tumors were detected, including four stage IA and 1 stage IB cancers. They calculated that the odds that a positive scan would detect an ovarian tumor was 1:2; an ovarian cancer, 1:37; and a primary ovarian cancer, 1:67. They had a false-positive rate of 2.3%; a specificity of 97.7%, and a PPV of 1.5%.

Transvaginal Sonography

TVS provides superior images (Fig. 32.1), and the results show strong interobserver agreement.[17] There is considerable interest in the potential of TVS for the early detection of ovarian cancer, when the ovarian morphology would differ only slightly from normal. In postmenopausal women, normal ovaries should have a volume of less than 8 cc and be homogeneously echogenic.[18] In a study of 1,300 asymptomatic postmenopausal women using these criteria, the specificity of TVS for detecting ovarian carcinoma was found to be 98.1% (CI, 97.4% to 98.8%).[19] In screening a high-risk patient population with at least one family member with ovarian cancer, Bourne et al.[20] detected 23 tumors and 32 tumor-like conditions in 776 screened asymptomatic women, with a predictive value of a positive screen of 7.7%, which was higher than from their previous population-based screening program. Van Nagell et al.[17] reported 1,000 patients screened for ovarian cancer using TVS. All patients were aged over 40 years. Thirty-one had abnormal scans (3.1%). Twenty-four elected to have surgical exploration, all having ovarian or fallopian tube tumors as predicted by the scan.

Difficulty with pelvic assessment by TVS was highlighted in a prospective study by DiSantis et al.,[21] who evaluated 113 ovaries in 59 women within 72 hours of surgery. The results were compared to the surgical findings. In 22 premenopausal patients, 16 (76%) histologically normal ovaries were identified on sonograms, but only 13 (59%) of the 22 confirmed adnexal masses were visualized. In 37 postmenopausal patients, only 12 (20%) of 59 normal ovaries were seen, and only 6 (54%) of 11 adnexal masses were identified. They conclude that their ability to detect normal postmenopausal ovaries and ovarian masses was often suboptimal. In another study using TVS in a group of postmenopausal women, they were able to image both ovaries in 60% cases and one ovary in 87% of cases. Their PPV was 96% and negative predictive value (NPV) was 92%.[22]

CA-125

The most promising monoclonal antibody for ovarian cancer serum screening is OC-125, which reacts to the CA-125 anti-

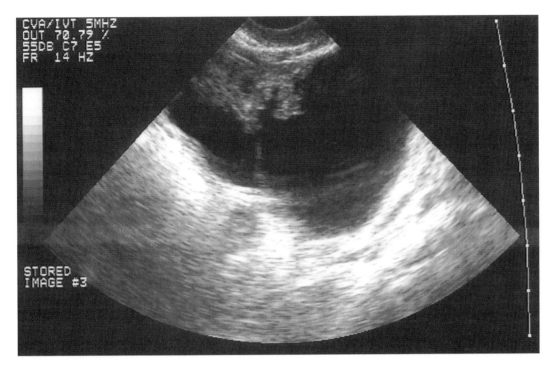

Figure 32.1 A papillary internal excrescence in this ovarian mass was morphologically highly suggestive on TVS. It proved to be an early ovarian carcinoma.

gen. CA-125 is an antigen present in the celomic fetal epithelium and its fetal and adult derivatives. It disappears early during normal development but reappears with ovarian pathology. Among apparently healthy individuals, 99% have a serum level less than 35 U/ml, and in 99.7%, the level is less than 65 U/ml. It was originally reported that serum CA-125 was greater than 35 U/ml in 83% of patients with epithelial ovarian cancer and 1% of presumably healthy patients,[23] but CA-125 has also been found to be elevated in pregnancy; endometriosis; pelvic inflammatory disease; uterine fibroids; peritonitis; hepatic, pancreatic, and renal conditions; as well as some nongynecologic cancers including hepatocellular carcinoma, breast, colon, and lung cancer. The sensitivity of CA-125 for ovarian cancer increases with the clinical stage at diagnosis, being only 50% for stage I and II disease, increasing to 90% for stage III and IV tumors. In a prospective study of 5,550 women greater than age 40, the specificity of CA-125 for ovarian cancer was 97.6%.[24]

To date, CA-125 is the best available tumor marker for ovarian cancer, but it is a poor marker for screening due to its low specificity.

Color Doppler Imaging

Color Doppler imaging and pulsed Doppler allow the localization of small blood vessels, the characterization of their flow-velocity waveforms, and determination of blood flow.

In 1972 Folkman[25] hypothesized and later reported the theory of tumor angiogenesis, whereby growing tumors develop new blood vessels to support their high metabolic demands. These new tumor blood vessels lack the normal vascular media, have an irregular course, much arteriovenous shunting, and low resistance to flow. They are peripheral and central. Ultrasound analysis of these vessels shows spectral broadening, increased diastolic flow, and resultant lowered pulsatility and resistive indices. Conversely, benign lesions have predominantly peripherally located vessels, that contain normal muscle fibers and are morphologically normal. The increased diastolic flow is demonstrated in Plates 32.1 to 32.3.

Reference ranges for normal pulsatility index (PI) and resistance index (RI) have been established.[26–29] Normal PI is greater than 1.0, while in malignant disease, PI is less than 1.0 and the RI is less than 0.5. Bourne et al.[28] found that the PI in 30 women with normal ovaries was 3.1 to 9.4, and in 9 with benign ovarian disease it was 3.2 to 7.0. Seven patients with ovarian cancer not only demonstrated increased flow with PI between 0.3 and 1.0, but all cancers also had evidence of neovascularization. In a much larger series, Kurjak and Zalud[30] detected 147 ovarian tumors in 5,000 screening examinations. Twenty-three were malignant (16%), and all had intratumoral blood flow. The RI was lowered (less than 0.4), indicating increased flow. There was only one false-positive, an inflammatory pseudocyst. The sensitivity was 100%, specificity 99.2%, and accuracy 99.3%.

To assess TVS and color flow Doppler in ovarian cancer screening, Bourne et al.[31] studied 1,601 self-referred asymptomatic women with a family history of ovarian cancer, aged 17 to 79 years (mean age 47). Sixty percent (959) were premenopausal. The authors found that a morphology score of 5 or more (a means of quantifying gray scale findings) or a PI of

1.0 or less maintained a high detection rate for ovarian cancer. In fact, all six cancers were detected by this algorithm and would have given 15 false-positive results with odds of 2:5. If both the morphologic score and the PI had been required to be abnormal, two of five cancers would have been missed. Use of a high morphologic score or a low PI increased the odds of finding ovarian cancer from 1 in 9 to about 2 in 5. Based on their results, Bourne et al. conclude that TVS rather than TAS enables a more detailed assessment of ovarian lesions. The addition of color flow Doppler can detect early ovarian cancer in women with a family history of the disease.

While some groups report high diagnostic accuracy in differentiating benign from malignant ovarian lesions by their resistance patterns alone, others feel that this is nonspecific. The diagnostic accuracy has varied from 70% to 90%.[32] Some of this variation can be due to lack of a defined level of positivity of the PI or RI.

Neovascularization also occurs in benign lesions such as corpora lutea, ectopic pregnancy, infection, and inflammation. These affect the specificity of the test. Impedances such as PI or RI may not be as reliable as a multiparameter analysis including PI or RI, vessel location, and other measurements, as proposed by Fleischer et al.[33] and Kurjak et al.[34]

Combined Modality Screening

It is clear from the above that vaginal examination, ultrasound, or CA-125 cannot be used alone for screening. In one study, 1,010 postmenopausal women were screened by vaginal examination and serum CA-125 with ultrasonography as a secondary procedure when indicated.[11] The specificities for ovarian cancer of CA-125 and vaginal examination were 97% and 97.3% respectively. The combination of serum CA-125 with ultrasound gave a specificity of 99.8%, while that of vaginal examination and ultrasound was 99%. When all three were combined, the specificity was 100%.

In a smaller series, 131 patients with an ovarian mass were examined before surgery using clinical examination, CA-125, original sonography, and reviewer sonography.[35] When used individually, the sensitivity and specificity of CA-125 were equal to those of a review ultrasound. The sensitivity and specificity of clinical examination and original ultrasound were poor. Sensitivity and specificity were highest for CA-125 assays in postmenopausal patients, especially when these were used as the second diagnostic test. All diagnostic tests had a low sensitivity in premenopausal women. The highest rate of sensitivity was 50% for both review ultrasound and CA-125.

Serum CA-125 measurement and TAS were used sequentially for prevalence screening by Jacobs et al.[36] Of 22,000 women screened, 41 had positive screening results. Eleven had ovarian cancer (true positives), and 30 either had no abnormality detected or had benign disorders (false-positive result). Of the 21,959 with a negative screen, 8 later presented with ovarian cancer (false-negative result) and 21,951 remain without evidence of ovarian cancer (apparent true-negative result). This screening protocol achieved a specificity of 99.9%, a PPV of 26.8%, and apparent sensitivity of 78.6% and 57.9% at 1-year and 2-years, respectively.

Karlan et al.[4] screened 597 asymptomatic women with a family history of ovarian cancer. This was the first report of screening using TVS, CA-125, and color flow Doppler combined. Positive ultrasounds were found in 6.2% of patients. A PI of less than 1.0 was found in 80% of premenopausal women and 24% of postmenopausal women, whereas an RI of less than 0.4 was found in 12% of premenopausal and 3% of postmenopausal women. An elevated CA-125 was found in 11.4% of women. One stage IA ovarian cancer and one endometrial cancer were detected. Although these were preliminary results, and the study small, a number of points were highlighted. First, no single test can be used for ovarian cancer screening. Second, due to the low prevalence of ovarian cancer, large numbers of patients need to be screened.

Who Should Be Screened?

It is unreasonable to expect to screen an entire population for ovarian cancer. This would certainly impose an enormous burden on the health care system, both monetarily and in physician time. It seems more prudent to focus on groups of women at increased risk. High-risk groups who may benefit from ovarian cancer screening are shown in Table 32.1.

Frequency of Screening

Twice-yearly screening from age 30 has been advocated for women from a family with an inherited cancer syndrome.[9,37] They may also need breast, corpus, and colorectal screening. For other women, yearly screening from age 40 appears appropriate.[38]

Prevention of Ovarian Cancer

Multiple studies have confirmed a 40% to 50% reduction in risk of developing ovarian cancer in women who take oral contraceptives, presumably because of the ovulation suppression. Their protective effect increases with their duration of use and may persist for 10 to 15 years after they have been discontinued.[39,40] Prophylactic oophorectomy at the completion of childbearing is

Table 32.1 High-Risk Groups Who May Benefit From Ovarian Cancer Screening

Family history of ovarian cancer

Family cancer syndrome

First-degree relative with colon or corpus cancer

Family history of breast cancer

History of breast cancer

Cancerophobia

an option for women who have a 50% risk of developing ovarian cancer. The risk of disease development far outweighs the risks of surgery.[41] Women of intermediate risk, with one first-degree or more than one second-degree relative with ovarian cancer, whose lifetime risk is in the order of 5% to 10% may also choose prophylactic oophorectomy and hormone replacement therapy rather than a lifetime of screening. Regular pelvic ultrasound examinations for screening are not performed after oophorectomy, but patients should be warned that oophorectomy will not reduce their risk of ovarian cancer to zero, as there have been cases reports of "ovarian-type cancer" developing in the peritoneal cavity of patients after oophorectomy.[41]

ENDOMETRIAL CANCER

Incidence

The incidence of endometrial cancer is increasing, and in the United States, it is now more frequent than cervical cancer. It is the most common malignancy of the female genital tract with 20 to 30 per 100,000 new cases diagnosed per annum.[6] It is the fourth most common cancer in females behind breast, bowel, and lung.

Rationale for Screening

Despite being more common than cervical and ovarian cancers, endometrial cancer will cause fewer deaths than both. This is because most patients present early with bleeding. Therefore, population-based screening for endometrial cancer may not be worthwhile. There are, however, a number of patient groups, at higher risk of development of endometrial cancer, who may benefit:

1. Patients on tamoxifen
2. Patients with a family history of breast, ovarian, or uterine cancer
3. Women taking unopposed estrogen

Methods of Screening

Bimanual Pelvic Examination

Historically, vaginal examination was used to diagnose gynecologic cancers. This could only detect lesions that were advanced enough to cause a palpable mass. The accuracy of these examinations has been questioned.[42]

The Papanicolaou Smear

The Pap smear is of limited use in screening for endometrial cancer. Only about 50% of women will have a positive smear. Six percent of postmenopausal patients with normal endometrial cells in smears will have endometrial carcinoma, and about 13% will have endometrial hyperplasia. If morphologically abnormal endometrial cells are present, about 25% of women will have endometrial carcinoma.[43]

Endometrial Sampling and Uterine Curettage

Endometrial biopsies can be easily performed in the office, with a biopsy catheter passed up through the cervix at the time of a speculum examination. However, very little of the endometrium is sampled, so the sensitivity and specificity of the test are poor.[44] Furthermore, this technique is not often used even in symptomatic patients because of the associated patient discomfort.[45]

While dilatation of the cervix and curettage of the uterus (D&C) has been the usual method of detecting of endometrial cancer in symptomatic patients, it does not always accurately diagnose cancer. Stovall and co-workers[46] found that D&C before hysterectomy missed 6% of hyperplasias and cancers. They also found that endometrial pathology was missed in 4% when the Novak biopsy was used. Stock and Kanbour[47] demonstrated the inaccuracy of prehysterectomy D&C both as a sampling technique and as a means of diagnosing endometrial cancer. In 30 of 50 patients (60%) undergoing D&C before hysterectomy, less than half of the surface of the cavity was sampled.

Transabdominal Sonography

On TAS, early endometrial cancer is seen as echogenic thickening of the endometrium. Less differentiated tumors may be hypoechoic due to the lower content of mucin.[48] Other sonographic findings that may be associated with endometrial carcinoma include a lobular endometrium, loss of the subendometrial halo with early invasion, an enlarged uterus with a heterogeneous echodensity, or the presence of fluid in the endometrial cavity.[49–51] The margins of the endometrial carcinoma may be difficult to distinguish from the adjacent myometrium when the echogenicity of each is similar, but bulky, benign endocavitary tumors may produce myometrial thinning and simulate an invasive tumor.[52] Requard et al.[53] found 94% of patients with stage I to II disease had a normal or bulky uterus and a normal or hypoechoic parenchymal pattern, while patients with a lobular uterus and/or mixed echo pattern had stage III to IV disease. Pre-existing conditions such as leiomyoma and adenomyosis also contribute to the difficulty in delineating the extent of myometrial invasion, and cervical involvement may be difficult to evaluate.

The effect of estrogen replacement therapy (ERT) on the endometrium, myometrium, and uterine blood flow in postmenopausal women was assessed by Zalud et al.,[54] who found that continuous ERT influences the thickness of the endometrium but not the myometrium or the uterine artery blood flow. Thus, the hormonal status, both endogenous and exogenous, should be considered when assessing endometrial thickness.

In view of the inferior resolution achieved with TAS, compared with TVS, it has no advantage as a screening test.

Transvaginal Sonography

TVS, which provides higher resolution images of the uterus and endometrium, has been proposed as a screening method for endometrial cancer.[55] Some reports have suggested that TVS is superior to TAS in evaluating most uterine pathology as well as determining local extension of endometrial carcinoma.[56]

One of the most important studies published, from Schulman and colleagues[57] addresses the prevalence of asymptomatic endometrial and ovarian cancer in a volunteer population aged 40 or greater. They offered a free volunteer screening program using vaginal sonography and color flow Doppler to screen for pelvic cancer. In the first 2 years, 2,117 women were examined, 51% of whom were postmenopausal. Thirty postmenopausal women, not on ERT, had an endometrial thickness of 6 mm or greater. Of the 20 patients who had endometrial biopsies performed, 3 had adenocarcinomas, 5 had hyperplasia, 7 had polyps, 2 had disordered endometrium, and 3 had atrophic endometrium.

Several studies have indicated that a thin endometrium as measured by TVS usually excludes endometrial pathology as the cause of postmenopausal bleeding.[58] An endometrial thickness of 4 mm or less as measured by TVS seems to exclude major endometrial pathology as the cause of postmenopausal bleeding.[59] Prevalence studies of endometrial cancer in asymptomatic women have supported reports on symptomatic women by finding that an endometrial thickness of greater than 5 mm may be discriminatory for neoplastic change.[60]

Endometrial carcinoma is usually seen as thickened endometrium of variable echogenicity. In a series of 18 patients with endometrial carcinoma, the average endometrial thickness was 17.7±5.8 mm.[61] However, endometrial carcinoma has been found in endometria as thin as 6 to 8 mm.[62] Other possible causes of a thickened endometrium include endometrial hyperplasia, endometrial polyps, ovarian carcinoma extending to the endometrium, hematometra, mucometra, and pyometra.[63]

The specificity and sensitivity of TVS was compared to endometrial cytology and D&C in discriminating between normal and pathologic endometrium. Karlsson et al.[64] studied 105 women and found a specificity of 81% and a sensitivity of 97% in detecting morphologic alterations by TVS compared with 81% specificity and 58% sensitivity for cytologic evaluation.

Tumor Markers

Carcinoembryonic antigen and CA-125 have been investigated as tumor markers for endometrial cancer. The sensitivity of each is low for screening, but when levels are found to be elevated in a symptomatic woman, they may be useful. Some 20% of patients with clinical stages I or II endometrial cancer have an elevated serum CA-125, which correlates with an increased risk of extra uterine disease.[65,66] Neither marker is useful as a screening test.

Color Doppler Imaging

While TAS and TVS are useful in identifying endometrial and uterine abnormalities, the signs of malignancy may be subtle and can mimic benign conditions. The addition of Doppler flow analysis may be of some value in such cases (Plates 32.4 to 32.6).

Over a 5-year period, Kurjak et al.[67] screened 5,013 asymptomatic women by transvaginal color and pulsed Doppler sonography. The screen was regarded as positive if the endometrial thickness was 10 mm or more in women not taking hormone replacement therapy or if there was abnormal blood flow (RI 0.43). Thirty four (0.68%) endometrial abnormalities were detected, due to 6 (0.12%) endometrial cancers, 18 (0.36%) endometrial hyperplasias, and 10 (0.12%) benign endometrial polyps. Of the 6 endometrial cancers, the mean endometrial thickness was 22 mm (range, 17 to 27 mm), and the mean RI was 0.38 (range, 0.34 to 0.40).

The impressive results obtained by the Kurjak group need to be tempered by less convincing data published by Chan et al.[68] and Carter et al.[69] Both found that color flow Doppler gives little if any additional information over that obtained from gray scale sonography.

Bourne et al.[70] have described the use of TVS and color flow Doppler in the detection of endometrial cancer in postmenopausal women. They measured the impedance to uterine arterial and intratumoral blood flow and found that a cutoff value of the PI of 2.00 would give a detection rate of 99.0% with a false-positive rate of 2.6%. In contrast, measurement of endometrial tumor thickness in the same group of patients (taking a cutoff value of 5 mm as the upper limit of normal) yielded a rate of detection of cancer of 99%, but a false-positive rate of 41%. In a follow-up study, Bourne and colleagues[71] prospectively evaluated whether changes in uterine blood flow could by used to detect endometrial cancer. One hundred and thirty eight postmenopausal women including 35 on ERT had their endometrial thickness measured and the PI of the uterine and intratumoral vessels recorded. There was an overlap in endometrial thickness between those women with endometrial cancer and those without, and the mean arterial PI value was lower in women with postmenopausal bleeding and endometrial cancer than in those patients with others reasons for uterine bleeding. They found a detection rate of 100% within the limitations of the study design, and the false-positive rate was 1% for all women not receiving ERT and 11% for those receiving ERT, with malignant tumors showing signs of altered vascularization and low PI (mean 0.49, range 0.29 to 0.92)

In the study by Chan et al.[68] of 67 patients, 17 had endometrial cancer, 12 had benign endometrial lesions, and 38 had no uterine pathology. The mean endometrial thickness in the patients with cancer was 10.08 mm standard deviation (SD 0.33), and the mean PI of the uterine artery was 2.17 (SD

0.80). They found that gray scale sonography was superior to color flow Doppler in the detection of pathologic conditions of the endometrium, but neither could significantly distinguish benign lesions from their malignant counterparts.

Color flow Doppler has been found to be unhelpful in diagnosing pathologic endometrial conditions in patients on tamoxifen. Among 39 asymptomatic postmenopausal women on tamoxifen, Tepper et al.[72] could find no pattern for the uterine artery PI that could be related to any endometrial lesion, nor were any changes seen in the PI with increasing severity of the endometrial pathology. They found no correlation between endometrial thickness and uterine artery PI. One criticism of this study is that their PI measurements were taken from the uterine artery, not within the myometrium or at the myometrial – endometrial interface, closer to the endometrial pathology.

In a preliminary report of the role of pelvic sonoangiography and color flow Doppler in the detection of endometrial cancer, Hata et al.[73] analyzed their color flow Doppler results in a group of 16 patients referred with postmenopausal bleeding. Using sophisticated ultrasound equipment, capable of measuring blood flow down to 0.77 cm/s, no flow was seen in their noncancer group (all with atrophic endometrium at curettage), while they were able to detect abnormal flow in all 9 patients with endometrial carcinoma, thus claiming 100% sensitivity and 100% specificity. Patient numbers are small in this series, so results must be viewed with caution. As ultrasound systems improve, lower blood flow velocities will be measured. This will undoubtedly include normal flow; thus, detecting a difference on the mere presence or absence of tumor flow may not be valid.

In a much larger series, with velocities at 1 to 2 cm/s, the sensitivity, specificity, and predictive value of color flow Doppler alone are significantly less than those obtained by Hata et al.[73] In our hands, color flow Doppler is able to give additional useful clinical information in only 15% of patients with suspected uterine tumors.[69]

REFERENCES

1. Campion MJ, Reid R. Screening for gynecologic cancer. Obstet Gynecol Clin North Am 1990;74:695–727
2. Wilson JMG, Jungner G. Principles and Practice of Screening for Disease. Public health papers 34. World Health Organization, Geneva, 1968
3. Devesa SS, Silverman DT, Young JL et al. Cancer incidence and mortality trends among whites in the United States 1947–1984. J Natl Cancer Inst 1987;79:701–770
4. Karlan BY, Raffel LJ, Crvenkovic G et al. A multidisciplinary approach to the early detection of ovarian carcinoma: rationale, protocol design, and early results. Am J Obstet Gynecol 1993;169:494–501
5. Boring CC, Squires TS, Tong T. Cancer Statistics 1991; 41:19–36
6. Platz CE, Benda JA. Female genital tract cancer. Cancer 1995;75:270–294
7. Miller BA, Ries LA, Hankey BF et al. Cancer statistics review 1973–1989. Ovary (vol. 20) NIH publication No. 92–2789. US Department of Health and Human Services, 1992, pp 1–7
8. Harlow BL, Cramer DW, Bell DA et al. Perineal exposure to talc and ovarian cancer risk. Obstet Gynecol 1992;45:20
9. Lynch HT, Harris RE, Guirgis HA et al. Familial association of breast/ovarian carcinoma. Cancer 1978;41:1543–1549
10. Lynch HT, Watson P, Bewtra C et al. Hereditary ovarian cancer. Hetereogeneity in age at diagnosis. Cancer 1991;67:1460–1466
11. Jacobs I, Stabile I, Bridges J et al. Multimodal approach to screening for ovarian cancer. Lancet 1988;1:268–271
12. Campbell S, Bhan V, Royston P et al. Transabdominal ultrasound screening for early ovarian cancer. Br Med J 1989;299:1363–1367
13. Carter J, Fowler J, Carlson J et al. Just how accurate is the pelvic examination? A prospective comparative study. J Reprod Med 1994;39:32–34
14. Frederick JL, Paulson RJ, Sauer MV. Routine use of vaginal ultrasonography in the preoperative evaluation of gynecologic patients. An adjunct to resident education. J Reprod Med 1991;36:779
15. Andolf E, Svalenius E, Astedt B. Ultrasonography for early detection of ovarian carcinoma. Br J Obstet Gynaecol 1986;93:1286–1289
16. Macfarlane C, Sturgis MC, Fetterman FS. Results of an experiment in the control of cancer of the female pelvic organs and report of a fifteen-year research. Am J Obst Gynecol 1955;69:294–298
17. van Nagell JR, Jr, DePriest PD, Puls LE et al. Ovarian cancer screening in asymptomatic postmenopausal women by transvaginal sonography. Cancer 1991;68:458–462
18. Rodriguez MH, Platt LD, Medearis AL et al. The use of transvaginal sonography for evaluation of postmenopausal ovarian size and morphology. Am J Obstet Gynecol 1988;159:810–814
19. Higgins RV, van Nagell JR, Jr, Donaldson ES et al. Transvaginal sonography as a screening method for ovarian cancer. Gynecol Oncol 1989;34:402–406
20. Bourne TH, Whitehead MI, Campbell S et al. Ultrasound screening for familial ovarian cancer. Gynecol Oncol 1991;43:92–97
21. DiSantis DJ, Scatarige JC, Kemp G et al. A prospective evaluation of transvaginal sonography for detection of ovarian disease. AJR Am J Roentgenol 1993;161:91–94
22. Fleischer AC, Gordon AN, Entmann SS. Transabdominal and transvaginal sonography of pelvic masses. Ultrasound Med Biol 1989;15:529–533
23. Bast RC, Klug TL, St John E et al. A radioimmunoassay using a monoclonal antibody to monitor the course of epithelial ovarian cancer. N Engl J Med. 1983;309:883–887
24. Einhorn N, Sjovall K, Knapp RC, Hall P et al. Prospective evaluation of serum CA-125 levels for early detection of ovarian cancer. Obstet Gynecol 1992;80:14–18
25. Folkman J, Watson K, Ingber D, Hanrahan D. Induction of angiogenesis during the transition from hyperplasia to neoplasia. Nature 1989;339:58–61
26. Taylor KJW, Burns PN, Woodcock JP, Wells PNT. Blood flow in deep abdominal and pelvic vessels: ultrasonic pulsed Doppler analysis. Radiology 1985;154:487–493
27. Farquhar CM, Rae T, Thomas DC et al. Doppler ultrasound in the nonpregnant pelvis. J Ultrasound Med 1989;8:451–457

28. Bourne T, Campbell S, Steer C et al. Transvaginal color flow imaging: a possible new screening technique for ovarian cancer. BMJ 1989;229:1367–1370

29. Kurjak A, Zalud I, Alfirevic Z. Evaluation of adnexal masses with transvaginal color ultrasound. J Ultrasound Med 1991;10:295–297

30. Kurjak A, Zalud I. Transvaginal color Doppler in the differentiation between benign and malignant ovarian masses. In: Sharp F, Mason W, Creasman W, Eds. Ovarian Cancer (vol. 2). Chapman and Hall, London, UK, 1992, pp 249–264

31. Bourne TH, Campbell S, Reynolds KM et al. Screening for early familial ovarian cancer with transvaginal ultrasonography and color flow imaging. BMJ 1993;306:1025–1029

32. Tekay A, Jouppila P. Validity of pulsatility and resistance indices in classification of adnexal tumors with transvaginal color Doppler ultrasound. Ultrasound Obstet Gynecol 1992; 2:338–344

33. Fleischer AC, Rodgers WH, Kepple DM et al. Color Doppler sonography of ovarian masses: a multiparameter analysis. J Ultrasound Med 1993;12:41–48

34. Kurjak A, Predanic M, Jupesic-Urek S, Jukic S. Transvaginal color and pulsed Doppler assessment of adnexal tumor vascularity. Gynecol Oncol 1993;50:3–9

35. Finkler NJ, Benacerraf B, Lavin PT et al. Comparison of serum CA-125, clinical impression, and ultrasound in the post-operative evaluation of ovarian masses. Obstet Gynecol 1988; 72:659–664

36. Jacobs I, Davies AP, Bridges J et al. Prevalence screening for ovarian cancer in postmenopausal women by CA-125 measurement and ultrasonography. BMJ 1993;306:1030–1034

37. Lynch HT, Albano WA, Lynch JF et al. Surveillance and management of patients at high genetic risk for ovarian carcinoma. Obstet Gynecol 1982;59:589–596

38. Carter J. An update on ovarian cancer screening. Aust NZ J Obstet Gynecol 1994;34:169–174

39. The Cancer and Steroid Hormone Study of the Centers for Disease Control and the National Institutes of Child Health and Human Development. The reduction in risk of ovarian cancer associated with oral contraceptive use. N Engl J Med 1987;316:650–655

40. Prentice RL, Thomas DB. On the epidemiology of oral contraceptives and disease. Adv Cancer Res 1987;49:285–410

41. Kerlikowske K, Brown JS, Grady DG. Should women with familial ovarian cancer undergo prophylactic oophorectomy? Obstet Gynecol 1992;80:700–707

42. Frederick JL, Paulson RJ, Sauer MV. Routine use of vaginal ultrasonography in the preoperative evaluation of gynecologic patients. An adjunct to resident education. J Reprod Med 1991;36:779

43. Ng ABP. The cellular detection of endometrial carcinoma and its precursors. Gynecol Oncol 1974;2:162–169

44. Iversen O, Segadal E. The value of endometrial cytology. A comparative study of the Gravlee Jet-Washer, Isaacs Cell sampler, and Endoscann versus curettage in 600 patients. Obstet Gynecol Surv 1985;40:14–20

45. Hacker NF, Moore JG, Eds. Essentials of Obstetrics and Gynecology. WB Saunders, Philadelphia, 1986, p 467

46. Stovall TG, Solomon SK, Ling FW. Endometrial sampling prior to hysterectomy. Obstet Gynecol 1989;73:405–409

47. Stock RJ, Kanbour A. Prehysterectomy curettage. Obstet Gynecol 1975;65:537–541

48. Conte M, Guariglia L, Benedetti Panici PB et al. Transvaginal ultrasound evaluation of myometrial invasion in endometrial carcinoma. Gynecol Oncol 1990;29:224–226

49. Chambers CB, Unis SJ. Ultrasonographic evidence of uterine malignancy in the postmenopausal uterus. Am J Obstet Gynecol 1986;154:1194–1199

50. Breckenridge JW, Kurtz AB, Ritchie WGM, Macht EL. Postmenopausal uterine fluid collection: indicator of carcinoma. AJR Am J Roentgenol 1982;39:529–534

51. Scott WW, Rosenshein NB, Siegelmann SS, Sanders RC. The obstructed uterus. Radiology 1981;141:767–770

52. Gordon AN, Fleischer AC, Dudley BS et al. Preoperative assessment of myometrial invasion of endometrial adenocarcinoma by sonography (us) and magnetic resonance imaging (MRI). Gynecol Oncol 1989;34:175–179

53. Requard CK, Wicks JD, Mettler FA. Ultrasonography in the staging of endometrial adenocarcinoma. Ultrasound 1981; 1140:781–785

54. Zalud I, Conway C, Schulman H, Trinca D. Endometrial and myometrial thickness and uterine blood flow in postmenopausal women: the influence of hormonal replacement and age. J Ultrasound Med 1993;12:737–741

55. Osmers R, Volksen M, Schauer A. Vaginosonography for early detection of endometrial carcinoma? Lancet 1990;335:1569–1 571

56. Sahakian V, Syrop C, Turner D. Endometrial carcinoma: transvaginal ultrasonography prediction of depth of myometrial invasion. Gynecol Oncol 1991;43:217–219

57. Schulman H, Conway C, Zalud I et al. Prevalence in a volunteer population of pelvic cancer detected with transvaginal ultrasound and color flow Doppler. Ultrasound Obstet Gynecol 1994;4:414–420

58. Osmers R, Volksen M, Rath W, Kuhn W. Vaginosonographic detection of endometrial cancer in postmenopausal women. Int J Gynecol Obstet 1990;32:35–37

59. Goldstein SR, Machtigall M, Snyder RJ, Nachtigall L. Endometrial assessment by vaginal ultrasonography before endometrial sampling in patients with postmenopausal bleeding. Am J Obstet Gynecol 1990;163:119–123

60. Klug PW, Leitner G. Comparison of transvaginal ultrasound and histologic findings of the endometrium. Geburtshilfe Frauenheilkd 1989;49:797–802

61. Granberg S, Wikland M, Karlsson B et al. Endometrial thickness as measured by endovaginal ultrasonography for identifying endometrial abnormality. Am J Obstet Gynecol 1991; 164:47–52

62. Karlsson B, Norstrom A, Granberg S, Wikland M. The use of endovaginal ultrasound to diagnose invasion of endometrial carcinoma. Ultrasound Obstet Gynecol 1992;2:35–39

63. Rubin D, Graham MF, Cronhelm C, Cooperberg PL. Echogenic hematometra mimicking endometrial carcinoma. J Ultrasound Med 1985;4:47–48

64. Karlsson B, Granberg S, Wikland M et al. Endovaginal scanning of the endometrium compared to cytology and histology in women with postmenopausal bleeding. Gynecol Oncol 1993;50:173–178

65. Duk JM, Aalders JG, Fleuren GJ et al. CA-125: a useful marker in endometrial cancer. Am J Obstet Gynecol 1986;155:1097

66. Patsner B, Mann WJ, Cohen H, Loesch M. Predictive value of preoperative serum CA-125 levels in clinically localized and advanced endometrial carcinoma. Am J Obstet Gynecol 1988;158:399

67. Kurjak A, Shalan H, Kupesic S et al. An attempt to screen

asymptomatic women for ovarian and endometrial cancer with transvaginal color flow and pulsed Doppler sonography. J Ultrasound Med 1994;13:295–301

68. Chan FY, Chau MT, Pun TC, Lam C et al. Limitations of transvaginal sonography and color flow Doppler imaging in the differentiation of endometrial carcinoma from benign lesions. J Ultrasound Med 1994;13:623–628

69. Carter JR, Lau M, Saltzman AK et al. Grey scale and color and flow characterization of uterine tumors. J Ultrasound Med 1994;13:835–840

70. Bourne TH, Campbell S, Whitehead MI et al. Detection of endometrial cancer in postmenopausal women by transvaginal ultrasonography and color flow imaging. BMJ 1990;301:369

71. Bourne T, Campbell S, Steer CV et al. Detection of endometrial cancer by transvaginal ultrasonography with color flow imaging and blood flow analysis: a preliminary report. Gynecol Oncol 1991;40:253–259

72. Tepper R, Cohen I, Altaras M et al. Doppler flow evaluation of pathologic endometrial conditions in postmenopausal breast cancer patients treated with tamoxifen. J Ultrasound 1994;13:640

73. Hata K, Hata T, Manabe A et al. New pelvic sonoangiography for the detection of endometrial carcinoma: a preliminary report. Gynecol Oncol 45:179–184, 1992

33

Ultrasonography of Neoplasms Metastatic to the Female Genital Tract

JONATHAN CARTER

Secondary or metastatic tumors to the female genital tract, while uncommon, pose diagnostic and therapeutic dilemmas. Metastases to the female genital tract can arise from either genital or extragenital sites. In a review of 325 cases of tumors metastatic to the female genital tract, Mazur et al.[1] attempted to define the frequency and patterns of metastases. They found that the ovary and vagina were the most frequent metastatic sites for both extragenital and genital primaries. The majority of the extragenital metastases were adenocarcinomas from the gastrointestinal tract, but other primaries did spread occasionally to the genital tract. Twenty-seven percent of the metastases presented as possible primary gynecologic lesions and hence were a source of possible diagnostic confusion, and 75% of these tumors had an extragenital origin. Only in the vulva did genital metastases account for lesions that could mimic a primary tumor.

OVARIAN METASTASES

While the term *Krukenberg* has been linked in perpetuity with epithelial cancers metastatic to the ovary, Krukenberg's original description was of six tumors that he thought were of connective tissue origin. He described these tumors as "fibrosarcoma ovarii mucocellulare." It was Schlagenhaufer in 1902 who correctly analyzed Krukenberg's original tumor as being epithelial in origin and metastatic, probably from the gastrointestinal tract. For most clinicians, however, any secondary cancer in the ovary remains synonymous with the "Krukenberg tumor." Ovarian metastases may originate from genital or extragenital primaries. It may occur from direct extension of another pelvic neoplasm, by hematogeneous or lymphatic spread or by transcelomic dissemination with surface implantation of cells that spread in the peritoneal cavity.

Genital Primaries

Spread to the ovaries from genital primaries occurs through direct extension or via the lymphatics. Tubal carcinomas involve the ovaries in 13% of cases, usually by direct extension.[2] It is common that the site of origin between the ovary and tube is not identified, and by convention the ovary is labeled as the primary tumor. Advanced adenocarcinoma of the endometrium often involves the ovaries by direct extension and sometimes via the lymphatics. Such involvement upstages the primary uterine tumor to FIGO (International Federation of Gynecology and Obstetrics) stage IIIA. Cervical cancer rarely spreads to the ovaries, and in those cases reported, most were advanced or were the relatively uncommon adenocarcinomas.[3]

Extragenital Primaries

Nongynecologic primaries that may metastasize to the ovaries include breast, gastrointestinal primaries including pseudomyxoma peritonei, carcinoid tumors, the lymphomas and leukemias, and melanomas.[4] The frequency with which breast carcinoma metastasizes to the ovaries depends on the method of diagnosis. In autopsy data of women who die of metastatic breast cancer, the ovaries are involved in 24% of cases, and in 80% of them, the ovaries are involved bilaterally.[5,6]

Incidence

It has been estimated that between 10 and 30% of ovarian cancers are not primaries, and almost any cancer can establish secondary growth in the female gonad.[7] The gastrointestinal tract, breast, and uterus account for about 75% of patients with cancer metastatic to the ovary. These patients are younger than patients with primary epithelial ovarian cancer, and the younger the patient is, the more likely the ovarian cancer is to be metastatic (after excluding germ cell tumors). In a review of 12 cases, Young et al.[8] concluded that ovarian

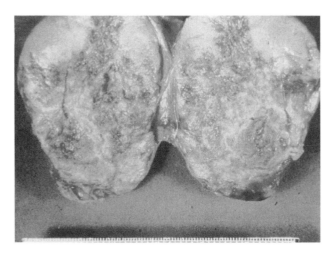

Figure 33.1 Gross picture of Krukenberg tumor. The ovary is bisected, demonstrating its solid consistency.

metastases from cervical cancer are uncommon but that occasionally striking examples with clinical manifestations of ovarian involvement occur.

Clinical Picture

Patients with metastatic ovarian cancer, like those with primary ovarian cancer, may be asymptomatic or may present with vague symptoms. In the series of Young et al.,[8] patients presented with abdominal swelling or distension, vaginal bleeding, an abnormal Papanicolaou smear, or an otherwise asymptomatic mass discovered during routine pelvic examination.[8] Patients may also complain of weakness or lethargy,

nausea or diarrhea, or weight loss, increasing abdominal distension secondary to peritoneal fluid accumulation, or a palpable mass.

The diagnosis is suspected in any patient with a history of cancer, particularly gastrointestinal or breast, who presents with or is found to have bilateral ovarian enlargement. In the report by Young et al.[8] of ovarian metastases from primary cervical tumors, the ovarian and cervical cancers were synchronous in eight patients, discovered in the post-treatment surveillance period up to 3 years later in three patients, and in one patient was not discovered until autopsy. The macroscopic appearance of metastatic or Krukenberg tumors is that of bilateral symmetrically enlarged ovaries that retain the overall ovarian outline[9] (Fig. 33.1) In tumors metastatic to the ovary from the cervix, the ovarian tumors were bilateral in 6 of the 12 reported cases and averaged 9 cm in diameter in all but one patient, whose tumor was microscopic.[8]

Histologically, the picture can be confusing. In general, the presence of intracellular mucin-producing signet ring cells and a diffuse stromal reaction resembling a sarcomatoid response is characteristic of secondaries from the gastrointestinal tract (Fig. 33.2). Features implicating metastatic disease from the cervix include extensive extracervical disease, bilateral ovarian masses, and certain histologic features.[8] Mucous cell predominant areas and the presence of a transition from benign, endocervical-like foci to carcinoma are emphasized by Scully[10] as the most helpful features in distinguishing primary mucinous cervical carcinomas from metastatic colonic carcinoma. Scully[10] also states that metastatic intestinal carcinoma may contain no goblet cells and cause confusion with endometrioid carcinoma.

The possible mechanisms of spread of cancer cells to the ovary include (1) direct extension from a local pelvic tumor,

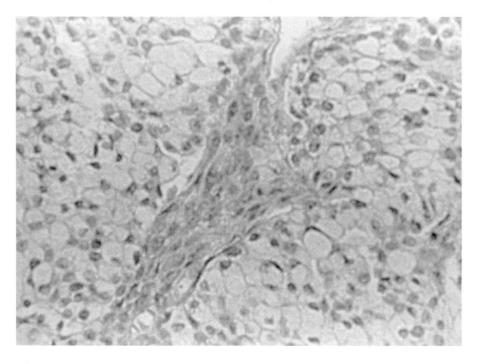

Figure 33.2 Typical microscopic appearance of Krukenberg tumor.

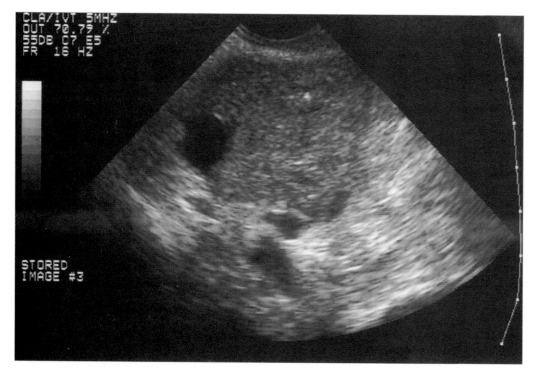

Figure 33.3 Transvaginal ultrasound of an enlarged, predominantly solid metastatic ovarian tumor with a homogeneous internal consistency.

commonly uterus or colon; (2) dissemination through peritoneal fluid of exfoliated viable tumor cells that are able to establish metastatic foci; (3) dissemination through the fallopian tube from an endometrial or, less likely, cervical primary; (4) lymphatic metastases either antegrade or retrograde through the extensive lymphatic system of the ovary; (5) hematogeneous spread from a distant focus; and (6) iatrogenic metastasis through surgical manipulation or during culdocentesis or paracentesis.

In contrast to Krukenberg tumors, which are usually bilateral and have a solid and multinodular appearance, ovarian metastases from large bowel are usually solid and cystic, with a smooth outer surface. Hemorrhage and "dirty necrosis" are also seen in most cases and, along with a garland pattern with cribriform areas, are the most distinctive features that help differentiate these tumors from primary endometrioid ovarian carcinomas.[11]

Ultrasound

Ultrasound is the preferred investigation for the evaluation of ovarian masses, although the features of metastatic ovarian cancer are nonspecific.[12,13] The ovaries tend to be bilaterally enlarged, due to apparently well-encapsulated solid masses, but cystic change with internal septa is not uncommon, and thus complex tumors may be seen.[14] There may be ascites.[15] The differential diagnosis includes early stage epithelial ovarian cancers, germ cell tumor, and sex cord stromal tumors. Patient age, menopausal status, and history may help in this dif-

ferentiation (Fig. 33.3 and Plate 33.1). Neither sonography nor computed tomography is accurate in predicting tumor type nor for differentiating between primary and metastatic disease.[16,17]

SPECIFIC TUMORS METASTATIC TO THE OVARY

Pseudomyxoma Peritonei

Pseudomyxoma peritonei is an uncommon clinical entity. It is characterized by massive abdominal distension by a gelatinous material, produced by mucous-secreting peritoneal implants secondary usually to an ovarian or appendiceal primary. Although remaining localized to the peritoneal cavity and hence thought to be a benign process, the clinical course of the disease, its association with a malignant primary and the report of a small number of cases with extraperitoneal spread all lend support to the concept that it is a malignancy. The 5-year survival is 68%, and the 10-year survival is 52%. Despite numerous adjuvant therapies, the mainstay of treatment remains complete surgical debulking initially followed by palliative debulking for symptomatic relief.[18] Radiographic findings are nonspecific and usually indicate massive ascites. Contrast studies show displacement of the intra- and retroperitoneal organs and localized areas of indentations of the intestinal tract produced by the different-sized cystic structures implanted over the peritoneal surfaces.[19] A more specific although uncommon sign is annular calcification in the walls of numerous opaque globules, similar to the ring-like calcifications reported in appendiceal mucoceles, termed *myxoglobulosis*.[20,21]

Ultrasound may show homogeneous nodular deposits and scalloping of the liver margin, but massive loculated ascites is characteristic. Semisolid cystic lesions may be seen throughout the abdominal and pelvic cavity and may indent and displace the bowel.[22,23] Although ascites could be confused with pseudomyxoma peritonei, there are differences. Bowel floats freely to the anterior abdominal wall and shifts with position when surrounded by ascites. In pseudomyxoma peritonei, the gelatinous mass is fixed in position and anterior between bowel and peritoneum.[24]

Lymphoma and Leukemia

Lymphoma and leukemia rarely involve the ovary and genital tract. Lymphomas may be primary or secondary. Secondary ovarian involvement tends to be bilateral and associated with advanced clinical disease.[25]

Carcinoid

Ovarian carcinoid tumors may be primary or metastatic. Primary tumors are classified as monodermal, highly specialized germ cell tumors. Metastatic carcinoids are rare, representing less than 2% of metastatic lesions to the ovaries. The discovery of an ovarian carcinoid should prompt a careful search for a primary intestinal lesion.

UTERINE CORPUS METASTASES

The uterine corpus is more commonly involved in metastatic spread from other gynecologic sites, rather than from nongynecologic sites. Cervical tumors may involve the corpus either by direct extension or from lymphatic and hematogeneous spread. Similarly, the corpus may be involved in spread from an ovarian primary through local extension, transperitoneal spread, and lymphatic and vascular spread. Rarely, the corpus can be the site of metastatic spread from extrapelvic sites by embolization from the breast, gastrointestinal tract, or the reticulo endothelial system (Fig. 33.4).[26,27]

Incidence

The incidence of metastatic spread to the uterus is difficult to determine, and less than 300 cases have been reported in the English literature.[28] Spread to the uterus alone is very rare, as the ovaries are usually involved also. Rarely, the uterine corpus and cervix may be the only site of spread from breast, colon, rectum, stomach, lung, kidney or pancreatic cancers, as well as melanoma and lymphoma.[29] There is a controversy as to whether the endometrium or myometrium is more com-

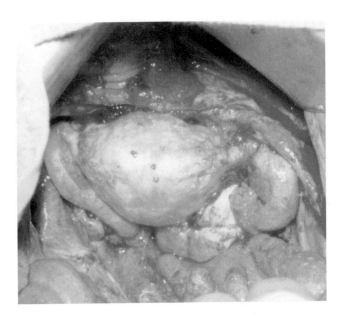

Figure 33.4 Intraoperative diagnosis of metastatic uterine spread from a colonic primary. The uterine corpus is completely replaced by tumor.

monly involved in secondary disease. According to Weingold and Boltuch,[30] the myometrium is less commonly affected by secondaries than the endometrium, and occasionally tumor can be localized to an encapsulated leiomyoma. In contrast, Kumar and Hart[31] believe that the myometrium is more commonly involved than the endometrium, but they report that endometrial curettings often contain metastatic tumor.

Clinical Picture

Patients may by asymptomatic or have nonspecific symptoms referable to the primary tumor site or only related to the uterus. Abnormal uterine bleeding or discharge or the presence of a uterine enlargement or a mass effect may be found on physical examination.[32]

The diagnosis is difficult to make preoperatively. Metastatic spread is likely to be intramyometrial and not involve the endometrium till late in the disease course, and thus a preoperative endometrial biopsy or curettage may be negative. More commonly, a patient undergoes hysterectomy for abnormal bleeding or discharge and an unexpected metastasis is found.

Ultrasound

The ultrasound findings are nonspecific and rarely diagnostic. They include an enlarged uterus with thickened myometrial walls. Rarely, foci of echoic or hypoechoic tumor may be apparent within the myometrium. Depending upon the size of the tumor, this may involve the endometrium (Fig. 33.5). Color flow Doppler allows the visualization and quantification of flow in the uterine vascular bed as well as within the

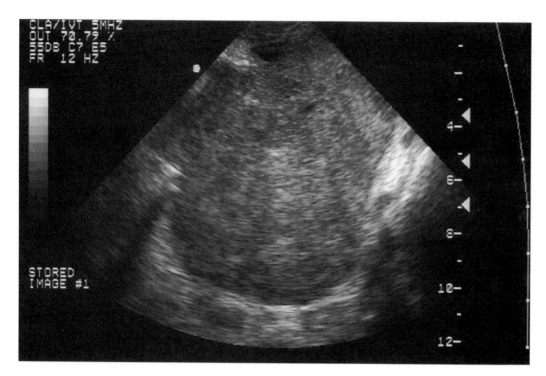

Figure 33.5 An enlarged, uterine corpus replaced by an homogenous isoechoic tumor, obliterating the endometrial stripe.

tumor bed. Color flow Doppler helps to detect malignant gynecologic lesions and shows promise in the screening of ovarian cancer.[33] Spectral analysis of intratumoral vessels shows lower systolic and increased diastolic velocities, confirming an increased blood flow in the tumor bed. The increased diastolic flow implies abnormal vascularity confirmed by the pulsatility indices.[34] The flows between the uterine artery and intratumoral vessels are different.[35]

UTERINE CERVIX METASTASES

The uterine cervix, like the corpus, is more commonly involved in metastatic spread from other gynecologic sites, than from extra pelvic sites. Cervical tumors may be involved by direct extension or from lymphatic and hematogeneous spread from adjacent organs such as the corpus, tubes, and ovaries and from nongynecologic organs such as the rectosigmoid. Rarely, the cervix can be the site of metastatic spread from breast, gastrointestinal, and lung tumors[36] and also can be involved in lymphoproliferative disorders such as lymphoma.[37]

Incidence

The incidence of metastatic spread to the cervix is difficult to determine but is probably rare. Spread to the corpus alone is very uncommon, and thus spread only to the cervix is very rare, as the corpus, cervix, and ovaries are usually involved in a large conglomerate mass. Metastases to the cervix from distant primary foci are rare, the most common sites being the gastrointestinal tract,[38,39] ovary, and breast.[40,41] Rarely, metastatic carcinoma of the kidney, gallbladder, pancreas, lung, thyroid, and melanoma have been described.[42]

Clinical Picture

When the cervix is the only site of spread, the symptoms and signs are similar to that of primary squamous cell carcinoma of the cervix. The patient may present with an abnormal smear or a history of serosanguinous discharge. Pelvic examination confirms an enlarged cervix which may have an exophytic or endophytic tumor. Autopsies of women who have died of leukemia confirm that infiltration of the cervix, especially of the granulocytic type, is common.[43] Secondary lymphomatous involvement of the cervix is reported in 6% of women dying with generalized disease.[44]

The diagnosis may not be suspected on preoperative clinical grounds. As outlined above, the signs and symptoms may be the same as for a primary cervical tumor, and it is not until the preoperative or staging biopsies are analyzed that the nature of the tumor is determined. Unusual morphology or histology such as signet ring cell carcinoma or clear cell carcinoma may provide a clue to the possibility of origin in a distant primary site.

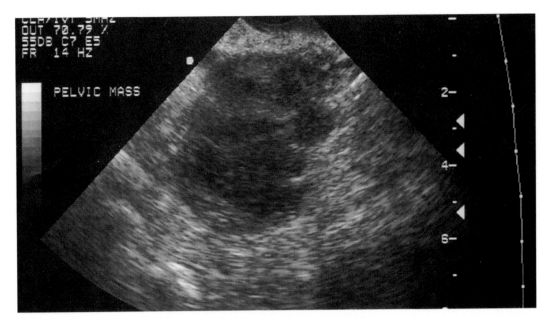

Figure 33.6 A solid, homogeneous, irregular vaginal apex mass confirmed to be recurrent tumor. Distinguishing between primary and secondary tumor is not possible.

Ultrasound

The majority of cervical tumors are hypoechoic, although hyperechoic masses have also been reported. The maximal depth of invasion may be graded according to whether the carcinoma is confined to the inner, middle, or outer third of the cervical wall, and vaginal infiltration can be assessed.[45] Parametrial involvement can also be assessed with transvaginal and transrectal sonography.[46] The normal parametria should be equal on both sides, with smooth margins, and taper off laterally in width. Features suggestive of infiltration include unilateral shortening or widening and, in particular, the presence of irregular parametrial margins.

VAGINAL METASTASES

Like the other anatomic sites discussed above, the vagina can be involved with metastatic tumor spread from gynecologic or nongynecologic origins. The incidence of such occurrence is extremely low and mainly based upon autopsy studies. The endometrium and cervix are the most common sources of metastases. Tumors of the ovary, rectum, and kidney may also metastasize to the vagina, as can choriocarcinoma.[47]

Clinical Picture

Symptoms may vary from none to vaginal discharge or bleeding or the presence of a lump or nodule. The extent of disease and its location may determine the type of symptomatology present. The diagnosis may be confirmed by evaluation of biopsy material. As with cancer of the cervix, the diagnosis may not be appreciated at the presentation. Implants from uterine corpus adenocarcinomas may reach the vagina by submucosal lymphatics or implantation. They are usually seen in the upper third and on the anterior wall. The metastases may be small and at times can resemble granulation tissue. The microscopic appearance is similar to that of the original tumor.

Ultrasound

Due to the location of metastatic tumor in the vagina, ultrasound and other imaging modalities have a limited role in the diagnosis of metastatic disease. It is usually not possible to distinguish between primary and secondary tumor (Fig. 33.6). Ultrasound is helpful in excluding spread to other pelvic organs.

REFERENCES

1. Mazur MT, Hsueh S, Gersell DJ. Metastases to the female genital tract. Analysis of 325 cases. Cancer 1984;53:1978–1984
2. Sedlis A. Primary carcinoma of the fallopian tube. Obstet Gynecol 1961;16:209–216
3. Woodruff JD, Murthy YS, Bhaskar JN et al. Metastatic ovarian tumors. Am J Obstet Gynecol 1970;107:202–209
4. Young RH, Scully RE. Malignant melanoma metastatic to the ovary. A clinicopathologic analysis of 20 cases. Am J Surg Pathol 1991;15:849–860
5. Kasilag FB, Rutledge FN. Metastatic breast carcinoma to the ovary. Am J Obstet Gynecol 989–996

6. Lee YN, Hori JM. Significance of ovarian metastasis in therapeutic oophorectomy for breast cancer. Cancer 1971;27:1374–1385

7. Webb MJ, Decker DG, Mussey E. Cancer metastatic to the ovary. Obstet Gynecol 1975;45:391–396

8. Young RH, Gersell DJ, Roth LM, Scully RE. Ovarian metastases from cervical carcinomas other than pure adenocarcinomas. A report of 12 cases. Cancer 1993;71:407–418

9. Ulbright TM, Roth LM, Stehman FB. Secondary ovarian neoplasia. a clinicopathologic study of 35 cases. Cancer 1984;53:1164–1174

10. Scully RE. Tumors of the ovary and maldeveloped gonads. In: Atlas of Tumor Pathology (series 2, fascicle 16). Armed Forces Institute of Pathology, Washington, DC, 1979, pp 323–352

11. Daya D, Nazerali L, Frank GL. Metastatic ovarian carcinoma of large intestinal origin simulating primary ovarian carcinoma. A clinicopathologic study of 25 cases. Am J Clin Pathol 1992;97:751–758

12. Moyle JW, Rochester D, Sider L et al. Sonography of ovarian tumors: predictability of tumor type. AJR Am J Roentgenol 1983;141:985–991

13. Requard CK, Mettler FA, Jr, Wicks JD. Preoperative sonography of malignant ovarian neoplasms. AJR Am J Roentgenol 1981;137:79–82

14. Shimizu H, Yamasaki M, Ohama K et al. Characteristic ultrasonographic appearance of the Krukenberg tumor. J Clin Ultrasound 1990;18:697–703

15. Choi BI, Choo IW, Han MC et al. Sonographic appearance of Krukenberg tumor from gastric carcinoma. Gastrointest Radiol 1988;13:15–18

16. Walsh JW, Rosenfield AT, Faffe CC et al. Prospective comparison of ultrasound and computed tomography in the evaluation of gynecologic pelvic masses. AJR Am J Roentgenol 1978;131:955–960

17. Cho KC, Gold BM. Computed tomography of Krukenberg tumors. AJR Am J Roentgenol 1985;145:285–288

18. Carter J, Moradi MM, Elg S et al. Pseudomyxoma peritonei—experience from a tertiary referral center. Aust N Z J Obstet Gynecol 1991;31:177–178

19. Carter J, Moradi MM, Adcock LL et al. Pseudomyxoma peritonei: a local disease causing systemic effects. A review and treatment recommendations. Int J Gynecol Cancer 1991;1:243–247

20. Lubin J, Berle E. Myxoglobulosis of the appendix. Arch Pathol 1972;94:533–536

21. Felson B, Wiot JF. Some interesting right lower quadrant entities. Myxoglobulosis of the appendix, ileal prolapse, diverticulitis, lymphoma, endometriosis. Radiol Clin North Am 1969;8:83–95

22. Hayashi N, Tamaki N, Yamamoto K et al. Sonography of pseudomyxoma peritonei. J Ultrasound Med 1986;5:401–403

23. Seale WB. Sonographic findings in a patient with pseudomyxoma peritonei. J Clin Ultrasound 1982;10:441–443

24. Hann L, Love S, Goldberg RP. Pseudomyxoma peritonei: preoperative diagnosis by ultrasound and computed tomography. Cancer 1983;52:642–644

25. Freeman C, Berg JW, Cutler SJ. Occurrence and prognosis of extranodal lymphomas. Cancer 1972;29:252–264

26. Kumar A, Schneider V. Metastasis to the uterus from extrapelvic primary tumors. Int J Gynecol Pathol 1983;2:134–140

27. Leiberman J, Chaim W, Choen A, Czernobilsky B. Primary carcinoma of stomach with uterine metastasis. Br J Obstet Gynaecol 1975;82:917–921

28. Kim SH, Hwang HY, Choi BI. Uterine metastasis from stomach cancer: radiological findings. Clin Radiol 1990;42:285–286

29. Stemmermann GN. Extrapelvic carcinoma metastatic to the uterus. Am J Obstet Gynecol 1961;82:1261–1266

30. Weingold AB, Boltuch SM. Extragenital metastases to the uterus. Am J Obstet Gynecol 1961;82:1267–1272

31. Kumar NB, Hart WR. Metastases to the uterine corpus from extragenital cancers. A clinicopathologic study of 63 cases. Cancer 1982;50:2163–2169

32. Pradhan SA, Jussawalla DJ. Mammary carcinoma metastasizing to the endometrium. Indian J Cancer 1979;16:70–71

33. Carter JR. Early detection of ovarian cancer by transvaginal ultrasound. Clin Dev Women Cancer 1991;5(1):1–4

34. Taylor KJW, Schwartz PE, Kohorn EI. Gestational trophoblastic neoplasia: diagnosis and Doppler US. Radiology 1987;165:445–448

35. Carter JR, Fowler JM, Carlson JW et al. Prediction of malignancy using transvaginal color flow Doppler in patients with gynecologic tumors. Int J Gynecol Cancer 1993;3:59–64

36. Takeda M, King DE, McHenry MJ et al. Lung cancer metastatic to the uterine cervix. [Abstract.] Acta Cytol 1981;25:442

37. Brady, LW, O'Neill EA, Farber SH. Unusual sites of metastasis. Semin Oncol 1977;4:59–63

38. Lemoine NR, Hall PA. Epithelial tumors metastatic to the uterine cervix. A study of 33 cases and review of the literature. Cancer 1986;57:2002–2005

39. Zhang YC, Zhang PF, Wei YH. Metastatic carcinoma of the cervix uteri from the gastrointestinal tract. Gynecol Oncol 1983;15:287–295

40. Korhonen M, Stenback F. Adenocarcinoma metastatic to the uterine cervix. Gynecol Obstet Invest 1984;17:57–65

41. Way S. Carcinoma metastatic to the cervix. Gynecol Oncol 1980;9:298–302

42. Twombley GH, DiPalma S. Growth and spread of cancer of cervix uteri. Am J Roentgenol 1951;65:691–695

43. Lucia SP, Mills H, Lowenhaupt E, Hunt ML. Visceral involvement on primary neoplastic disease of the reticuloendothelial system. Cancer 1952;5:1193–1199

44. Lathrop KC. Views and reviews' malignant pelvic lymphomas. Obstet Gynecol 1967;30:137–146

45. Bernaschek G, Deutinger J, Kratochwil A. Endosonography in Obstetrics and Gynecology. Springer-Verlag, Berlin, 1990, pp 97–122

46. Yuhara A, Akamatsu N, Sekiba K. Use of transrectal radial scan ultrasonography in evaluating the extent of uterine cervical cancer. J Clin Ultrasound 1987;15:507–517

47. Nordrum TA. Vaginal metastases of hypernephroma: report of 3 cases. Acta Obstet Gynecol Scand 1966;45:515–520

Computed Tomography and Magnetic Resonance Imaging of Neoplasms Metastatic to the Female Genital Tract

ERIC K. OUTWATER

Metastases to the genital tract from extragenital sites are an infrequent cause of pelvic masses when compared with the number of primary genital malignancies. They are important, however, because they can pose a diagnostic dilemma for radiologists and pathologists. Pathologically and clinically, tumors metastatic to the ovaries, uterus, and vagina can mimic primaries. The only evidence of a metastasis in the genital tract may be from images obtained before surgery. Occasionally, the radiologist is in the best position to make the preoperative diagnosis that a mass in the pelvis is metastatic. There are two broad clinical and pathologic groups. These are metastases from nearby primary genital malignancies and metastases from extragenital sites. Metastases to the ovaries, fallopian tubes, uterus, and vagina from primary genital malignancies are relatively frequent. These neoplasms are part of the FIGO (International Federation of Gynecology and Obstetrics) staging system for gynecologic cancer and therefore are included when considering treatment and prognosis. Metastases to the female genital tract from extragenital sites, on the other hand, are less common, but those to the ovaries are more frequent than expected, considering their size.

OVARIAN METASTASES

Incidence

Metastases From Primary Extragenital Tumors

It is difficult to establish the incidence of extragenital metastases to the genital tract. In a series of autopsies on women dying from cancer of the breast, the incidence of metastatic disease to the ovaries was approximately 30%, but about two-thirds of them were only evident microscopically and were unlikely to have been demonstrable radiologically during life.[1] About 5% to 10% of ovarian malignancies are found to be metastatic on histopathology after their removal[2–5]

with an incidence of 6.6% in seven clinical series (Table 34.1).[6–12] Secondaries in the ovaries arise mostly from primary carcinomas in the stomach, colon, or breast,[13] and therefore it is important to evaluate the abdomen and breast for the presence of an asymptomatic neoplasm before performing a laparotomy for an ovarian mass. Metastases to the ovaries are bilateral in 60% to 80% of cases.[4,13,14] This does not help to differentiate ovarian secondaries from ovarian primaries, because primaries can also be bilateral. Up to two-thirds of serous epithelial malignancies are bilateral at the time of diagnosis, but this is not so frequent with other cell types.[14] Signet ring cell carcinomas of the stomach, primary breast carcinomas (approximately one-third), colon carcinomas (2% to 10%), and melanomas (15% to 20% at autopsy) develop ovarian metastases.[4]

Metastases From Primary Genital Tumors

In women with known endometrial carcinoma, secondaries are found in the ovaries of 34% to 40% at autopsy and in approximately 7% at surgery.[3,15] Choriocarcinoma involves the ovary in up to 22% of patients with primary uterine choriocarcinoma[3], and the vagina in 16% to 30% of patients.[16,17] It is unusual for advanced cervical squamous cell carcinomas to metastasize to the ovary. The ovary is commonly involved with fallopian tube carcinomas, usually by direct extension or by peritoneal seeding. Leiomyosarcomas of the uterus rarely metastasize to the ovary, but endometrial stromal sarcomas do occasionally.[3]

Pathology

Metastases From Primary Extragenital Tumors

In most patients with metastases in the ovaries (approximately 86%), the diagnosis is obvious because there is already a history of carcinoma outside the genital tract.[13] The metastases

Table 34.1 Proportion of Metastases to Ovaries to Malignant Lesions in Adnexal Masses Removed by Laparotomy

Number of Patients	Benign	Malignant	Metastases (% of Malignant Lesions)	Reference
380	297	83	2 (2.4%)	Ovadia and Goldman[6]
63	36	27	2 (7.4%)	Hata et al.[7]
124	87	37	1 (2.7%)	Davies et al.[8]
149	121	28	2 (7.1%)	Valentin et al.[9]
33	17	16	1 (6.2%)	Stevens et al.[10]
83	54	29	4 (13.7%)	Kurjak and Predanic[11]
90	68	22	4 (18.1%)	Scout et al.[12]
922	680	242	16 (6.6%)	Total

will microscopically (although often not macroscopically) resemble the primary. Features suggesting that the tumor is metastatic include extensive areas of necrosis, multifocal patterns, and areas of vascular invasion. The presence of multiple solid nodules and surface involvement of the ovary without significant involvement of the underlying ovarian stroma is also suggestive.[14,18] When a neoplasm which is thought to be an ovarian primary spreads atypically, such as to the lung or liver, diagnosticians should be aware that the ovarian mass could actually be a metastasis and that the primary is yet to be found. Metastases in the ovary are often cystic, and it should not be assumed that, because they are cystic, they are primary.

The incidence of ovarian metastases at initial surgery for an intestinal neoplasm is 3% to 4%.[18] Microscopically, metastases from gastrointestinal adenocarcinomas may be impossible to distinguish from primary ovarian mucinous adenocarcinoma.[5] Tumors metastatic from the large intestine may be solid but are usually partly cystic.[4,5,19] If mucinous (goblet) cells predominate in the histologic specimen or if there is a gradual transition from benign epithelium to frankly malignant epithelium, then the lesion is more likely to be a primary ovarian neoplasm than a metastasis.[5,19] Carcinoid (argentaffin) tumors arise predominantly in the appendix, rectum, or other parts of the gastrointestinal tract, but they can originate in the gallbladder, bronchi, or ovary. They secrete serotonin and other vasoactive substances, which have little effect because they are metabolized by the liver. If, however, metastases form in the liver, high levels of serotonin can be released into the systemic circulation, producing a "carcinoid syndrome." This is characterized by (often postprandial) episodic flushing of the skin, mottled cyanosis, telangiectasia, bronchospasm, and borborygmi with diarrhea. Manifestations of the syndrome can also be produced without hepatic secondaries if the carcinoid occurs primarily or secondarily in the ovary because the serotonin passes directly into the systemic

circulation via the ovarian veins and the inferior vena cava rather than the portal circulation. For this reason, oophorectomy usually cures the syndrome when the primary is in the ovary but not when there are liver metastases.[20–22] The diagnosis of "carcinoid syndrome" can be made preoperatively by demonstrating an increase in urinary 5-hydroxyindolacetic acid, a metabolite of serotonin.

Metastases from breast carcinoma to the ovaries are frequently bilateral and usually appear as multiple nodules of solid tissue or as complete replacement of the ovaries with lobulated masses on gross inspection.[5,18] It is rare for metastatic breast carcinoma to be predominantly cystic in appearance, and it is unlikely that it will be initially identified by ovarian histopathology,[1,13] because most ovarian metastases are diagnosed after detection of the breast primary.[4] The histology of metastatic breast carcinoma usually resembles that of the primary, however, if the breast primary is undiagnosed, it may then be confused with an undifferentiated primary ovarian carcinoma.

At autopsy, 15% to 20% of patients with malignant melanoma are found to have ovarian metastases, but identification before death is much less frequent.[3,23] Melanomas metastatic to the ovary are usually completely solid and may be bilateral or unilateral.[24] Microscopically, metastatic melanoma must be distinguished from rare melanomas arising within a teratoma, or from a lipid-poor steroid cell tumor.[3,24]

Krukenberg Tumors

Krukenberg originally described tumors that he believed arose from the ovary. They were later identified as metastatic from primary extragenital adenocarcinomas.[18] The term *Krukenberg* has since been applied variously to any ovarian metastasis, to any ovarian metastasis from a primary gastric carcinoma, to any ovarian metastasis from a primary intestinal carcinoma, and, most narrowly, to ovarian metastases from signet ring cell carcinomas. It is this last interpretation that is most commonly accepted in pathology textbooks today and is the interpretation used here. Microscopically, Krukenberg tumors are formed of mucin-containing containing epithelial signet ring cells set in a dense cellular stroma.[10] Extracellular pools of mucin may also be present. The stroma is of an ovarian type and may give the tumor a "pseudosarcomatous" pattern.[18] They are usually solid and involve both ovaries in over 80% of patients.[3,18,25] An occasional Krukenberg tumor may be predominantly cystic. The vast majority are metastases from gastric primaries. Less commonly, signet ring cell carcinomas arising in the colon, breast, or gallbladder may metastasize to the ovary and present an identical histologic appearance.[18] Signet ring cell carcinomas have a predilection for spread to the ovary, and the incidence of the primary sites reflects the incidence of primary sites for signet ring cell carcinomas. In contrast, gastric adenocarcinomas do not metastasize to the ovary as readily.[13] Signet ring cell tumors rarely arise as primary neoplasms of the ovary. This diagnosis should be made cautiously, because identification of a distant primary may not occur for years after the removal of the Krukenberg tumor. Only 20% to 30% of patients with a Krukenberg tumor have a history of extragenital malignancy. Patients with Krukenberg tumors are usually younger than those with metastatic adenocarcinoma, with nearly half being below the age of 40 years.[3,18]

Pseudomyxoma Peritonei

Metastatic neoplasms from the appendix include mucinous adenocarcinomas, signet ring cell carcinomas, and mucinous carcinoids. Extension of a low-grade mucinous neoplasm from the appendix and occasionally the ovary may result in pseudomyxoma peritonei.[26–29] This enigmatic condition is very rare. Mucus-secreting cells spread over the peritoneum and produce gelatinous material in the peritoneal cavity. Most patients are between 50 and 70 years of age, but it can occur in younger people. The patient experiences painless abdominal distension due to accumulation of large quantities of mucinous fluid that does not demonstrate shifting dullness. At laparotomy, the peritoneal cavity is filled with yellow jelly-like liquid, often encysted. About 80% of patients gradually succumb to inanition and infection following repeated bouts of intestinal obstruction.[28] Survival rates are 45% to 50% at 5 years and 18% at 10 years. Time between diagnosis and death ranges from 3 months to 24 years.[29,30] Neither intraoperative rupture of a mucinous ovarian tumor nor needle aspiration before removal have been shown to lead to pseudomyxoma peritonei.[31]

Metastases From Primary Genital Tumors

The simultaneous development of carcinoma of the ovary and carcinoma of the endometrium is fairly common. One-third of endometrioid ovarian carcinomas may have coexistent carcinomas of the endometrium.[3] Many of these are thought to be independent primary tumor sites;[3,18,32] however, distinguishing between independent primary sites and metastases from one site to another may be impossible (Fig. 34.1), as the histopathology can be similar.[3] When endometrial carcinoma involves the adnexa, it is frequently microscopic and not apparent on imaging.[15,33]

COMPUTED TOMOGRAPHY AND MAGNETIC RESONANCE IMAGING

Unfortunately, with the possible exception of pseudomyxoma peritonei, there are no specific imaging features that distinguish metastases to the female genital tract from primary tumors. Computed tomography (CT) offers advantages over ultrasound and magnetic resonance imaging (MRI) because the entire abdomen, including the gastrointestinal tract, can be more easily evaluated at the time the adnexal masses are imaged, and a primary, for instance in the stomach or colon may be identified. MRI can also be used to demonstrate the upper abdomen, but lack of bowel distension, lack of bowel contrast, and bowel peristalsis limit its general effectiveness for the gastrointestinal tract.

Metastases From Primary Extragenital Tumors

Primary lesions in the intestine, breast, and stomach are rarely, if ever, truly cystic, although they may show central necrosis. A curious characteristic of their ovarian metastases is that they often become partially, or wholly, cystic.[3,18,25,34,35] The common primary epithelial neoplasms of the ovary (serous, mucinous, clear cell, and endometrioid) are also usually wholly or partially cystic, so it is often difficult to differentiate between the two on gross or radiologic appearance.[3,36–38] The CT appearance of metastases in the ovaries is similar to that of primary ovarian carcinoma. Typically, large, bilateral, lobulated, multicystic masses with enhancing soft tissue components are seen. Cho and Gold[35] reported three patients with metastases from colon adenocarcinomas to the ovary, each with large cystic components. Megibow and colleagues[25] described predominantly cystic metastases in 9 of 20 patients with colon cancer, 3 of 6 patients with breast cancer, and 1 of 5 patients with stomach cancer. A mixed solid and cystic appearance occurred in 9 of 20 patients with colon cancer and in 2 of 6 patients with breast cancer. Four of five patients with gastric carcinoma had predominantly solid metastases, an appearance noted by others.[39] A mainly solid appearance was seen in a small minority of patients with metastatic colon and breast adenocarcinoma (Fig. 34.2). Ascites and peritoneal implants were present in 4 of 20 patients with metastatic colon carcinoma, 2 of 6 patients with breast carcinoma, and 3 of 5 patients with stomach adenocarcinoma. Mata and co-workers[40] found predominantly cystic tumors in 6 of 7 patients with gastrointestinal tumors metastatic to the ovary. The appearance of the abdomen in these was not substantially different from that in patients with ovarian carcinoma metastatic to the peritoneum. Metastases to the ovary have not been described as simple cysts, so they should not be confused with benign functional cysts. Mucinous neoplasms from the gastrointestinal tract can calcify when metastatic to the ovary.[41] This may be indistinguishable from the psammatous calcification, which occurs in primary ovarian papillary serous neoplasms.

The features of MRI of metastases in the ovaries, like CT, are not specific. The multicystic nature of metastases mimics primary ovarian neoplasms so that differentiation based on morphologic criteria is usually impossible. Takemori and colleagues[42] and Togashi[37] have shown that the MRI appearance of Krukenberg tumors is mostly solid, with small areas of cyst formation and necrosis. Soft tissue contrast is high with MRI. Ovarian details such as small follicles, medulla, and cortex can be resolved on T2-weighted images.[42] Small masses within the ovary or masses that are partly replacing the ovary can be identified. Papillary projections within the cystic spaces can be demonstrated on T2-weighted images.[36–38,43] The presence of true papillary projections suggests a primary

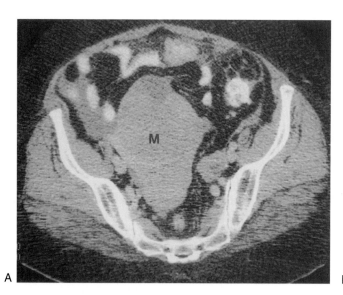

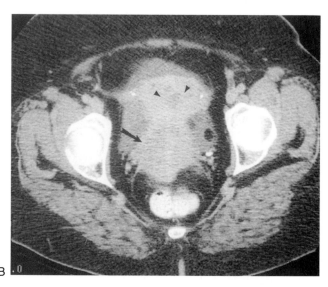

Figure 34.1 Ovarian metastases from malignant mixed mesodermal tumor of the cervix. The pattern of the ovarian and uterine metastases is more commonly produced by primary uterine and ovarian neoplasms and less commonly by extragenital neoplasms. **(A)** CT scan at the level of the ovaries shows a large right ovarian mass, which has cystic and solid components (M). **(B)** CT scan at the level of the cervix. There is a small amount of fluid and tumor in the uterine cavity (arrowheads) as well as enlargement of the lower segment and cervix (arrow), which is the primary site of the mixed mesodermal tumor.

Figure 34.2 Breast carcinoma metastatic to uterus and ovaries. **(A)** CT scan of a patient with breast carcinoma before the development of metastases to the uterus and ovaries. **(B)** CT scan after development of metastases. There are solid masses involving the right and left ovaries (arrows). Note the enlarged irregular and heterogeneous enlargement to the uterus in the interim. In the absence of relevant history of metastatic ovarian carcinoma, this appearance would be indistinguishable from endometrial carcinoma.

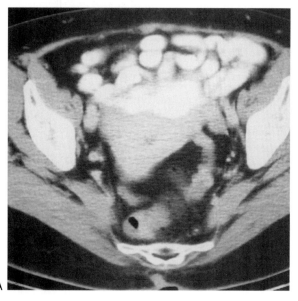

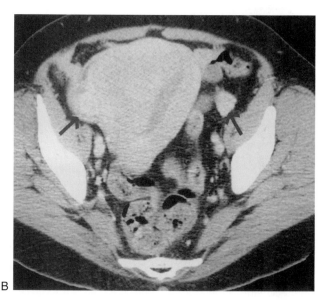

ovarian neoplasm rather than a metastasis. On T1-weighted images, metastases to the ovaries have a signal intensity similar to normal ovaries or myometrium. Foci of hemorrhagic necrosis that are common in metastases appear as ill-defined areas of higher signal intensity. On T2-weighted images, portions of solid tumor have intermediate to slightly high signal intensity. Very high signal intensity on the T2-weighted images indicates necrosis, cyst formation, or mucin. The mucinous component of mucinous neoplasms has very high signal intensity on T2-weighted images, often as high, or sometimes higher than that of simple fluid such as urine (Fig. 34.3). Despite the presence of cyst-like signal intensity on T2-weighted images, appreciable enhancement throughout is frequent on gadolinium-enhanced images. Intravenous gadolinium often

Figure 34.3 Ovarian metastases from mucinous rectal carcinoma. **(A)** T1-weighted spin echo image showing a large predominantly cystic mass in the right ovary (M). **(B)** T2-weighted fast spin echo (FSE) image showing right ovarian mass (M) and a simple functional cyst in the left ovary, which also contains small follicles (white arrow). **(C)** Fat-saturated gadolinium-enhanced image shows marked enhancement in portions of the right ovarian mass (arrow) indicating that it is mostly solid. Very high signal intensity in a solid mass is characteristic of mucinous neoplasms. **(D)** Axial image at the level of the rectum shows a tumor with similar signal characteristics as the right ovarian mass. Pathology showed a mucinous adenocarcinoma of the rectum metastatic to the right ovary.

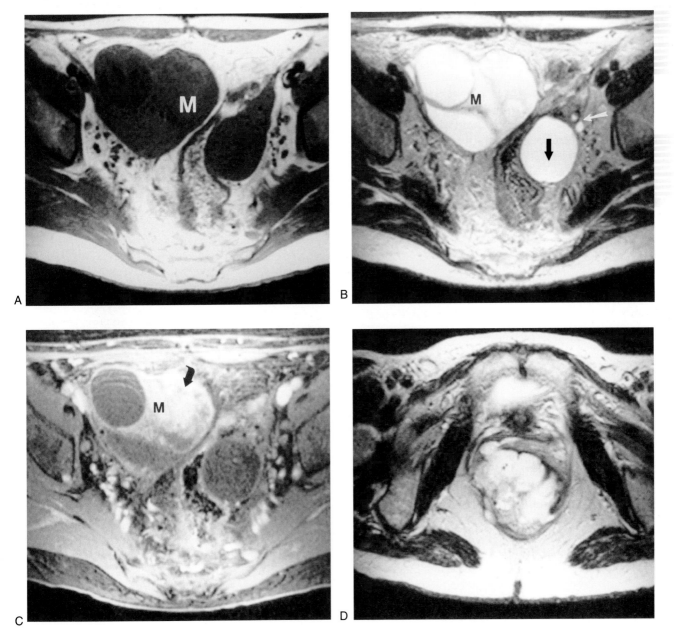

helps to distinguish adnexal masses. In particular, vascularity of areas that are not clearly fluid or solid, based on signal intensity, can be characterized with gadolinium enhancement.[10,42,44] Irregular debris adherent to the wall of the cyst can often be difficult to distinguish from a solid nodule or projections or vegetations arising from the cyst wall, and gadolinium can help diagnose such lesions[36–38,45] (Fig. 34.3). After gadolinium injection, it is useful to obtain T1-weighted fat-saturation images either with fast spin echo (also known as turbo spin echo) or gradient echo techniques. As with CT scanning or ultrasonography, metastases in the ovaries are unlikely to be mistaken for benign lesions. The solid tissue and necrosis associated with malignant tumors distinguish the mass from benign masses. Compared with primary ovarian carcinomas, metastatic lesions are more likely to be well defined and to contain necrosis and less likely to show papillary proliferations and irregular cyst formation.[34]

Metastases to the female genital tract from neoplasms other than intestinal primaries do not have any particular characteristic features. Carcinoid metastases are frequently of very high signal intensity on T2-weighted images when they appear in the liver, although the primary site in the small bowel mesentery as well as metastases elsewhere may have a low signal intensity (Fig. 34.4). Mucinous carcinoids, an unusual variant of carcinoid tumor, will have a much higher signal, reflecting the mucin content of the tumor (Fig. 34.5).

Melanoma may present with a characteristic appearance because of hemorrhage or melanin, both of which shorten T1, and as a result, appear as slightly hyperintense masses on T1-weighted images.

Pseudomyxoma Peritonei

One condition that may be distinctive on radiographic imaging is pseudomyxoma peritonei. These typically appear on CT as widespread loculations of low attenuation throughout the abdomen.[46–49] Mucinous deposits on MRI have a low signal intensity on T1-weighted images and very high signal intensity on T2-weighted images.[50] Fine septa separate the locules of mucin, and considerable mass effect on adjacent organs causes prominent scalloping of the capsular surface of the liver and spleen[46,50] (Fig. 34.6). Fine mottled attenuation within the locules may be seen by CT, reflecting fine septa or papillary projections within the mucinous areas. In typical ascites, bowel loops tend to float anteriorly to the midline when the patient is supine, but in pseudomyxoma peritonei, the bowel loops are displaced from the midline by the viscous and loculated mucinous material.[46] A similar appearance has been reported for a peritoneal mesothelioma,[51] but with considerably more solid tissue present.

Calcification of pseudomyxoma peritonei following intraperitoneal chemotherapy has been reported. It may be diffuse and amorphous or annular in appearance, or it may show extensive punctate or nodular calcification.[47] Presumably, the propensity of the tumor implants to calcify explains the uptake of bone-seeking agents (technetium 99M-MDP) by

pseudomyxoma peritonei;[52] however, similar uptake has been reported in noncalcified peritoneal implants.

Metastases From Primary Genital Tumors

MRI and CT are comprehensive in evaluation of gestational trophoblastic disease. MRI can assess the depth of penetration of invasive moles and choriocarcinoma[53] and metastases to the ovaries[54,55] because it can image sagittal and coronal planes. Unlike theca-lutein cysts, which are frequently associated with the condition, gestational trophoblastic disease in the uterus and ovaries typically appear heterogeneous with very high signal intensity on the T2-weighted images with a periphery of punctate signal voids due to enlarged vasculature.[53–56] Hemorrhage is frequent.[53,54] The appearance of the adnexal mass is not sufficiently specific however, to distinguish between metastases and other adnexal masses associated with an elevated β-human chorionic gonadotropin level such as ectopic pregnancy.[54]

CT scanning of the chest, abdomen, and pelvis provides the most sensitive evaluation of patients with choriocarcinoma.[16,17,57,58] Primary tumor and adnexal disease are not assessed as well as with MRI, but, more importantly, CT scanning can demonstrate the tumor in the liver and chest.[57] Both the primary tumor and hepatic metastases may show vascularity in the form of intense enhancement and large feeding vessels. Up to one-third of patients with endometrioid ovarian carcinomas have a coexistent endometrial adenocarcinoma of the uterus.[3] Features that suggest metastasis from an endometrial primary include a multinodular pattern in the ovarian mass, a relatively small ovarian metastasis, and bilateral involvement. Deep myometrial invasion or vascular invasion of a high-grade endometrial primary also supports a diagnosis of secondary disease.[32] MRI is better suited than CT to assess myometrial invasion by endometrial carcinoma. Heterogeneous signal intensity or low signal intensity nodules on the T2-weighted sequences may indicate the presence of endometrial tumor associated with adnexal masses (Fig. 34.7). Gadolinium helps to enhance the tumor and determine its extent.[2,45,59]

UTERINE METASTASES

Metastases to the uterus are rare. The incidence of extragenital neoplasms metastatic to the uterus is thought to be about 6% of the incidence of ovarian metastases.[13] In one autopsy series of patients with uterine metastases from extragenital malignancy, the metastases were the presenting sign of tumor in only 5 of 63 women.[60] Lesions of the breast and colon accounted for 75% of primary tumors whose metastases were discovered in the uterus at surgery (Fig. 34.7). Breast carcinoma accounted for 43% of all primary tumors metastatic to the uterus, with colon, stomach, and pancreas being other common primary tumors.

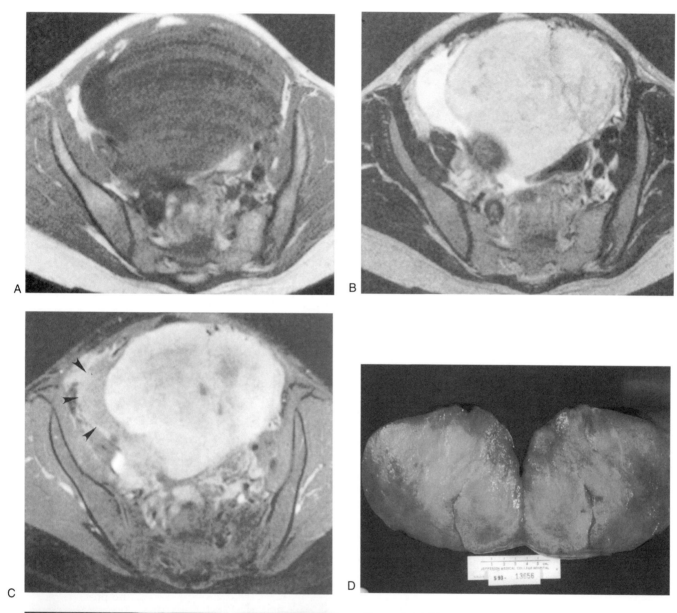

Figure 34.4 Metastatic appendiceal mucinous carcinoid in a 42-year-old. **(A)** Spin echo T1-weighted image shows a large mass of intermediate signal intensity in the left pelvis. **(B)** T2-weighted FSE image demonstrates nearly homogeneous high signal. Ascites lies in the right paracolic gutter. **(C)** T1-weighted, fat-saturated, gadolinium-enhanced image shows enhancement throughout the mass, indicating solid vascularized tumor. Note that the ascites, which has lower signal intensity than muscle on the T1-weighted image, shows enhancement, suggesting peritoneal disease that has allowed leakage of the gadolinium into the peritoneal fluid (arrowheads). **(D)** Photograph of the bihalved tumor at the same level shows a homogeneous tumor with a glistening mucoid surface. Pathology showed a mucinous carcinoma metastatic from a small appendiceal lesion. **(E)** T2-weighted FSE image at the level of the ovaries shows the tumor in the left pelvis arising from the left ovary to be marked by small follicles (black arrow). A fibroid (F) is present in the uterus. The right ovary (straight white arrow) appears to have a 1-cm cyst in the posterior pole (curved white arrow). (*Figure continues.*)

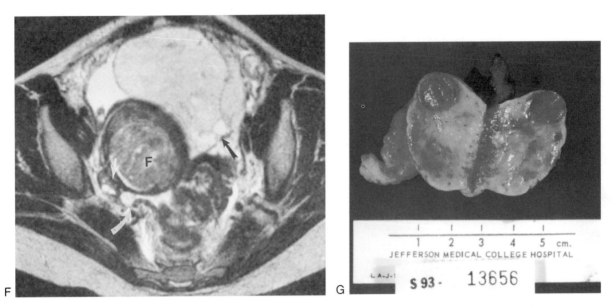

Figure 34.4 *(Continued)*. **(F)** Fat-saturation, gadolinium-enhanced T1-weighted image shows that what appeared to be a 1-cm cyst in the posterior pole of the right ovary in (D) is diffusely enhancing (curved arrow), similar to the tumor in the left pelvis, indicating that this is bilateral spread of tumor. Note enhancing ovarian stroma (white arrow). **(G)** Photograph of the bihalved right ovary shows the 1-cm nodule seen in images (Figs. E & F).

Figure 34.5 Metastatic carcinoid to the right ovary. **(A)** Axial T2-weighted spin echo image showing a low signal intensity mass (M) in the pouch of Douglas. The mass shows some high signal intensity components consistent with necrosis. This mass proved to be carcinoid metastatic to the ovaries. Signal intensity on T2-weighted images is atypical for carcinoid and suggests a benign ovarian lesion such as ovarian fibroma. **(B)** Sagittal T2-weighted image. M; mass.

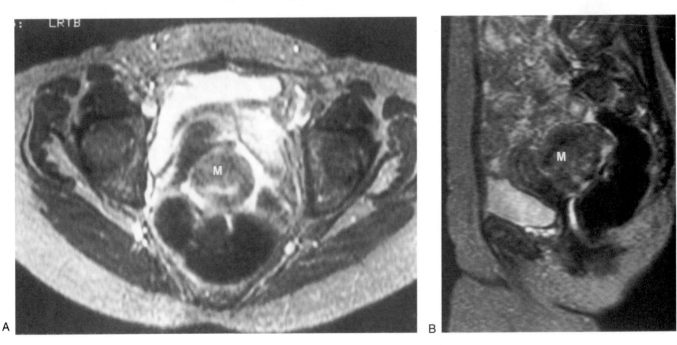

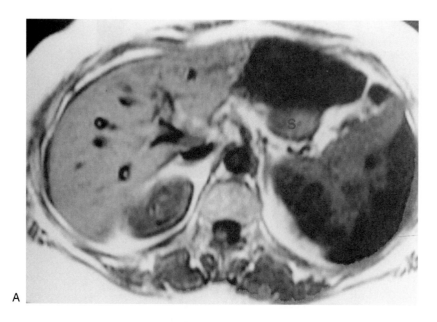

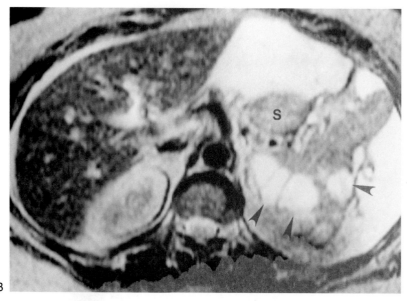

Figure 34.6 Pseudomyxoma peritonei due to ovarian carcinoma. (**A**) Axial T1-weighted spin echo image. (**B**) T2-weighted spin echo (TR2,500/TE80) showing numerous locules of fluid surrounding the spleen in this patient and mucinous borderline tumors of the ovaries. Notice the prominent indentations of the fluid deposits into the splenic parenchyma (arrowheads) Additional deposits lie anterior to the stomach (S).

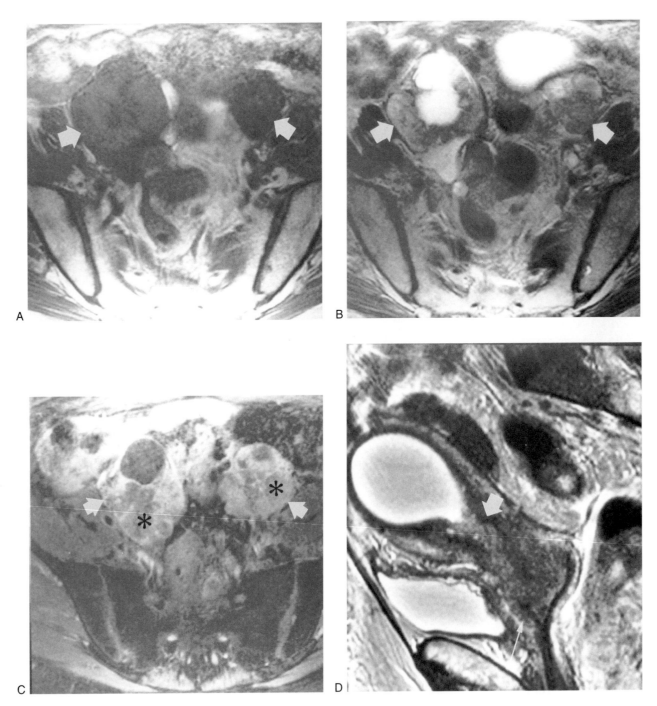

Figure 34.7 Coexistent bilateral ovarian and endometrial papillary cystadenocarcinoma. **(A)** Axial T1-weighted spin echo image. **(B)** T2-weighted FSE image. **(C)** Gadolinium-enhanced T1-weighted image with fat saturation, showing bilateral ovarian masses with cystic and solid components (white arrows). Solid components of the mass have irregular enhancement indicating tumor necrosis (asterisk), suggesting that the masses are likely to be malignant. **(D)** Sagittal T2-weighted FSE of the uterus shows T2-weighted irregular intermediate signal intensity tumor (large arrow) obstructing the endocervix with resulting hematometra. The cervical stroma is infiltrated with tumor, causing obliteration of zonal layers in the cervix and lower uterine segment. (*Figure continues.*)

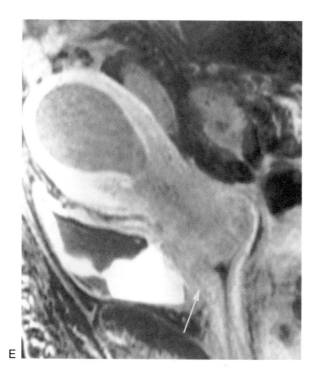

Figure 34.7 (*Continued*). **(E)** Gadolinium-enhanced sagittal image demonstrates that the endocervical canal tumor enhances, although less than the normal myometrium. The hematometra does not enhance. Thickened enhancing tissue along the anterior vaginal wall indicates vaginal wall invasion (long arrow). Pathology showed papillary cystadenocarcinoma, probably of an endometrial primary.

Most patients with metastases to the uterus also have metastases to the ovaries[60,61] (see Fig. 34.2). The most frequent locations of malignant cells in the uterus have been variously reported in the endometrium[13,61] and the myometrium,[60] and they can also spread to uterine myomas.[62] Metastases tend to be infiltrative and may closely mimic endometrial stromal sarcoma on histologic examination.[63] There is little in the literature concerning the CT appearance of metastases to the uterus, because they are difficult to image with CT or ultrasound. Metastases to the uterus tend to mimic leiomyoma, adenomyosis, or primary endometrial or cervical neoplasm. Clues to the diagnosis include enlargement of the uterus or progressive focal enlargement in a portion of the myometrial wall on serial studies (Fig. 34.2). Uterine enlargement with calcifications in mucinous metastases has been reported.[64] The identification of any irregularly enhancing mass within the myometrium suggests the diagnosis (Fig. 34.8), although leiomyomas are commonly heterogeneously enhancing. In general, soft tissue contrast between tumor and myometrium is inferior with CT compared to MRI.

With MRI, the normal morphology of the layers of myometrium is characteristic, so that tumor infiltration into the myometrium can easily be appreciated. The myometrium generally displays a very low signal intensity inner "junctional zone" and a slightly higher signal intensity outer myometrium. Leiomyomas, which constitute the majority of the masses encountered within the myometrium, usually appear as very low signal intensity, well-circumscribed masses. In contrast, infiltrating tumors appear as ill-defined higher signal intensity tissue[64] (Fig. 34.9). The enhancement pattern in metastases may be variable, but areas of nonenhancement are to be expected. Multiplanar imaging, particularly in the sagittal and parasagittal plane, is useful for displaying the uterine anatomy (Fig. 34.8). Endometrial secondaries may be impossible to distinguish from endometrial primaries.

VAGINAL METASTASES

Most malignancies involving the vagina result from direct spread of cervical or endometrial carcinoma.[65] The vagina is a common site for metastases from endometrial carcinomas. In a study of 325 cases of genital tract metastases, the vagina was the most frequent site, with most arising from endometrial carcinomas (85 of 109 cases) and the remainder resulting from ovarian and gestational trophoblastic primaries.[13] The cervical vaginal cuff is a common site for recurrence following hysterectomy for treatment of primary endometrial carcinoma. MRI is better suited than CT for evaluation of vaginal metastases.[65] Intermediate to high signal intensity tumor causing disruption of the low signal intensity vaginal muscular wall is typical. The vaginal wall is best displayed in axial and sagittal images.[65]

LYMPHOMA

At autopsy, approximately 25% of patients who have succumbed to non-Hodgkin's lymphoma are found to have involvement of the ovaries.[3,66] Patients who present with ovarian lymphoma are rare, comprising less than 1% of patients with lymphoma.[67] In one series of 39 patients with lymphoma presenting as an ovarian mass, 54% of the lymphomas were Burkitt's type, and only 4 patients had what were considered primary ovarian neoplasms. The tumors in these patients were detected incidentally and were asymptomatic at the time.[67] Lymphomas arising in association with acquired immunodeficiency syndrome show a strong tendency to manifest themselves in extranodal locations, but still they rarely appear in the genital tract.[15] Ovarian lymphomas appear grossly as smooth or lobulated fleshy masses, although necrosis and hemorrhage may sometimes be present.[61,66] It is common for ovarian lymphoma to be more solid than other metastases.[5] Uterine lymphoma may be confused with chronic endometritis or endometrial stromal sarcoma histologically. Leukemia in the uterus is much less common than lymphoma and is usually granulocytic in type.[63]

CT of pelvic lymphoma may show nonspecific ovarian or uterine enlargement. More importantly, lymphadenopathy can reveal the disseminated nature of the disease which is present

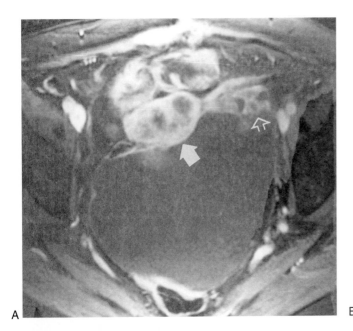

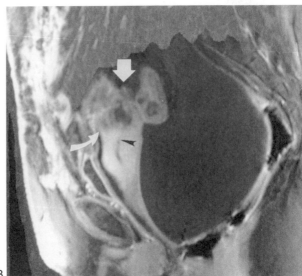

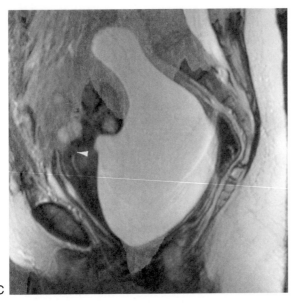

Figure 34.8 Metastatic carcinoma to the uterus and left ovary. (**A**) Axial fat-saturatied, gadolinium-enhanced image. An irregular cystic left ovary can be seen (open arrow). (**B**) Sagittal fat-saturated, gadolinium-enhanced images show a large fluid collection in the pouch of Douglas with peritoneal enhancement consistent with peritoneal spread. A mass (large arrows) involves the fundal surface of the uterus and invades the myometrium (curved arrow). (**C**) T-2 weighted FSE images showing the uterine anatomy and the myometrium invasion more clearly than in the axial plane. Tumor invading almost down to the endometrium (arrowhead) is seen. Surgical findings included metastases to the uterine fundus and left ovary as well as elsewhere in the pelvis.

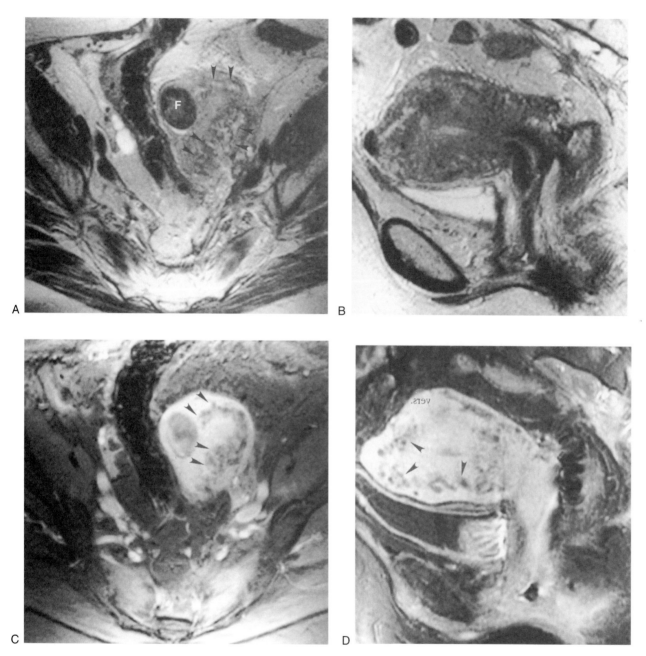

Figure 34.9 Metastatic mucinous colon carcinoma to the uterus. **(A)** Axial T2-weighted FSE image through the uterus shows a typical appearance of a uterine fibroid (F), which is low signal and well defined. There is irregular infiltrating high signal intensity in the myometrium (arrowheads), which is distorting and obliterating the junctional zone of the uterus on the sagittal image. **(B)** Sagittal T2-weighted FSE image. **(C)** Axial fat-saturation, gadolinium-enhanced, T1-weighted gradient echo image. **(D)** Sagittal fat-saturation, gadolinium-enhanced T1-weighted gradient echo image through the same levels as in Figures A and B shows that the high signal intensity tissue in the uterine myometrium in the T2-weighted FSE images is poorly enhancing (arrowheads) in contrast to the markedly enhanced myometrium in the gadolinium-enhanced scan. The signal intensity pattern of this infiltrating tissue is reminiscent of adenomyosis; however, adenomyosis usually shows enhancement and does not cause the finger-like extensions seen on the postgadolinium images. Surgical resection of the uterus showed diffusely infiltrating mucinous adenocarcinoma.

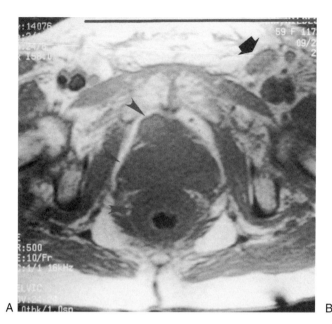
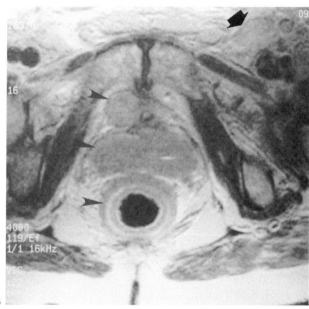

Figure 34.10 Diffuse lymphomatous infiltration. **(A)** T1-weighted spin echo series shows diffuse infiltration of the periurethral tissues, vagina, and rectum (arrowheads) as well as left common femoral adenopathy (arrow). **(B)** T2-weighted FSE image shows the general high signal intensity of the tumor. Note that the low signal intensity of the vaginal muscular wall is completely obliterated and there is expansion of the rectal muscular layers. (Courtesy of Dr. Evan Siegelman, Philadelphia, Pennsylvania.)

in 90% of patients. The MRI signal intensity characteristics of lymphoma are nonspecific; however, the excellent display of pelvic anatomy with MRI (Fig. 34.10) shows that the pelvic mass does not arise from the endometrium, cervix, or ovaries.[68]

SUMMARY

The majority of metastases to the female genital tract from nongynecologic sources arise from the gastrointestinal tract, while the gynecologic cancer with the greatest propensity to metastasize to other gynecologic organs is endometrial adenocarcinoma. Radiologic diagnosis of patients with metastatic lesions to the ovaries is limited by the nonspecific appearance of these tumors, which show a striking tendency to adopt gross cystic appearance different from the primary tumor. CT scanning may be of use in identifying a distant primary. MRI displays intrinsic soft tissue contrast better than CT to identify metastases to the uterus and vagina and to distinguish these from benign lesions.

REFERENCES

1. Lee YT, Hori JM. Significance of ovarian metastasis in therapeutic oophorectomy for advanced breast cancer. Cancer 1971;27:1374–1378
2. Hricak H, Hamm B, Semelka RC et al. Carcinoma of the uterus: use of gadopentetate dimeglumine in MR imaging. Radiology 1991;181:95–106
3. Young RH, Clement PB, Scully RE. The ovary. In: Sternberg SS, Ed. Diagnostic Surgical Pathology (vol. 2). Raven Press, New York, pp. 1655–1734
4. Petru E, Pickel H, Heydarfadai M et al. Nongenital cancers metastatic to the ovary. Gynecol Oncol 1992;44:83–86
5. Ulbright TM, Roth LM, Stehman FB. Secondary ovarian neoplasia. A clinicopathologic study of 35 cases. Cancer 1984;53:1164–1174
6. Ovadia J, Goldman GA. Ovarian masses in postmenopausal women. Int J Gynecol Obstet 1992;39:35–39
7. Hata K, Hata T, Manabe A et al. A critical evaluation of transvaginal Doppler studies, transvaginal sonography, magnetic resonance imaging, and CA 125 in detecting ovarian cancer. Obstet Gynecol 1992;80:922–926
8. Davies AP, Jacobs I, Woolas R et al. The adnexal mass: benign or malignant? Evaluation of a risk of malignancy index. Br J Obstet Gynecol 1993;100:927–931
9. Valentin L, Sladkevicius P, Marsal K. Limited contribution of Doppler velocimetry to the differential diagnosis of extrauterine pelvic tumors. Obstet Gynecol 1994;83:425–433
10. Stevens SK, Hricak H, Stern JL. Ovarian lesions: detection and characterization with gadolinium-enhanced MR imaging at 1.5T. Radiology 1991;181:481–488
11. Kurjak A, Predanic M. New scoring system for prediction of ovarian malignancy based on transvaginal color Doppler sonography. J Ultrasound Med 1992;11:631–638
12. Scoutt LM, McCarthy SM, Lange R et al. MR evaluation of clinically suspected adnexal masses. J Comput Assist Tomogr 1994;18:609–618

13. Mazur MT, Hsueh S, Gersell DJ. Metastases to the female genital tract: Analysis of 325 cases. Cancer 1984;53:1978–1984

14. Young RH, Scully RE. Metastatic tumors in the ovary: a problem-oriented approach and review of the recent literature. Semin Diagn Pathol 1991;8:250–276

15. Boronow RC, Morrow CP, Creasman WT et al. Surgical staging in endometrial cancer: clinical-pathologic findings of a prospective study. Obstet Gynecol 1984;63:825–832

16. Berkowitz RS, Goldstein DP. Gestational trophoblastic disease. Semin Oncol 1989;16:410–416

17. Hunter V, Raymond E, Christensen C et al. Efficacy of the metastatic survey in the staging of gestational trophoblastic disease. Cancer 1990;65:1647–1650

18. Fox H. Metastatic tumours of the ovary. In: Fox H, Ed. Haines and Taylor Obstetrical and Gynaecological Pathology (3rd ed.). Churchill Livingstone, New York, 1987, pp 714–723

19. Daya D, Nazerali L, Frank GL. Metastatic ovarian carcinoma of large intestinal origin simulating primary ovarian carcinoma: a clinicopathologic study of 25 cases. Am J Clin Pathol 1992;97:751–758

20. Robboy SJ, Scully RE, Norris HJ. Carcinoid metastatic to the ovary. A clinicopathologic analysis of 35 cases. Cancer 1974;33:798–811

21. Climie ARW, Health LP. Malignant degeneration of benign cystic teratomas of the ovary. Cancer 1968;22:824

22. Haines M. Carcinoid tumours of the ovary. J Obstet Gynacol Br Commonw 1971;78:1123

23. Fitzgibbons PL, Martin SE, Simmons TJ. Malignant melanoma metastatic to the ovary. Am J Surg Pathol 1987;11:959–964

24. Young RH, Scully RE. Malignant melanoma metastatic to the ovary. A clinicopathologic analysis of 20 cases. Am J Surg Pathol 1991;15:849–860

25. Megibow AJ, Hulnick DH, Bosniak MA, Balthazar EJ. Ovarian metastases: computed tomographic appearances. Radiology 1985;156:161–164

26. Seidman JD, Elsayed AM, Sobin LH, Tavassoli FA. Association of mucinous tumors of the ovary and appendix. A clinicopathologic study of 25 cases. Am J Surg Pathol 1993;17:22–34

27. Kahn MA, Demopoulos RI. Mucinous ovarian tumors with pseudomyxoma peritonei: a clinicopathological study. Int J Gynecol Pathol 1992;11:15–23

28. Cariker M, Dockerty MB. Mucinous cystadenomas and mucinous cystadenocarcinomas of the ovary: a clinical and pathological study of 355 cases. Cancer 1954;7:302

29. Fernandez RN, Daly JM. Pseudomyxoma peritonei. Arch Surg 1980;115:409

30. Long RTL, Spratt JS, Jr, Dowling E. Pseudomyxoma peritonei: new concepts in management with a report of seventeen patients. Am J Surg 1969;117:162

31. Hart WR, Norris HJ. Borderline and malignant mucinous tumors of the ovary: histologic criteria and clinical behaviour. Cancer 1973;31:1031

32. Ulbright TM, Roth LM. Metastatic and independent cancers of the endometrium and ovary: a clinicopathologic study of 34 cases. Hum Pathol 1985;16:28–34

33. Morrow CP, Bundy BN, Kurman RJ et al. Relationship between surgical-pathologic risk factors and outcome in clinical stage I and II carcinoma of the endometrium: a Gynecologic Oncology Group study. Gynecol Oncol 1991;40:55–65

34. Shimizu H, Yamasaki M, Ohama K et al. Characteristic ultrasonographic appearance of the Krukenberg tumor. J Clin Ultrasound 1990;18:697–703

35. Cho KC, Gold BM. Computed tomography of Krukenberg tumors. AJR Am J Roentgenol 1985;145:285–288

36. Togashi K, Konishi J. Magnetic resonance imaging in the evaluation of gynecologic malignancy. Magn Reson Q 1990;6:250–275

37. Togashi K. MRI of the Female Pelvis. Igaku-Shoin, Tokyo, 1993, pp 227–280

38. Hricak H, Carrington BM. MRI of the Pelvis: A Text Atlas. Appleton & Lange, Norwalk, CT, 1991

39. Choi BI, Choo IW, Han MC, Kim CW. Sonographic appearance of Krukenberg tumor from gastric carcinoma. Gastrointest Radiol 1988;13:15–18

40. Mata JM, Inaraja L, Rams A et al. CT findings in metastatic ovarian tumors from gastrointestinal tract neoplasms (Krukenberg tumors). Gastrointest Radiol 1988;13:242–246

41. Ferrozzi F, Castriota-Scanderbeg A, Bova D, Piazza N. Calcified ovarian metastases from mucinous carcinoma of the colon. Clin Imaging 1993;17:17–18

42. Takemori M, Nishimura R, Obayashi C, Sugimura K. Magnetic resonance imaging of Krukenberg tumor from gastric cancer. Eur J Obstet Gynecol Reprod Biol 1992;47:161–163

43. Outwater EK, Dunton CJ. Imaging of the ovary and adnexa: clinical issues and applications of MR imaging. Radiology 1995;194:1–18

44. Thurnher SA. MR imaging of pelvic masses in women: contrast-enhanced vs unenhanced images. AJR Am J Roentgenol 1992;159:1243–1250

45. Yamashita Y, Harada M, Sawada T et al. Normal uterus and FIGO stage I endometrial carcinoma: dynamic gadolinium-enhanced MR imaging. Radiology 1993;186:495–501

46. Yeh HC, Sharif MK, Slater G et al. Ultrasonography and computed tomography in pseudomyxoma peritonei. Radiology 1984;153:507–510

47. Miller DL, Udelsman R, Sugarbaker PH. Calcification of pseudomyxoma peritonei following intraperitoneal chemotherapy: CT demonstration. J Comput Assist Tomogr 1985;9:1123–1124

48. Hann L, Love S, Goldberg RP. Pseudomyxoma peritonei: preoperative diagnosis by ultrasound and computed tomography. A case report. Cancer 1983;52:642–644

49. Masaryk TJ, Chilcote WA. CT of pseudomyxoma peritonei: case report. Comput Radiol 1984;8:43–47

50. Weigert F, Lindner R, Rohde U. Computed tomography and magnetic resonance of pseudomyxoma peritonei. J Comput Assist Tomogr 1985;9:1120–1122

51. Gupta S, Gupta RK, Gujral RB et al. Peritoneal mesothelioma simulating pseudomyxoma peritonei on CT and sonography. Gastrointest Radiol 1992;17:129–131

52. Tumeh SS, Polak JF, Kaplan WD. Uptake of 99mTc MDP by pseudomyxoma peritonei: a case report. Eur J Nucl Med 1983;8:364–366

53. Hricak H, Demas BE, Braga CA et al. Gestational trophoblastic neoplasm of the uterus: MR assessment. Radiology 1986;161:11–16

54. Barton JW, McCarthy SM, Kohorn EI et al. Pelvic MR imaging findings in gestational trophoblastic disease, incomplete abortion, and ectopic pregnancy: are they specific? Radiology 1993;186:163–168

55. Mirich DR, Hall JT, Kraft WL et al. Metastatic adnexal trophoblastic neoplasm: contribution of MR imaging. J Comput Assist Tomogr 1988;12:1061–1067

56. Szolar DH, Ranner G, Lax S, Preidler K. MRI appearance of ges-

tational choriocarcinoma within the myometrium. Eur J Radiol 1994;18:61–63

57. Sanders C, Rubin E. Malignant gestational trophoblastic disease: CT findings. AJR Am J Roentgenol 1987;148:165–168

58. Davis WK, McCarthy S, Moss AA, Braga C. Computed tomography of gestational trophoblastic disease. J Comput Assist Tomogr 1984;8:1136–1139

59. Sironi S, Colombo E, Villa G et al. Myometrial invasion by endometrial carcinoma: assessment with plain and gadolinium-enhanced MR imaging. Radiology 1992;185:207–212

60. Kumar NB, Hart WR. Metastases to the uterine corpus from extragenital cancers: a clinicopathologic study of 63 cases. Cancer 1982;50:2163–2169

61. Weingold AB, Boltuch SM. Extragenital metastases to the uterus. Am J Obstet Gynecol 1961;82:1267–1272

62. Beattie GJ, Duncan AJ, Paterson AJ et al. Breast carcinoma metastatic to uterine leiomyoma. Gynecol Oncol 1993; 51:255–257

63. Kempson RL, Hendrickson MR. Pure mesenchymal neoplasms of the uterine corpus. In: Fox H, Ed Haines and Taylor Obstetrical and Gynaecological Pathology (3rd ed.). Churchill Livingstone, New York, 1987, pp 411–456

64. Kim SH, Hwang HY, Choi BI. Uterine metastasis from stomach cancer: radiological findings. Clin Radiol 1990;42:285–286

65. Chang YC, Hricak H, Thurnher S, Lacey CG. Vagina: evaluation with MR imaging: Part II. Neoplasms. Radiology 1988;169:175–179

66. Ioachim HL, Dorsett B, Cronin W et al. Acquired immunodeficiency syndrome-associated lymphomas: clinical, pathologic, immunologic and viral characteristics of 111 cases. Hum Pathol 1991;22:659–673

67. Monterroso V, Jaffe ES, Merino MJ, Medeiros LJ. Malignant lymphomas involving the ovary a clinicopathologic analysis of 39 cases. Am J Surg Pathol 1993;17:154–170

68. Kimura I, Togashi K, Tsutsui K et al. MR imaging of gynecologic lymphoma. J Comput Assist Tomogr 1991;15:500–501

Color Doppler Ultrasonography in Gynecologic Malignancy

ASIM KURJAK

SANJA KUPESIC

Ultrasound is inexpensive compared to computed tomography or magnetic resonance imaging when assessing the extent and occurrence of gynecologic malignancy and its response to therapy. The boundaries of the malignancy, its echogenicity, the presence of septa, vegetations, ascites, omental caking, and fixation to the surrounding structures are markers of malignancy. Ultrasound is highly sensitive but has poor specificity in the differentiation of benign from malignant, and vice versa.[1,2] This has improved with the addition of color and pulsed Doppler,[3] which offer a qualitative picture of blood flow in the vascular system (Plate 35.1). This is better understood if we consider the process of angiogenesis.

ANGIOGENESIS (NEOVASCULARIZATION)

It is now over 100 years since the first observation that tumors have an increased vascularity compared to normal tissues.[4] It was long believed that simple dilatation of existing host vessels accounted for this tumor hyperemia.[5] Vasodilation was generally thought to be a "side effect" of tumor metabolites or of necrotic tumor products escaping from the tumor. However, some suggested that tumor hyperemia is related to new blood vessel growth, that is, neovascularization, and not to dilatation of existing vessels. A 1945 report revealed that new vessels in the neighborhood of a tumor implant arose from host vessels and not from the tumor itself.[6] A debate then continued for two decades about whether tumors were supplied by existing vessels or new vessels.[7] A new concept that tumor growth is restricted in the absence of the vascular response developed in the 1960s. Experiments with isolated perfused organs revealed that tumor growth was severely restricted in these organs because of the absence of neovascularization.[8–11] Over the following decade, it was shown that tumors implanted into animals consistently induced growth of new capillary vessels. This process was called *angiogenesis*, a term coined in 1935 by Hertig[12] to describe the proliferation of new vessels in the placenta. Viable tumor cells release dif-

fusible angiogenic factors, which stimulate new capillary growth and endothelial mitosis in vivo,[13–15] even when tumor cell proliferation has been arrested by irradiation.[16] Necrotic tumor products were found not to be angiogenic. From these observations, Folkman et al.[15] proposed that once tumor "take" occurs, every further increase in tumor cell population must be preceded by an increase in new capillaries that converge on the tumor. According to this concept, a small focus of tumor cells (containing $<10^{17}$ cells in a volume of a few milliliters) could not increase indefinitely without the induction of angiogenesis. Angiogenesis occurs during embryonic development and during several physiologic and pathologic conditions in adult life. For example, ovulation and wound healing could not take place without angiogenesis, which is also associated with chronic inflammation and with certain immune reactions. Many nonmalignant diseases of unknown cause are dominated by angiogenesis. For example, neovascularization associated with retrolental fibroplasia or with diabetic retinopathy may lead to blindness; new capillaries may invade the joints in arthritis; and solid tumors induce angiogenesis. Tumor angiogenesis differs at least in a temporal manner from the other types of angiogenesis described. In physiologic situations, as in the development of the corpus luteum or in ovulation, angiogenesis subsides once the process is completed. In certain nonmalignant processes, angiogenesis is abnormally prolonged, although still self-limiting, as in pyogenic granuloma or keloid formation. In contrast, tumor angiogenesis is not self-limiting. Once tumor-induced angiogenesis starts, it continues indefinitely until the host dies or the tumor is eradicated.[8–11]

Recent evidence suggests that the development of metastases also depends on angiogenesis. Before vascularization, tumors are generally unable to shed cells into the circulation. Tumor cells must gain access to the vasculature in the primary tumor, survive in the circulation, settle in the microvasculature of the target organ,[17,18] escape from this vasculature,[19] grow in the target organ, and induce angiogenesis.[20] Angiogenesis is necessary at the beginning as well as at the end of these events. Tumor cells can enter the circulation by penetrating the proliferating capillaries. Growing capillaries have fragmented basement membranes and are "leaky."[21] Angiogenesis is necessary but is insufficient for continued tumor growth.[13] While the absence of angiogenesis will severely limit tumor growth, the onset of angiogenic activity in a tumor permits, but does not guarantee, continued expansion of the tumor population.[22] Angiogenesis is not necessary for certain tumor cells such as leukemic cells and tumor cells that grow in ascitic fluid, because they neither form a "solid" tumor nor grow in a three-dimensional tightly packed cell population. It may not be necessary for certain other cells capable of growth as a flat sheet between membranes, that is, gliomatosis in the meninges.[13] Tumor-induced vessels are often dilated and saccular and may even contain tumor cells within the endothelial lining.[23] Tumors may contain giant capillaries and arteriovenous shunts without intervening capillaries. Newly formed vessels contain no smooth muscle in their walls but instead contain only a small amount of fibrous connective tissue.[24] Quantitative morphometric studies in induced animal tumors show that vascular volume, length, and surface area increase during the early stages of tumor growth and then decrease after the onset of necrosis. The number of vessels of large diameter increases in the later stages of growth.[25] New vessels in a tumor arise from existing vessels and contain a relative paucity of smooth muscle in their walls in comparison to their caliber. Since most of the resistance to flow occurs at the level of the muscular arterioles, vessels deficient in these muscular elements offer reduced resistance to blood flow and transmit larger volume flow than vessels with high resistance (Plate 35.2). Indeed, the evidence for the regulatory role of angiogenesis in tumor growth is strong, but it is still not clear what part the phenomenon does play in the process of cancer metastasis.[26–28] Transvaginal color and pulsed Doppler ultrasound give us a new insight into the behavior of the vascularity of pelvic tumors.

CERVICAL CARCINOMA

Ultrasound with or without color Doppler is not suitable for screening for cervical cancer or for the further investigation of declared cervical cancer. Cervical flow measurement is inadequate, as blood flow within the cervix is not detectable in many healthy women as well as in many women with cervical malignancy. The newly formed vessels in early cervical carcinoma are very small, and the velocity within is below the resolving power of available equipment. Of the four types of spread (direct invasion, lymphatic metastasis, blood-borne and peritoneal implantation), invasion directly into the stroma and/or corpus is the only one that can be seen on color Doppler.

ENDOMETRIAL CARCINOMA

Color Doppler studies[29–34] have attempted to improve the sensitivity and specificity of transvaginal sonography (TVS) for diagnosing endometrial carcinoma. Color and pulsed Doppler features of the tumor can be used in addition to the morphology in the diagnosis of malignancy. It has been shown[35–37] that areas of endometrial neoplasia could be missed in 2% to 6% of cases at cervical dilatation and uterine curettage (D&C). Therefore, the use of color flow imaging along with TVS may help in the investigation of endometrial abnormalities. Transvaginal color and pulsed Doppler were performed on 750 postmenopausal women 1 day before hysterectomy for different gynecologic indications.[29] Arterial blood flow was not present in normal or atrophic endometria or in 92% of hyperplastic endometria. Thirty-five cases of endometrial carcinoma were diagnosed histologically, while 32 (91%) of them were detected by Doppler ultrasonography. In these women, intratumoral or peritumoral blood flow was seen (Plate 35.3). The mean resistance index (RI) was 0.42 +/- 0.02 (Plate 35.3). The peak systolic velocities were relatively high; for intratumoral vessels the mean velocity was 12.04 +/- 3.1 cm/s, whereas that of peritumoral vessels was 17.12 +/- 2.7 cm/s. The difference between both velocities and vascular impedance was significant ($P<0.05$). Three asymptomatic women with endometrial carcinoma (two stage IA and one stage IB) were detected. On B mode they had thick (>10 mm) inhomogeneous endometria with an intact subendometrial halo. Color flow revealed areas of vascularization within the endometrial echo, waveform analysis of which showed low impedance to flow (RI<0.42).

The application of transvaginal color Doppler to the general population for screening of endometrial carcinoma may be viable if combined with ovarian screening. This could reduce the number of D&C operations, eliminating the risk of anesthesia and reducing the cost. Newly formed vessels in endometrial carcinoma can be classed as intratumoral or peritumoral. Extensive flow at the periphery of the tumor is commonly present in patients with an interrupted subendometrial halo and myometrial invasion. Direct extension to adjacent structures can be precisely assessed by analysis of the abundant flow within the myometrial portion of the uterus. Other types of spread (transtubal, lymphatic, and hematogeneous) cannot be assessed and analyzed by color Doppler imaging.

UTERINE SARCOMA

Another possible application of color and pulsed Doppler is the in vivo recognition of uterine sarcoma. This tumor is rare and characterized by extremely aggressive behavior, which leads to an early pattern of widespread dissemination. It is expected to be more common in the future as conservative treatment of uterine myomas becomes more common.[38,39] We assessed blood flow in primary (uterine artery) (Plate 35.4) and secondary vessels (intratumoral neovascularization) (Plates 35.5 and 35.6) in 11 cases of uterine sarcoma.[40] The typical finding of sarcoma was that of irregular, thin, and randomly dispersed vessels in the peripheral and/or central area of the tumor, with very low impedance shunts. In those patients with sarcoma, both uterine arteries showed low resistance compared to those in normal or myomatous uteri. In the group of healthy volunteers, uterine artery RI approximated 0.88. Decreased values, such as 0.74 ($P<0.05$) were found in patients with uterine leiomyomas and 0.63 ($P<0.001$) in those with uterine sarcomas. There was no difference ($P>0.05$) between RI in right and left uterine arteries in each group. Color Doppler showed areas of neovascularization (at the border and/or in the center of the tumor) in all patients with sarcoma (100%), while only 61% of myomas were vascularized. Diastolic flow was present in all the uterine lesions and was increased compared to the uterine artery blood flow. The mean RI in sarcomas was 0.37 +/− 0.03 (Plate 35.7) ($P<0.05$) compared with that of myomas (0.54 +/− 0.08) (Plate 35.8). The mean Pourcelot* RI of myometrial blood flow in normals was 0.68 and was higher ($P<0.05$) when compared with controls (healthy volunteers) and women with uterine myomas.

The vascularization of benign uterine masses is largely dependent on tumor size, position, and the extent of secondary degeneration.[39] Large and laterally positioned leiomyomas, especially those with necrosis and inflammatory changes, may show increased diastolic flow and, consequently, low RI using an RI cut off of 0.40. We found an overlap among three cases of uterine myomas with that of uterine sarcomas. A multiparameter sonographic approach including morphology and size on TVS and color flow imaging with pulsed Doppler analysis of neovascular signals could help with the diagnosis of uterine sarcomas in high-risk groups (e.g., postmenopausal patients with a rapidly enlarging uterus).

The huge diastolic flow present in uterine sarcomas had a mean RI = 0.37 +/− 0.03, which was different ($P<0.001$) from that seen in myomas (RI = 0.54 +/− 0.08). The uterine arteries were different as well: An RI of 0.62 was found in patients with uterine sarcomas, while an RI of 0.74 and 0.88 was seen in patients with uterine leiomyomas and healthy volunteers, respectively. The conclusion was that color Doppler has the potential to distinguish uterine sarcomas from benign uterine lesions.[42] Transvaginal color Doppler examination of uterine tumors should include morphologic changes and analysis of vascularization (brightness of color, vascular location [see Plate 35.5], and type of vascularization) (see Plates 35.6 and 35.7). Malignant uterine masses have bright color signals from randomly dispersed vessels, while pulsed Doppler analysis has low vascular impedance (mean RI = 0.37 +/− 0.03). In huge necrotic leiomyomas, areas of neovascularization within the central parts usually have low velocity and low impedance

due to vasoactive compounds, while the ring of angiogenesis has a moderate impedance.

OVARIAN MASSES

Several studies have used transabdominal sonography and TVS to assess those features such as size and presence of septa or solid components that might suggest that an ovarian mass is malignant.[1,2,43] Simple adnexal cysts less than 5 cm in diameter with a normal CA-125 and without detectable areas of neovascularization can be observed safely by ultrasound. However, in patients with larger complex ultrasound masses, as well as in those with prominent diastolic flow, specificity and sensitivity of ultrasound for malignancy are insufficient to be solely relied upon, and a histologic diagnosis is required.

Small simple ovarian cysts provide the greatest diagnostic dilemma, since the vast majority of them are innocent. Cytologic examination of needle-aspirated fluid is not reliable. Laparoscopy allows inspection of the pelvis, abdomen, and excrescences on the surface of the ovary. It also allows cytologic examination of the cyst aspirate and peritoneal washings as well as excision of the cyst wall for frozen section, but it requires general anesthesia.

Whether Doppler analysis improves the accuracy in differentiating benign from malignant ovarian tumors is controversial. It is known that vessels may be present in any part of a malignant ovarian tumor. They may be within the sonographically heterogeneous central part of the mass (Plate 35.9), on its periphery, at the base, or within large papillary projections (Plate 35.10), in close proximity to cystic masses (Plate 35.11), and within the septa (Plate 35.12). Malignant breast tumors have low vascular impedance compared to normal tissue, which can be demonstrated on pulsed Doppler.[44–46] It seems reasonable that malignant ovarian vasculature has low-impedance Doppler waveform signals (Plate 35.13).

In 1989 transvaginal Doppler sonography of ovarian tumors suggested that this mode of imaging might be diagnostically helpful.[3,47] Low-impedance intratumoral flow was found in malignant ovarian lesions and other pelvic tumors. In five malignant ovarian tumors, the mean RI was 0.33 +/− 0.08.[3] Low impedance suggested malignancy. In another series, among 18 women with ovarian tumors, 8 were malignant. The pulsatility index (PI) was below 1.0 (0.3 to 0.9) in 7 of 8 malignant tumors.[4] Low PI values (0.4 and 0.8) were obtained from bilateral dermoid cysts, however, and if a value below 1.0 was used as an indicator of malignancy, these would be false-positives (Plate 35.14).

In another study of 14,317 asymptomatic or minimally symptomatic women, there were 680 adnexal masses of which 624 were benign and 56 malignant.[48] Using an RI of less than 0.41 a sensitivity of 97% and a specificity of 100% were attained in distinguishing malignant from benign. This suggested that high impedance could be used to exclude invasive primary ovarian cancer.

---

*The Pourcelot index is used for expressing blood flow impedance distal to the point of sampling. Each velocity parameter depends on the angle of measurement, but once they are in a proper relationship, the RI becomes independent of the angle between vessels under investigation and the emitted ultrasound beam. The RI is used as a calculation measurement of the flow velocity waveform, peak systolic flow minus end diastolic flow divided by the peak systolic flow. The increased value of RI is believed to result from increased peripheral vascular resistance, and vice versa.[41]

There were, however, simultaneous reports of malignant tumors with RI values higher than 0.40 and of benign masses such as endometrioid cysts (Plate 35.15), luteal cysts (Plate 35.16), and ovarian inflammatory masses (Plate 35.17) with low values. Hata and colleagues found moderate vascular impedance in 16 ovarian cancers (mean RI = 0.50), as well as in four benign lesions.[49,50] Even when a PI of 0.5, 1.0, or 1.25 was used, there was an overlap between benign and malignant.[51–55] Similar results were presented by Valentin et al.,[56] who found that ultrasound morphology of the tumor is a better discriminator between benign and malignant than any Doppler variable. The ultrasound morphology correctly identified all the malignant tumors with a false-positive rate of 27% in 149 women with 28 malignant and 121 benign ovarian masses. Color and pulsed Doppler were useful only in discrimination between benign and malignant multilocular cysts with some solid components. They claim that the present technique of Doppler velocimetry adds little to the diagnosis of extrauterine pelvic masses.

Others have also suggested that in an assessment of tumor angiogenesis, there are no cutoff values for either the PIs or RIs that differentiate malignant from benign lesions. Tekay and Jouppila,[57] in a group of 72 patients, with 51 benign, 8 malignant, and 3 borderline tumors, found a mean PI of tumor vessels was 1.2, 0.7 and 0.6, respectively. The corresponding mean RI values were 0.6, 0.5, and 0.5. The differences were not significant, and the overlap between the malignant and benign lesions was large.[57] The diagnosis of ovarian malignancy based on Doppler measurements of vascular impedance alone may be unreliable.

Fleischer and colleagues[51] suggested that, macroscopically, tumor vasculature is peripheral, central, and septal. In malignant masses, they found peripheral arteries had a mean PI of 1.1 (range 0.4 to 2.0), central arteries had a mean PI of 0.6 (range 0.5 to 0.9), and septal arteries had a mean PI of 0.5. They suggested that peripheral vessels of a tumor originate from pre-existing host vasculature, while central vessels develop as a response to angiogenic activity of tumor cells and/or due to necrotic processes. Vessels within septa (Plate 35.17) or papillae (Plate 35.18) represent specific intratumoral branches. Benign adnexal masses are mostly vascularized peripherally, while in malignant tumors, central vascularization with low RI values are more frequent[51,58,59] (Plate 35.19).

Arrangement of tumor vessels may be important. If tumors are classified into those that have no vessels (Plate 35.20), those that have regularly separated (single) vessels (Plate 35.21), and those that have randomly dispersed (diffuse) vessels (Plate 35.22), there appears to be a difference in the arrangement between malignant and benign. In malignant ovarian masses, diffuse arrangements of vessels, mostly localized centrally, are more frequent than in benign lesions. In benign masses, single vessels are mostly peripherally and pericystically located. A combination of vessel location, arrangement, and RI has been the basis of a color and pulsed Doppler scoring system achieving a sensitivity of 97% and a specificity of 100% compared with 92% and 95%, respectively, when morphologic features alone were used.[58,59] It seems safe to say that a cystic ovarian mass is more likely to be malignant if it contains solid components and more likely again if the central (papillary or septal) vasculature is of low resistance. If the vasculature is of high resistance, it is unlikely to be malignant.

SUMMARY

The addition of color Doppler flow analysis of tumor vessels to the assessment of morphologic features has the potential to improve our understanding of benign and malignant disease processes. It may prove beneficial in screening for ovarian and endometrial cancer as well as for the further evaluation of established disease. Further work needs to be done, however, as at this stage, its value is still controversial.

REFERENCES

1. Sassone AM, Timor Tritsch IE, Artner A et al. Transvaginal sonographic characterization of ovarian disease: evaluation of a new scoring system to predict ovarian malignancy. Obstet Gynecol 1991;78:70–76
2. Granberg S, Wikland M, Jansson I. Macroscopic characterization of ovarian tumors and their relation to the histological diagnosis: criteria to be used for ultrasound evaluation. Gynecol Oncol 1989;35:139–144
3. Kurjak A, Zalud I, Jurkovic D et al. Transvaginal color Doppler for the assessment of pelvic circulation. Acta Obstet Gynecol Scand 1989;68:131–135
4. Warren BA. The vascular morphology of tumors. In: Peterson HI, ed. Tumor Blood Circulation: Angiogenesis, Vascular Morphology and Blood Flow of Experimental Human Tumors, CRC Press, Boca Raton, FL, 1979, pp 1–47
5. Coman DR, Sheldon WF. The significance of hyperemia around tumor implants. Am J Pathol 1946;22:821–826
6. Algire GH, Chalkley HW, Legallais FY, Park HD. Vascular reactions of mice to wounds and to normal and neoplastic transplants. J Natl Cancer Inst 1945;6:73–85
7. Day ED. Vascular relationships of tumor and host. Prog Exp Tumor Res 1964;4:57–59
8. Folkman J, Long D, Becker F. Growth and metastasis of tumor in organ culture, Tumor Res 1963;16:453–467
9. Folkman J, Cole P, Zimmerman S. Tumor behaviour in isolated perfused organs: in vitro growth and metastasis of biopsy material in rabbit thyroid and canine intestinal segment. Ann Surg 1966;164:491–502
10. Folkman J, Gimbrone M. Perfusion of the thyroid. Acta Endocrinol 1972;4:237–248
11. Folkman J. The intestine as an organ culture. In: Burdette J, Thomas CC, Eds. Carcinoma of the Colon and Antecedent Epithelium. Charles C Thomas, Springfield, IL, 1970, pp 113–127
12. Hertig A. Angiogenesis in the early human chorion and in the primary placenta of the Macaque monkey. Contrib Embryol 1935;25:37–82

13. Folkman J, Shing Y. Angiogenesis. J Biol Chem 1992;267:10931–10934

14. Klagsbrun M, D'Amore PA. Regulators of angiogenesis. Annu Rev Physiol 1991;53:217–239

15. Folkman J, Melrel E, Abernethy C, Williams G. Isolation of a tumor factor responsible for angiogenesis. J Exp Med 1971;133:275–278

16. Auerbach R. Angiogenesis-inducing factors: a review. In: Pick E, ed. Lymphokines (vol.4). Academic Press, London, 1981, pp 69–88

17. Netland P, Letter B. Organ-specific adhesion and metastatic tumor cells in vitro. Science 1984;224:113–115

18. Nicholson GL. Organ specificity of tumor metastasis: role of preferential adhesion, invasion and growth of malignant cells at specific secondary sites. Cancer Metastasis Rev 1988;7:143–188

19. Boxberger HJ, Paweletz N, Speiss E, Kniehuber R. An in vitro model study of BS p 73 rat tumor cell invasion into endothelial monolayer. Anticancer Res 1989;9:1777–1786

20. Weidner N, Semple JP, Welch WR, Folkman J. Tumor angiogenesis and metastasis—correlation in invasive breast carcinoma. N Engl J Med 1991;324:1–8

21. Dvorak HF, Nagy JA, Dvorak JT, Dvorak AM. Identification and characterization of the blood vessels of solid tumors that are leaky to circulating macromolecules. Am J Pathol 1988;133:95–109

22. Ribbati D, Vacca A, Bertossi M et al. Angiogenesis induced by B-cell nonHodgkins lymphomas. Lack of correlation with tumor malignancy and immunological phenotype. Anticancer Res 1990;10:401–406

23. Jain RK. Determinants of tumor blood flow. Cancer Res 1988;48:2641–2658

24. Gammill SL, Shipkey FH, Himmelfarb EH et al. Roentgenology–pathology correlation study of neovascularization. Am J Radiol 1976;126:376–385

25. Jain RK, Ward-Hartley KA. Dynamics of cancer cell interaction with microvasculature and interstitium. Biorheology 1987;24:117–123

26. Folkman J. Tumor angiogenesis. Adv Cancer Res 1985;43:175–203

27. Furcht LT. Critical factors controlling angiogenesis products, cells matrix and growth factors. Lab Invest 1986;55:505–509

28. Mahdevan V, Hart IR. Angiogenesis and metastasis. Eur J Cancer 1991;27:679–680

29. Kurjak A, Shalan H, Sosic A et al. Endometrial carcinoma in postmenopausal women: evaluation by transvaginal color Doppler ultrasonography. Am J Obstet Gynecol 1993;169:1597–1603

30. Bourne TH, Campbell S, Whitehead MI et al. Detection of endometrial cancer in postmenopausal women by transvaginal ultrasonography and color flow imaging. Br Med J 1990;301:369–374

31. Hata K, Hata T, Manabe A et al. New pelvic sonoangiography for detection of endometrial carcinoma: a preliminary report. Gynecol Oncol 1992;45:179–184

32. Hata K, Hata T, Manabe A, Kitao M. Transvaginal Doppler ultrasound assessment of intratumoral hemodynamic change before and during hypertensive intra-arterial chemotherapy for uterine cancer. Obstet Gynecol 1992;80:801–804

33. Bonilla F, Ballesteros A, Ballesteros MJ. Transvaginal color Doppler in the diagnosis of endometrial adenocarcinomas. Ultrasound Obstet Gynecol 1993;3 (suppl 2):23

34. Rudigoz RC, Gaucherand P. Vaginal sonography and color Doppler in postmenopausal abnormalities. Ultrasound Obstet Gynecol 1993;3 (suppl 2):42

35. Stovall TG, Solomon SK, Ling FW. Endometrial sampling prior to hysterectomy. Obstet Gynecol 1989;73:405–409

36. Bistoletti P, Hjerpe A, Mollerstrom G. Cytological diagnosis of endometrial cancer and preinvasive endometrial lesions. A comparison of the Endo-Pap sampler with fractional curettage. Acta Obstet Gynecol Scand 1988;67:343–345

37. McKenzie IZ, Bibby JG. Critical assessment of dilatation and curettage in 1029 women. Lancet 1978;332:566–568

38. Meyer WR, Mayer AR, Diamond MP et al. Unsuspected leiomyosarcoma: treatment with a gonadotropin-releasing hormone analogue. Obstet Gynecol 1990;75:529–534

39. Kurjak A, Kupesic-Urek S, Miric D. The assessment of benign uterine tumor vascularization by transvaginal color Doppler. Ultrasound Med Biol 1992;18:645–649

40. Kurjak A, Kupesic S, Shalan H et al. Uterine sarcoma: A report of 10 cases studied by transvaginal color and pulsed Doppler sonography. Gynecol Oncol 1995;59:342–346

41. Pourcelot L. Applications clinique de l'examen Doppler transcutane. In: Peronneau P, Ed. Velocimetre ultrasonare Doppler (vol. 34). Inserm, Paris, 1974

42. Kurjak A, Kupesic S, Shalan H et al. Uterine sarcoma: a report of 10 cases studied by transvaginal color and pulsed Doppler sonography. Gynec Oncol 1995;59:342–346

43. Levine D, Gosink BB, Wolf SI et al. Simple adnexal cysts: the natural history in postmenopausal women. Radiology 1992;184:653–659

44. Wells PNT, Halliwell M, Skidmore R et al. Tumor detection by ultrasonic Doppler blood flow signals. Ultrasonics 1977;15:231–234

45. Burns PN, Halliwell M, Wells PNT, Webb AJ. Ultrasonic Doppler studies of the breast. Ultrasound Med Biol 1982;8:127–132

46. Minasian M, Bamber JC. A preliminary assessment of an ultrasonic Doppler method for the study of blood flow in human breast cancer. Ultrasound Med Biol 1982;8:357–362

47. Bourne T, Campbell S, Steer C et al. Transvaginal color flow imaging: a possible new screening technique for ovarian cancer. BMJ 1989;299:1367–1370

48. Kurjak A, Zalud I, Alfirevic Z. Evaluation of adnexal masses with transvaginal color ultrasound. J Ultrasound Med 1991;10:295–297

49. Hata T, Hata K, Senoh D et al. Doppler ultrasound assessment of tumor vascularity in gynecologic disorders. J Ultrasound Med 1989;8:309–314

50. Hata K, Makihara K, Hata T et al. Transvaginal color Doppler imaging for hemodynamic assessment of reproductive tract tumors. Int J Gynecol Obstet 1991;36:301–308

51. Fleischer AC, Rodgers WH, Rao BK et al. Assessment of ovarian tumor vascularity with transvaginal color Doppler sonography. J Ultrasound Med 1991;10:563–568

52. Fleischer AC, Rodgers WH, Rao BK et al. Transvaginal color Doppler sonography of ovarian masses with pathological correlation. Ultrasound Obstet Gynecol 1991;1:275–278

53. Weiner Z, Thaler I, Beck D et al. Differentiating malignant from benign ovarian tumors with transvaginal color flow imaging. Obstet Gynecol 1992;79:159–162

54. Timor-Tritsch IE, Lerner JP, Monteagudo A, Santos R. Transvaginal sonographic characterization of ovarian masses by

means of color flow-directed Doppler measurements and a morphological scoring system. Am J Obstet Gynecol 1993;168:909–913

55. Kawai M, Kano T, Kikkawa F et al. Transvaginal Doppler ultrasound with color flow imaging in the diagnosis of ovarian cancer. Obstet Gynecol 1992;79:163–167

56. Valentin L, Sladkevicius P, Marsal K. Limited contribution of Doppler velocimetry to the differential diagnosis of extrauterine pelvic tumors. Obstet Gynecol 1993;83:425–433

57. Tekay A, Jouppila P. Validity of pulsatility and resistance indices in classification of adnexal tumors with transvaginal color Doppler ultrasound. Ultrasound Obstet Gynecol 1992; 2:338–344

58. Kurjak A, Predanic M. New scoring system for prediction of ovarian malignancy based on transvaginal color Doppler sonography. J Ultrasound Med 1992;11:631–638

59. Kurjak A, Predanic M, Kupesic-Urek S, Jukic S. Transvaginal color and pulsed Doppler assessment of adnexal tumor vascularity. Gynecol Oncol 1993;50:3–9

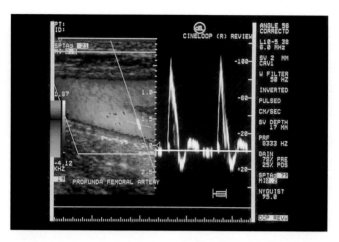

Plate 1.1. Spectral display and color Doppler image of the blood flow in a femoral artery.

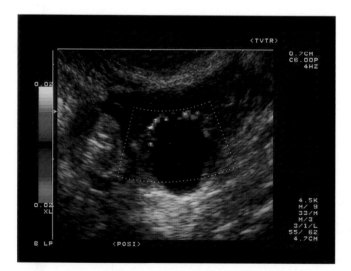

Plate 5.1. Color Doppler of preovulatory perifollicular new blood vessel growth (see also Fig. 5.15).

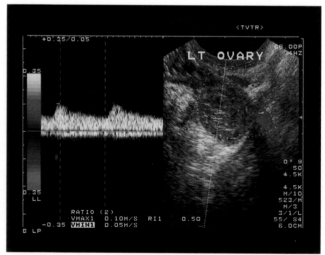

Plate 5.2. Color Doppler of the early corpus luteum, with invasion of new blood vessels into the luteal substance (see also Fig. 5.16).

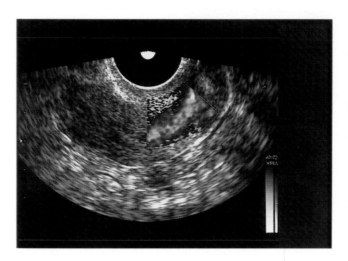

Plate 10.1. Color flow mapping of a large hypoechoic cervical polyp, showing increased vascularity (see also Fig. 10.6).

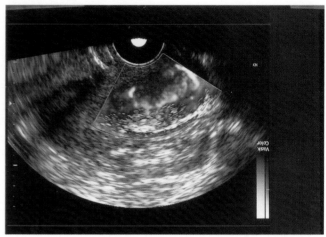

Plate 10.3. Color flow mapping of a hypoechoic cervical cancer, showing marked vascularization (see also Fig. 10.20).

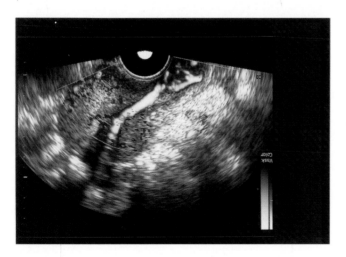

Plate 10.2. Color flow mapping of a hypoechoic fast-growing pedunculated fibroid in the cervix. Note vascularization of the peduncle (see also Fig. 10.10).

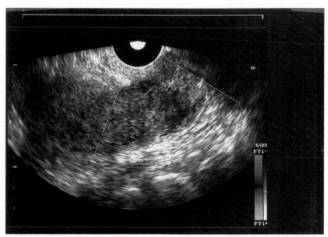

Plate 10.4. Color Doppler imaging of a large cervical carcinoma of the uterus showing increased vascularity within the cancer (see also Fig. 10.23).

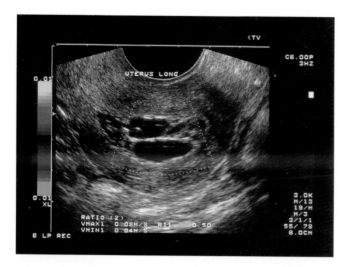

Plate 12.1. A 78-year-old woman after 10 months of receiving tamoxifen because of previous breast cancer. Note the large cystic spaces. The endometrium is not vascular, another example of the effect of tamoxifen.

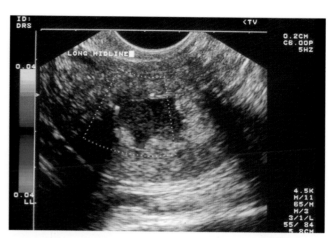

Plate 12.2. Transvaginal color Doppler sonogram of the uterus of a 61-year-old woman who presented with postmenopausal bleeding. There is a small hematometra due to bleeding coincidentally with an existing partially stenosed cervix. Color Doppler shows adjacent neovascularization. The patient had a FIGO stage IB carcinoma of the endometrium.

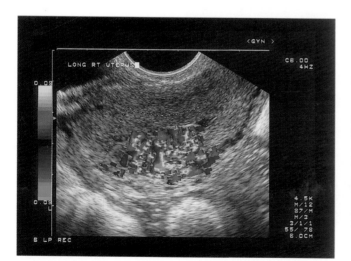

Plate 16.1. Hemangioma of the myometrium. This 30-year-old woman presented with persistent bleeding despite progestogen therapy. Sagittal TVS of the uterus shows a highly vascular lesion in the myometrium. The cavity was empty.

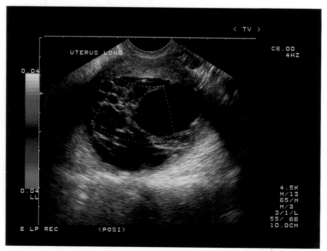

Plate 16.2. A 34-year-old woman presented in early pregnancy with occasional bleeding. A CT scan showed a blighted pregnancy and complex cyst (see Fig. 16.7A & B). Three months later the complex cyst was unchanged. Vessels can be seen in the mural components. The diagnosis of lymphangioma was made after surgical excision. (Courtesy of Dr. Mark Beale, Sydney, Australia.)

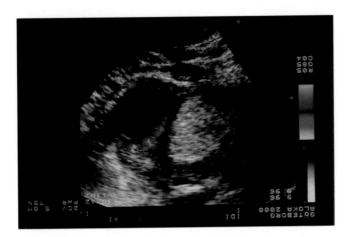

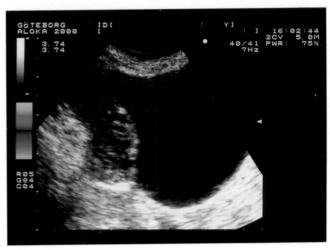

Plate 22.1. This ovary contains both a dermoid cyst and a corpus luteum. On the right, the dermoid can be seen as an echogenic mass. To the left is a just discernible cystic structure ringed by vascularity, the corpus luteum. It is easy to misinterpret low-impedance, high-velocity blood flow signals from the corpus luteum as originating from the benign dermoid cyst.

Plate 22.2. This ovary contains a simple cyst, but in the wall is an irregular thickened area that can be seen on the left of the image. The morphologic appearances are characteristic of a corpus luteum, and the surrounding ring of ordered vascularity supports this.

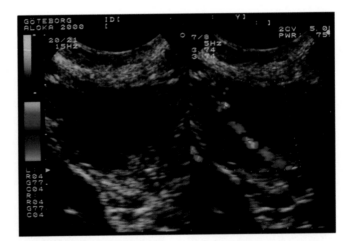

Plate 22.3. This split-screen image shows a benign physiologic cyst. In the B-mode image, the thin septum is barely if at all visible. Color Doppler makes the septum obvious and demonstrates blood flow within. The velocity range is set at its most sensitive, and yet there is still no aliasing of the color, which is clearly of low velocity. Tissues are perfused, and so low-impedance but low-velocity flow is normal and must not be confused with carcinoma.

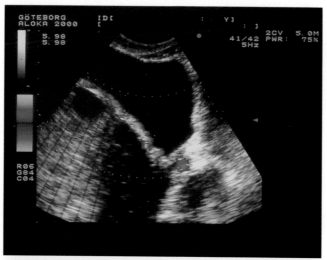

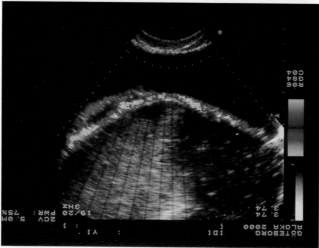

Plate 22.4. This image can be contrasted with Figure 22.3. There is a thick septum and florid blood flow. Again, the velocity range is at the most sensitive setting, and yet the color bar shows that the velocities present here are higher. This lesion was a serous cystadenocarcinoma.

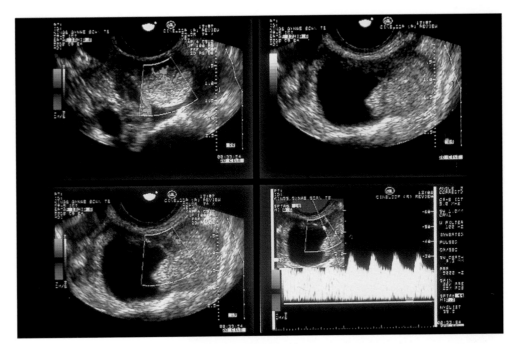

Plate 22.5. These four images of the same lesion show almost all the features of malignancy. There is an irregularly enlarged cystic ovary. Color Doppler shows a disordered and irregular arrangement of blood vessels over the solid part of the tumor, and pulsed Doppler demonstrates low-impedance high-velocity blood flow.

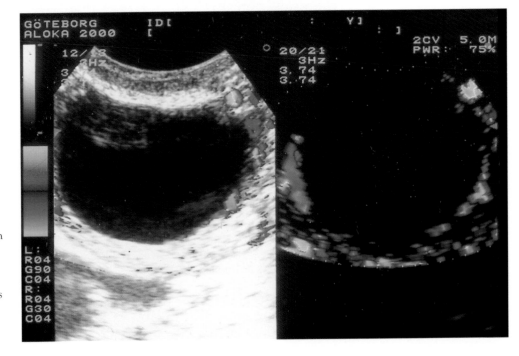

Plate 22.6. This split-screen image shows the clear regular margins of a normal follicle. In the right B-mode, gain has been turned off to leave only the color Doppler image on screen. This shows the extensive regular arrangement of blood vessels that are present, particularly after the luteinizing hormone (LH) peak.

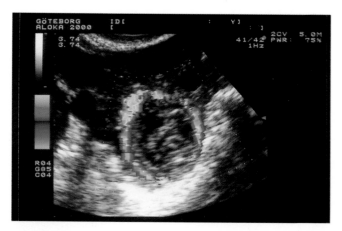

Plate 22.7. A "solid" corpus luteum. This appearance is most usual immediately after ovulation. Color Doppler has been used to delineate the margins.

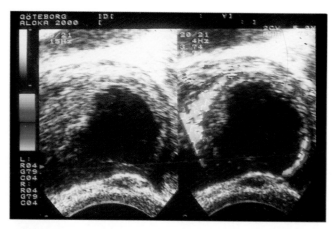

Plate 22.8. A vascular cystic corpus luteum. The ovary in this circumstance has a cystic area with a markedly irregular border and what almost looks like a papillary projection. The ovary is also highly vascular. It is not surprising that there are false-positive diagnoses of ovarian cancer when the normal appearance of the ovary in young women can be so relatively complex.

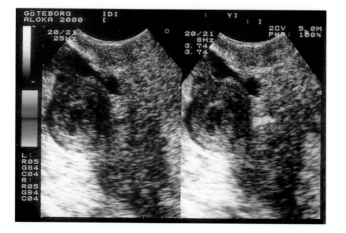

Plate 22.9. The B-mode image on the left of the split screen shows a solid lesion adjacent to the uterus. The central area of the lesion has a slightly cystic appearance. Bimanual examination, to elicit a "sliding organ" sign, suggested it was attached to the uterus. The color Doppler image on the right demonstrates a vascular connection and supports the diagnosis of a pedunculated fibroid.

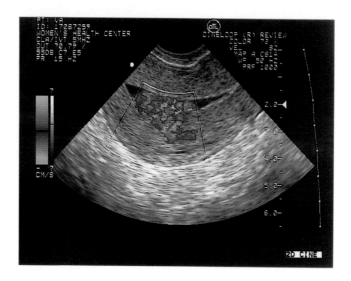

Plate 27.1. Residual trophoblastic tumor within the uterine cavity easily seen on gray scale sonography and eloquently outlined in color flow Doppler.

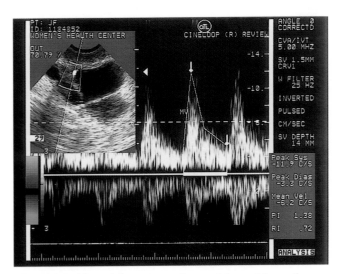

Plate 32.1. Normal flow measured around the periphery of an ovarian tumor. On TVS, this ovarian mass was highly suspicious morphologically.

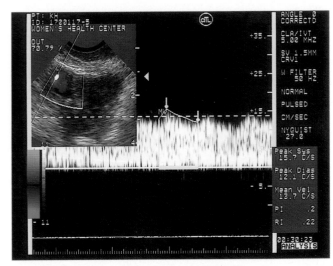

Plate 32.3. Significant increase in diastolic flow measured from within a region of increased color flow. The resulting low PI and RI, while not diagnostic, are suggestive of malignancy.

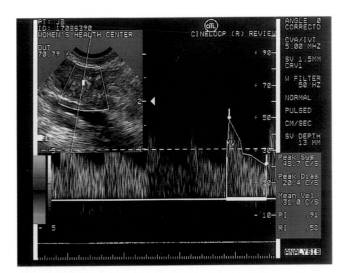

Plate 32.2. An increase in the diastolic flow.

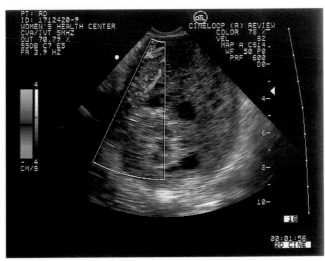

Plate 32.4. Neovascularization at the periphery of this uterine cancer.

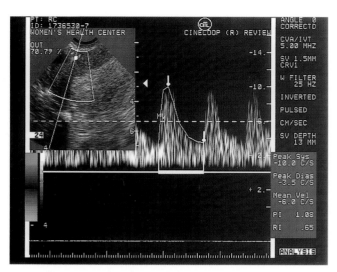

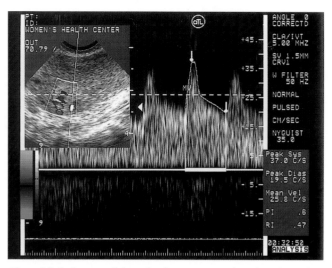

Plate 32.5. Spectral analysis of the arcuate artery confirms normal waveform and normal flow indices.

Plate 32.6. Increased diastolic flow on spectral analysis from this uterine tumor.

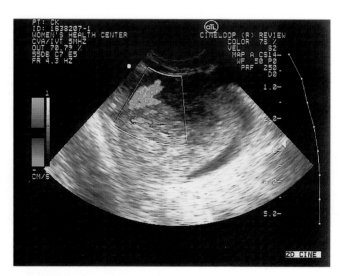

Plate 33.1. Color flow Doppler of a predominantly solid metastatic ovarian tumor.

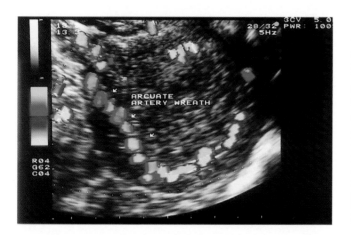

Plate 35.1. TVS of the uterus demonstrating a uterine vascular network containing an arcuate wreath encircling the uterus and radial arteries that are directed toward the uterine lumen.

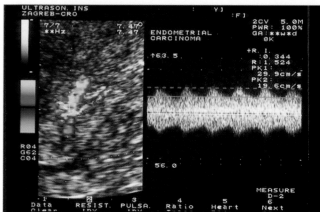

Plate 35.3. Doppler analysis demonstrates low impedance to blood flow (RI = 0.34). Endometrial malignancy was confirmed by histopathology.

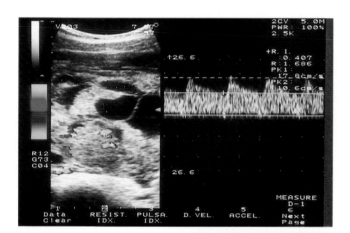

Plate 35.2. Abundant perfusion of the malignant tumor. Pulsed Doppler sonogram shows huge diastolic flow and, consequently, low impedance value.

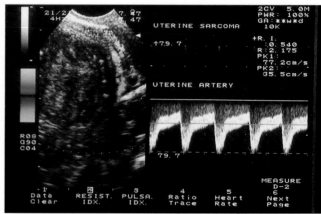

Plate 35.4. Blood flow velocity waveforms from the uterine artery in a postmenopausal patient with rapidly growing uterine tumor (left). Note increased end-diastolic flow velocity and decreased impedance to flow (RI = 0.54).

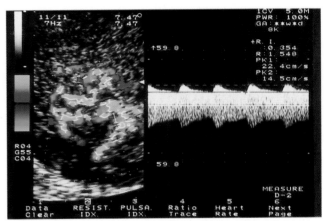

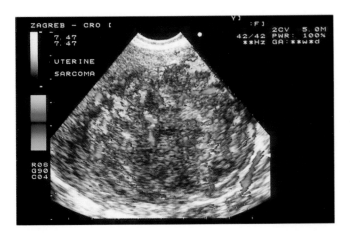

Plate 35.5. Uterine tumor demonstrating richly vascularized areas. The mass proved to be a sarcoma.

Plate 35.7. "Hot" area within the myometrial portion of the uterus, representing newly formed tumoral vessels in a case of uterine sarcoma (left). Pulsed Doppler velocity waveform analysis demonstrates low vascular impedance (RI = 0.35) (right).

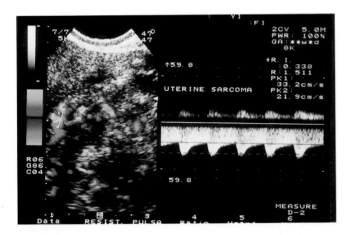

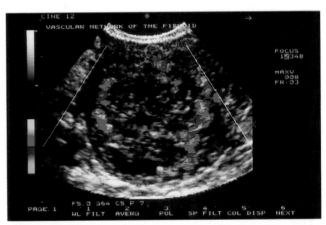

Plate 35.6. The same patient as in Plate 35.5. Areas of neovascularization with low impedance to flow (RI = 0.33) indicate tumoral malignancy.

Plate 35.8. Posterior leiomyoma showing peripheral vascularization. Note that vascularization of this benign tumor is supported by normal existing (arcuate and radial) arteries.

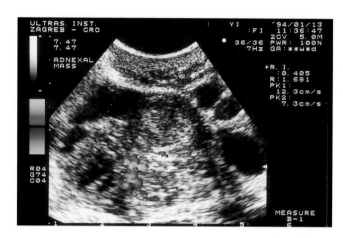

Plate 35.9. An example of central tumoral vascularization. Vessels are located within the two inner thirds of tumor. The malignant nature of the lesion was confirmed by histopathology.

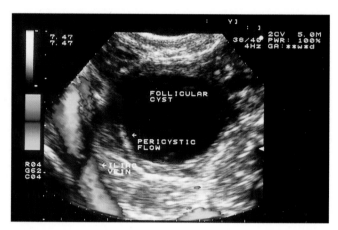

Plate 35.11. Solitary ovarian cyst demonstrating peripheral ring of angiogenesis. Iliac vessels are demonstrated below the ovary.

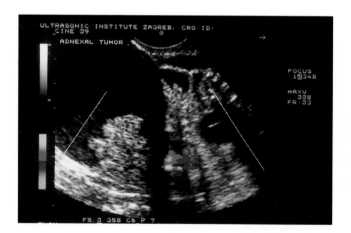

Plate 35.10. Malignant ovarian tumor with its characteristic image, which is created by papillary projections and septa. At the very base of the papilla there is a single blood vessel.

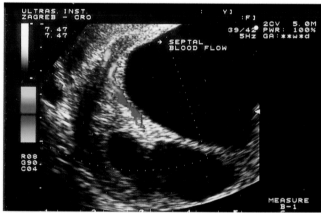

Plate 35.12. Septal neovascular signals visualized by color Doppler.

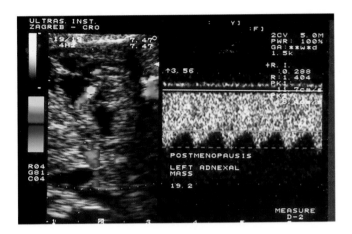

Plate 35.13. Huge peripheral and central vascularization of a malignant ovarian tumor. Richly vascularized areas represent the advancing tumor front and region of tumor hyperemia. Pulsed Doppler signal demonstrates low impedance to flow (RI = 0.28).

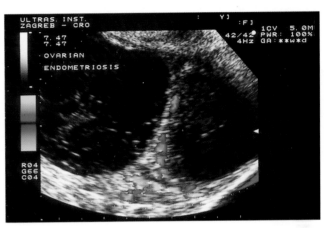

Plate 35.15. Ovarian endometrioma. Note homogeneous high-level internal echoes and prominent vascularization demonstrated by color flow at the level of the ovarian hilus.

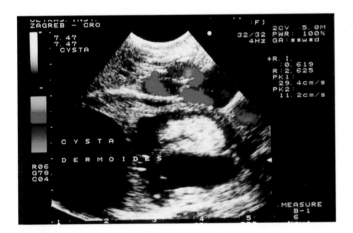

Plate 35.14. TVS of a complex adnexal tumor. Note the echogenicity of the solid tumor parts and color-coded area. This peripheral flow is typical for cystic teratomas with actively dividing cells.

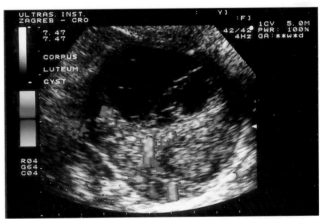

Plate 35.16. TVS of the corpus luteum cyst. Note greatly dilated vascular channels penetrating the hemorrhagic cavity of the ruptured follicle.

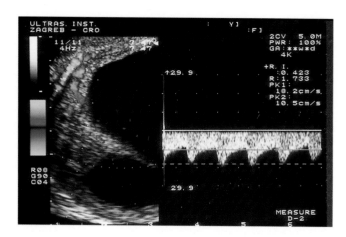

Plate 35.17. Neovascular signals detected in septal branches (left). Pulsed Doppler (right) shows low to moderate resistance blood flow (RI = 0.42). Borderline mucinous tumor was confirmed by histopathology.

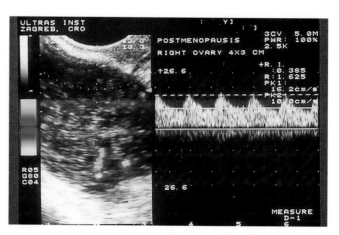

Plate 35.19. Richly vascularized area located within the central part of the enlarged ovarian stroma, with low vascular impedance to blood flow (RI = 0.38).

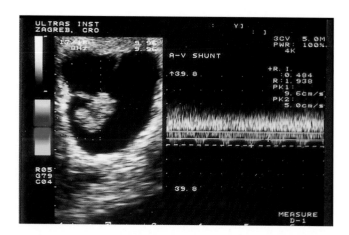

Plate 35.18. TVS of a small cystic structure with a papillary proliferation. At the base of a papilla, pulsed Doppler signal demonstrates atrioventricular shunt.

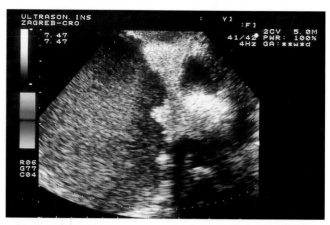

Plate 35.20. Multilocular voluminous tumor with thick septa, papillary projections, and some solid components. Color Doppler does not show increased vascularity; benign cyst was confirmed by histopathology.

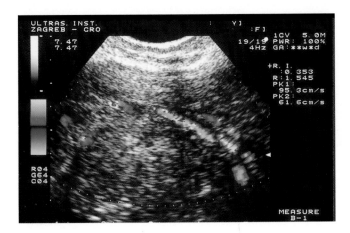

Plate 35.21. Solid tumor demonstrating regularly separated peripheral vessels. Such a vessel arrangement is typical for benign growths and represents vessel recruited from the pre-existing host vascular network.

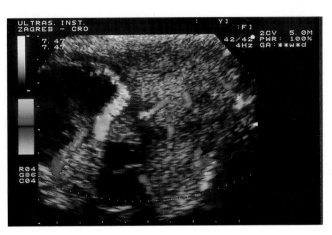

Plate 35.22. Huge adnexal mass containing vascular arrangement suggests high angiogenic activity typical for malignant tumors.

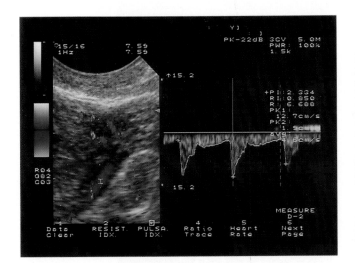

Plate 40.1. Longitudinal image of the uterus, showing the ascending branch of the left uterine artery as a blue coloration at the level of the cervical os.

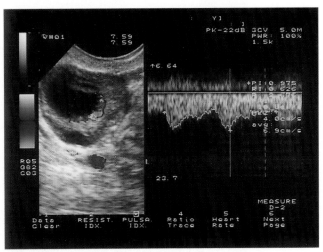

Plate 40.2. Preovulatory ovarian follicle showing peripheral low impedance flow (PI = 0.97).

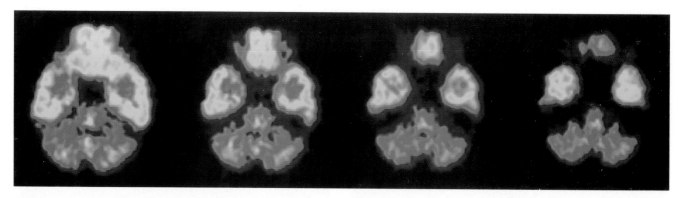

Plate 43.1. Transaxial neurologic FDG-PET images show marked cerebellar hypometabolism consistent with paraneoplastic cerebellar involvement (regions of high glucose metabolism appear as red-yellow and regions of low glucose metabolism are blue-green).

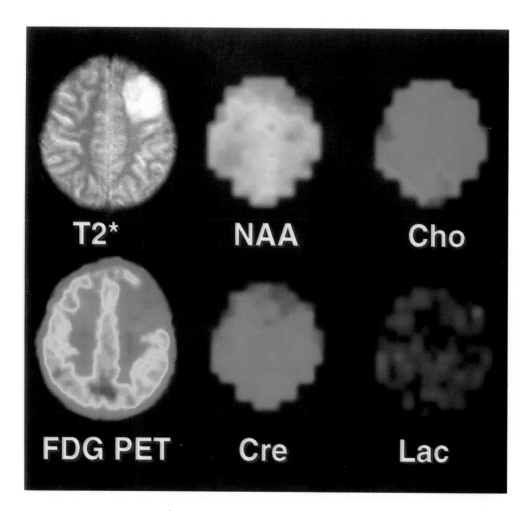

Plate 43.2. Single slice from ^{1}H-MRSI study in patient with a brain tumor shows T2-weighted MRI, FDG-PET scan, and individual metabolite maps of the distribution of choline-containing and creatine-containing compounds, lactate and N-acetyl-aspartate (NAA).

Computed Tomography and Magnetic Resonance Imaging in the Investigation of Gynecologic Malignancy

MATTI VARPULA

Assessment of treatment of gynecologic malignancies is based on the FIGO (International Federation of Gynecology and Obstetrics) staging system.[1] Physical examination with or without general anesthesia, fractional curettage, hysteroscopy, colposcopy, cystoscopy, proctoscopy, excretory urography, barium enema, and chest radiography have been used to stage malignancy but do not correlate well with the spread of disease.[2–4] The FIGO staging system is now based on surgical findings in the case of some gynecologic malignancies, such as those of the ovary and uterus.[1]

Computed tomography (CT) and magnetic resonance imaging (MRI) are not in use for staging, since they are not included in the FIGO system. However, they may be helpful in planning treatment.

MRI has a better soft tissue contrast than CT and displays multiplanar sections. MRI provides information about the local growth of tumors, but it is expensive and has a long examination time. Only the pelvis and lower abdomen can be imaged in a short time. Although only axial sections are available with CT, it is a short examination. When the entire abdomen, or in some cases the entire body, have to be imaged, CT is preferred. Respiratory and bowel movements do not disturb the image quality as seriously as those in MRI. The lack of ionizing radiation makes MRI a valuable complement to sonography in the evaluation of pelvic masses in pregnant patients.[5]

vault. The urinary bladder should be full. Contiguous 5-mm sections through the pelvis give better visualization of tumor extension. Contiguous 10-mm sections are then taken cephalad to the diaphragm. This extensive scanning is needed for ovarian carcinoma, which may send tumor implants under the diaphragm. After the abdominal study, additional 3 to 5-mm sections can be taken through the pelvic tumor. The interfaces between tumor, bladder, and ureters are then delineated.[6]

In MRI examination of the pelvis, images obtained with a standard body coil are often adequate, but the use of external or endorectal surface coils is recommended.[7,8] Surface coils are particularly important for the assessment of the local tumor growth of uterine cancers. Fast spin echo (also known as turbo spin echo) sequences are preferable to standard spin echo sequences.[7] The pelvis should be scanned with 5 to 7-mm slices at least in two directions using T1- and T2-weighted sequences to visualize the extent of the tumor. For assessment of pelvic and para-aortic adenopathy, T1-weighted 10-mm axial scans are recommended.[7] The limited size of the homogeneous magnetic field of the MRI device, the limited slice number, and the use of surface coils restrict the body volume available to image with a single acquisition. Intravenous contrast enhancement is essential for the characterization and staging of ovarian tumors[9] and may be helpful in gauging the extent of uterine tumors.[7] Contrast medium combined with fat suppression may be particularly helpful.[7,10]

IMAGING TECHNIQUE

For CT examination, the use of gastrointestinal and intravenous contrast is essential. A vaginal tampon should used when uterine tumors are scanned to help identify the vaginal

CERVICAL CARCINOMA

The size of tumor, histologic grade, and the extent of invasion into the cervical stroma, endometrium, and parametrium influence the outcome of cervical carcinoma. They increase the incidence of nodal metastases and recurrences.[11] Preoperative suggestion of lymph node metastases increases the incidence of radical surgery. When lymphatic or other metastases are extensive, surgery is not attempted or abandoned.

The overall accuracies of CT and MRI in the staging of cervical cancer are reported to be 66% to 69% and 76% to 81%, respectively.[12–15] They are not clearly more accurate than clinical staging (accuracy 66% to 79%).[2,13,15] However, MRI is the most useful tool for pretreatment staging of cervical carcinoma, because it shows the tumor itself. This makes the evaluation of local tumor extension possible (Fig. 36.1). Tumor volume and the depth of cervical stromal invasion can be measured,[12–14,16] except for cases limited to microinvasion. Knowing the tumor size and site helps in making the decision between surgery alone or surgery with radiation. Bulky tumors (> 3 to 4 cm) with or without parametrial infiltration may be treated with chemotherapy to reduce tumor size. Response to treatment and operability can be assessed accurately with MRI.[17,18] Invasion of the vaginal wall can be evaluated[12–14] but usually is easily assessed clinically.

The greatest benefit of MRI is the assessment of parametrial tumor growth. Bimanual pelvic examination under anesthesia is not accurate in assessing parametrial tumor. Underestimation is the most common error.[2,13] Parametrial tumor extension can be excluded with great certainty with MRI (negative predictive value 89% to 99%). The problem of MRI is a relatively high false-positive rate (positive predictive value 43% to 81%) in differentiating stage Ib from IIb. Parametrial extension is difficult to exclude when there is a full-thickness stromal invasion, and microscopic invasion cannot be detected with MRI.[12–14,19] With the use of an endorectal surface coil, the number of false-positives can be diminished.[8]

The value of CT in the examination of stages I to IIIa tumors is minimal, because tumor volume and vaginal and parametrial growth cannot be assessed adequately.[12,15,20,21] The accuracy of CT and MRI does not differ noticeably when evaluating more advanced cervical cancers (stages IIIb to IVb) (Fig. 36.2), although the results are limited due to the small number of positive cases.[12–15,20,21] The invasion of bladder or rectum is best seen in sagittal MRIs.[13,14] Ureteral obstruction and hydronephrosis can be seen on CT and MRI (Fig. 36.2), and excretory urography can be obviated. Distant metastases to lung, liver, and bone are easily and quickly detected with CT. In more advanced disease, when the accuracy of clinical staging decreases,[2] CT and MRI are indicated.[13,20,21]

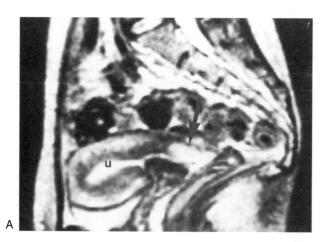

Figure 36.1 Squamous cell carcinoma of the cervix, surgical stage Ib. **(A)** Sagittal T2-weighted MRI. **(B)** Axial T2-weighted MRI. The tumor is the high signal intensity lesion in the low signal intensity normal cervical stroma (arrow). u, uterine body. **(C)** Axial CT image of the uterine cervix after intravenous contrast administration. Tumor cannot be delineated from the normal cervix tissue (arrow).

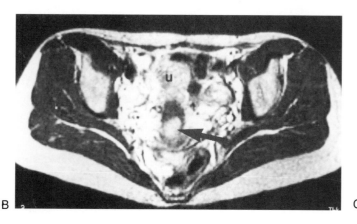

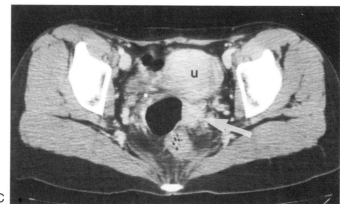

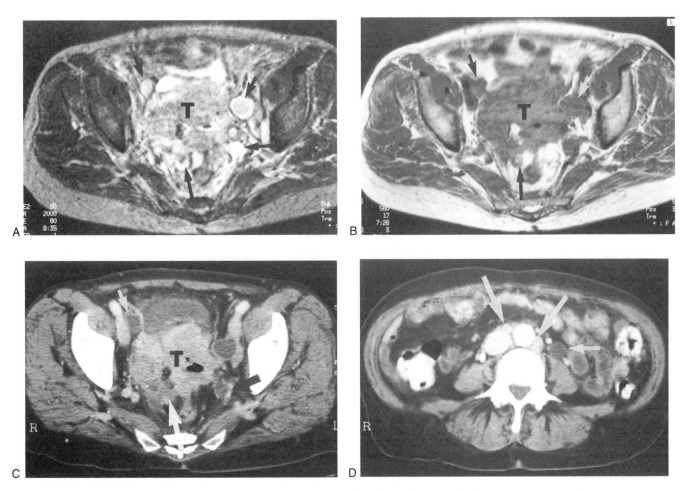

Figure 36.2 Squamous cell carcinoma of the cervix, clinical stage IIIb. Chemotherapy and radiotherapy, no histologic verification. CT images are obtained after intravenous contrast. **(A)** Axial T2-weighted MRI. **(B)** Axial T1-weighted MRI. **(C)** Axial CT image. Cervical tumor (T) is large, inhomogeneous, and ill defined. Its margins and infiltration into the perirectal fat (long arrow) are best seen on T1-weighted MRI and on CT scan. The left-sided hydroureter (small arrow) and two necrotic lymph node metastases with rimlike enhancement on CT image (arrowheads) indicates stage IIIb disease. **(D)** CT image at the level of the middle abdomen. Left-sided hydroureter is seen (small arrow). Para-aortic lymph node metastases (large arrows) will raise the stage to IVb. In the evaluation of advanced cervical carcinoma, MRI is not clearly more accurate than CT.

Staging principles of cervical carcinoma with CT and MRI are presented in Table 36.1.

ENDOMETRIAL CARCINOMA

The most important prognostic factors of endometrial carcinoma are the histologic grade of the tumor (grades 1 to III), the depth of invasion, and tumor growth to the cervix.[11] Substantial risk of lymph node metastases exists when tumor invades the outer half of the myometrium or extends to cervix. In the FIGO staging system, these are assessed postoperatively, and the usefulness of preoperative CT or MRI has not yet been demonstrated.

Histologic grading and assessment of cervical extension cannot be accurately assessed from a curettage specimen.[4] It is therefore difficult to base informed treatment upon such information. If the depth of myometrial and cervical invasion were known before surgery, the patient might benefit from treatment more appropriate to her disease. Those at risk of nodal metastases would be eligible for more extensive lymph node dissection, and aggressive surgery could be avoided in those not at risk.

The accuracy of CT and MRI in staging endometrial carcinoma is reported to be 84% to 89% and 85% to 92%, respectively.[3,22–24] Both are more accurate than clinical staging (49% to 73%).[4,22,23] Staging principles with CT and MRI are shown in Table 36.2.

MRI is preferable for pretreatment imaging of endometrial

Table 36.1 FIGO Staging of Cervical Carcinoma With CT and MRI Criteria

Stage	FIGO Classification	CT Criteria	MRI Criteria
0	Carcinoma in situ	Tumor not visible	Tumor not visible
Ia	Preclinical microscopic tumor	Tumor not visible	Tumor not visible
Ia1	Minimal stromal invasion	Tumor not visible	Tumor not visible, or abnormal signal intensity in cervix
Ia2	Stromal invasion ≤5 mm horizontal spread ≤7 mm	Tumor not visible	
Ib	Lesions of greater dimension than stage Ia2, confined strictly to the cervix	Tumor not visible, or cervix is enlarged, or hypodense area in cervix; well-defined cervix margins; tumor may be large without parametrial extension	Tumor of abnormal signal intensity is enveloped by normal cervical stroma; stromal invasion can be estimated; tumor may be large without parametrial extension
IIa	Tumor involves upper two-thirds of the vagina	Vaginal wall thickening or eccentric mass, upper two-thirds	Disruption of normal signal intensity vaginal wall, upper two-thirds
IIb	Obvious parametrial involvement	Irregular cervix margins, parametrial-strands, periureteral fat obliteration eccentric parametrial mass	Parametrial tumor protrusion through disrupted normal signal intensity cervical stroma
IIIa	Tumor involves lower third of the vagina	Vaginal wall thickening of eccentric mass, lower third	Disruption of normal signal intensity vaginal wall, lower third
IIIb	Tumor extends onto the pelvic wall or hydronephrosis or nonfunctioning kidney	Tumor infiltration to pelvic sidewall muscles, hydronephrosis pelvic lymph node enlargement (MIAD >10 mm)	Tumor infiltration to pelvic sidewall muscles, hydronephrosis, pelvic lymph node enlargement (MIAD >10 mm)
IVa	Tumor growth to adjacent organs	Loss of perivesical/perirectal fat, thickening/nodularity/serration of bladder or rectal wall	Disruption of normal signal intensity bladder or rectal wall
IVb	Distant metastases	Distant lymph node enlargement; lung, liver, omental, serosal, or peritoneal metastases	Distant lymph node enlargement; lung, liver, omental, serosal, or peritoneal metastases

MIAD, minimum axial diameter.

carcinoma, because it confidently excludes deep myometrial invasion (positive predictive value 50% to 80% and negative predictive value 72% to 88%),[3,25,26] and cervical tumor growth can be assessed accurately on sagittal images.[22,27] The evaluation of myometrial invasion is equally accurate with transvaginal ultrasound and MRI, but the latter has the advantage of imaging the entire pelvis and the lower abdomen.[26] MRI has a problem in differentiating the tumors confined entirely to the endometrium from those invading the inner half of the myometrium.[3,22,25,26] This is not, how-

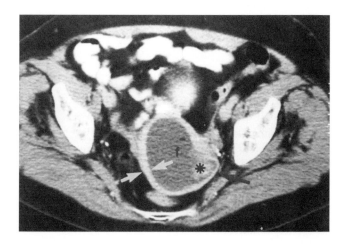

Figure 36.3 Endometrial adenocarcinoma, surgical stage Ib. Axial CT image after intravenous contrast. The endometrial cavity is filled with fluid (f), stretching the myometrium to a thin layer (arrows). At curettage, 500 ml of mucous fluid poured out. In the left uterine cornu, a small tumor (asterisk) is seen, enhanced with contrast medium. The myometrium next to the tumor is thin (arrow), indicating deep myometrial invasion. At histologic examination after surgery, only minimal myometrial invasion was detected. If the endometrial cavity is large due to exophytic tumor or fluid, CT and MRI may overestimate the myometrial invasion.

Table 36.2 FIGO Staging of Endometrial Carcinoma With CT and MRI Criteria

Stage	FIGO Classification	CT Criteria	MRI Criteria
Ia	Tumor limited to endometrium	Cannot be evaluated with CT; central hypodense area (tumor and secretion) enveloped by hyperdense myometrium is often small or invisible: tumor may be large and myometrium thin without myometrial invasion	Junctional zone is intact, or if not visible, endometrium–myometrium interface is smooth and sharp: tumor may be large and myometrium thin without myometrial invasion
Ib	Invasion to $<\frac{1}{2}$ myometrium	Central hypodense area is not visible or the ratio of minimum/maximum thickness of normal myometrium enveloping central hypodense area is $>\frac{1}{2}$, or myometrium with uniform thickness is >7 mm	Segmental interruption of junctional zone, or endometrium–myometrium interface is irregular, tumor of abnormal signal intensity extends at most into the inner half of the myometrium
Ic	Invasion to $>\frac{1}{2}$ myometrium	The ratio of minimum/maximum thickness of normal myometrium enveloping central hypodense area is $<\frac{1}{2}$, or myometrium with uniform thickness is <7 mm	As in Ib, but tumor of abnormal signal intensity extends into the outer half of myometrium; the residual myometrium may be thin
IIa	Endocervical glandular involvement only	Cannot be evaluated with CT	Cannot be evaluated with MRI
IIb	Cervical stromal invasion	Central hypodense area extends into the cervix	Tumor of abnormal signal intensity extends to the cervix (sagittal image)
IIIa	Tumor invades serosa and/or adnexa and/or positive peritoneal cytology	Tumor infiltration to parametrium or pelvic sidewall muscles; metastatic adnexal mass	Transmyometrial invasion is demonstrated by disruption of continuity of residual myometrium: tumor infiltration to parametrium or pelvic sidewall muscles; metastatic adnexal mass
IIIb	Vaginal metastases	Vaginal wall thickening or mass	Disruption of normal signal intensity vaginal wall, or vaginal mass
IIIc	Metastases to pelvic and/or para-aortic lymph nodes	Pelvic or para-aortic lymph node enlargement (MIAD >10 mm)	Pelvic or para-aortic lymph node enlargement (MIAD >10 mm)
IVa	Tumor invasion of bladder and/or bowel mucosa	Loss of perivesical/perirectal fat, thickening/nodularity/serration of bladder or rectal wall	Disruption or normal signal intensity bladder or rectal wall
IVb	Distant metastases including intra-abdominal and/or inguinal lymph nodes	Distant lymph node enlargement; lung liver, omental, serosal, or peritoneal metastases	Distant lymph node enlargement; lung, liver, omental, serosal, or peritoneal metastases

ever, important in clinical practice, because both tumors have a low risk of nodal metastases.

CT is not useful in the assessment of stage I to II endometrial carcinomas. It detects cervical tumor growth poorly,[24] and although differentiation between deep and superficial myometrial invasion is possible,[28] it is not accurate (Figs. 36.3).

The place of CT and MRI for staging of more advanced tumors (stages III to IV) is less clear because the number of patients reported is small. The accuracy of CT and MRI seem similar (Fig. 36.4), and they are probably more accurate than clinical examination.[3,22–24] Detection of ovarian or omental metastases is difficult.[3,22,28]

OVARIAN CARCINOMA

CT and MRI are not used for staging of ovarian carcinoma, because they are not available in most places in the world. Laparotomy identifies the primary site of the disease, determines tumor spread, provides histologic analysis, and allows debulking of tumor. No imaging method can replace surgery, because microscopic or small peritoneal, omental, and bowel implants cannot be detected.[9,29,30] CT and MRI do not differ in the accuracy of tumor staging,[10] but they are better than sonography.[31]

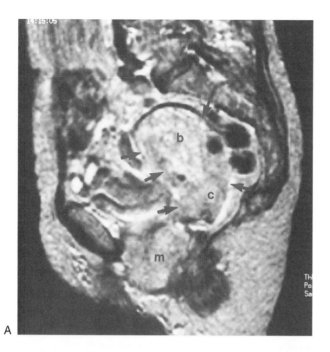

Figure 36.4 Endometrial adenocarcinoma with vaginal metastases, clinical stage IIIb. Radiation therapy. Histologic verification was obtained at autopsy. CT images are obtained after intravenous contrast administration. **(A)** Sagittal T2-weighted MRI. The uterine body (b) and cervix (c) are almost entirely infiltrated by carcinoma, but the outer margin of the uterus is well delineated (arrowheads), excluding tumor growth outside the uterus. Histologically, the carcinoma invaded almost through the myometrium. Normal low signal intensity vaginal walls are replaced by metastatic tumor (m). **(B)** Axial CT image of the vagina. The vaginal walls are thick, indicating tumor growth (small arrows). Urinary catheter (large arrow). **(C)** Axial CT image at the level of uterine body. A large endometrial tumor (t) infiltrates deeply into the myometrium, leaving the residual myometrium to a thin layer (compare with Fig. 36.3). Anteriorly, the myometrium entirely disappears (arrow), and tumor growth outside the uterus cannot be excluded with certainty.

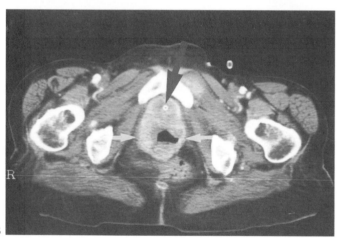

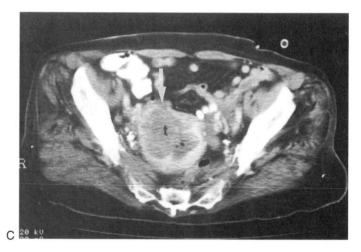

If clinically the diagnosis of ovarian cancer is in little doubt, the use of CT and MRI is not indicated. Preoperative cross-sectional imaging is justified (1) when the diagnosis is uncertain, (2) if an overall assessment of the extent of the disease is required to plan surgery, (3) to determine the amount and extent of cytoreductive surgery required to optimize subsequent chemotherapeutic response, and (4) when satisfactory pelvic examination is not possible because of obesity, previous surgery, radiotherapy, pelvic inflammatory disease, and in children.[6,32,33]

Preoperative knowledge of the potential nature of an adnexal mass (benign or malignant) might be helpful for management. CT and MRI can mostly discriminate benign from malignant ovarian lesions (positive predictive value 82% to 96%, negative predictive value 83% to 100%), but intravenous contrast enhancement is essential.[9,29,31,34] They do not yet replace histologic examination. MRI has not been shown to be practically superior to CT in tumor

characterization[29] (Fig. 36.5), but both are better than ultrasound.[31,34] Ultrasound provides sufficient characterization of most adnexal masses, but in cases with an indeterminate finding, MRI or CT can be more specific. Characteristics of malignant ovarian tumors are presented in Table 36.3.

CT is more practical than MRI in the staging of the ovarian malignancies, because the entire abdomen can be scanned in a reasonable time. If needed, the thoracic region can be scanned in the same session. The entire abdomen should be evaluated because ovarian cancer sends tumor implants through the abdominal cavity, often to the subphrenic region (Fig. 36.6). Retroperitoneal lymph node metastases are also frequent. Psammomatous tumor calcifications can be seen easily in CT images (Fig. 36.7). With the new-generation CT and MRI scanners, implants smaller than 5 mm can be detected, but intravenous contrast enhancement is essential.[30,35] Implants in the omentum (Fig. 36.8), pelvic peritoneum, peri-

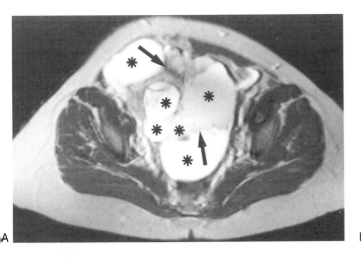

A

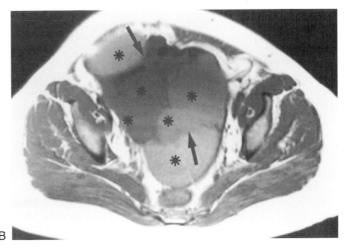

B

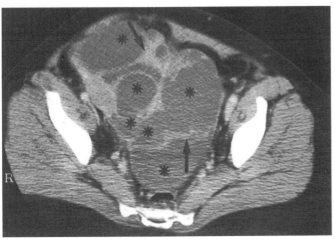

C

Figure 36.5 Undifferentiated cystadenocarcinoma of the ovary, surgical stage IIIc. (**A**) Axial T2-weighted MRI. (**B**) Axial T1-weighted MRI. (**C**) Axial CT image after intravenous contrast administration. The tumor is large, with multiloculated cysts (asterisks) and thick septa (small arrows). These properties indicate likely malignant tumor (see Table 36.3). On MRIs, the signal intensities of the cysts are different, indicating different liquid contents. On CT, this differentiation cannot be made, since the densities of the cysts are similar. At operation, the tumor originated from both ovaries and infiltrated largely into the side walls of the pelvis. That was not evident on MRI and CT examinations.

toneum, covering the colon or small bowel, and in the uterine and ovarian ligaments may be most difficult to identify.[29,30,35] Ascites adjacent to the implants tends to improve their detection.[30,35] The accuracy of CT can be increased with intraperitoneal contrast.[36] Staging principles of ovarian carcinoma with CT and MRI are presented in Table 36.3.

OTHER MALIGNANT TUMORS

There are many rare gynecologic malignant tumors, such as sarcoma of the uterus: carcinomas of the fallopian tube, vagina, and vulva; and gestational trophoblastic disease. If imaging is necessary, MRI is probably the most effective

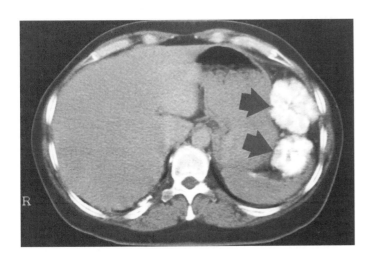

Figure 36.6 Serous cystadenocarcinoma of the ovary, surgical stage IIIc. Axial CT image without intravenous contrast enhancement. In the left subphrenic region, there are two calcified tumor implants (arrows).

Table 36.3 FIGO Staging of Ovarian Carcinoma With CT and MRI Criteria

Stage	FIGO Classification	CT/MRI Criteria
Ia	Tumor limited to one ovary, no ascites, no tumor on the external surfaces, capsules intact	Tumor is potentially malignant when (a) size >4 cm, (b) solid mass or large solid component, (c) wall thickness >3 mm, (d) septa >3 mm thick and/or presence of vegetations or nodularity, (e) necrosis, (f) amorphous coarse calcifications
Ib	Tumor limited to both ovaries, no ascites, no tumor on the external surface, capsule intact	Differentiation between Ia and Ib is often impossible
Ic	Tumor either Ia or Ib, but with tumor on surface of one or both ovaries, or with capsule ruptured, or with ascites present containing malignant cells, or with positive peritoneal washings	Ascites in the abdominal cavity usually means disseminated disease; ascites in the pelvic region is a nonspecific finding
IIa	Tumor involving one or both ovaries with extension and/or metastases to the uterus and/or fallopian tubes	Implants on the surface of the uterus or tubes
IIb	Tumor involving one or both ovaries with extension to other pelvic tissues	Implants on the pelvic peritoneum, on the uterine and ovarian ligaments, in the pouch of Douglas
IIc	Tumor either IIa or IIb, but with tumor on surface of one or both ovaries, or with capsule(s) ruptured, or with ascites present containing malignant cells, or with positive peritoneal washings	As IIa and IIb with ascites
IIIa	Tumor involving one or both ovaries, tumor grossly limited to the true pelvis with negative nodes but with histologically confirmed microscopic seeding of abdominal peritoneal surfaces	Microscopic seeding is undetectable
IIIb	Tumor involving one or both ovaries with histologically confirmed implants of abdominal peritoneal surfaces, none exceeding 2 cm in diameter, nodes are negative	Implants (≤2 cm) on the surface of abdominal peritoneum, omentum, mesenterium, and bowel; implants in subphrenic and subhepatic spaces
IIIc	Tumor involving one or both ovaries; abdominal implants >2 cm in diameter and/or positive retroperitoneal or inguinal nodes	As IIIb but implants are greater, and/or retroperitoneal or inguinal lymph node enlargement (MIAD >10 mm)
IV	Tumor involving one or both ovaries with distant metastases; pleural effusion with positive cytology; parenchymal liver metastases	Distant metastases in liver, lungs, and pleura

method of assessing local tumor growth.[37–39] MRI may be useful in detecting invasion of trophoblastic disease and in assessing the response to chemotherapy.[40] In more advanced neoplasms, such as metastatic trophoblastic diseases, CT is more useful because it can screen the brain, chest, abdomen, and pelvis quickly and accurately.[6]

LYMPH NODE METASTASES

Although MRI may be better than CT in detecting metastatic lymph nodes,[12,41] CT is more practical for their assessment. It offers convenient and rapid imaging of the pelvis and abdomen. Detection of lymph node metastases by CT and MRI is based on the size of the lymph node. The most reliable criterion is the minimum axial diameter (MIAD) of the lymph node measured from transverse scans. When MIAD is over 10

mm, metastatic involvement is probable.[42] (Figure 36.2D). With this criterion, a positive predictive value of 82% and a negative predictive value of 94% have been reported with MRI.[42] The false-positive rate may be decreased when the anatomic location of the lymph node is taken into consideration, because internal iliac and obturator nodes with a diameter of 8 to 10 mm may be metastatic.[43] Peripheral enhancement usually means a necrotic lymph node metastatis in spite of its size (Figure 36.2).

Neither CT nor MRI can distinguish lymph node enlargement due to reactive hyperplasia from metastatic disease, nor detect small tumor deposits in normal sized nodes.[42] Lymphography can demonstrate tumor deposits in lymph nodes of normal size. Because large nodes totally replaced by tumor may fail to opacify, and the hypogastric or internal iliac and the presacral nodes are only occasionally seen, lymphography has no advantage nowadays. Normal-sized lymph node metastases can also be overlooked by the surgeon.[44]

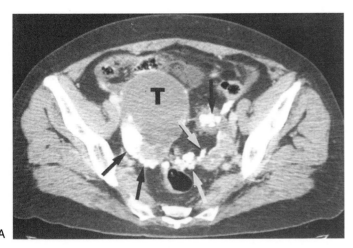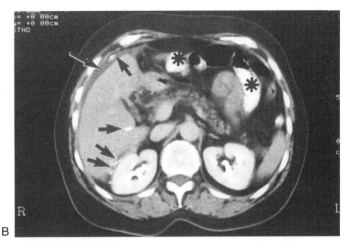

Figure 36.7 Serous cystadenocarcinoma of the ovary, surgical stage IIIc. **(A)** Axial CT image at the level of the pelvic tumor. **(B)** Axial CT image at the upper abdomen. CT images are obtained after the administration of gastrointestinal and intravenous contrast. The primary tumor is cystic (T). There are multiple psammomatous calcifications (small arrows) in the tumor wall, in the peritoneal surface of the intestine, and on the liver surface. A small amount of ascites is present around the liver (large arrow). Only palliative surgery was possible. Psammomatous tumor calcifications are typical of serous cystadenocarcinoma. They are well delineated with CT, but gastrointestinal contrast medium (asterisks) may be confusing. CT examination without contrast is advisable for the staging of serous cystadenocarcinoma.

No imaging is as accurate as histologic examination in the assessment of lymph node metastasis. For this reason, preoperative MRI examination of endometrial and cervical carcinomas is important, making it possible to identify high-risk patients. It is better to perform extensive lymphadenectomy and histologic lymph node examination than postoperative imaging to assess lymph nodes. With postoperative CT or MRI, it is not possible to exclude lymph node metastasis with certainty. Patients without risk factors and without evidence of nodal metastasis in preoperative CT and MRI can be managed with more conservative surgery.

ASSESSMENT OF TREATMENT AND RECURRENCE OF TUMORS

CT and MRI are effective in the assessment of chemotherapy or radiation therapy, but it is important to use the same imaging modality consistently. MRI is the method of choice when the cervical carcinoma is thought to be regressing locally.[17,18] CT is valuable in advanced disease when the entire abdomen should be examined (Fig. 36.9).

CT is preferred for cross-sectional imaging to detect persistent or recurrent tumors. The accuracies of CT and MRI do

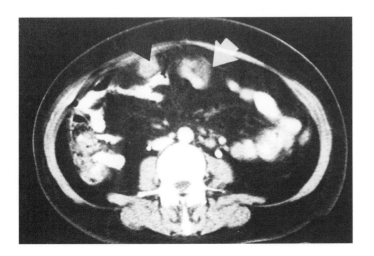

Figure 36.8 Omental implants (arrows) of anaplastic adenocarcinoma of the ovary. Axial CT image after intravenous contrast.

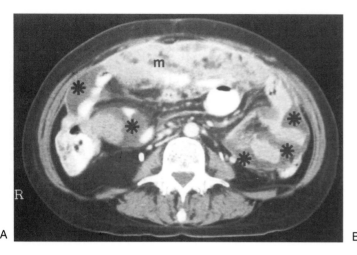
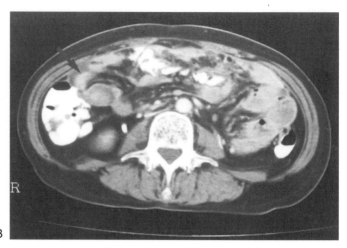

Figure 36.9 Serous cystadenocarcinoma of the ovary, surgical stage III. At exploratory laparotomy, adhesive peritoneal carcinosis was detected. **(A)** Axial CT image. Large omental cake (m) and ascites (asterisks) are seen. **(B)** Axial CT image at the corresponding level after chemotherapy of 7 months. Omental cake is reduced noticeably, and only a small amount of ascites is left (arrow).

not differ markedly, but MRI may be slightly more specific than CT.[45–47] When CT is equivocal, MRI can be helpful. Baseline examination after surgery or radiation is useful, decreasing the number of false-positives. Differentiation of recurrent tumors from post-treatment fibrosis, granulation tissue, and inflammatory changes is particularly difficult, because they enhance similarly after intravenous contrast.[45,48] Late post-treatment fibrosis (>12 months after the first treatment) is more easily differentiated from the tumor recurrence on heavily T2-weighted MRIs than early fibrosis (1 to 6 months after first treatment).[49] The sensitivity (82% to 92%) and specificity (78% to 95%) of CT and MRI in de-

tecting recurrence of uterine carcinoma are relatively high[45,46,48] (Fig. 36.10), and they appear to be superior to physical examination or ultrasound.[48] Sensitivity (42% to 78%) and specificity (75% to 93%) in detecting recurrence of ovarian carcinoma are lower.[47,50,51] The poor sensitivity identifying minimal abdominopelvic disease and carcinomatosis precludes the use of CT and MRI as a substitute for the second-look surgery.

CT and MRI are not useful when used routinely to detect recurrence of ovarian carcinoma. In patients in whom recurrent tumor is clinically suspected or in those who have an increased CA-125, cross-sectional imaging is useful to deter-

Figure 36.10 Recurrence of endometrial adenocarcinoma, stage Ia. **(A)** Axial CT image at the true pelvis. A large, inhomogeneously enhanced tumor is seen between bladder and rectum (arrows). **(B)** Axial CT image at the level of the middle abdomen. The mesenteric structures are thickened (curved arrows), indicating carcinosis, which was found at laparotomy.

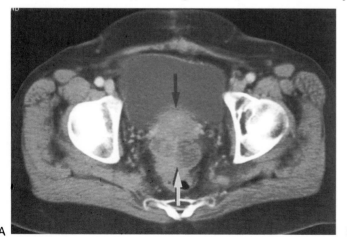
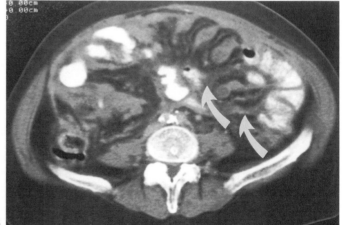

mine the location and extent of the tumor. In some patients, this may allow changes to treatment without laparotomy.[50]

SUMMARY

The soft tissue contrast of MRI is good, and multiplanar sections are available. It is the best method for the assessment of early cervical and endometrial carcinomas. In cervical carcinoma, the parametrial tumor growth, tumor volume, and macroscopic cervical stromal invasion can be evaluated. In endometrial carcinoma, myometrial invasion and cervical tumor growth can be assessed. All these factors increase the risk of nodal metastases and recurrences. The value of the preoperative MRI is its ability to identify high-risk patients. It is better to perform extensive lymphadenectomy and histologic lymph node examination than postoperative imaging to assess lymph nodes.

MRI is also effective in assessing local tumor growth of other malignancies, like carcinomas of the fallopian tube, vagina, and vulva, invasive trophoblastic disease, and ovarian carcinoma. MRI is slightly better than CT for detecting metastatic lymph nodes and persistent or recurrent tumors. However, MRI has a long examination time, and the body volume available to image with a single acquisition is restricted. In contrast, CT is a short examination, and the entire body can be imaged. The value of CT in the assessment of local tumors, like stage I to III cervical and endometrial cancers is minimal because of inferior soft tissue contrast. Fast CT examination is preferable in the assessment of more advanced tumors. In these cases, MRI is not more accurate than CT, which is also preferred for detection of persistent or recurrent tumors, and MRI can be used when CT is equivocal.

REFERENCES

1. Shepherd JH. Revised FIGO staging for gynaecological cancer. Br J Obstet Gynecol 1989;96:889–892
2. van Nagell JR, Jr, Roddick HW, Jr, Lowin DM. The staging of cervical cancer: inevitable discrepanices between clinical staging and pathologic findings. Am J Obstet Gynecol 1971;110:973–978
3. Hricak H, Rubinstein LV, Gherman GM, Karstaedt N. MR imaging evaluation of endometrial carcinoma: results of an NCI cooperative study. Radiology 1991;179:829–832
4. Cowles TA, Magrina JF, Masterson BJ, Capen CV. Comparison of clinical and surgical staging in patients with endometrial carcinoma. Obstet Gynecol 1985;66:413–416
5. Kier R, McCarthy SM, Scoutt LM et al. Pelvic masses in pregnancy: MR imaging. Radiology 1990;176:709–713
6. Walsh JW. Computed tomography of gynecologic neoplasms. Radiol Clin North Am 1992;30:817–830
7. Outwater EK, Mitchell DG. Magnetic resonance imaging techniques in the pelvis. MRI Clin North Am 1994;2:161–188
8. Kaji Y, Sugimura K, Kitao M, Ishida T. Histopathology of uterine cervical carcinoma: diagnostic comparison of endorectal surface coil and standard body coil MRI. J Comput Assist Tomogr 1994;18:785–792
9. Stevens SK, Hricak H, Stern JL. Ovarian lesions: detection and characterization with gadolinium-enhanced MR imaging at 1.5 T. Radiology 1991;181:481–488
10. Semelka RC, Lawrence PH, Shoenut JP et al. Primary ovarian cancer: prospective comparison of contrast-enhanced CT and pre- and postcontrast, fat-suppressed MR imaging with histologic correlation. J Magn Reson Imaging 1993;3:99–106
11. Boronow RC. Advances in diagnosis, staging, and management of cervical and endometrial cancer, stages I and II. Cancer 1990;65 (3 suppl):648–659
12. Kim SH, Choi BI, Han JK et al. Preoperative staging of uterine cervical carcinoma: comparison of CT and MRI in 99 patients. J Comput Assist Tomogr 1993;17:633–640
13. Hricak H, Lacey CG, Sandles LG et al. Invasive cervical carcinoma: comparison of MR imaging and surgical findings. Radiology 1988;166:623–631
14. Togashi K, Nishimura K, Sagoh T et al. Carcinoma of the cervix: staging with MR imaging Radiology 1989;171:245–251
15. Whitley NO, Brenner DE, Francis A et al. Computed tomographic evaluation of carcinoma of the cervix. Radiology 1982;142:439–446
16. Lien HH, Blomlie V, Kjørstad K. Clinical stage I carcinoma of the cervix: value of MR imaging in determining degree of invasiveness. AJR Am J Roentgenol 1991;156:1191–1194
17. Sironi S, Belloni C, Taccagni G, Del Maschio A. Invasive cervical carcinoma: MR imaging after preoperative chemotherapy. Radiology 1991;180:719–722
18. Kim KH, Lee BH, Do YS et al. Stage IIb cervical carcinoma: MR evaluation of effect of intraarterial chemotherapy. Radiology 1994;192:61–65
19. Lien HH, Blomlie V, Iversen T et al. Clinical stage I carcinoma of the cervix. Value of MR imaging in determining invasion into the parametrium. Acta Radiol 1993;34:130–132
20. Walsh JW, Goblerud DR. Prospective comparison between clinical and CT staging in primary cervical carcinoma. AJR Am J Roentgenol 1981;137:997–1003
21. Newton WA, Roberts WS, Marsden DE, Cavanagh D. Value of computerized axial tomography in cervical cancer. Oncology 1987;44:124–127
22. Hricak H, Stern JL, Fisher MR et al. Endometrial carcinoma staging by MR imaging. Radiology 1987;162:297–305
23. Balfe DM, Van Dyke J, Lee JKT et al. Computed tomography in malignant endometrial neoplasms. J Comput Assist Tomogr 1983;7:677–681
24. Walsh JW, Goplerud DR. Computed tomography of primary, persistent, and recurrent endometrial malignancy. AJR Am J Roentgenol 1982;139:1149–1154
25. Scoutt LM, McCarthy SM, Flynn SD et al. Clinical stage I endometrial carcinoma: pitfalls in preoperative assessment with MR imaging. Work in progress. Radiology 1995;194:567–572
26. Del Maschio A, Vanzulli A, Sironi S et al. Estimating the depth of myometrial involvement by endometrial carcinoma: efficacy of transvaginal sonography vs MR imaging. AJR Am J Roentgenol 1993;160:533–538
27. Murakami T, Kurachi H, Nakamura H et al. Cervical invasion of endometrial carcinoma—evaluation by parasagittal MR imaging. Acta Radiol 1995;36:248–253
28. Dore R, Moro G, D'Andrea F et al. CT evaluation of myometrial

invasion in endometrial carcinoma. J Comput Assist Tomogr 1987;11:282–289

29. Ghossain MA, Buy JN, Ligneres C et al. Epithelial tumors of the ovary: comparison of MR and CT findings. Radiology 1991;181:863–870

30. Buy JN, Moss AA, Ghossain MA et al. Peritoneal implants from ovarian tumors: CT findings. Radiology 1988;169:691–694

31. Buy JN, Ghossain MA, Sciot C et al. Epithelial tumors of the ovary: CT findings and correlation with US. Radiology 1991;178:811–818

32. Nelson BE, Rosenfield AT, Schwartz PE. Preoperative abdominopelvic computed tomographic prediction of optimal cytoreduction in epithelial ovarian carcinoma. J Clin Oncol 1993;11:166–172

33. Johnson RJ. Radiology in the management of ovarian cancer. Clin Radiol 1993;48:75–82

34. Yamashita Y, Torashima M, Hatanaka Y et al. Adnexal masses: accuracy of characterization with transvaginal US and precontrast and postcontrast MR imaging. Radiology 1995;194:557–565

35. Low RN, Sigeti JS. MR imaging of peritoneal disease: comparison of contrast-enhanced fast multiplanar spoiled gradient-recalled and spin-echo imaging. AJR Am J Roentgenol 1994;163:1131–1140

36. Frasci G, Contino A, Iaffaioli RV et al. Computerized tomography of the abdomen and pelvis with peritoneal administration of soluble contrast (IPC-CT) in detection of residual disease for patients with ovarian cancer. Gynecol Oncol 1994;52:154–160

37. Chang YC, Hricak H, Thurnher S, Lacey CG. Vagina: evaluation with MR imaging. Part II. Neoplasms. Radiology 1988;169:175–179

38. Kawakami S, Togashi K, Kimura I et al. Primary malignant tumor of the fallopian tube: appearance at CT and MR imaging. Radiology 1993;186:503–508

39. Shapeero LG, Hricak H. Mixed müllerian sarcoma of the uterus: MR imaging findings. AJR Am J Roentgenol 1989;153:317–319

40. Smith RC, McCarthy S. Magnetic resonance staging of neoplasms of the uterus. Radiol Clin North Am 1994;32:109–131

41. Dooms GC, Hricak H, Crooks LE, Higgins CB. Magnetic resonance imaging of the lymph nodes: comparison with CT. Radiology 1984;153:719–728

42. Kim SH, Kim SC, Choi BI, Han MC. Uterine cervical carcinoma: evaluation of pelvic lymph node metastasis with MR imaging. Radiology 1994;190:807–811

43. Vinnicombe SJ, Norman AR, Nicolson V, Husband JE. Normal pelvic lymph nodes: evaluation with CT after bipedal lymphangiography. Radiology 1995;194:349–355

44. Varpula M, Klemi P. Staging of uterine endometrial carcinoma with ultra low field (0.02 T) MRI: a comparative study with CT. J Comput Assist Tomogr 1993;17:641–647

45. Williams MP, Husband JE, Heron CW et al. Magnetic resonance imaging in recurrent carcinoma of the cervix. Br J Radiol 1989;62:544–550

46. Weber TN, Sostman HD, Spritzer CE et al. Cervical carcinoma: determination of recurrent tumor extent versus radiation changes with MR imaging. Radiology 1995;194:135–139

47. Prayer L, Kainz C, Kramer J et al. CT and MR accuracy in the detection of tumor recurrence in patients treated for ovarian cancer. J Comput Assist Tomogr 1993;17:626–632

48. Heron CW, Husband JE, Williams MP et al. The value of CT in the diagnosis of recurrent carcinoma of the cervix. Clin Radiol 1988;39:496–501

49. Ebner F, Kressel HY, Mintz MC et al. Tumor recurrence versus fibrosis in the female pelvis: differentiation with MR imaging at 1.5 T. Radiology 1988;166:333–340

50. Ngan HYS, Wong LC, Chan SY, Ma HK. Role of CA125 and abdominal pelvic computerized axial tomogram in the monitoring of chemotherapy treatment of ovarian cancer. Cancer Invest 990;8:467–470

51. Pectasides D, Kayianni H, Facou A et al. Correlation of abdominal computed tomography scanning and second-look operation findings on ovarian cancer patients. Am J Clin Oncol 1991;14:457–462

Ultrasonography of the Lower Urinary Tract

MARTIN QUINN

MICHAEL W. BOURNE

Ultrasound has been applied to the evaluation of urinary problems to improve on imaging techniques of the lower urinary tract. Early imaging depended on indirect techniques, such as bead-chain cystourethrography (BCUG) to image the bladder and urethra and their response to an increase in intra-abdominal pressure such as a Valsalva maneuver. This was superseded by cinefluoroscopy, enabling direct evaluation of the bladder outlet, and the effects of a cough on the continence mechanism, which were subsequently combined with urodynamic techniques to establish synchronous video-cystourethrography (VCU). Abdominal, perineal, rectal, urethral, and vaginal ultrasound have been applied to specific clinical problems with varying degrees of success. For reasons of image quality and patient acceptance, vaginal and perineal ultrasound have proven to be the most consistent techniques in the evaluation of the female continence mechanism. Both may be combined with traditional urodynamic techniques to enable evaluation without the requirement for x-ray facilities.

Perineal ultrasound does not distort the distal urethra, but vaginal ultrasound produces improved resolution and has been more widely used in this application.

Observations using BCUG have established the pathoanatomy of stress incontinence to include posterior and inferior rotation of the urethrovesical junction with an increase in intra-abdominal pressure.[1-4] The term *anatomic stress incontinence* was adopted to describe these observations and remains in widespread use in North America, though the *precise* anatomic lesions caused by vaginal delivery have not been described. Further studies with BCUG have established that successful surgical treatment of genuine stress incontinence by retropubic urethropexy prevented downward displacement of the urethrovesical junction when an increase in intra-abdominal pressure occurred.[4] "Genuine" stress incontinence (GSI) is defined in urodynamic terms as "the involuntary loss of urine with an increase in intra-abdominal pressure in the absence of an increase in intravesical pressure."[5-8] Some clinicians prefer concurrent imaging using fluoroscopic techniques to establish the diagnosis of GSI,[9-11]

although ultrasound techniques are being increasingly applied to the evaluation of the lower urinary tract. Few urodynamic investigations have been subjected to randomized evaluation, though retrograde filling cystometry contributes to an improved understanding of the dynamics of the urinary tract.[12] For clinical investigations, such studies depend on reproducing the symptoms in the urodynamic laboratory to confirm the relationship between test result and symptoms.

THE FEMALE CONTINENCE MECHANISM

Female continence depends on appropriate function of the *intrinsic components* of the continence mechanism, that is, the internal and external urethral sphincters, and their *extrinsic support* including the anterior vaginal wall, the anterior suspensory mechanism of the vesical neck, the arcus tendineus fasciae pelvis, the pubococcygeus, and the uterine cervix.[13,14]

Early theories of female continence have emphasized "pressure transmission to an intra-abdominal urethra" where an increase in intra-abdominal pressure is transmitted to the proximal (intra-abdominal) urethra contemporaneously to maintain continence.[12] Loss of support of the proximal urethra is associated with displacement of the urethrovesical junction from the intra-abdominal pressure zone, reduced urethral closure pressure, and urinary stress incontinence. The central objections to the pressure transmission theory are the lack of an anatomic feature to separate the intra-abdominal from the extra-abdominal urethra and the observation of continence in many patients with displacement of the urethrovesical junction outside the abdominal cavity in an isolated cystocoele. The hammock hypothesis represents another anatomic view that depends on the stability of the anterior vaginal wall and pubocervical fascia preventing downward displacement of the urethrovesical junction, and this hypothesis sustains a consistent explanation of the etiology, diagnosis, and surgical treatment of urinary stress incontinence.[15] The limited mobility of the nulliparous urethra results from the lateral at-

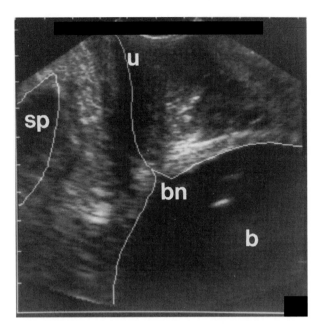

Figure 37.1 Successful colposuspension. The urethrovesical junction is supported by the fixation of the vaginal fornices to the iliopectineal ligaments by nonabsorbable sutures. An increase in intra-abdominal pressure is associated with no displacement of the urethrovesical junction. u, urethra; b, bladder; bn, bladder neck; sp, symphysis pubis.

tachments of the anterior vaginal wall to the arcus tendineus and pubococcygeus.

GSI is associated with disruption of the lateral vaginal attachments, permitting increased mobility of the urethrovesical junction. Retropubic urethropexy[16] restores urethral support and prevents downward displacement (Fig. 37.1). Over-elevation of the bladder neck may account for some of the postoperative morbidity associated with retropubic operations including voiding difficulties, frequency-urgency syndrome, and postoperative detrusor instability.[17–19]

The objective of suprapubic surgery is to prevent downward displacement rather than to elevate the bladder neck, although the two may occur together to some extent in many operations. Evidence to support either theory is limited, and the anatomic differences between increased mobility of the urethrovesical junction, GSI, and genital prolapse are unclear, since many other structures contribute to pelvic support. For example, the role of the anterior suspensory mechanism of the vesical neck is controversial, though it is apparent that all nulliparous subjects possess these anatomic features (Fig. 37.2).

The etiology and successful surgical treatment both depend on alterations to the anatomy of the lower urinary tract that may be seen on vaginal scanning. Interested readers are referred to the detailed summaries of DeLancey[15] and Nicholls[20] that provide extensive bibliographies of knowledge of individual anatomic features.

ULTRASOUND IMAGING OF THE LOWER URINARY TRACT

Abdominal, vaginal, perineal, and rectal ultrasound have been used to image the lower urinary tract.[21–28] At present, the vaginal and perineal approaches provide adequate resolution of the anatomic features in a noninvasive, patient-acceptable fashion. Perineal ultrasound may be limited by the acoustic impedance of the symphysis, lack of a consistent relationship of the transducer to the anatomic features, and the inability of the technique to be used for dynamic studies with the patient in the sitting position, though it is a simple method of observing the effects of retrograde filling cystometry on the bladder neck and proximal urethra.

Vaginal sonography (TVS) may be used with the patient in either the supine or sitting position to image the consequences of provocative maneuvers and suprapubic surgery. A disadvantage is that it can displace the anterior vaginal wall in patients with genital prolapse, preventing their true position from being seen. The enhanced resolution and patient acceptance are advantages. TVS is optimal for evaluating patients after suprapubic surgery. The role of vaginal ultrasound for imaging the female lower urinary tract is to demonstrate the anatomy of the lower urinary tract, the dynamic imaging of GSI, and the results of suprapubic surgery for GSI.

Figure 37.2 An oblique plane of the anterior pelvis demonstrating the hyperechoic appearances of the anterior suspensory mechanism of the vesical neck. The craniocaudal axis of the patient is indicated, since the transducer is offset at 45 degrees to the horizontal. P, pubis; B, bladder; BN, bladder neck.

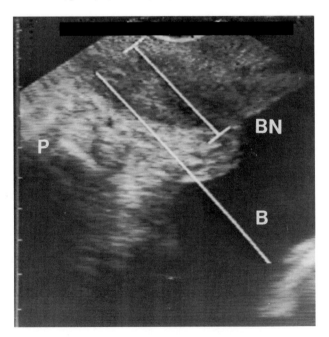

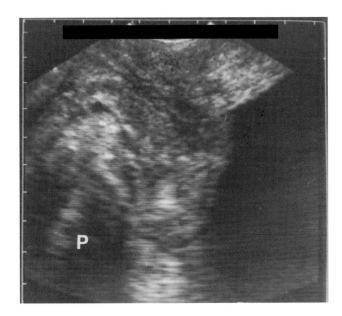

Figure 37.3 The midline sagittal plane of the pelvis demonstrated with vaginal ultrasound. The symphysis pubis (P) is a hyperechoic feature that appears in the same midline plane as the urethrovesical junction and the urethra.

The Ultrasound Anatomy of the Lower Urinary Tract

Ultrasound appearances of the lower urinary tract depend on the acoustic impedances of the adjacent tissues including cartilage (symphysis pubis), bone (pubic rami), urine, and soft tissues (Fig. 37.2 to 37.4). Additional information may be obtained by catheterization or by combining ultrasound with concurrent measurement of intravesical and intraurethral pressures (videocystosonography). Imaging in both clinical applications—that is, preoperative evaluation of the incontinent patient and evaluation of the postoperative anatomic result—has been consistently achieved with a high-frequency (7 MHz), mechanical sector scanner (Bruel & Kjaer 8537) that has reduced external dimensions (diameter 18 mm) and a wide-angle field of view (112 degrees), which enables imaging in supine and sitting positions, at rest, and during provocative maneuvers (Fig. 37.5).

Ultrasound Imaging of GSI

Clinical history, physical examination, and noninvasive investigations including urine culture, frequency–volume chart, urinary flow rate, and perineal pad weighing may contribute to an overall evaluation of the lower urinary tract. Urodynamic studies including filling cystometry may be carried out with or without ultrasound (videocystosonography). The investigation may be completed by voiding to completion to establish the bladder volume, urine flow rate, and final ultrasound evaluation to estimate residual volume.

In patients without symptoms, ultrasound demonstrates minor downward and posterior rotation of the urethrovesical junction; there is no demonstrable urinary leakage in either supine or sitting positions. In patients with GSI, ultrasound demonstrates passive opening of the bladder neck and proximal urethra when the patient coughs (Fig. 37.5) Few patients have these signs in the supine position, though they may be conveniently demonstrated in the sitting position. Almost invariably, there is posteroinferior rotation of the urethrovesical junction that is characteristic of "anatomic" stress incontinence, which has been demonstrated using indirect radiologic techniques including BCUG.[1–4] Patients with a "fixed" urethra are rare and have invariably had multiple unsuccessful surgical procedures. Patients with neurologic symptoms require formal evaluation with cystometry and concurrent measurement of intravesical and intra-abdominal pressures.

The sagittal plane of the pelvis is defined by the symphysis pubis, the urethra, and the urethrovesical junction. The symphysis pubis is a secondary cartilaginous joint with sonographic appearances that are determined by the pad of cartilage connecting the pubic bones (See Fig. 37.3). Cartilage is homogeneous and hyperechoic and is differentiated from adjacent connective tissue by the shape of its inferior border and its immobility during provocative maneuvers. The inferior border of the symphysis pubis is a fixed reference point from which reproducible anatomic observations may be made. The sagittal plane is clearly defined and is distinguished from the pubic bones by its characteristic appearance. The pubic bones are composed of trabecular bone that has a hypoechoic appearance with a dense inferior edge that has a contrasting hyperechoic appearance (see Fig. 37.4). In the oblique plane, the pubovesical component of the anterior suspensory mechanism of the neck may be seen between the anterior surface of

Figure 37.4 The parasagittal plane of the anterior pelvis demonstrating the same anatomic features as Figure 37.6 except for the hypoechoic appearance of the pubic ramus in a plane adjacent to the midline sagittal plane. PR, pubic ramus.

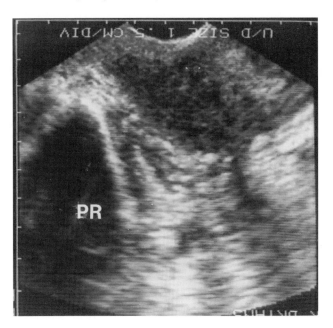

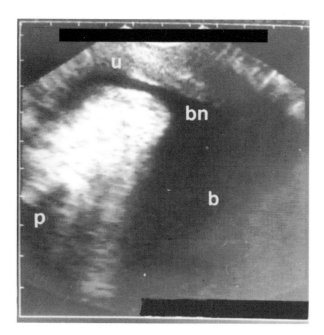

Figure 37.5 GSI: Concurrent opening of the bladder neck and proximal urethra with urinary leakage concurrent with a cough. Urinary incontinence is almost invariably associated with posteroinferior rotation of the urethrovesical junction. u, urethra; bn, bladder neck; b, bladder; p, pubis.

the bladder and the inferior border of the pubic ramus (see Fig. 37.2). The bladder is easily defined. The urethrovesical junction is identified by its characteristic shape, and the course of the urethra, by the appearances of the apposed epithelial surfaces.

Evaluation of the lower urinary tract requires ultrasound equipment that is capable of dynamic imaging in real time with the patient supine and sitting, at rest, and during a cough or valsalva maneuver in order to image urinary leakage as in GSI.[6] Many vaginal transducers do not have this ability, though most systems may be used for the evaluation of suprapubic operations such as colposuspension and bladder neck operations.

Incontinence associated with detrusor instability may be differentiated from GSI by the nature and timing of urinary leakage relative to the cough (see Fig. 37.6). Urinary leakage is delayed relative to the cough and is associated with active contraction of the detrusor muscle that accounts for the phasic increase in intravesical pressure. In a prospective comparison of traditional urodynamic techniques and vaginal ultrasound, the ultrasound technique was both sensitive and specific for the diagnosis of GSI without the necessity for urethral and rectal catheterization.[28] Imaging studies to detect the effects of detrusor instability on the continence mechanism have not been performed, since additional provocative maneuvers including retrograde bladder filling may be required to provoke detrusor activity, the clinical significance of which remains uncertain.

Ultrasound Imaging of Postoperative Surgical Anatomy

Surgery of GSI includes many procedures principally divided into three approaches: colposuspension, needle suspension operations, and sling procedures. Laparoscopic techniques for colposuspension are becoming more popular, since they combine increased surgical accuracy with reduced morbidity.[29] The principle of suprapubic surgery for GSI—elevation of the bladder neck—has been based on theories of pressure transmission so that a displaced urethrovesical junction is restored to an intra-abdominal pressure zone. This approach has been associated with successful treatment of primary stress incontinence, though it has been accompanied by significant rates of postoperative detrusor instability and voiding difficulties.[17–19]

Clinical and experimental observations indicated potential problems with this hypothesis; there is no anatomic feature that differentiates the intra-abdominal urethra from the extra-abdominal urethra; there are many continent patients with genital prolapse, and successful surgery is often associated with pressure transmission ratios in excess of 100% of the preoperative value. The hammock hypothesis proposes that the condition commonly results from loss of support of the urethrovesical junction and that successful surgery, particularly for primary stress incontinence, restores the support of the urethrovesical junction. The prevention of downward displacement of the urethrovesical junction by the interposition of a vaginal shelf, needle suspension, or sling is a subtle, but important, shift in surgical approach that may have compara-

Figure 37.6 Detrusor incontinence: The nature and timing of urinary incontinence associated with detrusor instability are different from that associated with GSI. Urinary incontinence is delayed relative to the cough. b, bladder; u, urethra.

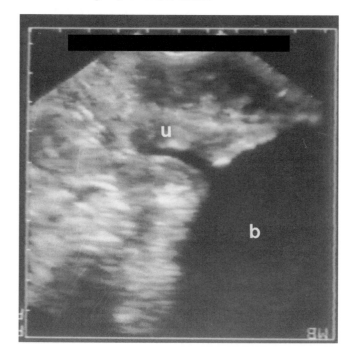

ble success rates without the additional morbidity associated with voiding difficulties and postoperative detrusor instability. In practical terms, this approach entails avoidance of overtightening the supporting sutures between the vaginal fornices and the iliopectineal ligament at colposuspension or overtightening an interposed sling. Other approaches may be required in patients with recurrent stress incontinence.

Preceding longitudinal studies in the medium term, with preoperative and postoperative urodynamic evaluation, have demonstrated that suprapubic operations appear both to cure and cause detrusor instability with equal facility.[17,19] The predictive value of the test in the determination of postoperative detrusor instability has a sensitivity and specificity of 32% and 36%, respectively.[30] Long-term postoperative evaluation of suprapubic surgery shows that detrusor instability produced by such procedures persists and continues to cause irritating symptoms to the patient in the long term.[31] Persistent symptoms may be caused by inaccurate suprapubic surgery or overzealous approximation of the vaginal fornices to the iliopectineal ligaments. Few postoperative patients have objective evidence of bladder outflow obstruction following suprapubic surgery (reduced flow rates in association with elevated detrusor pressures). Postoperative irritating symptoms and voiding dysfunction have been described in patients with normal outflow characteristics following suprapubic surgery, suggesting another explanation for their origin.[32]

Vaginal ultrasound of the postoperative results of suprapubic surgery is a simple, noninvasive method of confirming that the objectives of the operation have been achieved. Reproducible anatomic observations in the sagittal plane are independent of bladder volume, since the vaginal fornices have been permanently fixed, preventing downward displacement of the urethrovesical junction. Accurate configurations following colposuspension show that the urethrovesical junction is not displaced downward when there is an increase in intra-abdominal pressure and absence of fixed indentations of the trigone or bladder base (Fig. 37.1).

Abnormal postoperative configurations following colposuspension may be identified by mobility of the urethrovesical junction or fixed indentations of the trigone and bladder base. Abnormal mobility of the urethrovesical junction may be seen in association with recurrent stress incontinence (RSI), whereas fixed indentations are associated with frequency–urgency syndrome, postoperative detrusor instability, or persistent stress incontinence (PSI). RSI may occur in the immediate postoperative period or be delayed until the climacteric. In both cases, excessive mobility of the urethrovesical junction (> 10 mm with a Valsalva maneuver occurs with an increase in intra-abdominal pressure. Fixed indentations of the bladder base occur if there has been inaccurate placement of the supporting sutures (and possibly excessive elevation of the vaginal fornices toward the iliopectineal ligaments). If the sutures are placed at the level of the vaginal vault, then no support is afforded to the urethrovesical junction, and the patient has PSI; suture placement beneath the trigone can result in persistent urge syndrome and postoperative detrusor instabil-

ity. These observations regarding surgical technique may explain the variable incidence of postoperative detrusor instability in several series describing the long-term results of colposuspension[17,19] and also the persistent and intractable symptoms that have been described in the medium term.[31]

SUMMARY

Contemporary investigations based on retrograde filling cystometry remain the cornerstone of urodynamic evaluation, particularly for patients with neurologic problems. Fluoroscopy of the continence mechanism during synchronous VCU may be the best investigation to confirm a diagnosis of GSI, though it is invasive, time-consuming, and has limited patient acceptance. Traditional concepts of continence based on theories of pressure transmission to an intra-abdominal urethra are under increasing scrutiny, and anatomic concepts are being re-examined. Vaginal ultrasound enables dynamic study of the effects of provocative maneuvers on continence and high-resolution views of the postoperative anatomy following suprapubic surgery. The technique is simple, noninvasive, and acceptable to patients. Further studies using biplanar and three-dimensional ultrasound techniques to examine the etiology and pathoanatomy of urinary stress incontinence and genital prolapse are anticipated.

REFERENCES

1. Green TH. Development of a plan for the diagnosis and treatment of urinary stress incontinence. Am J Obstet Gynecol 1962;83:632–648
2. Green TH. Urinary stress incontinence: differential diagnosis, pathophysiology and management. Am J Obstet Gynecol 1975;122:368–400
3. Hodgkinson CP. Relationships of the female urethra in urinary incontinence. Am J Obstet Gynecol 1953;65:560–573
4. Hodgkinson CP. Urethrocystogram: metallic bead-chain technique. Clin Obstet Gynecol 1958;1:668–677
5. Bates CP, Bradley WE, Glen E et al. First report on the standardisation of terminology of lower urinary tract function. Urinary incontinence. Procedures related to the evaluation of urinary storage: cystometry, urethral closure pressure profile, units of measurement. Br J Urol 1976;48:39–42
6. Bates CP, Glen E, Griffiths D et al. Second report on the standardisation of terminology of lower urinary tract function. Procedures related to the evaluation of micturition: flow rate, pressure measurement, symbols. Br J Urol 1977;49:207–210
7. Bates CP, Bradley WE, Glen E et al. Third report on the standardisation of terminology of lower urinary tract function. Procedures related to the evaluation of micturition: pressure–flow relationships, residual urine. Br J Urol 1980;52:348–350
8. Bates CP, Bradley WE, Glen E et al. Fourth report on the standardisation of terminology of lower urinary tract function. Terminology related to neuromuscular dysfunction of the lower urinary tract. Br J Urol 1981;52:333–335

9. Bates CP, Whiteside CG, Turner-Warwick R. Synchronous cine/pressure/flow cystourethrography with special reference to stress and urge incontinence. Br J Urol 1970;42:714–723

10. Bates CP, Corney CE. Synchronous cine-pressure-flow cystography: a method of routine urodynamic investigation. Br J Radiol 1971;44:44–50.

11. Benness CJ, Barnick CG, Cardozo L. Is there a place for routine videocystourethrography in the assessment of lower urinary tract dysfunction? Neurourol Urodynam 1989;8:291–297

12. Enhorning G. Simultaneous recording of intravesical and intraurethral pressure. Acta Chir Scand Suppl 1961;276:1–6

13. Klutke C, Golomb J, Barbaric Z, Raz S. The anatomy of stress incontinence: magnetic resonance imaging of the female bladder neck and urethra. J Urol 1990;143:563–566

14. Huddleston HT, Dunnihoo DR, Huddleston PM, 3rd Meyers PC, Sr. Magnetic resonance imaging of defects in DeLancey's vaginal support levels I, II & II. Am J Obstet Gynecol 1995;172:1778–1782

15. De Lancey JO. Structural support of the urethra as it relates to stress urinary incontinence: the hammock hypothesis. Am J Obstet Gynecol 1994;170:1713–1720

16. Burch JC. Urethrovaginal fixation to Cooper's ligament for correction of stress incontinence, cystocoele and prolapse. Am J Obstet Gynecol 1961;117:805–813

17. Cardozo LD, Stanton SL, Williams JE. Detrusor instability following surgery for genuine stress incontinence. Br J Urol 1979;51:204–207

18. Galloway NT, Davies N, Stephenson TP. The complications of colposuspension. Br J Urol 1987;60:122–124

19. Eriksen BC, Hagen B, Eik-Nes S et al. Long-term effectiveness of the Burch colposuspension in female urinary stress incontinence. Acta Obstet Gynaecol Scand 1990;69:45–50

20. Nicholls DH. Pelvic anatomy of the living. In: Nicholls DH, Ed. Vaginal Surgery. Williams & Wilkins, Baltimore, MD, 1989, pp 1–45

21. Bergman A, McKenzie CJ, Richmond J et al. Transrectal ultrasound versus cystography in the evaluation of anatomical stress urinary incontinence. BJ Urol 1988;62:228–234

22. Bhatia NN, Ostergard DR, McQuown D. Ultrasonography in urinary incontinence. Urology 1987;29:90–94

23. Brown MC, Sutherst JR, Murray A, Richmond DH. Potential use of ultrasound in place of X-ray fluoroscopy in urodynamics. Br J Urol 1985;57:88–90

24. Clark AL, Creighton SM, Pearce JM, Stanton SL. Localisation of the bladder neck by perineal ultrasound; methodology and applications. Neurourol Urodynam 1990;9:394–395

25. Creighton SM, Pearce JM, Stanton SL. Perineal video-ultrasonography in the assessment of vaginal prolapse: early observations. Br J Obstet Gynaecol 1992;99:310–313

26. Quinn MJ, Beynon J, Mortensen NJ, Smith PJ. Transvaginal endosonography: a new method to study the anatomy of the lower urinary tract in urinary stress incontinence. Br J Urol 1988;62:414–418

27. Quinn MJ, Beynon J, Mortensen NN, Smith PJB. Vaginal endosonography in the post-operative assessment of colposuspension. Br J Urol 1989;63:295–300

28. Quinn MJ, Fransworth B, Pollard W et al. Vaginal ultrasound in the diagnosis of stress incontinence: a prospective comparison to urodynamic investigations. Neurourol Urodynam 1989;8:291

29. Lyons T. Laparoscopic retropubic colposuspension. In Garry R, Reich H, Eds. Laparoscopic Hysterectomy. Blackwell Science, Cambridge, MA, 1993, pp 142–147

30. Aagard J, Bruskewitz R. Are urodynamic studies useful in the evaluation of female incontinence? A critical review of the literature. Probl Urol 1991;5:12–22

31. Steel SA, Cox C, Stanton SL. Long term follow-up of detrusor instability following the colposuspension operation. Br J Urol 1985;58:138–142

32. Webster GD, Kreder KJ. Voiding dysfunction following cysoturethropexy: its evaluation and management. J Urol 1990;144:670–673

Magnetic Resonance Imaging of the Lower Urinary Tract

MARTIN QUINN

MICHAEL W. BOURNE

Sophisticated magnetic resonance imaging (MRI) techniques have overcome many of the limitations associated with ultrasound.[1-5] Computed tomography has a limited role in the investigation of the lower urinary tract and has been superseded by MRI, which provides an important account of nulliparous anatomy without the need for cadaveric dissection.[6-10]

The original description of the anatomy of stress incontinence used indirect imaging techniques (bead-chain cystourethrography) to describe the anatomic features of increased intra-abdominal pressure, that is, posterior and inferior rotation of the urethrovesical junction.[11-14] The loss of anatomic support of the urethrovesical junction was originally termed *anatomic stress incontinence*, though the anatomic lesion could not be imaged directly.[11,12] The anatomy of genital prolapse has been similarly elusive. Vaginal delivery, hysterectomy, the menopause, and advancing age are etiologic in the development of urinary stress incontinence, though their relative contributions are unclear. Comparative studies using improved MRI will enhance our understanding of the anatomy of the lower urinary tract in vivo together with an appreciation of the anatomy of urinary stress incontinence and genital prolapse.

THE ANATOMY OF THE FEMALE CONTINENCE MECHANISM

Traditional views of female continence have depended on the "pressure transmission theory of female continence."[15] The urethra is divided into intra-abdominal and extra-abdominal portions by the pelvic floor (Fig. 38.1). Any increase in intra-abdominal pressure is transmitted to the proximal urethra contemporaneously, and continence is preserved. Unfortunately, there is no anatomic feature related to the urethra that serves this function (Figs. 38.2 and 38.3), and there are many patients with prolapse of the anterior vaginal wall who remain continent despite displacement of the urethrovesical junction. DeLancey[10] proposed the "hammock hypothesis" of fe-

male continence. The urethra is compressed against a stable layer of the anterior vaginal wall and pubocervical fascia by increased intra-abdominal pressure. Stability of the supporting layer prevents downward displacement of the urethrovesical junction and is preserved by its attachments:

1. Laterally, to the pelvic side wall by virtue of insertions into the arcus tendineus fasciae pelvis and the pubococcygeus
2. Anteriorly, to the pubis via the anterior suspensory mechanism of the vesical neck and the arcus tendineus fasciae pelvis (Fig. 38.4).
3. Posteriorly, to the uterine cervix and the uterosacral–cardinal ligament complex of endopelvic fasciae, via the pericervical connective tissue

Variations in the nomenclature have contributed to the confusion that has arisen in discussions of this topic, and therefore DeLancey's nomenclature[6] will be used here.

The bladder is lined with transitional epithelium, and its wall consists of bundles of smooth muscle (the detrusor muscle). Extensions of the detrusor contribute to the pubovesical musculature (sometimes termed *pubovesical ligaments*) and to two specialized arrangements of smooth muscle in the region of the bladder neck that are U-shaped though their function remains controversial. The musculature of the trigone forms a ring around the urethra at the level of the vesical neck (trigonal ring), and the trigonal plate is a column of smooth muscle that extends along the dorsal aspect of the urethra, leading to its characteristic "horseshoe" appearance on MRI, where the urethral musculature may be incomplete posteriorly. The innervation of the trigone is different from that of the vesical neck and may contribute to an independent function of the trigonal ring in closing the vesical neck. The *internal* urethral sphincter describes the trigonal ring of smooth muscle at the level of the vesical neck and two loops of detrusor fibers that form specialized structures in the region of the vesical neck. The *external* sphincter (striated sphincter, or rhabdosphincter) describes the striated muscle of the lower urinary tract including the circular muscle of the urethra, the

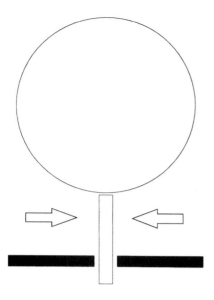

Figure 38.1 The pressure transmission hypothesis of female continence states that any increase in intra-abdominal pressure is transmitted to the intra-abdominal proximal urethra to maintain continence. There is no anatomic feature that separates the intra-abdominal urethra from the extra-abdominal urethra.

compressor urethrae, and the urethrovaginal sphincter (Fig. 38.5). The external sphincter is supplied by the pudendal nerve and is under voluntary control.

The urethra is approximately 3 cm in length and extends from the trigone to the external urethral meatus. Anatomic descriptions of the urethra and its adjacent supporting structures have been produced from serial postmortem dissection.[6–10] Some of the important features of the continence mechanism are described in stylized format in Figure 38.5. The urethra is primarily composed of an outer circular layer of striated muscle and an inner longitudinal layer of smooth muscle with an estrogen-dependent, stratified squamous epithelium that extends to the transitional epithelium of the trigone. The position of the junction between stratified squamous and transitional epithelium is variable, particularly in postmenopausal subjects. The submucosa contains a prominent, organized vascular plexus that may assist with hermetic closure of the urethral surfaces.

The anatomy of the retropubic space in a nulliparous cadaver illustrates the complex of supporting structures that comprises the anterior suspensory mechanism of the vesical neck (Fig. 38.4). This complex of structures includes a pubourethral component (sometimes termed the *pubourethral ligaments*), a pubovesical component (sometimes termed the

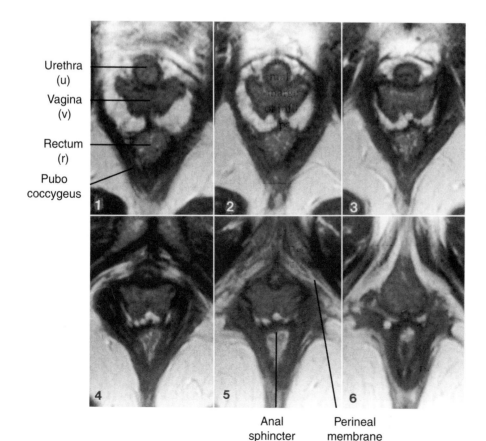

Urethra (u)

Vagina (v)

Rectum (r)

Pubo coccygeus

Anal sphincter

Perineal membrane

Figure 38.2 Serial sections of the anterior pelvis at 4-mm intervals from the vesical neck (**1**) to the perineal membrane (**5**) in a nulliparous subject. The hammock of the anterior vaginal wall provides inferior support for the proximal urethra by virtue of its lateral attachments to the arcus tendineus fasciae pelvis (**2**) and the pubococcygeus (**3 and 4**). Components of the anterior suspensory mechanism are demonstrated in Figures 1 to 4.

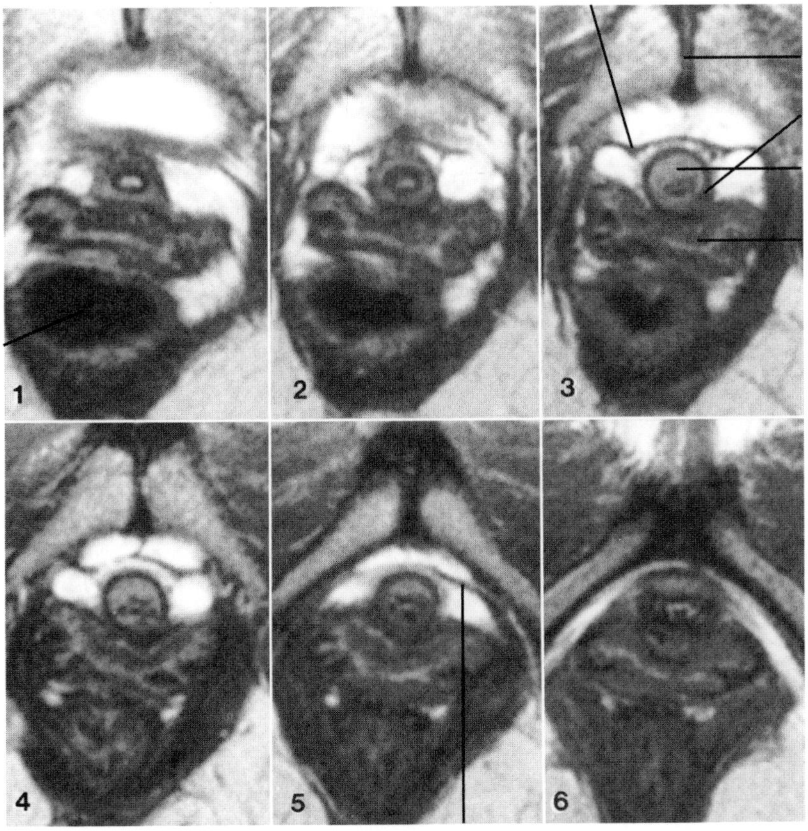

Anterior suspensory mechanism
of vesical neck (see 38.4)

Symphysis pubis (SP)

Urethra (circular striated)

Urethra (longitudinal
smooth)

Vagina

Rectum

Compressor urethrae

Figure 38.3 Serial sections of the anterior pelvis at 4-mm intervals from the vesical neck (2) to
the perineal membrane (6) in a nulliparous subject. The proximal urethra is identified by the ratio
of smooth to striated urethral muscle (3), the compressor urethrae passes anterior to the urethra
between the ischiopubic rami (5), and the urethrovaginal sphincter is a minor feature (6).

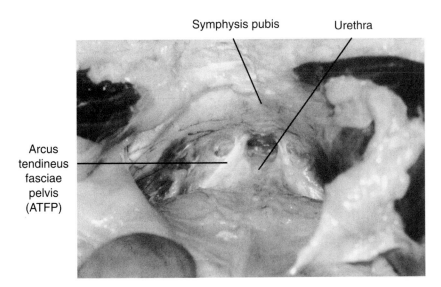

Symphysis pubis   Urethra

Arcus
tendineus
fasciae
pelvis
(ATFP)

Figure 38.4 The retropubic space of a nulliparous cadaver. The anterior suspensory mechanism of the vesical neck connects the posterior surface of the pubis, the anterior surface of
the vesical neck, the urethra, and the pubococcygeus. The pubovesical component extends
posteriorly to the ischial spines as the arcus
tendineus fasciae pelvis, otherwise known as
the white line over the obturator internus.

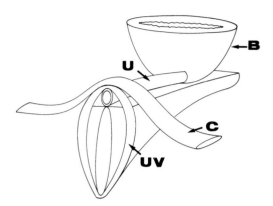

Figure 38.5 The external urethral sphincter (striated sphincter or "rhabdosphincter") comprises the outer circular layer of urethral striated muscle, the compressor urethrae, and the urethrovaginal sphincter. The compressor urethrae extends between the ischiopubic rami over the anterior surface of the distal urethra, and the urethrovaginal sphincter is a fine layer that encloses both the urethra and vagina at the level of the perineal membrane. (B, bladder; U, urethra; C, compressor urethrae; UV, uterovaginal sphincter.)

pubovesical ligaments), and its continuation as the arcus tendineus fasciae pelvis (white line over the obturator fascia). The precise function of the anterior suspensory mechanism remains speculative, though it is a substantial feature in nulliparae and seems appropriately placed to prevent downward

displacement of the urethrovesical junction during an increase in intra-abdominal pressure. Downward displacement of the urethrovesical junction will also be prevented by the hammock of the anterior vaginal wall with its lateral attachments that are demonstrated in an axial section of the proximal urethra (Fig. 38.6). The prominent feature of the nulliparous pelvis is the butterfly shape of the vagina; the anterior "wings" are maintained in position by the lateral attachments of the anterior vaginal wall to the arcus tendineus fasciae pelvis and the pubococcygeus, and the posterior wings connect to the rectum via the rectal pillars. The lateral attachments of the anterior vaginal wall form a `hammock' for the proximal urethra that prevents its downward displacement when the intra-abdominal pressure increases. There is no physical feature of the urethra dividing it into intra-abdominal and extra-abdominal portions to support the pressure transmission theory of continence.

MRI OF THE LOWER URINARY TRACT

Normal anatomy of the lower urinary tract has been defined in vivo on MRI in asymptomatic nulliparous women (Figs. 38.3 and 38.6 to 38.10). Some features of stress incontinence have been described, though controlled studies of the anatomic effect of vaginal delivery are awaited.[16–20] Serial ax-

Figure 38.6 (A & B) An axial section of the anterior pelvis at the level of the proximal urethra. The urethra, vagina, and rectum are enclosed within the sling of pubococcygeus. The anterior suspensory mechanism occupies the retropubic space and inserts between the pubococcygei anterior to the urethra. The prominent feature is the butterfly shape of the nulliparous vagina that is formed by the insertion of the anterior horns into the pubococcygei and the posterior horns into the rectum.

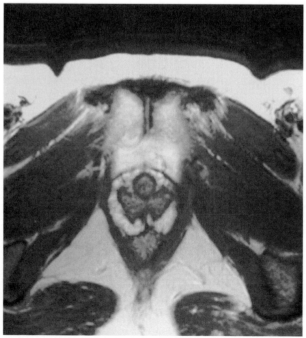

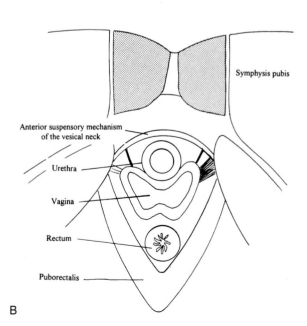

A

B

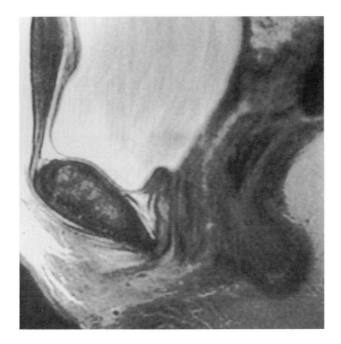

Figure 38.7 Midline sagittal section of the anterior female pelvis. The symphysis pubis is a cartilaginous joint with a pad of cartilage between the two bony surfaces. The urethral mucosa and the circular and longitudinal layers of urethral muscle are apparent. Components of the anterior suspensory mechanism are visible in the retropubic space.

Figure 38.8 Parasagittal section of the anterior pelvis 8 mm to the left of the midline. The pubis ramus is demonstrated with an outer layer of cortical bone and the pubovesical and pubourethral components of the anterior suspensory mechanism in the retropubic space.

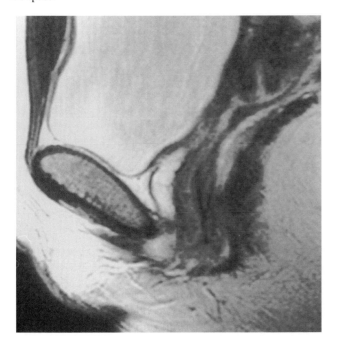

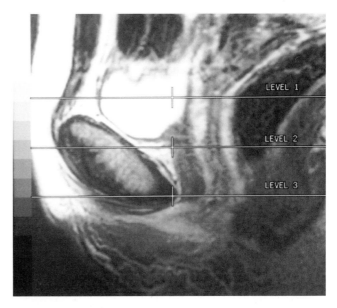

Figure 38.9 The important axial landmarks of the lower genital tract are the ischial spines (level 1), the proximal urethra (level 2), and the perineal membrane (level 3).

ial and sagittal images of 4 mm thickness show the urethra and its adjacent soft tissue and supporting structures in nulliparous subjects.

The levels of the ischial spines, the proximal urethra, and the perineal membrane are three important axial sections (Figs. 38.6 and 39.9 to 38.11). The proximal urethra is identified by the increased ratio of longitudinal smooth muscle to circular striated muscle (Fig. 38.6). The prominent soft tissue associated with the distal urethra is the perineal membrane that provides a platform for the external genitalia and serves as the distal anchor for the midline viscera (Fig. 38.11).

Figure 38.10 An axial section of the lower genital tract at the level of the ischial spines featuring the cervix and vagina. B, bladder; V, vagina; L, levator ani; R, rectum; I Sp, ischial spine. The uterosacral ligaments insert into the posterosuperior vagina.

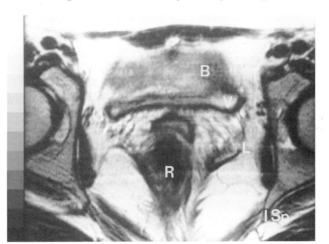

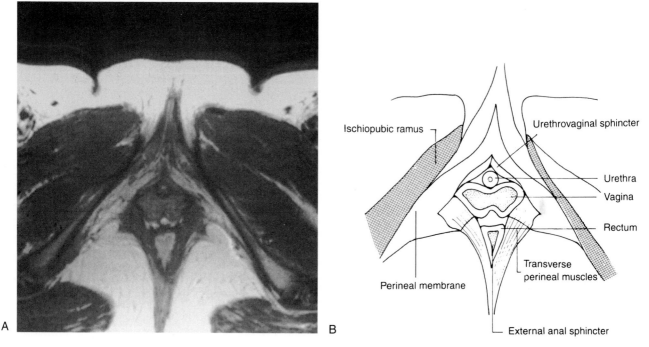

Figure 38.11 (A & B) An axial section of the anterior pelvis at the level of the perineal membrane. The urethra, vagina, and rectum penetrate the triangular perineal membrane whose posterior free edge is on each side of the rectum. The bulbocavernosi occupy the lateral edge of the perineal membrane adjacent to the ischiopubic rami. The perineal body is not a prominent feature, and the transverse perineal muscles arise from the external anal sphincter and insert into the posterior edge of the perineal membrane.

The prominent anatomic feature of the lower female pelvis is the characteristic H shape of the nulliparous vagina that is formed by the anterior attachments to the medial border of pubococcygeus and the posterior attachments to the rectum via the rectovaginal pillars. The important supports of the vagina are the cardinal ligaments at the level of the cervix at its upper extent and the perineal membrane at its lower extent. Between these attachments, it is connected to the arcus tendinei by the suburethral endopelvic fasciae and medial part of the pubococcygeus. These lateral attachments, together with the vaginolevator attachment, stabilize the anterior vaginal wall and pubocervical fascia to present a layer against which the urethra may be compressed.

The pubococcygeus provides a platform for the pelvic viscera, though it only supports the urethra indirectly by the insertion of the lateral vaginal fornices into the medial border of the muscle. MRI provides a reliable and consistent view of the levator ani at different levels, with the sling of pubococcygeus prominent in all sections of the lower pelvis. Relaxation of the pubococcygeus prior to voiding causes opening of the vesical neck and proximal urethra by virtue of the direct connection between the vagina and the proximal urethra. Contraction of the detrusor muscle and the longitudinal smooth muscle of the urethra causes bladder emptying through an open urethra. Pudendal neuropathy from vaginal delivery may disturb the function of the levator ani, and presents with altered urinary or bowel function. Previously, invasive techniques have been re-

quired to demonstrate these effects, and the literature remains controversial on their precise impact.

The perineal membrane separates the pelvic viscera from the external genitalia and extends between the medial borders of the ischiopubic rami to occupy a horizontal plane with the patient in an erect position. Direct support is provided for the distal vagina and urethra, and the posterior fibers insert into the perineal body. Both the compressor urethrae and the urethrovaginal sphincter are paraurethral structures that are composed of striated muscle and occupy a position immediately proximal to the perineal membrane. Their significance is uncertain, though they may act as secondary components in the female continence mechanism in some circumstances. Important anatomic features in the posterior compartment of the pelvis include the external anal sphincter and some striated fibers that insert into the perineal membrane. The perineal body is not a substantive feature of perineal anatomy and has a limited role in the prevention of prolapse (see Figs. 38.2 and 38.3).

The precise anatomy of the anterior suspensory mechanism (ASM) of the vesical neck has been a controversial subject for many years.[21,22] There have been few opportunities to study the retropubic space in continent nulliparous subjects, and it is rare to see significant remnants of the ASM at retropubic urethropexy, since they have been disrupted or attenuated by vaginal delivery. Anatomic features of the ASM have been awarded various terms, including the pubourethral liga-

Traditional treatment of urinary stress incontinence has depended on pelvic floor exercises or retropubic urethropexy. Objective evidence of benefit from pelvic floor exercises remains elusive. The pressure transmission hypothesis calls for elevation of the urethrovesical junction into an intra-abdominal pressure zone. In surgical terms, this translates into apposition of the iliopectineal ligaments to the vaginal fornices, though this approach may be associated with excessive rates of voiding difficulties, detrusor instability, and genital prolapse. The hammock hypothesis supports correction of the anatomy to prevent downward displacement of the urethrovesical junction with an increase in intra-abdominal pressure (Figs. 38.12 and 38.13). Randomized comparisons of these two surgical techniques have not been completed, though anatomic imaging may have a role in postoperative evaluation.

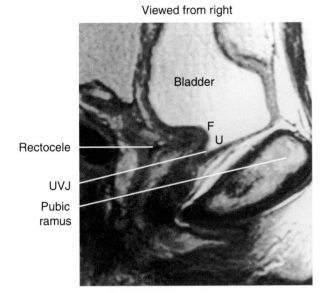

Viewed from right

Figure 38.12 Sagittal MRI of successful laparoscopic colposuspension. The vaginal fornices have been secured to the iliopectineal ligaments to support the urethrovesical junction and prevent its downward displacement with an increase in intra-abdominal pressure. The anterior vaginal wall is forked anteriorly, and the posterior vaginal wall shows a developing rectocoele following the operation.

SUMMARY

Many questions regarding the function of the female continence mechanism remain unanswered though MRI has provided new insights into the anatomy of the soft tissues. *Structure* and *function* are distinct entities, though an understanding of the anatomic features will form the basis for new hypotheses regarding the function of the female continence mechanism that can be tested in appropriate clinical

ments, pubovesical ligaments, pubovesical muscle, and urethropelvic ligaments. Parasagittal sections confirm the presence of bilateral structures arising from the anterior surface of the bladder and inserting into the posterior surface of the pubis (see Fig. 38.5). Axial sections show their close association with the proximal urethra (see Figs. 38.2 and 38.3) and the component that inserts into the medial border of pubococcygeus (Fig. 38.2). The function of the ASM is controversial, since it contains predominantly smooth muscle fibers, and when the patient is erect, the origin is above the insertion, making it unlikely that the bladder neck is suspended from the inferior border of the pubis.[8] It seems ideally placed to prevent downward displacement of the vesical neck with an increase in intra-abdominal pressure, though the anterior vaginal wall and pubococcygeus will also contribute to that function. Disruption of the ASM following traumatic vaginal delivery causes excessive mobility of the entire urethra and early onset of stress incontinence in the puerperium, though both lateral and suburethral supports may also be disrupted in such circumstances.

Occupying symmetric positions in the pelvis in similar fashion to the ASM are two additional pairs of ligaments that insert into the uterine cervix: the lateral cervical (cardinal) ligaments and the uterosacral ligaments. Removal of the cervix at hysterectomy has been associated with onset of incontinence and genital prolapse.

Figure 38.13 Axial MRI of successful laparoscopic colposuspension. The vaginal fornices have been secured to the iliopectineal ligaments (IPL) to support the urethrovesical junction (UVJ) and prevent its downward displacement with an increase in intra-abdominal pressure. There is an inflammatory response in the paravaginal space associated with the suture insertions.

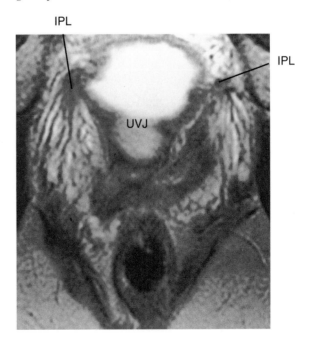

settings. One of the benefits of improved anatomic imaging may include the adoption of consistent anatomic terms enabling radiologic, gynecologic, and urologic clinicians to discuss overlapping problems using the same vocabulary. MRI has provided an important description of the soft tissue anatomy of the lower urinary tract in nulliparous women, although it may also be possible to demonstrate much of the detailed anatomy using advanced ultrasound techniques.

REFERENCES

1. Quinn MJ, Beynon J, Mortensen NJ, Smith PJ. Transvaginal endosonography: a new method to study the anatomy of the lower urinary tract in urinary stress incontinence. Br J Urol 1988;62:414–418

2. Quinn MJ, Beynon J, Mortensen NN, Smith PJB. Vaginal endosonography in the post-operative assessment of colposuspension. Br J Urol 1989;63:295–300

3. Quinn MJ, Farnsworth BA, Pollard WJ et al. Vaginal ultrasound in the diagnosis of stress incontinence: a prospective comparison to urodynamic investigation. Neurourol Urodynam 1989;8:291

4. Quinn MJ. Vaginal Ultrasound of the Lower Urinary Tract. MD thesis, University of Bristol, UK, 1994

5. Quinn MJ. The anatomy of female continence. In: O'Brien PMS, Ed. Yearbook of Obstetrics and Gynecology (vol 5). RCOG Press, 1997, pp 20–32

6. De Lancey JO. Correlative study of paraurethral anatomy. Obstet Gynecol 1986;68:91–97

7. De Lancey JO. Structural aspects of the extrinsic continence mechanism. Obstet Gynecol 1988;72:296–301

8. De Lancey JO. Pubovesical ligament: a separate structure from the urethral supports (pubourethral ligaments). Neurourol Urodynam 1989;8:53–61

9. De Lancey JO. Anatomy of the urethral sphincters and supports. In: Drife JO, Hilton P, Stanton SL, Eds. Micturition. Springer-Verlag, New York, 1990, pp 3–16

10. De Lancey JO. Structural support of the urethra as it relates to stress urinary incontinence: the hammock hypothesis. Am J Obstet Gynecol 1994;170:1713–1723

11. Green TH. Development of a plan for the diagnosis and treatment of urinary stress incontinence. Am J Obstet Gynecol 1962;83:632–648

12. Green TH. Urinary stress incontinence: differential diagnosis, pathophysiology and management. Am J Obstet Gynecol 1975;122:368–400

13. Hodgkinson CP. Relationships of the female urethra in urinary incontinence. Am J Obstet Gynecol 1953;65:560–573

14. Hodgkinson CP. Urethrocystogram: metallic bead-chain technique. Clin Obstet Gynecol 1958;1:668–677

15. Enhorning G. Simultaneous recording of intravesical and intraurethral pressure. Acta Chir Scand Suppl 1961;276:1–6

16. Klutke C, Golomb J, Barbaric Z, Raz S. The anatomy of stress incontinence: magnetic resonance imaging of the female bladder neck and urethra. J Urol 1990;143:563–566

17. Huddleston HT, Dunnihoo DR, Huddleston PM, 3rd, Meyers PC, Sr. Magnetic resonance imaging of defects in De Lancey's vaginal support levels I, II and III. Am J Obstet Gynecol 1995;172:1778–1784

18. Hricak H, Secaf E, Buckely DW et al. Female urethra: MR imaging. Radiology 1991;178:527–535

19. Kirschner-Hermanns R, Wein B, Niehaus S et al. The contribution of magnetic resonance imaging of the pelvic floor to the understanding of urinary incontinence. Br J Urol 1993;72:715–718

20. Plattner V, Leborgne J, Heloury Y et al. MRI evaluation of the levator ani muscle: anatomic correlations and practical applications. Surg Radiol Anat 1991;13:129–131

21. Zacharin RF. The suspensory mechanism of the female urethra. J Anat 1963;97:423–427

22. Zacharin RF. The anatomic supports of the female urethra. Obstet Gynecol 1968;32:754–759

39

Imaging in Gynecologic Infertility

ROBERT P.S. JANSEN

PHILIPPA A. RAMSAY

Pelvic imaging and the management of infertility are linked in several ways. An abnormality disclosed by an image of a pelvic structure can be a cause of infertility. Alternatively, an abnormal image can be a sign of a physiologic disturbance that is causing both the infertility and the image. Noninvasive imaging, especially ultrasound, can also be used to guide an endoscopic procedure for diagnosis or treatment. Finally, transvaginal sonography can be used for outpatient egg collection from the ovaries for in vitro fertilization (IVF).

This chapter will enable the ultrasonologist or radiologist to;

- acquire a working knowledge of the basis of the normal cycle control.
- understand the nature and causes of infertility.
- appreciate the underlying functional abnormalities that disrupt both fertility and imaged pelvic structure.
- appreciate which imaged pathology within the female pelvis reflects a direct cause of infertility.

ACHIEVING NORMAL PREGNANCY

For pregnancy to happen, four criteria need to be met. Sperm must reach the external cervical os; ovulation must occur; there must be no impediment to sperm and egg reaching each other in the fallopian tube; and implantation in the uterus must be permitted by both a metabolically sound pre-embryo and by a receptive endometrium. A total deficit of any of these criteria will cause *sterility*—an inability to conceive that will resist any amount of sexual intercourse. A partial abnormality within these criteria will cause a delay in conception, called *relative infertility*, or *subfertility*.

Timing of Crucial Events

Of the millions of sperm deposited in the vagina during intercourse, perhaps fewer than 200 reach the tube. There might not be more than 10 sperm in the outer part of the tube, the ampulla, at the time the egg is fertilized. We know (from scintigraphic studies using labeled albumin microspheres) that contractions of the myometrium steer sperm toward the side of ovulation,[1] in response to ipsilaterally high concentrations of ovarian steroids at midcycle.

In association with a postcoital test (a test for the presence of sperm in cervical mucus after intercourse), ultrasound can confirm that a woman is preovulatory and that the mucus is under the influence of ovarian estradiol unopposed by progesterone. A preovulatory follicle should be seen, with an endometrium that is more than 7 mm in thickness, usually with a triple-line pattern. Cervical mucus need not be identified ultrasonographically. Additional confirmation of proper midcycle timing of the test comes from serum levels of estradiol, high luteinizing hormone, and low progesterone.

At ovulation, the mature ovarian follicle discharges its contents, including the cumulus-enclosed oocyte. This is a sticky mucus-based structure several millimeters across that adheres first to the surface of the ovary then to the ciliated, fimbrial end of the fallopian tube. Within 30 minutes, the cumulus mass has been brought down the wide, thin-walled ampulla of the tube to the point where it narrows to become the thick-walled isthmus—the ampullary–isthmic junction, about two thirds of the way toward the uterus.[2] Fertilization takes place at the ampullary–isthmic junction and needs to occur within about 10 hours of ovulation for the embryo to develop normally (so it is best if sperm can reach the tube before the egg arrives).

The developing embryo (or more accurately, "pre-embryo") passes down to the endometrial cavity 3 days after ovulation and fertilization. It will soon be a *blastocyst*, a hollow ball of cells surrounding a cyst-like cavity, and consisting of a hundred or more cells. Six days after ovulation and fertilization, the blastocyst eases its way out of its surrounding zona pellucida, which by now is stretched and thinned. By this time, a few cells off to one side have become dedicated to forming the embryo; the rest of the cells (by far the majority) constitute the trophoblast and will form the placenta and supporting membranes for the pregnancy. The pre-embryo is now manufacturing human chorionic gonadotropin (hCG)—the hormone that causes the corpus luteum to persist in the ovary and to keep producing progesterone. A little later, several days before the menstrual period is missed, hCG is measurable in the blood (constituting the usual basis for testing for pregnancy).

To imagine how the blastocyst attaches to the endometrium, think of the triangular endometrial cavity as only

Table 39.1 Causes of Sterility

1. Azoospermia, a complete absence of sperm
   Diagnosis: Sperm count
2. Anovulation, especially anovulation due to ovarian follicular depletion
   Diagnosis: Persistently elevated serum follicle stimulating hormone
3. Obstruction of the female genital tract
   Diagnosis: Imaging and patency testing
4. Embryopathy and implantation failure[a]
   Diagnosis: By inference

---

[a] The pre-embryo consistently fails to display the genetic and metabolic power to implant (most commonly caused by fertilization of eggs that are past their "use-by" date: women over 40–42 years of age).

a potential space. The endometrial surfaces are in contact. The blastocyst, having shed the zona, attaches to the endometrial glycocalyx, then penetrates the surface layer to lie within the endometrial stroma. Attachment and penetration together constitute the process of implantation. Nutrition comes from secretions of the endometrial glands. The outer layer of the blastocyst, the trophoblast, is in touch with the mother's blood, so oxygen passes to the developing embryo. Sometimes as the blood first bathes the embryo (on about day 26 of the cycle), a small amount of blood leaks out of the uterus into the vagina—implantation bleeding. By day 28, a pregnancy test, set to measure hCG levels greater than 50 U in blood, will be positive. The general echogenicity of secretory phase endometrium unfortunately masks all these events ultrasonically, and positron emission tomography is required to image the implantation site within the endometrium.

The stroma of the endometrium reacts to the pregnancy and to the continued production of progesterone from the corpus luteum in the ovary by forming a thick, cell-filled, decidua (so-named because, like the leaves of a deciduous tree, it will be shed from the uterus at delivery). Ultrasonically, the decidua is a continuation of the echogenic state of secretory phase endometrium.

Infertility and Sterility

Getting pregnant is never certain. At the best of times (and perhaps at the worst of times), conception in humans is a matter of chance. When there is *sterility*, this chance of conception is zero. Sterility can have four general causes, with gynecologic imaging responsible for distinguishing these possibilities and diagnosing tubal blockage (Table 39.1).

More often, the chance is more than zero—a situation we refer to as *relative infertility*, or *subfertility*, and which is present when more than an arbitrary period, such as 12 months, has elapsed during which pregnancy has not occurred. Projecting how long it ought to take to conceive depends on compounding a statistic referred to as fecundability (f), the monthly probability of conception (in lay terms, monthly fertility). Like every statistic in biology, fecundability has a wide distribution of values (Fig. 39.1), and consequently the accumulating chance of having conceived over 12, 24, or 36 months (Fig. 39.2) will vary according to what the fecundability might be when attempting to conceive. In practice, we can establish fecundability only in retrospect: it will have a maximum practical value that is inversely proportional to the duration of the infertility, and it might be inferred to be lower still, depending on the pathology disclosed on infertility investigations. The more substantial such pathology is, the more likely it is to be the true cause of the infertility—and conversely, the more probable it is that treating the pathology will be followed by pregnancy.[3] Table 39.2 lists the abnormalities that can occur.

Investigation might reveal no abnormality: so-called unexplained infertility. Gynecologic imaging has an important role to play in making this diagnosis of exclusion. When normal experience with assisted conception procedures has taught us that subtle problems with sperm function are probable when the female is less than 38 years of age, whereas among women older than 38, embryopathy from metabolic and genetic limitations of oocytes is increasingly likely to be at fault. When no cause is found for infertility, it is the duration of infertility that is the chief prognostic determinant for conception.

Figure 39.1 Monthly probability of conception (fecundability) shows a wide normal range, with an average of 0.2 (20% per month—interrupted line). Zero fecundability is abnormal (S = sterility, accounting for about 3% to 4%). Relative infertility (RI) can arbitrarily be defined as the lower tail of the distribution. (From Jansen,[4] with permission.)

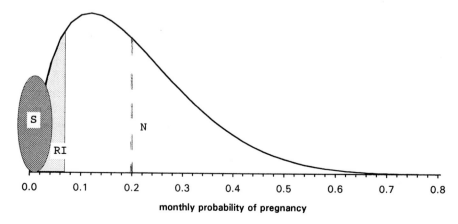

monthly probability of pregnancy

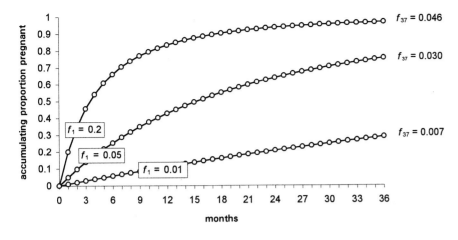

Figure 39.2 The accumulating chance of achieving pregnancy with time according to different fecundability values at commencement. Failure to conceive within 12 months is arbitrarily defined as infertility. Average fertility among couples not conceiving declines with time: residual fecundabilities after 36 months are given on the right of the figure. (From Jansen,[4] with permission.)

TREATING INFERTILITY

The last decade has seen a transformation in the physician's approach to treating infertility. The development of IVF has so improved the capacity for overcoming this disability that we have had to overhaul our ideas on the causes of infertility.[4] The more substantial the pathology, the stronger the case is for treating the pathology and expecting this pathology-based treatment to resolve the infertility. On the other hand, the weaker the pathology diagnosed—and especially in cases of unexplained infertility—the more we rely on the duration of the infertility to give a maximum estimate of the intrinsic fecundability.

Increasingly, this intervention means assisted conception with IVF or one of its related therapeutic modalities (Table 39.3). Although IVF commenced in the 1970s to circumvent inoperably damaged fallopian tubes, by the early 1980s it was found that it was just as effective with other causes of infertility.

Imaging has become inseparable from all modern assisted conception practices and has a special role in detecting pathology that might still act despite assisted conception—particularly the recognition of endometrial and ovarian pathology as well as hydrosalpinx fluid, any of which can thwart conception naturally or by IVF.

Table 39.2 Contributing Causes of Relative Infertility

1. Oligospermia and/or antibodies to sperm
2. Infrequent ovulation, including oligomenorrhea
3. Follicular phase or luteal phase defects
4. Abnormal cervix
5. Uterine cavity abnormalities, including fibroids, polyps, and adhesions
6. Partial or unilateral fallopian tube disease, including peritubal adhesions
7. Endometriosis

Table 39.3 Acronyms Used in Assisted Conception

IVF	In vitro fertilization Recovered eggs are fertilized with prepared sperm in the laboratory and transferred back to the genital tract after usually several days' culture.
GIFT	Gamete intrafallopian transfer Recovered eggs are almost immediately transferred, with prepared sperm, into the fallopian tubes, so that fertilization and early development occur in the normal situation; generally, a higher pregnancy rate than after IVF, provided the tube used is normal and normal sperm function can be assumed.
ZIFT	Zygote intrafallopian transfer IVF in which 1-day fertilized eggs, or zygotes, are transferred to the fallopian tube.
Uterine ET	Uterine embryo transfer Conventional procedure with IVF: 2-day pre-embryos are transferred through the cervix to the endometrial cavity.
FET, or FrET	Frozen embryo transfer Transfer of IVF pre-embryos previously cryostored.
TEST	Tubal embryo-stage transfer 2-day IVF pre-embryos are transferred to the tube instead of to the uterus.
ICSI	Intracytoplasmic sperm injection Laboratory refinement for IVF in cases of severely depressed sperm function, in which a single sperm is selected and microinjected into each egg.
MESA	Microepididymal sperm aspiration A means of obtaining sperm for ICSI in men with obstructive azoospermia.
TESE	Testicular sperm extraction A means of obtaining sperm cells from testicular tubules for ICSI in some men with nonobstructive azoospermia.

STRUCTURE DISRUPTING FUNCTION

Ovarian Endometriotic Cysts

"Chocolate cysts" of the ovary form the most conspicuous part of endometriosis, a benign condition in which tissue with the characteristics of endometrium grows outside the cavity of the uterus. Endometriosis rarely causes anatomic sterility but contributes chemically to infertility by shortening the survival time of sperm and perhaps by limiting the effectiveness of cumulus pickup mechanisms by the tube's fimbrial end.

Peritoneal endometriosis is almost always beyond the resolving power of ultrasound, computed tomographic scanning and magnetic resonance imaging. When endometriosis affects the ovaries, it typically begins to do so on the ovary's undersurface, with an ingrowth of endometrioid tissue that then forms a cyst.[5] Periodic stimulation by and withdrawal of the ovarian steroids estradiol and progesterone lead to growth of the cyst and to accumulation within it of old blood product. A diagnostic distinction from the varied appearances a normal corpus luteum might take is best achieved by scanning for endometriomas in the follicular phase, at or soon after completion of menstruation, when endometriomatous pathology will be most active and when there should not be a corpus luteum present.

Ovarian Endocrine Tumors

The primary sex-cord stromal ovarian tumors capable of disrupting the ovarian cycle vary in their mixture of stromal and sex-cord elements, with either element predominating and sometimes present in pure form. The age incidence of the classic varieties is shown in Figure 39.3.[6]

Normal tissues are usually more efficient in producing steroid hormones than abnormal, particularly neoplastic tissues. For example, if a preovulatory follicle has a diameter of 2 cm, one might suppose that a granulosa cell tumor would need to be several times this size to secrete a comparable amount of estrogen. A stromal tumor with clinical endocrine consequences will need to be bigger than a corpus luteum, for the same reasons. This means that the great majority of ovarian sex hormone-producing tumors cause obvious enlargement of the ovary, detectable on palpation or vaginal ultrasonography.[6] The exception is the hilus cell tumor, which is composed of differentiated Leydig or Leydig-like cells that produce close to adult male levels of testosterone without the presence of testicular tubules to push the size of the tumor to that typical of a normal testis. Hilus cell tumors, almost all of which occur after the menopause (Fig. 39.3), can be microscopically sized;[7,8] the differential diagnosis is generally a subcapsular adrenal testosterone-producing adenoma, which can be sensitive to hCG and luteinizing hormone[9,10] and which likewise can be too small to reliably detect with ultrasound, CT, or MRI. Almost alone among the steroid producing tumors, preoperative localization of hilus or adrenal Leydig-like tumors can require selective catheterization of adrenal and ovarian veins to detect the source of high testosterone production.

Congenital Anatomic Obstructions of the Genital Tract

Acquired Fallopian Tube Abnormalities: Hysterosalpingography

The hysterosalpingogram (HSG) is conventionally performed in the first 10 days of the cycle (counting the first day of menstruation as day 1), usually some days after cessation of bleeding, so that the possibility of inadvertent disruption of a pregnancy is avoided. A well-performed HSG (Fig. 39.4) is of immense value in the establishment of internal tubal normality or abnormality.[11]

When the fallopian tube is affected by salpingitis, occlusion occurs first either laterally, at the fimbrial end (distal oc-

Figure 39.3 Age distribution of ovarian sex-cord stromal tumors capable of secreting ovarian steroids that disrupt ovulation and fertility. These tumors are rare. Abbreviations: S-L: Sertoli-Leydig cell tumors; G: granulosa cell tumors; Th: thecomas; H-L: Hilus-Leydig cell tumors (From Jansen,[6] with permission.)

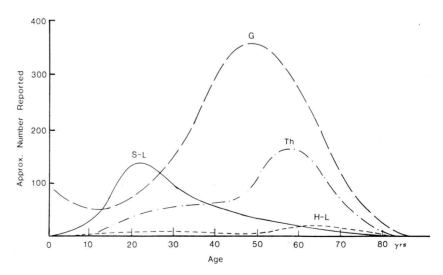

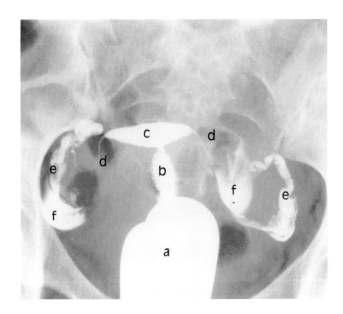

Figure 39.4 Normal HSG. Marked are (a) the speculum; (b) the endocervical canal with filling of endocervical crypts; (c) the triangular uterine cavity, with a smooth endometrial surface; (d) the fine, smooth tubal isthmic lumen; (e) the ampullary lumen, with evidence of normal longitudinal mucosal folds; and (f) spill of contrast medium among the intestines in the the peritoneal cavity. (From Jansen,[43] with permission.)

clusion, with formation of a hydrosalpinx) or medially, in the interstitial or isthmic segment (proximal occlusion). Proximal occlusion unaccompanied by the slightest sign of salpingitis isthmica nodosa can be confusing, as the differential diagnosis is a normal tube, anatomically narrow or physiologically contracted. Uterine spasm (Fig. 39.5) causes tubal spasm and risks a false diagnosis of isthmic (cornual) occlusion. This can be minimized by administration of a nonsteroidal anti-inflammatory drug 30 minutes before the HSG. More puzzling is the increase in muscular tone of the isthmus that occurs with rising estradiol as the follicular phase progresses.[2] A variety of administered agents, including intravenous glucagon[12] as well as nonsteroidal anti-inflammatory drugs have been suggested to overcome tubal spasm. A progestogen can overcome increased preovulatory isthmic contractility. In doubtful cases, selective salpingography can be used to increase pressure of the distending medium at the uterotubal junction.[13]

Short of palpating the fallopian tube, there is no more sensitive indicator of chronic salpingitis of the tubal isthmus than HSG. This is particularly so with salpingitis isthmica nodosa (SIN), in which fine diverticula are seen radiologically (Fig. 39.6A) and, after excision, histologically (Fig. 39.6B). SIN can be associated with tubal patency or with tubal obstruction. Even a single, small diverticulum in the tubal isth-

Figure 39.5 Uterotubal spasm during HSG. Note the varied size of the uterus and the absence of tubal filling. Painful cramps were experienced by the patient.

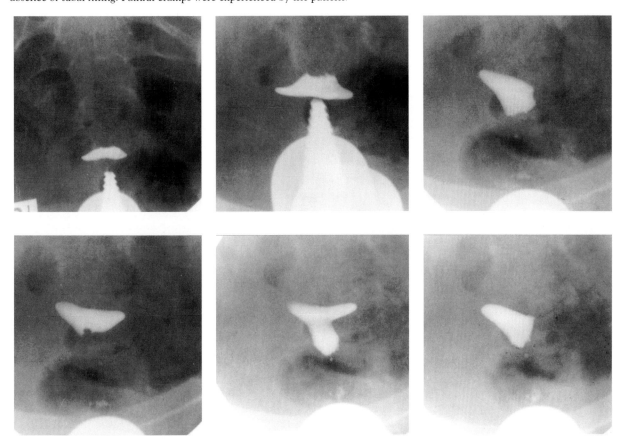

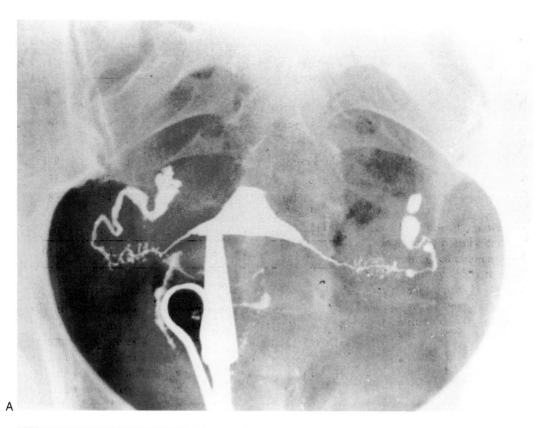

A

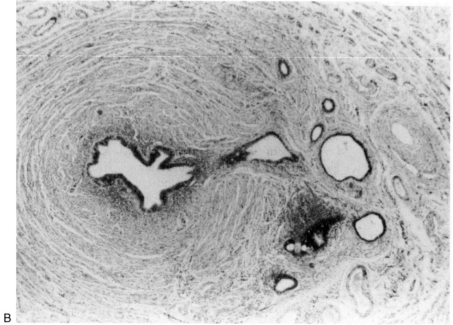

B

Figure 39.6 Salpingitis isthmica nodosa. (**A**) Diverticula on salpingography. Isthmic patency is still present. (**B**) Histologic correlation, with small accessory lumina representing the diverticula. (*Figure continues.*)

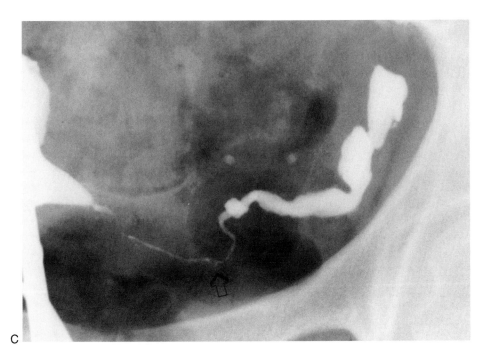

C

Figure 39.6 (*Continued*). (**C**) A single diverticulum—sufficient for diagnosing SIN.

mus (Fig. 39.6C) should be sufficient to make a confident diagnosis of SIN. (Tuberculous salpingitis, in which diverticula are typically florid and present for an extensive length of the tubes, constitutes the differential diagnosis among patients who come from countries where tuberculosis is endemic.)

In cases of hydrosalpinx (Fig. 39.7), early films exposed before the tubes are forcibly distended are useful to define the quality of the longitudinal endosalpingeal folds (in Fig. 39.7A these are seen to be partially preserved). The value of the HSG in such cases can be to forecast the degree of tubal damage and to indicate whether the hydrosalpinx might be best treated by a microsurgical salpingostomy, aimed at restoring tubal function, or by salpingectomy. Figure 39.8 reveals a hydrosalpinx with viscid contents on HSG and on ultrasound, such as might be seen with a partially resolved pyosalpinx. There is a high risk of acute salpingitis complicating salpingography in this circumstance.[14]

More direct imaging of the state of the endosalpinx can be accomplished endoscopically. Examinations of the mucosa of the fallopian tube with a 0.5-mm flexible scope passed from the uterus through the uterotubal junction is called *falloposcopy*.[15] *Salpingoscopy*[16] refers to the use of a rigid 3-mm scope passed through the abdominal wall at laparoscopy and then through the fimbrial end of the tube, if open (Fig. 39.9A), or through a slit made in the tubal wall, if a hydrosalpinx (Fig. 39.9B).[17] The value of falloposcopy and salpingoscopy in comparison with the much cheaper HSG is still to be proven. Combined forms of imaging in difficult cases can be useful.

Isolated occlusion of the tube in its midportion, near the ampullary–isthmic junction, is rare. In the absence of SIN, it most commonly results from surgery (for ectopic pregnancy or sterilization) or from endometriotic scarring and is amenable usually to microsurgical repair. In the presence of SIN, it is an indication of severe tubal damage.

Finally, there is sound evidence that an HSG performed with a fat-soluble medium is capable of improving fertility for several months afterward in cases of unexplained infertility or infertility due to endometriosis and/or oligospermia. It seems likely that it inhibits peritoneal and tubal luminal macrophages,[18] increasing sperm survival and so enhancing the chance of pregnancy.

Acquired Anatomic Obstructions of the Fallopian Tube: Ultrasound

It is uncommon to visualize the normal fallopian tube by ultrasound (except by passage of an echogenic medium such as Ecovist), but there is a particularly important exception among abnormal fallopian tubes: the hydrosalpinx.

A hydrosalpinx might be visible on ultrasound, distended with fluid, only at midcycle, under the estrogenic influence of a pre-ovulatory follicle, yet even a unilateral hydrosalpinx is capable of disrupting natural fertility and preventing the success of IVF.[19,20] The mechanism of this lies in the cyclical response of the tubal isthmus to ovarian estradiol and progesterone. Estradiol, produced by the preovulatory and ovulating follicle, stimulates both ampullary transudation of fluid and isthmic secretion of dense mucus, which with an estrogen-mediated increase in isthmic myosalpingeal tone functionally occludes the tube's communication with the cavity of the uterus.[2] Thus, the hydrosalpinx gathers fluid. With ovulation, rising progesterone secretion from the luteinizing postoperative follicle relaxes the isthmus, allowing passage of accumu-

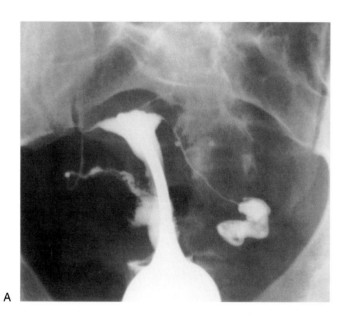

A

Figure 39.7 Distal tubal occlusion (hydrosalpinx) on salpingography. (**A**) Partial preservation of endosalpingeal folds in the ampulla. Salpingography or falloposcopy is required to resolve the severity of mucosal damage. (**B**) Loss of endosalpingeal folds (a), plus distal compartmentalization of contrast due to intraluminal adhesions (b), plus proximal SIN (c), indicative of end-to-end tubal damage.

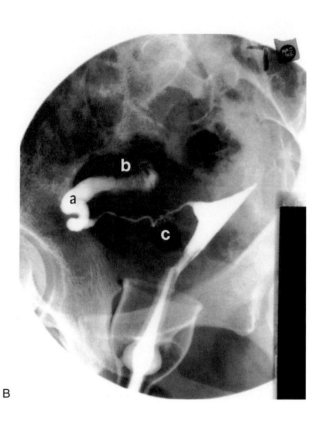

B

Figure 39.8 Possible pyosalpinx. (**A**) Salpingography reveals distal occlusion and globulization of contrast. (**B**) Sonography reveals slightly echogenic contents within the hydrosalpinx on transverse and longitudinal sections.

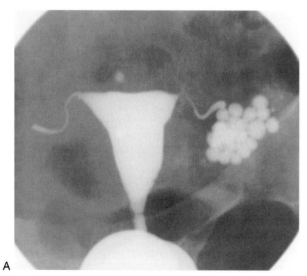

A

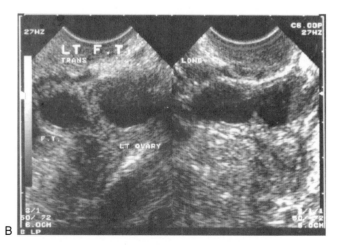

B

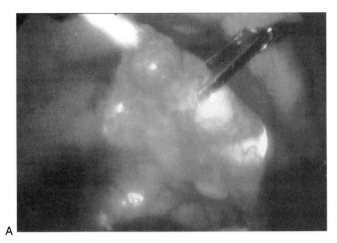

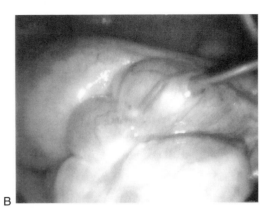

Figure 39.9 Salpingoscopy, using a 3-mm rigid endoscope. (**A**) Through the fimbrial end of an open tube. (**B**) Through the wall of a hydrosalpinx.

lated hydrosalpinx fluid down through the endometrial cavity just at the time that a normal tube allows passage of the pre-embryo to the uterus. This cascade from even just one tube is therefore likely to displace any pre-embryos that might have reached the uterus through a contralateral patent one, or through IVF and transcervical transfer. Treatment consists of salpingectomy, permanent salpingostomy, or occlusion of the abnormal tube's isthmus with a laparoscopically placed clip.

Endometrial Cavity Pathology and Implantation Failure

Three forms of endometrial pathology are of concern to the infertility specialist:

1. endometrial atrophy, either due to endometrial adhesions after trauma[21] or from chronic inflammation as in tuberculous endometritis[22] (often accompanied by amenorrhea or hypomenorrhea)

2. an endometrial space-occupying lesion such as an endometrial polyp[23] or submucous fibroid[24] (perhaps accompanied by menorrhagia, intermenstrual bleeding, or premenstrual spotting)

3. untreated endometritis (also a cause of abnormal bleeding, but often asymptomatic).[25]

Because these causes of infertility are equally applicable when IVF is used for treatment, and because they can be otherwise unsuspected, the ultrasonologist or radiologist should maintain a high level of suspicion.

Amenorrhea from traumatically induced adhesions is known as Asherman syndrome and is a cause of infertility because of both genital tract occlusion and a lack of adequate responsive endometrium for implantation. HSG is best for revealing the location of the adhesions (Fig. 39.10A), whereas ultrasound is best for indicating the amount of residual en-

dometrial mucosa (Fig. 39.10B). Pregnancy sometimes becomes established despite a very restricted amount of endometrium, as it does in the occasional pregnancy reported after endometrial ablation,[26] but with untreated intracavity adhesions, there is a high prevalence of spontaneous miscarriage and premature delivery.[27] There is also a risk of placenta accreta—a cause of potentially life-threatening postpartum hemorrhage. Pregnancy is even less likely in atrophic endometritis from chronic infections such as tuberculosis.

Nontuberculous endometritis is an enigmatic condition of uncertain persistence from one menstrual cycle to the next and often of uncertain bacterial origin.[25,28] Mycoplasmas have been implicated. The diagnosis is usually made histologically after curettage, but florid cases can present on ultrasound with a thin echogenic endometrium that does not thicken as the follicular phase advances (Fig. 39.11).

The mechanism for infertility with an endometrial polyp or with fibroids is different. Here, the mass lies within the cavity, probably preventing the anterior and posterior endometrium pressing effectively upon the hatching blastocyst. There can also be a secondary endometritis, comparable to the presence in the cavity of an intrauterine device, diagnosed at hysteroscopy, resection, and curettage.

Intrauterine adhesions and intrauterine space-occupying lesions are both well diagnosed on hysterography or on hysteroscopy, but some infertile patients starting treatment will not have had these investigations done. Ultrasound findings can be equivocal unless considered carefully in relation to endometrial appearances normal for the particular stage of the endometrial cycle. Atrophy and intrauterine adhesions might be inferred only by showing patchy endometrial development (Fig. 39.10C) despite late follicular phase activity in an ovary.

Endometrial polyps should be suspected ultrasonographically when there is focal or general echogenicity of the endometrium at times in the follicular phase of the cycle when

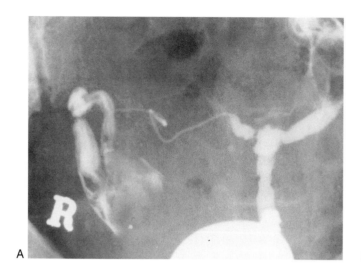

A

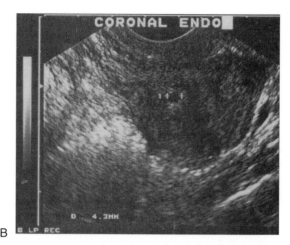

B

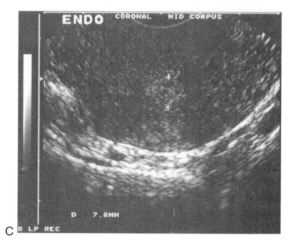

C

Figure 39.10 Endometrial atrophy in Asherman syndrome. (**A**) HSG showing extent of intrauterine adhesions. (**B**) Ultrasound revealing residual islands of endometrium. (**C**) Endometrial islands limited despite maximum exposure to estrogen.

Figure 39.11 Nontuberculous endometritis preventing pregnancy with IVF. Ultrasound shows persistence of thin echogenic endometrium despite ovarian stimulation and substantial exposure to estrogen.

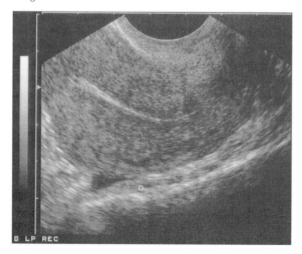

the endometrium is ordinarily relatively lucent. Figure 39.12A and 39.12B show a thickened echogenic follicular phase endometrium, with a sonohysterogram (Fig. 39.12C) clearly demonstrating a polyp—a diagnosis then confirmed at the hysteroscopy used for its resection (Fig. 39.12D).

Fibroids are usually obvious ultrasonographically even when small (Fig. 39.13), although it is only those that approach the endometrium or that substantially disrupt the myometrium (and with it the vascular supply to the endometrium) that are likely to cause infertility or spontaneous miscarriage.

Finally, most experienced infertility specialists will have come across instances of unwittingly retained intrauterine contraceptive devices causing persistent difficulty with conception. Diagnosis is usually straightforward radiologically, as they should be radio-opaque plastic, but we have seen a long-standing case no longer radio-opaque yet retaining characteristically highly reflective echoes within the endometrial cavity on ultrasound.

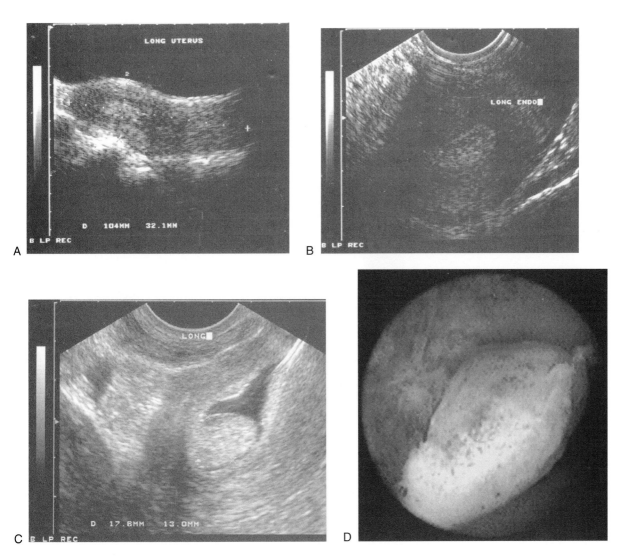

Figure 39.12 Endometrial polyp preventing pregnancy with IVF. (**A**) Nondescript echogenic endometrium on transabdominal sonographic scanning—normal for the secretory phase but abnormal (as here) in the mildfollicular phase of the ovarian cycle. (**B**) Transvaginal sonographic scanning indicates a possible endometrial polyp. (**C**) Sonohysterogram, with introduction of saline, clearly reveals the polyp. (**D**) Hysteroscopy confirms the diagnosis and permits treatment.

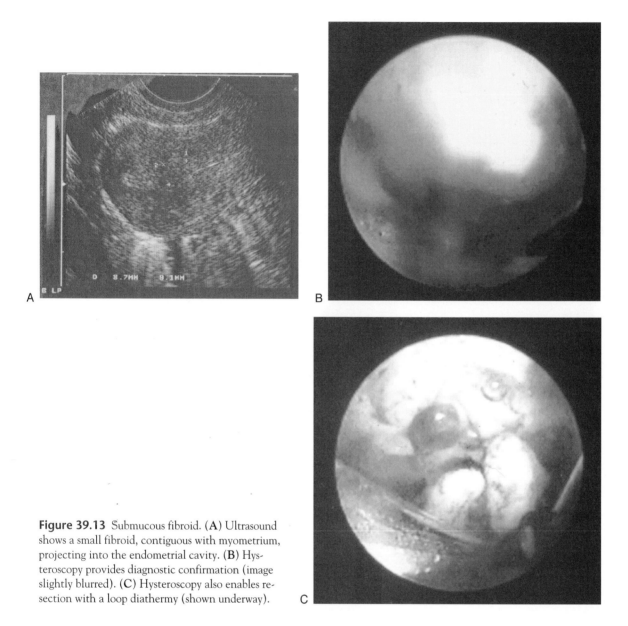

Figure 39.13 Submucous fibroid. (**A**) Ultrasound shows a small fibroid, contiguous with myometrium, projecting into the endometrial cavity. (**B**) Hysteroscopy provides diagnostic confirmation (image slightly blurred). (**C**) Hysteroscopy also enables resection with a loop diathermy (shown underway).

FUNCTION-DISRUPTING STRUCTURE

Disorders of Ovulation

Best known of the ovulatory disorders detectable ultrasonographically is the polycystic ovary syndrome.[29] Ultrasound is regarded as the most sensitive diagnostic indicator of this condition—surpassing an elevated serum luteinizing hormone/follicle stimulating hormone ratio and an elevation of serum androgens.[30–32] The typical ultrasound picture of polycystic ovaries, with cortical accumulation of mid-sized lucent follicles around an echogenic stroma and an increased ovarian volume, can be seen despite regular ovulatory cycles in some women, and even in women receiving oral contraceptives.[32] The diagnosis is an important one to make, as it predicts a susceptibility among infertile women to ovarian hy-

perstimulation syndrome should they be given gonadotropic drugs.

Distinct from polycystic ovaries are the more chaotically distributed multiple follicles seen in what has come to be called *multifollicular ovaries*.[33–36] The ovulatory pattern in these patients is often irregular, reminiscent of the postmenarcheal or premenopausal states, and premature menopause is common among these patients. Their response to ovarian stimulation for assisted conception can be unpredictable; many respond poorly. The ultrasound appearance of variably sized follicles, irregularly dispersed, and often larger than usually seen, is not always convincingly different from normal. Nonetheless, there is a continuum of such appearances with fewer and fewer follicles, still of uneven size, seen with incipient ovarian failure.

Isolated functional ovarian cysts can form as a result of failure of an estradiol-secreting follicle to ovulate (a follicular cyst), from partial luteinization of a follicle (the luteinized unruptured follicle), or from failure of a cystic corpus luteum to regress fully (a luteal cyst); each is in turn capable of temporarily disturbing the ovarian cycle. Persistence for several months is likely among cysts greater than 4 cm in diameter[37] and such cysts can be drained by ultrasound-guided transvaginal aspiration.

Endometrial Hyperplasia

In the endometrium, the chief structural consequence of disordered ovarian function is endometrial hyperplasia, with thickened, echogenic endometrium on ultrasound, complicating the unopposed estrogens produced in anovulatory states, and with a long-term risk of endometrial neoplasia.[38,39] The ultrasonologist might distinguish echogenic hyperplastic endometrium from similar-looking secretory endometrium by noting the absence of a corpus luteum on simultaneous scanning of the two ovaries. When ovulation is to be induced, it is probably important for fertility not to build on accumulated proliferative endometrium[40,41] but to cause its shedding, first by administering, and then withdrawing, a course of a progestogen, or by performing a curettage.

ULTRASOUND-ASSISTED ENDOSCOPIC IMAGING

Ultrasound is useful to guide safe placement of endoscopes for diagnosis and treatment. Laparoscopy can be hazardous after an earlier abdominal operation because intestines can be adherent to the anterior parietal peritoneum, risking bowel damage on placing the insufflation needle and trochar just below the umbilicus for passage of the laparoscope. Real-time ultrasound can confirm or exclude such adhesions by measuring the excursion of intestinal echoes with deep respiratory excursion. Free movement of intestines for 5 cm or more immediately below the umbilicus indicates conventional levels of safety.

Transabdominal, transvesical scanning of the endometrial cavity for islands of residual endometrium can be most useful in placing a hysteroscope through a badly scarred endocervical canal or among dense intrauterine adhesions in treating Asherman syndrome or recovering a lost intrauterine contraceptive device.[42]

REFERENCES

1. Kunz G, Beil D, Deininger H et al. The dynamics of rapid sperm transport through the female genital tract: evidence from vaginal sonography of uterine peristalsis and hysterosalpingoscintigraphy. Hum Reprod 1996;11:627–632

2. Jansen RPS. Endocrine response in the fallopian tube. Endocr Rev 1984;5:525–551

3. Jansen RPS. Relative infertility: modeling clinical paradoxes. Fertil Steril 1993;59:1041–1045

4. Jansen RPS. Elusive fertility: fecundability and assisted conception in perspective. Fertil Steril 1995;64:252–254

5. Brosens IA, Puttemans P, Deprest J, Rombauts L. The endometriosis cycle and its derailments. Hum Reprod 1994; 9:770–771

6. Jansen RPS. Oncological endocrinology. In: Coppleson M, Ed. Gynecologic Oncology. Fundamental Principles and Clinical Practice (2nd ed.). Churchill Livingstone, Edinburgh, 1992, pp 135–171

7. Casthely S, Diamandis HP, Pierre-Louis R. Hilar cell tumor of the ovary: diagnostic value of plasma testosterone by selective ovarian vein catheterization. Am J Obstet Gynecol 1977; 129:108–110

8. Dunnihoo DR, Grieme DL, Woolf RB. Hilar-cell tumors of the ovary. Report of 2 new cases and a review of the world literature. Obstet Gynecol 1966;27:703–713

9. Horvath E, Chalvardjian A, Kovacs K, Singer W. Leydig-like cells in the adrenals of a woman with ectopic ACTH syndrome. Hum Pathol 1980;11:284–287

10. Wong T-W, Warner NE. Ovarian thecal metaplasia in the adrenal gland. Arch Pathol 1971;92:319–328

11. Siegler AM. Hysterosalpingography. Fertil Steril 1983; 40:139–158

12. Gerlock AJ, Hooser CW. Oviduct response to glucagon during hysterosalpingography. Radiology 1976;119:727–728

13. Gleicher N, Pratt D, Parrilli M et al. Standardization of hysterosalpingography and selective salpingography: a valuable adjunct to simple opacification studies. Fertil Steril 1992;58:1136–1141

14. Pittaway DE, Winfield AC, Maxson W et al. Prevention of acute pelvic inflammatory disease after hysterosalpingography: efficacy of doxycycline prophylaxis. Am J Obstet Gynecol 1983;147:623–626

15. Kerin JF, Pearlstone AC, Williams DB et al. Falloposcopic classification and treatment of fallopian tube lumen disease. Fertil Steril 1992;57:731–741

16. Brosens I, Boeckx W, Delattin P, Puttemans P. Salpingoscopy: a new preoperative diagnostic tool in tubal infertility. Br J Obstet Gynaecol 1987;94:768–773

17. Jansen RPS. Medicine and surgery inside the fallopian tube. Med J Aust 1993;158:799–800

18. Johnson JV, Montoya IA, Olive DL. Ethiodol oil contrast medium inhibits macrophage phagocytosis and adherence by altering membrane electronegativity and microviscosity. Fertil Steril 1992;58:511–517

19. Strandell A, Waldenstrom U, Nilsson L, Hamberger L. Hydrosalpinx reduces in-vitro fertilization/embryo transfer pregnancy rates. Hum Reprod 1994;9:861–863

20. Andersen AN, Yue Z, Meng FJ, Petersen K. Low implantation rate after in-vitro fertilization in patients with hydrosalpinges diagnosed by ultrasonography. Hum Reprod 1994;9:1935–1938

21. Yaffe H, Ron M, Polishuk WZ. Amenorrhea, hypomenorrhea, and uterine fibrosis. Am J Obstet Gynecol 1978;130:599–601

22. Bazaz-Malik G, Maheshwari B, Lal N. Tuberculous endometritis: a clinicopathological study of 1000 cases. Br J Obstet Gynaecol 1983;90:84–86

23. Syrop CH, Sahakian V. Transvaginal sonographic detection of endometrial polyps with fluid contrast augmentation. Obstet Gynecol 1992;79:1041–1043

24. Buttram VCJ, Reiter RC. Uterine leiomyomata: etiology, symptomatology, and management. Fertil Steril 1981;36:433–445

25. Czernobilsky B. Endometritis and infertility. Fertil Steril 1978;30:119–130

26. Edwards A, Tippett C, Lawrence M, Tsaltas J. Pregnancy outcome following endometrial ablation. Gynaecol Endosc 1996;5:349–351

27. Jansen RPS. Spontaneous abortion incidence in the treatment of infertility. Am J Obstet Gynecol 1982;143:451–473

28. Greenwood SM, Moran JJ. Chronic endometritis: morphologic and clinical observations. Obstet Gynecol 1981;58:176–184

29. Jansen RPS. Ovulation and the polycystic ovary syndrome. Aust NZJ Obstet Gynaecol 1994;34:277–285

30. Polson DW, Wadsworth J, Aams J, Franks S. Polycystic ovaries—a common finding in normal women. Lancet 1988;i:870–872

31. Robinson S, Rodin DA, Deacon A et al. Which hormone tests for the diagnosis of polycystic ovary syndrome. Br J Obstet Gynaecol 1992;99:232–238

32. Clayton RN, Ogden V, Hodgkinson J et al. How common are polycystic ovaries in normal women and what is their significance for the fertility of the population. Clin Endocrinol 1992;37:127–134

33. Adams J, Franks S, Polson DW et al. Multifollicular ovaries: clinical and endocrine features and response to pulsatile gonadotropin releasing hormone. Lancet 1985;ii:1375–1379

34. Treasure JL, Gordon PAL, King EA et al. Cystic ovaries: a phase of anorexia nervosa. Lancet 1985;ii:1379–1382

35. Anonymous. Follicular multiplicity. Lancet 1985;ii:1404

36. Futterweit W, Yeh H-C, Mechanick JI. Multifollicular ovaries in weight-loss-related amenorrhoea. Lancet 1986;i:796

37. Zanetta G, Lissoni A, Torri V et al. Role of puncture and aspiration in expectant management of simple ovarian cysts: a randomised study. Br Med J 1996;313:1110–1113

38. Grattarola R. Misdiagnosis of endometrial adenocarcinoma in young women with polycystic ovarian disease. Am J Obstet Gynecol 1969;105:498–502

39. Fechner RE, Kaufman HK. Endometrial adenocarcinoma in Stein-Leventhal syndrome. Cancer 1974;34:444–452

40. Younis JS, Mordel N, Lewin A et al. Artificial endometrial preparation for oocyte donation: the effect of estrogen stimulation on clinical outcome. J Assist Reprod Genet 1992; 9:222–227

41. Michalas S, Loutradis D, Drakakis P et al. A flexible protocol for the induction of recipient endometrial cycles in an oocyte donation programme. Hum Reprod 1996;11:1063–1066

42. Fraser IS, Song J-Y, Jansen RPS et al. Hysteroscopic lysis of intra-uterine adhesions under ultrasound guidance. Gynaecol Endosc 1995;4:35–40

43. Jansen R, Overcoming Infertility. WH Freeman, New York, 1997

40

Color Doppler Ultrasonography in Gynecologic Infertility

CHRISTOPHER STEER

Despite improvements in fertilization rates and stimulation regimens, the probability of implantation per embryo transferred remains low in assisted conception program (10% to 15%).[1] The most promising application of color Doppler could be in this field. Changes in ovarian and uterine perfusion can be measured with color Doppler, and it may be that embryo replacement could be better timed to improve implantation rates.[2]

The probability of an embryo implanting depends on three variables: embryo transfer efficiency, embryo quality, and endometrial receptivity.[3] Endometrial receptivity is diminished in stimulated cycles and is the principal limiting step in assisting conception. Mathematically derived values, from the data of four in vitro fertilization units, expressed the importance of embryo quality and endometrial receptivity to successful implantation.[4] The contribution of embryo quality ranged from 21% to 32% and for endometrial receptivity from 31% to 64%. A noninvasive assessment of uterine receptivity might therefore be useful in deciding whether embryos should be transferred or cryostored until the uterus became more receptive.

METHODS OF ASSESSING UTERINE RECEPTIVITY

The search for an indicator of uterine receptivity has ranged from histologic dating of peri-implantation endometrial biopsies to the electrophoretic patterns of uterine secretory proteins.[5,6] Ultrasound was first used to measure the growth of follicles[7] and has since been used in assisted reproduction programs to assess endometrial characteristics. Endometrial thickness on the day before oocyte recovery may be greater in cycles that result in pregnancy.[8] A multilayered endometrial pattern, due to glandular edema, may be associated with a higher pregnancy rate.[9] Its absence could indicate suboptimal conditions for implantation.

COLOR DOPPLER OF THE UTERINE ARTERY IN THE NORMAL CYCLE

Transvaginal color Doppler can be used to obtain flow-velocity waveforms from the uterine arteries in healthy women (Plate 40.1).[10] With color, the ascending branch of the uterine artery can be located just lateral to the cervix. The times of lowest impedance to uterine flow occur at the start of rapid follicular growth 6 days before the luteinizing hormone (LH) peak and later during peak luteal function, around the time of implantation (Fig. 40.1). There is a short increase in resistance to blood flow around the LH peak plus 3 days (i.e, the time of fertilization). The peak impedance to uterine blood flow around menstruation may be part of the mechanism that regulates the breakdown of the endometrium. Similarly, the increasing impedance to uterine blood flow during the development of a preovulatory follicle may reflect the complex interorgan regulatory mechanisms, which lead to ovulation.

When flow-velocity waveforms in the midluteal phase of the menstrual cycle in women with known causes of infertility were compared with those of normal women, it was found that all categories of infertility had a different pulsatility index (PI). Figure 40.2 shows the ranges of the midluteal PIs and the percentage of women in each of the four groups of infertility who were outside the normal PI range. A possible explanation for the increased PI in patients with tubal damage or endometriosis is that the associated scarring and inflammation inhibits the increase in uterine perfusion that normally occurs in the midluteal phase. In the case of patients with anovulatory infertility, the likely explanation for the raised PI is the subnormal hormone levels on day 21 of the cycle. In patients with "unexplained" infertility, 23% had PI values outside the normal range. This suggests that decreased uterine artery perfusion might be the cause.[11]

COLOR DOPPLER OF THE UTERINE ARTERY IN ASSISTED CONCEPTION CYCLES

The effect of perfusion on uterine receptivity in women undergoing embryo transfer has been studied.[12–14] The PI was measured in 82 women during the hour before embryo transfer.[12] There was a difference in PI between those who became pregnant and those who did not (P<0.007). The PI was divided into three (low, 1.00 to 1.99; medium, 2.00 to 2.99; and high, >3.0). There was a probability of conception of 0.47

% of Maximum

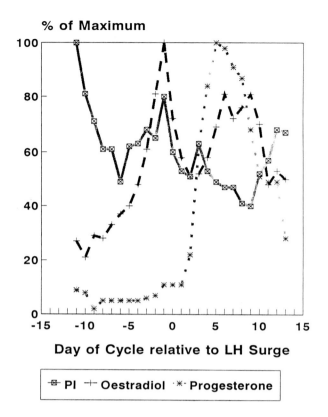

Figure 40.1 Daily changes in the pulsatility index (PI), and the concentrations of plasma estradiol and progesterone, relative to the day of peak urinary LH.

Figure 40.2 Median midluteal PI (with ranges) observed in each category of infertile women compared with fertile women. The figures indicate the proportion of infertile patients in each category with PI values outside the normal range.

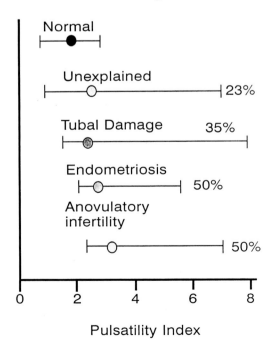

when the PI was between 2.00 and 2.99. Nineteen women (23.2%) had a PI higher than 3.00, and none became pregnant. The pregnancy rate was 44.4% in the 63 women who had a PI less than 3.00. If a PI of 3.00 was taken as the upper limit for the transfer of embryos, then the sensitivity for predicting a nonreceptive uterus was 35.2%, the specificity 100%, and the predictive value of a positive scan was 100%. The uterine arterial PI can be used to predict uterine receptivity. A mean PI higher than 3.0 before transfer would predict up to 35% of nonconception cycles.

OVARIAN COLOR DOPPLER

The preovulatory blood flow around the follicles is seen in Plate 40.2. This can be used to measure peak flow velocity, which increases before ovulation.[15] Intraovarian flow has been studied in the luteal phase of an in vitro fertilization cycle, and a correlation was found between conception and the impedance of the corpus luteal blood supply.[16] There is an increase in velocity of blood around follicles as they increase in size.[17] Little or no change in velocity occurred when the response to ovarian stimulation was poor. Thus, color Doppler might be useful to cancel poor responders or those at risk of severe hyperstimulation.

It has also been suggested that pulsed Doppler analysis of individual pre-ovulatory follicles (at the time of ovom harvest in an IVF program) may provide an indication of the potential of the enclosed oocyte to produce a pregnancy.[18]

SUMMARY

Maximum uterine receptivity occurs at a PI between 2.00 and 3.00. Transvaginal color Doppler could improve the pregnancy rate to 50% per embryo transfer. Women with optimal uterine receptivity are at high risk of multiple pregnancy after embryo transfer and may be better to have only two embryos transferred. Some form of assessment of endometrial receptivity will probably help management of assisted conception. Color Doppler should be superior to other imaging techniques, as it could be used to monitor endometrial receptivity and ovarian response.

REFERENCES

1. Edwards RG, Craft I. Development of assisted conception. Br Med Bull 1990;46:565–579
2. Fleischer AC. Ultrasound imaging-2000: assessment of utero-ovarian blood flow with transvaginal color Doppler sonography; potential clinical applications in infertility. Fertil Steril 1991;55:684–691

3. Paulson RJ, Sauer MV, Lobo RA. Factors affecting embryo implantation after human in vitro fertilization: a hypothesis. Am J Obstet Gynecol 1990;163:2020–2023

4. Rogers PA, Milne BJ, Trounson AO. A model to show human uterine receptivity and embryo viability following ovarian stimulation for in vitro fertilization. J In Vitro Fertil Embryo Transf 1986;3:93–98

5. Graf MJ, Reyniak JV, Battle-Mutter P, Laufer N. Histologic evaluation of the luteal phase in women following follicle aspiration for oocyte retrieval. Fertil Steril 1988;49:616–619

6. Beier-Hellwig K, Sterzik K, Bonn B, Beier HM. Contribution to the physiology and pathology of endometrial receptivity: the determination of protein patterns in human uterine secretions. Hum Reprod 1989;4:115–120

7. Queenan JT, O'Brien GD, Bains LM et al. Ultrasound scanning of ovaries to detect ovulation in women. Fertil Steril 1980;34:99–105

8. Gonen Y, Casper RF, Jacobson W, Blankier J. Endometrial thickness and growth during ovarian stimulation: a possible predictor of implantation in in vitro fertilization. Fertil Steril 1989;52:446–450

9. Welker BG, Gembruch U, Diedrich K et al. Transvaginal sonography of the endometrium during ovum pickup in stimulated cycles for in vitro fertilization. J Ultrasound Med 1989;8:549–553

10. Steer CV, Campbell S, Pampiglione JS et al. Transvaginal colour flow imaging of the uterine arteries during the ovarian and menstrual cycles. Hum Reprod 1990;5:391–395

11. Goswamy RK, Williams G, Steptoe PC. Decreased uterine perfusion—a cause of infertility. Hum Reprod 1988;3:955–959

12. Steer CV, Campbell S, Tan SL et al. The use of transvaginal color flow imaging after in vitro fertilization to identify optimum uterine conditions before embryo transfer. Fertil Steril 1992;57:372–376

13. Favre R, Bettahar-Lebugle K, Grange G et al. Predictive value of transvaginal uterine Doppler assessment in an in vitro fertilization program. Ultrasound Obstet Gynecol 1993;3:350

14. Strohmer H, Herczeg C, Plockinger B et al. Prognostic appraisal of success and failure in an in vitro fertilization program by transvaginal Doppler at the time of ovulation induction. Ultrasound Obstet Gynecol 1991;1:1–3

15. Collins W, Jurkovic D, Bourne T et al. Ovarian morphology, endocrine function and intra-follicular blood flow during the periovulatory period. Hum Reprod 1991;6:319–324

16. Baber RJ, McSweeney MB, Gill RW et al. Transvaginal pulsed Doppler ultrasound assessment of blood flow to the corpus luteum in IVF patients following embryo transfer. Br J Obstet Gynaecol 1988;95:1226–1230

17. Balakier H, Stronell RD. Color Doppler assessment of folliculogenesis in in vitro fertilization patients. Fertil Steril 1994;62:1211–1216

18. Van Blerkom J, Antczak M, Schrader R. The developmental potential of the human oocyte is related to the dissolved oxygen content of follicular fluid: association with vascular endothelial growth factor levels and perifollicular blood flow characteristics. Hum Reprod 1997; 12:1047–1055

Transvaginal Sonography in an Assisted Conception Program

LYNDON M. HILL

The potential for assisted reproductive technology arose when fiberoptics were introduced to the endoscope in 1954[1] and when gonadotropins were extracted from human postmenopausal urine in 1964.[2] The combination of fiberoptics and endoscopy spawned the laparoscope, which allowed oocytes to be collected under general anesthesia but without open surgery. Fertilization could be carried out in vitro and the resulting embryo returned to the cavity of the uterus. In vitro fertilization (IVF) with embryo transfer to the uterus was developed to bypass damaged fallopian tubes and resulted in the first successful IVF-assisted birth in 1978.[3] The availability of gonadotropins made it possible to stimulate the ovary to produce more than one oocyte per cycle, which increased pregnancy rates from IVF in the 1980s. The improvement in resolution that resulted when transvaginal sonography (TVS) became available in 1984 was such that it was embraced for monitoring follicle development and, with a biopsy guide, oocyte retrieval. Transvaginal oocyte retrieval does not usually require a general anesthetic. Assisted reproductive technologies have expanded rapidly in the last two decades and not only have improved the pregnancy rates with damaged fallopian tubes but have also enabled treatment of other causes of infertility.

FOLLICLE DEVELOPMENT

Sonography has become important in the monitoring of follicle development. An understanding of follicular development is, therefore, crucial for those involved with ultrasound tracking of the follicles of women undergoing assisted reproduction.

Follicle growth has been described as a continuum.[4] At 20 weeks of gestation, the female fetus has approximately 6 million germ cells. From then on, the numbers will irretrievably decrease at a rate proportional to the numbers remaining. A massive loss of germ cells between 20 weeks and birth occurs as a result of several mechanisms. Before follicle growth and atresia become common, some oocytes regress during meiosis, and those oocytes that fail to be enveloped by follicle cells undergo degeneration. By birth, all oocytes—numbering approximately 2 million—have long been enclosed in follicles. The further decrease in numbers will only occur through atresia, leaving about 300,000 by puberty (Fig. 41.1).[5] The number of follicles then declines biexponentially.[6] When just 25,000 or so are left, at an average age of 37.5 years, the rate of attrition increases by more than twofold. The follicle population falls to the menopause-linked threshold of 1,000 at a median age of 51 years.

Follicles begin to grow and then to undergo atresia in all physiologic conditions. Growth and atresia are not interrupted by pregnancy, ovulation, anovulation, or oral contraception. This applies at all ages, including infancy, until after the menopause, when the follicle numbers are eventually exhausted.

An eight-stage process for follicular growth and maturation taking 85 days has been proposed.[7] A follicle that finally ovulates has gone through the stages illustrated in Figure 41.2. According to this concept, the follicle ultimately destined to ovulate is thus one of a number whose early growth occurs over several cycles. A cohort of these is selected during the late luteal phase of the preceding cycle for further development. The follicle destined to ovulate is singled out by the end of the first week of the ovulatory cycle.

The early growth of primordial follicles is not initiated by gonadotropins, although in the absence of follicle stimulating hormone (FSH), atresia is inevitable. Further growth of the follicle takes it through the stage of a primary follicle (one layer of follicle cells) to the preantral stage of a secondary follicle. The oocyte becomes surrounded by a developing zona pellucida and by the follicle cells, which continue to proliferate. Specific FSH receptors are present on the follicle cells and, in the presence of FSH, produce estrogens from androgens, thereby creating their own estrogen environment.[8] The success of a follicle depends on this ability. Together, FSH and estrogen increase the FSH-receptor content of the follicle. Estrogen and FSH are synergistic in their ability to increase the production of follicular fluid in the intercellular spaces of the follicle. These spaces coalesce to form the antrum that characterizes the tertiary, or antral, follicle. With attainment of a diameter of a few millimeters (achieved by the

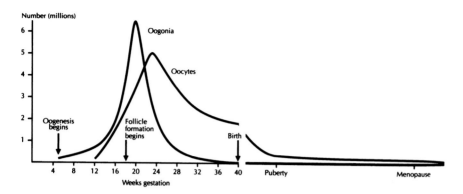

Figure 41.1 The number of available follicles by year. (From Speroff L et al.,[5] with permission.)

start of the ovulatory cycle), tertiary follicles can first be seen on ultrasound (Figs. 41.3 and 41.4). The fluid in a growing, healthy follicle is rich in estrogen, which along with FSH is required for sustained division of follicle cells. The success that a follicle has in maintaining this situation determines whether it will become the dominant (preovulatory) follicle. Estrogen has a positive effect locally on FSH action within the follicle, and has (in concert with the protein hormone inhibin) a negative effect on FSH production at the hypothalamic–pituitary level. This means that, as growth of a group of tertiary follicles takes place in the early follicular phase of the cycle, FSH production declines and support is withdrawn from the less developed follicles. This limits estrogen production in them, and results sooner or later in atresia.

This internal hormonal struggle results in one follicle (sometimes two, rarely three) achieving dominance by the end of the first week of the cycle, and the remaining follicles being suppressed and undergoing atresia.[9,10] Among the sub-

Figure 41.2 Follicular growth and development based on nonprimate and primate data. (From Speroff et al.,[100] with permission.)

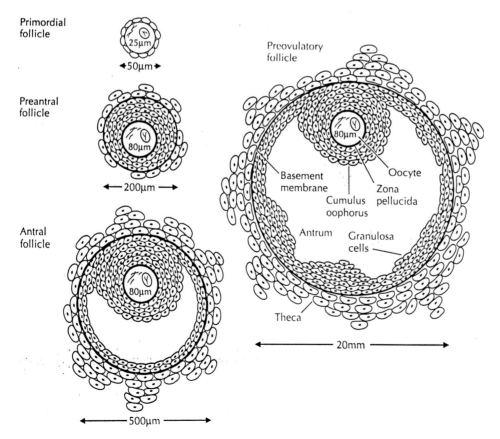

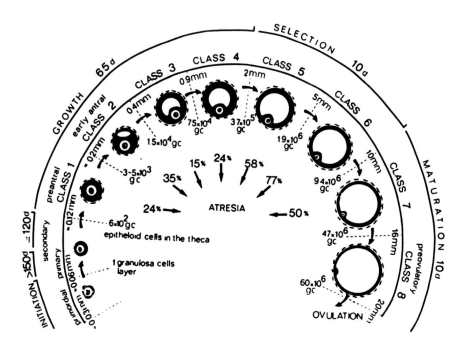

Figure 41.3 Stages of folliculogenesis in the adult human ovary and level of atresia in the eight classes of growing follicles. The granulosa cell (9c) numbers and their corresponding estimated follicle diameter indicate the limits of each class. (From Gougeon,[7] with permission.)

Figure 41.4 Stages of folliculogenesis by Gougeon. (**A**) Class 5, 3 mm. (**B**) Class 6, 6 mm. (**C**) Class 8, 19 mm. (From Gougeon.[7] With permission of Oxford University Press.) (*Figure continues.*)

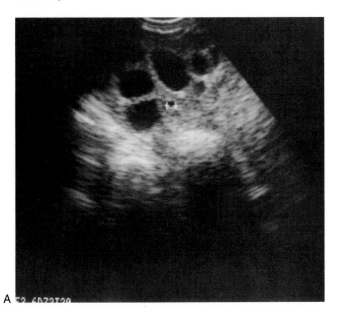

A

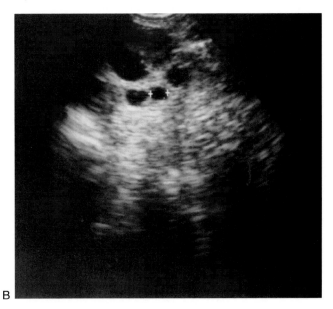

B

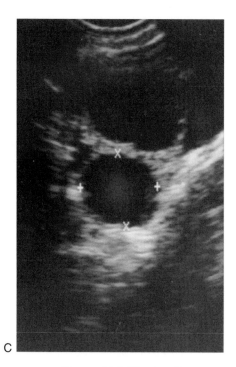

C

Figure 41.4 (*Continued*).

ordinate, nondominant follicles, the diameter of the two largest is greater than the lower-order follicles in the contralateral ovary (Fig. 41.5); it thus appears that the dominant follicle exerts a local supportive effect on the development of neighboring follicles.[10] The diameter of nondominant folli-

cles is nearly always less than 11 mm.[11] The side of ovulation in subsequent cycles is a random event that is not influenced by the location of the dominant follicle in the previous cycle.[12]

The mean follicular diameter increases by 2.5 mm per day until a mean of 2.0 cm is attained; further growth in the absence of ovulation then slows to 1.3 mm per day.[13] The highest pregnancy rates are associated with follicles that reach ovulatory size after 6 days of dominant growth.[14] Figure 41.6 illustrates the frequency distribution of the maximum follicular diameter during 158 natural cycles. The average maximum mean follicle diameter was 21.8, while the range varied between 16 and 33 mm.[15] Silverberg et al.[16] reported their experience with follicular size and the incidence of ovulation. The percentage of ovulating follicles varied from 0.5% for those smaller than 1.4 cm to 95% for those over 2.0 cm. Conception during a spontaneous cycle is at best rare if the mean measured diameter of the dominant follicle is less than 16 mm.[17]

At midcycle, when the dominant follicle is mature, a surge of luteinizing hormone (LH) from the pituitary gland initiates the process of ovulation. The presence of plasmin within the follicular fluid activates a collagenase, which weakens the wall of the follicle and leads to its physical rupture (Fig. 41.7).[18] There is considerable variation in the rate of follicular fluid evacuation[19] (Fig. 41.8). After the initial sudden loss, the remaining fluid drains at a variable rate. The time required for a follicle to evacuate completely its follicular fluid ranges from 6 seconds to more than 18 minutes[20] (Fig. 41.9).

Ultrasound Doppler studies reveal an increase in blood

Figure 41.5 The daily growth of the dominant, second-order, third-order, and fourth-order follicles in each ovary from day −4 to day 0 can be seen. The values are shown as mean ± SEM (From Kerin JF et al.,[94] with permission.)

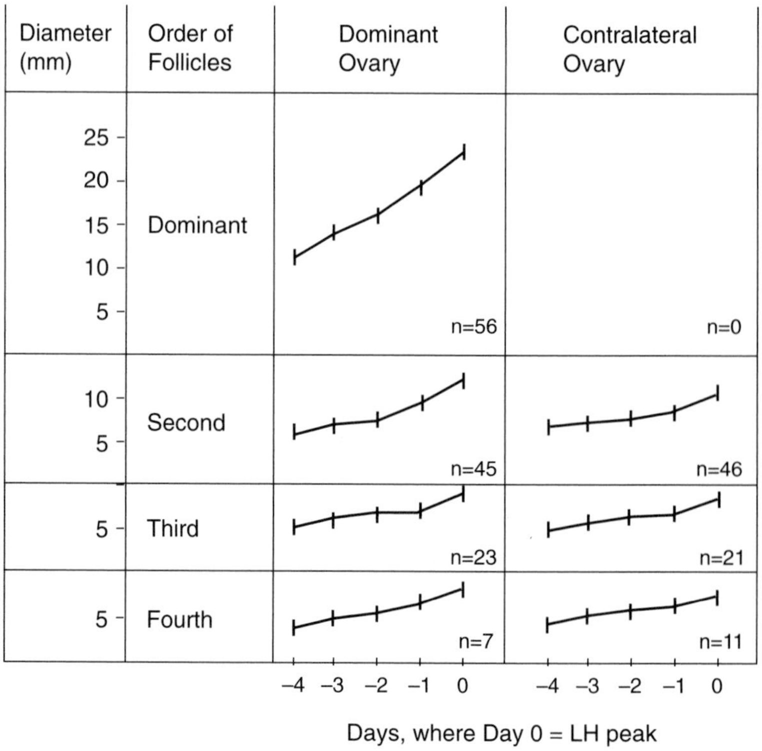

Diameter (mm)	Order of Follicles	Dominant Ovary	Contralateral Ovary
25 20 15 10 5	Dominant	n=56	n=0
10 5	Second	n=45	n=46
5	Third	n=23	n=21
5	Fourth	n=7	n=11
		−4 −3 −2 −1 0	−4 −3 −2 −1 0

Days, where Day 0 = LH peak

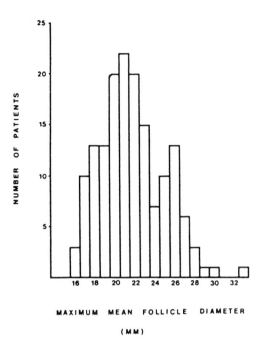

Figure 41.6 Frequency distribution of the maximum mean preovulatory follicle diameter in 158 spontaneous menstrual cycles of 158 infertility patients. (From Hamilton et al.[15] With permission of Oxford University Press.)

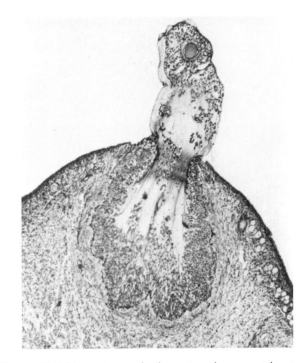

Figure 41.7 Photomicrograph of a section of an ovary taken just after rupture of a mature ovarian follicle during ovulation. The follicular cells adhering to the secondary oocyte constitute the corona radiata. (From Moore,[95] with permission.)

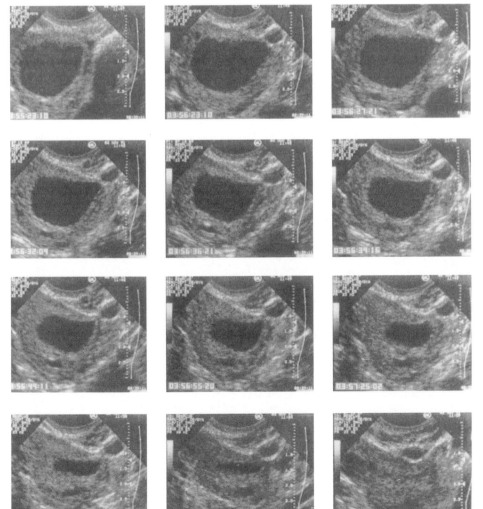

Figure 41.8 Sequence of images recorded during ovulation. This ovulation took 11 minutes from onset to complete apposition of the follicular walls. Images range from 1 minute prior to the onset, to ovulation, to complete follicular evacuation. Time-code values are visible in the left lower corner of each image, displaying hours, minutes, seconds, and video frame. (From Hanna et al.,[20] with permission.)

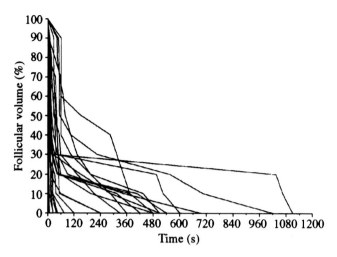

Figure 41.9 Graphic representation of the individual profiles of follicular evacuation over time for the 23 ovulations in which complete follicular evacuation was reached. All follicles displayed an initial burst of fluid, usually representing more than half their volume. (From Hanna et al.,[20] with permission.)

flow to the ovary carrying the dominant follicle (and later, the corpus luteum)—an increase that precedes other indicators of follicular dominance.[21,22] With maturation of the follicle, increased flow is directed to the follicle itself within the dominant ovary.[23] Intrafollicular neovascularization occurs over the hours preceding ovulation[24] and becomes massive after follicular collapse as blood vessels invade the luteinizing follicular (or granulosa) cells and the corpus luteum forms. The increase in blood flow to the corpus luteum is important for the delivery of steroid hormone precursors to the ovary and the release from the ovary of progesterone. A week or more into the luteal phase, there is a difference in the mean resistance index (RI) of luteal vessels among women who conceive (RI = 0.46) compared with those who do not (RI = 0.83).[23,25]

MONITORING OVARIAN RESPONSE

Baseline Ultrasound

Before commencing expensive and time-consuming IVF treatment, it is useful to carry out baseline TVS of the pelvis. This is meant to exclude pathology that might cause or contribute not just to the infertility but to a lack of success with IVF. Endometrial polyps, submucous fibroids, or hydrosalpinges can usually be diagnosed by ultrasound. Sometimes a patient starts a cycle of treatment only to discover that a misplaced intrauterine contraceptive device is still in place in the cavity of the uterus. These conditions are demonstrated in other chapters of this book. At the time of baseline ultrasound, it is also useful to establish whether the ovaries are accessible to pickup by the transvaginal route and whether the uterus is anteverted or retroverted for the embryo transfer.

Follicle Tracking

The first successful IVF cycles resulted from oocytes that were recovered in natural cycles after monitoring follicle development by measuring LH every 3 hours. Oocyte collection required a laparoscopy and therefore general anesthesia, so it became preferable to stimulate the ovaries with clomiphene citrate and/or exogenous FSH to stimulate development of more than one dominant follicle destined to ovulate. This meant that more than one embryo could be transferred, improving the pregnancy rate per cycle (Fig. 41.10). Because human chorionic gonadotropin (hCG) is biologically and chemically similar to LH, it can be given to time precisely the oocyte retrieval, provided that the endogenous surge of LH has not commenced. Ovulation occurs about 37 to 39 hours after administration of hCG, so retrieval of the oocyte is scheduled 34 to 36 hours later, to maximize the recovery of mature oocytes while minimizing the chance of losing oocytes due to completed ovulation. Now, an agonist analog of gonadotropin releasing hormone (GnRH), such as leuprolide or nafarelin, is used to suppress endogenous FSH and LH production, avoiding the LH surge and preventing it from spoiling the IVF treatment cycle because of premature ovulation.[26–28] When a GnRH agonist is used this way, the dose of FSH has to be increased to stimulate the ovaries, so the cost is increased, but this is offset by the security achieved in timing oocyte retrieval, and GnRH agonists are used by most IVF programs today.

The attainment of follicular maturity can be difficult to predict by follicle size alone. Consequently, it is usual to monitor follicular development with both ultrasound and assays of estrogens.[15,29–31] The aim of stimulation is to achieve a lead follicle of at least 1.7 cm, with at least three or four other follicles whose diameter is 1.4 cm or more, with an estradiol level of approximately 740 pmol/L (200 pg/ml) for each such follicle. Individual programs have developed their own stimulation protocols, and each has its own criteria for adequacy of follicle size and estradiol levels. When this point is reached, hCG (5,000 to 10,000 U) is administered to induce final maturation of the follicle and its oocyte by initiating the ovula-

Figure 41.10 Comparison of results from unstimulated, natural-cycle IVF[14] and stimulated IVF in the Norfolk program.[15] ART, assisted reproductive technologies; clin preg, clinical pregnancies; term preg, term pregnancies; # ova retr, ovum retrieved. (From Toner and Hodgen,[96] with permission.)

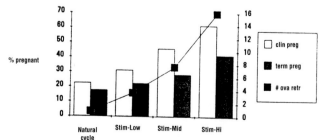

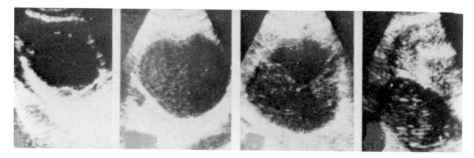

Figure 41.11 A luteinized unruptured follicle on TVS. (**A**) Mature follicle (21 to 27 mm) on day 14 of the menstrual cycle. (**B**) Luteinized unruptured follicle (29 to 39 mm) on day 16 of the cycle. (**C**) Enlarged luteinized unruptured follicle (36 to 37 mm) with intrafollicular echogenicity on day 18 of the cycle. (**D**) Reduced size of luteinized unruptured follicle (30 to 36 mm) with increasing intrafollicular echogenicity on day 22 of the cycle

tory process, with the precise time of injection being determined by subtracting 36 hours from the scheduled time of intended oocyte retrieval.

Luteinized Unruptured Follicle Syndrome

Although not directly relevant to ultrasound for IVF, it is useful to appreciate what happens to mature follicles that fail to respond fully to an endocrine signal to ovulate, whether endogenous LH or exogenous hCG. The term *luteinized unruptured follicle syndrome* was first used by Jewelewicz[32] to describe infertile women with regular menses and presumptive evidence for ovulation (i.e., evidence of subsequent progesterone production), but in whom ovum release did not occur (Fig. 41.11). It is estimated that luteinized unruptured follicles occur in approximately 5% of natural menstrual cycles.[33] Aspiration of a luteinized unruptured follicle will often retrieve a degenerate or postmature oocyte.[34]

Endometrial Response

Reports concerning endometrial thickness and the functional receptivity of the endometrium are conflicting. Some authors have found an association between an endometrial thickness of 6 mm and successful pregnancy,[35–37] while others have not found such a relationship.[38–40] Clomiphene citrate, if it has been used (now rare in IVF treatment cycles), has an antagonistic effect on the endometrium; there is an absence of diastolic flow in the uterine arteries,[41] the endometrial lining is reduced in thickness,[42] and the histology of the glands and stroma can be out of phase.[43] Ovarian stimulation with FSH thickens the endometrium in 24% of women who, during a preceding natural cycle, had a thin endometrium.[44] Ultimate endometrial thickness is otherwise not affected by the markedly elevated estradiol levels that result from induced ovulation with FSH. This suggests that the maximum endometrial response to estrogen is usually achieved during the normal menstrual cycle.[42,45]

Myometrial Contractility

The inner third of the myometrium—the layer immediately adjacent to the endometrium—exhibits wavelike contractions with a frequency of one to two per minute (Fig. 41.12).[46] This contractility can be more easily appreciated if the endometrium is recorded on videotape during TVS and then played back at a faster speed. Myometrial contractions are at their peak during the preovulatory phase of the menstrual cycle.[47] Anderson and colleagues[48] recorded endometrial motion in 378 transvaginal follicle scans on 137 women undergoing frozen embryo transfer cycles. The video recordings taken on days 5, 8, 11, 15, and 21 were assessed later by different observers who were unaware of the circumstances in which the recordings had been made. The amplitude of the contractions increased slightly from the early to the late follicular stage and then fell after ovulation until it was almost gone by the midluteal phase (Fig. 41.13). The frequency of contractions showed a similar pattern of change throughout the cycle (Fig 41.14). The direction in the follicular phase was not specific (Figs. 41.15). In the early luteal phase, the contractions were almost without exception directed toward the fundus (Figs. 41.15), presumably to ensure that the embryo, upon reaching the uterine cavity, remained in the upper part of the uterus. Implantation is less obviously affected by the direction of propagation,[46] at least as revealed by present methodology, than by the presence of myometrial motion, which seems to be crucial to success.

Ovarian Hyperstimulation Syndrome

Ovarian hyperstimulation syndrome (OHSS) occurs when there is marked enlargement of the ovaries with ascites. In more severe cases, ascites, pleural effusions, hypovolemia, oliguria, and hemoconcentration can occur, with a risk of thromboembolism. A clinical classification of OHSS[49] is shown in Table 41.1. Polycystic ovaries are predisposed to the hyperstimulated state.

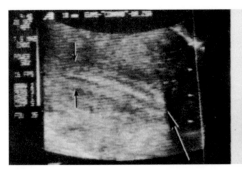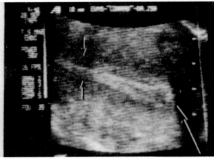

Figure 41.12 Peristaltic movements of the endometrium (midsagittal TVS). The small double arrow represents "muscular" contraction. The large arrow represents the top of the endometrial cavity. Four-second interval between Figures A and B. (From Abramowicz and Archer.[97] With permission of the American Society for Reproductive Medicine.)

TVS can detect those of patients prone to develop hyperstimulation during the follicular phase of superovulatory cycles. Tal and co-workers[50] noted an increase in hyperstimulation when three or more secondary follicles were observed before ovulation, but this state is often a goal in IVF treatment cycles. Women with more than 10 follicles between 4 and 8 mm per ovary—follicles large enough to contribute steroid and polypeptide secretory products but too small to yield oocytes usable for IVF—are at special risk for hyperstimulation.[51] Blankstein et al.[52] further refined the sonographic signs associated with OHSS; they noted an increase in intermediate follicles (9 to 15 mm) with mild hyperstimulation and a predominance of smaller follicles (under 9 mm) in women in whom severe hyperstimulation subsequently developed (Fig. 41.16). If the dose of FSH is increased during a cycle in which the ovaries are already responding, subordinate follicles are recruited, resulting in OHSS.

Rogue Ovarian Cysts at Commencement of Ovarian Stimulation

Reports are conflicting as to whether the presence of ovarian cysts during an IVF cycle impairs pregnancy rates. Such cysts are particularly prevalent (about 10% of cycles) when the GnRH agonist used to downregulate endogenous pituitary gondotropic function is commenced well before the start of the ovulatory cycle being stimulated. Some authors have reported a decreased success rate,[53] whereas others claim pregnancy rates are unaffected.[54,55] In practice, it depends on whether the cyst is functional (producing estrogen) or nonfunctional, with the latter usually being innocuous.[56] In the past, when one or more cysts 3.0 cm in diameter were discovered sonographically, the treatment cycle was delayed until they had resolved; after successfully aspirating 32 unilocular

Figure 41.13 Amplitude of subendometrial myometrium at different stages of the menstrual cycle. Amplitude was assessed as 2 if the endometrium changed greatly, 1 if it barely changed, and 0 if it did not change. Results were averaged. Observers had no knowledge of the patients. Scans were carried out on days 5 (EF, early follicular), 8 (MF, mid follicular), 11 (LF, late follicular), 15 (EL, early luteal) and 21 (ML, mid luteal). Amplitude can be seen to increase slightly toward the ovulatory phase.

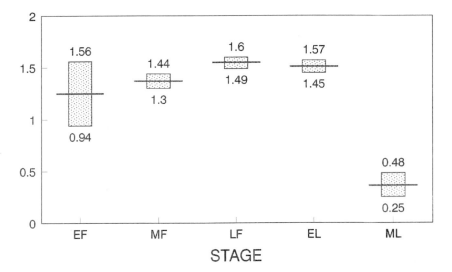

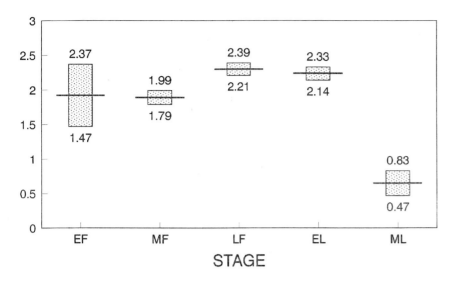

Figure 41.14 Frequency of calculations at different stages of the menstrual cycle. Frequency was calculated in waves per minute from a video that was replayed at eight times the normal speed, making observations easier.

cysts with an average diameter of 4.5 cm, Waegemakers et al.[57] concluded that ovarian cyst puncture in the early follicular phase of the menstrual cycle would diminish the cancellation rate of IVF cycles without affecting the pregnancy rate.

PROCEDURES

Transvaginal Oocyte Retrieval

Lenz and co-workers,[58] in 1982, were among the first to describe an ultrasonically guided alternative to laparoscopic oocyte retrieval for IVF, with a transabdominal–transvesical follicle aspiration procedure. In 1982 Dellenbach and colleagues[59] showed that oocytes could be collected using a transabdominal transducer to guide a needle in the vagina.

Two operators were required for this method. Transvaginal probes could be operated by one person and improved the yield from sonographically directed oocyte retrieval procedures (Table 41.2).[60–62] Either a transvaginal biopsy guide (Fig. 41.17)[62] or an automated puncture device[64] is now used to direct a 30-cm 16 or 18-gauge needle through the vaginal wall into each individual follicle (Fig. 41.18). The follicular fluid is then aspirated. If an oocyte is not obtained with aspiration, the follicle may be flushed with culture medium in order to dislodge the cumulus and oocyte from the follicle wall. Such flushing is not usually required in a properly preovulatory follicle, but the technique is necessary to secure intentionally immature oocytes from 2- to 10-mm follicles for women in the midfollicular phase of their natural cycles—an alternative to ovarian stimulation—the recovered oocytes then being matured in vitro before IVF is attempted.[65]

Figure 41.15 Direction of contractions at different stages of the menstrual cycle. Direction was nonspecific until after ovulation, when it became predominantly toward the fundus.

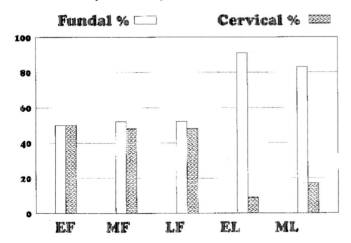

Table 41.1 Clinical Classification of OHSS

Classification	Grade	Symptoms
Mild	1	Abdominal distension
	2	Nausea, vomiting, diarrhea, ovarian enlargement <12 cm
Moderate	3	Mild + ascites evident by ultrasound
Severe	4	Moderate + hydrothorax
	5	Hemoconcentration, coagulation and electrolyte disorders, renal failure, ovarian enlargement > 12 cm

(Modified from Golan A. Ron-El R, Herman A et al. Ovarian hyperstimulation syndrome. An update review. Obstetrical and Gynecological Survey. 1989;44:430–432, with permission.)

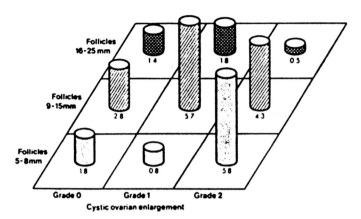

Figure 41.16 The representation of ovarian follicles on day of assumed ovulation in relation to the development of hyperstimulation. (From Blankstein et al.[52] With permission of the American Society for Reproductive Medicine.)

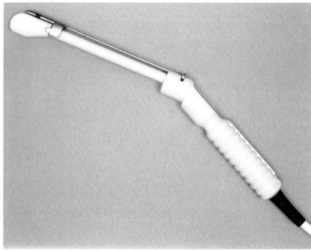

Figure 41.17 A transvaginal probe with an attached biopsy guide.

With the incorporation of ultrasound into IVF programs, the original use of laparoscopy for oocyte retrieval is restricted to laparoscopic gamete intrafallopian transfer (GIFT) treatments, during which oocyte retrieval is followed immediately by transfer of several recovered eggs together with previously prepared sperm directly into one or other fallopian tube, through its laparoscopically secured fimbrial end.[66] Even then, the oocyte retrieval part of the procedure is often undertaken transvaginally, guided by ultrasound.

Complications associated with transvaginal oocyte retrieval are infrequent. In a consecutive series of 3,656 transvaginal oocyte retrievals, Dicker and co-workers[67] reported 9 (0.24%) tubo-ovarian or pelvic abscesses and 3 patients (0.08%) with severe intra-abdominal bleeding. Abscess formation appears to be more frequent in patients with large ovarian endometriotic cysts entered during the follicle aspiration procedure.[63] Inad-

vertent puncture of a pelvic vein or adherent bowel may occur, most often without serious sequelae.[68,69]

Uterine Transfer

Transfer of early embryos to the uterus is a critical last step in the IVF treatment cycle.[70] Such embryos may be produced in the same cycle, or they may have been stored during a previous cycle of treatment. Inaccurate placement of the embryos within the uterus can lead to unsuccessful implantation. Hurely et al.[71] have used TVS guidance for intrauterine embryo transfer (Fig. 41.19). This technique not only ensures that the tip of the catheter is appropriately positioned but also assists the operator when submucous myomas or uterine anomalies make anatomically correct embryo transfer difficult.

Table 41.2 Oocyte Retrieval and Pregnancy Rates by Retrieval Method

	Combined	Laparoscopic	Transvesical	Transvaginal
No. of cycles	40	117	116	43
Mean No. of follicles aspirated	6.44	5.96	5.53	9.14
Mean No. of oocytes retrieved	3.82	4.98	3.43	5.17
Ratio of oocytes to follicles	.59	.83	.62	.56
Mean No. of embryos transferred with pregnancy resulting	1.25	3.0	2.8	3.1
Patients (%) with at least one embryo transferred	85	93.2	91	97.7
No. of cycles resulting in clinical pregnancy	4(10)	16(13.7)	24(20.7)	12(27.9)
No. of live births	3(7.5)	13(11.1)	15(12.9)	7(16.3)

Note: Percentages in parentheses.
(From Wiseman et al.,[99] with permission.)

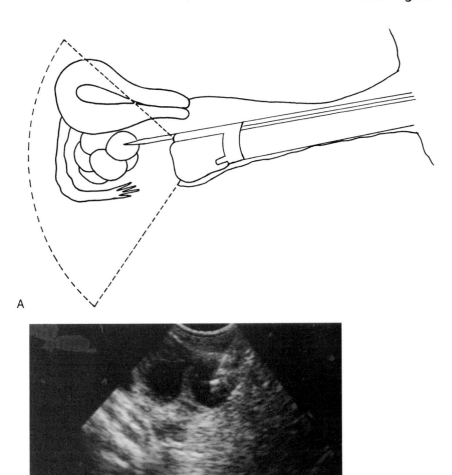

A

B

Figure 41.18 Transvaginal oocyte retrieval with TVS guidance. (**A**) Diagram illustrating the retrieval technique. (From Hill et al.,[98] with permission.) (**B**) Needle tip in a mature follicle.

Figure 41.19 Diagram illustrating intrauterine embryo transfer. Once the catheter is introduced into the cervix, the speculum is withdrawn and the transvaginal probe introduced. (From Hurley et al.[71] With permission of the American Society for Reproductive Medicine.)

Figure 41.20 Diagram illustrating TVS-guided surgical embryo transfer. (From Parsons et al.[73] With permission of the American Society for Reproductive Medicine.)

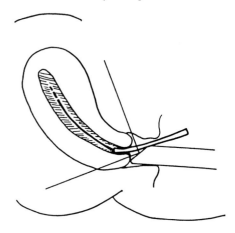

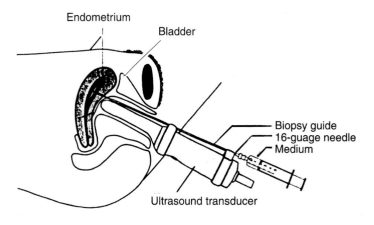

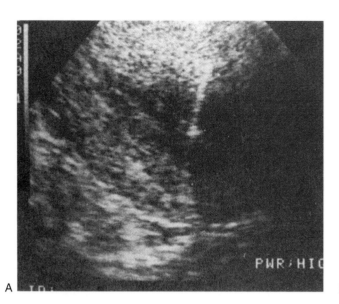
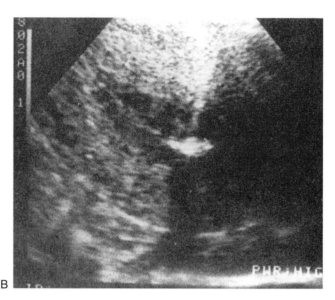

Figure 41.21 Transmyometrial embryo transfer by TVS. (**A**) Introduction of the needle through the anterior fornix of the vagina into the myometrium and endometrium. (**B**) Injection of the embryos and high-contrast media in the middle layer of the endometrium. (From Kato et al.,[74] with permission.)

Transfundal embryo transfer under transabdominal[72] or transvaginal[73,74] ultrasound has also been reported (Figs. 41.20 and 41.21). Either of these methods can be used when transfer through the cervix is not possible. Three-dimensional transvaginal scanning has recently been used to confirm the "landing site" of transferred embryos.[75]

Fallopian Tube Catheterization

Transvaginal fallopian tube catheterization has been used, not only to assess individual tubal patency,[76] but also to transfer spermatozoa, oocytes, or early embryos,[77-80] (Fig. 41.22). Both transvaginal (GIFT) and tubal embryo transfer have been performed. However, the pregnancy rates reported with transvaginal GIFT (20%) are lower than those with the la-

paroscopically directed transabdominal approach (35%).[81,82] It has been shown that the rate of injection is of major importance in determining the pregnancy rate associated with transvaginal transfer of gametes or embryos.[83] An injection rate of 50 μL/min is associated with a higher rate of peritoneal spillage,[84] with, theoretically, a wider dispersion of gametes or embryos along the fallopian tube; and with a greater risk of losing them out through the tube's fimbrial end.

SAFETY CONSIDERATIONS
Ovum Bioeffects of Ultrasound

The universal utilization of repeated ultrasound examinations to evaluate follicular development and to guide ovum re-

Figure 41.22 (**A**) A metal obturator is used to guide the cannula through the curve of the cervix into the uterus. (**B**) As the obturator is withdrawn, the cannula regains its lateral curve and is advanced to the uterotubal junction. (**C**) The catheter is passed down the cannula and through the isthmus of the fallopian tube (From Jansen and Anderson,[77] with permission of the The Lancet Ltd.)

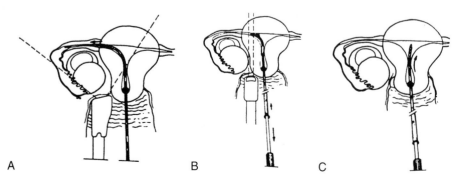

trieval has raised inevitable concerns about the bioeffects of ultrasound upon the ovum. Under normal diagnostic conditions, there have been no reports of any adverse effects of ultrasound upon human preovulatory oocytes.[85–89] There is also no evidence that the use of fertility drugs, in vitro fertilization, and embryo transfer, gamete intrafallopian transfer, or embryo cryopreservation are associated with an increased risk of congenital malformations.[90]

Ultrasound Coupling Gels

Ultrasound coupling gels have a detrimental effect on sperm motility[91] and are embryotoxic.[92,93] Hence, they should not be used during retrievals or for replacement of gametes or embryos into the uterus or fallopain tubes.

SUMMARY

TVS has a number of uses in cycles of treatment involving IVF and related forms of assisted conception. It is indispensable for monitoring of follicular growth with administration of FSH and it is usually used for aspirating follicuar fluid for oocyte retrieval. It has uses in improving the accuracy of embryo replacement into the uterus or, via the uterus, into the fallopian tubes.

REFERENCES

1. Hopkins HH, Kapany NS Letter. Nature 1954;173:39
2. Donini P, Puzzuoli D, Montezemolo R. Purification of gonadotropin from human menopausal urine. Acta Endocrinol (Kbh) 1964;45:321–328
3. Steptoe PC, Edwards RG. Birth after reimplantation of a human embryo. Lancet 1978;2:366
4. Peters H, Byskiv AG, Himelstein-Graw R, Faber M. Follicular growth: the basic event in the mouse and the human ovary. J Repord Fertil 1975;45:559
5. Speroff L, Glass RH, Kase NG. (eds) Clinical Gynecologic Endocinology and Infertility (5th ed.). Williams & Wilkins, Baltimore, MD, 1994, p 98
6. Faddy MJ, Gosden RG, Gougeon A et al. Accelerated disappearance of ovarian follicles in mid-life: implications for forecasting menopause. Hum Reprod 1992;7:1342–1346
7. Gougeon A. Dynamics of follicular growth in the human: a model from preliminary results. Hum Reprod 1986;1:81–87
8. McNatty KP, Makris A, DeGrazia C et al. The production of progesterone, androgens, and estrogens by granulosa cells, thecal tissue, and stromal tissue from human ovaries in vitro. J Clin Endocrinol Metab 1979;49:687
9. Pache TD, Wladimiroff JW, deJong FH et al. Growth patterns of nondominant ovarian follicles during the normal menstrual cycle. Fertil Steril 1990;54:638–642
10. Mendelson EB, Friedman H, Neiman HL et al. The role of imaging in infertility management. AJR Am J Roentgenol 1985;144:415–420
11. DiZerega GS, Hodgen GD. Folliculgenesis in the primate ovarian cycle. Endocr Rev 1981;2:27–49
12. Check JH, Dietterich C, Houck MA. Ipsilateral versus contralateral ovary selection of dominant follicle in succeeding follicle. Obstet Gynecol 1991;77:247–249
13. Rossavik IK, Gibbons WE. Variability of ovarian follicular growth in natural menstrual cycles. Fertil Steril 1985;44:195–199
14. Coulam CB, Bustillo M, Soenksen DM, Britten S. Ultrasonographic predictors of implantation after assisted reproduction. Fertil Steril 1994;62:1004–1010
15. Hamilton CJCM, Evers JLH, Tan FES, Hoogland HJ. The reliability of ovulation prediction by a single ultrasonographic follicle measurement. Hum Reprod 1987;2:102–107
16. Silverberg KM, Olive DL, Burns WN et al. Follicular size at the time of human chorionic gonadotropin administration predicts ovulation outcome in human menopausal gonadotropin—stimulated cycles. Fertil Steril 1991;56:296–300
17. Smith DH, Picker RH, Sinosich M, Saunders DM. Assessment of ovulation by an ultrasound and estradiol levels during spontaneous and induced cycles. Fertil Steril 1980;33:387–390
18. Bateman BG, Kolp LA, Nunley WC et al. Oocyte retention after follicle luteinization. Fertil Steril 1990;54:593–598
19. Yaron Y, Botchan A, Amit A et al. Endometrial receptivity in the light of modern assisted reproductive technologies. Fertil Steril 1994;62:225–232
20. Hanna MD, Chizen DR, Pierson RA. Characteristics of follicular evacuation during human ovulation. Ultrasound Obstet Gynecol 1994;4:488–493
21. Campbell S, Bourne TH, Waterstone J et al. Transvaginal colour blood flow imaging of the periovulatory follicle. Fertil Steril 1993;60:433–438
22. Taylor KJW, Wells PNT, Conway PI. Ultrasound Doppler flow studies of the ovarian and uterine arteries. Br J Obstet Gynaecol 1985;92:240–246
23. Deutinger J, Reinthaller A, Bernaschek G. Transvaginal pulsed doppler measurement of blood flow velocity in the ovarian arteries during cycle stimulation and after follicle puncture. Fertil Steril 1989;51:466–470
24. Collins W, Jurkovic D, Bourne T et al. Ovarian morphology, endocrine function and intra-follicular blood flow during the peri-ovulatory period. Hum Reprod 1991;6:319–324
25. Baber RJ, McSweeney MB, Gill RW et al. Transvaginal pulsed Doppler ultrasound assessment of blood flow to the corpus luteum in IVF patients following embryo transfer. Br J Obstet Gynaecol 1988;95:1226–1230
26. Thanki KH, Schmidt CL. Follicular development and oocyte maturation after stimulation with gonadotropins versus leuprolide acetate/gonadotropins during in vitro fertilization. Fertil Steril 1990;54:656–660
27. Kubik CJ, Guzick DS, Berga SL, Zeleznik AJ. Randomized prospective trial of leuprolide acetate and conventional superovulation in first cycles of in vitro fertilization and gamete intrafallopian transfer. Fertil Steril 1990;54:836–841
28. Hughes EG, Fedorkow DM, Daya S et al. The routine use of gonadotrophin-releasing hormone agonists prior to in vitro fertilization and gamete intra-fallopian transfer: a meta-analysis of randomized controlled trials. Fertil Steril 1992;58:888
29. Grinsted J, Jacobsen JD, Grinsted L et al. Prediction of ovulation. Fertil Steril 1989;52:388–393
30. Leader A, Wiseman D, Taylor PJ. The prediction of ovulation:

a comparison of the basal body temperature graph, cervical mucus score and real-time pelvic ultrasonography. Fertil Steril 1985;43:385–348

31. DeCherney AH, Laufer N. The monitoring of ovulation induction using ultrasound and estrogen. Clin Obstet Gynecol 1984;27:993–1002

32. Jewelewicz R. Management of infertility resulting from anovulation. Am J Obstet Gynecol 1975;122:909–220

33. Kerin JF, Kirby C, Morris D et al. Incidence of the luteinized unruptured follicle phenomenon in cycling women. Fertil Steril 1983;40:620–626

34. Mio Y, Toda T, Harada T, Terakawa N. Luteinized unruptured follicle in the early stages of endometriosis as a cause of unexplained infertility. Am J Obstet Gynecol 1992;167:271–273

35. Bakos O, Lundkvist O, Bergh T. Transvaginal sonographic evaluation of endometrial growth and texture in spontaneous ovulatory cycles—a descriptive study. Hum Reprod 1993;8:799–806

36. Abdalla HI, Brooks AA, Johnson MR et al. Endometrial thickness: a prediction of implantation in ovum recipients. Hum Reprod 1994;9:363–365

37. Shapiro H, Cowell C, Casper RF. The use of vaginal ultrasound for monitoring endometrial preparation in a donor oocyte program. Fertil Steril 1993;59:1055–1058

38. Welker BG, Gembruch U, Diedrich K et al. Transvaginal sonography of the endometrium during ovum pickup in stimulated cycles for in vitro fertilization. J Ultrasound Med 1989;8:549–553

39. Thickman D, Arger P, Tureck R et al. Sonographic assessment of the endometrium in patients undergoing in vitro fertilization. J Ultrasound Med 1986;5:197–201

40. Strohmer H, Obruca A, Radner KM, Feichtinger W. Relationship of the individual uterine size and the endometrial thickness in stimulated cycles. Fertil Steril 1994;61:972–975

41. Kupesic S, Kurjak A. Uterine and ovarian perfusion during the periovulatory period assessed by transvaginal color Doppler. Fertil Steril 1993;60:439–443

42. Fleischer AC, Pittaway DE, Beard LA et al. Sonographic depiction of endometrial changes occurring with ovulation induction. J Ultrasound Med 1984;3:341–346

43. Forrest TS, Elyadareni MK, Muilenburg MI et al. Cyclic endometrial changes: ultrasound assessment with histologic correlation. Radiology 1988;167:233–237

44. Sher G, Dodge S, Maassarani G et al. Management of suboptimal sonographic endometrial patterns in patients undergoing in-vitro fertilization and embryo transfer. Hum Reprod 1993;8:347–349

45. Imoedembe DAG, Shaw RW, Kirkland A, Chan R. Ultrasound measurement of endometrial thickness on different ovarian stimulation regimens during in vitro fertilization. Hum Reprod 1987;2:545–547

46. Narayan R, Gowamy R. Subendometrial–myometrial contractility in conception and nonconception embryo transfer cycles. Ultrasound Obstet Gynecol 1994;4:499–504

47. Chalubinski K, Deutinger J, Bernaschek G. Vaginosonography for recording of cycle-related myometrial contractions. Fertil Steril 1993;59:225–228

48. Anderson, JC, Ramsay, PA, Jansen, RPS. Subendometrial motility of the endometrium: its effects on embryo transfer to the uterus. Presented at the 6th World Congress on IVF, Kyoto, Japan, 1992

49. Golan A. Ron-El. R, Herman A et al. Ovarian hyperstimulation syndrome: An update review. Obstet Gynecol Surv 1989;44: 430–432

50. Tal J, Paz B, Sanberg I et al. Ultrasonographic and clinical correlates of menotropin versus sequential clomiphene citrate: menotropin therapy for induction of ovulation. Fertil Steril 1985;44:342–349

51. Ritzk B, Smitz J. Ovarian hyperstimulation syndrome after superovulation using GnRH agonists for IVF and related procedures. Hum Reprod 1992;7:320–327

52. Blankstein J, Shalev J, Saadon T et al. Ovarian hyperstimulation syndrome: prediction by number and size of preovulatory ovarian follicles. Fertil Steril 1987; 47:597–602

53. Thatcher SS, Jones E, DeCherney AH. Ovarian cysts decrease the succuss of controlled ovarian stimulation and in vitro fertilization. Fertil Steril 1989;52:812–816

54. Hornstein MD, Barbieri RL, Ravnikar V, mcShane PM. The effects of baseline ovarian cysts on the clinical response to controlled ovarian hyperstimulation in an in vitro fertilization program. Fertil Steril 1989;52:437–440

55. Goldberg JM, Miller FA, Friedman CI et al. Effect of baseline ovarian cysts on in vitro fertilization and gamete intrafallopian transfer cycles. Fertil Steril 1991;55: 319–323

56. Jenkins JM, Davies DW, Anthony F et al. The detrimental influence of functional ovarian cyst during in vitro fertilization cycles. Hum Reprod 1992;7:776–780

57. Waegemakers CT, Berg-Helder A, Blankhart A, Naaktgeboren N. Transvaginal ovarian cyst puncture in the early follicular phase of an IVF cycle, indications and results. Hum Reprod 1988;3(suppl 1):80

58. Lenz S, Lauritsen JG, Kjellow M. Collection of human oocytes for in vitro fertilization by ultrasonically guided follicular puncture. Lancet 1981;1:1163–1164

59. Dellenbach P, Nisand I, Moreau L et al. Transvaginal, sonographically controlled ovarian follicle puncture for egg retrieval. Lancet 1984;1(8392):1467

60. Levy G, Restrepo-Candelo H, Diamond M et al. Laparoscopic and transvaginal ova recovery: the effect on ova quality. Fertil Steril 1988;49:1002–1006

61. Barlow D, Bromwich P, Wiley M et al. Transvaginal compared with transvesical ultrasonography for recovery of oocytes for in vitro fertilization. Br Med J 1988;296:751

62. Wiseman D, Short WB, Pattinson HA et al. Oocyte retrieval in an in vitro fertilization–embryo transfer program: comparison of four methods. Radiology 1989; 173:88–102

63. Baber R, Porter R, Picker R et al. Transvaginal ultrasound directed ooctye collection for in vitro fertilization: successes and complications. J Ultrasound Med 1988;7:377–379

64. Kemeter P, Feichtinger W. Transvaginal oocyte retrieval using a transvaginal sector scan probe combined with an automated puncture device. Hum Reprod 1986;1:21–24

65. Trounson A, Wood C, Kausche A. In vitro maturation and the fertilization and developmental competence of oocytes recovered from untreated polycystic ovarian patients. Fertil Steril 1994;62:353–362

66. Asch RH, Elsworth IR, Balmaceda JD, Wong PC. Pregnancy after translaparoscopic gamete intrafallopian transfer. Lancet 1984;2:1034–1035

67. Dicker D, Ashkenazi J, Feldberg D et al. Severe abdominal complications after transvaginal ultrasonographically guided retrieval of oocytes for in vitro fertilization and embryo transfer. Fertil Steril 1993;59:1313–1315

68. Riddle AF, Sharma V, Mason BA et al. Two years experience of ultrasound-directed oocyte retrieval. Fertil Steril 1987; 48:454–458

69. Dellenbach P, Nisand I, Moreau L et al. Transvaginal sonographically controlled follicle puncture for oocyte retrieval. Fertil Steril 1985;44:656–662

70. Leston J, Embryo transfer. In: Trounsou A, Wood C, Eds. In Vitro Fertilization and Embryo Transfer. Churchill Livingstone, Edinburgh, 1984, p 127

71. Hurley VA, Osborn JC, Leoni MA, Leeton J. Ultrasound-guided embryo transfer: a controlled trial. Fertil Steril 1991;55:559–562

72. Lenz S, Leeton J. Evaluating the possibility of uterine transfer by ultrasonically guided transabdominal puncture. J In Vitro Fertil Embryo Transf 1987;4:18–22

73. Parsons JH, Bolton VN, Wilson L, Campbell S. Pregnancies following in vitro fertilization and ultrasound-directed surgical embryo transfer by periurethral and transvaginal techniques. Fertil Steril 1987;48:691–694

74. Kato O, Takatsuka R, Asch RH. Transvaginal-transmyometrial embryo transfer: the Towako method; experience of 104 cases. Fertil Steril 1993;59:51–53

75. Feichtinger W. Transvaginal three-dimensional imaging. Ultrasound Obstet Gynecol 1993;3:375–378

76. Kumpe DA, Zwerdlinger SC, Rothbarth LJ et al. Proximal fallopian tube occlusion: diagnosis and treatment with transcervical fallopian tube catheterization. Radiology 1990; 177:183–187

77. Jansen RPS, Anderson JC. Catheterisation of the fallopian tubes from the vagina. Lancet 1987;2:309–310

78. Jansen RPS, Anderson JC, Radonic I et al. Pregnancies after ultrasound-guided fallopian insemination with cryostored donor semen. Fertil Steril 1988;49:920–922

79. Jansen RPS, Anderson JC, Sutherland PD. Nonoperative embryo transfer to the fallopian tube. N Engl J Med 1988;319:288–291

80. Schodtes MCW, Roozenburg BJ, Alberda A, Zeilmaker GH. Transcervical intrafallopian transfer of zygotes. Fertil Steril 1990;54:283–286

81. Strowitzki T, Korrell M, Seehaus D, Hepp H. "Blind" transvaginal gamete intra-fallopian transfer in distal tubal and peritubal pathology: an evaluation in respect to the laparoscopic approach. Hum Reprod 1993;8: 1703–1707

82. Jansen RPS, Anderson JC. Transvaginal versus laparoscopic gamete intrafallopian transfer: a case control retrospective comparison. Fertil Steril 1993;59:836–840

83. Woolcott R, Stranger J, Cohen R, Silber S. Refinements in the methodology of injection for transvaginal gamete intra-fallopian transfer. Hum Repord 1994;9:1466–1468

84. Woolcott R, Stranger J. The fluid dynamics of injection: variables as they relate to transvaginal gamete intra-fallopian transfer and tubal embryo transfer. Hum Reprod 1994; 9:1670–1672

85. American Institute of Ultrasound in Medicine. Safety Considerations for Diagnostic Ultrasound. AIUM publication No. 316. American Institute of Ultrasound in Medicine, Bioeffects Committee, Bethesda, MD, 1984, pp 1–15

86. Demoulin A, Bologne R, Hustin J, Lambotte R. Is ultrasound monitoring of follicular growth harmless? Ann NY Acad Sci 1985;442:146–152

87. Lenz S, Lindenberg S, Fehilly C, Petersen K. Are ultrasonic-guided follicular aspiration and flushing safe for the oocyte? J In Vitro Fertil Embryo Transf 1987;4:159–161

88. Daya S, Wakland M, Nilssan L, Enk L. Fertilization and embryo development of oocyte obtained transvaginally under ultrasound guidance. J In Vitro Fertil Embryo Transf 1987; 4:338–342

89. Williams SR, Rothchild I, Wesolowski D et al. Does exposure of preovulatory oocytes to ultrasonic radiation affect reproductive performance? J In Vitro Fertil Embryo Transf 1986; 5:18–21

90. Shoham Z, Zosmer A, Insler V. Early miscarriage and fetal malformations after induction of ovulation (by clomiphere citrate and/or human menotropins), in vitro fertilization, and gamete intrafallopian transfer. Fertil Steril 1991;55:1–11

91. Schwimer SR, Rothman CM, Lebovic J, Dye DM. The effect of ultrasound coupling gels on sperm motility in vitro. Fertil Steril 1984;42:946–947

92. Sheean LA, Goldfarb JJ, Kiwi R, Utian WH. Arrest of embryo development by ultrasound coupling gels. Fertil Steril 1986;45:568–571

93. Carver-Ward JA, DeVol EB, Evers JLH. A method to prevent arrest of embryo development by ultrasound coupling gels after transvaginal ultrasound-guided oocyte retrieval. Hum Reprod 1987;2:611–614

94. Kerin JF et al. Morphological and functional relations of Graafian follicle growth to ovulation in women using ultrasonic, laparoscopic and biochemical measurements. Br J Obstet Gynaecol 1981;88:81–90

95. Moore KL. The Developing Human. Clinically Oriented Embryology (4th ed.). WB Saunders, Philadelphia, 1988, p. 25

96. Toner J, Hodgen GD. Future development in reproductive biology. In: Behrman SJ, Patton GW, Holtz G, Eds. Progress in Infertility (4th ed.). Little, Brown, Boston, 1990, pp 3

97. Abramowicz JS, Archer DF. Uterine endometrial peristalsis–a transvaginal ultrasound study. Fertil Steril 1990;54:451–454

98. Hill LM, Nyberg DA. Transvaginal sonography–guided procedures. In: Nyberg DA, Hill LM, Böhm-Velez M, Mendelson EB, Eds. Mosby-Yearbook, St. Louis, 1992

99. Wiseman DA, Short WB, Pattinson HA et al. Oocyte retrieval in an in vitro fertilization—embryo transfer program: comparison of four methods. Radiology 1989:173:88–102

100. Speroff L, Glass RH, Kase NG. Regulation of the Menstrual Cycle. In: Speroff L, Glass RH, Kase NG, (eds). Clinical Gynecologic Endocrinology and Infertility (5th ed.) William & Wilkins, Baltimore 1994, p. 185

Interventional Radiology in Gynecology

RICHARD WAUGH

Interventional radiology has gained wide acceptance since its emergence in the mid 1970s. Tremendous advances have been made in radiographic fluoroscopy, ultrasound, computed tomography allowing precise placement of needles and catheters into selected areas of the body. Training programs for interventional radiologists are available in most countries, and dedicated angiographic suites are now available with full resuscitative facilities and trained staff. Most interventional procedures are performed under local anesthesia aided by intravenous drugs for sedation such as medazalam and narcotics for pain relief. All patients are monitored with a pulse oximeter, and cardiac monitoring is available when required.

Great advances have also been made in the design of equipment used to perform interventional radiology including very flexible hydrophilic guidewires, small catheters with good torque control withstanding high injection pressures, and a large array of drainage catheters, biopsy needles, and embolic equipment including detachable balloons and stainless steel coils to occlude blood vessels.

Many interventional procedures now have replaced conventional surgical operations, and these have become well established in the treatment of many illnesses.

Interventional radiology has low complication rates, although major complications can occur with the more complex procedures. In general, the patient's in-hospital stay is shorter than with alternative surgical methods, and the cost is less than surgery, although the cost of consumables has risen dramatically in the last few years. Guidewires and catheters can cost up to $100 each, dilatation balloon catheters are in the order of several hundred dollars, and implants such as inferior vena cava (IVC) and intravascular stents usually cost several thousand dollars.

The main procedures relevant to gynecology follow:

1. Fine needle aspiration biopsy and core biopsy of lesions in the pelvis
2. Drainage of collections and abscesses
3. Percutaneous nephrostomy and internal ureteric stenting
4. Inferior vena caval filters and investigation of deep venous thrombosis
5. Fallopian tube recanalization
6. Thrombose the arteriovenous (A-V) malformations and bleeding vessels in the pelvis

FINE NEEDLE ASPIRATION BIOPSY

The most common indication for fine needle aspiration biopsy is to confirm malignant disease related to a mass seen on ultrasound or CT. Percutaneous aspiration biopsy can be performed in any region of the body, but pelvic masses, para-aortic lymphadenopathy, liver, and lung lesions are the most common sites related to gynecologic malignances.

Most procedures are performed under ultrasound or fluoroscopy guidance, which are quicker than under CT guidance. A 22- or 23-gauge needle is usually used to obtain tissue for cytologic evaluation. Rapid staining allows the material to be examined within minutes, and further passes can be made if the tissue is undiagnostic or if tissue is required for special stains or electronmicroscopy. Improvements in Trucut needles allow a rapid-fire action automated handle to be attached to needles, varying from 22 to 14 gauge to obtain tissue for histologic evaluation. The success rate of obtaining tissue varies according to the size, location, and the type of lesion but is in the order of 60% to 90% with very low complication rates if 22-gauge aspiration needles are used.[1–3] Minor bleeding and localized sepsis have been reported, but needle spread of malignancy is considered very rare.

The procedure is performed under local anesthesia with intravenous sedation if required, usually on an outpatient basis (Fig. 42.1).

Aspiration of cystic collections such as ovarian cysts or lymphocysts can also be performed with the same technique. Small catheters can be introduced using specially designed one-stick sets, and full aspiration of the liquid contents is usually performed. If a lymphocyst has recurred, introduction of sclerosing agents such as tetracyclines or 100% alcohol can be performed in an attempt to prevent recurrence.

DRAINAGE OF PELVIC COLLECTIONS

Almost all pelvic collections that have been demonstrated on ultrasound or CT can be drained by percutaneous means.[4] CT is best in allowing a safe access route to be planned. It is im-

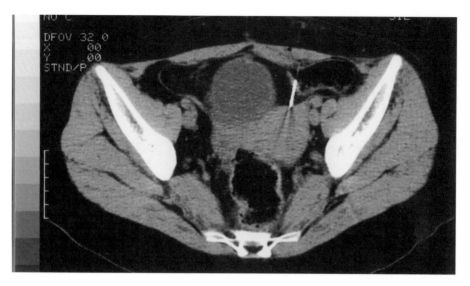

Figure 42.1 Fine needle (22-gauge) aspiration under CT control of soft tissue mass in a patient with previous resection of a germ cell tumor.

portant to avoid the tract passing through the bowel, and in many situations it is necessary to plan a transgluteal route.[5] Aspiration is initially performed with a 22-gauge needle, and once infected fluid or pus has been removed (and sent to the laboratory), an appropriate-size drainage catheter is inserted over a larger wire. The tract needs to be dilated up to the appropriate-size catheter. Usually, 8- to 12-French drainage catheters are sufficient to drain abscess cavities (Fig. 42.2). The catheters are flushed with saline regularly, and a follow-up CT or ultrasound is performed to ascertain complete resolution of the collections. It may be necessary to reposition the catheter or even to place a second catheter where there are locules that are not being adequately drained by the first catheter.

Antibiotics are chosen according to the organism isolated from culture. Even though a transgluteal approach is often required to drain pelvic abscesses, it is very rare for the sciatic nerve to be injured. However, the catheter position may prove uncomfortable for the patient, but it can usually be removed after several days. Hematomas cannot be readily evacuated by percutaneous means, unless they are liquid in nature. Occasionally, it is possible to instill urokinase solution in an attempt to lyse nondrainable clot.

The potential complications of percutaneous drainage of pelvic collections include the following:

1. *Localized bleeding.* This is usually of a mild nature, but in cases where a major vessel is traumatized, the catheter should be clamped. If bleeding persists, percutaneous embolization of the bleeding artery can be performed to arrest the bleeding.

2. *Bacteremia.* The patient will invariably respond to normal resuscitative measures including intravenous fluids, antibiotics, and drainage of the affected collection.

PERCUTANEOUS NEPHROSTOMY AND URETERIC STENTING

The main indications for percutaneous nephrostomy in the gynecologic setting are to relieve obstructions of the ureter in malignancies such as carcinoma of the cervix or to divert urine when there is leakage from trauma or surgery.[6] In general, an attempt is made to place a retrograde stent, but if extensive metastasis is demonstrated on CT, it is likely a retrograde attempt will be unsuccessful, and a percutaneous nephrostomy is the preferred treatment.

The procedure is performed under local anesthesia with intravenous sedation and analgesia.[7] Using ultrasound or fluoroscopic guidance, entry is made through a lower pole calyx using a needle and catheter system (one-stick set) (Fig. 42.3). It is almost always possible to pass a guidewire and subsequently a catheter down through the ureteric obstruction, which usually consists of a short severe stricture in the lower ureter, and at the same attendance, place a 6- to 8-French internal ureteric stent via a long sheath such that the stent is positioned from the renal pelvis to the bladder. External drainage is maintained with a nephrostomy catheter, and providing there has been no bleeding, the catheter can be clamped and removed within 24 hours if there is no leakage or pain. The catheter is left on free drainage if there has been bleeding, and a follow-up nephrostogram will determine when the nephrostomy catheter can be removed. The stent usually needs to be changed endoscopically within 3 to 6 months due to encrustation and blockage. In cases of ureteric trauma or leakage, the stents usually remain in situ for approximately 3 months before removal, allowing healing to occur.[8] Recurrent benign strictures can be balloon dilated, although this has proven to be of good long-term benefit in less than about 50% of cases. There have been some reports of the use of metal stents for severe malignant obstructions where ureteric stenting does not lead to drainage. These stents are expensive but do offer better long-term patency rates, although they will ultimately block due to tumor growth.

The main complication of percutaneous nephrostomy is bleeding that requires embolization. This procedure is performed by selective catheterization of the relevant second- or third-order branch of the renal artery. Small stainless coils or polyvinylalcohol particles are placed via a coaxial catheter system. After occlusion of this vessel, depending on its size, about 1/10 or less of the kidney tissue will be infarcted. The other major complication is sepsis, particularly if there is underlying infected urine or pus. The patient almost always responds to the usual resuscitative measures with antibiotics and intravenous fluids. In rare situations, a patient may require intensive care unit monitoring due to severe shock.

INFERIOR VENA CAVA (ENDOCAVAL) FILTERS

The use of IVC filters is now standard treatment (1) for patients who have a deep venous thrombosis (DVT), usually extending above the popliteal vein, and who have recurrent pulmonary emboli despite adequate anticoagulation or (2) for patients who have a DVT with a pulmonary embolus and who have contraindications to anticoagulation (Fig 42.4).[9]

The DVT is diagnosed by duplex Doppler ultrasound, but occasionally femoral venography is required to delineate the extent of the thrombus into the iliac veins or IVC. Pulmonary angiography can be performed at the same time if there is an equivocal lung scan, which can clarify whether there has been a pulmonary embolus.

IVC filters are placed via the right or left femoral veins, or,

Figure 42.2 Pelvic abscess in a 53-year-old following vaginal repair and colpopexy. **(A)** CT scan shows a pelvic collection before drainage. **(B)** Transgluteal draining with 12-French catheter. CT shows complete resolution of the abscess 2 days later.

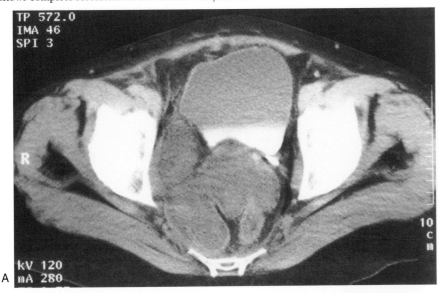

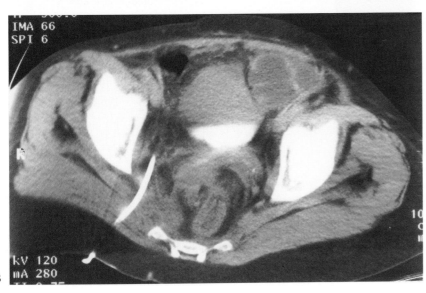

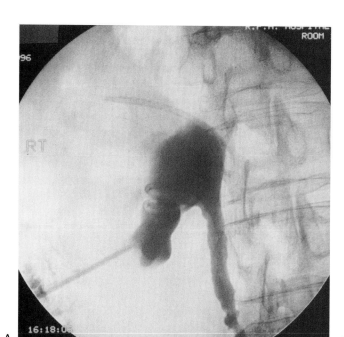

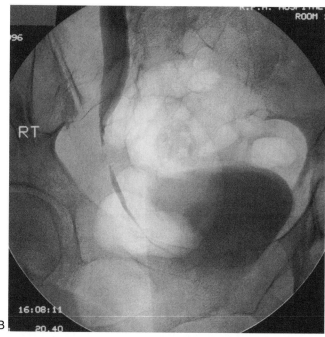

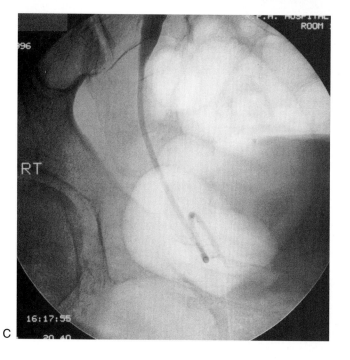

Figure 42.3 Percutaneous nephrostomy by fluoroscopy. **(A)** Percutaneous nephrostomy via the lower pole calyx in an obstructed kidney caused by ureteric narrowing in a 49-year-old with metastatic carcinoma of the ovary following chemotherapy. **(B)** Narrowing of the lower ureter is demonstrated. **(C)** A 7-French polyurethane stent has been placed to provide satisfactory drainage.

in cases where the thrombus occupies the iliac veins, the right jugular vein can be used as access. A 12-French sheath is introduced into the IVC, and the conical shaped filter is pushed through the sheath and positioned usually at the L2–L4 level in the IVC just below the renal veins.

Several different types of filters are available. The Greenfield filter has been available for over 30 years and has small struts projecting to tether themselves to the wall of the IVC. The filters have a high capture rate of clot and a very low long-term IVC thrombosis rate. It is very rare for these filters to migrate.[10]

FALLOPIAN TUBE RECANALIZATION

Fallopian tube recanalization is a simple procedure that has become a standard method of assessing the patency of fallopian tubes in the treatment of infertility. The procedure is performed on an outpatient basis under mild sedation. An initial hysterogram is performed by an occluding balloon catheter, which is placed under direct vision through the os. If either fallopian tube is shown to be occluded, gentle probing with a selective catheter and hydrophilic 35 guidewire is

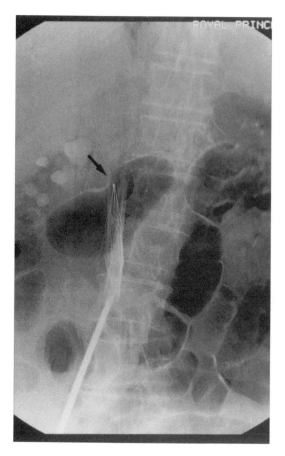

Figure 42.4 IVC filter seen at fluoroscopy. A Greenfield filter (arrow) placed percutaneously via the right femoral vein into the inferior vena cava. This patient was 36 years old with a history of endometrial carcinoma and subsequent recurrent pulmonary emboli and deep venous thrombosis despite adequate anticoagulation.

EMBOLIZATION OF ARTERIO-VENOUS MALFORMATION OR BLEEDING VESSELS

With the wide array of catheters and guidewires, it is now possible by using coaxial catheter systems to place small catheters into third and fourth-order branches of vessels such as the internal iliac artery. When significant arterial bleeding occurs after manipulation or surgery in the pelvis,[12–14] it has become standard practice to place a small catheter percutaneously via the femoral artery into the bleeding vessel and deposit some small particles such as polyvinylacohol or small stainless steel coils to occlude the vessel (Fig. 42.6). Control angiograms monitor the progress of the procedure, but it may be necessary to occlude several vessels, particularly in cases of trauma from a penetrating injury. Larger vessels are occluded by the use of larger coils or, occasionally, detachable silicon balloons.

Congenital A-V malformations are notoriously very difficult to eradicate completely, but palliation can be undertaken by the use of percutaneous embolization. If a small catheter can be placed into the nidus of the malformation, 0.5 ml of History (a liquid polymer) can be introduced to occlude the central component of the malformation. Occluding the main feeding vessels only achieves temporary success due to the large number of potential collaterals that quickly open up to keep the A-V malformation open. Patients with large A-V malformations can present with high cardiac output states, and initial angiography is necessary to define the exact anatomy of the feeding arteries and draining veins. The procedure may have to be performed on multiple occasions, but

Figure 42.5 Fallopian tube recanalization under fluoroscopic guidance. A 35 hydrophilic guidewire was placed through the left fallopian tube in a 38-year-old with a blocked fallopian tube on hysterosalpingogram.

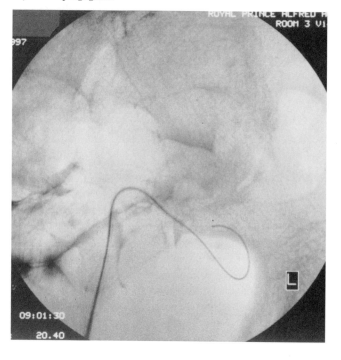

performed. The blockage is usually in the proximal part of the tube, and by gentle manipulation, the guidewire can readily be passed down the tube for at least 5 cm. The subsequent injection of dye confirms patency of the tube with free spillage of contrast into the peritoneal cavity. If there has been previous surgery to the tubes, it can be very difficult to pass points of anastomotic stricturing, and a variety of different catheters and wires can be tried to pass the blockage (Fig. 42.5). Occasionally, it may be necessary to use a small balloon to dilate recurrent areas of occlusion or tight strictures. In cases of hydrosalpinx, distension of the fallopian tube can be quite painful, but usually a point is reached where the contrast suddenly is released into the peritoneal cavity.

With this technique pregnancy has been reported in up to 30% of patients who have primary occlusion of the fallopian tubes.[11] This procedure is virtually complication free, but a small amount of bleeding can occur, and very rarely localized infection may result from the manipulation, which can be readily managed by antibiotics.

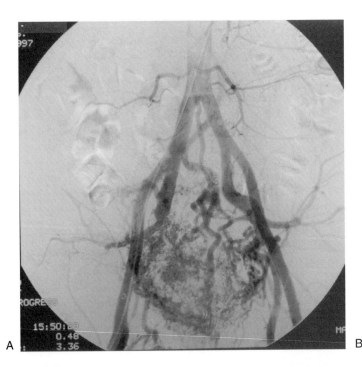

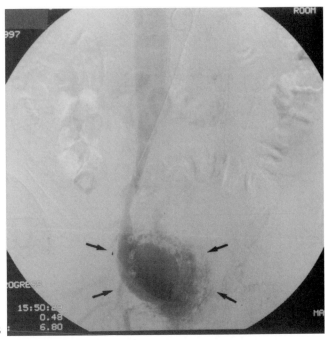

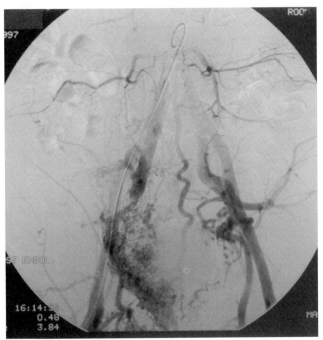

Figure 42.6 (A) Angiogram of a patient with pelvic A-V malformation with multiple feeding arteries. (B) Early venous filling with a large venous aneurysm (arrows). (C) A significant decrease in vascularity is seen following embolization with polyvinylalcohol particles.

it is almost always possible to lessen the degree of shunting. Care must be taken to avoid embolization of other vascular territories, particularly when using the liquid polymers, which can readily infarct tissues.

Bleeding arising from malignant tumors can also be treated by percutaneous embolization, although this is usually only of a medium-term success in control of the hemorrhage. Embolization of feeding vessels from the ovarian artery can be performed in the pelvic congestion syndrome if the clinical index of suspicion is high and diagnostic angiography is performed to make the diagnosis.

The major complication of percutaneous embolization is infarction on non target vessels, which can cause localized tissue necrosis or organ infarction. These procedures should be performed by skilled vascular radiologists in centers with extensive experience in treating such lesions.

SUMMARY

Interventional radiology plays an important role in the treatment of a variety of conditions seen in gynecologic practice.

Many of these procedures need to be performed on an urgent basis and occasionally out of hours. Direct communication between the gynecologist and radiologist is essential, and the procedures offer high success rates with low complications and often the avoidance of further surgery in an already compromised patient. Most obstetricians and gynecologists have become fully aware of the role of interventional radiology. The use of high-resolution ultrasound and CT and more lately magnetic resonance imaging has increased the role of interventional radiology due to the more accurate means of diagnosis.

REFERENCES

1. Layfield LJ, Berek JS. Fine-needle aspiration cytology in the management of gynecologic oncology patients. Cancer Treat Res 1994;70:1–13

2. Zanetta G, Brenna A, Pittell M et al. Transvaginal ultrasound-guided fine needle sampling of deep cancer recurrences in the pelvis: usefulness and limitations. Gynecol Oncol 1994;54:59–63

3. Dordoni D, Zaglio S, Zucca S, Favalli G. The role of sonographically guided aspiration in the clinical management of ovarian cysts. J Ultrasound Med 1993;12:27–31

4. Fabiszewski NL, Sumkin JH, Johns CM. Contemporary radiologic percutaneous abscess drainage in the pelvis. Clin Obstet Gynecol 1993;36:445–456

5. Yeung EY, Ho CS. Percutaneous radiologic drainage of pelvic abscesses. Ann Acad Med Singapore 1993;22:663–669

6. Hoe JW, Tung KH, Tan EC. Re-evaluation of indications for percutaneous nephrostomy and interventional uroradiological procedures in pelvic malignancy. Br J Urol 1993; 71:469–472

7. Lu DS, Papanicolaou N, Girard M et al. Percutaneous internal ureteral stent placement: review of technical issues and solutions in 50 consecutive cases. Clin Radiol 1994;49:256–261

8. Cormio L, Battaglia M, Traficante A, Selvaggi FP. Endourological treatment of ureteric injuries Br J Urol 1993;72:165–168

9. Midy D, Pheline P, Baste JC. Another percutaneous endocaval filter. Multicenter evaluation based on 300 cases. J Mal Vasc 1994;19:308–313

10. Ferris EJ, McCowan TC, Carver DK, McFarland DR. Percutaneous inferior vena caval filters: follow-up of seven designs in 320 patients. Radiology 1993;188:851–856

11. Thurmond AS, Rosch J. Nonsurgical fallopian tube recanalisation for treatment of infertility. Radiology 1990;174:371–374

12. Joseph JF, Mernoff D, Donovan J, Metz SA. Percutaneous angiographic arterial embolization for gynecologic and obstetric pelvic hemorrhage. A report of three cases. J Reprod Med 1994;39:915–920

13. Yamashita Y, Harada M, Yamamoto H et al. Transcatheter arterial embolization of obstetric and gynecological bleeding: efficacy and outcome. Br J Radiol 1994;67:530–534

14. Bazsa S. Transcatheter embolization of the hypogastric artery as a hemostatic method in obstetrics and gynecology. Orv Hetil 1994;135:2867–2869

Functional Imaging in Gynecologic Disease: The Role for Positron Emission Tomography, Single-Photon Emission Computed Tomography, Echo-Planar Imaging, and Magnetic Resonance Spectroscopy

MICHAEL J. FULHAM

It is just over a century ago that Roentgen discovered the x-ray and thus the medical specialty of radiology. The penetrating ability of this new ray was first used to localize bullets in the calvarium and indirectly provided the first insights into the morphology of the living brain. However, the bony skeleton remained a formidable barrier to direct visualization of body organs for over 75 years. Instead, the anatomic status of organs was inferred from other observations such as bony erosion on plain x-ray, displacement of arteries and veins with angiography, or the outline of tissues after oral radio-opaque material. When Hounsfield introduced x-ray computed tomography (CT) in 1972, he revolutionized anatomic imaging. In the brain, for the first time, a noninvasive modality could separate grey from white matter, outline the deep nuclei, and recognize pathologic changes in the cerebral parenchyma. It was not long before CT provided similar insights into anatomy of the chest, abdomen, and pelvis, and not only was it able to portray fine anatomic detail, but it also introduced a fundamentally new technique of true tomography (imaging of slices) through mathematic reconstruction of data obtained from multiple projections. This breakthrough was made possible by computer technology, which also accelerated the development of the other major three-dimensional imaging modalities: emission computed tomography (ECT) in its two forms, positron emission tomography (PET) and single-photon emission computed tomography (SPECT), and magnetic resonance imaging (MRI).[1-4] A fundamental aspect of three-dimensional imaging and the basis of all reconstruction techniques is the synthesis of a three-dimensional image from a series of two-dimensional images (projections) taken at various angles around the subject. The reconstructed image is a quantitative measure of some property of the tissue. In CT, the tissue property is the x-ray attenuation coefficient. PET and SPECT measure the tissue concentration of a radioisotope (tracer) in counts or nanoCuries (nCi) per milliliter and for MRI the property being measured is the transverse magnetization density.

The current accepted noninvasive imaging evaluation for patients with gynecologic disease in most centers is anatomic imaging (CT, MRI) and ultrasound. Medical imaging, however, is a dynamic field, and in the last few years, there have been rapid developments, most of which were not predicted 5 years ago. It can be expected that in the future some of what we currently regard as essential elements of gynecologic imaging may be surpassed. It is in this context that the concept of functional imaging (PET, SPECT, MRI spectroscopy and echo-planar MRI) for the evaluation of gynecologic conditions will be presented.

PET AND SPECT

Physics and Instrumentation

PET and SPECT utilize the principles of the tracer kinetic assay method and tomographic image reconstruction. In the tracer method, a radiolabeled, biologically active compound is injected into a subject in minute quantities. The tracer then participates in, but does not perturb, the biochemical process of interest. The tomograph (PET or SPECT scanner) detects the tissue concentration of the tracer, and a mathematical model can then be derived to describe the kinetics of the process, and in some instances it is possible to convert raw counts to a unit of physiologic function such as the metabolic rate for glucose or blood flow. In Table 43.1 there is a list of common PET and SPECT radiotracers. The list is not exhaustive, but it is noteworthy that radioactive isotopes of some of the most important elements in biology are positron emitters (^{15}O, ^{13}N, ^{11}C).

Despite some shared characteristics there are a number of fundamental differences between PET and SPECT. PET radioisotopes have very short half-lives (^{18}F with $t_{1/2} = 110$ minutes; ^{11}C, $t_{1/2} = 20$ minutes; ^{13}N, $t_{1/2} = 10$ minutes; ^{15}O, $t_{1/2} = 2$ minutes), and they are produced in charged particle accelerators called *cyclotrons*. The short half-lives of PET radiotracers generally mean that the PET scanner must be in close proximity to the cyclotron. SPECT isotopes are much longer-lived, and they can be transported long distances. They are produced in reactors except for ^{123}I and ^{201}TI, which are cyclotron produced. Positron emitters decay to a stable state by emitting a positron (positive electron) from the nucleus. The positron travels a small distance (1 to 2 mm) in tissue before colliding with a surrounding electron, and the masses of the positron and electron are converted to energy in the form of two high-energy photons or γ-rays that are emitted 180 degrees apart (Figs. 43.1). The simultaneous production of annihilation photons in opposite directions and their coincident detection by the crystals of the PET scanner provide the basis for the localization of the PET radiotracer in tissue.[5,6] The PET detectors scintillate when struck by photons, and photomultiplier tubes convert the light energy into a digital

signal, using sophisticated electronics, to provide a three-dimensional distribution of the tracer. The physics of PET also allows for the correction of scattered and attenuated photons and enable quantification of a particular physiologic process.

In SPECT, single photons are detected by rotating γ-cameras with single or multiple large crystal detectors (Figs. 43.2). Multidetector γ-cameras (double- and triple-headed cameras) have enabled improved resolution through the detection of a greater proportion of unscattered photons. However, the problems of scatter and attenuation correction in SPECT have not yet been satisfactorily resolved, which has limited SPECT's ability to provide quantitative data. Instead, ratios of regional counts within a study are used to compare data. In addition, the resolution in SPECT is inferior to that in PET. The latest generation PET scanners have resolution in the order of 2 to 3 mm full width at half maximum (FWHM) whereas for triple-headed SPECT cameras, resolution approximates 8 to 10 mm FWHM and 14 to 17 mm FWHM for single-head systems. Ring-detector SPECT devices, similar to PET scanners, have resolution in the 7 to 8-mm FWHM range, but these devices are not widely available. A new detector material called *lutetium oxyorthosilicate (LSO)* which has more efficient fluorescence, is currently under development for PET and SPECT cameras. Cherry et al. recently showed images from a PET device, using LSO detectors, that was built within an MRI scanner and provides an image 10 times sharper than current PET devices.[7] It is likely that the next generation of PET/SPECT scanners will approach the theoretical finite in-plane spatial resolution which for PET is of the order of less than 2 mm.

The first PET scan in a human was reported in 1979, but its

Table 43.1 Some PET and SPECT Radiotracers

Technique	Radiotracer	Radioisotope and Half-life	Biologic Parameter/Receptor
PET			
	[^{18}F]fluorodeoxyglucose (FDG)	^{18}F ~ 108 min	Glucose metabolism
	[^{18}F]-6-fluorodopa		Presynaptic DOPA uptake
	[^{11}C]-methionine	^{11}C = 20 min	Amino acid uptake
	[^{11}C]-raclopride		D2 receptor binding
	[^{11}C]-nomifensine		Catecholamine re-uptake
	[^{11}C]-flumazenil		Central benzodiazepine
	[^{11}C]-PK 11195		Peripheral benzodiazepine
	^{15}O-water	^{15}O ~ 2 min	Blood flow
SPECT			
	^{99m}Tc-hexamethyl propylene amine oxime (HMPAO)	^{99m}Tc = 6 hr	Blood flow
	^{201}Thallium	^{201}Tl = 73.1 hr	K$^+$ analog-cellularity
	^{133}Xenon	^{133}Xe = 5.25 days	Blood flow
	^{123}I-iodoamphetamine	^{123}I ~ 13 hr	Blood flow
	^{123}I-iodo-a-methyl tyrosine		Amino acid transport
	^{123}I-QNB		Muscarinic cholinergic
	^{123}I-iodobenzamide		Dopamine D2
	^{123}I-iomazenil		Central benzodiazepine
	^{123}I-iododexetimide		Muscarinic cholinergic
	^{111}In-CYT	^{111}In = 2.8 days	TAG-72

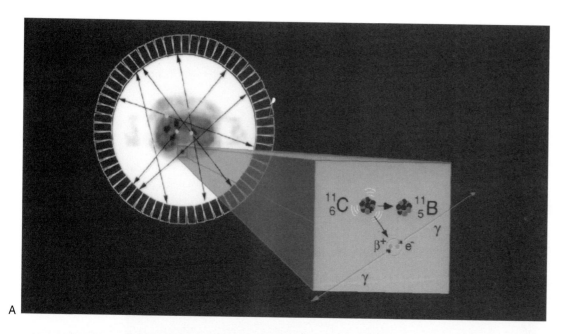

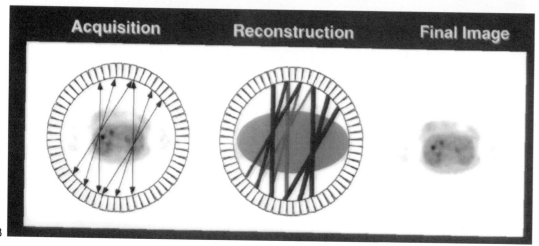

Figure 43.1 (**A**) Cross-sectional images through PET scanner showing ring of detectors, body in center of field of view, positron emission with detection of coincident γ-rays by detectors. (**Inset**) A cartoon of positron emission, annihilation, and emission of two γ-rays 180 degrees apart. (*Note*: For all PET images, the patient's left is on the viewer's right). (**B**) Steps in image production in PET. Depiction of positron emission, coincidence detection, and lines of response (LoRs) (center panel) used to produce final image (far-right panel).

role was limited to research in the neurosciences for much of the 1980s because of the cost incurred in building a large aperture device that could image the body.[8–10] Overall, PET has proved more fruitful than SPECT by virtue of its superior resolution and the capability for quantification. PET has been employed for the evaluation of blood flow, blood volume, oxygen utilization and metabolism, glucose metabolism, tissue hypoxia, amino acid transport and metabolism, protein synthesis, and the measurement of tissue receptor concentrations mainly in the brain. However, improvements in instrumentation in the late 1980s enabled the production of affordable wide-aperture PET scanners that permitted the whole body (WB-PET) to be imaged and thus heralded the investigation of malignant dis-

ease with PET. It should be emphasized that the study of cancer with PET is a relatively new field internationally, and data from large series of patients with a variety of tumors are only now beginning to appear. Nevertheless, as studies from our own center at Royal Prince Alfred Hospital (RPAH) indicate, the evaluation of cancer with WB-PET is assuming a major role in clinical management.[11,12]

Clinical Applications: PET

The majority of the WB-PET work in cancer has focused on staging a variety of cancers using [^{18}F] fluoro-2-deoxyglucose (FDG) and is based on three independent observations.

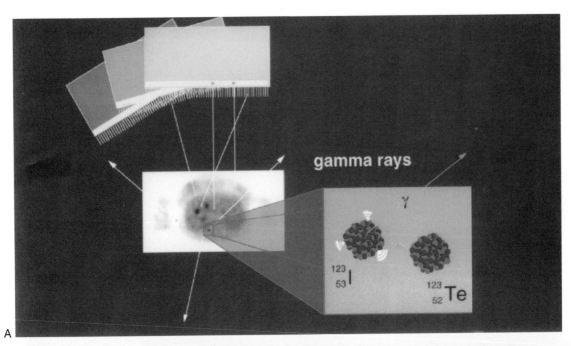

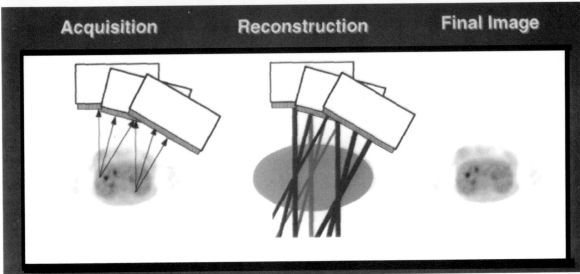

Figure 43.2 (A) Cross-sectional images of SPECT: rotating crystal detector, single-photon emission and detection. (**Inset**) Single-photon emission. (**B**) Steps in image production in SPECT. Center panel shows LoRs used in final image.

Figure 43.3 The three-compartment model for FDG (applies also to deoxyglucose). Rate constants k_1, k_2, k_3 describe movement of FDG between plasma and tissues, k_4 describes dephosphorylation of FDG-6-phosphate.

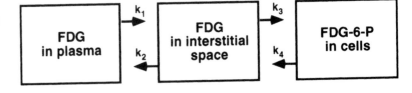

1. Warburg demonstrated, in the 1930s, that as tumors become malignant there is enhanced "aerobic glycolysis" when compared to benign tissue.[13,14]

2. Sokoloff et al.,[15] at the National Institutes of Health demonstrated in 1977 that [14C] deoxyglucose (DG) autoradiography could be used to measure cerebral glucose metabolism in the albino rat brain. Deoxyglucose is an analog of glucose and is taken up by cells via the glucose transporter and then phosphorylated in the cytosol by hexokinase to deoxyglucose-6-phosphate (DG-6-P). However, DG-6-P cannot participate in subsequent steps of the glycolytic cycle and so is effectively trapped in the cell. Thus, uptake and phosphorylation of DG reflect cellular glucose utilization (Fig. 43.3).

3. This work was later validated in humans using FDG.[16] Then, Di Chiro and co-workers,[17–19] from the NIH, showed that the measurement of glucose metabolism with FDG-PET could separate benign from malignant cerebral-gliomas and differentiate recurrent tumor from treatment (radiation- and chemotherapy-induced necrosis) effects noninvasively.

These findings were later translated to cancer in the body and the ability of FDG-PET to separate benign from malignant disease, to separate recurrent tumor from the effects of treatment (e.g., recurrent rectal carcinoma from scar tissue), and to detect tumor in lymph nodes that are morphologically normal on CT/ MRI, which have led to its increasing role in the noninvasive staging/detection of malignancy.) Preliminary data have appeared on the role of FDG-PET in staging cancer of the lung (non-small cell lung), head and neck, skin (melanoma), liver (colorectal hepatic metastases), breast, ovary, and prostate, and in lymphoma.[11,12,20,21] In these situations FDG-PET has been compared to standard staging with anatomic imaging (CT, MRI), and in most situations PET has proven superior for the detection of disease. There are no data on the role of PET in detecting or staging endometrial cancer, and the data presented below refer to ovarian malignancy.

The PET Procedure

For FDG-PET scans patients are studied after a 6-hour fast to reduce fluctuations in serum glucose levels. FDG uptake can be affected by serum glucose alterations. For example, changing levels of blood glucose and serum insulin levels after a meal can increase FDG uptake into muscle. Approximately 5.3 MBq/kg of FDG is injected intravenously, and an uptake period of 50 minutes is allowed before scanning commences. The scanning period generally lasts 60 minutes. At Royal Prince Alfred Hospital, a major improvement in image quality for WB-PET studies has been developed.[22] This technique involves the simultaneous measurement of photon attenuation while emission data are being acquired, and then image reconstruction is carried out using an expectation-maximization technique. This technique has been called simultaneous omission and transmission using ordered subsets expectation maximization (SET-OSEM).[23] It eliminates artifacts that result from image reconstruction using filtered back projection (the generally accepted method) and the lack of attenuation correction and at the same time improves lesion detection (Fig. 43.4).

FDG-PET in Ovarian Cancer

The role and value of anatomic imaging in the staging of ovarian cancer are controversial, notwithstanding the concern regarding the role of second-look laparotomy.[24–30] Nevertheless, there are preliminary PET data in three situations:

Figure 43.4 Transaxial WB-PET slices in a patient with hepatic metastases. Far-left image is emission-only study reconstructed with filtered back projection (FBP). Right panel of images all have attenuation correction, but there is progressive improvement in image quality with segmented attenuation correction to the RPAH method (far-right panel) with segmented attenuation correction and reconstruction with OSEM. The RPAH method reveals three rather than one hepatic metastasis.

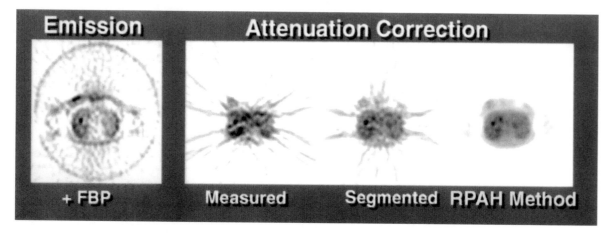

Emission
+ FBP

Attenuation Correction

Measured   Segmented   RPAH Method

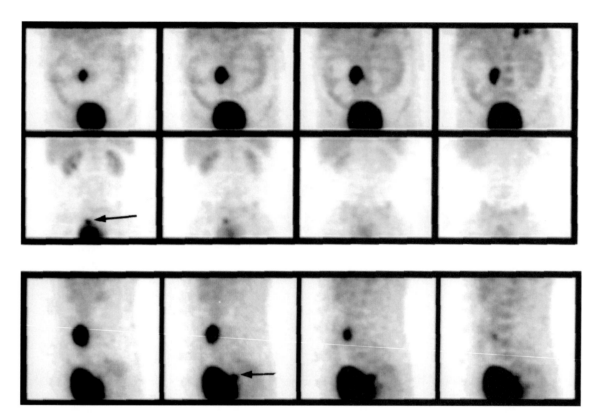

Figure 43.5 Clinical study. This 52-year-old woman presented with a 12-month history of cerebellar ataxia (positive antineuronal antibodies to Purkinje cells) as the initial manifestation of ovarian carcinoma. Pelvic ultrasound and CT were normal. Abdominal CT suggested a midline mass at L3. (**A**)Coronal (both panels, from anterior to posterior) FDG-PET study shows a large rounded region of FDG due to pooling in bladder at the bottom of the field of view. A large para-and prevertebral mass is seen to the right of midline due to tumoral involvement of para-aortic nodes (upper panel). Lower panel shows the ovarian primary as a small focus of increased FDG uptake posterosuperior to bladder (arrow). (**B**) Sagittal (from left to right of midline) FDG-PET images show small glucose-avid ovarian tumor posterior to bladder (arrow) and a large prevertebral nodal mass (see also Plate 43.1).

(1) detection of ovarian cancer in patients who present with an ovarian mass, (2) detection of suspected recurrent disease, and (3) the role of FDG-PET in monitoring response to treatment.

Hubner et al.[31,32] in the largest series to date, reported the University of Tennessee experience in the detection of local and metastatic ovarian cancer in 90 patients. In patients with a pelvic mass suspected of harboring ovarian cancer, prior to laparotomy, there was an 89% sensitivity and 92% specificity for detection of the tumor, with a positive predictive value of 94% and negative predictive value of 85%. For CT and MRI, accuracy for detection varies from 70% to 90%.[26,29] FDG-PET also identified sites of occult disease not detected on CT, and a patient who presented with a paraneoplastic syndrome is shown in Figure 43.5 and Plate 43.1. Hubner et al.[32] also reported a high sensitivity and specificity (94% and 100%) in 44 patients with recurrent disease. Karlan et al.[33] reported findings in a much smaller group of patients (n=12) prior to second-look laparotomy. They found disease in six patients that was later confirmed at surgery; in six patients with nor-

mal PET scans, microscopic disease was found pathologically in five of six. These data emphasize the limitations of all imaging modalities in detecting microscopic disease. FDG-PET is better able to detect disease in lymph nodes that are not enlarged (Fig. 43.6) but lesions less than 5 mm in size pose problems for all PET devices with resolution greater than 2 mm. Although data are not yet available in the detection of peritoneal disease, our own experience with advanced gastric carcinoma suggests that FDG-PET is also not able to detect small peritoneal tumors in the 1 to 5 mm range.

Measurement of tumoral glucose metabolism with FDG-PET after treatment is an active area of research. In our own center, there are a number of active protocols to evaluate the role of FDG-PET in this setting. WB-PET scans are done early and/or at the completion of a course of chemotherapy to determine if a reduction in tumoral glucose metabolism predicts tumor response. Two examples are shown in Figures 43.6 and 43.7. These cases illustrate how PET may be used to tailor chemotherapy in an individual case but perhaps more importantly how PET can be

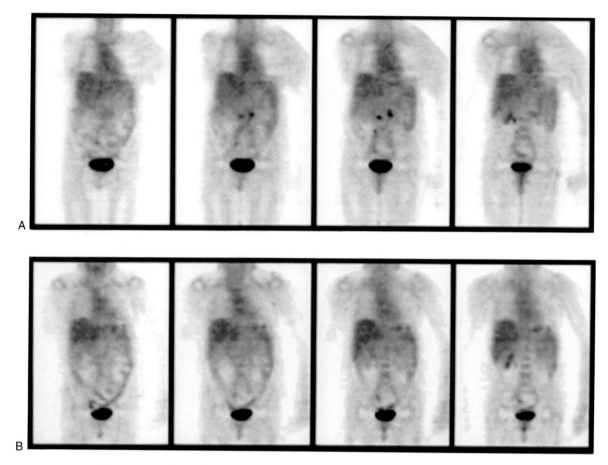

Figure 43.6 Clinical study. Serial FDG-PET scans in a 57-year-old woman with recurrent ovarian carcinoma after surgery and chemotherapy. Coronal FDC-PET scans show identical image planes from each of the four PET scans performed over a period of 25 months. (**A**)Study 1. Patient clinically well, normal abdominal CT, but elevated CA-125 (reference range <35 IU/ml). Coronal FDG-PET images show bilateral paravertebral foci of increased FDG uptake, which became apparent on CT 8 weeks after PET scan. (**B**) Study 2. FDG-PET scan 8 months later shows a marked reduction of glucose metabolism in nodal foci consistent with a complete response after chemotherapy. CA-125 is normal. (*Figure continues*)

used to evaluate newer agents in the phase I/II setting. Although the bulk of current PET work has been performed with FDG, as outlined above, increasingly, tumoral biology is under investigation with a variety of radiotracers: (1) tumoral DNA synthesis through [^{11}C]-thymidine, (2) estrogen and progesterone receptors through [^{18}F]-estradiol, (3) tumor hypoxia through [^{18}F]-misonidazole[34–38] (4) several cytotoxic drugs that have been radiolabeled and undergone preliminary evaluation in the clinical setting for example, [^{18}F]-5-fluorouracil in the evaluation of its distribution/ metabolism. There is also early work examining the impact of a variety of established and novel modulators of its metabolism.[39] The ability of PET to evaluate plasma pharmacology makes it an ideal candidate for the real-time prediction of a patient's handling of a chemotherapeutic drug and thus avoids undue toxicity.

Clinical Applications: SPECT

Thus far the role of SPECT and general nuclear medicine techniques (planar imaging) in gynecologic disease has been limited to the detection of local and disseminated disease using radiolabeled monoclonal antibodies. This technique, referred to as radioimmunoscintigraphy has promised much for diagnosis and treatment but unfortunately has failed to deliver in the clinical setting for many conditions. A variety of monoclonal antibodies have been evaluated,[40] but the most promising agent was CYT-103 labeled with [111]indium. CYT-103 reacts with TAG-72, which is an antigen that is highly expressed in ovarian adenocarcinomas. A multicentre trial of [111] In-CYT-103 reported a higher sensitivity (69% vs. 44%) and lower specificity (57% vs. 79%) than CT imaging for detecting local and disseminated disease. However, the detection rate for CT was lower than

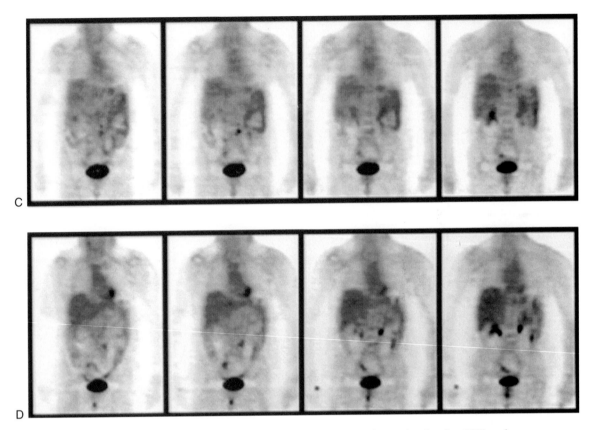

Figure 43.6 *(Continued)* **(C)** Study 3. Third FDG-PET scan 19 months after first PET study when CA-125 was rising (=42); clinically well and normal CT. Coronal FDG-PET scans show new foci of increased FDG uptake in para-aortic nodes. **(D)** Study 4. Fourth FDG-PET at 25 months after first PET scan. CA-125 = 16. CT normal but PET shows persistent FDG uptake in nodes despite further chemotherapy consistent with a submaximal response to treatment.

other studies mentioned above.[41] It is unlikely that radioimmunoscintigraphy will play a major role in diagnosis, and as ever, a more promising role lies in targeting therapy. The translation of developments in PET chemistry using ^{11}C to SPECT with ^{123}I may see a broader role for SPECT in the future.

FUNCTIONAL MRI

The nuclear magnetic resonance (NMR) phenomenon was originally described in 1946 but it was nearly 30 years before this discovery was translated into medical imaging. The physics of MRI are complex, however in routine clinical MRI the signal used to create an image arises from water proton nuclei (^{1}H). Early in the development of MRI it was apparent that the image quality surpassed that of CT, particularly for the brain. It was also appreciated that despite the greater sensitivity of MRI when compared to CT, major weaknesses included poor specificity and marked image degradation with patient motion. In an effort to improve these deficiencies, together with a desire to explore and push the technology to its limits, a bewildering number of advances have been made in the past few years: (1) improvements in surface coils; (2) the introduction of high magnetic field strength devices (4.0 Tesla [T]); (3)

software and pulse sequence developments with acronyms such as STEAM, FLASH, FLAIR, MPRAGE, and ISIS that appear almost monthly in the literature; (4) techniques such as magnetization transfer and tensor imaging; (5) pulse sequences to image blood flow and hence MR angiography; and (6) a group of MRI techniques known as functional MRI.[3,4,42]

The term *functional* MRI refers to MRI techniques that provide data about aspects of metabolism rather than anatomy such as tissue metabolite concentrations, perfusion, and blood flow. The term encompasses MR spectroscopy (MRS), those techniques that rely on the change in blood oxygenation levels, referred to in some circles as fMRI, and rapid scanning techniques such as echo-planar imaging. This is an exciting area of development, because it means that functional data, formerly the exclusive domain of PET and SPECT can now be obtained with MRI scanners without the associated ionizing radiation. There are few data for the role of these techniques in clinical gynecologic practice at present, and the role of these exciting techniques has yet to be clarified.

Echo-Planar Imaging

All MRI techniques depend to some extent on a homogeneous magnetic field and patient co-operation for good image quality.

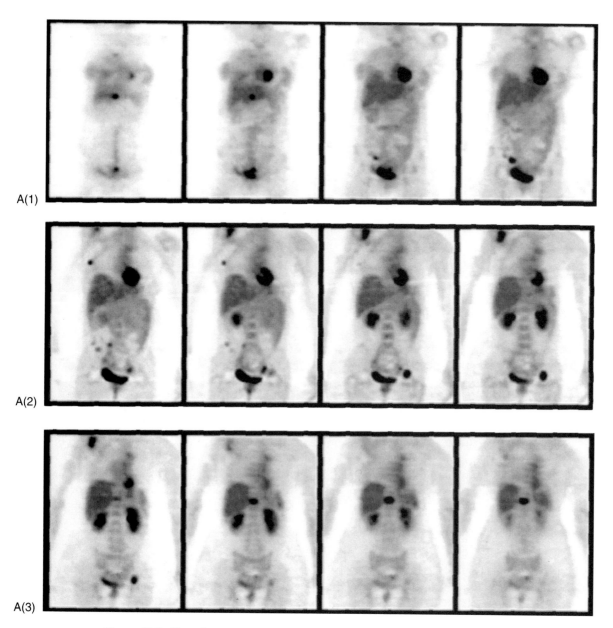

A(1)

A(2)

A(3)

Figure 43.7 Clinical study. A 48-year-old woman with stage 1C clear cell ovarian carcinoma diagnosed 6 months prior to the PET scan. PET scan was done after three cycles of adjuvant chemotherapy to check for residual disease. (**A**)Coronal FDG-PET scans (panels 1 to 3) show multiple foci of markedly increased FDG uptake consistent with disseminated disease in the liver, proximal right humerus, para-aortic and iliac nodes, ribs, left ilium and pelvis, and body of T10 vertebra. (Note: Physiologic FDG uptake in myocardium, FDG excretion by kidneys, and sausage-shaped bladder in pelvis due to compression from omental tumor.) (*Figure continues*)

The signal-to-noise ratio is improved by longer data acquisition, but then the trade-off is the increased likelihood of patient motion during an acquisition of several minutes' duration. There is an additional problem of physiologic motion from respiration, the circulation, and peristalsis in the bowel and ureters. In 1977 Mansfield[43] reported a technique, called echoplanar imaging (EPI), where imaging times of 30 to 100 ms were possible. The physics of EPI are beyond the scope of this chapter but, in summary, k-space is sampled in a single continuous trajectory, and this technique effectively freezes anatomic motion. Blood flow in large vessels can still be problematic, but there is the added advantage of utilizing contrast agents to provide dynamic data in the first 2 minutes after infusion to provide tissue contrast in pathologic states. EPI has been utilized in a number of centers to evaluate cardiac function, mapping tissue water diffusion and temperature, mapping the blood pool and perfusion, cerebrospinal fluid flow, the liver and the mobile fetus in utero.[44] Diffusion is a measure of Brownian motion, and

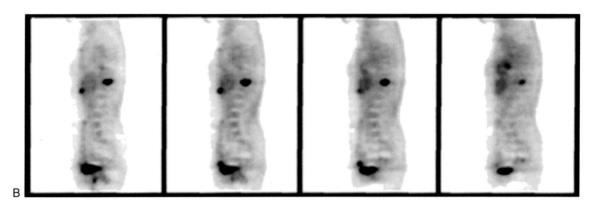

Figure 43.7 *(Continued)* **(B)** Sagittal images PET scan show liver metastases and T10 metastasis. The detection of vertebral involvement predated neurologic symptoms by 1 month and was later confirmed by MRI.

some authors believe that it may be a sensitive parameter to charactize tissues at a microscopic level. Using echo-planar techniques, a measurement of molecular diffusion called the *apparent diffusion coefficient (ADC)* can be obtained for different organs. Until recently, these developments were restricted to research sites, but vendors now provide hardware and software upgrades to clinical 1.5 T magnets, and the technique has been refined for clinical imaging. Muller et al.[45] reported preliminary findings for abdominal diffusion mapping in 10 normal volunteers in 1994. They measured ADCs in liver, spleen, kidney, and muscle, and although the image quality was poor and there was wide scatter in the ADCs for kidney, the authors speculated that "ADCs in vivo could prove helpful in the identification and classification of abdominal disease."

Magnetic Resonance Spectroscopy

In MRS, signals are obtained from nuclei that are constituents of molecules other than water. These signals are generated by non radioactive nuclei that are parts of other solutes or metabolites and are much weaker than the signals arising from water. The solutes that produce them occur in concentrations of 0.5 mM. Nonwater ^1H, ^{31}P, ^{13}C, ^{23}Na, and ^{19}F are the most important nuclei in MRS. The signals are analyzed and the radiofrequencies emitted by the sample of interest appear as peaks on a plot of signal intensity against signal frequency, thus producing an NMR, spectrum.[46–48] The horizontal or frequency axes are normalized to the frequency of a strong signal of known origin, and the location of peaks are given as parts per million relative to the known signal (Fig. 43.8). The signal strength (the vertical axis) is proportional to a number of factors including the number of nuclei in the tissue volume being studied. Signals from different isotopes are distinguisable because they occur at different frequencies in any given magnetic field, and nuclear signals from different solutes can also be separated from one another by the property of chemical shift. Chemical shift refers to the fact that within a molecule containing magnetic nuclei, the electron clouds in the chemical bonds surrounding the nuclei change the local magnetic field, so that nuclei of the same species spin at different frequencies.

Figure 43.8 **(A)** ^{31}P MRS spectrum from normal volunteer shows peaks detected. **(B)** ^1H-MRS spectrum from a patient with a brain tumor. Upper trace is the normal hemisphere and the lower trace is from the hemisphere containing the tumor.

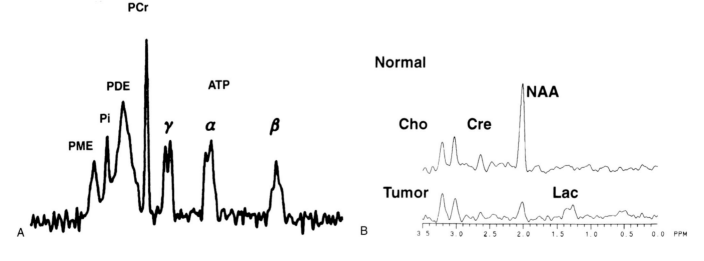

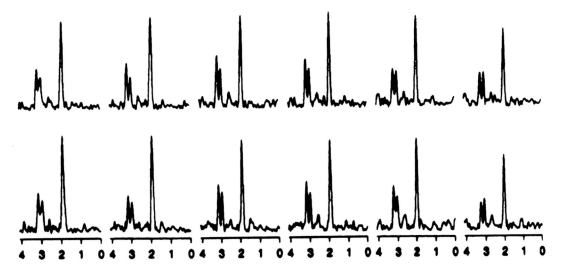

Figure 43.9 Multiple ^{1}H-MRS spectra from multiple voxels in spectroscopic imaging technique (see also Plate 43.2).

The impact of these weak signals is that (1) MRS has poorer sensitivity and resolution when compared to clinical imaging, and (2) some solutes cannot be measured with MRS. In addition, molecular motion is required for a solute to be detected with MRS, and most macromolecules (proteins, nucleosides, phospholipids) are inaccessible because of their limited mobility. For most clinical situations ^{1}H-MRS has been preferred over ^{31}P-MRS because of its inherently stronger signal, better resolution, and greater sensitivity. The metabolites of interest include (1) choline-containing compounds (Cho) involved in membrane synthesis and degradation; (2) creatine-containing compounds (Cre) sources of high- and low-energy phosphates; (3) lactate (Lac) the terminal metabolite of aerobic glycolysis; and (4) possibly citrate levels, because epithelial cancer adenocarcinoma cells have a reduced capacity to synthesize citrate.[49] Initial ^{1}H-MRS studies involved acquisition of data from single voxels of varying sizes, so effectively, only a small region could be sampled at once. Developments with gradient-based phase-encoding techniques allowed the simultaneous acquisition of data from multiple voxels in a single tissue slab and so instead of interpreting an NMR spectrum, an image of the topographic distribution of metabolites, spectroscopic imaging (MRSI), is produced (Fig. 43.9 and Plate 43.2). Further pulse sequence enhancements led to the development of multislice spectroscopic imaging.

Much of this work has been developed in the neurosciences and, in particular, in brain tumours.[50–57] The main findings from these studies are that in malignant tumors there are increased choline and often creatine metabolite levels, relative to normal tissues, reflecting increased cell membrane turnover and energy requirements in malignant tissue. Lactate levels are also often increased from the inability of malignant tumors to shunt glucose through the more efficient tricarboxylic acid cycle instead of relying upon the relatively inefficient production of adenosinetriphosphate through pyruvate and lactic acid production. Furthermore, brain tumors replace the normal neuronal framework and so levels of another metabolite, N-acetyl-aspartate, which is a neuronal marker, are reduced. Work is now appearing in other cancers, and the application of endorectal and vaginal coils makes the investigation of gynecologic and urologic malignancy feasible. To my knowledge there are no preliminary data in gynecologic disease. However, the recent work of Kurhanewicz et al.[49] indicate that ^{1}H-MRSI in the pelvis is feasible. They reported data from 99 male subjects—9 normal volunteers, 5 patients with benign prostate disease, and 85 patient with prostate cancer—using endorectal and phased-array coils and a spatial resolution between 0.24 and 0.7 cm^3.

MRSI has a number of limitations that should be considered. Spectroscopic imaging places more stringent demands upon the quality and strength of the magnetic field than does clinical imaging. Whereas clinical MRI can be performed quite satisfactorily at 0.5 T, stronger fields are needed for MRSI. Poor field homogeneity manifests as difficulty in resolving signals from one another and from noise. Unfortunately, ^{1}H-MRSI is still limited to a few centers that have the resources and personnel to fine tune the MRI hardware and develop acquisition and analysis software. Further technical developments will shorten data acquisition times and data analysis procedures so that ^{1}H-MRSI will be available on clinical MRI scanners within a few years. MRSI offers greater potential for tissue characterization than clinical or diffusion MRI both for ovarian and endometrial disease, and reports of the first comparative studies will be eagerly awaited.

Acknowledgment I thank Patrick K. Hooper, BAppSci, Chief Technologist, and Kim M. Silver, BAppSci, Senior Technologist, in the PET Department for expert help with the illustrations in this chapter.

REFERENCES

1. Phelps ME, Mazziotta JC, Schelbert HR, Eds. Positron Emission Tomography and Autoradiography. Raven Press, New York, 1986

2. Fulham MJ, Di Chiro G. Neurological PET and SPECT. In: Harbert JC, Eckelman WC, Neumann RD, Eds. Nuclear Medicine: Diagnosis and Therapy. Thieme, New York, 1996, pp 361–386

3. Prichard JW. Magnetic resonance spectroscopy of cerebral metabolism in vivo. In: Asbury AK, McKhann GM, McDonald WI, Eds. Diseases of the Nervous System: Clinical Neurobiology (vol. 2). WB Saunders, Philadelphia, 1992, pp 1589–1605

4. Radda GK. The use of NMR spectroscopy for the understanding of disease. Science 1986;233:640–645

5. Ter-Pogossian MM, Phelps ME, Hoffman EJ et al. A positron emission transaxial tomograph for nuclear medicine imaging (PETT). Radiology 1975;114:39–93

6. Phelps ME, Hoffman EJ, Mullani NA, Ter-Pogossian MM. Application of annihilation coincidence detection to transaxial reconstruction tomography. J Nucl Med 1975;16:210–223

7. Service RF. New dynamic duo: PET, MRI, joined for the first time. Science 1996;272:1423

8. Reivich M, Kuhl D, Wolf A et al. The [18F] fluorodeoxyglucose method for the measurement of local cerebral glucose utilization in man. Circ Res 1979;44:127–137

9. Phelps ME, Mazziotta JC. Positron emission tomography: human brain function and biochemistry. Science 1985; 228:799–809

10. Phelps ME. Positron emission tomography (PET). In: Mazziotta JC, Gilman S, Eds. Clinical Brain Imaging: Principles and Applications. FA Davis, Philadelphia, 1992, pp 71–107

11. Damian D, Fulham MJ, Thompson E, Thompson JF. Positron emission tomography in the detection and management of metastatic melanoma. Mel Res 1996;6:325–329

12. Lai DT, Fulham MJ, Stephen M et al. The role of whole body positron emission tomography with [18F] fluorodeoxyglucose in identifying operable colorectal liver metastases. Arch Surg 1996;31:703–707

13. Warburg O. Metabolism of Tumors Arnold & Constable, London, 1930

14. Warburg O. On the origin of cancer cells. Science 1956;123:309–314

15. Sokoloff L, Reivich M, Kennedy C et al. The 14C-deoxyglucose method for the measurement of local cerebral glucose utilization: Theory procedure and normal values in the conscious and anesthetized albino rat. J Neurochem 1977;28:897–916

16. Phelps ME, Huang SC, Hoffman EJ et al. Tomographic measurement of local cerebral glucose metabolic rate in humans with [18F]2-fluoro-2-deoxy-d-glucose: validation of method. Ann Neurol 1979;6:371–388

17. Di Chiro G, DeLaPaz R, Brooks RA et al. Glucose utilization of cerebral gliomas measured by [18F] fluorodeoxyglucose and positron emission tomography. Neurology 1982;32:1323–1329

18. Di Chiro G. Positron emission tomography using [18F] fluorodeoxyglucose in brain tumors: a powerful diagnostic and prognostic tool. Invest Radiol 1987;22:360–371

19. Di Chiro G, Oldfield E, Wright DC et al. Cerebral necrosis after irradiation and/or intraarterial chemotherapy for brain tumors: PET and neuropathologic studies. Am J Neuroradiol 1987;8:1083–109

20. Conti PS, Lilien DL, Hawley K et al. PET and [18F]-FDG in oncology: a clinical update. Nucl Med Biol 1996;23:717–735

21. Rigo P, Paulus P, Kaschten BJ et al. Oncological applications of positron emission tomography with fluorine-18 fluorodeoxyglucose. Eur J Nucl Med 1996;23:1641–1674

22. Meikle SR, Hutton BF, Bailey DL et al. Accelerated EM reconstruction in total body PET: potential for improving tumour detectability. Phys Biol Med 1994;39(10): 1689–1704

23. Meikle SR, Bailey DL, Hooper PK et al. Simultaneous emission and transmission measurements for attentuation correction in whole-body PET. J Nucl Med 1995;36:1680–1688

24. NIH Consensus Conference. Ovarian cancer. Screening, treatment and follow-up. NIH Consensus Development Panel on Ovarian Cancer. JAMA 1995;273:491–497

25. Friedman JB, Weiss NS. Second thoughts about second-look laparotomy in advanced ovarian cancer. N Engl J Med 1990;322:1079–1082

26. Johnson RJ. Radiology in the management of ovarian cancer. Clin Radiol 1993;48:75–82

27. Jacquet P, Jelinek JS, Steves MA, Sugarbaker PH. Evaluation of computed tomography in patients with peritoneal carcinomatosis. Cancer 1993;72:1631–1636

28. Shiels RA, Peel KR, MacDonald HN et al. A prospective trial of computed tomography in the staging of ovarian malignancy. Br J Obstet Gynaecol 1985;92:407–412

29. Forstner R, Hricak H, Occhipinti KA et al. Ovarian cancer: staging with CT and MR imaging. Radiology 1995;197:619–626

30. Forstner R, Hricak H, Powell CB et al. Ovarian cancer recurrence: value of MR imaging. Radiology 1995;196: 715–720

31. Hubner KF, McDonald TW, Niethammer JG et al. Assessment of primary and metastatic ovarian cancer by positron emission tomography (PET) using 2-[18F] deoxyglucose (2-[18F]FDG). Gynecol Oncol 1993;51: 197–204

32. Hubner KF, Smith GT, Hunter K et al. Assessment of primary and recurrent cancer of the ovary using F-18-FDG PET. In: Proceedings of the 6th Annual Meeting of Institute of Clinical PET, Washington, DC, 1994

33. Karlan BY, Hawkins R, Hoh C et al. Whole body positron emission tomography with 2-[18F]-fluoro-2-deoxy-D-glucose can detect recurrent ovarian carcinoma. Gynecol Oncol 1993;51:175–181

34. Valk PE, Mathis CA, Prados MD et al. Hypoxia in human gliomas: demonstration by PET with fluorine-18-fluoromisonidazole. J Nucl Med 1992;33:2133–2137

35. Moulder JE, Rockwell S. Hypoxic fractions of solid tumors: experimental techniques, methods of analysis and a survey of existing data. Int J Radiat Oncol Biol Phys 1984;10:695–712

36. Mottram JC. Factors of importance in the radiosensitivity of tumors. Br J Radiol 1936;9:606–614

37. Yang DJ, Wallace S, Cherif A et al. Development of F-18-labeled fluoroerythronitroimidazole as a PET agent for imaging tumor hypoxia. Radiology 1995;194:795–800

38. Bush RS, Jenkins RDT, Allt WC et al. Definitive evidence for hypoxic cells influencing cure in cancer therapy. Br J Cancer 1978;37 (suppl 3):302–306

39. Findlay M, Young H, Cunningham D et al. Non-invasive monitoring of tumour metabolism using fluorodeoxyglucose and

positron emission tomography: correlation with tumour response. J Clin Oncol 1996;14 (3):700–708

40. Neal CE, Swenson LC, Fanning J, Texter JH. Monoclonal antibodies in ovarian and prostate cancer. Semin Nucl Med 1993;23:114–126

41. Gallup DG. Multicenter clinical trial of 111-In-CYT-103 in patients with ovarian cancer. In: Maquire RT, Van Nostrand D, Eds. Diagnosis of Colorectal and Ovarian Carcinoma. Marcel Dekker, New York, 1992, pp 111–124

42. Prichard JW, Brass LM. New anatomical and functional imaging methods. Ann Neurol 1992;32:395–440

43. Mansfield P. Multi-planar image formation using NMR spin echoes. J Phys 1977;C10:L55–58

44. Stehling MK, Turner R, Mansfield P. Echo-planar imaging: magentic resonance imaging in a fraction of a second. Science 1991;254:43–50

45. Muller MF, Prasad P, Siewert B et al. Abdominal diffusion mapping with use of a whole-body echo-planar system. Radiology 1994;190:475–478

46. Maudsley AA, Hilal SK, Perman WH, Simon HE. Spatially resolved high resolution spectroscopy by "four dimensional" NMR. J Magn Reson 1983;51:147–152

47. Miller BL. A review of chemical issues in 1H NMR spectroscopy: N-acetyl-l-aspartate, creatine and choline. NMR Biomed 1991;4:47–52

48. Negendank W. Studies of human tumors by MRS: a review. NMR Biomed 1992;5:303–324

49. Kurhanewicz J, Vigneron DB, Hricak H et al. Three-dimensional H-1 spectroscopic imaging of the in situ human prostate with high (0.24–0.7-cm^3) spatial resolution. Radiology 1996;198:795–805

50. Aisen AM, Chenevert TL. MR spectroscopy: clinical perspective. Radiology 1989;173:593–599

51. Alger JR, Frank JA, Bizzi A et al. Metabolism of human gliomas: assessment with H-1 MR spectroscopy and F-18 fluorodeoxyglucose PET. Radiology 1990;177:633–641

52. Arnold DL, Shoubridge EA, Villemure JG, Feindel W. Proton and phosphorus magnetic resonance spectroscopy of human astrocytomas in vivo. Preliminary observations on tumor grading. NMR Biomed 1990;3:184–189

53. Bottomley PA. Human in vivo NMR spectroscopy in diagnostic medicine: clinical tool or research probe. Radiology 1989;170:1–15

54. Bottomley PA. The trouble with spectroscopy papers. Radiology 1991;181:344–350

55. Fulham MJ, Bizzi A, Deitz MJ et al. Metabolite mapping of brain tumors with proton MR spectroscopic imaging: clinical relevance. Radiology 1992;185:675–686

56. Fulham MJ, Dietz MJ, Duyn JH et al. Transsynaptic reduction in N-acetyl-aspartate in cerebellar diaschisis: a proton MR spectroscopic imaging study. J Comput Assist Tomogr 1994;18:697–704

57. Weiner MW. The promise of magnetic resonance spectroscopy for medical diagnosis. Invest Radiol 1988;23: 253–261

44

Radionuclide Imaging in Gynecology

MARIO P. ITURRALDE

Advances in medical imaging have resulted from developments in computer science and applied mathematics. There has been an increasing realization that the identification of human disease depends on early biochemical characterization of local organ dysfunction, rather than just on clinical detection of disease or of destroyed tissue structures. Although structural imaging is important, nuclear medicine procedures allow us to conceptualize abnormality rather than visualize it.

As with other imaging modalities, nuclear medicine technology has the ability to make nondestructive measurements, but there are important differences. While the former provide information about body structure, radioactive tracers bring together structure and function, allowing the reconstruction of anatomy from measurements of function.

Using a variety of radioactive tracers, each measuring a specific process, a mosaic of quantitative measurement of regional function can be constructed with sufficient spatial and temporal resolution to provide an image of every organ or system. An example of such an image is the portrayal of the rate of change of regional concentrations of radioactivity rather than the concentration at a single moment. By measuring these spatial distributions at various times, determinations can be made within the body with respect to specific physiologic or biochemical processes, as well as how fast and where such processes are occurring. The result has been increasing precision in the perception, measurement, and definition of biologic phenomena.

GENERAL PRINCIPLES

Nuclear medicine imaging combines the administration and detection of γ-ray emissions from radiopharmaceutical agents having a specific distribution in the body and in vivo reconstruction of radiotracer tissue concentrations. An ever-increasing array of instruments, radioactive tracers, and techniques based upon physical principles has extended the exploration of living materials to the molecular level. Tools of this sort facilitate the identification, measurement, isolation, and characterization of the components of living systems.

RADIOPHARMACEUTICALS

The imaging techniques described in this chapter use a radionuclide linked to a suitable chemical (radiopharmaceutical) to study the particular tissue, organ, or area of interest. In radionuclide scintigraphy, radiopharmaceuticals are used in trace amounts and do not have pharmacologic or toxic actions.

An ideal radiopharmaceutical is one that is safe to handle and administer, suits the purpose for which it is intended, and is readily available and affordable. In choosing a radiopharmaceutical, consideration must be given to the physical properties of the radionuclide and the chemical and biologic properties of the radiopharmaceutical. The two most important characteristics of a radioisotope are the nature of the emissions and the physical and biological half-life of the incorporated radionuclide. For nuclear imaging procedures, the optimal radionuclide emits a single γ-ray of 80 to 300 keV energy with no charged particle emissions. It localizes in the area of interest and is eliminated from the body with a half-life similar to the duration of the examination.

Organs and body systems may (selectively) concentrate a radiopharmaceutical and eliminate it by means of a specific metabolic pathway, or otherwise deal with it depending on its chemical and physical constitution. Some substances (notably iodine) go to the thyroid, while colloids are taken up by the reticuloendothelial system, and phosphates are concentrated in the skeleton. The mechanisms of localization for radionuclide imaging are based on active cellular transport, specific receptor binding of antigens to membrane proteins, phagocytosis, cellular sequestration, capillary blockade, simple diffusion, physiochemical absorption, compartmental localization, bulk flow, or a combination of these mechanisms. The radioactive atom incorporated into the pharmaceutical is only a means of tracing its distribution in the body. It is chosen because its radiation has suitable characteristics for diagnostic procedures and because its physical half-life is similar to the time required for the test to be performed.

Pathology can be recognized with these radiopharmaceuticals by the following:

1. Detecting areas of increased concentration of the radiopharmaceutical within an area of relative homogeneous distribution of the radioactive tracer ("hot spot"). Exam-

ples of this are seen in certain brain tumors, bone metastases, and myocardial infarctions.

2. Detecting areas of decreased concentration of the tracer within a uniform radioactive organ ("cold spot"). Examples of this are seen in liver tumors or secondaries and renal or thyroid cysts.

3. Monitoring the arrival and departure of the radiopharmaceutical over an area of interest. Examples of this are time activity curves over the kidneys in renography, the brain in cerebral perfusion studies, the fallopian tubes in radionuclide hysterosalpingography (HSG), or the heart in left ventricular volume curves.

The most widely used radioactive tracer used is technetium (Tc); the specific isotope being technetium-99m (^{99m}Tc). ^{99m}Tc agents have progressed from those with crude, largely uncharacteristic chemistry to those based on a solid structural chemistry foundation. These second-generation agents are handled by biologic transport mechanisms for which a basic structure distribution relationship now exists because of the physicochemical properties of ^{99m}Tc complexes and not because they are simply bound to biochemicals.[1]

Advances have also occurred for radiopharmaceuticals based on positron and radiohalogen radionuclides. These include radiopharmaceuticals for the heart, brain, and adrenal glands. Exciting results have been obtained with radiolabeled compounds of high specific activity that bind to tissue receptors, and the feasibility of imaging neuroreceptors in the brain has been demonstrated.

The ability to image sites of disease using radiolabeled antibodies, termed radioimmunodetection, has been demonstrated. Immunoscintigraphy shows cell-bound antigens and, in contrast to other imaging methods, is a functional, not a morphologic, imaging procedure. It is possible to detect tumors immunoscintigraphically, even when x-ray, computed tomography (CT), magnetic resonance imaging (MRI), or sonographic results are completely normal. It is also possible to detect recurrences in patients with normal tumor markers. Additionally, immunoscintigraphy allows the topographic localization of the disease, if the antigen is known (e.g., by immunohistochemistry of the primary tumor or by the presence of the tumor-associated antigen in serum). Thereafter, occult lesions can be studied in detail radiologically or by biopsy. The same principle of targeting radionuclides to cancers by specific antibodies is being investigated and used as a means of radioimmunotherapy to destroy tumors.[2]

Radionuclides that are suitable for immunoscintigraphy include iodine-131 (^{131}I), iodine-123 (^{123}I), indium-111 (^{111}In) and ^{99m}Tc. ^{131}I is readily available and inexpensive. ^{123}I and ^{111}In provide high count rates and simple chemistry, but they are more expensive. ^{99m}Tc produces high count rates, it is readily available and inexpensive, and the radiation dose to the patient is low. The disadvantage of ^{99m}Tc for immunoscintigraphy is its short physical half-life.[3]

INSTRUMENTS

The Anger scintillation γ camera has been perfected over the years and has been particularly adapted for imaging the 140-keV γ-rays emitted by ^{99m}Tc. The combination of this radioisotope and the Anger camera has provided the nuclear medicine physician with a powerful tool that has contributed to the continued growth in the field of nuclear medicine.

When γ-rays emitted by a radioisotope strike the collimator front on the head of a scintillation camera, they are projected on to the thin thallium-activated sodium iodide (NaI-T1) scintillation crystal. The light emitted in the crystal travels in all directions and is detected by an array of photomultipliers, which converts the light distribution into a set of electronic signals. The summing network combines these signals into X and Y position signals by finding the centroid of the light distribution. These signals are then normalized in the radiocircuit, which divides them by the energy signal, Z. In addition, a single-channel analyzer selects those events that fall into the energy range corresponding to the γ-ray energy of the injected radiopharmaceutical. Finally, the normalized position signals are used to form an image of the radioisotope distribution in a readout device, which may consist of either a cathode ray tube and film or a digital memory and display. This last feature permits recall, processing, and storage of the image.

Planar radionuclide imaging has some limitations. Not only are the exact location and size of abnormalities unattainable, but the quantification of scintigraphic data within an organ is limited by activity from over- and underlying tissues and by attenuation.

Single-photon emission computed tomography (SPECT) with rotating camera head(s) provides data where attenuation problems are considerably reduced. Its essential goals are enhancement of the image detectability and the extraction of quantitative data from a true three-dimensional scintigram.

Another method of physiologic tomography is positron emission tomography (PET). This radionuclide imaging modality was immediately perceived as a powerful diagnostic technique and basic tool to study in vivo metabolism and physiology. There were two primary reasons for this perception. First, the isotopes used in PET (carbon, nitrogen, oxygen, and fluorine for hydrogen) are chemically identical to atoms within the building blocks of biologic compounds. These isotopes can therefore be used as integral parts of biologic molecules, thus allowing PET to function with almost any number of compounds. Once in the body, these compounds take the place of similar, naturally occurring stable compounds, and replicate their activity. The isotopes themselves decay by the emission of subatomic particles called positrons. The positrons, in turn, combine with electrons, each time producing two γ-photons. The photons are emitted at a 180-degree angle to one another. As a result, γ-detectors surrounding the patient can detect these events, while a computer records only those events that are opposite one another and simultaneous. The resulting information is processed to produce images representing activity within a few millimeters of its location. Second, the physical properties of PET allow the quantitative measurement of the three-dimensional distribution of a positron emitter in the human body.

The advantage of PET over other cross-sectional, anatomically based imaging techniques is its ability to characterize tumor physiology and anatomy, thus having clinical value in evaluating cancer patients. Compared to healthy tissues, malignant tumors have higher proliferative and glycolytic rates, so tumors demonstrate increased glucose, or deoxyglucose utilization as well as heightened incorporation of amino acids. Using PET, ^{18}fluorodeoxyglucose (^{18}FDG) accumulation in a wide variety of primary and metastatic malignant tumors has been demonstrated, including carcinomas of the breast and ovaries.

^{18}FDG, a structural analog of glucose, is trapped across cell membranes by glucose-transfer molecules in a manner similar to glucose and then phosphorylated to ^{18}FDG-6-phosphate by hexokinase. Most malignant cells are deficient in glucose-6-phosphorylase, so ^{18}FDG-phosphate is trapped intracellularly. This results in progressive uptake of ^{18}FDG in tumor cells compared to normal cells. The proposed mechanisms for ^{18}FDG accumulation in malignant cells include increased expression of glucose-transfer molecules at tumor cell membranes and elevated levels of hexokinase.

An increased ^{18}FDG uptake and increased standard uptake ratio are reliable indicator of viable malignancy, while benign or low-grade neoplasms generally have lower or normal ^{18}FDG uptake and standard uptake ratios. PET is the only technology that offers a physiologic view of pathologic as well as normal processes throughout the body (W. Martin, personal communication, Key Biscayne, FL, 1996).

IMAGING PROCEDURES

Diagnostic nuclear medicine imaging usually involves the intravenous injection, deposition, or oral ingestion of a radiolabeled agent and the acquisition of static images of areas of the body at fixed times after the delivery of the radioisotope. Ventilation studies require inhalation of the radionuclide as a gas or aerosol, while radionuclide HSG requires the deposition of radiolabeled particles in the vagina. Dynamic studies usually involve the tracing of a radiopharmaceutical and the collection of images at various times within the organ of interest. These images can be digitized for quantitative data processing, display, and storage. In some studies, physiologic and pharmacologic intervention may be used before, during, or after administration of the radiopharmaceutical, to achieve or to enhance the differential distribution of radioactivity necessary to obtain the desired information.

RELEVANT STRUCTURE AND PHYSIOLOGY OF THE FALLOPIAN TUBES

Although the fallopian tubes appear to be modest passive uterine appendages, functionally, they are extremely sensitive organs responding to hormonal, biochemical, and neural stimulation that facilitate the process of fertilization.

The existence of upward transportation processes at the time of conception implies that the motility of spermatozoa may not be the only relevant factor for their ascension. The union of spermatozoon and oocyte depends on the active role of spermatozoa and the actions of the ciliated epithelium of the female reproductive tract.

The simple columnar epithelial lining of the uterine tube is made up of ciliated cells interspersed with intercalated (indifferent) and nonciliated secretory cells that are believed to produce a nutritive secretion. Ciliated cells in the tube are most prominent in the epithelial surface of the fimbriated infundibulum, where they form dense arrays, while a large number of cilia may also be found in the ampulla. In general, ciliated cells are less frequent in the isthmus.

The ciliated cells of the fallopian tubes have a common structural and functional pattern of internal tubules, with propulsive action similar to that of the respiratory tract, some of the tympanic cavity and auditory tube, efferent ductules of the testis, and spermatozoid flagellum.

Growth of the ciliated epithelium appears to be under the influence of ovarian hormones. The rate of cilial beat and muscular contraction seem to be the greatest just at or after the time of ovulation, thereby ensuring effective transport of eggs to the site of fertilization. Ciliated and secretory cells begin to increase in height shortly after menstruation, and by the time of ovulation are approximately $30\mu m$ high. Treatment with progesterone, by contrast, antagonizes motility and the estrogen-driven cell growth.[4]

Paltieli[5] described a method for measuring the beat frequency of fallopian tube cilia, using a laser light-scattering technique as part of the laparoscopic evaluation in infertile women. They determined a normal ciliary beat frequency to be about 5.6 Hz. These measurements revealed changes in the ciliary beat frequency at different stages of ovulation as the fallopian tubes prepare for ovum pickup and transport. In the fimbria, the highest frequency, 6.0 Hz, was measured during the late follicular phase before ovulation. This figure dropped to 4.9 Hz after ovulation.

Measurements of ciliary beat frequency also correlated with the percentage of ciliated cells in the fallopian tubes (known as the "ciliary index"). The ciliary index was determined in 19 women. In 12 of the 13 women whose ciliary beat frequency was normal, the ciliary index was normal as well, above 50%. In 5 of the 6 whose ciliary beat frequency was below normal, the ciliary index was also below normal.

The role of a simple nuclear medicine procedure, based on these structural and physiologic concepts, became clinically apparent in eliciting, if not answers, perhaps questions about

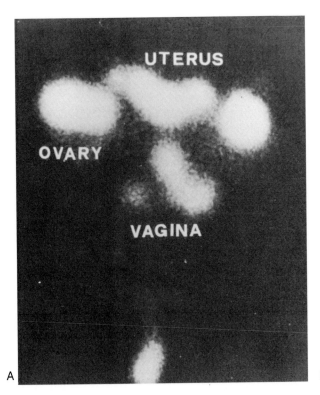

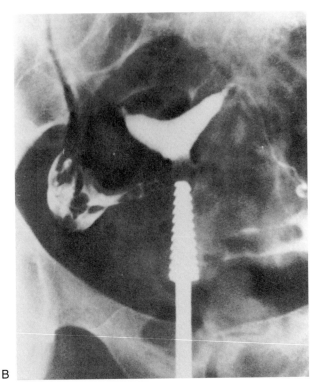

Figure 44.1 (**A**) Normal HERS portraying the pattern of flow of radiolabeled microspheres from the vagina, through the uterus, to the fimbriated peritoneal opening of patent fallopian tubes. (**B**) Contrast spillage into the peritoneal cavity during HSG.

the transport mechanisms with special interest in the aspect of tubal ciliary motion and its relationship to infertility.

HYSTEROSALPINGORADIONUCLIDE SCINTIGRAPHY

To demonstrate the upward migration of nonmotile, inert chemical substances, we described a radionuclide imaging and counting technique.[4,6] The images reflected the dynamic state of the tube and could be used for evaluating fallopian tube function. Hysterosalpingoradionuclide scintigraphy (HERS) was assessed in a study of 53 women.[6] Patients were divided into two groups: Group I consisted of 24 adult white women admitted for elective gynecologic operations; group II consisted of 29 adult white women referred for evaluation of their tubal patency.

In patients from group I, 24 hours after deposition of the radioactive tracer in their vaginas, in vitro counts were performed on removed surgical specimens using a well-scintillation detector. The uterus and each of the fallopian tubes was counted separately, as were the fimbria and ovaries. In two cases, a piece of the anterior peritoneum, fluid from the pouch of Douglas, peripheral blood, and lymphatic glands were also counted to determine the possibility of reabsorption of the radionuclide into the blood stream or lymphatic drainage from the vaginal mucosa.

Radioactivity levels of the surgical specimens substantially higher than background levels were regarded as evidence of migration of the ^{99m}Tc human albumin microspheres (^{99m}Tc-HAM) from the vagina to the uterus or the tubes and ovaries. However, if radioactivity levels were similar to background levels, it was assumed that there had been no migration, and the cause for possible obstruction was investigated.

For the imaging procedure, patients were placed in the supine gynecologic examination position with the buttocks slightly elevated or in the Trendelenburg position. Commercially available HAM was labeled with ^{99m}Tc (half-life 6 hours). The size of more than 95% of HAM ranged between 10 and 40μm with an average diameter 20μm. This approximates the size of a human sperm. Then 370 MBq (10 mCi) (for patients of group I) and 70 MBq (2 mCi) (for patients of group II) of ^{99m}Tc-HAM was deposited close to the os.

Images were obtained 1, 2, 3, and 24 hours after deposition of the radioactive tracer. Scans were interpreted as abnormal if there was no activity in one or both tubes and specially if the distal focal area of high activity in the fimbria did not appear within 3 hours. The course and migration of ^{99m}Tc-HAM were the transit time from deposition in the vagina until appearance in either fimbria. In healthy females with patent tubes, the transit time varies from 1 to 3 hours (Figs. 44.1 to 44.5).

Although the ^{99m}Tc-HAM molecules are biochemically and immunologically different from human spermatozoa,

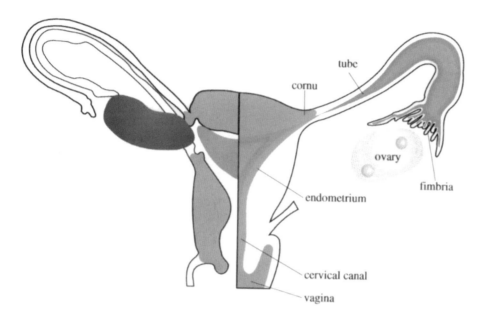

Figure 44.2 Composite image: left, diagrammatic anatomic description, right, HERS.

their diameter approximates that of human spermatozoa. It is suggested that the radiolabeled molecules are transported by the same mechanisms that support spermatozoal migration and that migration of the radionuclide reflects that of spermatozoa.

All patients of group II had contrast HSG and laparoscopic chromopertubation after HERS. The three diagnostic procedures were compared.

Radiation exposure to patients of group I was not relevant, since the target organs had been surgically removed. However, this was not the case for patients of group II. For this reason, in patients from group II, the dose of ^{99m}Tc-HAM was reduced to 70 MBq.

In 14 of 21 cases, it was possible to measure high radioactivity levels in the adnexa separately from the uterus. Nine of

these showed marked radioactivity in the tubes (most of it localized in the fimbria). In five cases, radioactivity in the tubes was not much higher than the background. In these patients, severe tubal occlusion was confirmed after surgery. In the two patients where pieces of the anterior peritoneum, peripheral blood, and lymphatic glands were counted, the radioactivity levels in the samples were as low as that of the background. This showed that the ^{99m}Tc-HAM had not reached the adnexa through the blood supply, owing to local reabsorption or lymphatic drainage from the vaginal mucosa (Fig. 44.6).

When HERS was compared with HSG and laparoscopy in patients from group II, it was found that in 21 patients there was complete accordance among the three modalities,

Figure 44.3 Normal HERS with bilateral visualization of the fimbria.

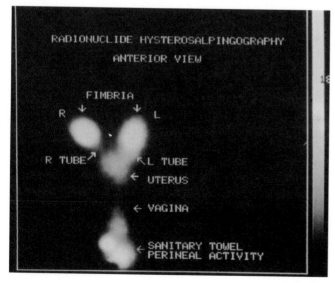

Figure 44.4 Normal HERS at 30, 60, 90 and 180 minutes with asymmetric migration of radiolabeled microspheres appearing early in the left fimbria at 3 hours, finally showing bilateral tubal patency.

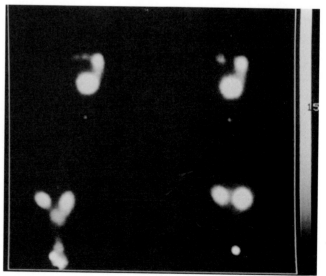

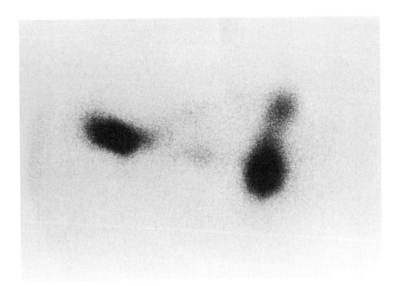

Figure 44.5 HERS image (anterior view) obtained at 6 hours after deposition of ^{99m}TC-HAM in the vagina with normal migration through a patent left tube and decreased migration through the functionally impaired right tube. (HSG showed bilateral tubal patency.)

whether the tubes were patent or occluded. In six cases there was no agreement between HERS and HSG and laparoscopy. In five, both HSG and laparoscopy showed that the tubes were patent. In these cases, HERS showed no evidence of migration in one or other tube (Fig. 44.7). In two cases, the results were equivocal because at least two of the three diagnostic procedures were technically deficient (Figs. 44.8 and 44.9).

The results from this study with HERS in patients from group I show the upward migration of a particulate radioactive tracer such as ^{99m}Tc-HAM from the vagina through the uterus and tubes into the peritoneal cavity and ovaries. This correlated with findings on surgical specimens, proving the accuracy of the procedure. HERS, when compared to laparoscopy in 77 infertile females, showed a sensitivity for detection of tubal patency of 93% and a specificity of 94%. For the detection of tubal obstruction, the sensitivity was 94% and the specificity 93%. The overall predictive value for tubal patency was 96% and for tubal obstruction 90%. The overall efficiency (percent of tubes correctly diagnosed) of HERS was 97%.

HERS is a simple procedure that could be used to confirm the success of a reanastomosis or tubal ligation[7] (Fig. 44.10).

A number of other studies have since suggested that HERS be accepted, with the other imaging procedures, as part of the investigation of infertility.[8–16] If a woman is found to have pelvic adhesions, but HERS shows normal ciliary function, she may require surgery. However, if HERS indicates that tubal ciliary function is abnormal, then gamete intrafallopian transfer or zygote intrafallopian transfer may not be appropriate. In vitro fertilization and embryo transfer to the uterine cavity could be preferable.

CILIARY FUNCTION IN INFERTILE CIGARETTE-SMOKING FEMALES

In numerous studies, cigarette smoking has been shown to affect the humoral and cellular systems.[17–19] These changes might affect tubal epithelial behaviour with altered tubal

Figure 44.6 Abnormal HERS with patent left tube and obstructed right tube. HSG showed normal bilateral spilling of contrast into the peritoneum.

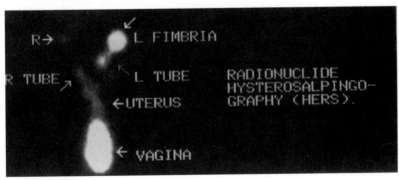

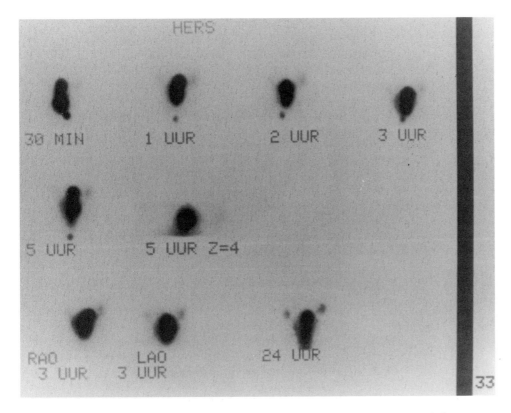

Figure 44.7 Abnormal HERS with images obtained for up to 24 hours. Bilateral tubal obstruction (faint activity is seen bilaterally in the ampulla of the fallopian tubes).

Figure 44.8 (A) HSG showing hydrosalpinx in the left tube and patency on the right. (B) HERS shows intense activity in the hydrosalpinx of the left tube and functional obstruction of the right tube.

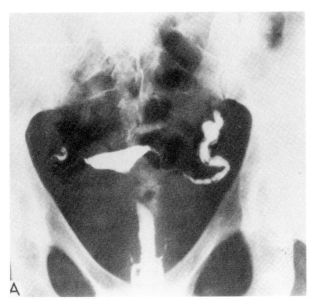

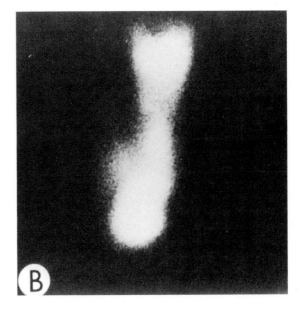

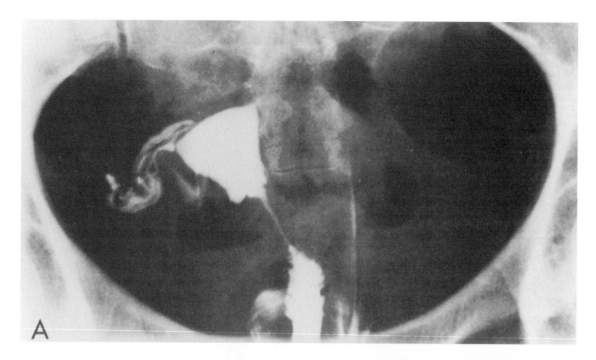

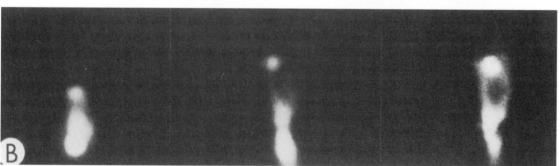

Figure 44.9 **(A)** HSG. **(B)** HERS demonstrating left tubal occlusion and normal patent right tube. Partial migration of radiolabeled microspheres is present on the right.

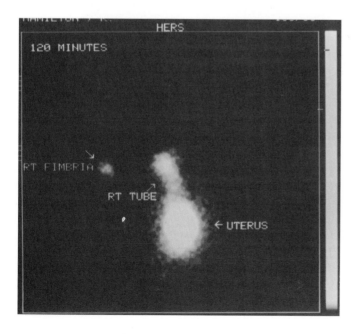

Figure 44.10 HERS of a patient who underwent tubal ligation, showing radiolabeled microspheres migration through the right tube to the fimbria beyond the level of ligation.

transport and decreased ciliary motility.[19] This is supported by epidemiologic evidence showing that women who smoke suffer from bronchial disease and have a greater chance of being infertile or take longer to conceive than nonsmokers.[20–23] This observation suggested that there was connection between ciliary damage between the respiratory system and the fallopian tubes due to cigarette smoking.

The fact that fertility is adversely affected by smoking is presumably related to the ciliotoxic effects of cigarette smoke that cause bronchial damage. Iturralde and Venter tested this hypothesis,[24–26] based on the principle that cilia of the respiratory tract and fallopian tubes have a common structural and functional pattern of internal tubules.[27,28]

Two procedures were used to show the tracheobronchial and oviductal ciliary function in infertile cigarette smokers.[29,30] The scintigraphic display of tracheobronchial function following radioaerosol inhalation of ^{99m}Tc-colloid particles was used for the visualization of the mucociliary function of the lungs, while HERS was used to evaluate the cilia of the fallopian tubes.

Radioaerosol Lung Cinescintrigraphy

The cinescintigraphic display of the lungs following radioaerosol inhalation of monodispersed particles is a useful procedure for the visual and qualitative assessment of mucociliary clearance in the tracheobronchial tree.[29] In non-smokers, radioaerosol particle deposition is homogeneous throughout the lungs and airways. The transport of mucus in the airways is always cephalad in direction, fast and steady in its progress. In smokers, radioaerosol transport showed stagnation, with up and down motion of mucus in the trachea or bronchi or migration into the opposite bronchus. All subjects had slow mucociliary clearance[30] (Fig. 44.11).

A further study using an analog light contrast enhancement technique similar to that described by Paltieli and co-workers[5] for measuring the beat frequency of the fallopian tube cilia was used to assess nasal ciliary beat frequency in smokers and nonsmokers.[31,32]

Normal values were obtained from eight healthy non-smoking volunteers who had an average cilia beat frequency of 11.7 Hz. In 12 of the smokers who underwent nasal brushings, the cilia beat frequency dropped to 6.5 Hz. After stopping smoking for 3 weeks, they recovered to an average beat frequency of 9.8 Hz.

Fallopian Tube Ciliary Function

Of the 28 tubes examined in 14 cigarette smokers, 8 were found to be obstructed, while the rest were patent on HSG and laparoscopy. However, when studied by HERS, all the tubes showed delayed or absent tubociliary migration. In those patients who stopped smoking, after 3 months, ciliary function of the tracheobronchial tree and fallopian tubes had improved (Fig. 44.12).

Figure 44.11 Tracheobronchial mucociliary clearance with curves during cigarette smoking and after stopping cigarette smoking.

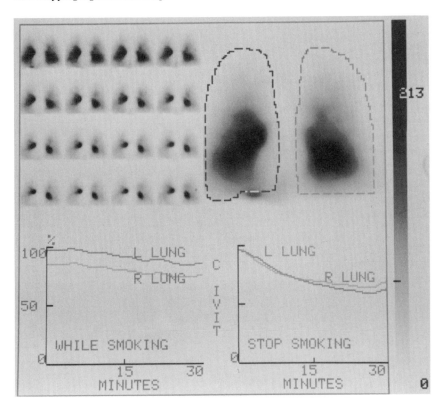

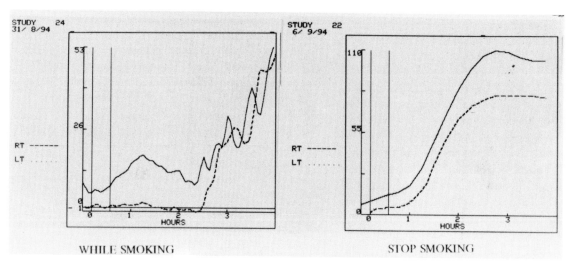

Figure 44.12 HERS tubociliary clearance of same woman as Figure 44.11 showing curves of arrival of radiolabeled activity (^{99m}Tc-HAM) in the fimbria for up to 4 hours, during cigarette smoking, and after stopping smoking. This apparently infertile woman conceived after stopping smoking.

BREAST CANCER IMAGING

All conventional breast imaging techniques have inherent limitations, since they are based on anatomic considerations. The biologic localization of radionuclide techniques offers another method of studying variables in planning treatment of breast carcinoma. A number of different nuclear medicine techniques have been used for breast cancer imaging including thallium 201[33], ^{99m}Tc-sestamibi,[34] monoclonal antibodies,[2] and PET with[18]FDG.[35]

Scintimammography with ^{99m}Tc-Sestamibi

^{99m}Tc-sestamibi is a lipophilic ^{99m}Tc organometallic cationic chemical complex that accumulates in myocardial tissue with some properties similar to those of thallium (^{201}T1) chloride. The exact mechanism of cellular uptake of ^{99m}Tc-sestamibi in cancer cells is unknown.

Khalkhali and co-workers[36] evaluated the complementary role of ^{99m}Tc-sestamibi scintimammography in the detection of carcinoma of the breast. Scintimammograms were obtained at 5, 10, and 60 minutes after injection of ^{99m}Tc-sestamibi in 127 women with 153 lesions that warranted histologic or cytologic analysis. There were 113 palpable and 40 nonpalpable lesions. Each patient had 740 MBq (20 mCi) of ^{99m}Tc-sestamibi intravenously in the arm contralateral to the affected breast. Scintimammography was true-positive in 47 carcinomas, true-negative in 91 benign lesions, false-positive in 11 benign lesions, and false-negative in four infiltrating duct carcinomas.

This study had a sensitivity of 92.2%, a specificity of 89.2%, a positive predictive value of 81.0%, and a negative predictive value of 95.8% for scintimammography in the detection of carcinoma of the breast. The authors concluded that scintimammography has a high sensitivity and specificity compared with conventional mammography and that scintimammographic findings resulted in correct identification of malignant or benign lesions in patients with indeterminate mammography (Figs. 44.13 and 44.14).

PET Scintimammography

Using ^{18}F-fluoroestradiol, PET has detected primary and metastatic lesions with a sensitivity of 93% in patients with estrogen receptor positive tumors. The sensitivity for the detection of estrogen receptor negative tumours is presumably low.[35] In several reports of ^{18}FDG PET, primary breast can-

Figure 44.13 Normal ^{99m}Tc-MBI scan of breasts and axilla of patient with breast carcinoma (myocardium is visualized in the left anterior thorax).

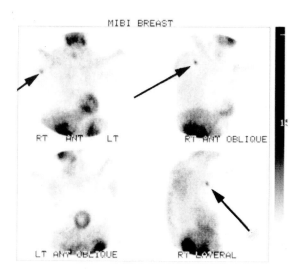

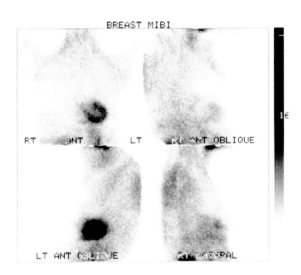

BREAST MIBI

RT   ANT   LT   RT ANT OBLIQUE

LT ANT OBLIQUE   RT LATERAL

Figure 44.14 ^{99m}Tc-MBI scan showing focal right axillary lymph node metastasis (non palpable) in a patient with breast carcinoma. (The myocardium visualized in the left anterior thorax.)

cers were detected with a sensitivity of 86% to 100%. Staging of metastatic disease to the axillae has been mixed.[37] As with sestamibi and thallium scintigraphy, initial reports using ^{18}FDG Single-photon emission computed tomography are encouraging, but larger series are required before clinical usefulness is known.

Antibody Imaging of the Breast

Radioimmunolocalization of breast cancer has been studied using different mucin antigen directed monoclonal antibodies. Anti-human milk fat globule antibodies, tumour-associated antigen, and anticarcinoembryonic antibodies were used in clinical trials. Anticarcinoembryonic antigen (anti-CEA) is one of the most extensively studied antibodies.[2] Reactivity for CEA in ductal carcinoma of the breast is 70% to 90%, but normal breast, fibroadenomas, and fibrocystic disease show virtually no CEA reactivity.

Anti-CEA immunoconjugates have been investigated since 1978 and have evolved from polyclonal antibodies to monoclonal antibody fragments, using first iodine and indium isotopes and now ^{99m}Tc. The application of radioimmunoscintigraphy (RIS) with ^{99m}Tc-IMMU-4 Fab' fragment (CEA-scan, Immunomedics, Inc., Morris Plains, NJ) in breast carcinoma might allow definition of stromal extension of the disease and determination of axillary nodal status.[38]

Serafini and co-workers[39] described RIS using ^{99m}Tc-labeled anti-CEA Fab' fragments on 36 patients with suspected or diagnosed breast cancer in a clinical trial. The patients received 1 mg of antibody labeled with 900 MBq (25 mCi) ^{99m}Tc. Planar and SPECT images of the thorax and axillae were taken 5 to 8 hours after injection. Nineteen patients proved to have breast cancer, and axillary metastases were found in 8 of the 14 patients undergoing axillary node dissec-

tion. CEA-scan correctly diagnosed primaries in 17 of 19 patients (89%) and axillary node involvement in 4 of 8 patients (50%). RIS had a sensitivity, specificity, positive predictive value, and negative predictive value of 89%, 63%, 85%, and 71%, respectively. These suggest that RIS using ^{99m}Tc-labeled anti-CEA Fab' promises to be sensitive and noninvasive for breast cancer diagnosis. Radioimmunostaging potentially makes selective rather than routine use of axillary lymph node dissection feasible in patients with early breast cancer.

Receptor Imaging of the Breast

The physiopathology of somatostatin receptor expression in breast cancer is unknown. However, somatostatin has been shown to inhibit tumor growth by binding to specific cell surface receptors.[40] Studies of somatostatin-receptor scintigraphy (OctreoScan, Mallinckrodt, St. Louis, Missouri) showed a high sensitivity in the imaging of breast cancer. However, the specificity has yet to be determined, and its clinical applications remain to be defined.[40] Serafini (personal communication, Key Biscayne, FL, 1996) studied 22 patients suspected of having primary or recurrent or metastatic breast cancer. OctreoScan was positive in 20 patients. Sixteen had cancer on histopathology. Three cases of occult metastatic disease were first detected by OctreoScan. Somatostatin-receptor imaging was found to be equally sensitive in revealing both node and bone metastases. These suggest that somatostatin-receptor expression is a frequent feature in breast cancer. However, receptor expression may also be seen in some nonmalignant breast lesions with proliferative activity. Clinical applications of somatostatin-receptor imaging may include detection of occult recurrent/metastatic disease.

OVARIAN CANCER IMAGING

RIS in the Detection of Ovarian Carcinoma

Since the development of monoclonal antibody (MAb) technology, many MAbs reactive with ovarian tumour-associated antigens have been studied. The first clinical results of radioimmunodetection of ovarian cancer were obtained with ^{131}I-labeled anti-CEA polyclonal antibodies. The antibodies had been developed against γ-fetoprotin and human chorionic gonadotropin. Applications for these MAbs include RIS for tumor imaging, intraoperative detection, and immunotherapy (M, W. Method, personal communication, Key Biscayne, FL, 1996).

A number of studies have demonstrated the usefulness of RIS with ^{111}In-satumomab pendetide in patients with ovarian cancer. Surwit et al.[41] reported the results of 103 patients undergoing surgery for diagnosis of primary or recurrent disease. The sensitivity of RIS was 68% and the accuracy was 64%. Recent studies have shown RIS to be even more accurate and sensitive. Low, Carten, et al.[42] compared the accuracy of breath-hold contrast-enhanced MRI, CT, and ^{111}In-Cyt-103 immunoscintigraphy for detecting pelvic and abdominal tumors in 16 patients with primary, residual, or recurrent ovarian cancer. They found that the sensitivity of immunoscintigraphy was 92%. Radioimmunodetection is an evolving technique that may allow noninvasive detection of persistent or recurrent ovarian cancer. The above suggests that CT is of limited value in the assessment of patients with negative physical examinations and normal CA-125 levels.

Intraoperative Localization

Intraoperative localization of radiolabeled MAbs uses sterilizable, collimated γ-detection probes. Studies in patients with ovarian cancer showed that the procedure had a high sensitivity for detection of subclinical tumor after injection of ^{131}I-labeled anti-CA-125 antibodies. It was found that 94.4% of all specimens taken from regions with increased count were tumor-involved. The probe is also promising for increasing the number of tumor-positive biopsies taken at second-look surgery. Seventy-four of 144 biopsies taken when guided by the probe were tumor-involved compared with 4 of 197 biopsy specimens obtained at random.[3]

REFERENCES

1. Iturralde MP. Nuclear medicine procedures in surgical diagnosis. In: Mieny CL, Mennen U, Eds. Principles of Surgical Patient Care. Academica, Pretoria, South Africa, 1990, pp. 57–78

2. Goldenberg DM, Larson SM. Radioimmunodetection in cancer identification. J Nucl Med 1992;33:803–814

3. Haberkorn U, Baum PR, Hör G. Breast and ovary. In: Wagner HN, Szabo Z, Buchanan JW, Eds. Principles of Nuclear Medicine. WB Saunders, Philadelphia, 1995, pp. 1065–1082

4. Venter PF, Iturralde MP. Migration of a particulate radioactive tracer from the vagina to the peritoneal cavity and ovaries. S Afr Med J 1979;55:917–919

5. Paltieli Y. New laser technique can help pinpoint infertility due to fallopian tube pathology. Med Chronicle 1994; March 7

6. Iturralde MP, Venter PF. Hysterosalpingo-radionuclide scintigraphy (HERS). Semin Nucl Med 1981;11:301–314

7. Strauss SA. Unsuccessful sterilisation of woman—doctor liable for child-raising cost. S Afr Med J 1990;75:557

8. Brundin J, Dahlborn M, Ahlber-Ahre E, Lundberg HJ. Radionuclide hysterosalpingography for measurement of human oviductal function. Int J Gynecol Obstet 1989;28:53–59

9. Uzler M, Jacobson A, Warnich A, Nassor G. Radionuclide hysterosalpingography—Appropriate for the new assisted reproduction techniques. J Nucl Med 1993;164:P797

10. McQueen D, McKillop JH, Gray HW et al. Investigation of tubal infertility by radionuclide migration. Hum Reprod 1991;6:529–532

11. Steck T, Wurfel W, Becker W, Albert PJ. Serial scintigraphic imaging for visual passive transport processes in the human fallopian tube. Hum Reprod 1991;6:1186–1191

12. Barrada M, Buxbaum P, Schatten C et al. Hystero-salpingo scintigraphy: a routine investigation in sterile women? Nucl Med Commun 1995;16:447–451

13. Hyznar V, Heczko P, Husak V et al. Indication and clinical application of radionuclide hysterosalpingography using ^{99m}Tc-pertechnetate. Acta Univ Palacki Olomuc Fac Med 1984;107:185–193

14. Mojiminiyi OA, Kennedy SH, Saper NDW et al. Clinical application of radionuclide hysterosalpingography in the management of female infertility. Nucl Med Comm 1991; 12:310–311

15. McKillop JA, Mc Queen D, Gray HW et al. Radionuclide hysterosalpingography in infertility (Abstract 754). Proceedings of the 5th World Congress of Nuclear Medicine, Montreal, 1990

16. McQueen D, Gray HW, McKillop JH et al. Radionuclide evaluation of fallopian tube patency in 80 infertile women. Nucl Med Commun 1988;9:169

17. Panayiotis M, Zavos EDS. Cigarette smoking and human reproduction: effects on female and male fecundity. Infertility 1989;12:35–46

18. Stillman RJ, Rosenberg MJ, Sachs BP. Smoking and reproduction. Fertil Steril 1989;46:545–566

19. Weathersbee PS. Nicotine and its influence on the female reproduction system. J Reprod Med 1980;25:243–250

20. Dalhamn T. In vivo and in vitro ciliotoxic effects of tobacco smoke. Arch Environ Health 1970;21:633–634

21. Kokuhata GK. Smoking in relation to infertility and fetal loss. Arch Environ Health 1968;17:353–359

22. London Press Service. Smoking can harm fertility. Specialist Med 1993;15:44

23. Howe GH, Westhoff C, Vessey M, Yeates D. Effects of age, cigarette smoking, and other factors on fertility: findings in a large prospective study. Br Med J 1985;290:1697–1700

24. Elliason R, Mossberg B, Camner P, Afzelius B. The immotile-cilia syndrome. N Engl J Med 1977;297:1–6

25. Parker GS, Mehlum DL, Bacher-Westmore B. Ciliary dyskinesis: the immotile cilia syndrome. Laryngoscope 1983;93:5 73–577

26. Iturralde MP, Venter PF. Radionuclide studies of fallopian tubes ciliary function in infertile cigarette-smoking females. [Abstract 179.] Eur J Nucl Med 1994;21:547

27. Evans HJ, Fletcher J, Torrance M, Hargreave TB. Sperm abnormalities and cigarette smoking. Lancet 1981;1:627–629

28. Berry EM. Sperm abnormalities and cigarette smoking. Lancet 1981;1:1159

29. Agnew JE, Bateman JRM, Pavia D, Clarke SW. A model for assessing bronchial mucus transport. J Nucl Med 1984;24:170–176

30. Iturralde MP. Mucociliary clearance mechanism in cigarette smokers. S Afr Med J 1987;72:814

31. Yager J, Chen T-M, Dulfano MJ. Measurement of frequency of ciliary beats of human respiratory epithelium. Chest 1978; 73:627–633

32. Rutland J, Griffin W, Cole P. Nasal brushing and measurement of ciliary beat frequency. Chest 1981;80:865–867

33. Waxman AD, Ramanna L, Memsic LD et al. Thallium scintigraphy in evalation of mass abnormalities of the breast. J Nucl Med 1993;34:18–23

34. Khalkhali I, Mena I, Jouanne E et al. Prone scintimammography in patients with suspicion of carcinoma of the breast. J Am Coll Surg 1994;178:491–497

35. McGuire AH, Dehdashti F, Siegel BA et al. Positron tomographic assessment of 16-alpha-(18F)-Fluoro-17-beta-estradiol uptake in metastatic breast carcinoma. J Nucl Med 1991; 32:1526–1531

36. Khalkhali I, Cutrone JA, Mena IG et al. Scintimmamography: The complemetary role of ^{99m}Tc sestamibi prone breast imaging for the diagnosis of breast carcinoma. Radiology 1995;196: 421–426

37. Adler LP, Crowe JP, al-Kasis NK, Sunshine JL. Evaluation of breast masses and axillary lymph nodes with (F-18)2-deoxy-2-fluoro-D-glucose PET. Radiology 1993;187:743–750

38. Kuhajda FP, Offut LE, Mendelsonn G. The distribution of carcinoembryogenic antigen in breast carcinoma. Diagnostic and prognostic implications. Cancer 1983;52:1257

39. Serafini AN, Goldenbberg DM, Higgibotham-Ford EA et al. A multicenter trial cancer imaging with fragments of CEA antibodies. J Nucl Med 1989;30:748

40. Krenning EP, Kwekkeboom DJ, Reubi JC et al. ^{111}In-octreotide scintigraphy in oncology. Metabolism 1992;41;83–86

41. Surwit EA, Childers JM, Krag DN et al. Clinical assessment of ^{111}In-CYT-103 immunoscintigraphy in ovarian cancer. Gynecol Oncol 1993;48:285–292

42. Low RN, Carter WD, Saleh F, Sigeti JS. Ovarian cancer: comparison of findings with perfluorocarbon-enhanced MR imaging. In-III-CYT-103 immunoscintigraphy, and CT. Radiology 1995;195:391–400

45

Three-Dimensional Ultrasound in Gynecology

KATHARINA GRUBOECK

DAVOR JURKOVIC

Three-dimensional ultrasound has two advantages over conventional ultrasound. The first is the ability to store and then reconstruct ultrasound images. This enables the visualization of an infinite number of planes, including those not often seen during B-mode examination. The second is three-dimensional reconstruction of anatomy and the assessment of spatial relationships. In this respect, three-dimensional ultrasound is similar to computed tomography and magnetic resonance imaging.

TECHNIQUE OF THREE-DIMENSIONAL SONOGRAPHY

Scans are performed using a B-mode scanner, which monitors spatial orientation of images and stores them as a volume set in a computer. When performing a volume scan, conventional two-dimensional B-mode transvaginal ultrasound examination is usually performed first. The organ of interest is then centered on the screen, and a large number of consecutive tomograms are obtained by moving the transducer. They are stored in the computer memory. The acquired volume is analyzed using computer-generated planar reformatted sections. They are usually displayed in three orthogonal planes. These views provide the operator with improved spatial evaluation of the organ of interest and allow reconstruction of an unlimited number of planes (Fig. 45.1). Reconstruction can be achieved by moving the two-dimensional images, which are confined in the three planes, concomitantly. Their relative positions are indicated by reference lines on the other two planes on the monitor, and any section can be reconstructed. Sections of the organ of interest that were not visualized during data acquisition may also be generated.

Volume measurements can be performed by showing all three perpendicular planes on the screen. One plane is chosen for volume measurements. The other two planes are used to ensure that the whole object of interest has been included in the measurement. The measurement is performed by delineating the whole of the object in a number of parallel sections 1 to 2 mm apart. The volume is then calculated by the computer software. This enables accurate volume measurements of organs or tissues regardless of their shape.

THREE-DIMENSIONAL ULTRASOUND OF THE UTERUS

Congenital Uterine Anomalies

The accuracy of three-dimensional ultrasound for the diagnosis of congenital uterine anomalies has been investigated.[1] High-risk patients with a history of recurrent miscarriage or infertility were studied. All had a hysterosalpingogram in the previous 6 months. Using three-dimensional ultrasound, all cases of congenital uterine anomalies were correctly identified, and there were no false-positives or false-negatives. This made it superior to two-dimensional ultrasound, which detected all cases of anomalies but had a number of false-positives.

The most useful plane was the transverse section through the whole length of the uterus from the fundus to the cervix. This enabled the measurement of both the fundal cleft and the length of the uterine septum. This plane, being perpendicular to the ultrasound beam, cannot be seen on a conventional two-dimensional transvaginal scan, making it impossible to distinguish between arcuate, subseptate, and bicornuate uterus (Figs. 45.2 and 45.3).

Endometrial Cancer

Three-dimensional ultrasound enables endometrial volume measurement. Endometrial thickness and volume were mea-

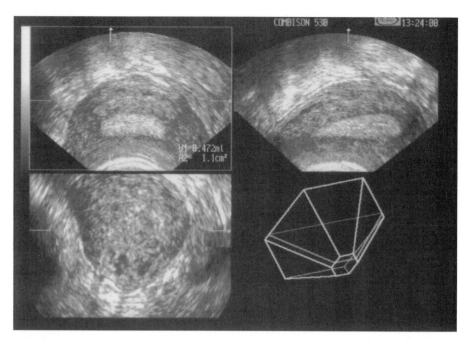

Figure 45.1 A display of three perpendicular planes through the uterus. The measurement of endometrial volume using planer reformatted sections is illustrated. The whole uterine cavity is displayed in numerous parallel sections, and the volume is calculated by the internal computer program.

sured in women with postmenopausal bleeding.[2] Volume was successfully measured in 95% of patients. In patients with atrophic or normal endometrium, the mean thickness and volume were 5.3 mm and 0.9 ml, respectively. The endometrial thickness and volume were both lower in patients with benign pathology such as polyps or hyperplasia. However, there was an overlap between benign and malignant that was much less with volume than with thickness. Above 13 ml, all cancers were diagnosed, and there was only one false-positive in a patient with endometrial hyperplasia.

Figure 45.2 A normal uterus shown in the transverse section through the whole of the uterine cavity. The myometrium as well as the endometrium are intact, and there is no fundal cleft.

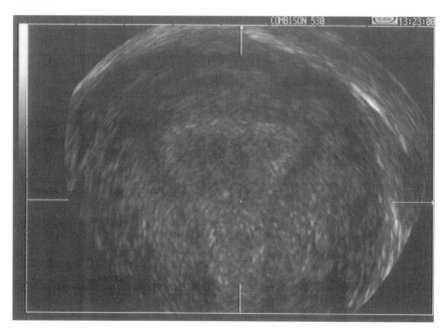

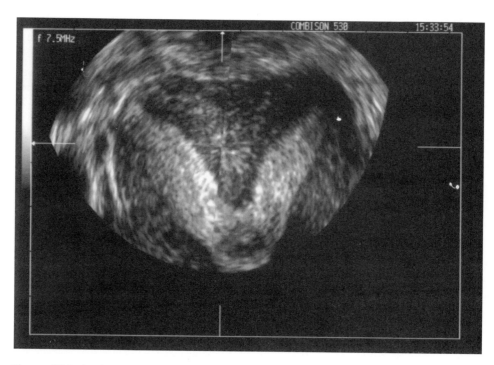

Figure 45.3 A subseptate uterus with normal fundal appearance. A thick septum is seen partially dividing the uterine cavity.

THREE-DIMENSIONAL ULTRASOUND OF THE ADNEXA

Follicular Monitoring

The accuracy of follicular volume measurements by two- and three-dimensional ultrasound has been measured.[3] Volumes were calculated either by the formula for an ovoid from three follicular diameters measured by two-dimensional ultrasound or by three-dimensional ultrasound using the same method as previously described for endometrium. The results were compared to the volume of aspirate at ovum harvest. Three-dimensional measurements were more accurate, especially in the clinically important range of 3 to 7 ml.

Diagnosis of Polycystic Ovaries

It has been shown that the pretreatment total ovarian volume, calculated by the use of the formula for an ovoid, is increased in women who subsequently developed ovarian hyperstimulation syndrome.[4] Kyei-Mensah et al.[5] used three-dimensional ultrasound to measure ovarian volume. Their method proved to be reliable and reproducible with a minimal measurement error. It remains to be seen whether the prediction of ovarian hyperstimulation syndrome will be more accurate than with two-dimensional ultrasound.

Ovarian Masses

The ability of three-dimensional ultrasound to measure ovarian volume and to produce an unlimited numbers of tomo-graphic planes of the ovaries may also be helpful in the morphologic analysis of ovarian tumors. The value of two- and three-dimensional ultrasound for the diagnosis of ovarian cancer has been examined.[6] Three-dimensional ultrasound provided more information about papillary projections, characteristics of the cyst wall, and the extent of capsular infiltration. This enabled the diagnosis of cancer in one case that would be missed on two-dimensional scanning.

THREE-DIMENSIONAL ULTRASOUND IN UROGYNECOLOGY

Three-dimensional ultrasound enables the visualization of pelvic floor structures in planes not possible with two-dimensional scanning. This provides better images of the lower urinary tract and pelvic floor. It is also possible to measure the volume of the sphincter and other pelvic floor structures to assess their functional competence.

The Urethra

With three-dimensional ultrasound, the urethra and the striated urethral sphincter can be visualized. Stored three-dimensional images enable detailed morphologic assessment of the urethra at different levels. The size and the morphology of the urethral sphincter assessed by three-dimensional ultrasound have been studied in patients with urinary incontinence undergoing urodynamic investigations. By using

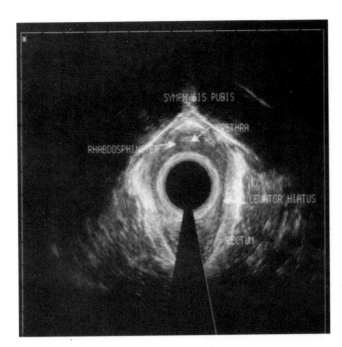

Figure 45.4 A transverse section of the pelvis at the level of the pubococcygeus muscle.

transperineal and transvaginal approaches, the authors showed that patients with urethral sphincter incompetence had smaller urethral sphincters than women with competent urethral mechanisms[7,8] (Fig. 45.4).

CONCLUSION

The experience with three-dimensional ultrasound in gynecology is still limited. However, studies published so far indicate that there are a few conditions such as congenital uterine anomalies, urogynecology, and infertility, where three-dimensional scanning offers advantages.

REFERENCES

1. Jurkovic D, Geipel A, Gruboeck K et al. Three-dimensional ultrasound for the assessment of uterine anatomy and detection of congenital anomalies: a comparison with hysterosalpingography and two-dimensional sonography. Ultrasound Obstet Gynaecol 1995;5:233–237
2. Gruboeck K, Jurkovic D, Lawton F et al. The diagnostic value of endometrial thickness and volume measurements by three-dimensional ultrasound in patients with postmenopausal bleeding Ultrasound Obstet Gynaecol 1996;8:272–276
3. Kyei-Mensah A, Zaidi J, Pittrof R et al. Transvaginal three-dimensional ultrasound: accuracy of follicular volume measurements. Fertil Steril 1995;65:371–376
4. Oyesanya OA, Parsons JH, Collins WP, Campbell S. Ultrasound estimation of total ovarian volume before the administration of hCG in IVF cycles: correlation with serum oestradiol levels and prognostic implications. Ultrasound Obstet Gynaecol 1994;4:114–118
5. Kyei-Mensah A, Zaidi J, Pittrof R et al. Transvaginal three-dimensional ultrasound: accuracy and reliability of ovarian and endometrial volume measurements. Hum Reprod 1995;10:109–112
6. Bonilla-Musoles F, Raga F, Osborne NG. Three-dimensional ultrasound evaluation of ovarian masses. Gynecol Oncol 1995;59:129–135
7. Khullar V, Salvatore S, Cardozo LD et al. Three-dimensional ultrasound of the urethra and the urethral sphincter—a new diagnostic technique. Neurol Urodyn 1994;13:352–353
8. Athanasiou S, Hill S, Cardozo LD et al. Three-dimensional ultrasound of the urethra, periurethral tissues and pelvic floor. Int Urogyn J 1995;6:239–241

Imaging of the Breast

SECTION

IV

46

Mammography and Ultrasound of the Breast

MARY T. RICKARD

NORMAL ANATOMY

The distinguishing feature of the breast is the glandular tissue contained within a capsule of fascia (Fig. 46.1). A layer of fat surrounds the fascia and lies between it and the skin and the muscles of the the chest wall. Connective tissue strands, called Cooper's ligaments, traverse the fat from the fascia to the chest wall muscles and to the skin. Within the fascia are 15 to 20 poorly defined lobes in a radial pattern. The long axis of the breast extends toward the axilla where the tissue is called the *axillary tail.*

Within each lobe is a major duct opening onto the nipple. Peripherally, the ducts branch many times, ending in the terminal ductulolobular unit (TDLU). This is made up of extra- and intralobular terminal ducts and ductules or acini (Fig. 46.2). The smallest structural unit is the lobule, which contains the intralobular terminal duct, the ductules, and the surrounding intralobular fat, vessels, and connective tissue. Interlobular fat, vessels, and connective tissues are present between the lobules. The TDLU is approximately 500 μm in diameter in an adult and is the most important functional unit. The TDLU is modified by physiologic influences, and it is within the TDLU that carcinomas and most benign conditions arise.[1,2]

The major lymphatic drainage of the breast is to the axillary lymph nodes, with some drainage elsewhere, most importantly from the medial breast to the internal mammary nodes. Lymph nodes are frequently found within the breast itself, usually in the upper outer quadrant.

Developmental changes occur under hormonal influence at puberty, and the lobules, ducts, acini, and epithelium of the female breast proliferate and mature. With each menstrual cycle, there are proliferative and subsequent regressive changes. Functional development occurs most markedly during pregnancy and results in a fully differentiated state for lactation. With increasing age, from about the fourth decade, there is progressive atrophy of the parenchymal cells of the breast and replacement with fat (Fig. 46.3). These changes continue postmenopausally but may be altered by exogenous hormone therapy.

In the male breast, puberty does not lead to maturation of breast parenchyma, but some enlargement, or gynecomastia, is occasionally seen at puberty. It may also be induced at any age by exogenous hormones or by other causes of alteration to the normal hormone balance.[3]

IMAGING

Mammography and ultrasound are the two most widely used breast imaging modalities. A different range of information is obtained from each, and therefore the two examinations are best used in a complimentary fashion.

MAMMOGRAPHY

Technique

Breast positioning, image contrast, and resolution are critical in mammography. Correct technique is necessary to visualize the fine differences between normal and pathologic tissue. High contrast and resolution enable differentiation between the normal TDLUs, fat, and connective tissues and pathologic structures such as microcalcifications or spicules.

The major factors contributing to image contrast and resolution are the mammographic unit, the film–screen combination, and the film processing.[4,5] A dedicated mammographic unit allows the use of low kilovolt peaks (in the 22- to 30-kVp range) by featuring suitable target materials, filters, and windows. Accurate, reliable, automatic exposure control is essential to obtain consistent film optical densities. The best optical density for contrast resolution in mammography is about 1.6. The mammographic unit requires focal spots of approximately 0.3 mm for normal contact mammography, and approximately 0.1 mm for magnification views. An adequate milliampere output (e.g., 100 mA or greater for the larger focal spot), minimizes exposure times and reduces the risk of movement blur. Scatter is reduced by a moving grid and firm compression, which evens breast thickness and exposure. Dedicated film–screen combinations maximize contrast and spatial resolution while minimizing exposure. Pro-

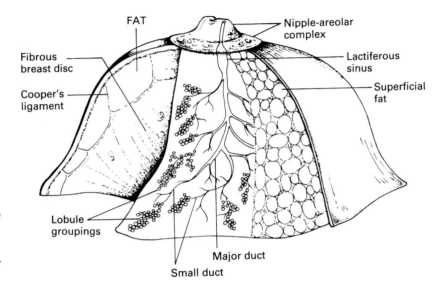

Figure 46.1 A schematic diagram of the mature breast components in sagittal section (left) and "window" view of duct and lobular system (center) connecting with the nipple–areolar complex. (From Page and Anderson,[1] with permission.)

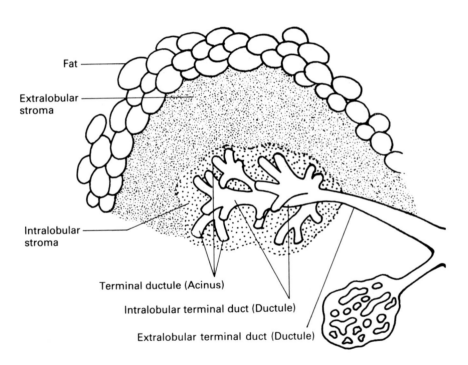

Figure 46.2 A schematic diagram of a mature resting lobular unit to show the TDLU components. (From Page and Anderson,[1] with permission.)

cessing the film under optimal dwell time and temperature conditions minimizes exposure while ensuring high image quality.

Fine radiographer skills are necessary to produce a well-positioned film. Films may be taken in many projections, but the most commonly used as standard projections are the medio-lateral oblique (MLO) and craniocaudal (CC) views. The x-ray beam passes obliquely upward from the medial to the lateral breast with the MLO projection. The MLO view, when well positioned, includes most of the breast tissue on the film (Fig. 46.4). The pectoral muscle is seen at the back of the breast down to the level of the nipple, which is projected in profile. With the CC projection, the beam passes superoinferiorly through the breast (Fig. 46.5). Not all breast tissue is in-

cluded on this projection, which may be varied to include more medial or lateral tissue by biasing the breast positioning appropriately. As the standard MLO and CC projections do not show all breast tissue, other projections can be used to visualize particular areas of the breast. For example, the "cleopatra" view is used for the axillary tail, and the cleavage view for the medial breast tissue (Fig. 46.6).

Coned compression and magnification are specially used separately or together for improved focal mammography.[6] With coned compression, contrast and spatial resolution are improved as overlying structures are pushed aside, the tissue is thinned, scatter is reduced, and the tissue of interest placed closer to the film. With magnification using a microfocal spot, the spatial resolution of a small area is increased and its image

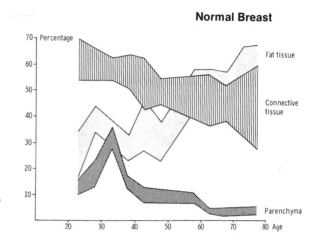

Figure 46.3 Age-dependent progression and regression of fat, connective, and glandular tissue determined from macrosections. (From Page and Anderson,[1] with permission.)

Figure 46.4 MLO projections of two different breasts show the range of normal mammographic appearances. (**A**) Considerable fibroglandular tissue is present (giving a dense breast appearance). (**B**) The fibroglandular tissue has been largely replaced by fat (giving a fatty breast appearance). Only a single axillary lymph node is visualized in Figure A, whereas many nodes, some with prominent fatty hila, are seen in Figure B. An incidental densely calcified fibroadenoma is seen in Figure B.

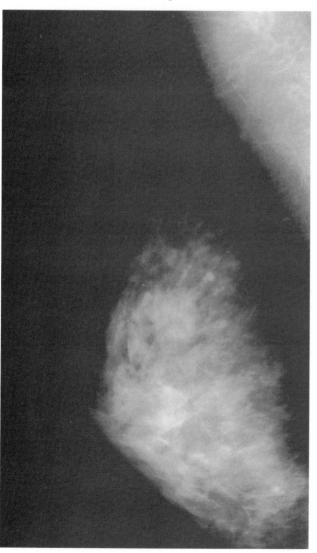

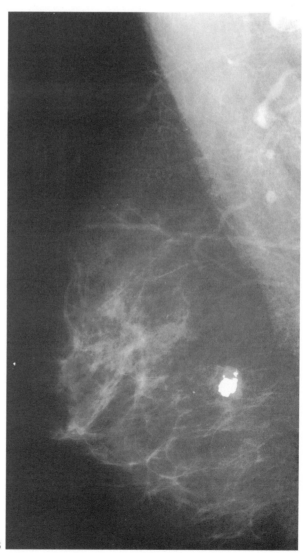

A

B

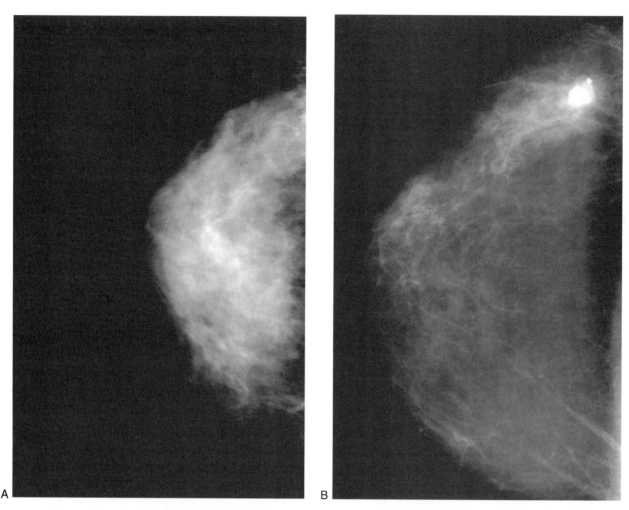

Figure 46.5 CC mammograms of the same two breasts as illustrated in Figure 46.4 show differing fibroglandular distributions. (**A**) Prominent fibroglandular tissue is present in both medial and lateral parts of the breast. (**B**) The medial and posterior (retromammary) portions of the breast are largely fatty in density.

enlarged. Coned compression and magnification used in combination achieve the advantages of both (Fig. 46.7).

When there is a silicone prosthesis or implant in the breast, films including and excluding the prosthesis can be taken in any projection. Because much of the breast tissue is obscured by the prosthesis, a special technique is needed to more completely visualize the breast.[7] The tissue that lies over the prosthesis is pinched off the prosthesis and then compressed in the standard way. Coned, magnification, or combined coned–magnification films can be taken with this technique.

Appearance and Interpretation

On a mammogram, the glandular and fibrous tissue and ducts of the breast appear white, the fat grey, and the chest wall muscles white. The skin and nipple–areolar complex are white, but, because of exposure factors, a bright light must be used to see these. Many normal anatomic structures, such as

TDLUs and Cooper's ligaments, can be identified on a normal image. The ease with which these are seen depends on the relative amounts of glandular, fibrous, and fatty tissue, as well as image quality. Typically, the young adult female breast contains more glandular tissue and is mammographically denser than the older adult breast, which shows increasing fatty replacement with age, particularly after the menopause (Figs. 46.4 and 46.5).

The three main mammographic findings that indicate pathology are mass (asymmetric density), architectural disturbance, and microcalcification. These can be further evaluated using combined coned- magnification, coned compression, or magnification alone. There is a wide range of normal mammographic appearances, but it is usual for the breasts of an individual to be similar in appearance. This forms one of the bases of interpretation, that is, comparison of the same area of the two breasts (Fig. 46.8). When the breasts have been symmetrically positioned, they can be compared using a masking technique to concentrate vision on a particular area of the

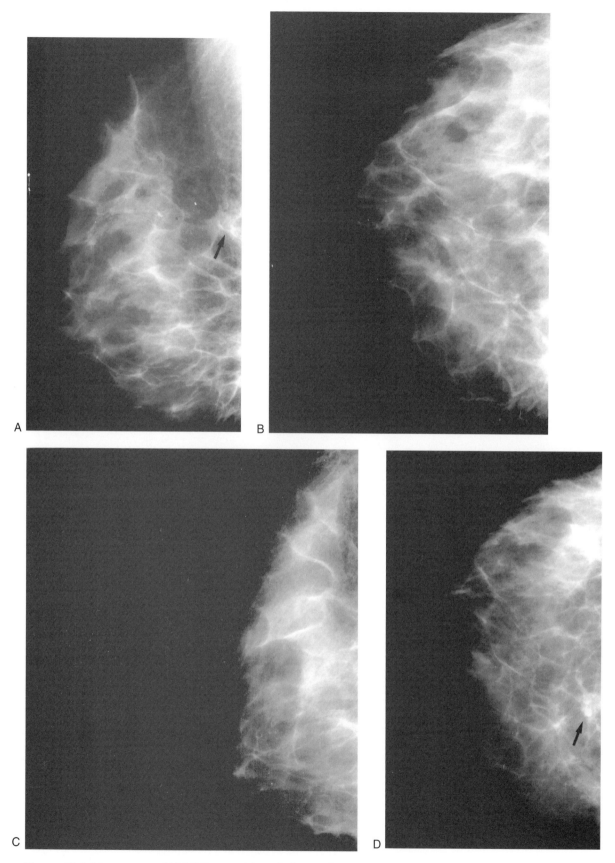

Figure 46.6 Mammograms. (**A**) MLO view of the right breast of a 55-year-old shows a 1-cm spiculated lesion (arrow) posteriorly, overlying the inferior margin of the pectoral muscle. (**B**) The lesion cannot be identified on the standard CC view. (**C**) A CC view with lateral bias also shows no abnormality. (**D**) A cleavage view shows the lesion, which lies medially and posteriorly (arrow). Histopathology showed a 10-mm (grade I) tubular carcinoma.

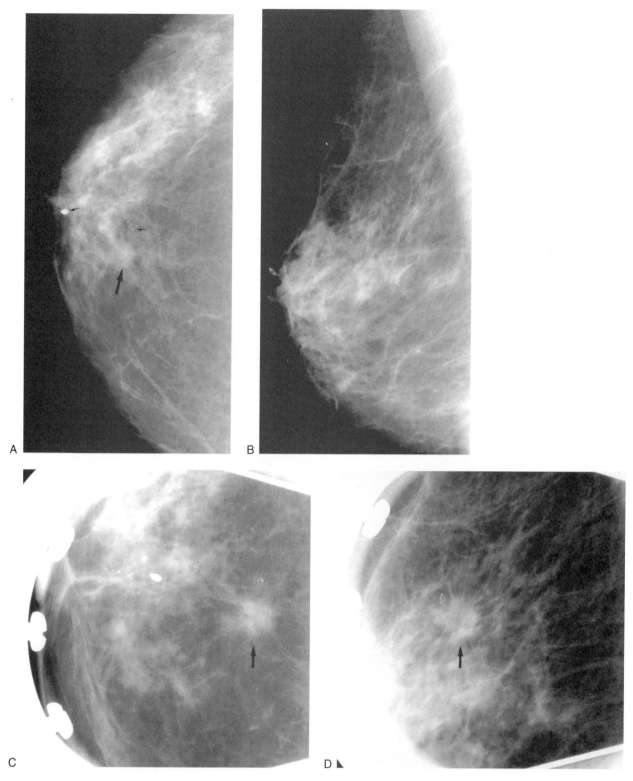

Figure 46.7 Mammograms. (**A**) CC view of the right breast of an asymptomatic 60-year-old shows a small, irregular mass lying medially on the posterior aspect of the fibroglandular tissue (arrow). Incidental benign calcifications due to fat necrosis and lobular secretions are noted centrally (small arrows) (**B**) MLO view. The lesion is not seen. (**C**) CC coned–magnification view clearly shows the features of the lesion, which has spiculated margins (arrow). (**D**) MLO coned–magnification view of the upper breast shows the location of the lesion (arrow) and confirms its malignant features. Histopathology showed a 10-mm (grade 2) infiltrating ductal carcinoma. There was also an associated, mammographically occult, in situ carcinoma.

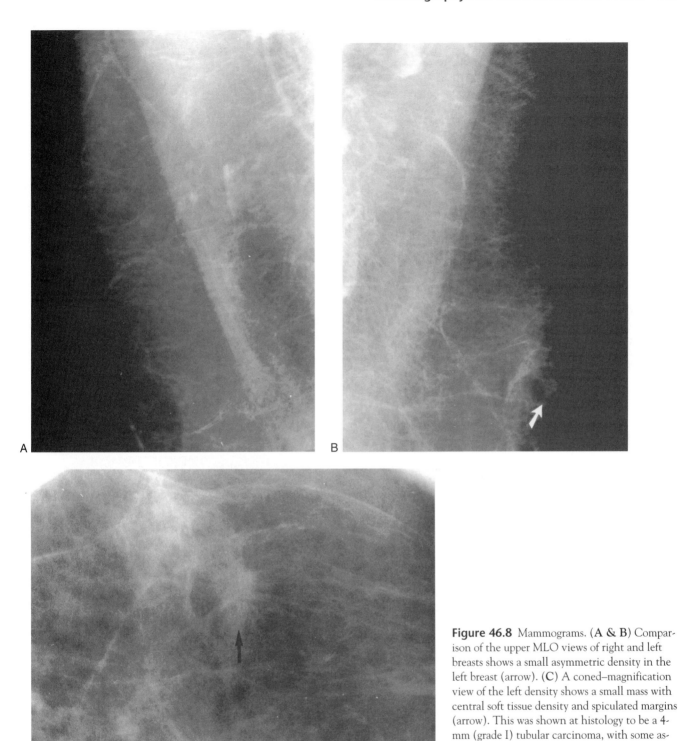

A

B

C

Figure 46.8 Mammograms. (**A & B**) Comparison of the upper MLO views of right and left breasts shows a small asymmetric density in the left breast (arrow). (**C**) A coned–magnification view of the left density shows a small mass with central soft tissue density and spiculated margins (arrow). This was shown at histology to be a 4-mm (grade I) tubular carcinoma, with some associated in situ carcinoma.

breasts.[8] Pathology can be found anywhere within the breast, but there are "check" areas to be evaluated when interpreting a mammogram. These include the retromammary areas (i.e., the fatty area deep to the greater mass of glandular tissue); the retroareolar areas; the contours of the glandular tissue; and, on the MLO projection, the inferior angle of the breast (Fig. 46.9). The skin and nipple–areolar complex should be examined for thickening, distortion, and inversion by using a

bright light (Fig. 46.10). A magnifying glass is needed to check for microcalcifications. While comparison with previous mammograms is always valuable, it must be appreciated that both change with time and lack of change can be seen in both malignant and benign conditions.

Careful analysis of the mammographic features of a lesion is the key to accurate diagnosis. The main features that should be analysed are the type of lesion, its shape, margins, density,

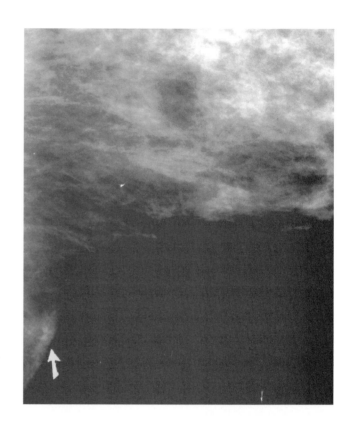

Figure 46.9 The inferior angle of the left breast (MLO projection) is shown in detail in this mammogram. A density can be seen at the junction of the breast and abdominal wall tissues (arrow), and this was a small invasive carcinoma.

Figure 46.10 Mammograms. (**A & B**) Comparison CC projections of the right and left breasts of a 72-year-old woman who had recently noticed inversion of the right nipple. The right areolar tissue is thickened and the nipple inverted. (*Figure continues.*)

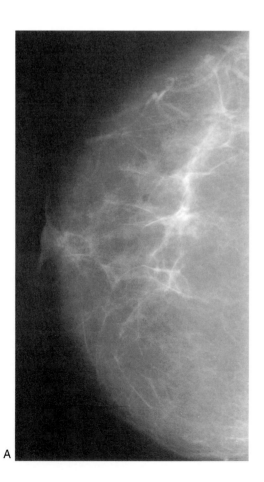

A

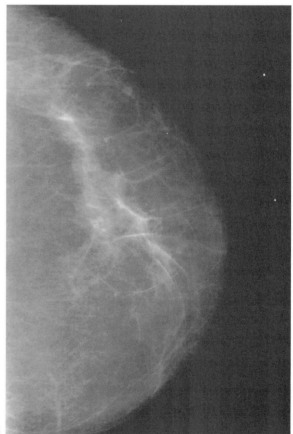

B

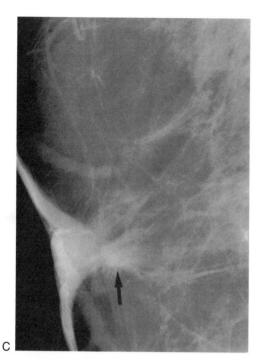

C

Figure 46.10 (*Continued*). (**C**) A coned–magnification film of the right nipple–areolar region shows that there is a small, spiculated mass just deep to the nipple (arrow). This lesion was also shown on ultrasound examination (see Fig. 46.12) and was confirmed on histologic examination to be a 9-mm infiltrating carcinoma.

changes in adjacent tissues, size, number, distribution/location, and associated calcifications.

ULTRASOUND

Technique

As with mammography, the quality of a breast ultrasound examination is dependent on the ultrasound equipment and the expertise with which it is used.[9] Even more so than with mammography, the image quality and the likelihood of demonstrating an abnormality and its features are operator dependent.

The ultrasound unit requires a high-quality, dedicated small parts probe with excellent surface coupling to avoid loss of detail in the cutaneous and immediate subcutaneous tissues. A hand-held probe that does not require any additional coupling material is preferred to one that requires a "stand-off gel pack." Many probes are now designed to cover a range of several megahertz and a range of focal zones. A probe ranging from 7.5 to 12.0 MHz will image most tissue within 5 cm of the probe. Image processing must be designed to optimize the grey scale differences between the soft tissue structures of the breast, particularly those differences between fibroglandular tissue and fat.

With ultrasound, unlike mammography, only small areas

of the breast can be imaged at any one time. Therefore, it is recommended that ultrasound be limited to the area of interest, be this clinical or mammographic, so that the study of the area is comprehensive.

The supine and supine-oblique are the most useful positions for ultrasound examination. In these positions, the arm on the side being examined is raised and rested above the head to spread the breast tissue and reduce breast movement. The approach used may differ with the indications for the examination. When evaluating an impalpable mammographic finding, the approximate location should be estimated from the mammogram, and the area should then be examined by moving the probe radially from the periphery of the breast toward the nipple, that is, in the orientation of the normal anatomy. This radial orientation assists in the perception of an abnormality that will disturb the predicted pattern of the normal anatomy. When evaluating a palpable lesion, it should be located under the patient's or the examiner's fingers and the probe placed directly upon it.

Appearance and Interpretation

The ultrasound appearance of the normal structures correlates well with those on the mammogram (Fig. 46.11). The fibroglandular tissue and skin are white on the mammogram and on the ultrasound image, and the fat is grey on both. Major ducts, identified on the mammogram as white tubular structures behind the nipple, are similarly identified on the ultrasound image where they are shown to contain varying amounts of low echo content. The chest wall muscles, which are white on the mammogram, vary in echogenicity on the ultrasound image, between white and grey depending on their internal structure and the angle at which the ultrasound beam traverses the muscle bundles. The normal ultrasound appearance is variable and, as with a mammogram, depends on the relative amounts of fibroglandular tissue and fat.

The main ultrasound appearances of pathology are a mass and an architectural disturbance. While microcalcifications are readily seen on a mammogram, they are often not seen at all on ultrasound. Interpretation of an ultrasound image, as with that of a mammogram, is two-stage. A feature must be first recognized and then analyzed. The ultrasound features are the type of lesion, its size, shape, margins, and comparative echogenicity; changes in through transmission; changes in adjacent tissues; the lesion size, number, and distribution; and the presence of associated calcifications. When both mammography and ultrasonography are carried out, the findings must be correlated (Fig. 46.12).

INDICATIONS FOR THE USE OF MAMMOGRAPHY AND ULTRASOUND

Imaging may be used to diagnose a clinical symptom or sign or to screen the breast to detect malignancy before it becomes palpable.

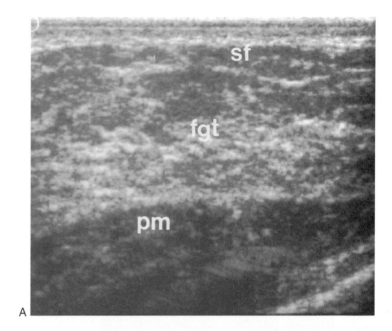

A

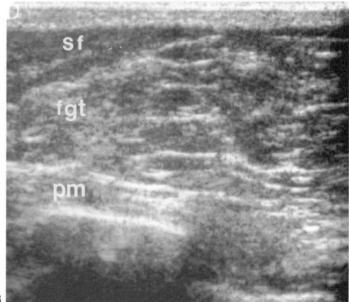

B

Figure 46.11 Normal sonographic appearances are illustrated in these images of two different breasts. (**A**) Dense fibroglandular tissue (fgt) is seen between a thin layer of subcutaneous fat (sf) and the pectoral muscle (pm). (**B**) Fat is seen interspersed throughout the fibroglandular tissue back to the pectoral muscle (pm).

Figure 46.12 Mammography correlates well with ultrasound of the same area as shown in Figure 46.10. The ultrasound shows a hypoechoic mass (arrows), which is the same size as the mammographic lesion. The margins are irregular and ill-defined and protrude into the normal subcutaneous fat (sf) and fibroglandular tissues (fgt), which are disrupted. Both mammographic and ultrasonographic features are consistent with invasive malignancy.

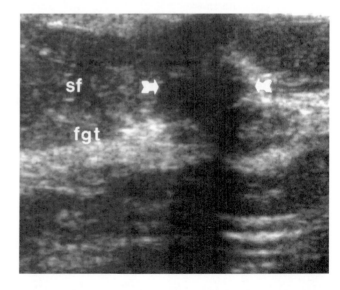

Whether mammography or ultrasound is used first in a clinical setting depends particularly on the age of the patient.[10] There is an age-related risk of radiation inducing breast cancer.[11] The younger the woman, the greater the risk. At the doses used in modern mammography, the risk of inducing breast cancer is remote, but it remains a reason to avoid mammography in young women unless it is expected to make an important contribution to the diagnosis. Mammography becomes more useful as a woman ages. The characteristics of benign and malignant conditions can be obscured by the density of fibroglandular tissue found in young women.[12] This is less likely to be the case in the fatty breasts of older women. On the other hand, the reverse applies in ultrasonography, where benign and malignant characteristics, except for microcalcifications, are more easily identified when surrounded by glandular tissue rather than fat. For diagnostic purposes, mammography is the first choice in women over 35. Below this age ultrasound is preferred. In every case, the initial imaging must be correlated with the clinical findings. If a clear diagnosis of normality or benign pathology is not established, then further investigation is indicated.

For screening, mammography has been shown to reduce mortality from breast cancer.[13–16] For women 50 years or older, the benefit is proven. For women 40 to 49, a benefit remains unproven. A number of studies have included women in the 40- to 49-year age group, but the numbers in individual studies are too small to show a statistical benefit or to prove a nil effect; however, a meta-analysis of the Swedish trials suggests limited benefit.[17] The lowest age at which the benefit of reduced mortality is achievable is unknown. The difficulties of analyzing the younger age group in part reflect the smaller number of breast cancers in these women and the statistical need for large numbers to be studied. The difficulties in part reflect the poorer sensitivity of mammography in younger women, for the reasons discussed above, and perhaps a faster growth rate of the disease.

Ultrasound screening has never been shown to affect breast cancer mortality in any age group, but ultrasound is valuable in the evaluation of lesions detected by mammographic screening.

Breast lesions, clinical or subclinical, are most effectively evaluated by the triple test, which is a combination of imaging (mammography and ultrasound), tissue sampling (cytology and core biopsy), and clinical examination.[18–21] The integrated result of the triple test determines further management. If cytology or core biopsy shows malignancy and this is consistent with the imaging and clinical findings, then the patient can be informed of the diagnosis and appropriate single-stage surgery carried out. If all tests suggest benign or normal findings, then unnecessary surgery can be avoided. If any one test suggests malignancy, then further investigation, such as open surgical biopsy, is required. It may be that all three components of the triple test are not necessary in every patient. If, for example, a mammographic or a clinical finding suggests a benign mass, and ultrasound shows this to be a simple cyst, then further investigation by tissue sam-

pling is unnecessary. Judicious use of the triple test should minimize false-positive and false-negative diagnoses.

USE OF IMAGING GUIDANCE FOR TISSUE SAMPLING

Tissue diagnosis can be made by nonoperative sampling of a lesion by fine needle cytology and/or core biopsy. For cytology sampling, the typical needle size is 25 gauge and for core biopsy is 14 gauge. The sampling procedure can be guided by palpation, ultrasound, or stereotactic mammography.[22–25] Imaging guidance ensures precise placement of the needle in relation to the tissue to be sampled and is therefore accurate for both palpable and nonpalpable lesions.

Irrespective of the method of guidance, the quality of the tissue sample reflects the operator's skill, and the experience of the cytologist or pathologist affects the interpretation of the sample. This is particularly true of the interpretation of a cytology sample where a diagnosis is made without the assistance of the histologic architecture.

When imaging guidance is required, excellent results can be obtained with both ultrasonographic and stereotactic techniques. With ultrasonographic guidance, the biopsy is visualized in real time. It is quicker to perform than biopsy with stereotactic guidance and is comfortable for the patient and easy for the clinician. Biopsy with stereotactic guidance takes longer than that with ultrasound guidance even when digital acquisition and display are used. Stereotactic technique may be less comfortable than ultrasound for the patient, particularly when an upright stereotactic add-on device is used rather than a dedicated prone table.

For ultrasound-guided biopsy, the patient is usually positioned as for ultrasound examination, although any angle or direction of approach may be used. The shortest length of approach to the region of interest is preferable. The needle (for both cytology and core biopsy) should always be visualized along its length so that the position of the needle tip is constantly identified and the full biopsy procedure monitored in real time (Fig. 46.13).

For stereotactic localization, the angle of approach may follow the direction of the x-ray beam or may be at right angles to it, depending on the attachments used. All directions of approach are possible, and the shortest route to the target is preferable. Stereotactic exposures showing the needle tip before (for both cytology and core biopsy) and after sampling (for core biopsy) are used to confirm the accuracy of positioning (Fig. 46.14A–D).

Monitoring by imaging will improve adequacy of sampling. If cytology is performed, then immediate microscopy will indicate whether the sample is adequate. If core biopsy has been carried out and the lesion is calcified, then core specimen radiography can be used to show whether representative calcification is present in the specimen (Fig. 46.14E).

Results of tissue sampling must be correlated with the

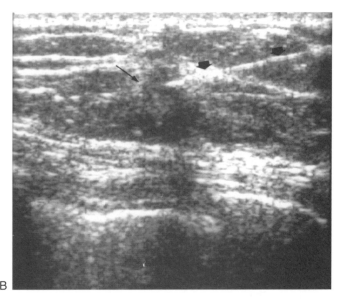

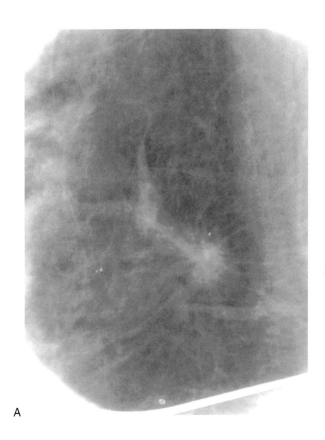

A

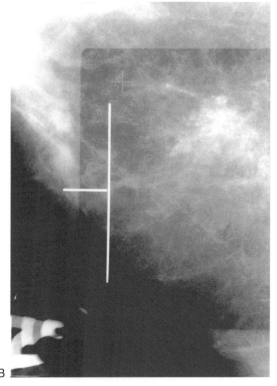

B

Figure 46.13 (**A**) Coned–magnification mammogram of the upper right breast shows an impalpable, spiculated lesion, characteristic of invasive malignancy. Tissue sampling is required for confirmation of diagnosis and could be carried out either with mammographic (stereotactic) guidance or, as in this case, with ultrasound guidance. (**B**) Ultrasound image of the needle in position shows the full length of the fine needle (arrowheads) and confirms that the needle tip lies within the lesion (arrow). The procedure should be monitored in real time to enhance the quality of the tissue sampling.

Figure 46.14 (**A**) A coned–magnification mammogram shows a cluster of microcalcifications with some surrounding, ill-defined, soft tissue opacity. (**B**) Ninety-degree stereotactic control mammogram shows that the area of interest is located for tissue sampling under the window of the perspex plate. (*Figure continues.*)

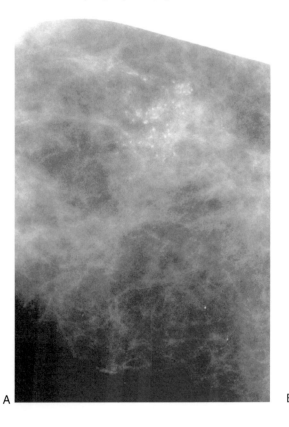

A

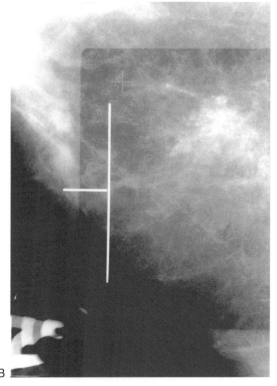

B

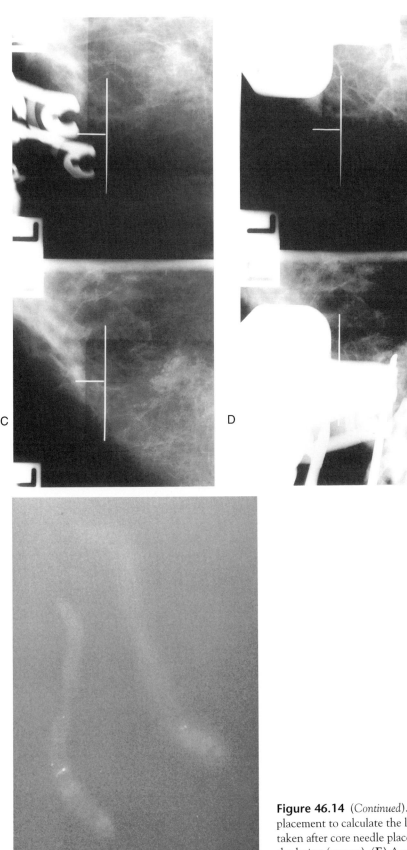

Figure 46.14 (*Continued*). (**C**) Stereotactic mammograms are taken before needle placement to calculate the location of the lesion. (**D**) Stereotactic mammograms taken after core needle placement ensure accurate positioning of the needle within the lesion (arrows). (**E**) A specimen radiograph of core biopsy tissue samples confirms that representative calcifications have been obtained from the mammographic area of interest. Core histology confirmed a diagnosis of ductal carcinoma in situ.

imaging and clinical findings so that an integrated approach is taken to diagnosis and management.

BENIGN CHANGES

Fibrocystic Change

Fibrocystic change covers a wide spectrum of histologic findings including adenosis, fibrosis, sclerosing adenosis, epithelial hyperplasia with and without atypia, lobular carcinoma in situ, papillomatosis, duct ectasia, granulomatous mastitis, radial scar, papilloma, cyst formation, and fibroadenoma. These are now regarded as a spectrum of normal changes within breast tissue. The previously used term *disease* has been replaced by *change* to reflect the histologic changes, only a few of which are associated with an increased risk of development of breast cancer.[26,27]

Many of the histologic changes that are included under this title are microscopic only and not detectable clinically or by imaging. From an imaging point of view, fibrocystic change results in mass, nonspecific density, and microcalcifications. These may be typically benign or they may be difficult to differentiate from malignancy.

Sclerosing Adenosis

Adenosis is a condition in which the glandular-units or TDLUs of the breast enlarge and the number of their acini increases.[28] The epithelium of the TDLUs remains normal. If there is a fibrous alteration of the surrounding stroma, the condition is termed *sclerosing adenosis*, and the TDLUs become distorted. Typically, the changes are impalpable. If this condition is focal, it may present as an irregularly shaped lump, an adenosis tumor, or sclerosing adenoma, which may mimic carcinoma both clinically and on imaging. Sclerosing adenosis is not a premalignant condition.

The imaging appearances in sclerosing adenosis are usually indistinguishable from those of normal parenchyma. Sometimes, the adenotic TDLUs may be identified on the mammogram as poorly defined, rounded, parenchymal densities, which are larger (approximately 4 to 5 mm in diameter) than the normal TDLUs (approximately 1 to 2 mm in diameter).

Calcification may deposit in the lumina of the acini and can be either solid concretions or suspended material. This accounts for the mammographic description of the calcifications as "pearls" and "teacups and saucers."[29] The pearls are solid concretions, which maintain their shape when viewed mammographically from any angle (Fig. 46.15). The "teacups and saucers" are the suspended calcifications, which are grav-

Figure 46.15 (A & B) Mammograms show benign, rounded calcifications, termed "pearls," are illustrated here in two different types of breast tissue. As they are solid and spheric, their appearance does not alter with a change in mammographic projection.

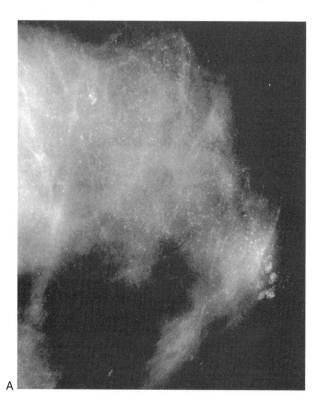
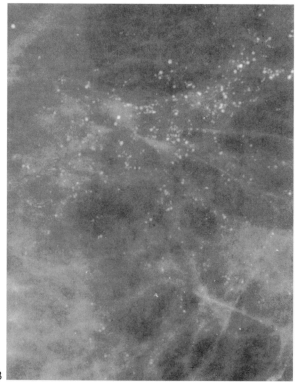

A

B

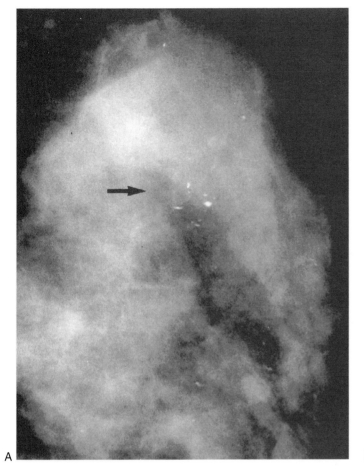 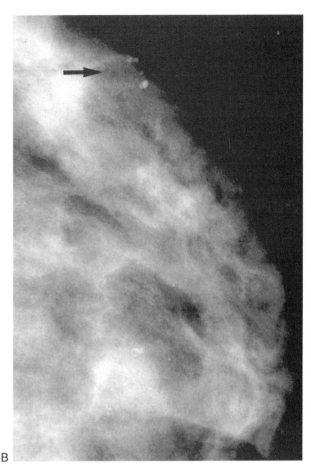

A   B

Figure 46.16 MLO (**A**) and CC (**B**) mammograms of the same patient showing an area of focal, benign calcifications in the shapes of "tea cups" (MLO) (arrow) and "saucers" (CC) (arrow). The calcifications are suspended in secretions within dilated acini and are therefore gravity dependent, varying in appearance from view to view.

ity dependent (Fig. 46.16). On a craniocaudal view, they are rounded with soft density edges, that is, "saucers." On the 90-degree mediolateral or lateromedial views, they appear as "cups," that is, aggregated in the dependent position of the acini with sharp curvilinear inferior margins and somewhat ill-defined horizontal superior margins.

When there is only minor distortion of the adenotic TDLU, then the radiographic appearances of the calcifications are typical and usually diagnostic. With increasing sclerosis and distortion, the shapes of the calcifications become less typical and more difficult to differentiate from the microcalcifications of ductal carcinoma in situ.

Duct Ectasia

Duct ectasia is part of a spectrum of conditions with various names including plasma cell mastitis and idiopathic granulomatous mastitis. Large- to medium-sized ducts are involved in

an inflammatory process that leads to both duct enlargement and obliteration. Amorphous debris may fill the ducts, and a chronic inflammatory cell infiltrate may encase the affected ducts, leading to periductal fibrosis. Both the intraductal contents and periductal fibrosis may calcify.

Clinically, the condition may be asymptomatic, or there may be nipple discharge or retraction, or discharging sinuses or fistulae. The condition is not a premalignant one.

Mammography varies with the clinical picture. Coarse, dense intraductal and periductal calcifications are a common incidental finding. The calcifications are typically well marginated and described as solid (intraductal) or hollow (periductal) (Fig. 46.17).[30] They may be seen anywhere in the breast but are typically associated with larger ducts and therefore oriented toward the nipple. The calcifications have a very typical mammographic appearance and rarely present a differential diagnostic dilemma. When sinuses or fistulae are present in the retroareolar region, ultrasound examination may be useful to check for abscess formation.

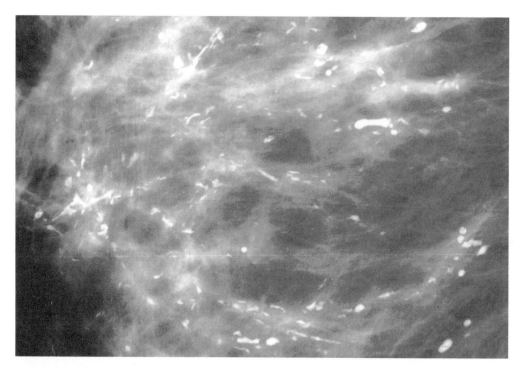

Figure 46.17 This mammogram shows numerous calcifications typical of plasma cell mastitis. The calcifications are either intraductal (solid, linear, and branching) or periductal (hollow and tubular). Some are associated with ill-defined periductal fibrosis, and most are oriented toward the nipple.

Fat Necrosis

In fat necrosis, lipid-filled spaces are walled off by histiocytes with foamy cytoplasm and occasional foreign body giant cells. Surrounding fibrosis may be conspicuous, or it may be absent.

Fat necrosis is often an asymptomatic condition found incidentally by imaging or histology. The cause may be unrecognized, or it may follow trauma or biopsy (see the following section entitled "Postsurgery/Trauma Changes").

On mammography, the most common appearance of incidental fat necrosis is that of a smooth, well-marginated round-to-oval fat density with rim or mural calcification.[30] The size may vary from millimeters to centimeters (Fig. 46.18). This appearance is not typically associated with any architectural disturbance. If it is poorly calcified, its appearance may be less specific, and tissue sampling may be required for diagnosis. If fibrosis is prominent, as may be the case after surgery, then it may have a stellate appearance (see Fig. 46.55). Even though a fatty density or low echogenicity center is typical, the differentiation from invasive malignancy may require tissue sampling.

Cyst

Cysts, which are collections of secretions within the terminal ductulolobular units of the breast, range in size from microscopic to macroscopic. Cysts may occur at any age, are typically hormone dependent and multiple, and may be asymptomatic or may present as nontender or tender lumps. They may increase or decrease in size and number over time, and on imaging they are a common incidental finding. Cysts may be palpable depending on their size and position within the breast and the degree of tension within them. When the cyst is tense, it may become tender, particularly if pressure is applied. This tension and tenderness can be relieved by aspiration. While a variety of epithelial changes and a variety of contents may be observed microscopically and chemically, these differences are not clinically relevant and not distinguishable on imaging. As they have no malignant potential, their diagnosis is important only to exclude more significant pathology. The typical mammographic features of a cyst are shown in Table 46.1 and Fig. 46.19.

The well-defined nature of the mass may be in part or totally obscured by the density of the adjacent parenchyma.[31] Even when all the described features are present, they are not diagnostic of a cyst. The solid or cystic nature of a mammographically benign mass requires ultrasound examination for clarification.

The ultrasound features of a simple cyst are seen in Table 46.2. If these criteria are fulfilled, then they are pathognomonic of a simple cyst (Fig. 46.20).[32] For a cyst to be simple, the interior does not need to be echo-free, and it may vary between different lesions or between different compartments of the one lesion, as in cysts containing septa (Fig. 46.21).

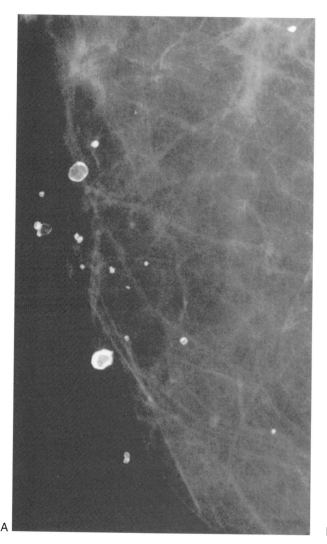 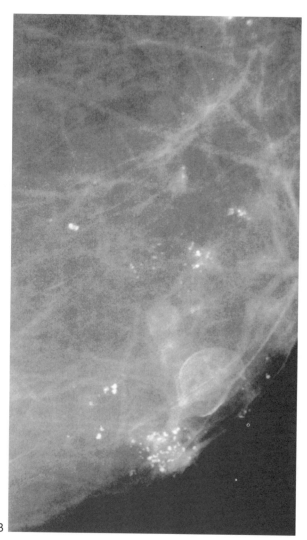

A   B

Figure 46.18 (A) Right mammogram shows typical fat necrosis calcifications. The calcifications, which vary in size, are mural or rim-like in position and round to oval in configuration. (B) Left mammogram of the same patient shows small clusters of dense calcifications and several low-density masses with faint rim calcification. These appearances are also those of old fat necrosis but are less typical than those seen in the right breast.

The aspirated contents of a cyst are rarely clear, and the echogenic appearances reflect the presence of proteinaceous material and cellular debris.

Aspiration of a simple cyst is indicated if the lesion is palpable and of clinical concern to the patient or if it is tender. The cyst can be aspirated using clinical or preferably ultrasound guidance to ensure that the needle tip is placed for complete emptying. Cytologic examination of the contents of a simple cyst is not necessary. If the cyst shows atypical ultrasound features or if the cyst contents are blood stained, then cytologic examination is indicated.

Simple cysts may be traumatized or become inflamed or infected.[33] If mural thickening is seen on ultrasound and the clinical picture is that of trauma or infection, aspiration and cytology and/or culture are indicated (Fig. 46.22). The lesion

can be treated clinically and monitored by ultrasound to confirm a return to normal appearances. Alternatively, if the features are suggestive of malignancy, then it can be surgically excised (Fig. 46.23).

Cysts may develop benign, macroscopic intracystic papillomas, which may rarely progress to papillary carcinomas. These papillomas are well-defined solid growths that extend into the lumen of the cyst and do not distort or thicken the wall (Fig. 46.24).[34] A tissue diagnosis is indicated by cytology or core biopsy of the solid component.

Rarely, cysts may be associated with carcinomas. A carcinoma may grow into an adjacent cyst, or the "cyst" may not be a true cyst but rather the "cystic" or necrotic component of a malignancy. The solid malignant component of such a lesion and the "cystic" component have the same irregular, ill-

Table 46.1 Mammographic Features

	Cyst	Fibroadenoma	Radial Scar	Phyllodes Tumor	Invasive Carcinoma
Type of lesion	Mass	Mass	Architectural disturbance ± minor or no central mass	Mass	Mass or architectural disturbance with minor mass
Shape	Round or ovoid ± lobulations	Oval or round ± few macrolobulations	Irregular, stellate, variable, and changing from view to view	Variable with micro- or macrolobulations	Variable, irregular, stellate, ± microlobulations
Margins	Sharp, smooth, and well defined	Sharp, smooth, and well defined	Spiculated, ill-defined	Predominantly sharp, typically smooth, may be ill-defined or irregular	Irregular, spiculated, ill-defined
Density	Equivalent to normal fibroglandular tissue	Equivalent to normal fibroglandular tissue	Variable with mixed fat and fibroglandular densities centrally	Variable but typically similar to fibroglandular tissues and increasing with increasing size	Variable but typically higher than normal fibroglandular tissue
Adjacent tissue	No disturbance	No disturbance	Disrupted	No disturbance	Disrupted
Size	Variable: several millimeters to many centimeters	Variable: several millimeters to centimeters	Variable: several millimeters to centimeters	Variable: may be very large	Variable
Number	Variable: one to many, typically multiple	Variable: one to many, commonly solitary	Typically single	Typically single, may be multifocal, multicentric, or bilateral	Typically single, but may be multifocal, multicentric, or bilateral
Distribution	Variable: unifocal to multifocal to multicentric and bilateral	Variable: unifocal to multifocal to multicentric and bilateral	Variable	Variable	Variable
Calcifications	Rare but typically mural or rim-like when present	May be present within the mass, typically being coarse, dense and of "popcorn" configuration	Common both centrally and peripherally within the lesion	Unusual	Common both within and/or adjacent to the mass

Table 46.2 Ultrasonographic Features

	Cyst	Fibroadenoma	Radial Scar	Phyllodes Tumor	Invasive Carcinoma
Type of lesion	Mass	Mass	Architectural disturbance ± minor or central mass	Mass	Mass or architectural disturbance with minor mass
Shape	Round or ovoid ± lobulations and septations	Ovoid with depth/width ratio of <1 ± a few macrolobulations	Irregular and variable	Round or ovoid with micro- or macrolobulations	Irregular and variable with variable depth/width ratio
Margins	Sharp, smooth, and well defined	Sharp, smooth, and well defined	Spiculated	Typically smooth and sharp, may be ill-defined or irregular	Irregular, ill-defined, and spiculated
Echogenicity	Variable: typically echo-free	Variable: Frequently equal to fat	Variable: Central echogenicity typically < fibroglandular tissue and >fat	Variable: Typically <fibroglandular tissue and >fat, cystic spaces uncommon	Variable: typically <fat
Through transmission	Increased	Variable	Variable	Variable	Variable but often decreased
Adjacent tissue	No disturbance	No disturbance	Disrupted or distorted	No disturbance	Disruption of architecture, alteration of echogenicity with echogenic rim between core of tumor and normal tissue
Size	Variable: several millimeters to many centimeters	Variable: several millimeters to many centimeters	Variable: central mass small compared to distortion	Variable but often large	Variable
Number	Variable: one to many, typically multiple	Variable: one to many, commonly solitary	Typically single	Typically single	Typically single
Distribution	Variable: unifocal, multifocal, multicentric, and bilateral	Variable: unifocal, multifocal, multicentric, and bilateral	Variable	Variable: may be multifocal, multicentric, or bilateral	Variable: may be multifocal, multicentric, or bilateral
Calcifications	Rare but typically mural	May be present in mass	Not usually seen	Unusual	Common within and/or adjacent to the mass

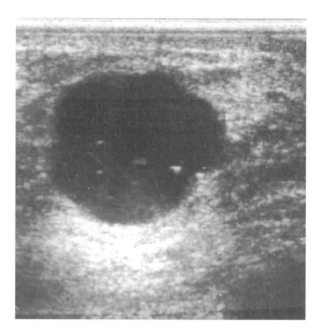

Figure 46.20 This ultrasound image shows that the retroareolar mass lesion seen in Figure 46.19 is a simple cyst. The margins of the lesion are smooth and well-defined with some lobulations. A few scattered echoes are present within the lumen of the cyst due to the presence of proteinaceous debris. Adjacent tissues are normal, and through transmission is increased.

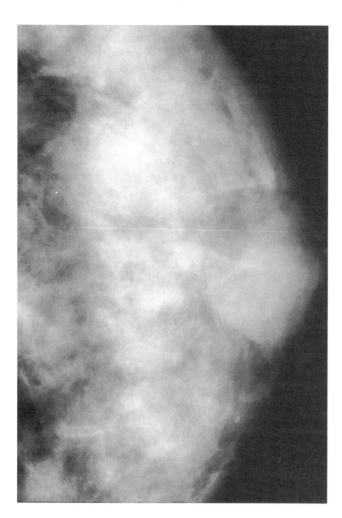

Figure 46.19 On this CC mammogram, a rounded mass of similar density to the surrounding fibroglandular tissue is seen in the retroareolar area. The lesion margins are mostly well-defined, and an incomplete halo is seen around the lesion due to the juxtaposition of the soft tissue density mass and the surrounding fat. The appearances are those of a benign lesion, and ultrasound was used to evaluate further the nature of the lesion.

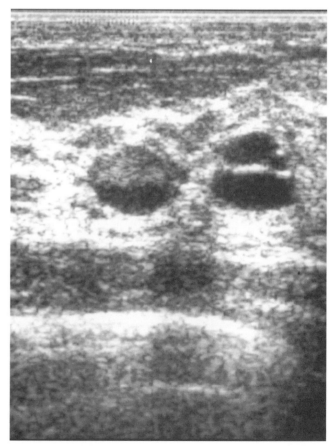

Figure 46.21 Ultrasound shows two adjacent simple cysts, both of which contain septa. The contents of one of the upper compartments are echogenic, but those of the other compartments are echo-free.

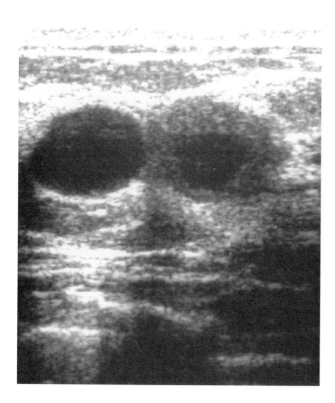

Figure 46.22 Ultrasound of an area of clinical tenderness shows two cysts. The left cyst has normal appearances. There are a few reverberation echoes seen anteriorly within it. On the other hand, the right cyst shows a thickened wall and loss of the sharp demarcation of the margin from the adjacent tissue. The features of the right cyst are consistent with inflammation or infection. Cytologic examination of a needle aspirate showed features of a cyst with proteinaceous fluid, macrophages, and cell debris. No malignant cells were identified. The abnormal features and symptoms resolved following antibiotic treatment.

Figure 46.23 (**A**) On this mammogram, a mass of parenchymal density (arrow) is seen bulging from the fibroglandular contour. The mass has benign features but cannot be fully characterized by mammography. (**B**) Ultrasound examination of the lesion shows its contents to be of variable echogenicity, and its margins to be partially ill-defined. Again, the mass is not definitively characterized. Histology showed the lesion to be a cyst containing altered blood and associated with some adjacent organizing inflammatory exudate. No malignancy was identified.

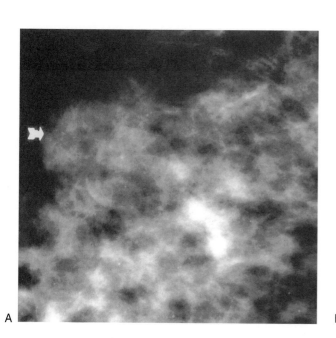

A

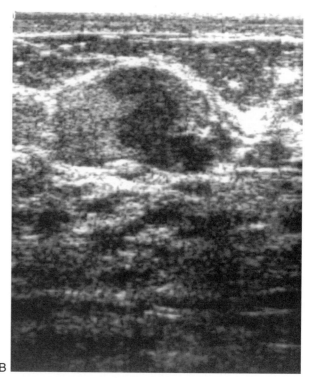

B

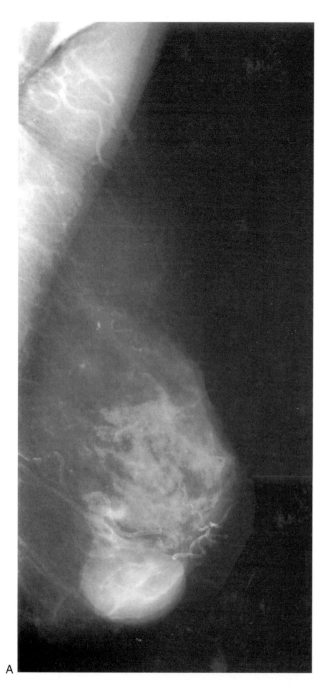

A

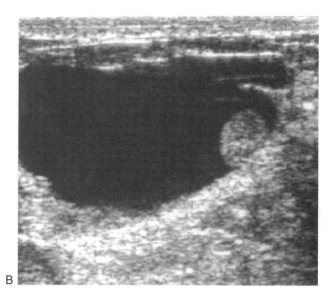

B

Figure 46.24 (**A**) This mammogram shows a prominent, well-defined mass in the inferior breast. The features are generally benign, but its size and its relatively high density (probably a reflection of its size) are suspicious and merit further assessment. (**B**) Ultrasound examination shows that it is a cyst with a mural nodule extending into the lumen. No mural thickening or other malignant features are identified. Part of a septum is seen above the nodule. Histology showed a cyst with a mural papilloma. No evidence of malignancy was identified.

defined appearance. Again, tissue sampling is indicated for diagnosis.

Fibroadenoma

Fibroadenomas are the most common benign, solid mass found in the breast.[35] It is thought that their development is hormone dependent and that most develop and grow in early adulthood. Composed of normal mesenchymal (fibrous) and epithelial (adenomatous) tissue, fibroadenomas are well- encapsulated masses. Arising from the TDLU, both intra-canalicular and pericanalicular forms are described histologically but are indistinguishable on imaging. Their natural history is to regress in size with age, particularly after the menopause. Development of de novo lesions and growth of previously recognized lesions have been described at all premenopausal ages and in post menopausal women taking hormones. As part of the aging or degenerative process, cyst formation may occur, or subcapsular or central hyalinization may develop. This hyalinized component may calcify to produce the characteristic high-density "popcorn" calcification seen on mammography. Infarction may also occur and can lead to irregularity of the margins, sometimes mimicking malignant change clinically and on imaging.

Clinically, a fibroadenoma can present as a palpable mass at any age. When palpable, it may have the typical characteristics of a soft rubbery mass that slips beneath the fingers, a so-called breast "mouse." Occasionally, a fibroadenoma may rapidly enlarge to become a giant fibroadenoma. In older women, it is an infrequent clinical finding but a common incidental finding at screening mammography. It is considered part of the spectrum of fibrocystic change and does not have any malignant potential. Carcinomas have been described in association with fibroadenomas either due to growth into a fibroadenoma by an adjacent carcinoma or due to true de novo in situ or invasive carcinoma development within the fibroadenoma, as might occur in other breast tissue. On mammography, fibroadenomas have an appearance typical of their benign nature (Table 46.1).[31]

If a fibroadenoma has characteristic calcifications within it, then the mammographic appearances are pathognomonic (Fig. 46.25). The calcifications may be absent or may be atypical in their early development and thus indistinguishable from other atypical benign or malignant calcifications. The noncalcified fibroadenoma may present a diagnostic dilemma, particularly if some of the margins are obscured by adjacent parenchyma, or if degenerative change has made the margins irregular. The mammographic appearances are then nonspecific (Fig. 46.26A).[36]

The most reliable diagnostic features on ultrasound are the sharp, smooth margins of the lesion, its ovoid shape, and the normal adjacent architecture (Fig. 46.26B).[37,38] The internal echogenicity and effect on through transmission are variable and not useful in differentiating a fibroadenoma from a malignancy. When the characteristic features are present, the ultrasound may be diagnostic (Table 46.2). Many authors believe the combined mammographic and ultrasonographic

features of noncalcified fibroadenomas are sufficiently nonspecific to make tissue sampling mandatory.[39]

Tissue sampling may be made by cytology or core biopsy, and these can be guided clinically or by ultrasound or stereotactic mammography. While cytology and core biopsy may both be diagnostic of fibroadenoma, it is often found that as fibroadenomas age and lose their cellularity, cytology becomes more difficult and atypical cells are more frequently seen. In this group of lesions, core biopsy will establish a definitive benign diagnosis.

Radial Scar/Complex Sclerosing Lesion

The *radial scar*, which is of unknown etiology, has been known by a variety of other terminologies, the most common of which is *complex sclerosing lesion*.[40] It is frequently found incidentally on histologic examination of breast tissue. It consists histologically of a central fibroelastic core, which contains obliterated ducts and entrapped tubular structures. From this core, ductules, lobules, and fibrosis extend outward in a radiating or stellate configuration. There are often associated elements of fibrocystic change, such as adenosis, sclerosing adenosis, and epithelial hyperplasia. The radial scar is of clinical interest because it is a marker for increased risk of malignancy and because of its possible progression to malignancy. Ductal carcinoma in situ and invasive tubular carcinoma have been found associated with radial scars, but it is not known how often this occurs.

Interest in radial scars also results from their spiculated or stellate imaging appearance, which may be difficult or impossible to differentiate from carcinoma (Fig. 46.27A). The typ-

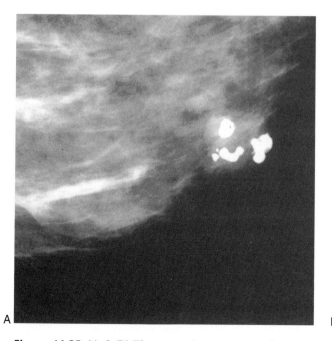

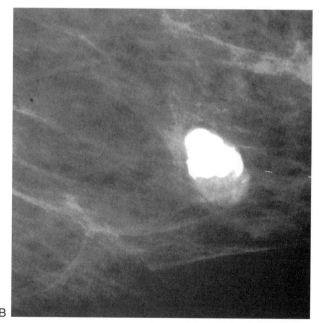

A   B

Figure 46.25 (A & B) These typical mammograms show examples of heavily but incompletely calcified fibroadenomas. The degenerative calcifications are sometimes described as popcorn-like in appearance.

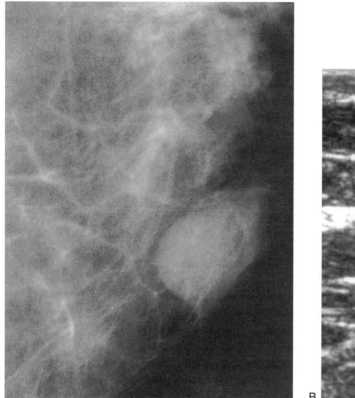

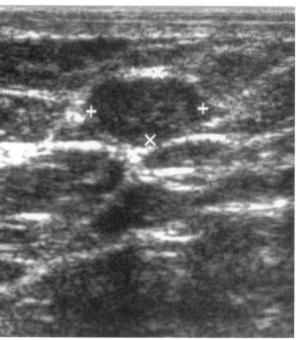

A

B

Figure 46.26 (A) The mammographic appearance is suggestive but not diagnostic of a fibroadenoma. The mass is well-defined, is of parenchymal density, and does not disturb adjacent tissues. (B) The ultrasound appearance is typical of a fibroadenoma. The lesion is ovoid, with its long axis parallel to the chest wall. Its margins are well-defined, and the adjacent tissues show a normal appearance right up to the edge of the lesion. Opinions differ as to whether tissue sampling of a lesion such as this is indicated, as the combined imaging appearances are characteristic of a fibroadenoma. If any diagnostic uncertainty exists, then cytology or core biopsy can readily confirm the diagnosis.

ical mammographic features are shown in Table 46.1.[41] Several mammographic features have been described to help distinguish radial scars from malignancy.[42,43] These include the density of the central area, which often includes fatty tissue in a radial scar. The shape of the spicules in radial scar tends to be curved, and in malignancy tends to be straight. The length of the spicules in radial scars may be very long when compared with the small or negligible size of the central mass, whereas with malignancy, the spicule length typically increases as the central mass increases. Also, because of its somewhat "plate-like" configuration, the overall mammographic appearance of the radial scar may vary considerably with change in mammographic projection, while that of the stellate malignancy tends to remain constant.

The ultrasound appearance of radial scars (Fig. 46.27B) is not well described in the literature, but the typical features are shown in Table 46.2.[44,45] The architectural distortion caused by radial scars is usually visible, but the central core may only be seen if it is of sufficient size. The ultrasound appearances are not specific enough to allow a radial scar to be differenti-

ated from a malignancy with associated stellate architectural distortion.

The role of cytology and core biopsy in the diagnosis of radial scar has been disputed.[46] As the imaging appearance is not pathognomonic, core biopsy is advised, primarily to exclude malignancy rather than to confirm the diagnosis of radial scar (Fig. 46.27C & D). Core diagnosis of radial scar does not eliminate the need for surgical excision, which is recommended because of the rare association of in situ and invasive malignancy, which may not be sampled by core biopsy.[47]

Papilloma

A papilloma forms in the main ducts as an intraluminal mass with a fibrovascular core covered by a layer of normal epithelium.[48] It may be microscopic or may measure several centimeters. Hemorrhagic infarction is commonly seen at histology. A papilloma usually develops centrally and may present with symptoms of bloody or serous nipple discharge or a retroareolar lump. It may also present as an asymptomatic, in-

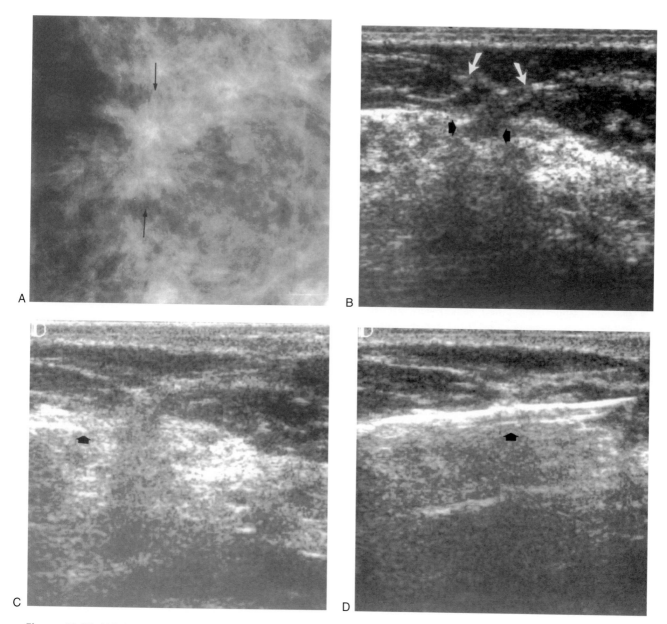

Figure 46.27 (A) A coned–magnification mammogram shows an area of disturbed architecture with a somewhat radiating pattern of spicules extending over several centimeters (arrows). There is no obvious central mass within the lesion, and the density is mixed and includes some fatty tissue. These appearances, particularly in an asymptomatic patient with a clinically normal breast and no history of breast surgery, are suggestive of a radial scar/complex sclerosing lesion. (B) The ultrasound appearance is also consistent with but not diagnostic of radial scar. The core of the lesion is seen breaking the normal contour of the fibroglandular tissue, drawing into it thickened fibrous strands from within the subcutaneous fat (arrows). The margins of the center of the lesion are ill-defined and irregular (arrowheads). The appearances are nonspecific but consistent with a radial scar. Tissue diagnosis is mandatory. (C & D) Pre- and postfire ultrasound images illustrate the core sampling of the lesion. Prefire, the tip of the core biopsy needle (arrowhead) is positioned several millimeters short of the central area. Postfire, the needle is seen to have traversed the central portion of the lesion (arrowhead). Microscopic examination of the core samples showed lobules with apocrine change, fibrosis and elastosis, and ducts with epithelial hyperplasia. The findings were consistent with a radial scar. Surgical excision of radial scars is required. The diagnosis of this lesion was confirmed following surgical removal, and no focus of malignancy was identified.

cidental finding on mammography or ultrasound, as an ovoid, round, or multilobulated mass close to the nipple. There may be an associated dilated duct, and degenerative calcification may be seen within the papilloma. There is no increased risk for development of a carcinoma.

Juvenile Papillomatosis

Juvenile papillomatosis is typically seen in young women and consists of a series of macroscopic papillomas within enlarged, peripherally rather than centrally located ducts. The mammographic appearance is of a "rosary bead"-like series of masses joined by dilated ducts. Epithelial proliferation occurs, and there appears to be an increased risk of malignant development.[49]

Fibroadenolipoma

Fibroadenolipomas, sometimes called *hamartomas*, are an anomaly of breast development. The three major components are those of normal breast tissue; fibrous, adenomatous, and lipomatous tissue. There is architectural derangement enclosed within a fibrous pseudocapsule of variable completeness. Fibroadenolipomas may be diagnosed clinically at any age but are commonly an asymtomatic mammographic finding. On mammography, they are of mixed soft tissue and fatty density. The margins may be more or less defined depending on the completeness of the pseudocapsule. The mammographic appearance is usually pathognomonic because of its relatively well-defined nature, the fat content, and the lack of disturbance of adjacent normal tissue architecture (Fig. 46.28).[50] The echogenicity is variable and reflects the mixed tissue content and its disorganized structure (Fig. 46.29).

Lipoma

A *lipoma* consists of encapsulated fat and may be seen as a fat density mass with clear margins on mammogram and may be recognized if it is displacing adjacent normal fibroglandular structures (Fig. 46.30A).[50] On a mammogram, a lipoma may be indistinguishable from other normal fatty structures in the breast. Ultrasound typically shows the lipoma to be a poorly marginated lesion with an echogenicity slightly greater than that of the normal breast fat (Fig. 46.30B). A diagnosis of lipoma may be confirmed by ultrasound examination when the lesion is mammographically occult.

Phyllodes Tumor

Phyllodes tumor, previously known as *cystosarcoma phyllodes*, is composed of epithelial tissues and stroma.[51] The stroma of this tumor is more cellular and hyperplastic than that of the fibroadenoma, which is its histologic cousin. Most phyllodes tumors are benign, but between 3% and 12% exhibit malignant behavior. The differentiation of benign from malignant

varieties can be impossible, clinically, on imaging or on cytology. The most common sarcomatous change is to fibrosarcoma, but malignant change of all stromal components has been described. Metastatic spread from malignant phyllodes tumors is typically hematogenous. Nodal spread and malignant epithelial change are rare.

The phyllodes tumor has a pseudocapsule that may be incomplete in both benign and malignant tumors. Microscopically multiple, small fingerlets of phyllodes stroma infiltrate into adjacent tissue, explaining the local recurrence seen with both benign and malignant varieties.

Clinically, the tumor may present at any age. It is typically palpable as a rubbery, mobile mass and varies from small, 1 to 2 cm, to very large.

The mammographic (see Table 46.1) and ultrasound (see Table 46.2) appearances of a benign phyllodes tumor are seen in Figure 46.31.[52,53] The incompletely encapsulated portions of the tumor may be difficult to identify. Cystic spaces or clefts containing serous or serosanguinous fluid may be seen on ul-

Figure 46.28 This close-up mammographic view shows a rounded mass, which is of mixed density, both fibroglandular and fatty. Its margins are relatively well-defined, with some macrolobulations. The appearances are typical of a fibroadenolipoma or hamartoma. This lesion is sometimes called "a breast within a breast," which reflects its normal breast tissue components.

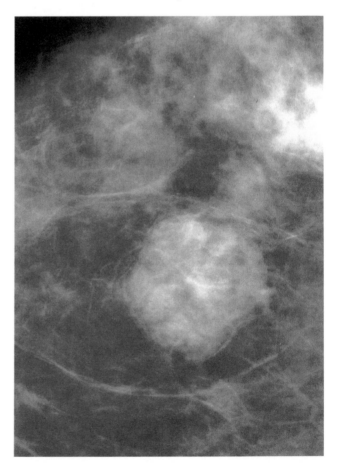

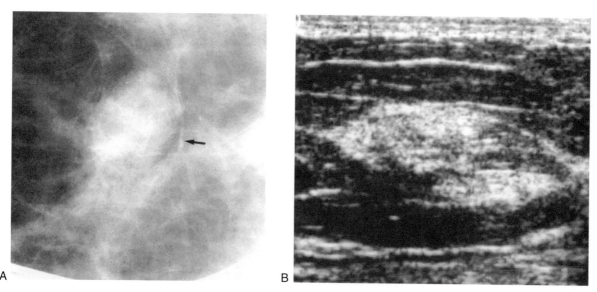

Figure 46.29 (A) The coned–magnification mammogram shows a mass of mixed parenchymal and fatty density with some obscuring of the margins (arrow). (B) The ultrasound examination similarly shows a relatively well-defined lesion, which is of mixed echogenicity consistent with parenchymal and fatty components. No disruption of normal tissues is seen on either examination, and the appearances on both examinations are typical of fibroadenolipoma.

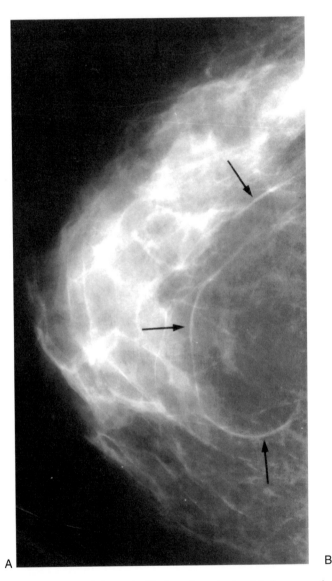

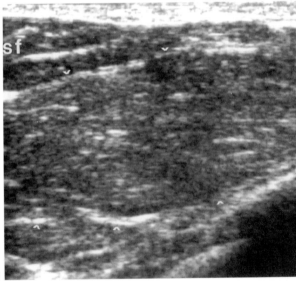

Figure 46.30 (A) A palpable 5-cm lump in the right breast can be correlated with the fatty density seen posteriorly on this right CC mammogram (arrows). The lesion is incompletely encapsulated and could be interpreted as normal retroparenchymal fat. (B) Ultrasound examination of the lump shows features typical of a lipoma (arrowheads). The echogenicity of the lipoma is slightly greater than that of the adjacent normal subcutaneous fat (sf), and the lesion appears incompletely encapsulated. In this case, because of its size, the whole mass is not demonstrated on this single image.

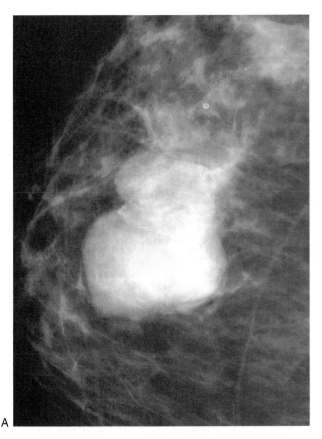

A

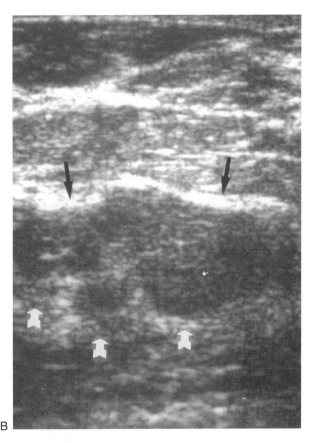

B

Figure 46.31 (A) This mammogram of an asymptomatic 55-year-old shows a 4-cm macrolobulated mass that is largely well-defined with an incomplete halo sign. The features are mostly benign, but the shape raises the possible diagnosis of phyllodes tumor. (B) Ultrasound shows a solid mass with large and small macrolobulations and margins that are in part ill-defined (arrows). These features again suggest a benign differential diagnosis including phyllodes tumor. Histology established a diagnosis of benign phyllodes tumor.

trasound but are not specific for phyllodes tumor. Hemorrhage, necrosis, and rarely calcification may be present. Fatty densities may be seen within the tumor on the mammogram if liposarcomatous change is present Liposarcoma is the only malignant breast condition that contains tissue of fatty density.

The mammographic and ultrasonographic appearances of phyllodes tumor are nonspecific.[54] Cytology and core sampling may be unhelpful in differentiating phyllodes tumor from fibroadenoma or in identifying malignant change, which may be focal within the tumor. Careful microscopic histologic examination is required for accurate diagnosis of both benign and malignant phyllodes tumors.

Infection

Breast infection or mastitis may be de novo or associated with lactation.[55] The most common organism is *Staphylococcus aureus*. The typical clinical signs of swelling, redness, and tenderness may be focal or widespread, and abscess development may occur if the infection is not controlled by antibiotic treatment. Establishing the diagnosis by needle aspiration is essen-

tial, as infection and abscess formation can be indistinguishable from inflammatory invasive carcinoma. The overlap in diagnostic features occurs because in both cases there is breakdown of normal tissue planes with surrounding edema (Fig. 46.32).

MALIGNANCY

Breast carcinoma is a common malignancy. In Western societies, it is the most common cancer occurring in women and the most common cause of cancer death in women. A number of genetic and lifestyle or environmental factors are known to affect the development of breast cancer.[56] Many of the lifestyle or environmental factors influence the breast's exposure to female sex hormones, and breast cancers are known to be hormone dependent. The cause remains unknown, but the most important single, identifiable risk factor is increasing age.

Breast carcinoma may be in situ (i.e., noninvasive), or it

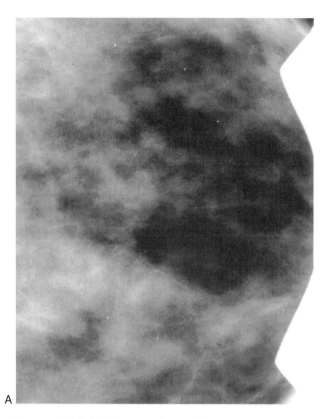

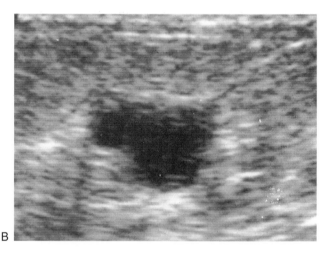

A   B

Figure 46.32 (A) This coned–magnification mammogram of an area that was red, tender, and swollen, showed no significant features. (B) Ultrasound examination of the same area of interest shows an irregular, hypoechoic mass surrounded by a loss of differentiation of the normal fatty and fibroglandular tissues due to edema. The appearances are consistent with abscess formation, but inflammatory malignancy is the main differential diagnosis. Culture of the needle aspirate confirmed an infective process requiring antibiotic treatment and drainage.

may be invasive. The imaging appearances of malignancy reflect the pathologic diversity of both noninvasive and invasive tumors. The imaging feature of ductal carcinoma in situ is microcalcification, and the features of invasive malignancy are a spiculated or ill-defined mass and/or an architectural disturbance.

In Situ Carcinoma

Pathologists describe both ductal carcinoma in situ (DCIS) and lobular carcinoma in situ (LCIS), with quite different malignant potential.[57] DCIS can progress directly to invasive malignancy, whereas LCIS does not develop directly into invasive tumor. LCIS is part of the spectrum of fibrocystic change. It is not clinically or mammographically detectable and is a chance histologic finding. It can be regarded as a marker for malignancy because its presence indicates a predisposition to the development in either breast of invasive carcinoma of either ductal or lobular type.

On mammogram, DCIS is typically seen as microcalcifications.[58] A surrounding, ill-defined density or minor architectural disturbance is sometimes found in association with ma-

lignant microcalcification and is due to a cellular and fibrotic inflammatory response, presumably immune generated, encasing the ducts involved by malignancy.[59] It is not indicative of invasive disease. Rarely, DCIS is identified as a mass or as an architectural disturbance without calcification. The detection of DCIS is more commonly mammographic than clinical, and its incidence is therefore increasing with increasing use of mammographic screening.[60] DCIS makes up approximately 10% to 20% of screen-detected cancers and approximately 5% of clinically detected cancers.

The understanding of the pathology classification of DCIS has altered as a result of screening experience. Classifications are now based on the grade of nuclear DNA and cytology characteristics and therefore on invasive malignant potential, rather than on microarchitecture. DCIS may be divided into three major categories (Table 46.3).[61–63] The first is low nuclear grade DCIS, typically with diploid DNA, small uniform cell size, micropapillary or cribriform architecture, and infrequent cellular necrosis. The second category is high nuclear grade DCIS, which typically has aneuploid DNA, large and variable cell size, solid microarchitecture, and frequent cellular necrosis. The third category lies between these two and is

Table 46.3 Cytonuclear Classification of DCIS

Nuclear Grade	Necrosis	Microscopic Architecture
Low	Rare	Usually cribriform or micropapillary, may be solid
Intermediate	Variable	Cribriform or micropapillary or solid
High	Frequent	Usually solid, may be cribriform or micropapillary

termed *intermediate nuclear grade*. In this category, there is a range of ploidy, cell size and architecture, and variable necrosis. The grade and associated necrosis are the important features in the classification, and the cell size and architecture may vary in each category. The purpose of such classification is to derive prognostic information. It is clear that DCIS represents a spectrum of disease, not one alone. At the borderlines, distinction of low-grade DCIS from atypical ductal hyperplasia and distinction of high-grade DCIS without invasion from that with microinvasion can be very difficult. The spectrum of pathology has a corresponding range of appearances, indicating a range of invasive malignant potentials and a range of management requirements.[64,65]

Features of the mammographic microcalcifications, to some extent, correlate with the different malignant subtypes.[66] The microcalcifications of DCIS are predominantly dystrophic and luminal in position. When only secretory material is present, calcifications are uncommon. The greater the necrosis, the more likely microcalcification is to occur and the more likely it is to take up the irregular shape of the luminal debris and therefore a recognizable malignant form.

The mammographic features of microcalcifications are its form (the most important), size, density, and distribution.[58] The degree of variability of each feature is important. Evaluation of the surrounding soft tissues also assists in the differential diagnosis (Table 46.4).

The descriptive terms commonly used for the form of malignant microcalcifications are *casting* and *granular*. *Casting* implies that the calcification takes the shape of the diseased duct that contains necrotic material. It is therefore typically linear or branching, with irregular margins and a variety of sizes. Casting calcification may be clustered or scattered in distribution and is pathognomonic of DCIS, usually of high nuclear grade (Fig. 46.33).[66] Granular calcifications are similar to the particles of a crushed stone. They vary in size, shape, and density, and the degree of variation tends to correlate with the nuclear grade of the tumor.[67] Microcalcifications in low nuclear grade DCIS are fine in pattern, that is, rather uniform in size, shape, and density. The greater uniformity reflects the lack of necrosis. These fine granular calcifications also tend more frequently to be clustered than the coarse granular microcalcifications of intermediate or high nuclear grade tumor, reflecting the more patchy calcification of low-grade tumor tissue (Fig. 46.34). When intermediate or high nuclear grade DCIS is present, the coarse granular calcifications show irregular margins and variability of form and size (Fig. 46.35). It is usual to see a mixture of casting and coarse granular calcifications in high-grade DCIS (Fig. 46.36).

DCIS starts in the TDLUs and progresses into the larger ducts and toward the nipple, an area that should always be examined with magnification films when DCIS is suspected. Some retrograde growth into acini may be seen microscopically. DCIS tends to occupy a lobe or lobes and to be multifocal rather than multicentric in origin. Although malignant microcalcifications are seen on the mammogram in a scattered or clustered distribution, the disease process tends to be more continuous pathologically, with calcifications being either absent in part or beyond mammographic resolution. Even with high-quality magnification, mammography tends to underestimate the extent of disease, particularly in the more poorly calcified low nuclear grade DCIS.[66]

Deposition of calcification in DCIS is not static. Progress mammographic examinations of DCIS may show increasing numbers and changing patterns of microcalcifications. Fine granular calcifications may coalesce to become coarse in appearance, and coarse granular calcifications may coalesce to form a casting pattern. It should be appreciated that malig-

Table 46.4 Differential Diagnostic Features of Mammographic Microcalcifications

	Malignant (Ductal)	Benign (Lobular)
Form	Variable, irregular, "fine" or "coarse granular" (like a crushed stone) or Linear or branching, "casting" (taking the shape of the diseased duct)	Uniform, round (solid) "pearls," similar appearance on all views or "Teacups" and "saucers" (gravity-dependant precipitate), changing appearance with changing views, i.e., rounded on CC view and semilunar on MLO view
Size and Density	High to low variability	Low variability
Distribution	Single or multiple clusters or scattered	Single or multiple clusters or scattered
Surrounding Soft Tissue Density	Fluffy, ill-defined, focal and irregular	Smooth, diffuse, and uniform

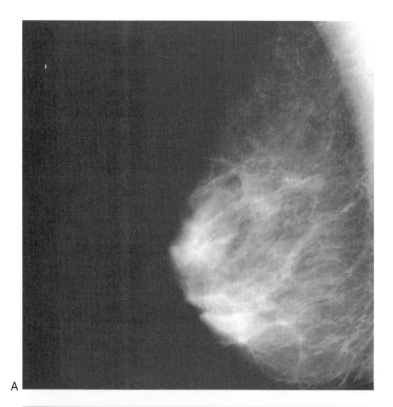

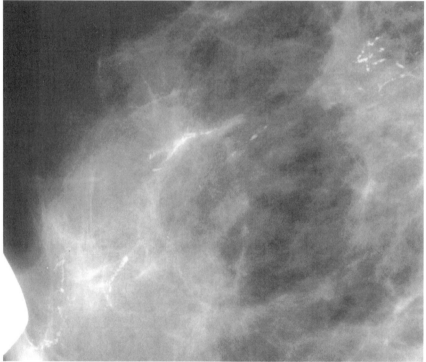

Figure 46.33 Full (**A**) and coned–magnification (**B**) MLO mammograms of a 62 -year-old asymptomatic woman show extensive microcalcifications. These have the shape of the ductal system, that is, casting appearance, and extend from the periphery of the breast to the nipple. No other change is evident. Histology showed high-grade intraduct carcinoma with central calcified necrosis.

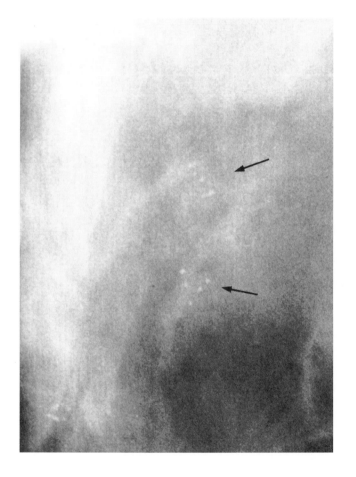

Figure 46.34 This coned–magnification mammogram of an asymptomatic 55-year-old shows multiple clusters of microcalcifications that have a fine granular form. Histology showed widespread ductal carcinoma in situ of low-to-intermediate nuclear grade with cribriform and solid patterns, some cytologic atypia, and infrequent necrosis. Calcification was present in luminal necrosis and secretions. Some areas of DCIS were uncalcified, and no infiltrative carcinoma was identified.

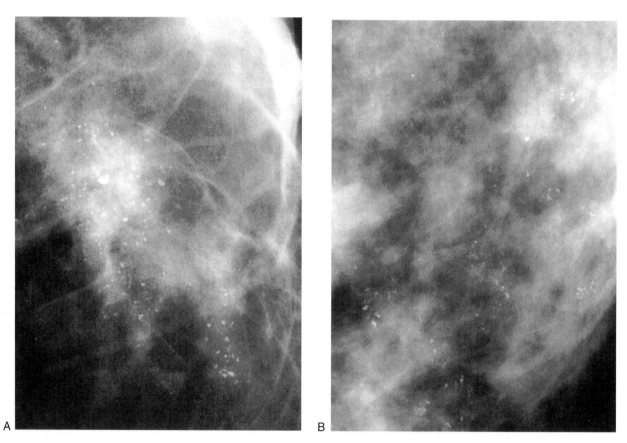

Figure 46.35 (**A**) This mammogram of an asymptomatic 55-year-old woman demonstrates widespread calcifications that vary considerably in shape, size, and density, that is, coarse granular in appearance. The microcalcifications are surrounded by marked, ill-defined, soft tissue opacities. (**B**) In this mammogram of an asymptomatic 59-year-old woman, multiple clusters of microcalcifications are seen with coarse granular and linear forms. Histology of both cases (Figs. A and B) showed intermediate to high nuclear grade DCIS of mixed papillary, cribriform, and solid patterns. Calcifications were present within luminal necrosis, and no definite invasive tumor was identified.

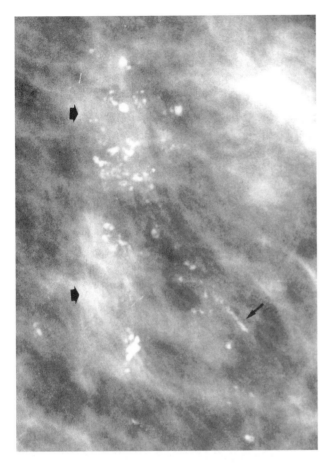

Figure 46.36 This magnification mammogram of a 60-year-old shows calcifications of irregular shape and variable size and density, that is, coarse granular in type. A focus of casting type calcification is also evident (arrow), and there is some surrounding, ill-defined, soft tissue density (arrowheads). Histology showed high nuclear grade DCIS with calcification in luminal necrosis. Some foci of early invasion were present.

nant microcalcifications may also decrease in size and number with progression of disease, particularly if invasive malignancy has developed (Fig. 46.37).

Knowledge of the underlying pathologic changes and of their mammographic presentations assists in differentiating malignant microcalcifications from those of benign fibrocystic change and in guiding management. The casting pattern is the only one that is pathognomonic of DCIS. Other appearances, particularly fine granular forms, may be seen in both benign and malignant processes. Tissue sampling, usually by core biopsy, and usually requiring stereotactic mammographic guidance, is necessary for preoperative diagnosis (Figs. 46.14 and 46.38).

Most microcalcifications cannot be seen on ultrasound. Mammography is much more sensitive and specific than ultrasound in demonstrating microcalcifications. On ultrasound, microcalcifications produce echogenic foci, which may be too small to shadow, and which may be indistinguish-

able from adjacent echogenic glandular tissue. A desmoplastic or inflammatory reaction may be seen around malignant microcalcifications. It is seen as an ill-defined density on the mammogram and as a reduction in the echogenicity of the periductal tissue involved by DCIS on ultrasound. The microcalcifications can then be seen against the hypoechoic background.[68] When visible in this way, the microcalcifications can be sampled or localized for removal using ultrasound guidance.

Mammography of DCIS may underestimate the extent and the type of disease. Microinvasion associated with DCIS will not be visible on mammography, and even a macroscopic focus of invasive disease may not be seen if obscured by the density of surrounding fibroglandular tissue. Ultrasound examination of an area of DCIS can sometimes show a mammographically occult focus of invasion as a typical hypoechoic and ill-defined mass in the midst of echogenic tissue (Fig. 46.39). Ultrasound core biopsy can establish a tissue diagnosis and influence surgery.

Figure 46.37 (A) A left screening mammogram shows a cluster of microcalcifications lying deep within the breast and a few scattered calcifications visible near the nipple (arrows). These calcifications were not further investigated. (*Figure continues.*)

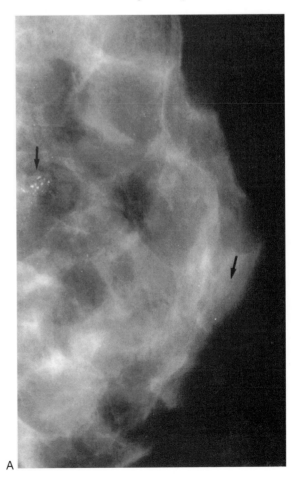

A

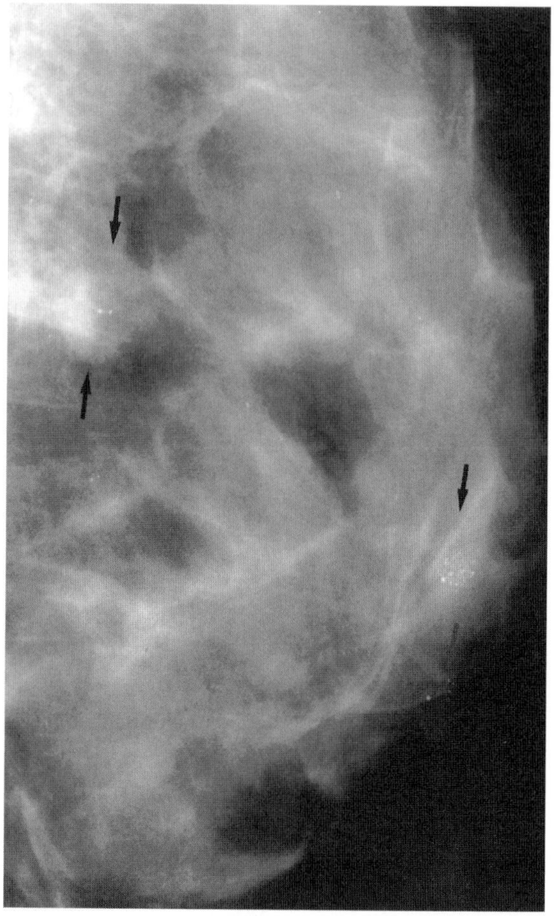

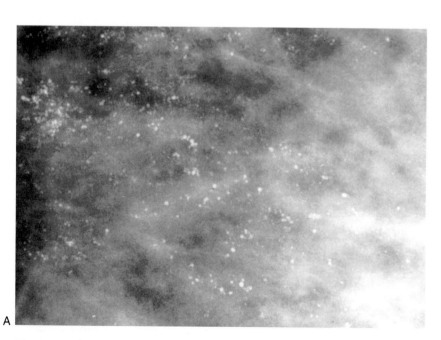

Figure 46.37 (*Continued*). (**B**) A mammogram of the same breast taken 30 months later shows that most of the microcalcifications previously seen deep within the breast have disappeared and are replaced by a mass (arrows). Clusters of microcalcifications are now clearly seen just deep to the nipple (arrows). At histologic examination, the mass was an infiltrating mucinous carcinoma with DCIS with necrosis of cribriform and comedo type both within and around the invasive mass. The microcalcifications near the nipple were present within similar DCIS in the subareolar ducts. This case illustrates that, with progression of disease, malignant microcalcifications may decrease in number.

Figure 46.38 (**A**) This magnification mammogram of a 61-year-old woman shows scattered microcalcifications that are regular in form but quite variable in size. The appearances favor a benign condition. (*Figure continues.*)

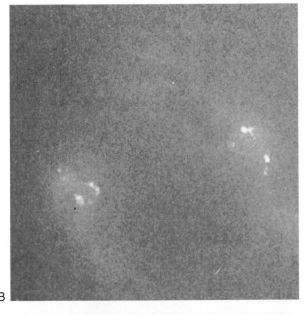

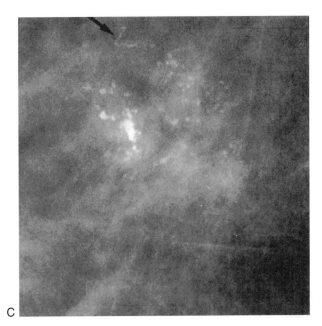

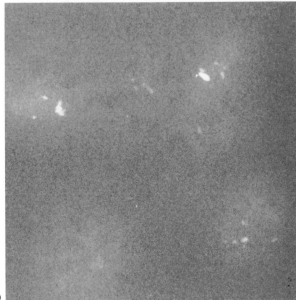

Figure 46.38 (*Continued*). (**B**) Core biopsy specimen radiograph of tissue taken from the area illustrated in Figure A confirms the presence of microcalcifications and therefore the adequacy of sampling. Histology of the core-tissue showed calcification in benign fibroadenotic tissue. (**C**) A 1-cm cluster of calcifications is seen in this magnification mammogram of an asymptomatic 46-year-old woman. The calcifications vary considerably in form and size, and an area of casting is present (arrow). The appearances are those of DCIS. (**D**) Core biopsy specimen radiograph of tissue taken from the area illustrated in Figure C shows microcalcifications in the core tissue. Core histology showed intraduct carcinoma of intermediate nuclear grade with a cribriform pattern and prominent intraluminal microcalcification.

Invasive Carcinoma

Invasive breast carcinoma is a disease with different behaviors and prognoses. All invasive tumors are believed to arise from the TDLU and to invade through the basement membrane into the surrounding tissues.[2,67] The principal pathologic division of invasive carcinomas is into ductal and lobular types, although some tumors have mixed features and do not easily fit into either category. The most common invasive tumor is a ductal type, not otherwise specified, but there are many subtypes of invasive ductal carcinoma, some of which are of prognostic significance and have distinguishing imaging features that reflect their histology.

The most typical mammographic and ultrasonographic appearance of invasive carcinoma, particularly of invasive ductal carcinoma, is that of a spiculated or stellate mass (Fig. 46.40).[41] The central body of the mass represents the bulk of the tumor growth. The spicules, which radiate out from the mass, contain malignant cells in their basal few millimeters where they are attached to the central mass, but are usually only fibrous beyond that point. The fibrous spicules are thought to be a histochemically generated, immune response to the tumor. They contract the adjacent normal fibroglandular tissues onto the tumor body, causing an architectural distortion.

When the central malignant tumor volume is small and

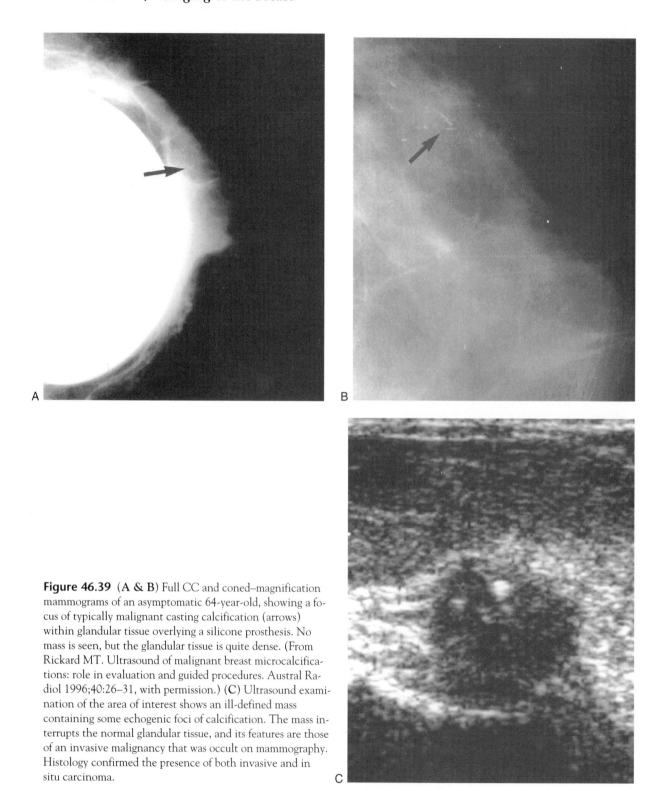

Figure 46.39 (**A & B**) Full CC and coned–magnification mammograms of an asymptomatic 64-year-old, showing a focus of typically malignant casting calcification (arrows) within glandular tissue overlying a silicone prosthesis. No mass is seen, but the glandular tissue is quite dense. (From Rickard MT. Ultrasound of malignant breast microcalcifications: role in evaluation and guided procedures. Austral Radiol 1996;40:26–31, with permission.) (**C**) Ultrasound examination of the area of interest shows an ill-defined mass containing some echogenic foci of calcification. The mass interrupts the normal glandular tissue, and its features are those of an invasive malignancy that was occult on mammography. Histology confirmed the presence of both invasive and in situ carcinoma.

dispersed, then the main imaging feature will be an architectural disturbance rather than a spiculated mass (Fig. 46.41).[41] An architectural disturbance is frequently the main feature of a lobular invasive cancer (Fig. 46.42). The malignant cells of a lobular invasive cancer may grow out into the adjacent tissues in a single-cell or "Indian file" pattern and infiltrate themselves between normal tissue structures. The resultant pattern is sometimes described as a spider's web, seen as an increased density and disturbed architecture without a dominant central mass.

At the other end of the spectrum of invasive cancers are those that grow in a rather well-contained manner (Fig.

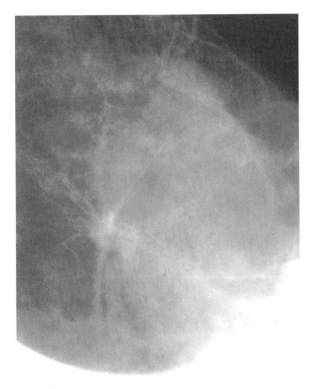

A

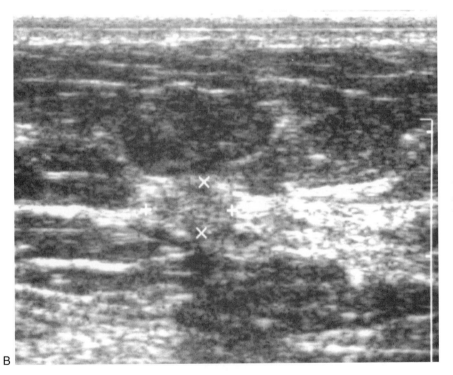

B

Figure 46.40 (**A**) This coned–magnification mammogram shows a small mass with straight spicules or fibrous strands extending radially from it into the adjacent tissues. The mammographic appearance is quite characteristic of an invasive carcinoma. (**B**) Ultrasound shows the margins of the lesion to be ill-defined and irregular (cursors). There is a break or interruption of the normal pattern of the surrounding fibroglandular tissues. These features are typical of an invasive malignancy. The echogenicity of malignancies, which in this case is greater than that of the fat, is variable but typically less than that of fat.

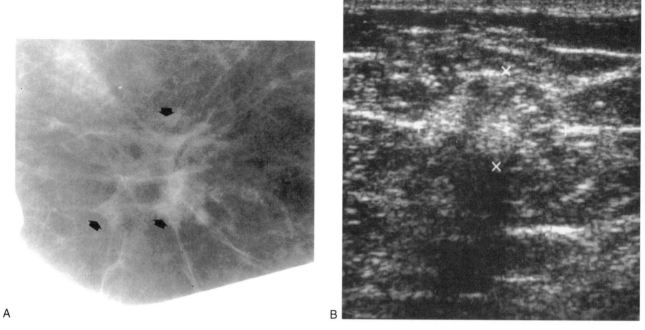

A   B

Figure 46.41 (**A**) This coned–magnification mammogram shows a small area of disturbed architecture with spiculations. There is no single central mass, although there is abnormal soft tissue change (arrowheads). This appearance is typical of invasive malignancy but is less common than the mass-like appearance seen in Figure 46.40. (**B**) Ultrasound shows interruption to the normal fibroglandular pattern (cursors). Corresponding to its mammogram appearance, the lesion is of nonuniform or mixed echogenicity. These appearances, like those of the mammogram, are probably due to malignancy. Some attenuation of the beam is shown, but this finding is unreliable in the differentiation of benign and malignant lesions. The histology of this lesion was that of infiltrating ductal carcinoma.

Figure 46.42 (**A**) CC mammogram of this 49-year-old patient shows an ill-defined architectural disturbance in the midportion of the left breast (arrowheads). (*Figure continues.*)

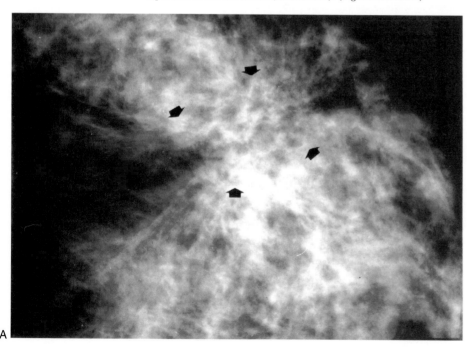

A

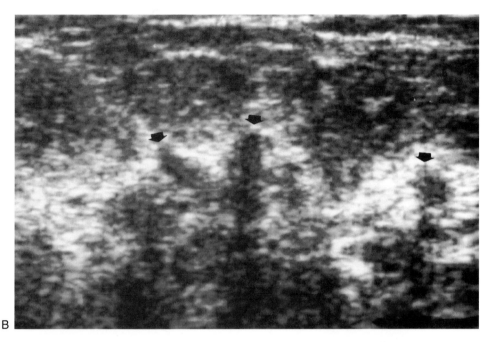

B

Figure 46.42 (*Continued*). (**B**) An ultrasound film shows corresponding small masses (arrowheads) and extensive disruption to the normal pattern of the fibroglandular tissue. The diffuse rather than focal imaging pattern of this lesion is characteristic of infiltrating lobular carcinoma. At histology, the tumor, an infiltrating lobular carcinoma, was shown to involve an area of at least 10 cm and to be associated with numerous foci of lobular carcinoma in situ.

46.43). The tumor tends to displace the adjacent tissues rather than infiltrate them. The image is then that of a well-defined mass with minimal adjacent tissue disruption. Other terms used to describe these tumors are circumscribed, knobby, or microlobulated.[31] Typical of this group of well-contained tumors are mucinous or colloid carcinoma and medullary carcinoma.

High-quality mammography and ultrasound are required to demonstrate malignancy as the features can be subtle. The primary mammographic features typical of an invasive carcinoma are shown in Table 46.1 and the ultrasound features are shown in Table 46.2.[37,41,69]

Secondary imaging signs include skin thickening, skin tethering or dimpling, nipple retraction, areolar thickening, interstitial infiltrate due either to blockage of lymphatic drainage or to direct malignant cellular infiltrate, and axillary lymph node enlargement (Fig. 46.44A). The same secondary malignant signs are seen on mammography and ultrasound.[70,71] Interstitial infiltrate is recognized as a loss of definition between the normal tissue structures and as an increase in breast mammographic density or ultrasonographic echogenicity (Fig. 46.44B).

A mammogram is likely to be the primary screening or diagnostic test except in young women. As with all lesions in the breast, the mammographic diagnosis of invasive malignancy is two stage. The lesion must be recognized then analyzed. Attention should be paid to mammographic asymmetry of contour, to architecture and density, and to any density not present on previous mammograms. Coned magnification films of any suggestive area must be examined before the mammogram can be called normal. Approximately 10% to 20% of clinical tumors are not identifiable on mammography.[72] Some cancers are mammographically occult because their features are obscured by overlying fibroglandular tissue. Others are simply not recognized, as their features are subtle or are not well-displayed because of poor technique.

The same false-negative results may occur with ultrasound examination. Mammography and ultrasound are complementary. Any clinical lesion that is occult on mammography, and any mammographically indeterminate mass, should be examined by ultrasound. A carcinoma can be difficult to see or occult on mammography because it is of parenchymal density (white) and therefore can be obscured by glandular tissue.

As it is typically hypoechoic (black) on ultrasound, it is easily seen within glandular tissue (Fig. 46.45). Ultrasound may show the malignant features of a growing margin or echogenic rim and of tissue disruption (Fig. 46.46), not evident on the mammogram.

For both mammography and ultrasound, the important features for the differentiation of benign from malignant are the shape and margins of the mass and the effect on adjacent

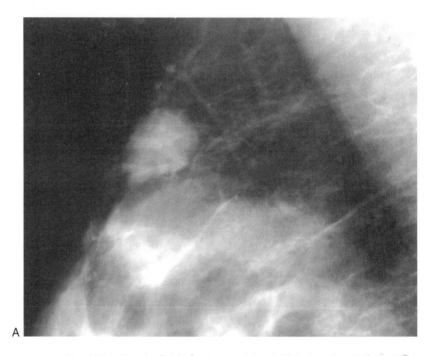

A

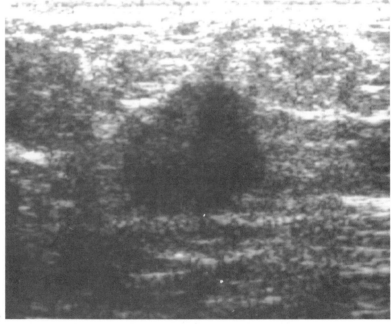

B

Figure 46.43 (**A**) On this close-up mammogram of an upper MLO view, there is a knobbly well-defined mass. No spicules are seen. This lesion is suggestive of a well-circumscribed carcinoma. (**B**) The ultrasound appearance is typical of an invasive malignancy. The lesion has ill-defined, irregular margins. It disrupts the normal fibroglandular pattern and extensively alters the echogenicity of the overlying fat. Histopathology was that of a (grade 2) ductal carcinoma with an apocrine appearance.

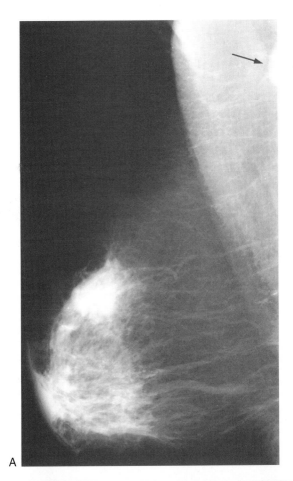

A

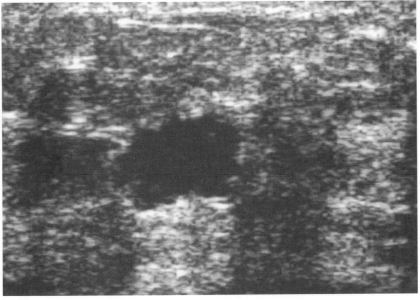

B

Figure 46.44 (**A**) This mammogram of a patient with clinically advanced breast carcinoma with peau d'orange shows a density in the upper breast. Also seen are thickening of the nipple–areolar complex and skin, and a diffuse coarsening of the normal fibroglandular pattern due to lymphatic obstruction. An enlarged, dense axillary lymph node is present (arrow). The picture is that of advanced breast carcinoma with axillary nodal involvement and secondary signs. (**B**) Ultrasound of the upper breast shows an echo-free area of central lucency, probably due to tumor necrosis. The extent of tumor tissue is not clearly identified, and the normal echogenicity distinctions between skin, fat, and fibroglandular tissue are lost due to the diffuse lymphatic infiltration involving all soft tissue structures.

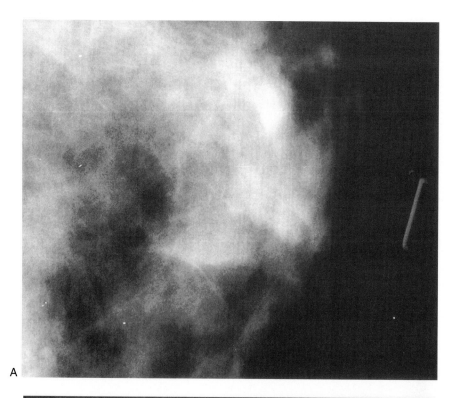

A

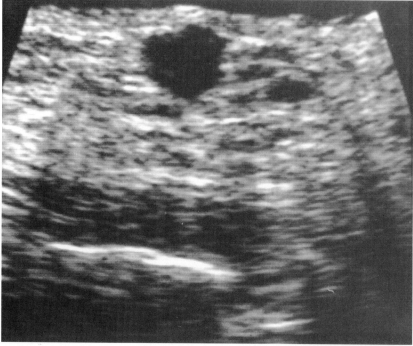

B

Figure 46.45 (**A**) A coned–magnification mammogram over a palpable lump (note skin marker) fails to reveal any significant abnormality. The fibroglandular tissue is mammographically dense and could obscure underlying pathology. (**B**) Ultrasound of the same palpable lump shows a low echogenicity mass with ill-defined margins that disrupt the adjacent normal tissue planes. The ultrasound features are those of an invasive malignancy, confirmed at histologic examination.

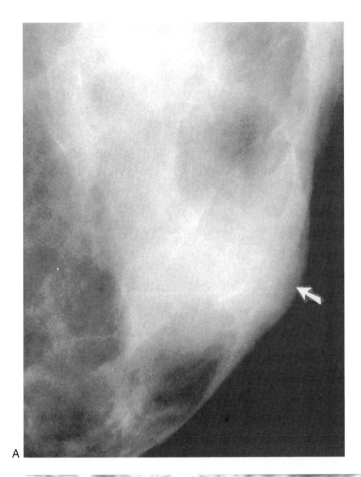

A

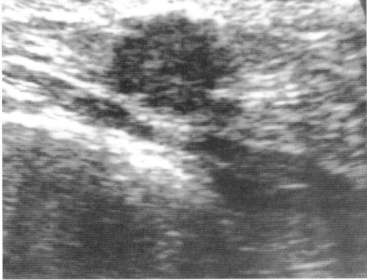

B

Figure 46.46 (**A**) A coned–magnification mammogram of a palpable mass in a 41-year-old woman shows a smooth bulge to the fibroglandular contour but no clearly defined mass. The mammographic features suggest a benign lesion, but a malignant lesion is not excluded. (**B**) Ultrasound of the lesion shows a mass with irregular margins that disrupt the normal fibroglandular pattern. These features are typical of a malignant lesion, which was confirmed by histology examination.

tissues. These features are not specific and, the major differential diagnoses to be considered follow:

1. Trauma with hematoma and/or fat necrosis (see Figs. 46.54 and 46.55)[50,73]

2. Infection with abscess formation (see Fig. 46.32)[50]

3. Radial scar or complex sclerosing lesion (see Fig. 46.27)[42,43,50]

The diagnosis is often evident from imaging when the clinical picture is known. For example, a stellate mass at the site of recent surgery for benign disease is typical of hematoma and/or fat necrosis and not of malignancy.

Even when the imaging is typical of malignancy, tissue diagnosis is imperative before definitive surgery. It is preferable to establish a preoperative diagnosis by cytology and/or core biopsy rather than by surgical biopsy. Tissue sampling may be guided by palpation, ultrasound, or stereotactic mammography. If clinical examination, imaging, and tissue sampling are all consistent with malignancy, then definitive single-stage treatment surgery can be undertaken. If tissue sampling is suggestive, atypical, or inconclusive, and the imaging or clinical picture is suggestive, then diagnostic surgical biopsy is indicated.

It is well recognized that breast malignancy is typically multifocal at pathologic examination.[74] This can be considered as a field change in which multiple sites in the one-duct system develop synchronously into malignancy. Although multifocality is underestimated by mammography, it should be looked for on coned and/or magnification views (Fig. 46.47). Multicentricity, that is, separate foci of synchronous malignancy in different duct systems or quadrants of the breast, is unusual (Fig. 46.48). Synchronous bilaterality is also unusual (Fig. 46.49). It is important to be aware of the possibility of multifocality, multicentricity, and bilaterality and to look for other foci of disease once the primary has been identified. One must also be aware that multiple synchronous tumors are not all necessarily of the same histologic subtype or of the same imaging appearance.

Multiple foci of invasive tumor or of a combination of both invasive tumor and ductal carcinoma in situ may be evidence of multifocality. DCIS may be present within an invasive mass but is also commonly found in adjacent tissues (Fig. 46.50). The amount of DCIS present both within and without an invasive mass is of prognostic importance.[75,76] If the DCIS content is considerable, then the tumor may be termed *extensive intraduct component positive* (EIC–positive). There are several definitions of EIC positivity. The two most widely accepted are

1. DCIS makes up 20% or more of the tumor mass and is also present in the surrounding tissues.

2. There are multiple foci of invasive disease within a tumor predominantly composed of DCIS.

Local recurrence following conservative surgery is increased in EIC-positive disease, regardless of whether adjuvant radiotherapy is used or not.

While multifocality may be evident on imaging, it may also be occult. Small invasive foci may not be identifiable, and in situ carcinoma may not be calcified. Careful imaging and histologic assessment of surgical margins are required for effective treatment by conservative surgery and adjuvent therapy.

Other Breast Malignancies

Paget's disease of the breast is characterized clinically by a cutaneous eczematoid change and pathologically by the presence of Paget's cells in the epidermis of the nipple and areola.[77] These changes are typically associated with underlying breast in situ carcinoma, or invasive carcinoma, or a combination of both. The underlying malignancy may be near the nipple, or it may also be located elsewhere in the breast.[77,78]

Inflammatory breast cancer is a variant of invasive ductal carcinoma that presents with an inflammatory clinical picture. Pathologically, this is usually due to tumor invasion of vascular spaces leading to edema.[79] It must be differentiated from infection and abscess using the triple test.

Primary breast malignancy other than carcinoma is extremely rare. Primary sarcoma may occur in isolation but is more frequently seen as part of a phyllodes tumor. Both primary and secondary lymphoma may involve breast tissue. The imaging appearances of sarcoma or lymphoma may be indistinguishable from those of carcinoma. Metastatic disease to the breast may have benign features, as the deposits are typically moderately circumscribed and multiple. The most common sites of origin for metastatic disease are from the contralateral breast, lung, and melanoma.

AXILLARY LYMPH NODE ENLARGEMENT

While breast carcinoma characteristically spreads to ipsilateral axillary nodes, contralateral spread is possible. When the lymph node enlargement is bilateral, nonbreast origins are more common. These may be malignant or inflammatory and include primary malignancies such as lymphoma and leukemia, secondary malignancies such as metastatic ovarian carcinoma, or inflammatory conditions such as rheumatoid arthritis and sarcoidosis (Fig. 46.51).[80] Clinical history and/or tissue sampling are needed for diagnosis.

PREOPERATIVE AND POST-TREATMENT IMAGING

It is necessary to have a knowledge of the type of tumor and its multifocality and extent, to manage the cancer conservatively. In many cases, these characteristics can be established

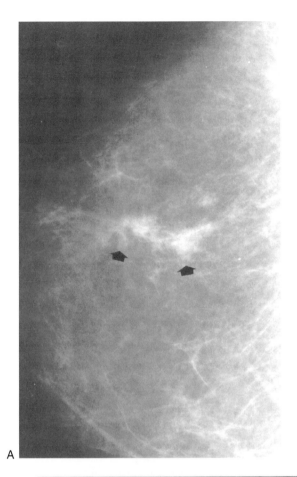

A

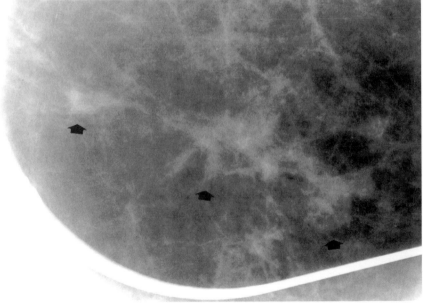

B

Figure 46.47 (A & B) Full and coned–magnification CC mammograms show multiple, irregularly shaped masses of varying size in the midbreast (arrowheads). These lesions represent multifocal ductal carcinoma with some associated, noncalcified, ductal carcinoma in situ.

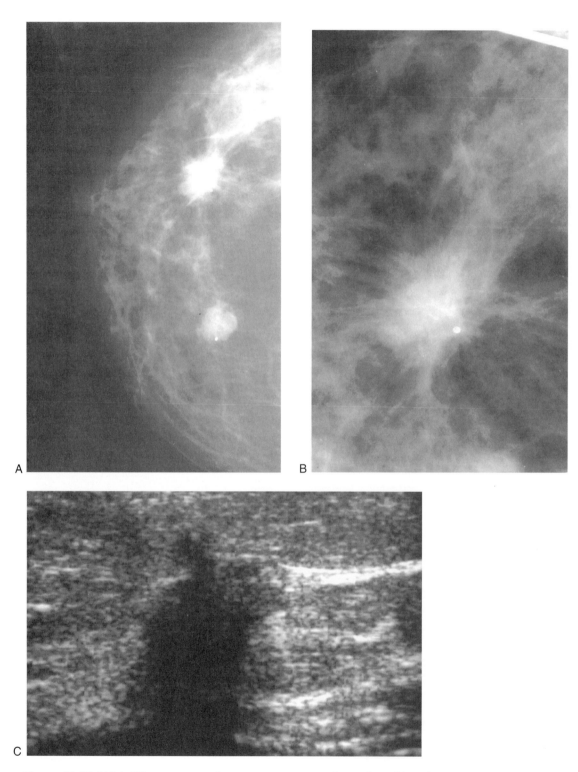

Figure 46.48 (A) A CC mammogram shows two masses, one with spicules and lying lateral to midline, and one knobbly and lying medially. These lesions represent synchronous, multicentric, invasive ductal carcinomas of not otherwise specified type. (B & C) Mammogram and ultrasound of the laterally placed lesion show it to have a highly spiculated (i.e., fibrous) margin on mammography and therefore to be irregularly marginated and attenuating on ultrasound. (*Figure continues.*)

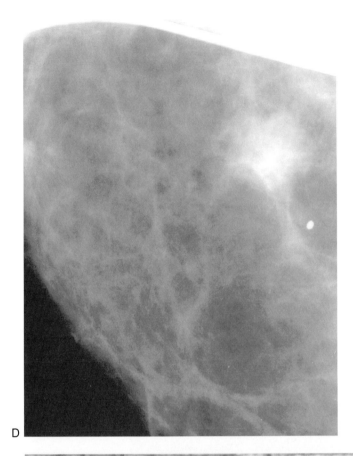

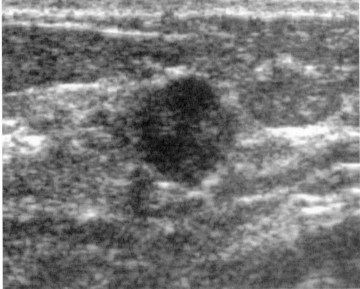

Figure 46.48 (*Continued*). (**D & E**) Mammogram and ultrasound of the medially placed lesion show it to be mammographically more knobbly than spiculated and therefore to be more smoothly marginated and less attenuating on ultrasound examination than the lateral lesion.

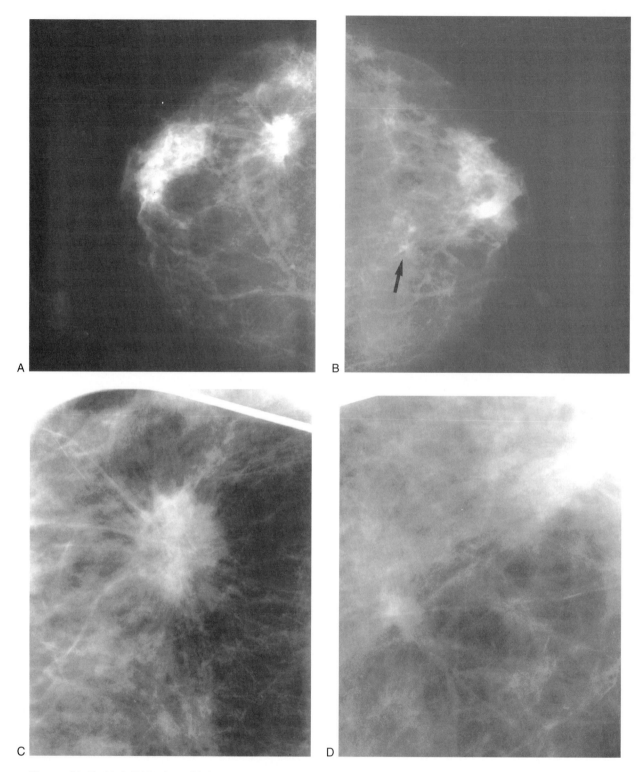

Figure 46.49 (**A & B**) Right and left CC mammograms of a 59-year-old show an obvious spiculated mass in the right lateral breast and a subtle irregular density in the left medial breast (arrow). (**C & D**) Coned–magnification mammograms of these two areas show that both have a central mass and spiculated margins, characteristic of malignancy. (*Figure continues*)

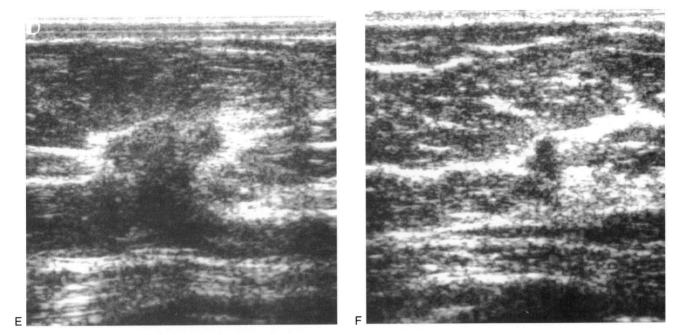

E   F

Figure 46.49 (*Continued*). (**E & F**) Ultrasound of the same two lesions shows central masses, irregular margins, and tissue disruption, again features characteristic of malignancy. These lesions were confirmed histologically as a right 18-mm, grade 1 ductal carcinoma and a left 5-mm, grade 2 ductal carcinoma with no evidence of axillary nodal involvement.

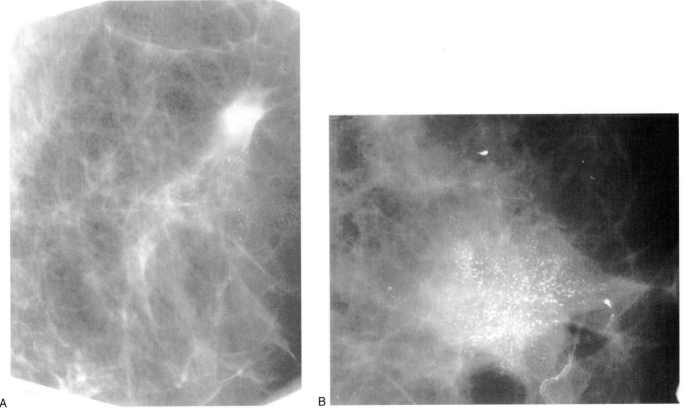

A   B

Figure 46.50 These two cases illustrate the characteristic radiographic appearances of carcinomas of mixed invasive and intraductal histologic types. (**A**) A small invasive ductal carcinoma (mass) with intraductal carcinoma (microcalcifications) both within the invasive tumor and extending for several centimeters beyond it. (**B**) A large invasive carcinoma (mass) with an extensive amount of intraductal carcinoma (microcalcifications) within the mass and a minor amount extending beyond its margins.

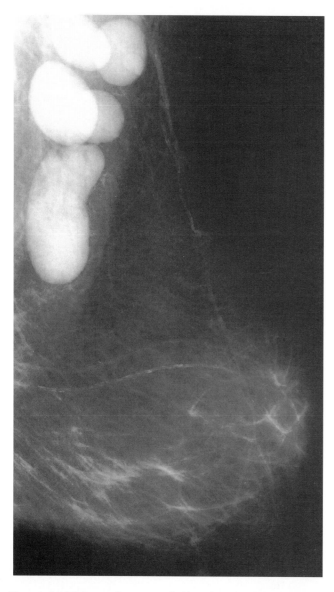

Figure 46.51 Large, dense, rounded lymph nodes that have lost their fatty hila are present in the axilla of this 82-year-old patient with lymphoma.

by a combination of imaging, clinical examination, and percutaneous tissue sampling. Based on the integrated results of these tests (the triple test), single-stage surgical management for breast cancer can be undertaken in most patients. In some, the histology of the surgical specimen may show that the tumor characteristics have been underestimated or that the resection margins are involved by tumor, and then further surgery may be necessary.

Preoperative Localization

The palpability of a tumor must be assessed before tissue sampling, to ensure accuracy prior to any soft tissue bruising or hematoma. An impalpable lesion requires preoperative localization if it is to be sampled surgically or if the planned treatment is local excision rather than mastectomy. The most common method of localization is by hookwire, but carbon tracking can also be used.[81] It is important to select the most suitable approach to the lesion. This is usually the shortest, so that only minimal disruption of normal tissues will result. The shortest approach is particularly important if the surgeon plans to follow the length of the hookwire (or carbon track). It is less important if the surgeon intends to cut down on to the hookwire near its tip. Some surgeons prefer that the radiologist insert the localization needle (or track) in a radial direction along a line that takes the nipple as the central point of a spoke wheel. This is best for a periareolar incision, which has cosmetic advantages.

It is important that the tip of the hookwire lies 1 to 2 cm distal to the lesion or that the carbon track lies within it. If the tip of the hookwire or carbon track falls short of the lesion, an inadequate excision may result.

Guidance for localization can be by stereotactic or grid mammography or by ultrasound. With all techniques, needle placement should be made parallel to the chest wall. To use the mammographic grid technique, a lesion must be visible in two right-angle (or near right-angle) views. The needle is inserted into the compressed breast at a position overlying the lesion. This position is indicated on a control film, which is marked with X and Y coordinate surface markers. Once a postpositioning film indicates that the inserted needle overlies the lesion, the compression is removed, and the breast containing the needle is imaged in the right-angle position. From this exposure, the depth of the needle can be adjusted, and when correctly positioned, the hookwire can be passed through the needle tip and into the tissue, and the needle removed.

With stereotactic technique, any mammographically visible lesion can be localized even if it is seen in one view only. The direction of needle placement can be from any angle. All three coordinates of the lesion (i.e., X, Y, and Z depth axes) can be calculated from the stereotactic control films. If a hookwire is used, then once the needle tip position is shown to be within the lesion on the postpositioning stereotactic views, it is advanced a further 1 to 2 cm in depth before the hookwire is passed through the needle tip into the tissues. This additional depth ensures that the hookwire tip is 1 cm or more distal to the lesion when compression is released. If the hookwire is released into the lesion without further needle advancement, there is the risk of the tip of the hookwire not opening in the lesion and of retracting and opening short of the lesion once the compression is removed.

Ultrasound is a very quick and easy method of localization for any lesion that can be seen by this technique. The hookwire-containing needle can be guided into and through the lesion by positioning the needle in line with the long axis of the probe. With this approach, the needle tip always remains visible and can be accurately positioned.

For clarification of the final hookwire position relative to the lesion and the skin entry point, a skin marker can be placed at the entry point, and two right-angled mammographic films taken after positioning (Fig. 46.52). Some hook-wires have distinguishing marks placed at various distances along their length. These are identifiable on final films and can be mentioned in the accompanying report in reference to the position of the lesion.

Specimen Radiography

A surgical specimen of breast tissue can be radiographed on normal mammographic equipment or on dedicated equipment. This radiograph should be taken for all lesions that require hookwire localization (Fig. 46.52C). A whole-specimen radiograph is used to indicate whether the lesion is adequately sampled or grossly removed. The orientation of the specimen should be indicated by surgical sutures placed to mark, for example, the nipple end, the distal end, and the deep and superficial surfaces. As the radiograph is two dimensional only, it is not possible to indicate accurately if the specimen margins are clear of the lesion. Microscopy of the oriented specimen is required to assess margin involvement. It is important not to compress the specimen when taking the radiograph or it may interfere with the surgical margins. A low-kilovolt peak technique without compression should give consistently good images.

Sliced specimen radiography can be used to guide the pathology examination of the tissue.[82] The whole specimen

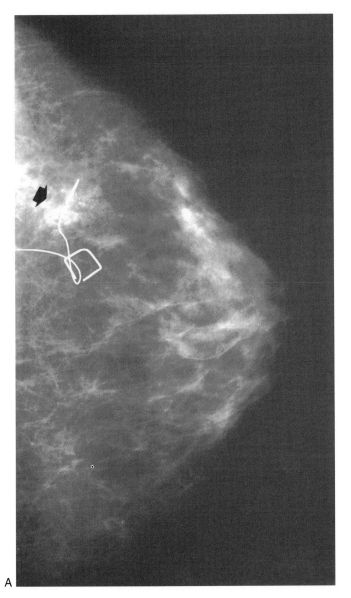

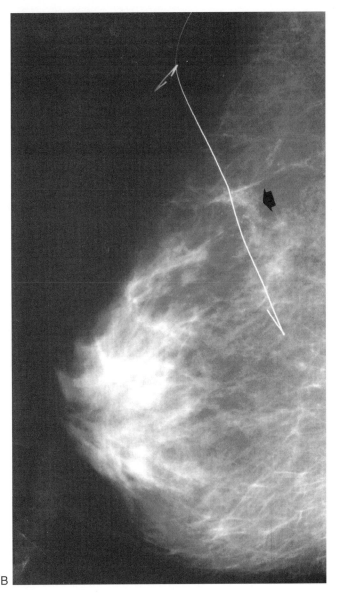

A

B

Figure 46.52 (A & B) Two right-angle mammograms, 90 degrees lateromedial and CC, show the position of the hookwire in relation to the mammographic abnormality of micro-calcifications and associated opacity of soft tissue density (arrowheads). The wire has passed through the microcalcifications, and its tip lies several centimeters distal to them. A surface marker indicates the skin entry point. (*Figure continues.*)

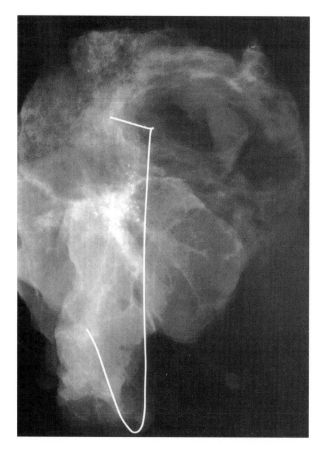

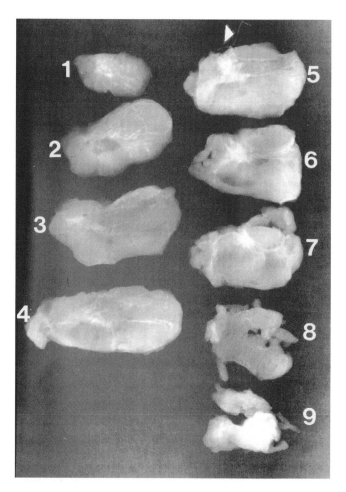

Figure 46.52 (*Continued*). (**C**) A specimen radiograph shows that the lesion has been macroscopically removed. Histology showed that the lesion, intermediate-grade DCIS without invasion, had been entirely removed. The nature of this lesion had been diagnosed by stereotactically guided core biopsy, as illustrated in Figure 46.14.

Figure 46.53 Sliced specimen radiograph of a small mass shows that the greater part of the lesion is in slices 5,6, and 7. One of the lesion margins abuts the edge of the specimen, which is marked by a single suture (arrow). Microscopic examination confirmed a 5-mm invasive ductal carcinoma extending to involve this excision margin.

should have its surfaces inked and then be chilled. When firm, the chilled specimen is cut into 5-mm slices, preferably transverse to the long axis of the main ducts, as indicated by the surgical sutures. The slices are placed in order, identified, and radiographed. The pathologist is then able to direct initial attention to the slices containing the mammographic abnormality (Fig. 46.53). Any pathology report should indicate that the mammographic abnormality has been identified, and its cause explained. If the imaged lesion is not identified on histology examination, then the paraffin blocks can be radiographed to see if the area of interest can be identified and further slices for microscopic examination taken from that area.

Postsurgery/Trauma Changes

Imaging changes may be seen in the skin, fat, and fibroglandular tissues after surgery or trauma to the breast.[83] These will modify with time and may resolve completely so that no imaging abnormality remains identifiable. In other cases, the changes may persist and be confused with other pathologic changes. Radiotherapy is often given to the breast following

conservative surgical management of carcinoma. Radiotherapy may exacerbate many of the changes produced by surgery.[84] The radiologist should be aware of any previous breast surgery and/or radiotherapy and should assess whether imaging changes can be explained on the basis of treatment or recurrence.

It is usual for some hemorrhage, serous fluid, or avascularized fat to accumulate at the site of surgical biopsy. Similar changes may occur following other forms of penetrating or blunt trauma, and fat necrosis may occur at the site of radiotherapy. Hematoma, seroma, and/or fat necrosis may be resorbed or may persist and become organized, with a fibrous response leading to an irregularly shaped mass. This mass may or may not be clinically evident. Typically, the lesion contracts with time, but change varies widely and may occur slowly over several years. Dystrophic calcification may deposit in the lesion. Skin thickening and/or tethering may develop at the cutaneous site of the scar.

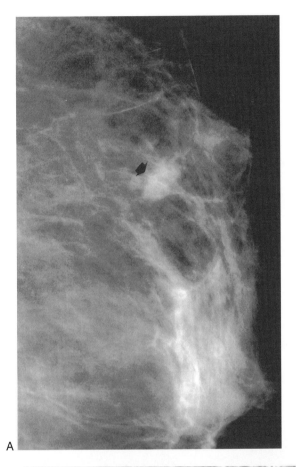

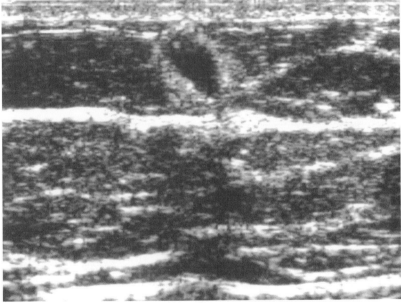

Figure 46.54 (A) This mammogram was taken several weeks following a knock to the left upper breast. The 46-year-old woman had noted a palpable pea-like lump and overlying bruising. The mammogram shows an irregularly shaped mass with ill-defined margins (arrowhead). The appearances could be due to an invasive carcinoma, but the clinical history suggests a hematoma. (B) An ultrasound shows a superficial hypoechoic area with a thick echogenic rim. These appearances are typical of a hematoma. The mass resolved without intervention.

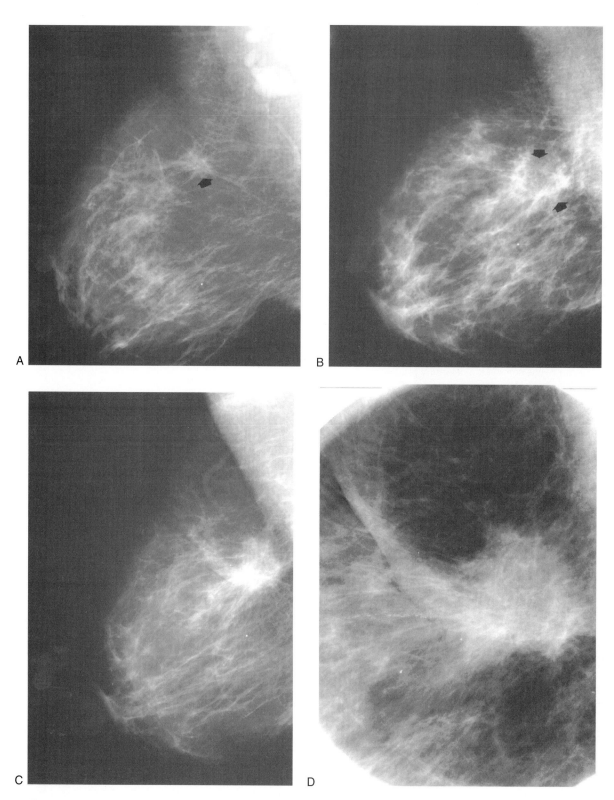

Figure 46.55 (A) The screening mammogram of this 57-year-old woman shows a 10-mm spiculated invasive carcinoma in the upper right breast (arrowhead). (B) At 12 months, after wide local excision and radiotherapy, there is, at the operative site, a spiculated deformity containing central fatty densities (arrowheads). Diffuse interstitial thickening of the breast tissue is also evident. The appearances are typical of those seen after conservative management of breast malignancy. (C & D) Two years after treatment, full and coned MLO mammograms show that the focal deformity appears denser and more contracted and that a central fatty lucency persists. There is also an adjacent skin fold due to deformity at the surgical site. (*Figure continues.*)

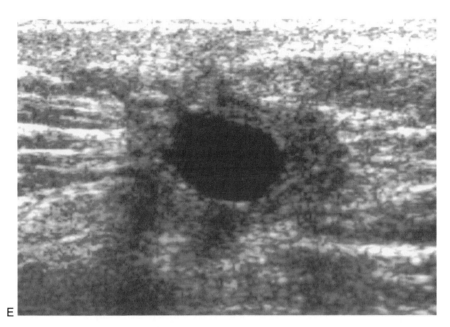

Figure 46.55 (*Continued*). (**E**) The focal area shown in Figures C and D was examined by ultrasound. There is a well-defined central echo-free collection of fat necrosis surrounded by hypoechoic scar tissue and some contraction deformity of adjacent normal tissues. The mammographic and ultrasonographic appearances are consistent with resolving fat necrosis and fibrosis. Films taken at 36 months showed further resolution and no evidence of recurrence.

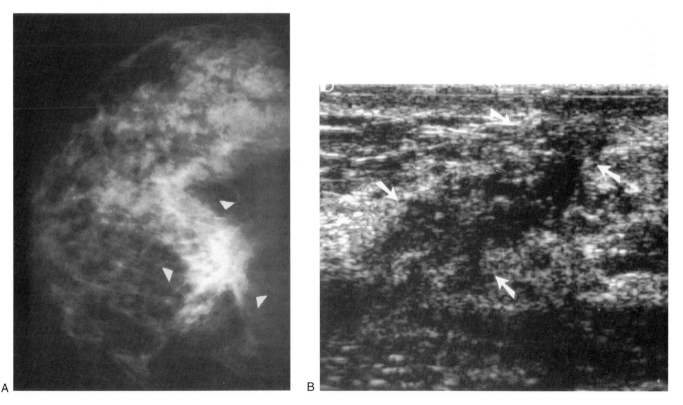

Figure 46.56 (**A**) This mammogram of a 52-year-old woman was taken several years post-surgical biopsy for a benign lesion. There is an area of increased density and distorted, contracted architecture at the site of previous surgery (arrows). (**B**) Ultrasound examination showed a corresponding serpentine, hypoechoic change extending from the skin surface deep into the glandular tissue (arrows). The appearances are those of fibrosis or scar tissue, which was confirmed by core biopsy histology.

Imaging of an immediate postoperative/traumatic site by mammography or ultrasound will show an ill-defined mass with irregular or spiculated or stellate margins (Fig. 46.54).[83–85] Fibrosis may develop later and trap areas of fat into the mass. On ultrasound, the mass has a thick irregular wall and contents of liquid or mixed echogenicity. It may be complex with thick, irregular septa. With time, the fibrous wall may thicken and contract, and the contents may reduce to be contained within one or two locules (Fig. 46.55). Calcific deposits in fat necrosis are typically mural in position and rim-like in appearance on both mammography (see Fig. 46.18) and ultrasound. Dystrophic stromal calcification may be more haphazard in location and position. A soft tissue density due to fibrosis may persist for years (Fig. 46.56).

The spiculated or stellate appearance may be difficult to differentiate on imaging from that of an invasive carcinoma. This differential diagnosis is of most concern when the surgery causing the appearance was carried out for a malignancy. Local recurrence of malignancy is not necessarily of the same histologic type as the original lesion, and therefore, for example, noninvasive carcinoma seen as microcalcifications may recur as a noncalcified stellate mass rather than as microcalcifications.

It should be appreciated that interpretation of not only the imaging findings but also of the clinical findings and of the cytology and core biopsy findings is made more difficult by previous surgery and/or radiotherapy. Close correlation of the imaging and clinical features and, if necessary, tissue sampling will ensure accurate diagnosis and early management of recurrent disease.

REFERENCES

1. Page DL, Anderson TJ. Diagnostic Histopathology of the Breast. Churchill Livingstone, New York, 1987, pp 4–10
2. Wellings SR. A hypothesis of the origin of human breast cancer from the terminal ductal lobular unit. Pathol Res Pract 1980;166:515–535
3. Kapdi CC, Parekh NJ. The male breast. Radiol Clin North Am 1983;21:137–148
4. Haus AG, Erickson L. Image quality factors and radiation dose in mammography. J Imaging Techn 1984;10:29–35
5. Yaffe MJ, Hendrick RE, Feig SA et al. Recommended specifications for new mammography equipment: report of the ACR-CDC Focus Group on mammography equipment. Radiology 1995;197:19–26
6. Tabar L. Microfocal spot magnification mammography. Recent Results Cancer Res 1984;90:62–68
7. Eklund GW, Busby RC, Miller SH, Job JS. Improved imaging of the augmented breast. AJR Am J Roentgenol 1988;151:469–473
8. Tabar L, Dean PB. Teaching Atlas of Mammography (2nd rev ed.). Georg Thieme Verlag, New York, 1985, pp 6–9
9. Jellins J. Concepts for breast surveillance. Challenges in quality assurance. In: Madjar H, Teubner J, Hackeloer BJ, Eds. Breast Ultrasound Update. Karger, Basel, 1994, pp 13–25
10. Dixon JM, Mansel RE. ABC of breast disease. Symptoms assessment and guidelines for referral. BMJ 1994;309:722–726
11. Feig SA. A new method for assessment of radiation risk from screening mammography Recent Results Cancer Res 1990;119:141–150
12. Feig SA, Shaber GS, Patchefsky A et al. Analysis of clinically occult and mammographically occult breast tumors. AJR Am J Roentgenol 1977;128:403–408
13. Tabar L, Fagerberg CJ, Gad A et al. Reduction in mortality from breast cancer after mass screening with mammography. Randomised trial from the Breast Cancer Screening Working Group of the Swedish National Board of Health and Welfare. Lancet 1985;1:829–832
14. Verbeek AL, Hendriks JH, Holland R et al. Reduction of breast cancer mortality through mass screening with modern mammography. First results of the Nijmegen project, 1975–1981. Lancet 1984;1:1222–1224
15. Shapiro S, Venet W, Strax P et al. Ten to fourteen-year effect of screening on breast cancer mortality. J Natl Cancer Inst 1982;69:349–355
16. Nystrom L, Rutqvist LE, Wall S et al. Breast cancer screening with mammography: overview of Swedish randomised trials. Lancet 1993;341:973–978
17. Klausner RD. Rimer BK. NCI adopts new mammography screening guidelines for women. Journal of the National Cancer Institute 1997: 89:538-540
18. Hermansen C, Skovgaard Poulsen H, Jensen J et al. Diagnostic reliability of combined physical examination, mammography, and fine-needle puncture ("triple test") in breast tumors. A prospective study. Cancer 1987;60:1866–1871
19. Giard RW, Hermans J. The value of aspiration cytologic examination of the breast. A statistical review of the medical literature. Cancer 1992;69:2104–2110
20. Ellis IO, Galea MH, Locker A et al. Early experience in breast cancer screening: emphasis on development of protocols for triple assessment. Breast 1993;2:148–153
21. Azavedo E, Svane G, Auer G. Stereotactic fine-needle biopsy in 2594 mammographically detected non-palpable lesions. Lancet 1989;1:1033–1036
22. Mouriquand J. In: Diagnosis of Nonpalpable Breast Lesions. Ultrasonographically Controlled Fine Needle Aspiration. Karger, Basel, 1993
23. Fajardo LL, Willison KM, Pizzutiello RJ, Eds. A Comprehensive Approach to Stereotactic Breast Biopsy. Blackwell Science, Cambridge, MA, 1995
24. Jackson VP. The status of mammographically guided fine needle aspiration biopsy of nonpalpable breast lesions. Radiol Clin North Am 1992;30:155–166
25. Fornage BD, Coan JP, David CL. Ultrasound-guided needle biopsy of the breast and other interventional procedures. Radiol Clin North Am 1992;30:167–185
26. Love SM, Gelman RS, Silen W. Sounding board. Fibrocystic "disease" of the breast: a nondisease? N Engl J Med 1982;307:1010–1014
27. Dupont WD, Page DL. Risk factors for breast cancer in women with proliferative breast disease. N Engl J Med 1985;312:146–151
28. Page DL, Anderson TJ. Diagnostic Histopathology of the Breast. Churchill Livingstone, New York, 1987, pp 51–61
29. Tabar L, Dean PB. Teaching Atlas of Mammography (2nd rev. ed.). Georg Thieme Verlag, New York, 1985, p 170

30. Tabar L, Dean PB. Teaching Atlas of Mammography (2nd rev. ed.). Georg Thieme Verlag, New York, 1985, p 12

31. Tabar L, Dean PB. Teaching Atlas of Mammography (2nd rev. ed.). Georg Thieme Verlag, New York, 1985, pp 18–19

32. Tohno E, Cosgrove DO, Sloane JP. Ultrasound Diagnosis of Breast Diseases. Churchill Livingstone, Edinburgh, 1994, pp 104–112

33. Tohno E, Cosgrove DO, Sloane JP. Ultrasound Diagnosis of Breast Diseases. Churchill Livingstone, Edinburgh, 1994, pp 112–117

34. Tohno E, Cosgrove DO, Sloane JP. Ultrasound Diagnosis of Breast Diseases Churchill Livingstone, Edinburgh, 1994, pp 94–96

35. Page DL, Anderson TJ. Diagnostic Histopathology of the Breast. Churchill Livingstone, New York, 1987, pp 72–79

36. Sickles EA. Nonpalpable, circumscribed, noncalcified solid breast masses: likelihood of malignancy based on lesion size and age of patient. Radiology 1994;192:439–442

37. Stavros AT, Thickman D, Rapp CL et al. Solid breast nodules: use of sonography to distinguish between benign and malignant lesions. Radiology 1995;196:123–134

38. Tohno E, Cosgrove DO, Sloane JP. Ultrasound Diagnosis of Breast Diseases. Churchill Livingstone, Edinburgh, 1994, pp 76–91

39. Jackson VP. Management of solid breast nodules: what is the role of sonography? Radiology 1995;196:14–15

40. Page DL, Anderson TJ. Diagnostic Histopathology of the Breast. Churchill Livingstone, New York, 1987, pp 89–103

41. Tabar L, Dean PB. Teaching Atlas of Mammography (2nd rev. ed.). Georg Thieme Verlag, New York, 1985, pp 88–90

42. Ciatto S, Morrone D, Catarzi S et al. Radial scars of the breast: review of 38 consecutive mammographic diagnoses. Radiology 1993;187:757–760

43. Frouge C, Tristant H, Guinebretiere JM et al. Mammographic lesions suggestive of radial scars: microscopic findings in 40 cases. Radiology 1995;195:623–625

44. Vega A, Garijo F. Radial scar and tubular carcinoma. Mammographic and sonographic findings. Acta Radiol 1993;34:43–47

45. Finlay ME, Liston JE, Lunt LG, Young JR. Assessment of the role of ultrasound in the differentiation of radial scars and stellate carcinomas of the breast. Clin Radiol 1994;49:52–55

46. Lamb J, McGoogan E. Fine needle aspiration cytology of breast in invasive carcinoma of tubular type and in radial scar/complex sclerosing lesions. Cytopathology 1994;5:17–26

47. Sloane JP, Mayers MM. Carcinoma and atypical hyperplasia in radial scars and complex sclerosing lesions: importance of lesion size and patient age. Histopathology 1993;23:225–231

48. Page DL, Anderson TJ. Diagnostic Histopathology of the Breast. Churchill Livingstone, New York, 1987, pp 104–119

49. Rosen PP, Holmes G, Lesser ML et al. Juvenile papillomatosis and breast carcinoma. Cancer 1985;55:1345–1352

50. Feig SA. Breast masses. Mammographic and sonographic evaluation. Radiol Clin North Am 1992;30:67–92

51. Page DL, Anderson TJ. Diagnostic Histopathology of the Breast. Churchill Livingstone, New York, 1987, pp 341–350

52. Cole-Beuglet C, Soriano R, Kurtz AB et al. Ultrasound, xray mammography, and histology of cystosarcoma phylloides. Radiology 1983;146:481–486

53. Buchberger W, Strasser K, Heim K et al. Phylloides tumour: findings on mammography, sonography and aspiration cytology in 10 cases. AJR Am J Roentgenol 1991;157:715–719

54. Auger M, Hanna W, Kahn HJ. Cystosarcoma phyllodes of the breast and its mimics. An immunohistochemical and ultrastructural study. Arch Pathol Lab Med 1989;113:1231–1235

55. Dixon JM. ABC of breast diseases. Breast infection. BMJ 1994;309:946–949

56. Hulka BS, Stark AT. Breast cancer: cause and prevention. Lancet 1995;346:883–887

57. Page DL, Steel CM, Dixon JM. ABC of breast diseases. Carcinoma in situ and patients at high risk of breast cancer. BMJ 1995;310:39–42

58. Tabar L, Dean PB. Teaching Atlas of Mammography (2nd rev. ed.). Georg Thieme Verlag, New York, 1985, p 138

59. Kinkel K, Gilles R, Feger C et al. Focal areas of increased opacity in ductal carcinoma in situ of the comedo type: mammographic–pathologic correlation. Radiology 1994;192:443–446

60. Ernster VL, Barclay J, Kerlikowske K et al. Incidence of and treatment for ductal carcinoma in situ of the breast. JAMA 1996;275:913–918

61. Page DL, Jensen RA. Ductal carcinoma in situ of the breast: understanding the misunderstood stepchild. JAMA 1996;275:948–949

62. Holland R, Peterse JL, Millis RR et al. Ductal carcinoma in situ: a proposal for a new classification. Semin Diagn Pathol 1994;11:167–180

63. Poller DN, Ellis IO. Ductal carcinoma in situ (DCIS) of the breast. In: Kirkham N, Lemoine NR, Eds. Progress in Pathology (vol. 2). Churchill Livingstone, London, 1995

64. Lagios MD, Margolin FR, Westdahl PR, Rose-MR. Mammographically detected duct carcinoma in situ. Frequency of local recurrence following tylectomy and prognostic effect of nuclear grade on local recurrence. Cancer 1989;63:618–624

65. Silverstein MJ, Poller DN, Waisman JR et al. Prognostic classification of breast ductal carcinoma-in-situ. Lancet 1995;345:1154–1157

66. Holland R, Hendriks JHCL, Vebeek AL et al. Extent, distribution, and mammographic/histological correlations of breast ductal carcinoma in situ. Lancet 1990;335:519–522

67. Rosen PP. Invasive mammary carcinoma. In: Harris JR, Lippman ME, Morrow M, Hellman S, Eds. Diseases of the Breast. Lippincott-Raven, Philadelphia, 1996, pp 393–426

68. Rickard MT. Ultrasound of malignant breast microcalcifications: role in evaluation and guided procedures. Austral Radiol 1996;40:26–31

69. Tohno E, Cosgrove DO, Sloane JP. Ultrasound Diagnosis of Breast Diseases. Churchill Livingstone, Edinburgh, 1994, pp 159–164

70. Voegeli DR. Mammographic signs of malignancy. In: Peters ME, Voegeli DR, Scanlan KA, Eds. Handbook of Breast Imaging. Churchill Livingstone, New York, 1989, pp 183–217

71. Tohno E, Cosgrove DO, Sloane JP. Ultrasound Diagnosis of Breast Diseases. Churchill Livingstone, Edinburgh, 1994, pp 165–166

72. Buchanan JB, Spratt JS, Heuser LS. Tumour growth, doubling times, and the inability of the radiologist to diagnose certain cancers. Radiol Clin North Am 1983;21:115–126

73. Bassett LW, Gold RH, Cove HC. Mammographic spectrum of traumatic fat necrosis: the fallibility of "pathognomonic" signs of carcinoma. AJR Am J Roentgenol 1978;130:119–122

74. Holland R, Veling SHJ, Mravunac M, Hendriks JHCL. Histologic multifocality of Tis, T1-2 breast carcinomas. Implications for clinical trials of breast-conserving surgery. Cancer 1985;56:979–990

75. Holland R, Connolly JL, Gelman R et al. The presence of an extensive intraductal component following a limited excision correlates with prominent residual disease in the remainder of the breast. J Clin Oncol 1990;8:113–118

76. Boyages J, Recht A, Connolly JL et al. Early breast cancer: predictors of breast recurrence for patients treated with conservative surgery and radiation therapy. Radiother Oncol 1990;19:29–41

77. Ascenso AC, Marques MS, Capitao-Mor M. Paget's disease of the nipple. Clinical and pathological review of 109 female patients. Dermatologica 1985;170:170–179

78. Ikeda DM, Helvie MA, Frank TS et al. Paget's disease of the nipple: radiologic–pathologic correlation. Radiology 1993;189:89–94

79. Rosen PP. Inflammatory carcinoma. In: Harris JR, Lippman ME, Morrow M, Hellman S, Eds. Diseases of the Breast. Lippincott-Raven, Philadelphia, 1996, pp 425–426

80. Tabar L, Dean PB. Teaching Atlas of Mammography (2nd rev. ed.). Georg Thieme Verlag, New York, 1985, p 213

81. Kopans DB, Smith BL. Preoperative imaging guided needle localisation and biopsy of nonpalpable breast lesions. In: Harris JR, Lippman ME, Morrow M, Hellman S, Eds. Diseases of the Breast. Lippincott-Raven, Philadelphia, 1996, pp 139–144

82. Holland R. The role of specimen x-ray in the diagnosis of breast cancer. Diagn Imag Clin Med 1985;54:178–185

83. Mendelson EB. Evaluation of the postoperative breast. Radiol Clin North Am 1992;30:107–138

84. Tohno E, Cosgrove DO, Sloane JP. Ultrasound Diagnosis of Breast Diseases. Churchill Livingstone, Edinburgh, 1994, pp 154–155

85. Tohno E, Cosgrove DO, Sloane JP. Ultrasound Diagnosis of Breast Diseases. Churchill Livingstone, Edinburgh, 1994, pp 140–147

47

Magnetic Resonance Imaging of the Breast

SHIH-CHANG WANG

MAGNETIC RESONANCE MAMMOGRAPHY FOR DETECTION OF BREAST CANCER
Development

It was the lure of finding breast and other cancers with in vivo spectroscopy that originally led Damadian to construct a whole body nuclear magnetic resonance (NMR) instrument. Lauterbur took the concept further and went on to invent a new type of imaging. Magnetic resonance imaging (MRI) of the breast was attempted in vivo almost immediately after the first commercial body MRIs became available. Earlier, Mansfield et al.[1] had first described the in vitro imaging of breast carcinoma using a prototype instrument. Thus, with the brain, the breast has the distinction of being one of the first organs to be studied with MRI.

Early breast MRI could only study three characteristics: lesion morphology, signal intensity, and tissue relaxation times. Although large carcinomas typically had a moderately prolonged T1 and T2, it soon became clear that many tumors could not be reliably detected. There was considerable overlap between the relaxation times of benign and malignant tissues,[2] and distinguishing between benign and malignant microcalcifications was unreliable.[3]

It was the introduction of gadolinium-based paramagnetic contrast agents that gave breast MRI (often called MR mammography, or MRM) new impetus. Early studies using T1-weighted spin echo scans had low spatial and temporal resolution. Bright signal from fat and enhancement of normal and benign tissues during the imaging time could obscure small foci of enhancement.[4] Kaiser et al.[5] introduced contrast-enhanced dynamic (i.e., rapid sequential) imaging using gradient recalled echo (GRE) scanning, performing multiple slices in about 1 minute with partial suppression of fat signal. Initially, this technique suggested that almost all invasive carcinomas enhanced strongly and rapidly. An exciting new tool for the investigation of breast disease had arrived.

MRM: Why and When?

Contrast-enhanced MRM has several highly desirable characteristics for problem solving in breast disease (Table 47.1);

generally accepted indications for MRM are listed in Table 47.2. However, despite the advantages, there are several factors that have constrained widespread adoption of MRM (Table 47.3).

Various MRM criteria for malignancy are listed in Table 47.4, and criteria predictive of a benign process are summarized in Table 47.5. The most important (although not the most specific) criterion suggesting a malignant process is strong, rapid contrast enhancement (suggestive enhancement) on early postcontrast sequences. Typical profiles of region of interest (ROI) enhancement against time for various breast tissues are shown in Figure 47.1.

A major limitation of MRM is its relatively low specificity; some benign lesions may enhance like malignancies (Table 47.6), and vice versa. A "washout" enhancement profile, with rapid enhancement to an early peak, followed by a slow fall in enhancement over the first 5 minutes (Fig. 47.1), is highly specific for carcinoma (Table 47.4). Unfortunately, this is uncommon, and typically there is overlap in enhancement profiles between benign and malignant lesions. Nonetheless, two developments that appear to improve the specificity of MRM have been recently reported.

First, a new interpretational model for high-resolution MRM has been devised by Nunes et al.[6] that appears to add greatly to the predictive value of individual image characteristics and the specificity of MRM overall.

Second, T2-weighted first-pass perfusion imaging has been used by Kuhl and co-workers[7] to differentiate benign from malignant enhancing lesions. This involves very rapid single-slice heavily T2-weighted scanning through a suspect lesion during an additional bolus injection of contrast agent. The initial passage of contrast produces a large difference in magnetic susceptibility between the capillary lumen and surrounding interstitium, causing a marked loss of signal in malignant tumors but apparently not in benign lesions (even those with suggestive enhancement). The technique as described has important technical limitations: Spatial resolution is poor, it uses partial k-space sampling,[8] only a single level can be studied, and there are the costs and side-effects of additional contrast agent. At present, the results apply only to large lesions.

Table 47.1 Advantages of MRM

No ionizing radiation
Any imaging plane possible
Superb three-dimensional lesion mapping
>90% sensitivity to invasive carcinoma
Accurate size estimation
Excellent spatial resolution
Good temporal resolution
Can image the entire breast volume

Table 47.2 Indications for MRM

Possible multifocal tumour or extensive intraduct component
Characterize indeterminate lesion after full triple assessment
Detection of recurrent breast cancer
Detection of occult breast carcinoma
Monitoring neoadjuvant chemotherapy

Table 47.3 Disadvantages of MRM

High equipment costs
Limited scanner availability
Requires expensive contrast agents
No agreed standard technique
Very large number of images[a]
Steep and long learning curve
Significant interobserver variability[58]
Relatively low specificity
Unreliable enhancement of in situ carcinoma
5–10% incidence of slowly/poorly enhancing invasive carcinomas[12]

[a] At our institution, a typical 40-minute examination produces over 300 images for a single breast study and over 350 for both breasts (including postprocessing)

Table 47.4 MRM Criteria for Malignancy

Criterion	Statistic[a]	Values[a]
Rapid contrast enhancement		
Peak reached in 60–90 s postinjection	Sensitivity	>90%
Peak >50% above baseline	Sensitivity	>90%
Peak >80% above baseline	Sensitivity	70–80%
"Washout" after peak with falling enhancement over 5 min	Specificity	>90%
Rim enhancement[6]	PPV	79%
Ductal enhancement[6]	PPV	80%
Spiculated borders[6]	PPV	88%
Irregular borders[6]	PPV	81%
Regional enhancement[6]	PPV	58%

Abbreviation: PPV, positive predictive value.

[a] Where the literature quotes a wide range of statistics, these figures are approximate and are synthesized from the literature as well as results from our own institution.

Table 47.5 MRM Criteria for a Benign Process

Criterion	Statistic	Values
Minimal enhancement[59]	Specificity	>95%
Centrifugal enhancement[24]	Specificity	Not assessed independently
Minimal enhancement[6]	NPV	92%
No enhancement[6]	NPV	100%
Smooth borders[6]	NPV	100%
Lobulated borders[6]	NPV	87%
Internal septations[6]	NPV	91%

Abbreviation: Negative predictive value.

Table 47.6 Benign Processes That May Mimic Malignancy on MRM

Fibroadenoma
Intraduct papilloma
Juvenile papillomatosis
Radial scar/complex sclerosing lesion
Sclerosing adenosis
Florid epithelial hyperplasia
Lobular carcinoma in situ
Infection
Fat necrosis
Post-treatment scarring/granulation tissue (see text)
Cyclic focal enhancement[37]

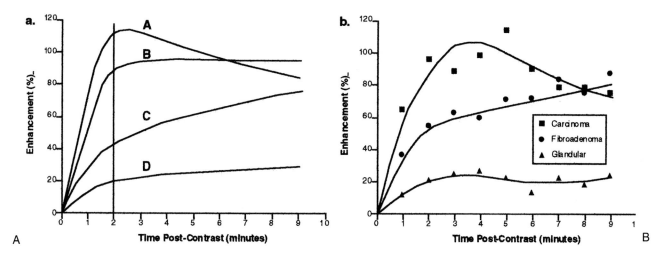

Figure 47.1 Breast time-enhancement curves. (**A**) Four typical curve types are shown. Curves A and B are typical of malignancy, with rapid strong enhancement peaking 2 minutes' postinjection. Curve A shows the "washout" phenomenon where enhancement falls soon after peaking, reflecting a high tumor vascularity. Curve B is seen in most breast malignancies and inflammatory conditions. Curve C, where enhancement gradually increases over several minutes, is typical of benign lesions (Table 47.6). This is uncommonly seen in ductal carcinoma in situ (DCIS) and invasive carcinomas. Curve D, with weak slow enhancement only, is typical of glandular tissue in postmenopausal women and after radiotherapy; it may be seen in occasional cases of DCIS and less than 1% of invasive carcinomas. (**B**) Plots derived from our patient data showing mean enhancement values for each of three tissue types. Curves for invasive carcinomas are similar to curve A, for fibroadenomas to curve C, and for glandular parenchyma to curve D.

Established Indications for MRM

Staging of Intramammary Malignancy

Triple assessment means the use of film-screen mammography, high-resolution ultrasound, and clinical examination. Carcinomas are known to have an extensive intraduct component (EIC) and multifocality quite commonly, with typical rates ranging from 20% to 60%. This variability leads to limitations of triple assessment: Only mammography can detect in situ carcinomas; 5% to 10% of malignancies are mammographically occult even in retrospect; and ultrasound is limited to small "windows" of tissue, limiting its value for preoperative lesion mapping. These factors may cause underestimation of the extent of intramammary malignancy and difficulty in obtaining histologically "clear margins" surgically.

MRM can detect and map the extent of intramammary neoplasm more accurately than either mammography or ultrasound,[9] although it may overestimate disease extent in some cases.[10] It is accepted that MRM is an adjunctive technique and should not be performed without conventional imaging. In our experience, apart from one case (see Fig. 47.1). MRM adds little if mammography shows a well-defined focal lesion surrounded by fat. When adjacent parenchymal density is present, the likelihood of multifocality or EIC is increased, and MRM is then probably warranted. MRM has a potentially important role to play in future when malignancy has already been diagnosed and multifocality or EIC are suspected.

Characterization of Indeterminate Lesions

MRM may have a cost-effective role in the management of lesions that are indeterminate on triple assessment by obviating surgery in some cases. About 10% to 15% of all mammographic lesions assessed at breast screening programs are indeterminate. While often benign, some eventually prove to be malignant, a situation that is not clarified by needle biopsy in up to 25% of cases.[11] These lesions are usually surgically excised, and about half then prove to be benign.

A completely negative MRM in this scenario is highly predictive of a subsequent benign biopsy (Fig. 47.2) and could safely be used to avert surgical biopsy. This use of MRM should be tempered by the observation that, rarely, fibrous invasive lobular carcinomas, highly scirrhous invasive ductal carcinomas, and low-grade carcinomas (papillary or tubular) may show minimal or slow weak enhancement.[12] MRM can also be used to characterize lesions adjacent to breast implants when needle biopsy may be undesirable (Fig. 47.3; see also Fig. 47.28).

Detection of Tumor Recurrence

MRM plays an important role in monitoring patients after local breast cancer treatment by lumpectomy and radiotherapy (Fig. 47.4), since the rate of local recurrence ranges from 3% to 19% even with radiotherapy after breast-conserving surgery.[13] Detection is often limited by scarring and distortion after treatment. MRM has been shown to be highly sensitive

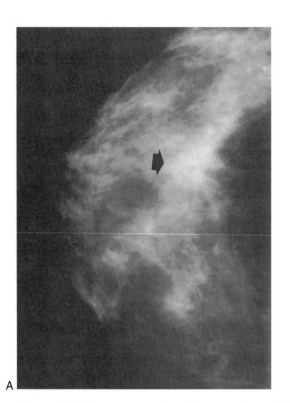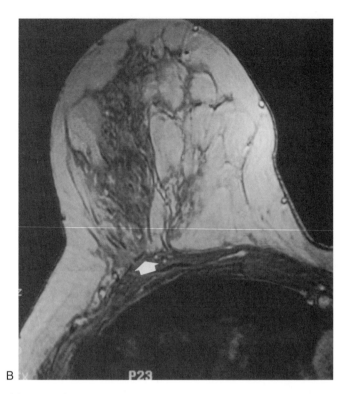

Figure 47.2 True-negative MRM. Fibrosis and normal glandular parenchyma in an asymptomatic 51-year-old. (**A**) Craniocaudal (CC) mammograms show architectural distortion and poorly defined increased density in the right breast laterally (arrow), unaltered on coned compression views. (**B**) Postcontrast axial three-dimensional GRE scan through the right breast showing nonenhancing distortion only near the chest wall (white arrow).

Figure 47.3 Silicone implant with adjacent mass. A small mass at the upper aspect of the right implant was palpable in this 38-year-old. MRM was requested, as needle biopsy might puncture the implant. The implant appeared normal on other scans. Pathology revealed florid epithelial hyperplasia, papillomatosis, and 8-mm central focus of DCIS only. This is an example of dysplastic enhancement surrounding and obscuring a small focus of malignancy. (**A**) Ultrasound of the mass shows a poorly defined solid lesion (arrows) with minor parenchymal distortion.(**B**) Sagittal high-resolution fat-suppressed (HR/FS) three-dimensional fast spoiled gradient echo sequence (FSPGR), postcontrast scan shows a strongly but inhomogeneously enhancing irregular 25-mm mass (long arrow), highly suggestive of malignancy. A focal "hot spot" at the inferior margin of the breast (short arrow) is a susceptibility artifact where the breast is closely applied to the edge of the breast coil.

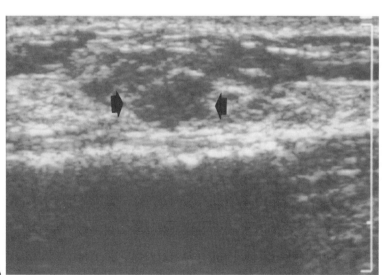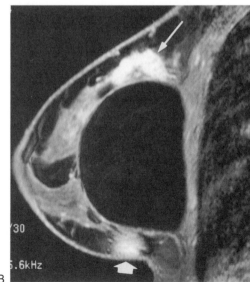

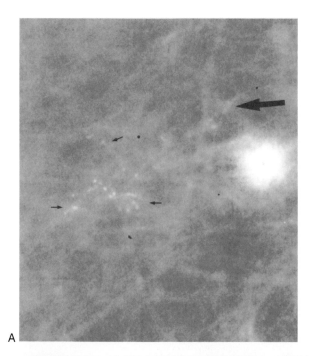

A

Figure 47.4 Recurrent DCIS in a 51-year-old 2 years after surgical excision of DCIS. Pathology showed comedo- and cribriform DCIS. (**A**) Magnification mammography shows pleomorphic and rounded calcifications (small arrows), and some "soft" lobular calcifications toward the nipple (long arrow) in the left breast inferiorly. (**B**) Four dynamic (two-dimensional GRE) images at the same level before (1), during (2), at 2 minutes (3) and at 3 minutes (4) postinjection through the suspect area. A focal nodule (short arrow) and an adjacent linear streak (long arrow) of strong enhancement are demonstrated 2 minutes after injection. This enhancement appears larger than the calcifications seen on mammography (about 50 mm).

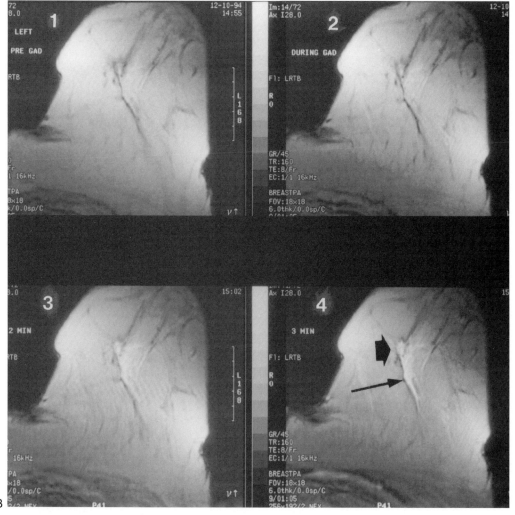

B

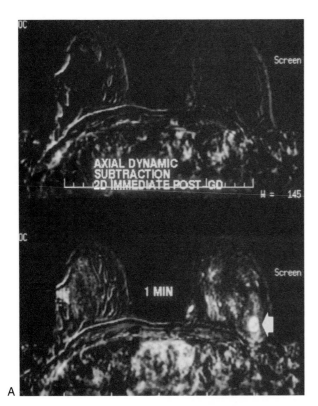

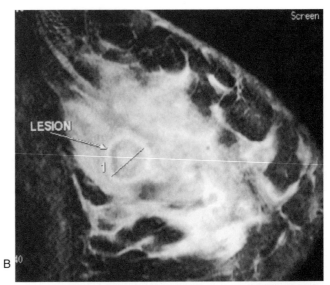

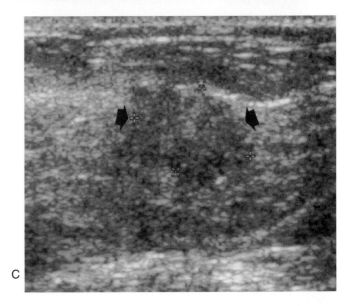

Figure 47.5 Occult invasive ductal carcinoma in a 46-year-old with palpable axillary lymphadenopathy that yielded adenocarcinoma cells on fine-needle aspiration biopsy (FNAB). Clinical examination, mammography, and ultrasound were normal. (**A**) Axial subtracted dynamic scans at the same level immediately and 1 minute after Gd-DTPA injection. A solitary rounded mass with intense, early, and inhomogeneous enhancement is seen on the left laterally (arrow). (**B**) Sagittal delayed HR/FS three-dimensional FSPGR image of the left breast. The lesion is surrounded by enhancing normal glandular tissue. There is a "target" appearance with inhomogeneous internal and rim enhancement (Table 47.4). (**C**) MRI-guided ultrasound was performed with close scrutiny of the left axillary tail. A poorly defined low echogenicity mass with adjacent distortion was identified (arrows) and biopsied under ultrasound guidance.

and specific for recurrent tumor 6 months after surgery alone[14] and 18 months after surgery and radiotherapy, even in the presence of breast implants.[15] While Mussurakis et al.[16] assert that dynamic scanning is essential for this purpose, the indicator with the best sensitivity and specificity for local recurrence analysis is peak lesion enhancement.

Detection of Occult Breast Carcinoma

Patients may present with axillary or distant metastases that are possibly from breast carcinoma. It is common for a primary breast carcinoma to be missed by conventional assessment in

this setting.[17] In most of these cases, MRM does find a primary breast lesion (75% of cases in a recent series[18]), permitting ultrasonic or MRI-guided biopsy and localization (Fig. 47.5).

Monitor Neoadjuvant Chemotherapy

MRM may also be used to monitor tumor response to neoadjuvant chemotherapy[19] in locally advanced malignancy. Assessment of response typically involves clinical palpation of the tumor, a procedure that has been shown to be highly inaccurate.[20] MRM can depict tumor response (or lack of it) by demonstrating tumor shrinkage and any residual abnormal enhancement before surgical excision.

Poor Indications for MRM

There are a few situations for which MRM is known to be either clinically unhelpful or potentially misleading. These include the following:

1. *Screening for carcinoma.* Limited high-speed dynamic scanning only could reduce the high cost of MRM. However, despite its high sensitivity to malignancy, this is impractical because of two factors: (a) the high incidence of focal suggestive enhancement seen in normal premenopausal[21] and to a lesser extent in postmenopausal women and (b) the inability of dynamic MRM to detect 30% to 40% of ductal carcinoma in situ (DCIS) and about 5% of invasive malignancies.[12]

2. *Characterization of clustered microcalcifications.* These are frequently indeterminate on mammography; while MRM may correctly diagnose DCIS in many cases, it may also either be falsely negative or produce false-positive enhancement if the calcifications arise in intraduct papilloma, ductal hyperplasia, or sclerosing adenosis.[12] At present, this is better dealt with by stereotactic biopsy or excision.

3. *Characterization of stellate lesions without a clearly defined central mass.* These are commonly due to radial scars; occasionally, they are due to invasive carcinomas or fat necrosis.[12] In any of these conditions, MRM may show suggestive enhancement with irregular borders. At this time, these lesions should be excised as a matter of course.

Technique and Instrumentation

Magnet and Coils

While MRM can be performed at field strengths below 1.0 Tesla (IT), there are three major reasons for not doing so today. First, low field magnets lack the gradient subsystems required for high-speed, high-resolution volumetric (three-dimensional) scans. Second, narrow separation of fat and water peaks at low field precludes effective fat suppression. Third, sensitivity to gadolinium enhancement is reduced at lower field strengths due to the inherently shorter, T1 of tissues.[22] However, this effect can be compensated for at 0.5 T by the use of three-dimensional GRE instead of multislice (two-dimensional) GRE sequences.[23]

A dedicated double breast coil, preferably of phased array design, is essential, as it permits high-resolution imaging of one breast or both breasts simultaneously. Such coils should have excellent homogeneity, or image shading and "hot spots" will be visible and fat suppression will be unpredictable and patchy.

Scan Sequences

With the introduction of dynamic MRM, it seemed that faster sequences were critical to diagnostic success. It was believed that the first postcontrast series should be finished within 60 to 90 seconds of injection, as "virtually all carcinomas" appeared to reach peak enhancement by this time.[5] Time-enhancement ROI analysis of these images was thought to provide very high levels of sensitivity and specificity for invasive malignancy.[5] However, many have found such high specificities difficult to replicate.

Further attempts have been made to image even more quickly, using techniques including single-slice turbo fast low-angle shot sequence (FLASH),[24] partial *k*-space sampling, or "keyhole" imaging;[8] half-Fourier imaging;[25] echo planar imaging;[26] and even functional parametric images that color-code pixels for slope, speed, and strength of enhancement.[27] These complex methods are no more sensitive or specific than previous methods, require special hardware and software, cannot survey the entire breast, may have inferior contrast sensitivity, and have uniformly poor spatial resolution. To detect suggestive contrast enhancement, imaging times shorter than 1 minute are generally unnecessary; 10% to 15% of carcinomas enhance quite slowly, reaching peak enhancement at 3 minutes or even longer.[12] Thus, the emphasis today is less on speed and more on spatial resolution. Some temporal information is still felt to be important by many workers, and a semidynamic dynamic protocol with repeated 90 to 120 second acquisitions is recommended by some,[12] while others use only nondynamic fat-suppressed high-resolution three-dimensional sequences with a temporal resolution of about 5 to 7 minutes.[28,29] Slice thickness should be as thin as practically possible (2 to 3 mm) to minimize the contrast-reducing effects of partial volume averaging, and the entire breast cone and its chest wall attachment should always be imaged, preferably without interslice gaps. Numerous protocols for MRM have been described. Some typical dynamic and semidynamic protocols are listed in Table 47.7. Successful MRM can be performed with any of these. We use a combination of high-speed and high-resolution imaging, performing serial dynamic three-dimensional acquisitions followed by high-resolution sagittal and axial fat-suppressed three-dimensional scans Table 47.8).

The acquisition plane and its impact on technique are important. Phase-direction motion artifacts from breathing and the heart are minimized by ensuring that the frequency-encoding direction is in the anteroposterior direction for axial and sagittal imaging. In the coronal plane, switching the phase direction cranio caudally allows the use of a rectangular field of view with reduced phase encoding, reducing acquisition time. However, intramammary mapping of lesions can be difficult in the coronal plane, and respiratory motion may produce unpredictable variations in signal across the images, making subtractions useless. For these reasons, we prefer the more robust axial and sagittal planes. These are also easier to correlate with mammographic projections.

Contrast Enhancement and Signal From Fat

Gadolinium-diethylenetriaminepentaacetic acid (Gd-DTPA) (Magnevist, Schering) is only one of a group of paramagnetic

Table 47.7 Some Dynamic and Semidynamic Sequences With Proven Efficacy

Author	Sequence	TR	TE	FA	Slices	FOV/Matrix	Time
Heywang-Köbrunner and Beck[12]	Three-dimensional turbo-FLASH, 1.5 T	9 ms	3.6 ms	25 degrees	64/2.5 mm	32 cm/112 × 256	63 s
Kaiser[60]	Two-dimensional FLASH, 1.5 T	100 ms	5.0 ms	80 degrees	9/4–8 mm	32 cm/not stated	60 s
Kerslake et al.[61]	Two-dimensional FSPGR, 1.5 T	11 ms	4.2 ms	?	1–4/5–7 mm	not stated/128 × 256	3–12 s
Heiberg et al.[62]	Three-dimensional FSPGR, 1.5 T	10.6 ms	2.2 ms	20 degrees	32/3–4 mm	20 cm/128 × 256	44 s

Both FLASH and FSPGR are spoiled T1-weighted GRE sequences.

Abbreviations: FLASH, Siemens' fast low-angle shot sequence; FA, GRE flip angle; FSPGR, General Electric's fast spoiled gradient echo sequence. FOV, field of view.

contrast agents with virtually identical pharmacokinetics and contrast-enhancement characteristics. Other agents that can be used equally well for MRM include Gd-DOTA (Dotarem, Guébet), Gd-DO3A (ProHance, Squibb) and Gd-DTPA-BMA (Omniscan, Nycomed). They all shorten T1 and increase tissue relaxation rates, thus increasing signal on T1-weighted or GRE imaging.

Contrast administration may be by infusion or bolus, but better peak enhancement is achieved by bolus injections.[30] These are delivered either by hand injection or MRI-compatible power injector. For two-dimensional GRE sequences a dose of 0.16 mmol/kg gives better sensitivity for lesion detection than the standard dose of 0.1 mmol Gd/kg at field strengths below 1.0 Tesla.[31] However, there is good evidence that if three-dimensional gradient echo sequences are used, the dose can be lowered to 0.1 mmol Gd/kg without loss of sensitivity.[6]

There has been some controversy over the optimal method of measuring contrast enhancement. Early papers advocated signal intensity normalized to fat, but this was too sequence- and instrument-specific to be used widely. Today, most quote percent enhancement above baseline, where all values are corrected to fat, using the formula:

$$\text{Enhancement (\%)} = \left[\frac{(SI_1/SI_{f1})}{(SI_0/SI_{f0})} - 1 \right] \times 100$$

where SI_1 is postcontrast signal, SI_0 is precontrast signal, SI_{f1} is postcontrast fat signal, and SI_{f0} is precontrast fat signal.

Threshold enhancement values from 50% to 90% above baseline have been reported as being specific for malignancy by various workers. In fact, such values will vary with field strength, pulse sequence, sequence timing, and contrast dose. It is now accepted that there is no fixed threshold below which one can invariably exclude invasive malignancy, though it is rare to have no enhancement in carcinomas.

Many lesions have inhomogeneous enhancement; if time-enhancement curves or enhancement thresholds for malignancy are to be used, the target lesion must be searched carefully to find the area of maximal enhancement. A large ROI size will average pixel intensities and may give falsely low enhancement values.

Detecting contrast enhancement requires high sensitivity to the T1-shortening effects of Gd-based contrast agents. This in turn leads to bright fat signal, which can then obscure small foci of enhancement. Four major approaches have been used to reduce or remove fat signal, in order to show enhancement more clearly:

1. Gradient echo scanning using carefully chosen TR, TE, and flip angles and a high dose of Gd-DTPA (0.16 to 0.2 mmol Gd/kg). However, high contrast cost and a tendency to "swamp" normal tissues with the contrast agent are undesirable.

Table 47.8 Protocol Using Dynamic and High-Resolution Fat-Suppressed MRM

Sequence	Plane	Suppression	TR	TE	FA	Slices	FOV/Matrix/NPW	Time
Three-dimensional FSPGR	Axial	Subtraction	32 ms	4 ms	30 degrees	28/3–4 mm	30 cm/160 × 256/On	0:55 s
Three-dimensional FSPGR	Sagittal	Spectral fat	26 ms	3 ms	30 degrees	28/3–4 mm	18 cm/192 × 512/Off	2:39 s
Three-dimensional FSPGR	Axial	Spectral fat	31 ms	3 ms	30 degrees	28/3–4 mm	18 cm/192 × 256/Off	6:23 s

This is our current protocol and is performed at 1.5 T on a GE Signa MRI unit.

All TEs are fractional echoes.

Abbreviation: NPW, no phase wrap option.

2. Pre- and post-contrast digital image subtraction. It is the only reliable method of fat suppression at low field strength and is the best means of canceling signal inhomogeneity across the breast. However, it is time-consuming and susceptible to motion artifacts. Worse, misregistration may actually cause a lesion to become less visible, so if subtraction is used, the source images must be carefully reviewed.

3. Spectral fat saturation using frequency-selective pulses. Below 1 T, the spectral separation of fat and water resonances is too narrow to use this technique reliably. Successful application requires careful shimming, good coil design, and frequently, manual prescan tuning. Even so, homogeneous fat suppression may not be possible with very large breasts.

4. Magnetization transfer suppression. This method reduces tissue signal by using detuned saturation pulses prior to the imaging sequence, shortening water relaxation by coupling it to macromolecular motion. The best known application of this method is rotating delivery of excitation off-resonance (RODEO),[32] which achieves excellent fat suppression and high contrast sensitivity. However, it is not widely available.

Patient Positioning and Scanning

The patient is positioned prone on the breast coil, which has a well for each breast. The breasts may be suspended free, constrained by a T-shirt or padded to minimize movement. An intravenous cannula is then inserted and connected to tubing for injection and saline flushing. If the patient is anxious or claustrophobic, sedation can be achieved with either oral benzodiazepines (20 to 30 mg temazepam) or parenteral midazolam (5 mg intramuscularly or 2 to 3 mg intravenously).

Our protocol (Table 47.8) is as follows. After one to two precontrast sequences, dynamic scans are performed. We perform one repetition precontrast and then inject the Gd as a rapid bolus (2 ml/s) followed immediately by a saline flush of 15 to 20 ml. The immediate postcontrast series starts with the injection. The remaining dynamic scans are then acquired for 4 minutes, followed by high-resolution scans as appropriate. A typical study takes 35 to 40 minutes at our institution.

Postprocessing

Another advantage of MRM is that images can be digitally postprocessed on graphics workstations, permitting analyses such as ROI signal measurement, digital subtraction MRM (see Figs. 47.5, 47.7, 47.10, 47.13, 47.20, 47.22, 47.23, and 47.25), multiplanar reformatting (see Fig. 47.17), and three-dimensional maximum intensity projection (MIP) models, which can be rotated and viewed from arbitrary angles (see Figs. 47.17 and 47.20). Complex, multiple, or large lesions can be more effectively visualized than by slice-by-slice viewing.

MRI-Guided Biopsy

The nature of unexpected foci of suspicious enhancement detected by MRM can be determined by various methods, including the following:

High-resolution MRI-guided ultrasound to search for a specific "lesion," once its approximate location is known. We and others have found malignancies previously missed by routine ultrasound in this way. Ultrasound-guided needle biopsy and/or localization for excision are then routine. However, even with care, ultrasound can miss small tumors.

In premenopausal patients, repeat MRM in mid-cycle reduces the incidence of false-positive foci and can show whether a "lesion" changes from one cycle to the next. This is characteristic of hormonally influenced benign tissue (see below).

Various techniques for MR-guided fine-needle biopsy or localization have been developed.[33,34] In each case, imaging coils are used with a perforated grid plate. After contrast, the suggestive lesion is punctured with an MRI-compatible (nonferromagnetic) needle, using repeated scanning for localization. Aspiration biopsy can then be performed. While time-consuming, this can confirm malignancy when all other tests have been negative. Unfortunately the dedicated coils required are not widely available.

Enhancement on MRM

Contrast enhancement of breast tissues is due to a combination of tumor angiogenesis and increased capillary permeability.[35] With MRM, microvascular contrast leakage is mapped in three dimensions, exploiting the fact that almost all invasive malignancies (and a majority of DCIS) produce a vascular endothelial growth factor that stimulates angiogenesis.[36] The relationship of enhancement to microvascular density, biologic aggression, and hence prognosis is the subject of active research.

Until recently, MRM aimed only to detect and measure suggestive enhancement, on the premise that time-enhancement profiles could distinguish benign from malignant tissues. This premise has been debunked; while strong rapid enhancement is typical of malignancy, benign processes may produce similar enhancement (see Table 47.6). Though extremely strong enhancement of greater than 150% to 200% is virtually diagnostic of malignancy, this is not common even in large carcinomas. There is no lower threshold that invariably distinguishes benign from malignant lesions. A small minority of invasive and many in situ malignancies may enhance slowly and/or weakly. Strong but slow diffuse enhancement may occur in patients with proliferative breast disease in patients with dense breasts under the age of forty, and in patients who are lactating.[12]

Attention has shifted to analysis of lesion appearances on

high-resolution fat-suppressed images. Although there is evidence that using architectural characteristics and enhancement criteria can markedly improve the specificity and accuracy of MRM,[6] systematic use of these criteria is not widespread. (see Tables 47.3 and 47.4).

Benign Conditions

Normal Glandular Parenchyma

On T1- and T2-weighted imaging, normal parenchyma appears as bland, dark gray tissue surrounded by bright fat, defining the glandular cone. The enhancement of normal parenchyma may have a number of patterns (Table 47.9), depending on the patient's age, stage of the menstrual cycle, and prior medical treatment. Normal parenchyma enhances more strongly in the 35- to 50-year age range, and least in the second and third weeks of the menstrual cycle[21] with nonspecific focal areas of enhancement on one examination fluctuating in size or resolving from month to month.[37] In practice, most women show minor or no enhancement on dynamic MRM, with variable amounts of parenchymal enhancement on delayed images. However, nonspecific regional enhancement may occur early and may be difficult to differentiate from malignancy[6] (Fig. 47.6).

Table 47.9 Patterns of Normal Parenchymal Enhancement

No enhancement

Minimal or mild enhancement

Diffuse slow enhancement

Slow or rapid regional enhancement

Slow or rapid patchy enhancement

Small focal areas of slow or rapid enhancement

Normal Nipple and Areola

The normal nipple frequently enhances intensely. Retroareolar ducts may enhance normally, though not as intensely. Mammary duct ectasia may be visible on pre-contrast T1-weighted scans as hyperintense dilated retroareolar ducts due to high protein inspissated secretions. Such ducts are readily overlooked. However, they mimic prominent enhancing ducts and are potentially misleading (Fig. 47.7). Unlike DCIS, they are always sharply defined on high resolution.

In contrast, the areola does not normally enhance and ap-

Figure 47.6 False-negative MRM. Diffuse contrast enhancement with DCIS was detected by screening in this 42-year-old asymptomatic woman. Pathology revealed extensive DCIS (>11 cm diameter) requiring mastectomy to achieve adequate resection. (**A**) Right mediolateral oblique (MLO) mammogram shows prominent clustered high-density microcalcifications inferiorly (arrows). (**B**) Sagittal delayed HR/FS right breast image. Strong but delayed enhancement involved most of the breast parenchyma, more intense inferiorly. This pattern was also seen in the contralateral breast and is indistinguishable from normal. Dynamic scans were of poor quality due to breathing artifact and were thus unhelpful.

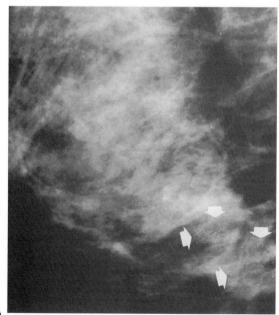
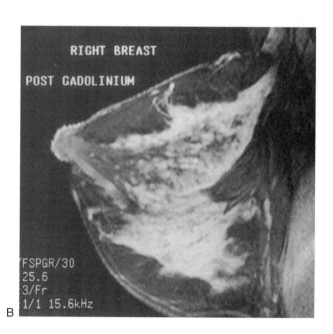

A   B

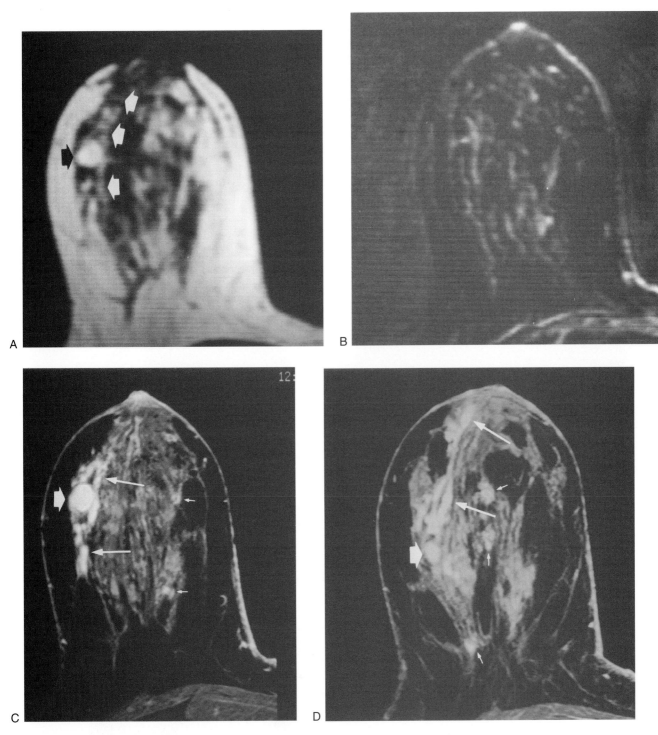

Figure 47.7 Mammary duct ectasia and hyperintense cysts. Mammography showed distortion and asymmetric density. (**A**) Axial two-dimensional FSPGR dynamic noncontrast scan of the right breast. Note the high signal cyst (black arrow) and several bright linear structures around it radiating toward the nipple (white arrows). These are high-signal ducts. (**B**) Subtraction image at the same level 4 minutes postcontrast shows no significant enhancement. (**C & D**) Axial HR/FS three-dimensional FSPGR delayed scans of the right breast. (Figure C) is at the same level as Figures A and B. The sharply circumscribed high-signal cysts are obvious (short arrows), and branching dilated hyperintense ducts are seen laterally (long arrows). A few foci of delayed weak benign glandular enhancement are seen (small arrows)

pears only slightly thicker than adjacent skin, permitting detection of areolar infiltration by malignancy.

Fibrocystic Disease

Perimenopausally, fibrocystic change is very common and is best detected with T2-weighted fast spin echo. Multiple, high-signal, sharply circumscribed cysts of variable size are the hallmark of this condition. They do not enhance and may appear as "holes" within enhancing parenchyma (Fig. 47.8). Sometimes they are hyperintense on T1-weighted scans, due to proteinaceous contents (Fig. 47.7).

Fibroadenoma

Fibroadenomas may enhance strongly when myxoid but are usually hyalinized and enhance more slowly and weakly than carcinomas. They almost always have sharply defined smooth or lobulated borders. Larger fibroadenomas may appear mod-

erately bright on T2-weighted precontrast imaging. Nonenhancing internal septa are due to fibrous bands between adjacent lobules are highly specific for a benign lesion and suggest a fibroadenoma.[6] Occasionally, they have minimal or no enhancement (Fig. 47.9; see also Fig. 47.16).

Proliferative Dysplasia

Proliferative dysplasias usually appear as foci or regions of slow moderate enhancement. However, a few patients with atypical ductal hyperplasia have associated angiogenesis, producing enhancement indistinguishable from carcinoma[12] (Fig. 47.10; see also Fig. 47.22).

Sclerosing Adenosis

Sclerosing adenosis typically enhances like normal glandular parenchyma. It may occasionally appear as an irregular area of strong focal enhancement. While this enhancement is usually

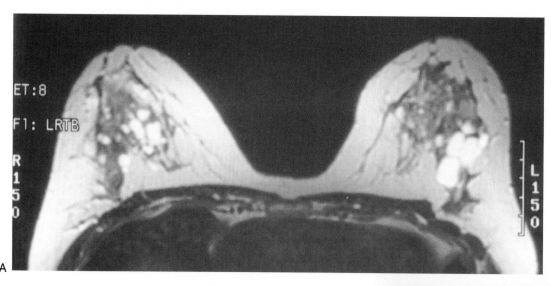

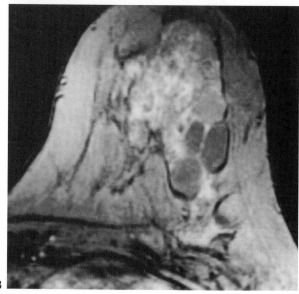

Figure 47.8 True-negative MRM. Fibrocystic disease in a 54-year-old with indeterminate microcalcifications at screening mammography. (**A**) Axial T2-weighted fast spin echo (FSE) scans showing multiple cysts appearing as bilateral sharply circumscribed hyperintense ovoid lesions. (**B**) Axial two-dimensional GRE scan through the left breast 3 minutes' postcontrast, showing diffuse low-level early glandular enhancement surrounding three nonenhancing cysts. No suspicious enhancing lesion was found.

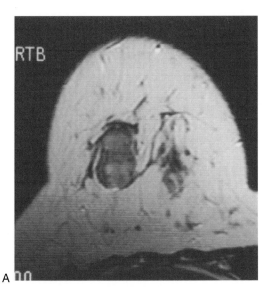

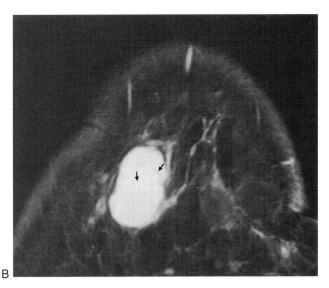

Figure 47.9 Large fibroadenoma in a 50-year-old with a palpable mass in the lower right breast. The mass appeared ovoid with smooth borders on mammography and heterogeneous on ultrasound. (**A**) Axial two-dimensional FSE scan through the right breast showing a sharply defined low signal mass with patchy mildly increased internal signal. (**B**) Axial three-dimensional FSPGR HR/FS scan. The lesion is homogeneously and brightly enhancing with very sharply circumscribed borders and nonenhancing internal septa (small arrows). These are characteristic of nonmalignant lesions (see text).

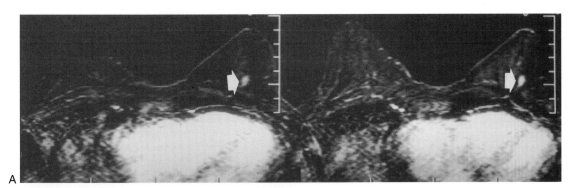

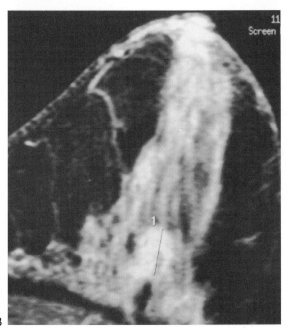

Figure 47.10 False-positive MRM. Florid epithelial hyperplasia with no malignancy in a 55-year-old with an 8-mm cluster of grouped microcalcifications in the lower left breast on mammography. (**A**) Axial dynamic three-dimensional FSPGR subtraction images through both breasts at 1 minute (left) and 2 minute (right) postcontrast showing a small focus of early intense enhancement (arrows). (**B**) Delayed axial HR/FS three-dimensional FSPGR scan through the same lesion (measured) showing persistent intense enhancement with fairly poorly defined borders, surrounded by delayed moderately intense benign enhancement. This lesion is indistinguishable from malignancy.

slow, it can appear suggestive, particularly if dynamic imaging has not been performed.

Radial Scar/Complex Sclerosing Lesion

Radial scar/Complex sclerosing lesions are stellate, irregular lesions on triple assessment that remain diagnostically difficult; MRM is unable to differentiate them reliably from carcinoma. Precontrast, they appear as an area of architectural distortion with a low signal central focus and long low signal spicules. They often have proliferative dysplasia centrally with resultant angiogenesis, and they may enhance exactly like carcinomas, with a strongly enhancing nodular center and spiculated irregular borders,[29] necessitating surgical removal in most cases. Occasionally, they appear as a stellate structure without a central nodule (Fig. 47.11); while this appearance might distinguish radial scar from malignancy, excision is still recommended.

Papilloma

Intraduct papillomas appear indistinguishable from fibroadenomas in many cases. They are typically low-signal nodules precontrast and may enhance strongly, moderately, or not at all. They usually have well-defined borders and can then be accurately classified as benign. Rim enhancement may be seen, which can confuse the diagnosis (Fig. 47.12).

Juvenile Papillomatosis

Juvenile papillomatosis is an uncommon condition seen in young women, producing an appearance of multiple nodules with marked distortion on mammography. On MRM, this may appear as a network of enhancing bead-like nodules connected together by enhancing ducts (Fig. 47.13) or as a lobulated enhancing mass with internal small cysts.[38]

Phyllodes Tumor

Phyllodes tumors are rare and are usually diagnosed with mammography and ultrasound. MRM adds little diagnostically. These lesions typically appear as large, well-circumscribed masses with rapid strong enhancement, often with internal lobulation and cystic spaces.[12]

Other Tumors

Lipomas and fibroadenolipomas (hamartomas) are readily diagnosed by other modalities and so are only imaged with MRM incidentally. The characteristic feature is fat within the lesion.

Infection

Infection may be acute or chronic, and MRM adds little to conventional assessment. Acute mastitis is a clinical diagnosis occasionally confused with inflammatory carcinoma. Chronic mastitis may be focal or diffuse. In both conditions, strong rapid enhancement may be present, usually with a poorly defined regional or diffuse pattern and cannot usually be distinguished from malignancy.

Malignant Lesions

Lobular Carcinoma In Situ

Lobular carcinoma in situ (LCIS) is generally a chance finding at surgical biopsy. It is usually indistinguishable from benign tissue on MRM. It may occasionally appear as a focus of suggestive enhancement indistinguishable from malignancy (see Fig. 47.22).

Ductal Carcinoma In Situ

DCIS has a variety of enhancement patterns on MRM, including minimal or no enhancement. Any combination of these patterns may be present, and commonly one or more is seen in association with invasive carcinoma. The patterns include the following:

1. *Ductal pattern.* This is a tree-like linear branching or reticular pattern, often with nodular foci within nodes of branches (Figs. 47.14 and 47.15). It is usually associated with comedocarcinoma or other high nuclear grade DCIS[30] and is due to periductal angiogenesis. The enhancement may extend to the nipple. Suggesting nipple involvement before the clinical signs of Paget's disease. The nodules may represent either foci of clumped DCIS, focal microinvasion, or small invasive carcinomas.

2. *Focal nodular pattern.* Many foci of DCIS appear mass-like and may be indistinguishable from invasive carcinomas (Fig. 47.14). The nodules are usually multiple and may be connected by enhancing ducts. This is a well-recognized but atypical pattern of DCIS and is frequently noncalcified. MRM may be the only modality that clearly displays these areas as malignant.

3. *Regional pattern.* Occasionally, a branching ductal pattern may be seen on dynamic scans, spreading into a broad region of strong enhancement on delayed images (Fig. 47.15). DCIS may also appear simply as a poorly defined region of strong enhancement, often surrounding an invasive malignancy. It may obscure the boundaries of a small invasive tumor, making it appear to be a single large lesion (Fig. 47.15).

4. *Benign pattern.* A minority (15% to 40%) of DCIS shows minimal to moderate enhancement indistinguishable from normal glandular tissues (see Fig. 47.6). This tends to occur in lower grades of DCIS[39] but has been seen in comedocarcinoma.[40]

The variability in DCIS enhancement is probably due to variable angiogenesis, which in turn is largely related to the histologic grade.[39] Linear and focal patterns of enhancement occur more often in comedocarcinoma, while noncomedo DCIS is more likely to have a diffuse enhancement pattern.[40]

Diffuse enhancement causes difficulties in measuring

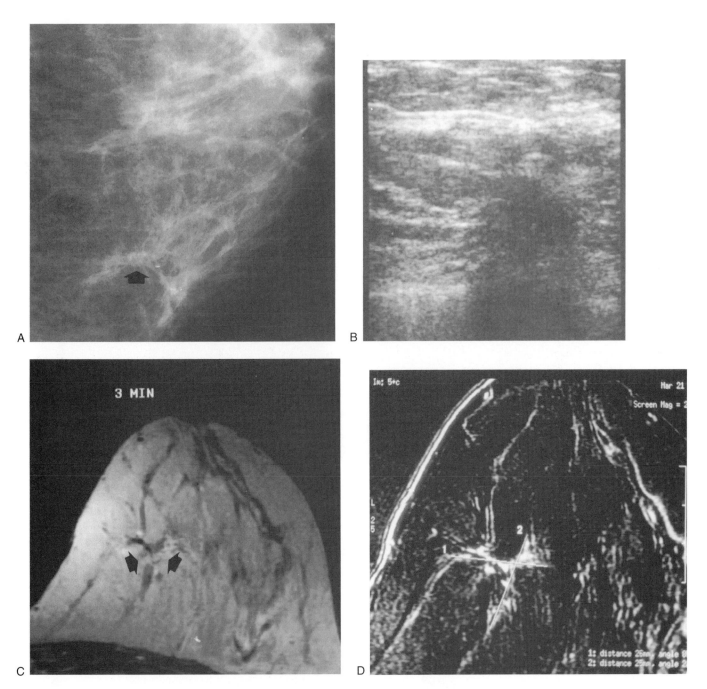

Figure 47.11 Radial scar/complex sclerosing lesion in a 49-year-old, found at screening. This was the only case of radial scar in our series without a central nodular focus. (**A**) Left breast mammogram, craniocaudal CC projection. Poorly defined stellate area of architectural distortion medially with a small possible central nodule (arrow). (**B**) Ultrasound shows a markedly hypoechoic lesion with architectural distortion and shadowing. FNAB showed benign atypia. (**C**) Axial two-dimensional GRE dynamic scan through left breast 3 minutes postcontrast showing triradiate early enhancement without a central nodule (arrows). (**D**) Axial three-dimensional FSPGR high-resolution subtracted image through the lesion showing an enhancing triradiate lesion with no central mass.

Figure 47.12 False-positive MRM. Intraduct papilloma in a 47-year-old who had left upper breast distortion and a cluster of indeterminate calcifications from previous benign surgery. A small poorly defined nodule was identified in the inferior left breast at 8 o'clock on mammography. (**A**) Ultrasound of lower breast showing an indeterminate rounded sharply circumscribed nodule with low-level internal echoes and posterior enhancement. Fine-needle biopsy showed epithelial proliferation. (**B**) High-resolution three-dimensional GRE axial scans through the lower left breast before (left) and 1 minute after (right) Gd-DTPA. The lesion appears as a rounded nodule with a slightly lobulated contour that shows early, moderate, and inhomogeneous enhancement. There is a rim enhancement pattern suspicious of malignancy and adjacent poorly defined parenchymal enhancement (arrow).

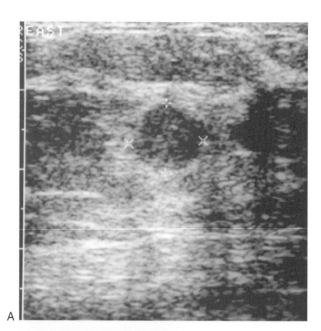

A

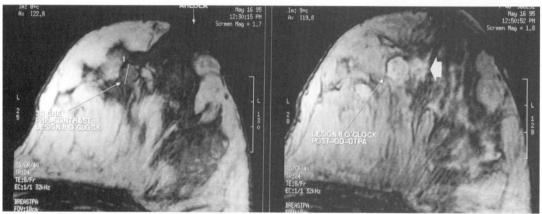

B

Figure 47.13 (Figure continues on opposite page.)

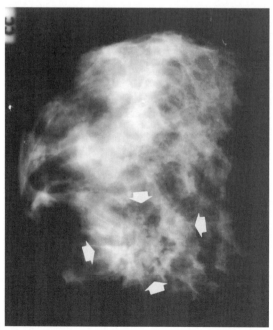

A

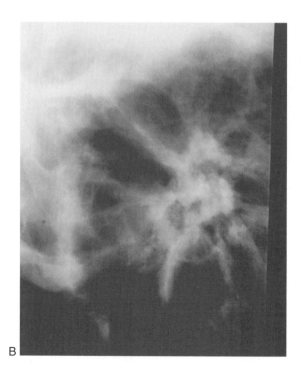

B

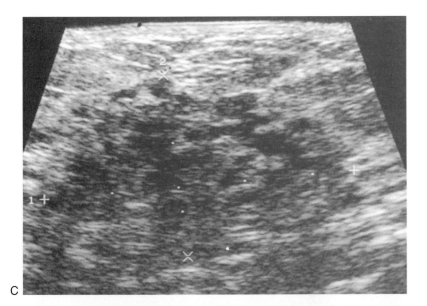

C

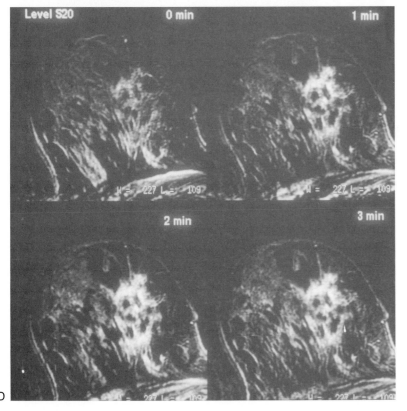

D

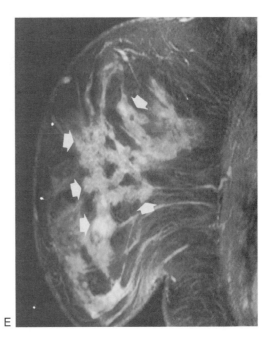

E

Figure 47.13 (*Continued*) Juvenile papillomatosis in a 27-years-old with palpable thickening in the medial right breast. Pathologic size of the lesion correlated well with the MRM measurement of 60 mm, with no evidence of malignancy. (**A**) Right mammogram (CC) shows a large area of architectural distortion in the upper right breast medially (arrows). (**B**) Compression CC view of the right breast lesion showing a bizarre lesion with internal nodular densities, fat, and extensive surrounding architectural distortion. (**C**) Ultrasound showing a large (4.6 cm × 2.7 cm) poorly defined hypoechoic area with heterogeneous shadowing. (**D**) Dynamic subtraction axial MRM using a high-resolution three-dimensional GRE technique. Four images at the same level at 0, 1, 2, and 3 minutes postinjection show a large area of early intense enhancement with a bizarre pattern of multiple confluent nodular areas and central areas of nonenhancing fat. (**E**) Sagittal delayed HR/FS image showing that the lesion comprises multiple well-defined nodular lesions, iso enhancing with glandular tissue (arrows). These are interspersed with fat and connected to each other by ductal "bridges."

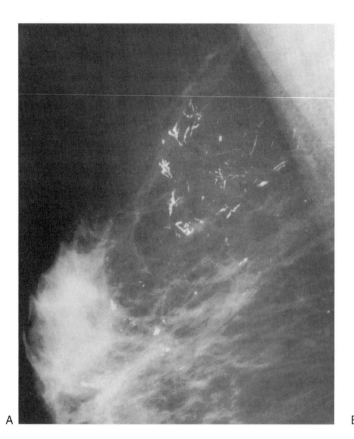
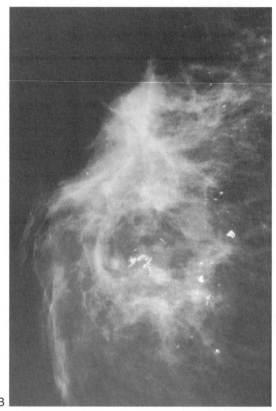

A

B

Figure 47.14 Comedocarcinoma with nipple involvement in a 67-year-old. Clinical examination revealed possible Paget's disease of the nipple and no other abnormality. Mammography and ultrasound markedly underestimated the extent of the disease in this case. MRI pathology correlation at mastectomy was excellent and showed extensive comedocarcinoma in all four quadrants, Paget's disease of the nipple, and multiple focal nodules of microinvasive carcinoma. (**A**) Right MLO mammogram showing casting malignant calcifications in the upper and central breast radiating toward the nipple. No masses are seen. (**B**) CC mammogram showing that the casting calcifications are lateral and central in distribution. No medial disease or focal masses are seen. (**C**) Axial dynamic two-dimensional GRE MRM series at one level through the nipple precontrast (1), and at 0,1, and 2 minutes postcontrast (2,3 and 4, respectively). There is intense early enhancement in a branching ductal pattern radiating to and involving the nipple and areola (short white arrows). There is medial breast involvement, which was not appreciated mammographically (small black arrows). (**D**) Axial dynamic two-dimensional GRE MRM series at one level above the nipple (timing as for Figure C). Two nodular areas of strong early enhancement are connected to a smaller posterior focus by a nonenhancing ductal "bridge" (arrows). These correspond to poorly defined density seen above the nipple on the MLO mammogram Though suggestive of invasive carcinoma, these were subsequently shown to be mass-like pure DCIS (*Figure continues.*)

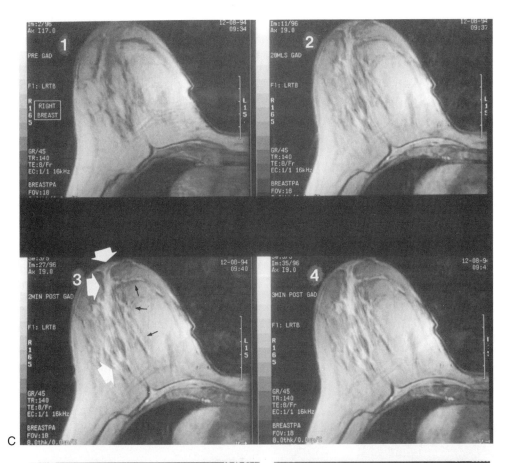

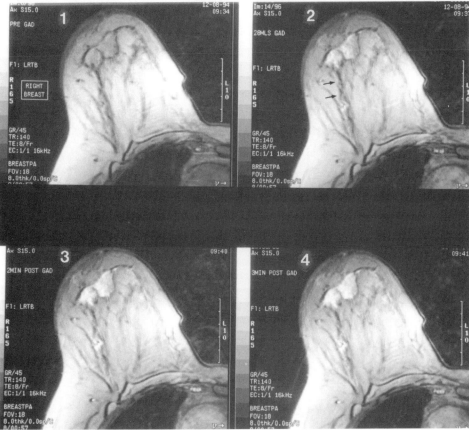

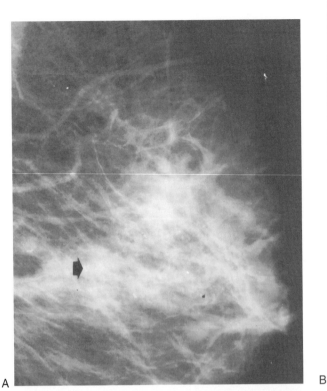

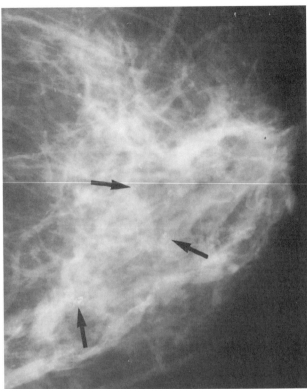

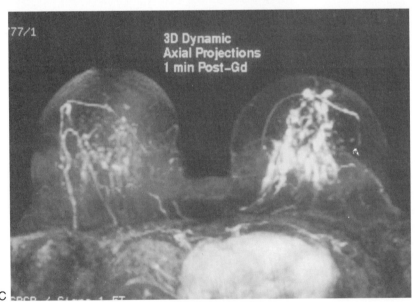

Figure 47.15 Extensive noncalcified DCIS and focal invasive ductal carcinomas (IDC) in an asymptomatic patient detected by screening. Mammography markedly understimated the extent of the disease in this case. Pathology confirmed extensive comedo and cribriform DCIS with involvement of retroareolar ducts, but not the nipple. There was also a 6 mm mass of IDC. (**A**) Left MLO projection. Poorly defined aysmmetric increased density is seen in the central and upper glandular cone A few clustered microcalcifications are noted posteriorly (arrow). (**B**) Left CC projection. Multiple clustered microcalcifications are seen centrally and posteromedially (arrows) on a background of diffuse moderately increased glandular density. (**C**) Axial MIP slab image reconstructed from dynamic three-dimensional subtraction MRM images 1 minute after contrast, depicting the entire thickness of both breast cones. An extensive intensely enhancing ductal pattern with diffuse intense enhancement is seen in the central left breast, corresponding to the mammographic area of increased density. Normal vascular and weak benign parenchymal enhancement are seen on the right.

lesions. Mass-like enhancement may contain only invasive tumor, only an area of pure DCIS, a small focus of invasive tumor surrounded by a "cloud" of DCIS, and occasionally a small invasive tumor surrounded by reactive glandular enhancement. While analysis of dynamic scans can help to clarify which is which, this must be tempered by the fact that some DCIS enhances strongly but slowly. About 40% of DCIS is not calcified, even when of high nuclear grade.[41] MRM may thus depict the extent of DCIS better than magnification mammography.[30] In some cases, this will alter management, leading directly to mastectomy instead of conservative surgery. The ultimate role of MRM in the management of DCIS requires further investigation.

Invasive Carcinoma

DUCTAL

Most invasive ductal carcinomas (IDCs) appear on MRM as an irregular nodular mass with strong rapid contrast enhancement at least 60% above baseline. Typically cancers have spiculated or lobulated borders, rim or inhomogeneous enhancement (Figs. 47.5, 47.16, and 47.17), and surrounding architectural distortion (Figs 47.16 and 47.17). Some appear as mutilobulated masses (Fig. 47.17). The exception is mucinous or colloid carcinoma, which may be well defined with a lobulated border and homogeneous enhancement, superficially resembling a large fibroadenoma. However, enhancing internal septa may be visible; if present, malignancy can be correctly

diagnosed.[6] A small proportion of these tumors enhance slowly and/or less strongly.

As described above, carcinomas can be associated with surrounding enhancement of variable intensity, representing either surrounding DCIS (Figs. 47.18 and 47.19), adjacent florid dysplasia (see Fig. 47.3), or benign parenchymal enhancement (see Fig. 47.5). In larger or multiple lesions, MRM may show nipple or chest wall involvement, which may not be otherwise evident (Figs. 47.14, and 47.16). Extensive neoplasia on MRM may be due to extensive intraduct carcinoma (Fig. 47.15), multifocality (Fig. 47.20), or both (Fig. 47.19).

LOBULAR

Invasive lobular carcinoma (ILC) comprises about 10% to 15% of breast carcinomas and can be mammographically occult or subtle in 20% to 40% of cases.[42,43] Up to 85% are isodense to glandular parenchyma, and a minority have malignant microcalcifications.[11] The incidence of multifocal, multicentric, and bilateral synchronous or metachronous involvement is higher with ILC than IDC, being found in up to 28% of cases. Mammography and ultrasound tend to markedly underestimate the extent of ILC. MRM has been shown to be much more accurate correctly demonstrating the extent of disease in about 85% of cases.[9]

In most cases, ILC shows strong rapid enhancement typical of malignancy. Single or multiple irregular masses in one or more quadrants are sometimes demonstrated (Figs. 47.21 and 47.22). and extensive diffuse enhancement may be seen.

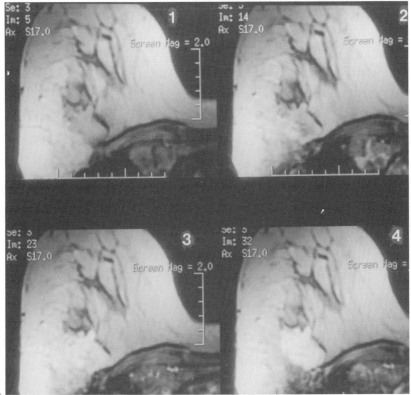

A

Figure 47.16 Ductal carcinoma with invasion of the pectoralis fascia and muscle correctly diagnosed preoperatively by MRM. This asymptomatic 57-year-old presented for screening. A large irregular spiculated mass was evident on mammography and ultrasound (not shown). It appeared clear of the chest wall on the MLO projection and was also not evident on ultrasound or clinical examination (**A**) Set of four images from a dynamic two-dimensional GRE axial series through the right breast (1) precontrast, (2) immediate, (3) 1-minute, and (4) 2-minute time points postcontrast. A large irregular mass with increased signal precontrast shows strong early rim enhancement and then enhances centrifugally. It is applied to the pectoralis fascia.(*Figure continues*)

Figure 47.16 (*Continued*). (**B**) Oblique multiplanar reformation image from HR/FS three-dimensional FSPGR sagittal data set. The initial scans did not show the full length of the mass in any single image. A large, 5-cm spiculated mass with intense inhomogeneous enhancement is seen. There is apparent invasion of the pectoralis fascia and possibly the muscle (arrows). (**C**) Four images from a three-dimensional MIP model of the 2-minute axial dynamic three-dimensional FSPGR subtraction data set showing varying degrees of rotation from the routine inferior projection used for axial scanning (0 degrees) to the anterior projection used for coronal imaging (90 degrees) as follows (1) 0 degrees, (2) 20 degrees, (3) 70 degrees, and (4) 90 degrees. A small sharply defined mass is noted on the right away from the main tumor, consistent with a fibroadenoma. No lesion is seen on the left.

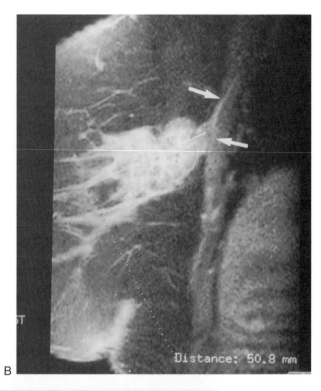

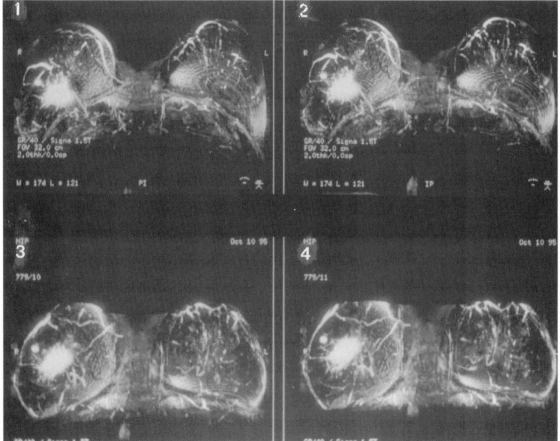

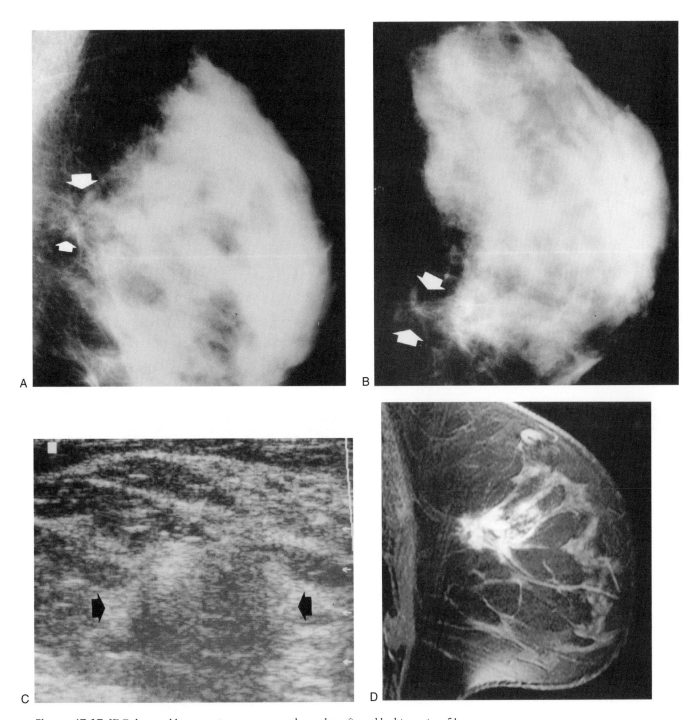

Figure 47.17 IDC detected by screening mammography and confirmed by biopsy in a 51-year-old. Clinically, no lesion was palpable, and FNAB was negative. (**A**) Left mammogram MLO projection. (**B**) CC projection shows a 15- to 20-mm area of architectural distortion in the posteromedial breast (arrows). No mass or microcalcifications is seen. (**C**) Ultrasound of medial left breast lesion shows a vague area of hypoechoic change with hyperechoic margins and poorly defined shadowing (arrows). (**D**) Left breast sagittal HR/FS three-dimensional FSPGR postcontrast image showing a multi-lobulated mass with marked enhancement, internal heterogeneity, spiculated borders, and adjacent architectural distortion, typical of malignancy.

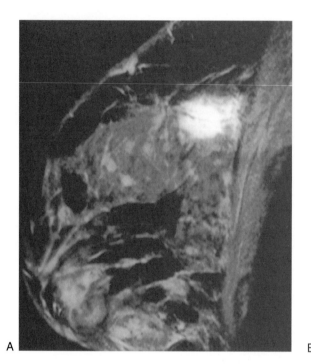

A

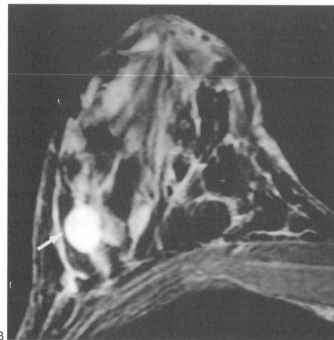

B

Figure 47.18 Fibroadenomas and focal IDC surrounded by DCIS. This 44-year-old had three known fibroadenomas and presented with new palpable thickening in the upper right breast. The palpable lesion was not visible on mammography; ultrasound showed a poorly defined hypoechoic mass. The upper lesion was excised, and histology showed a 20-mm area of DCIS with a central 10-mm focus of IDC. The DCIS could not be differentiated from IDC by MRM, which also slightly underestimated the size of the whole lesion. (**A**) Sagittal delayed HR/FS MRM of right breast showing focal nodular intense enhancement with irregular borders measuring 15 mm at the upper margin of the glandular cone. This lesion showed early intense enhancement on dynamic MRM. Several small foci of weak delayed benign enhancement are seen elsewhere in the breast. (**B & C**) Axial delayed HR/FS images through two of the known fibroadenomas. Both appear as sharply circumscribed enhancing masses (arrows). The lesion in Figure B shows homogeneous enhancement, while that in Figure C has a central area of lower enhancement.

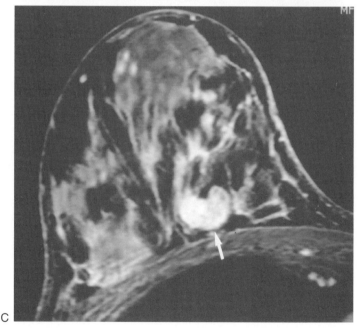

C

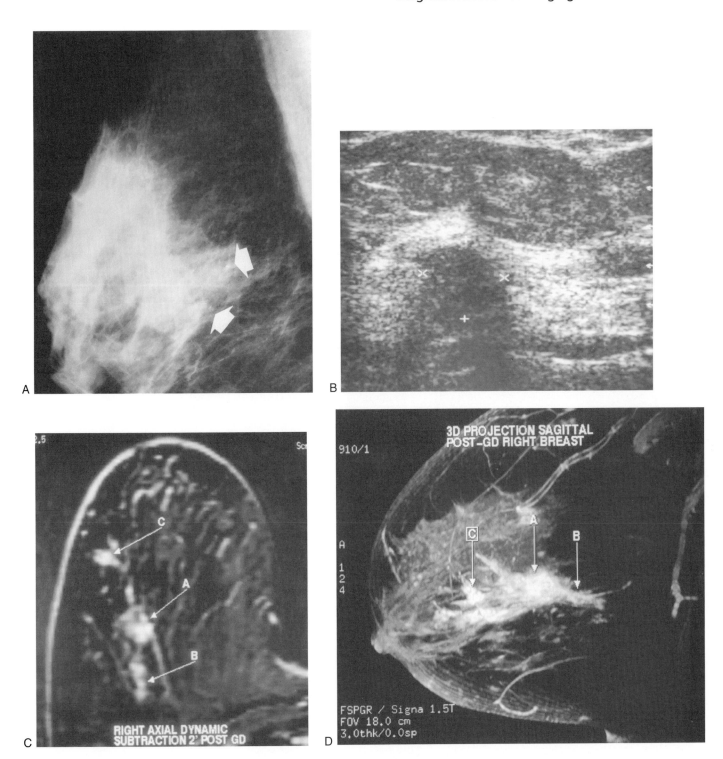

Figure 47.19 Multifocal carcinoma with surrounding EIC in a 51-year-old woman presenting for breast screening. Mammography and ultrasound failed to characterize fully the extent of disease preoperatively. Clinical examination normal. (**A**) Right MLO mammogram showing small foci of indeterminate clustered microcalcification posteriorly (arrows) with adjacent asymmetric increased density. (**B**) Ultrasound right breast laterally showing a suspicious 10-mm mass. FNAB yielded malignant cells. (**C**) Axial subtraction dynamic three-dimensional FSPGR image of the right breast at 2 minutes postcontrast shows three strongly enhancing nodular foci as marked. (**D**) Right breast sagittal MIP reconstruction from the delayed HR/FS data set showing an extensive area of malignant involvement. The lesions have been marked using computerized cross-referencing. There is marked confluent delayed enhancement between the lesions due to surrounding DCIS, while the uninvolved parenchyma shows no significant enhancement.

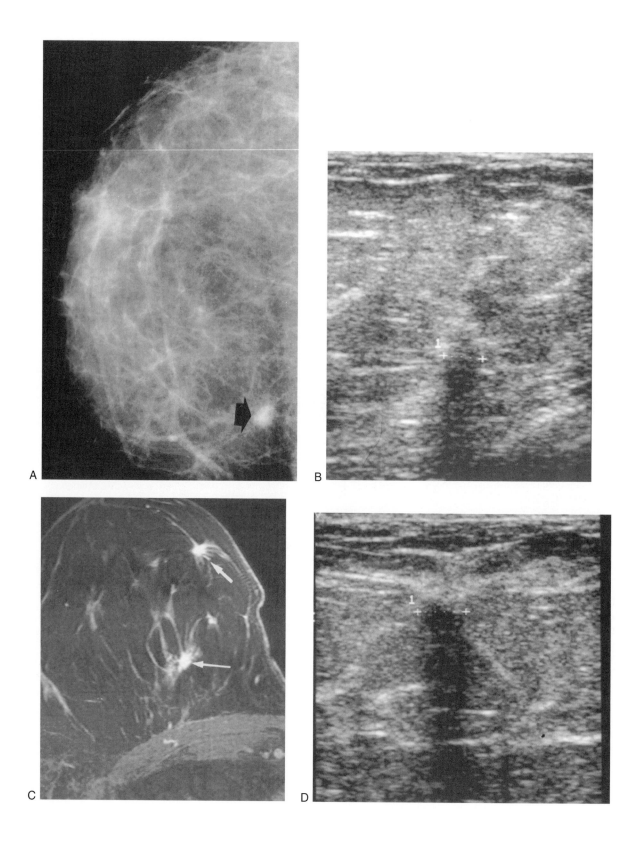

A

B

C

D

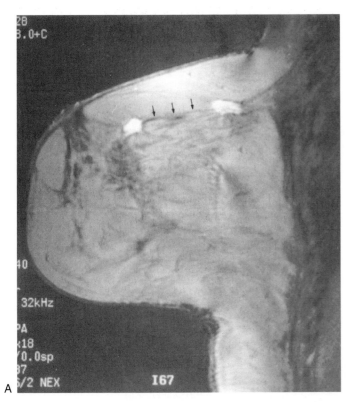

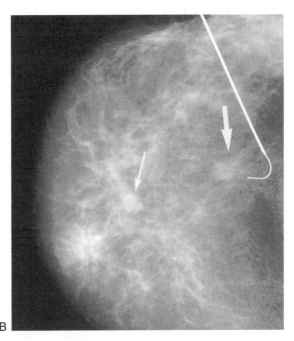

Figure 47.21 Multifocal recurrent ILC and scarring in a 70-year-old woman with a history of ILC 10 years earlier and a new mammographic density. (**A**) Sagittal scan of right breast after contrast showing deformity of the nipple due to previous surgery. There are two intensely enhancing irregular nodules, appear to be connected by a low signal duct (short arrows). The posterior lesion is the index lesion; the anterior lesion was not initially seen on mammography. (**B**) Right CC mammogram following hook wire localization of the more posterior lesion (thick arrow). The second lesion is now evident anteriorly (thin arrow).

Figure 47.20 Multifocal IDCs detected by MRM in a 60-year-old presenting for screening. A second 6-mm lesion seen on MRM was not visible on mammography on review (despite fatty breasts), and was only detected on ultrasound after MRM. (**A**) Right CC mammogram showing a small well-circumscribed high-density mass with spiculated borders posteromedially (arrow) consistent with malignancy. (**B**) Ultrasound showing index lesion found at mammography. The lesion is small with dense posterior shadowing. (**C**) Axial HR/FS three-dimensional FSPGR postcontrast image of the right breast shows the index lesion as a small irregular focus of strong enhancement posteriorly and medially (long arrow). In the same slice, there is a second lesion anteriorly (short arrow) with identical enhancement, irregular margins, and architectural distortion. On other slices, it was apparent that these lesions were in the one duct system (enhancing ducts connected the two). (**D**) Subsequent ultrasound of the anterior right breast shows a hypoechoic second lesion, with architectural distortion and dense posterior shadowing. Ultrasound-guided FNAB confirmed malignant cells.

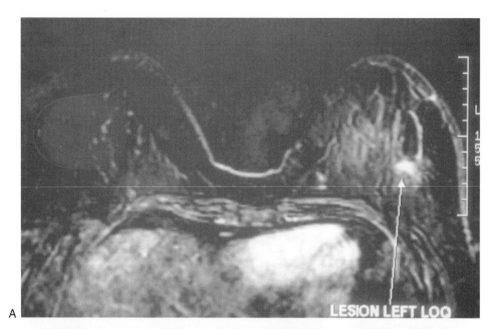

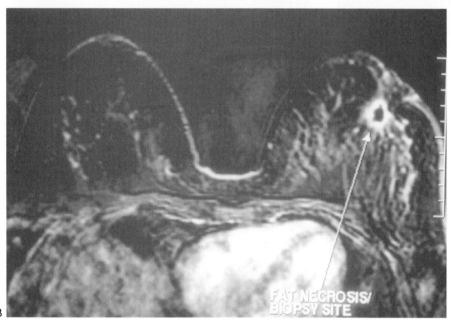

Figure 47.22 Multifocal ILC and early postoperative enhancement in a 42-year-old with palpable thickening in the left breast. Mammography showed minor asymmetric density. Ultrasound showed two suggestive mass lesions, at 12 o'clock, and 3 o'clock. Biopsy at 12 o'clock showed dysplasia and LCIS only. At 3 o'clock, a large mass of ILC with surrounding LCIS was removed without clear margins. MRM was performed 6 weeks after surgery to assess for residual disease and to exclude synchronous malignancy on the right. Serial section radiographs of the mastectomy specimen were correlated with MRM. (**A**) Axial subtraction 1 minute postcontrast dynamic three-dimensional FSPGR scan, below the nipple. A small enhancing focus is seen at the posterior margin of the 3 o'clock biopsy site. This contained florid atypical ductal hyperplasia (ADH) atypical lobular hyperplasia (ALH) and LCIS. (**B**) Axial subtraction 1 minute postcontrast dynamic three-dimensional FSPGR scan, level with the nipple. The 12 o'clock biopsy site is seen as a strongly enhancing ring-shaped lesion with spiculated margins, typical of fat necrosis and early scarring in the wall of a biopsy cavity. (*Figure continues.*)

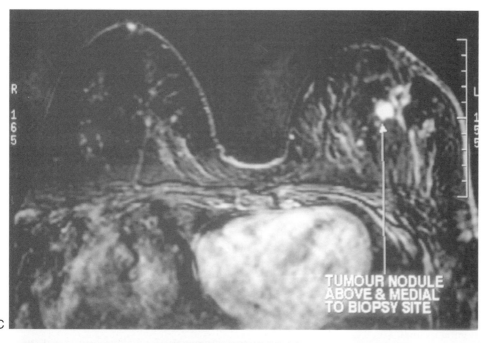

C

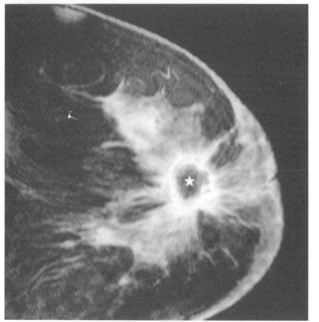

D

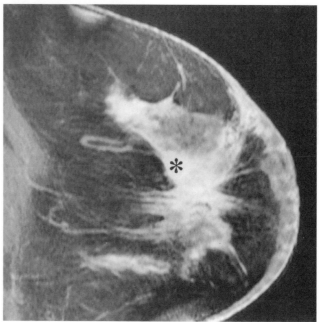

E

Figure 47.22 (*Continued*). (**C**) Axial subtraction dynamic three-dimensional FSPGR scan 1 minute postcontrast. A nodular mass is seen to enhance intensely immediately above and deep to the biopsy scar. This was a 13-mm invasive lobular carcinoma with adjacent LCIS and ALH; this lesion had been shown by ultrasound but was missed at the initial surgical biopsy. No other focal lesions were seen in either breast. (**D**) Sagittal delayed HR/FS three-dimensional FSPGR scan of the left breast level with the nipple. There is strong enhancement in the wall of the biopsy scar, with persistent nonenhancement of the central cavity (*). The wall of the cavity showed LCIS and ALH only. This appearance is typical of a resolving hematoma or seroma with associated fat necrosis. In contrast, the biopsy site at 3 o'-clock showed almost no surrounding mural enhancement. (**E**) Sagittal delayed HR/FS three-dimensional FSPGR scan medial to the biopsy scar. The nodular mass above and medial to the cavity is seen as a poorly defined ovoid area of enhancement (*) partially obscured by delayed glandular enhancement. There is also a poorly defined focal area of strong delayed enhancement at the upper margin of the breast cone; pathology showed LCIS and ALH.

In a small proportion of cases, ILC may have weak enhancement only;[12] close mammographic and ultrasonic correlation is important if this occasional finding is not to be misdiagnosed. Despite this limitation, MRM will usually provide more accurate preoperative breast staging than is possible with triple assessment.

OTHERS

Other less aggressive types of IDC, notably papillary and tubular carcinomas, generally do enhance suspiciously. Some of these tumors have low angiogenesis, reflecting their lower biologic aggression, and may then enhance relatively slowly and/or weakly.[12] Careful correlation with mammography and ultrasound will help to minimize errors with such lesions.

Other Breast Malignancies

Involvement of the nipple and areola by in situ or invasive carcinoma is reliably seen on MRM as localized areolar thickening with skin enhancement, universally in the presence of a subareolar mass or abnormal ductal enhancement (see Fig. 47.14). This appearance may not have frank histologic features of Paget's disease and may be demonstrated before involvement of the nipple is clinically detectable. This diagnosis is important as malignant involvement of the nipple–areola complex obviates conservative surgery.

Sarcomas are rare neoplasms and appear as an otherwise nonspecific focal mass with suspicious enhancement. Intramammary metastases are generally diagnosed clinically in conjunction with ultrasound and mammography, and MRM is of little value in assessing these lesions; they appear as sharply defined enhancing masses.

Non-Hodgkin's lymphoma of the breast is rare and usually secondary to extensive involvement elsewhere in the body. It appears as focal well-defined nodular mass(es) with suggestive enhancement.[12] Primary lymphoma of the breast is rare and may be synchronously or metachronously bilateral, in some cases growing rapidly to become very large (Fig. 47.23).

Lymph Node Assessment

MRM may detect enhancing malignant lymph nodes.[9,29] These may be normal in size or enlarged (>1 cm). As MRM routinely includes nodal regions of the chest wall, internal mammary chain and part of the axilla, it is attractive to consider routinely searching for metastatic lymphadenopathy. However, as reactive lymph nodes can enhance strongly, it seems unlikely that MRM could reliably differentiate these from involved nodes unless they were increased in size.

Breast Changes After Intervention

Postbiopsy

In general, tissues do not significantly alter their enhancement following needle biopsy (even with multiple 14-gauge core samples). Foci of hemorrhage or hypointense ferromag-
netic metal artifact may occasionally be seen at the biopsy site, particularly on GRE images. If seen, this confirms that the imaged lesion corresponds to the biopsy site, which is useful if MRM detects more extensive involvement than was previously suspected.

Postoperative Scarring

Postoperative scarring may be severe, producing marked architectural distortion, increased density on mammography (Fig. 47.24), and even an apparent mass. This causes significant clinical problems if recurrent malignancy is suspected, particularly as the appearance of the scar may evolve over 6 to 12 months.

Scar tissue generally appears as a low signal band or stellate irregularity, which enhances variably, depending largely on the interval since treatment. In the first few months after surgery, the borders of the surgical cavity may have very strong enhancement, particularly if hemorrhage or fat necrosis has occurred. A small focus of recent fat necrosis may appear similar to a focus of residual tumor.[12]

This reactive enhancement gradually subsides, and after 6 months following surgery without radiotherapy, most patients show minimal or no enhancement.[14] Occasionally strong, delayed enhancement may persist in fat necrosis (Fig. 47.25).

In the first 9 to 12 months after radiotherapy, there is an edematous reaction that causes a diffuse increase in capillary permeability. Initially, there is marked parenchymal enhancement, gradually becoming patchy and declining after about 18 months in the majority of women, reflecting the development of fibrosis.[15] This eventual response of bland enhancement of normal tissues is very helpful for detecting recurrent enhancing tumor, which may appear nodular (Fig. 47.21) or linear (see Fig. 47.4).[45]

The shape and architecture of reactive enhancement can differentiate it from malignancy. Some patients may benefit from MRM soon after surgery if there is strong suspicion of residual disease. Diffuse enhancement is of little diagnostic value; demonstration of one or more focal nodular lesions with enhancement typical for malignancy should prompt surgical re-excision or MRM-guided needle biopsy.

Chemotherapeutic Response

MRM has been used successfully following neoadjuvant chemotherapy to assess preoperative tumor response in advanced local malignancy, usually with excellent correlation between MRM and pathologic assessment of residual tumor.[19] Chemotherapy does not produce the initial edema response seen with radiotherapy, and parenchymal enhancement becomes bland soon after its administration, again helping the differentiation of normal from malignant tissues.

Conclusions

MRM is an exciting and rapidly evolving method of imaging breast pathology. It has numerous technical advantages over

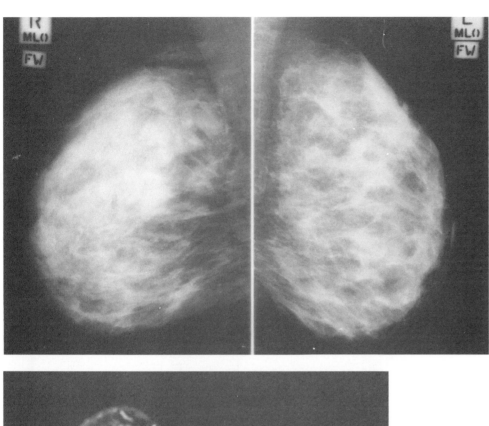

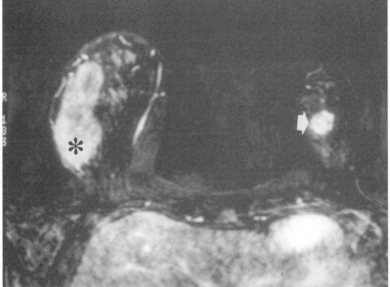

Figure 47.23 Primary lymphoma of the breast in a 42-year-old after left breast surgery and radiotherapy for "IDC" 2 years earlier. Shortly after commencing tamoxifen therapy the contralateral breast began rapidly increasing in size, beginning with a vague palpable thickening. MRM was performed 2 months later after further breast enlargement and repeat mammography and ultrasound, when "mastitis" had been diagnosed. (**A**) Bilateral MLO mammograms 2 months prior to the MRM showing asymmetric glandular density in the right breast but no focal lesion, despite a palpable thickening on the right. Ultrasound at this time was reported as normal. (**B**) Axial subtraction dynamic three-dimensional FSPGR scans 2 minutes after contrast through the inferior aspect of both breasts. On the left there is a rounded well-defined nodule (short arrow) with suggestive enhancement. On the right, there is a large mass (*) which enhances strongly but inhomogeneously. Multiple ultrasound-guided core needle biopsies of the right mass and the small left nodule yielded high-grade B-cell lymphoma. (*Figure continues.*)

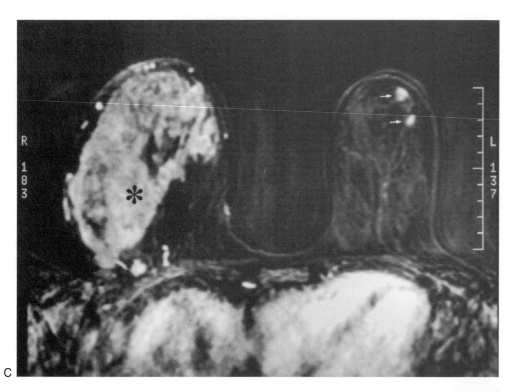

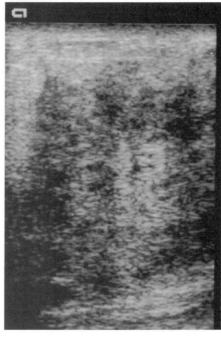

Figure 47.23 (*Continued*). (**C**) Axial subtraction dynamic three-dimensional FSPGR scans above the nipples 2 minutes after contrast. The huge heterogeneously enhancing mass on the right (*) almost occupies the whole breast. Two small suggestive nodular lesions are seen in the upper left breast (short arrows). These were not seen on subsequent ultrasound. (**D**) Ultrasound of the right breast laterally after MRM shows extensive thickening of the breast by heterogeneous predominantly hypoechoic tissue with poorly defined borders and posterior shadowing.

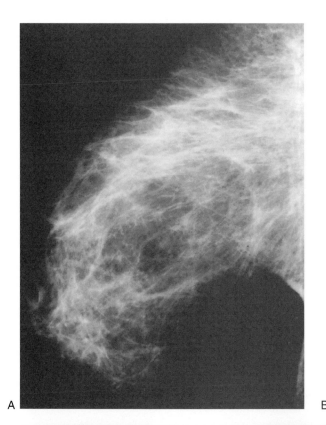

A

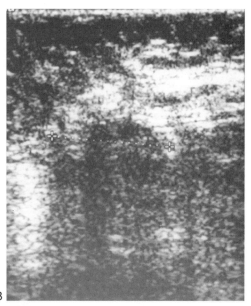

B

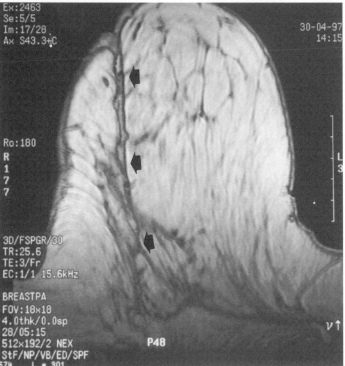

C

Figure 47.24 Simple postsurgical scarring in a 60-year-old after resection of IDC from the right breast superiorly 2 years earlier and subsequent radiotherapy. (**A**) Right MLO mammogram showing a band of increased density superiorly extending to the chest wall. This had developed recently, raising suspicion of recurrent malignancy. (**B**) Ultrasound showing right breast a poorly defined hypoechoic band with shadowing posteriorly. (**C**) Axial high-resolution three-dimensional FSPGR postgadolinium scan through the right upper breast showing a linear low-signal band of scarring extending right back to the chest wall (arrows). No abnormal enhancement was seen within the breast at any level.

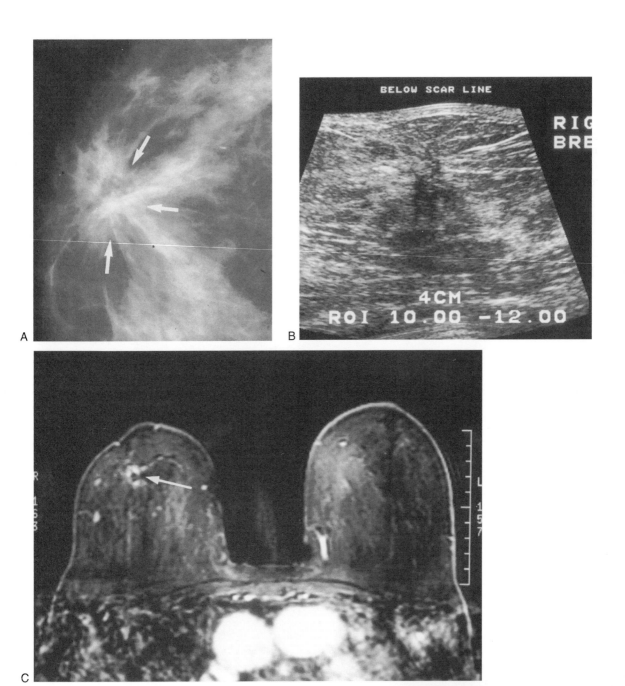

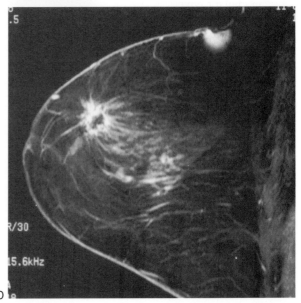

Figure 47.25 Fat necrosis and scarring in a 54-year-old with IDC
treated by excision and radiotherapy 2 years earlier. (**A**) Right CC
mammogram showing marked distortion and increased density in the
central upper breast (arrows), which had altered over 6 months. (**B**)
Ultrasound of the right breast showing hypoechoic distortion and
shadowing. (**C**) Axial subtraction dynamic three-dimensional FSPGR
2 minutes postcontrast. A ring-shaped moderately enhancing lesion is
seen in the right breast with associated distortion (arrow). (**D**) Sagittal
HR/FS three dimensional FSPGR delayed scan of the right breast
showing the cavity with spiculated rim enhancement at the biopsy
site. Biopsy confirmed benign tissue only. This is similar to the biopsy
cavity in Figure 47.22.

conventional assessment, although at present, it remains a costly test that still has problems with diagnostic specificity. It is the most sensitive method today of detecting invasive breast malignancy and uniquely permits depiction of the full extent of intramammary neoplasia. While it is gradually gaining acceptance, it is a technique that demands vigilance, scrupulous technique, and careful correlation with conventional imaging by the radiologist in order to minimize errors in interpretation.

MRI OF BREAST IMPLANTS
Background

Characteristics and Metabolism of Silicone

Silicons are forms of polydimethylsiloxane (PDMS— $[(CH_3)_2Si—O]n—$) that may be free (silicone oil), moderately cross-linked (gel), or heavily cross-linked (silicone elastomer). Only free PDMS is able to migrate freely across membranes and enter body fluids. The "gel" in most implants is actually a mixture of silicone gel (Å60—20%) and free silicone oil (Å40—80%), depending on the style and model of implant. Silicone oil is known to "bleed" freely across the semipermeable membrane of an implant's elastomer shell, while the actual gel polymer does not do so under normal circumstances.

There are long and short T1 and T2 components in various silicones. In implants, typically T1 and T2 are long because of low cross-linking, which results in the implants being of high signal on T2-weighted imaging. Conversely, the implant shell's elastomer has a short T2 and thus appears dark on T2-weighted scans.

The three-dimensional structure of the gel disintegrates in vivo over time (i.e., polymer chain rupture occurs), increasing the molecular mobility of the polymer, and consequently, increasing its proton T2 values.[46] There is also evidence from proton MRI spectroscopy (H_1-MRS) that, once silicone escapes the implant envelope, the gel can migrate locally and the oil component can also enter the blood stream via lymphatics to reach the liver, spleen, and other organs. In both rats and humans, H_1-MRS shows a silicone peak in the liver when an implant is present, though the amount is increased if the implant is ruptured.[47] Alterations in chemical shift of the silicone spectral peak suggest in vivo metabolization of the silicone.[48] Silicone eventually disappears from liver spectra once implants are removed.[47]

Development of Breast Implants

The silicone-filled implant was introduced by Dow Corning in the early 1960s. Early attempts at breast augmentation had included direct paraffin or silicone injection (a technique still used widely in Asia) and synthetic implants of various different sponges and plastics.[49] These older techniques suffered from various unacceptable complications including severe

scarring and inflammatory reactions. The new implants revolutionized cosmetic breast surgery. In the early 1990s, controversy arose over the long-term effects of silicone implants with allegations that they caused connective tissue diseases such as scleroderma. While this claim is disputed and in doubt, it has nevertheless become important to detect even asymptomatic implant ruptures, as there is an (as yet unproven) assumption that the risk of extracapsular rupture increases once intracapsular rupture has occurred.

Mammography is extremely insensitive to implant rupture, and ultrasound has been promoted as a cost-effective method of making the diagnosis. Some studies have suggested that MRI has no advantage over ultrasound for the detection of implant failure, both having good specificity but low prospective sensitivities ranging from 45% to 75%.[50,51] However, these studies used a low-resolution MRI technique, sometimes without a dedicated breast coil, and did not use silicone-selective sequences. With better equipment, optimized techniques, and better diagnostic criteria, newer studies clearly show the superiority of high-resolution multiplanar MRI for the detection of intracapsular implant rupture. Typical sensitivities and specificities of greater than 90% have been described.[52–54] Computed tomography also has good sensitivity and specificity[55] but uses an unacceptably high dose of ionizing radiation.

There are over 100 different types of implant, with numerous variations in envelope thickness, gel composition, and valve type. The major types which can be differentiated with MRI include the following:

Single-lumen silicone (with or without polyurethane coating, textured surface, etc.)

Single-lumen saline

Double-lumen (silicone-in-saline)

Others are rare (reverse double-lumen [saline-in-silicone], triple-lumen, multiple or stacked implants, saline injected into silicone, etc.).

The patient's surgical history, particularly the type of implant and its implanted position (subglandular or retropectoral), is often important for interpretation. For example, a double-lumen implant with a ruptured outer shell is indistinguishable from an intact single-lumen implant on MRI.

MRI Technique

A dedicated breast surface coil is essential. There are two basic methods of imaging implants with high sensitivity and specificity for implant rupture. These include the following:

high-resolution fast spin echo (FSE). This allows high-resolution images to be obtained in a reasonable time in order to detect subtle tears.

silicone-only imaging, The silicone-resonant peak is shifted - 22.3 parts per million (ppm), 320 Hz from water and 80 Hz from fat at 1.5 T. This chemical shift can be exploited to produce silicone-only imaging, most commonly using water-suppressed short term inversion recovery (STIR). This technique nulls the signal of fat by exploiting its short T1 and suppresses glandular parenchyma with spectral saturation pulses. Its main disadvantages are relatively long imaging times, lower signal-to-noise ratio and lower resolution than FSE, however, it is more reliable for detecting extracapsular silicone. Recently, fast STIR has been introduced by most scanner manufacturers. This uses echo trains similar to FSE, enabling high-resolution scanning without excessive acquisition times.

As with MRM, numerous scan sequence variations have been described. A typical protocol might include

High-resolution FSE of both breasts. TR 4,000/TE 140 to 200, echo train length 8 to 12. 512 × 256, 3 to 4 mm,, 32-cm-field of view (FOV) in the axial and coronal planes

Water-suppressed fast STIR of each breast individually, TR 4,000/TI 150/TE 30, echo train length 12, 256 × 192, 5 to 7 mm, 18-cm FOV in the sagittal plane

Findings

Normal Implants

After implantation, the thin fibrous capsule around the implant is usually imperceptible on MRI, though it may appear as a thin low signal line. The vast majority of implants are single lumen in type and appear as a high-signal single-compartment structure, frequently with low-signal internal radial folds (see Fig. 47.3). These are a double layered fold of implant shell projecting into the lumen, are very common, and are due to underfilling. It is important to differentiate them from a small tear producing partial collapse of the envelope; the multiplanar, multislice capabilities of MRI are very helpful for making this distinction. The collapsed shell of a ruptured implant has only one layer and tends to appear thinner than a radial fold (Figs. 47.26 and 47.27). Polyurethane-covered implants frequently have a moderate layer of reactive fluid around them.[56] This appears as a band of high signal around the implant on FSE scans, which is suppressed on silicone-selective sequences, distinguishing this from extracapsular silicone. Double-lumen implants usually have a silicone-filled implant within an outer shell filled with saline, or less commonly, an inner saline prosthesis inside an outer silicone-filled envelope. On FSE scans, the saline appears very bright while the silicone has a lower signal intensity. There is frequently a bright/dark chemical shift artifact at the junction between the two lumens (Fig. 47.28). Valves are generally seen as low-signal, rounded structures at the margin of the implant and may be in any position around the periphery (Fig. 47.28). Saline-filled implants are brighter on FSE scans than silicone-filled implants and appear dark on silicone-selective or fat-suppressed T1-weighted sequences (Fig. 47.29).

Rarely, a mass adjacent to an implant may be due to a granulomatous reaction to the implant shell or valve rather than to extracapsular silicone. Such masses can enhance markedly (Fig. 47.29), and it is difficult to distinguish them from malignancy.

Figure 47.26 Silicone implant with complex folds. (**A**) Ultrasound of inferior aspect of left breast implant shows apparent disruption of the implant envelope and shell with possible extracapsular silicone as indicated. This is later shown to be an artifact. (*Figure continues.*)

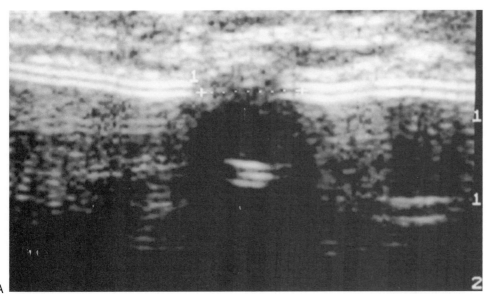

A

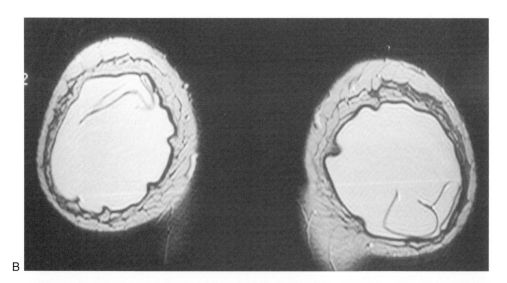

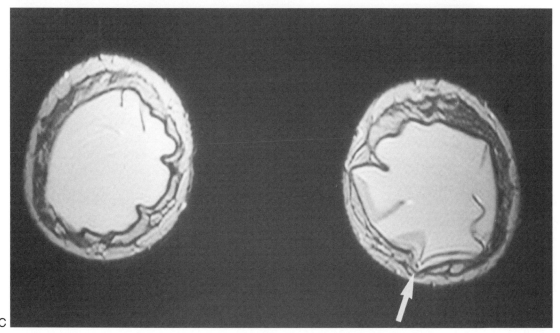

Figure 47.26 (*Continued*). (**B & C**) Coronal central (Fig. B) and anterior (Fig. C) high-resolution FSE scans. Complex radial folds are seen as low signal lines within the implant lumens. The borders of the implants are crinkled, suggesting that they were too large and underfilled at the time of surgery. The ultrasonic artifact is due to a small focal inferior bulge in the implant shell (arrow). Other silicone-specific scans did not show any free silicone.

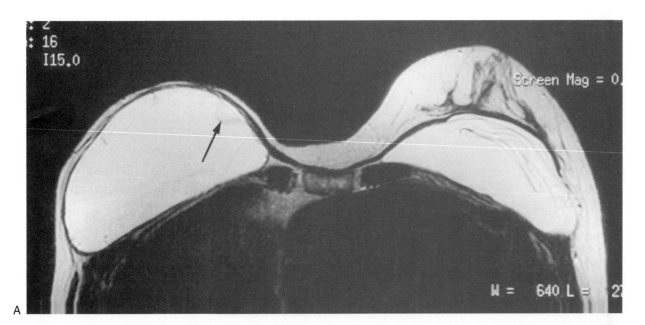

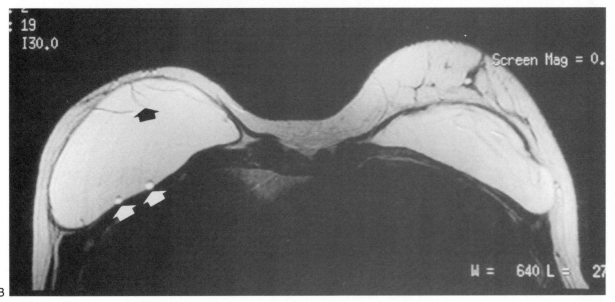

Figure 47.27 Bilateral implant ruptures following right breast surgery and a reconstruction with retropectoral silicone implants bilaterally, smaller on the left. (**A & B**) Axial high-resolution FSE scans through both breasts at the level of the nipple (Fig. A), and below the nipple (Fig. B). On the right, radial folds are seen within the implant. In addition, there is partial anterior separation of the shell from the capsule with gel on both sides of the shell, which was confirmed on examination of adjacent slices (long arrow). The "noose" sign is evident on the right (black arrow), and there are two droplets of high signal fluid within the implant posteriorly (white arrows). On the left, the "linguine" sign is evident at both levels as thin wavy lines within the implant, floating anteriorly (the dependent portion of the implant in the prone position). All these signs are highly specific for intracapsular implant rupture.

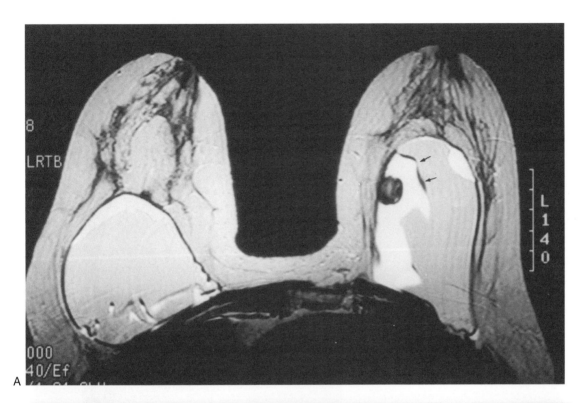

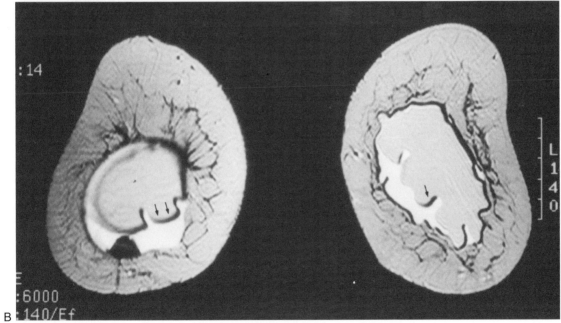

Figure 47.28 Intact, double-lumen, silicone-in-saline implants. (**A**) Axial high-resolution
FSE scan through both breasts showing bilateral retromammary silicone-in-saline double-lumen implants where the saline appears brighter than the silicone. (**B**) Coronal scan. Note
the chemical shift artifact (bright and dark bands along frequency-encoding direction) at
the boundaries of the silicone and saline lumens (small arrows), which is absent in the
phase-encoding direction. Each implant has a low-signal rounded valve, seen medially on
the left and inferiorly on the right.

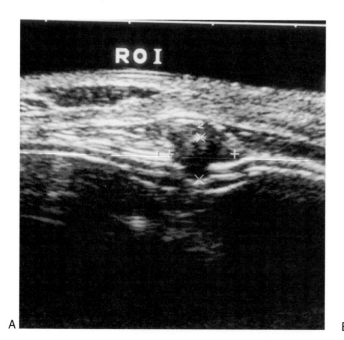

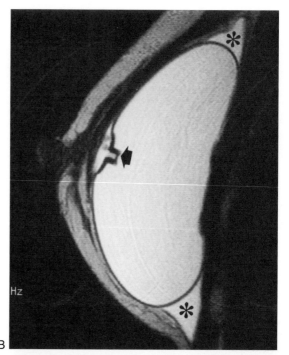

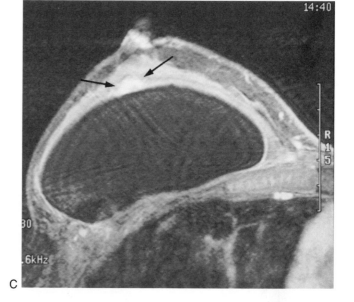

Figure 47.29 Saline breast implant with anterior granuloma in a 40-year-old. A small nodule became palpable anteriorly just behind the nipple 6 months after implantation. Pathology showed fibrous and granulomatous reactive tissue, presumably a reaction to the valve. (**A**) Ultrasound shows a small solid lesion indenting the anterior aspect of the implant, 1 cm from the nipple. (**B**) Sagittal T2-weighted FSE scan shows the retropectoral high-signal implant to be smoothly bounded and surrounded by a cuff of high signal fluid (*) The implant valve lies anteriorly (short arrow). (**C**) Axial contrast-enhanced FSPGR delayed scan shows a strongly enhancing nodule anterior to the implant, just above the nipple (arrows).

Implant Rupture

About 85% of implant ruptures are intracapsular, and 15% are extracapsular. Major signs of envelope disruption are listed in Table 47.10. Most signs rely on detecting gel on both sides of the implant envelope ("gel outside the shell"), and all have been shown to have excellent specificities of greater than 90% when seen.[53] In detail, these are as follows:

The "linguine" sign (10% to 15% of cases) represents envelope collapse, the shell floating within the silicone-filled capsule, and forming multiple thin low-signal lines (Fig. 47.27). The "noose" sign (also called the "keyhole" or "inverted teardrop" sign) appears as a small amount of gel

Table 47.10 MRI Signs of Silicone Implant Rupture

Sign	Specificity
"Linguine" sign	91–92%
"Noose," "inverted teardrop," or "keyhole" sign	96%
Partial shell-capsule separation	Unknown
"C" sign	96–99%
Fluid droplets within silicone	97–99%
Extracapsular silicone	Unknown

(Data from Quinn SF, Neubauer NM, Sheley RC et al. MR imaging of silicone breast implants: evaluation of prospective and retrospective interpretations and interobserver agreement. J Magn Reson Imaging 1996;6:213–218, with permission.)

trapped within a radial fold and thus positioned between the shell and the capsule (Figs. 47.27 and 47.30). This implies a tear without complete envelope collapse. These "gel bleeds" can be caused by gel with low cross-linking passing through the semipermeable shell,[56] but in most cases they are due to a tiny pinhole or tear in the envelope.

Partial shell-capsule separation appears as small wrinkles in the implant shell falling away from the capsule, usually anteriorly (Fig. 47.27), and must be distinguished from small radial folds. They are most reliably seen with high resolution MRI and are difficult to detect by ultrasound because impedance mismatch between breast tissue and the implant often produces anterior shadowing and noise, obscuring the separation.

The "C" sign is not widely used but has been described as a focal thickening of the posterior margin of the implant, which curves into a C-shape when collapsing away from the capsule.[53] This is a variant of partial shell–capsule separation.

Fluid and silicone are not miscible. Therefore, fluid droplets within the silicone are seen as globules of high signal within the implant on FSE scans and as dark globules on silicone-specific sequences. They are usually 1 cm or less in diameter (Fig. 47.27). The source of the droplets is unclear, but their presence is highly specific for implant rupture. The ex-

ception to this is when fluid has been deliberately injected into the implant at the time of surgery (usually to alter implant inflation). Typically, numerous and/or large globules of fluid are present when this has occurred.

Extracapsular silicone appears as moderately bright rounded blobs or plaques outside the main implant on FSE scans and may be of similar intensity to normal fat (Fig. 47.31). Silicone-selective sequences can detect these if they exceed about 1 cc in size. There is good evidence that, for smaller extracapsular leaks, sonography is more sensitive than MRI.[57] With previously ruptured implants that have been replaced, some free silicone is frequently present, which may be visible in the breast and axillary nodes (Fig. 47.32) in the presence of an intact implant. An appropriate clinical history is essential to avoid diagnostic error, as it is possible to have extracapsular silicone due to implant rupture even when an implant appears otherwise intact.

Pitfalls

A number of potential sources of errors in interpretation are detailed below:

Very complex folds in unruptured implants may be difficult to distinguish from the linguine sign, "C" sign, and partial

Figure 47.30 Bilateral implant ruptures with "noose" sign demonstrated with water-suppressed silicone-selective STIR. This is an inherently low-resolution technique. Bilateral "noose" signs are visible (arrows), indicating intracapsular implant shell rupture.

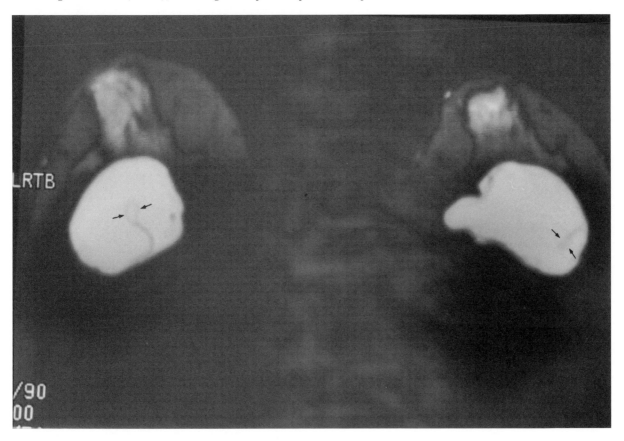

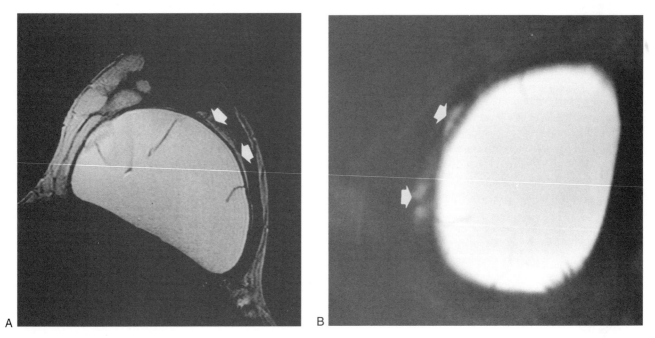

A

B

Figure 47.31 Extracapsular rupture with free silicone. (**A**) Axial FSE scan of the left breast showing internal radial folds and an apparently intact single-lumen retromammary implant. A thin band of high signal anterior to the implant (arrows) represents free extracapsular silicone. It is very similar in signal to fat on this sequence. (**B**) Sagittal silicone-selective STIR scan of the left breast showing multiple blobs of hyperintense extracapsular silicone (arrows). This is diagnostic of extracapsular implant rupture unless previous implants have been replaced.

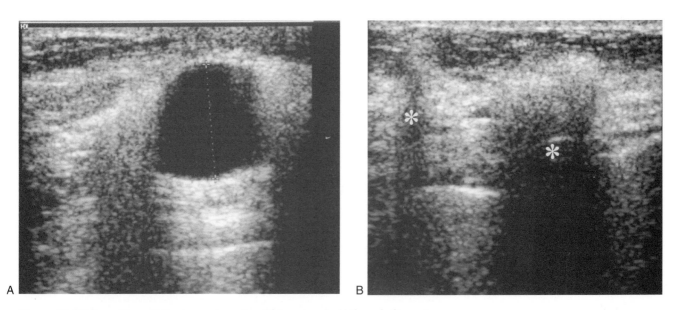

A

B

Figure 47.32 Free silicone following explantation. This patient had bilateral silicone implants removed with free spill of silicone into the left breast. (**A**) Ultrasound shows a large blob of anechoic silicone with characteristic specular reflections from anterior and posterior margins and "dirty" shadowing from the edges. (**B**) Ultrasound of the left lower outer quadrant showing more typical appearance of silicone granulomas with marked "dirty" shadowing from two poorly defined foci (*). (*Figure continues.*)

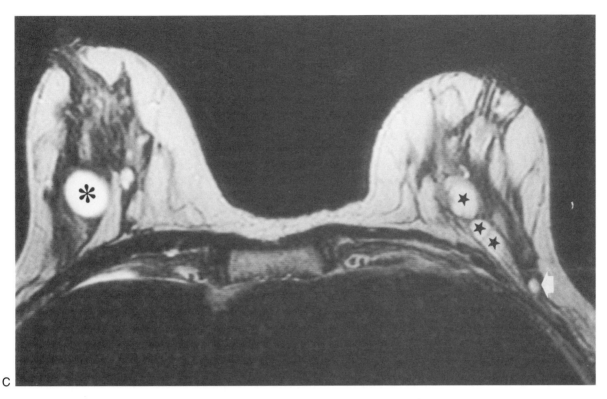

C

Figure 47.32 *(Continued).* (**C**) Axial FSE of both breasts at the level of the nipples show-ing very bright fluid-filled cysts on the right (*) and less hyperintense blobs of free silicone on the left (★). Note silicone within an axillary tail lymph node (arrow).

collapse of the shell. This is the most common cause of mis-diagnosis of implant rupture.

Prior intraimplant injection with fluid (see above).

A small silicone leak into the outer lumen of double lumen implant may be obscured by chemical shift artifact along the radial folds.

Implant herniation through a defect in the capsule may oc-cur without rupture, particularly after closed capsulotomy. A "tongue" of implant is then seen extending outward, with no other evidence of implant rupture.

Silicone oil bleed only. The oil within all silicone implants "bleeds" through the intact shell normally. This appears sim-ilar to the keyhole sign but is seen on one cut only and is no more than 1 to 2 mm in diameter.

Postoperative hematoma. If scans are performed within a few days to weeks after surgery, blood may appear bright due to methemoglobin. However, it will have the wrong chemi-cal shift for silicone and will be suppressed on silicone-se-lective scans.

Silicone may be at brachial plexus, down the arm, in axil-lary nodes, and in other ectopic locations. Using a large FOV and extending scan coverage into these regions may be helpful.

Conclusions

MRI is the best available noninvasive method for the detec-tion of implant rupture. However, it has limited availability and is expensive. If used suboptimally, it is no better than ul-trasound. Ultrasound may be more sensitive than MRI for the detection of small quantities of extracapsular silicone. It is im-portant to realize that even with the best techniques and close surgical correlation, 5% to 10% of implant ruptures are unde-tectable by MRI.

REFERENCES

1. Mansfield P, Morris PG, Ordidge R et al. Carcinoma of the breast imaged by nuclear magnetic resonance (NMR). Br J Ra-diol 1979;52:242–243

2. Powell DE, Stelling CB. Magnetic resonance imaging of the hu-man female breast. Current status and pathologic correlations. [Review]. Pathol Annu 1988;1:159–94

3. Heywang SH, Fenzl G, Hahn D et al. MR imaging of the breast; comparison with mammography and ultrasound. J Comput As-sist Tomogr 1986;10:615–620

4. Heywang SH, Hahn D, Schmidt H et al. MR imaging of the

breast using gadolinium-DTPA. J Comput Assist Tomogr 1986;10:199–204

5. Kaiser WA, Zeitler E. MR imaging of the breast: fast imaging sequences with and without Gd-DTPA. Preliminary observations. Radiology 1989 170;681–686

6. Nunes LW, Schnall MD, Orel SG et al. Breast MR imaging: interpretation model. Radiology 1997;202:833–841

7. Kuhl CK, Bieling H, Gieseke J et al. Breast neoplasms: T2* susceptibility-contrast, first-pass perfusion MR imaging. Radiology 1997;202:87–95

8. Plewes DB, Bishop J, Soutar I, Cohen E. Errors in quantitative dynamic three-dimensional keyhole MR imaging of the breast. J Magn Reson Imaging 1995;5:361–364

9. Rodenko GN, Harms SE, Pruneda JM et al. MR imaging in the management before surgery of lobular carcinoma of the breast: correlation with pathology. Am J Roentgenol 1996; 167:1415–1419

10. Boetes C, Mus RD, Holland R et al. Breast tumors: comparative accuracy of MR imaging relative to mammography and US for demonstrating extent. Radiology 1995;197:743–747

11. Logan-Young W, Hoffman N, Janus J. Fine-needle aspiration cytology in the detection of breast cancer in nonsuspicious lesions. Radiology 1992;184:49–53

12. Heywang-Köbrunner SH, Beck R. Contrast-enhanced MRI of the breast (2nd ed.). Springer-Verlag, Berlin, 1996

13. Harms SE, Flaming DP. Staging of breast cancer with MR imaging. MRI Clin North Am 1994;2:573–584

14. Heywang SH, Hilbertz T, Beck R et al. Gd-DTPA enhanced MR imaging of the breast in patients with postoperative scarring and silicon implants. J Comput Assist Tomogr 1990;14:348–356

15. Heywang-Köbrunner SH, Schlegel A, Beck R et al. Contrast-enhanced MRI of the breast after limited surgery and radiation therapy. J Comput Assist Tomogr 1993;17:891–900

16. Mussurakis S, Buckley DL, Bowsley SJ et al. Dynamic contrast-enhanced magnetic resonance imaging of the breast combined with pharmacokinetic analysis of gadolinium-DTPA uptake in the diagnosis of local recurrence of early stage breast carcinoma. Invest Radiol 1995;30:650–662

17. Leibman AJ, Kossoff MB. Mammography in women with axillary lymphadenopathy and normal breasts on physical examination: value in detecting occult breast carcinoma. Am J Roentgenol 1992;159:493–495

18. Beatty SM, Orel SG, Schnall MD et al. MR imaging of occult breast carcinoma manifesting as axillary metastases. In: Radiological Society of North America, Chicago. Radiology 1996;201:129

19. Abraham DC, Jones RC, Jones SE et al. Evaluation of neoadjuvant chemotherapeutic response of locally advanced breast cancer by magnetic resonance imaging. Cancer 1996;78:91–100

20. Davis PL, McCarty KS, Jr. Technologic considerations for breast tumor size assessment. Magn Reson Imaging Clin N Am 1994;2:623–631

21. Mueller-Schimpfe MP, Ohmenhauser K, Kurz S, Claussen CD. Influence of menstrual cycle and age on parenchymal contrast enhancement in MR mammography. In: Radiological Society of North America, Chicago. Radiology 1995;197:130

22. Hittmair K, Turetschek K, Gomiscek G et al. Field strength dependence of MRI contrast enhancement: phantom measurements and application to dynamic breast imaging. Br J Radiol 1996;69:215–220

23. Kuhl CK, Kreft BP, Hauswirth A et al. MR mammography at 0.5 tesla. I. Comparison of image quality and sensitivity of MR mammography at 0.5 and 1.5 T. Rofo Fortschr Geb Rontgenstr Neuen Bildgeb Verfahr 1995;162:381–389

24. Boetes C, Barentsz JO, Mus RD et al. MR characterization of suspicious breast lesions with a gadolinium-enhanced TurboFLASH subtraction technique. Radiology 1994;193:777–781

25. Perman WH, Heiberg EV, Herrmann VM. Half-Fourier, three-dimensional technique for dynamic contrast-enhanced MR imaging of both breasts and axillae: initial characterization of breast lesions. Radiology 1996;200:263–269

26. Hulka CA, Smith BL, Sgroi DC et al. Benign and malignant breast lesions: differentiation with echo-planar MR imaging. Radiology 1995;197:33–38

27. Knopp MV, Junkermann HJ, Hess T et al. Functional MR mammography for diagnostic workup of indeterminate breast lesions. In: Radiological Society of North America, Chicago. Radiology 1995:197:130

28. Harms SE, Flamig DP, Hesley KL et al. MR imaging of the breast with rotating delivery of excitation off resonance: clinical experience with pathologic correlation. Radiology 1993; 187:493–501

29. Orel SG, High-resolution MR imaging of the breast. Semin Ultrasound CT MR 1996;17:476–493

30. Tofts PS, Berkowitz BA. Measurement of capillary permeability from the Gd enhancement curve: a comparison of bolus and constant infusion injection methods. Magn Reson Imag 1994;12:81–91

31. Heywang-Köbrunner SH, Haustein J, Pohl C et al. Contrast-enhanced MR imaging of the breast: comparison of two different doses of gadopentetate dimeglumine Radiology 1994;191: 639–646

32. Pierce WB, Harms SE, Flamig DP et al. Three-dimensional gadolinium-enhanced MR imaging of the breast: pulse sequence with fat suppression and magnetization transfer contrast. Work in progress. Radiology 1991;181:757–763

33. Fischer U, Vosshenrich R, Bruhn H et al. MR-guided localization of suspected breast lesions detected exclusively by postcontrast MRI. J Comput Assist Tomogr 1995;19:63–66

34. Doler W, Fischer U, Metzger I et al. Stereotaxic add-on device for MR-guided biopsy of breast lesions. Radiology 1996;200:863–864

35. Brasch R, Pham C, Shames D et al. Assessing tumor angiogenesis using macromolecular MR imaging contrast media. J Magn Reson Imaging 1997;7:68–74

36. Gasparini G, Toi M, Gion M et al. Prognostic significance of vascular endothelial growth factor protein in node-negative breast carcinoma. J Nat Cancer Inst 1997;89:139–147

37. Kuhl CK, Kreft BP, Gieseke MS, Schild HH. Normal variants of dynamic contrast-enhanced MR mammography in healthy volunteers: range of "normal" contrast enhancement. In: Radiological Society of North America, Chicago. Radiology 1995;197:130

38. Mussurakis S, Carleton PJ, Turnbull LW. Case report: MR imaging of juvenile papillomatosis of the breast. Br J Radiol 1996;69:867–870

39. Orel SG, Mendonca MH, Reynolds C et al. MR imaging of ductal carcinoma in situ. Radiology 1997;202:413–420

40. Gilles R, Zarani B, Guinebretière J-M et al. Ductal carcinoma in situ: MR imaging—histopathologic correlation. Radiology 1995;196:415–419

41. Evans A, Pinder S, Wilson R et al. Ductal carcinoma in situ of the breast: correlation between mammographic and pathologic findings. AJR Am J Roentgenol 1994;162:1307–1311

42. Hilleren D, Andersson I, Lindholm K, Linnell F. Invasive lobular carcinoma mammographic findingss in a 10-year experience. Radiology 1991;178:149–154

43. Le Gal M, Ollivier L, Asselain B et al. Mammographic features of 455 invasive lobular carcinomas. Radiology 1992;185:705–708

44. Newstead G, Baute P, Toth H. Invasive lobular and ductal carcinoma: mammographic findings and stage at diagnosis. Radiology 1992;184:623–627

45. Gilles R, Guinebretiere JM, Shapeero LG et al. Assessment of breast cancer recurrence with contrast-enhanced subtraction MR imaging: preliminary results in 26 patients. Radiology 1993;188:473–478

46. Pfleiderer B, Ackerman JL, Garrido L. Migration and biodegradation of free silicone from silicone-gel-filled implants after long-term implantation. Magn Reson Med 1993;30:534–543

47. Pfleiderer B, Garrido L. Migration and accumulation of silicone in the liver of women with silicone gel-filled breast implants. Magn Reson Med 1995;33:8–17

48. Garrido L, Pfleiderer B, Papisov M, Ackerman JL. In vivo degradation of silicones. Magn Reson Med 1993;29:839–483

49. Gorczyca DP. MR imaging of breast implants. Magn Reson Imaging Clin N Am 1994;2:659–672

50. Reynolds HE, Buckwalter KA, Jackson VP et al. Comparison of mammography, sonography, and magnetic resonance imaging in the detection of silicone-gel breast implant rupture. Ann Plast Surg 1994;33:247–255

51. Berg WA, Caskey CI, Hamper UM et al. Diagnosing breast implant rupture with MR imaging, US, and mammography. Radiographics 1993;13:1323–1336

52. Samuels JB, Rohrich RJ, Weatherall PT et al. Radiographic diagnosis of breast implant rupture: current status and comparison of techniques. Plast Reconstr Surg 1995;96:865–877

53. Quinn SF, Neubauer NM, Sheley RC et al. MR imaging of silicone breast implants: evaluation of prospective and retrospective interpretations and interobserver agreement. J Magn Reson Imaging 1996;6:213–218

54. Hilbertz T, Patt R. Imaging of implant failure by MRI. In: Heywang-Köbrunner SH, Beck R, Eds. Contrast-Enhanced MRI of the Breast (2nd ed.). Springer-Verlag, Berlin, 1996, pp 207–218

55. Everson LI, Paratainen H, Detlie T et al. Diagnosis of breast implant rupture: imaging findings and relative efficacies of imaging techniques. Am J Roentgenol 1994;163:57–60

56. Mund DF, Farria DM, Gorczyca DP et al. MR imaging of the breast in patients with silicone-gel implants: spectrum of findings. Am J Roentgenol 1993;161:773–778

57. Middleton MS, McNamara MPJ. Detail blinded comparison of MR imaging and US by experienced observers for detection of residual breast soft-tissue silicone In: Radiological Society of North America, Chicago. Radiology 1996;201:347

58. Mussurakis S, Buckley DL, Coady AM et al. Observer variability in the interpretation of contrast enhanced MRI of the breast. Br J Radiol 1996;69:1009–1016

59. Heywang-Köbrunner SH, Viehweg P. Sensitivity of contrast-enhanced MR imaging of the breast. Magn Reson Imaging Clin N Am 1994;2:527–538

60. Kaiser WA. False-positive results in dynamic MR mammography. Causes, frequency, and methods to avoid. Magn Reson Imaging Clin North Am 1994;2:539–555

61. Kerslake RW, Carleton PJ, Fox JN et al. Dynamic gradient-echo and fat-suppressed spin-echo contrast-enhanced MRI of the breast. Clin Radiol 1995;50:440–454

62. Heiberg EV, Perman WH, Herrmann VM et al. Dynamic sequential 3D gadolinium-enhanced MRI of the whole breast. Magn Resonan Imaging 1996;14:337–348

Index

Note: Page numbers followed by f indicate figures; those followed by t indicate tables.